Nursing Theorists
and Their Work

Nursing Theorists
and Their Work

sixth edition

Ann Marriner Tomey, PhD, RN, FAAN

Professor
College of Nursing
Indiana State University
Terre Haute, Indiana

Martha Raile Alligood, PhD, RN

Professor and Director, PhD Program
School of Nursing
East Carolina University
Greenville, North Carolina

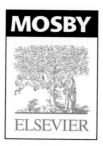

MOSBY

ELSEVIER

MOSBY
ELSEVIER

11830 Westline Industrial Drive
St. Louis, Missouri 63146

Notice

Previous editions copyrighted 2002, 1998, 1994, 1989, and 1986.

ISBN-13: 978-0-323-03010-6
ISBN-10: 0-323-03010-6

Senior Editor: Yvonne Alexopoulos
Associate Developmental Editor: Kristin Hebberd
Editorial Assistant: Sarah Vales
Publishing Services Manager: John Rogers
Project Manager: Doug Turner
Design Project Manager: Bill Drone

Printed in the United States of America

Last digit is print number: 9 8 7 6 5 4 3 2

Contributors

Martha Raile Alligood, PhD, RN
Professor and Director, PhD Program
School of Nursing
East Carolina University
Greenville, North Carolina

Herdis Alvsvåg, RN, Cand. Polit
Associate Professor
Department of Education and Health Promotion
University of Bergen
Bergen, Norway

Donald E. Bailey, Jr., PhD
Assistant Professor
John A. Hartford Foundation Scholar
School of Nursing
University of North Carolina
Chapel Hill, North Carolina

Sue Marquis Bishop, PhD, RN, FAAN
Professor and Dean Emeritus
College of Health and Human Professions
University of North Carolina, Charlotte
Charlotte, North Carolina

Nancy Brookes, PhD, RN, CPMHN(C)
Nurse Scholar
Royal Ottawa Hospital
Ottawa, Ontario, Canada

Janet Witucki Brown, PhD, RN
Assistant Professor
College of Nursing
University of Tennessee
Knoxville, Tennessee

Victoria M. Brown, PhD, RN, HNC
Professor
Division of Nursing and Health Sciences
Macon State College
Macon, Georgia

Karen A. Brykczynski, DNSc, RN, CS, FNP, FANP
Associate Professor
School of Nursing at Galveston
The University of Texas Medical Branch at
 Galveston
Galveston, Texas

Sherrilyn Coffman, DNS, RN
Associate Professor
Nevada State College
Henderson, Nevada

Doris D. Coward, PhD, RN
Associate Professor
School of Nursing
The University of Texas at Austin
Austin, Texas

Nellie S. Droes, DNSc, RN
Associate Professor
Department of Family and Community Nursing
School of Nursing
East Carolina University
Greenville, North Carolina

Thérèse Dowd, PhD, RN
Associate Professor
College of Nursing
The University of Akron
Akron, Ohio

Margaret E. Erickson, PhD
Holistic Healing Consultants
Executive Director
American Holistic Nurses Certification
 Corporation
Cedar Park, Texas

Barbara T. Freese, EdD, RN
Professor
School of Nursing
Lander University
Greenwood, South Carolina

Mary E. Gunther, PhD, RN
Assistant Professor
College of Nursing
University of Tennessee
Knoxville, Tennessee

Sonya R. Hardin, PhD, RN, CCRN, APRN
Associate Professor
Department of Adult Health Nursing
School of Nursing
College of Health and Human Services
University of North Carolina, Charlotte
Charlotte, North Carolina

Patricia A. Higgins, PhD, RN
Assistant Professor
Francis Payne Bolton School of Nursing
Case Western Reserve University
Cleveland, Ohio

Lisbet Lindholm
Associate Professor
Faculty of Social and Caring Sciences
Åbo Academy University
Vaasa, Finland

Unni Å. Lindström, PhD, RN
Professor
Faculty of Social and Caring Sciences
Åbo Academy University
Vaasa, Finland

Chin-Fang Liu, PhD, RN
Assistant Professor
College of Nursing
Kaohsiung Medical University
Kaohsiung (807), Taiwan

M. Katherine Maeve, PhD, RN
Veterans Administration Medical Center
Augusta, Georgia

Marilyn McFarland, PhD, RN, CTN
Adjunct Faculty
Crystal M. Lange College of Nursing and Health
    Sciences
Saginaw Valley State University
University Center, Michigan

Molly Meighan, PhD, RNC
Assistant Professor
Division of Nursing
Carson-Newman College
Jefferson City, Tennessee

Gail J. Mitchell, PhD, RN
Assistant Professor
York University
Atkinson Faculty
Toronto, Ontario, Canada

Ruth M. Neil, PhD, RN
Clinical Director
Julia Temple Center
Englewood, Colorado

Janice Penrod, PhD, RN
Assistant Professor of Nursing
School of Nursing
College of Health and Human Development
Associate Professor of Humanities
College of Medicine
Pennsylvania State University
University Park, Pennsylvania

Susan A. Pfettscher, DNSc, RN
Retired
Bakersfield, California

Kenneth D. Phillips, PhD, RN
Associate Professor
College of Nursing
University of South Carolina
Columbia, South Carolina

Marguerite J. Purnell, PhD, RN
Assistant Professor
Christine E. Lynn College of Nursing
Florida Atlantic University
Boca Raton, Florida

Teresa J. Sakraida, DNSc, MS, RN
Coordinator
RN Options Program
School of Nursing
University of Pittsburgh
Pittsburgh, Pennsylvania

Karen Moore Schaefer, DNSc, RN
Assistant Professor
Department of Nursing
College of Health Professions
Temple University
Philadelphia, Pennsylvania

Norma Jean Schmieding, EdD, RN
Professor
College of Nursing
University of Rhode Island
Kingston, Rhode Island

Ann M. Schreier, PhD, RN
Director, Alternate Entry to MSN
Assistant Professor
School of Nursing
East Carolina University
Greenville, North Carolina

Carrie Scotto, PhD, RN, CCRN
Assistant Professor
College of Nursing
Kent State University
Kent, Ohio

Christina L. Sieloff, PhD, RN, CAN
Associate Professor
School of Nursing
Oakland University
Rochester, Michigan

Janet L. Stewart, PhD, RN
Assistant Professor
Department of Health Promotion and
    Development
School of Nursing
University of Pittsburgh
Pittsburgh, Pennsylvania

Susan G. Taylor, PhD, RN, FAAN
Professor Emeritus
Sinclair School of Nursing
University of Missouri, Columbia
Columbia, Missouri

Ann Marriner Tomey, PhD, RN, FAAN
Professor
College of Nursing
Indiana State University
Terra Haute, Indiana

Danuta M. Wojnar, PhDc, RN
Doctoral Student and Research Associate CMHP
Department of Family and Child Nursing
School of Nursing
University of Washington
Seattle, Washington

Joan E. Zetterlund, PhD, RN
Paul W. Brandel Professor of Nursing
School of Nursing
North Park University
Chicago, Illinois

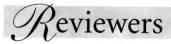# Reviewers

Minerva S. Guttman, EdD, RN
Director and Associate Professor
School of Nursing and Allied Health
Fairleigh Dickinson University
Teaneck, New Jersey

Susan Michael, DNSc, RN, CDE
Associate Professor
School of Nursing
University of Nevada, Las Vegas
Las Vegas, Nevada

Theorists

Faye Glenn Abdellah, EdD, ScD, LLD, RN, FAAN
Professor and Dean Emeritus
Graduate School of Nursing
Uniformed Services University of the Health Sciences
4301 Jones Bridge Road
Bethesda, MD 20814-4799

Evelyn Adam, MN, RN
Professor Emeritus
University of Montreal
6950 Côte Saint-Lue
Montreal, Quebec H4V 2Z9
Canada
(514) 484-0217
evelyn.adam@sympatice.ca

Phil Barker, PhD, RN, FRCN
Department of Nursing and Midwifery
School of Health Sciences
Trinity College
D'Olier Street
Dublin 2 Ireland
00 44 1382 542191
Phil_Barker@ukf.net

Kathryn E. Barnard, PhD, RN, FAAN
Charles and Gerda Spence Professor of Nursing
School of Nursing
Family and Child Nursing
University of Washington
Box 357920
Seattle, WA 98195
(206) 543-4152
kathyb@u.washington.edu

Cheryl Tatano Beck, DNSc, RN, CNM, FAAN
Professor
School of Nursing
University of Connecticut
231 Glenbrook Road
Storrs, CT 06269-2026
(860) 466-0547
cheryl.beck@uconn.edu

Patricia Benner, PhD, RN, FAAN
Professor and Thelma Cook Chair in Ethics and
    Spirituality
School of Nursing
University of California, San Francisco
San Francisco, CA 94143
(415) 476-4313
benpat@itsa.ucsf.edu

Anne Boykin, PhD, RN
Dean and Professor
Christine E. Lynn College of Nursing
Florida Atlantic University
777 Glades Road
Boca Raton, FL 33431
(561) 297-3206
Boykina@fau.edu

Mary Lermann Burke, DNSc, RN
Professor Emeritus
Department of Nursing
Rhode Island College
Providence, RI 02908

Marylin J. Dodd, PhD, RN, FAAN
Professor, Department of Physiological Nursing
Associate Dean, School of Nursing
Director, Center for Symptom Management
Sharon A. Lamb Endowed Chair in Symptom
    Management
School of Nursing
University of California, San Francisco
San Francisco, CA 94143-0610
(415) 476-0712
marylin.dodd@nursing.ucsf.edu

Georgene Gaskill Eakes, EdD, RN
Professor
School of Nursing
Department of Family and Community Nursing
East Carolina University
Greenville, NC 27858
eakesg@mail.ecu.edu

Helen C. Erickson, PhD, RN, AHN-BC, FAAN
Professor Emeritus
The University of Texas
Chair, Board of Directors
American Holistic Nurses Certification
    Corporation
406 Trail Ridge Drive
Cedar Park, TX 78613
(512) 250-0901

Katie Eriksson, PhD, RN
Professor of Caring Science
Åbo Academy University
Professor of Nursing Science
University of Helsinki
Director of Nursing
Helsinki University Central Hospital
Standgatan 2 B5, PO Box 311
FIN-65101
Vaasa, Finland
+358-6-3247501
kaerikss@abo.fi

Margaret A. Hainsworth, PhD, RN
Professor Emeritus
Department of Nursing
Rhode Island College
Providence, RI 02908

†Lydia Hall, MA, RN

†Virginia Henderson, MA, RN

Gladys L. Husted
Distinguished Professor of Nursing
Duquesne University
853 Sherwood Road
Pittsburgh, PA 15221-3723
(412) 731-0736
husted@duq.edu

James H. Husted, BA
Independent Scholar
853 Sherwood Road
Pittsburgh, PA 15221-3723
(412) 731-0736
husted@duq.edu

†Dorothy E. Johnson, MPH, RN

Imogene King, EdD, RN, FAAN
(Retired)
7400 Sun Island Drive
South Pasadena, FL 32168
(904) 360-1943
imkn@earthlink.net

**Katharine Kolcaba, PhD, RN,
    C(ANA, gerontology)**
Associate Professor
College of Nursing
The University of Akron
Akron, OH 44325-3701
Kolcaba@uakron.edu

Madeleine Leininger, PhD, RN, LhD, FAAN
TCN Consultant
1121 Woolworth Plaza
Omaha, NE 68144-1875
(402) 691-0791

†Myra Estrin Levine, MSN, RN, FAAN

**Winifred W. Logan (Gordon), MA, DNS (Educ),
    RGN, RNT**
54 Ellan Gowan Court
Allander Gardens
Milngavie
Glasgow G62 8pp
Scotland, United Kingdom

Kari Martinsen, PhD, RN
Professor
Department of Nursing Science
University of Bergen
Kalfarveien 31
Bergen, Norway
0047 55 58 61 60
kari.martinsen@isf.uib.no

Ramona T. Mercer, PhD, RN, FAAN
Professor Emerita
1809 Ashton Avenue
Burlingame, CA 94010
(650) 697-2324
1pmercer@juno.com

†Deceased.

Merle H. Mishel, PhD, RN, FAAN
Kenan Professor
School of Nursing
University of North Carolina, Chapel Hill
429 Carrington Hall
CB #7460
Chapel Hill, NC 27599
(919) 966-6610
mishel@email.unc.edu

Shirley M. Moore, PhD, RN, FAAN
Professor and Associate Dean of Research
Frances Payne Bolton School of Nursing
Case Western Reserve University
10900 Euclid Avenue
Cleveland, OH 44106
(216) 368-5978
smm8@po.cwru.edu

Betty Neuman, MS, RN, FAAN
Independent International Consultant
PO Box 77
Watertown, OH 45787
(740) 749-3322

Margaret A. Newman, PhD, RN, FAAN
Professor Emeritus
University of Minnesota
289 East Fifth #511
St. Paul, MN 55101
(651) 292-0437

†Florence Nightingale

Dorothea E. Orem, MNSE, RN
Savannah, GA

Rosemarie Rizzo Parse, PhD, RN, FAAN
Editor, *Nursing Science Quarterly*
President, Discovery International
Professor and Niehoff Chair, Loyola University,
    Chicago
320 Fort Duquesne Boulevard
Suite 251
Pittsburgh, PA 15222
(412) 391-8471
rparse@verizon.net

Ida Jean Orlando (Pelletier), MA, RN
111 Waverly
Belmont, MA 02178
(401) 783-2442
schmieding@uri.edu

Nola J. Pender, PhD, RN, FAAN
Professor Emeritus
University of Michigan
Distinguished Professor
Loyola University, Chicago
22838 Harbour Lane
Plainfield, IL 60544
(815) 436-9946
npender@umich.edu

†Hildegard E. Peplau, EdD, RN

Marilyn Anne Ray, PhD, RN, CTN
Professor
Christine E. Lynn College of Nursing
Florida Atlantic University
Boca Raton, FL 33431
(561) 297-2872
mray@fau.edu

Pamela G. Reed, PhD, RN, FAAN
Professor
College of Nursing
University of Arizona
1305 North Martin Street
Tucson, AZ 85721-0203
(520) 626-4038
preed@nursing.arizona.edu

†Martha E. Rogers, ScD, RN

†Nancy Roper, MPhil, RGN, RSCN, RNT

Sister Callista Roy, PhD, RN, FAAN
Professor and Nurse Theorist
Boston College
Cushing Hall
140 Commonwealth Avenue
Chestnut Hill, MA 02467
(617) 552-8811
careyab@bc.edu

†Deceased.

Cornelia M. Ruland PhD, RN
Director, Center for Shared Decision Making and
    Nursing Research
Rikshospitalet National Hospital
Forskningsvn, 2b
0027 Oslo
Norway
+47 23075460
FAX: +47 23075450
cornelia.ruland@rikshospitalet.no

Savina O. Schoenhofer, PhD, RN
Professor
School of Nursing
Alcorn State University
PO Box 18399
Natchez, MS 39122
(601) 948-6746
savibus@jam.rrr.com

Mary Ann P. Swain, PhD
Provost and Vice President for Academic Affairs
Binghamton University
PO Box 6000
Binghamton, NY 13902
(607) 777-2141
mswain@binghamton.edu

Kristen M. Swanson, PhD, RN, FAAN
Professor
Department of Family and Child Nursing
School of Nursing
University of Washington
Box 357262
Seattle, WA 98195
(206) 543-8228
kswanson@u.washington.edu

**Alison J. Tierney, PhD, DNurs(Hon), BSC, RN,
    FRCN, CBE**
Scotland, United Kingdom

Evelyn M. Tomlin, PhD, RN
(Retired)
1521 Kirkwood Drive
Geneva, IL 60134

†Joyce Travelbee, MS, RN

Jean Watson, PhD, RN, HNC, FAAN
Distinguished Professor of Nursing
Founder, Center for Human Caring
University of Colorado Health Sciences Center
School of Nursing
4200 East Ninth Avenue
Denver, CO 80262
(303) 384-7754
Jean.Watson@uchsc.edu

†Ernestine Wiedenbach, MS, RN

Carolyn L. Wiener, PhD
Research Sociologist and Adjunct Professor
Department of Physiological Nursing
Department of Social and Behavioral Sciences
School of Nursing
University of California, San Francisco
San Francisco, CA 94143-0610
(415) 476-0712
cwiener@scbglobal.net

†Deceased.

*P*reface

This book is a tribute to nursing theorists. It identifies major thinkers in nursing, reviews some of their important ideas, and lists their publications, what has been written about their publications, and the major sources the theorists used. Many publications before 1995 have been deleted from the sixth edition but are available in the fifth edition. The Web sites were correct at the time the book went to press.

Chapter 1 presents a brief history of nursing theory, its significance, and a framework for analysis of the theoretical works included in this volume. Other chapters in Unit I discuss the history and philosophy of science, logical reasoning, and the theory development process. Nine chapters from the fifth edition were condensed into chapter five in the sixth edition. Eleven theorists are discussed in Chapter 5 as nursing theorists of historical significance. They include Peplau, Abdellah, Wiedenbach, Hall, Henderson, Travelbee, Barnard, Adam, and Roper, Logan, and Tierney. Complete chapters about them are available in the fifth edition.

The philosophies of Nightingale, Watson, Ray, Benner, Martinsen, and Eriksson are presented in Unit II. Unit III includes nursing models by Levine, Rogers, Orem, King, Neuman, Roy, Johnson, and Boykin and Schoenhofer. The nursing theories of Orlando, Pender, Leininger, Newman, Parse, the Husteds, and Erickson, Tomlin, and Swain are presented in Unit IV. Unit V contains middle range theories by Mercer; Mishel; Reed; Wiener and Dodd; Eakes, Burke, and Hainsworth; Barker; Kolcaba; Beck; Swanson; and Ruland and Moore. Martha Alligood brings this sixth edition of the book to a close in Unit VI with a chapter that points to a bright future for nursing theory based on the current state of its art and science.

The following are identified for each theorist: credentials and background, theoretical sources for theory development, use of empirical data, major concepts and definitions, major assumptions, theoretical assertions, logical form, acceptance by the nursing community, further development, a critique of the work, and a summary. Case studies have been added, and the critical thinking activities and bibliographies have been updated for this edition. More theorists have been added to each unit, especially the unit that addresses middle range theories. There is more international work in this edition. There are differences in the alphabet in various languages. The Swedish alphabet has three letters that follow "z" in the English alphabet, and there are also differences in the Norwegian alphabet.

Baccalaureate students may be most interested in the concepts, definitions, and theoretical assertions. Graduate students will be interested in logical form, acceptance by the nursing community, the theoretical sources for theory development, and the use of empirical data. The extensive bibliographies should be particularly useful to master's and doctoral graduate students for locating primary and secondary sources.

In addition, students at all stages of learning may be interested in learning more about one or more of the theorists featured in this text. Although certain chapters list Web sites specific to that theorist, the following comprehensive Web sites in particular are excellent resources to learn more about any individual featured in this book:

- Nursing Theory link page, Clayton College and State University, Department of Nursing: *http://www.healthsci.clayton.edu/eichelberger/nursing.htm*
- Nursing Theory page, Hahn School of Nursing and Health Science, University of San Diego: *http://www.sandiego.edu/nursing/theory/*
- Nursing Theory page, Valdosta State University, College of Nursing: *http://www.valdosta.edu/nursing/history_theory/theory.html*

The theorists discussed in this book have enriched our professional lives by providing theoretical works to guide our research and practice. It is now our responsibility to analyze and synthesize their work, generate new ideas, and continue theory development and application.

We would like to thank the theorists for critiquing the original and some subsequent chapters about themselves to keep the content current and accurate. So that their omission does not appear to have been an oversight, it must be noted that the work of Paterson and Zderad has not been included at their request.

We thank the librarians who have helped us obtain obscure information and all the other people working behind the scenes. Dr. Martha Raile Alligood reordered the chapters, served as a contributing author, and edited for consistency with the new organization in the third edition. After Dr. Alligood coedited *Nursing Theory: Utilization & Application* with Dr. Marriner Tomey, and based on her expertise in nursing science theory, she became a coeditor and a contributing author for the fourth and fifth editions. She is a consultant and contributing author for the sixth edition.

We thank our loving husbands, Charlie K. Alligood and H. Keith Tomey, for enriching our private lives while supporting our professional activities.

Ann Marriner Tomey
Martha Raile Alligood

Contents

UNIT I

Evolution of Nursing Theories

1 **Introduction to Nursing Theory: Its History, Significance, and Analysis,** *3*
Martha Raile Alligood

2 **History and Philosophy of Science,** *16*
Sue Marquis Bishop and Sonya R. Hardin

3 **Logical Reasoning,** *25*
Sue Marquis Bishop and Sonya R. Hardin

4 **Theory Development Process,** *35*
Sue Marquis Bishop and Sonya R. Hardin

5 **Nursing Theorists of Historical Significance,** *50*
    Hildegard E. Peplau
    Faye Glenn Abdellah
    Ernestine Wiedenbach
    Lydia Hall
    Virginia Henderson
    Joyce Travelbee
    Kathryn E. Barnard
    Evelyn Adam
    Nancy Roper, Winifred W. Logan, Alison J. Tierney
Ann Marriner Tomey

UNIT II

Philosophies

6 **Florence Nightingale: Modern Nursing,** *71*
Susan A. Pfettscher

7   Jean Watson: Philosophy and Science of Caring, *91*
     Ruth M. Neil and Ann Marriner Tomey

8   Marilyn Anne Ray: Theory of Bureaucratic Caring, *116*
     Sherrilyn Coffman

9   Patricia Benner: From Novice to Expert: Excellence and Power in Clinical
     Nursing Practice, *140*
     Karen A. Brykczynski

10   Kari Martinsen: Philosophy of Caring, *167*
     Herdis Alvsvåg

11   Katie Eriksson: Theory of Caritative Caring, *191*
     Unni Å. Lindström, Lisbet Lindholm, and Joan E. Zetterlund

UNIT III
Nursing Models

12   Myra Estrin Levine: The Conservation Model, *227*
     Karen Moore Schaefer

13   Martha E. Rogers: Unitary Human Beings, *244*
     Mary E. Gunther

14   Dorothea E. Orem: Self-Care Deficit Theory of Nursing, *267*
     Susan G. Taylor

15   Imogene King: Interacting Systems Framework and Middle Range Theory
     of Goal Attainment, *297*
     Christina L. Sieloff

16   Betty Neuman: Systems Model, *318*
     Barbara T. Freese

17   Sister Callista Roy: Adaptation Model, *355*
     Kenneth D. Phillips

18   Dorothy E. Johnson: Behavioral System Model, *386*
Victoria M. Brown

19   Anne Boykin and Savina O. Schoenhofer: Nursing as Caring: A Model for Transforming Practice, *405*
Marguerite J. Purnell

UNIT IV
Nursing Theories

20   Ida Jean Orlando (Pelletier): Nursing Process Theory, *431*
Norma Jean Schmieding

21   Nola J. Pender: Health Promotion Model, *452*
Teresa J. Sakraida

22   Madeleine Leininger: Culture Care Theory of Diversity and Universality, *472*
Marilyn McFarland

23   Margaret A. Newman: Health as Expanding Consciousness, *497*
Janet Witucki Brown

24   Rosemarie Rizzo Parse: Human Becoming, *522*
Gail J. Mitchell

25   Helen C. Erickson, Evelyn M. Tomlin, and Mary Ann P. Swain: Modeling and Role-Modeling, *560*
Margaret E. Erickson

26   Gladys L. Husted and James H. Husted: Symphonological Bioethical Theory, *584*
Carrie Scotto

UNIT V
Middle Range Theories

27   Ramona T. Mercer: Maternal Role Attainment—Becoming a Mother, *605*
Molly Meighan

28 **Merle H. Mishel: Uncertainty in Illness Theory,** *623*
Donald E. Bailey, Jr. and Janet L. Stewart

29 **Pamela G. Reed: Self-Transcendence Theory,** *643*
Doris D. Coward

30 **Carolyn L. Wiener and Marylin J. Dodd: Theory of Illness Trajectory,** *663*
Janice Penrod and Chin-Fang Liu

31 **Georgene Gaskill Eakes, Mary Lermann Burke, and
     Margaret A. Hainsworth: Theory of Chronic Sorrow,** *679*
Ann M. Schreier and Nellie S. Droes

32 **Phil Barker: Tidal Model of Mental Health Recovery,** *696*
Nancy Brookes

33 **Katharine Kolcaba: Theory of Comfort,** *726*
Thérèse Dowd

34 **Cheryl Tatano Beck: Postpartum Depression Theory,** *743*
M. Katherine Maeve

35 **Kristen M. Swanson: Theory of Caring,** *762*
Danuta M. Wojnar

36 **Cornelia M. Ruland and Shirley M. Moore: Peaceful End of Life Theory,** *774*
Patricia A. Higgins

UNIT VI

Future of Nursing Theory

37 **State of the Art and Science of Nursing Theory,** *785*
Martha Raile Alligood

Evolution of Nursing Theories

- Searching for nursing substance to guide practice led to the evolution of nursing theories.

- Analysis is a process in learning and knowledge development that includes activities such as in-depth examination, inquiry, investigation, study, appraisal, estimation, evaluation, and judgment and ultimately leads to synthesis.

- In education, analysis is highly valued because it leads the student to new understandings of nursing through reflection and critical thinking.

- Analysis of theoretical works is based on knowledge of the theory development process, the history and philosophy of science, the nature of science within the discipline, the state of progress in the various theoretical endeavors, and logic.

- Nursing history demonstrates the significance of theory for nursing as a division of education (the discipline) and a specialized field of practice (the profession).

Introduction to Nursing Theory: Its History, Significance, and Analysis

Martha Raile Alligood

The literature has never been more replete with examples of nursing theory–based practice and research. The number of doctorally prepared nurse scholars with a commitment to nursing theories has never been higher. The challenge today is to translate the knowledge base nurtured and grown in the world of scholarship into practice in the worlds of nurses' direct experiences. (Cody, 1997, p. 5)

This text is designed to introduce the reader to nursing theorists and their work. Nursing theory has been a prevalent theme in the nursing literature for the past 35 years and has stimulated phenomenal growth in the nursing profession. Selected nursing theorists are included to familiarize the reader with a wide range of nursing theoretical works. Although many nurses of early eras delivered excellent care to patients, much of what was known about nursing was not written down, nor was research documenting the effectiveness of their care practices recorded. Therefore nurses began to move

toward the goal of developing nursing knowledge upon which to base their practice, and that goal served to direct the nursing profession throughout the twentieth century. The history of nursing clearly documents that efforts were sustained over time toward the goal of developing a substantive body of nursing knowledge to guide nursing practice (Alligood, 2002a; Chinn & Kramer, 2004; George, 2002; Johnson & Webber, 2001; McEwen & Willis, 2002; Parker, 2001).

This chapter introduces the reader to nursing theory under three major headings: history, significance, and analysis. A brief history presents the movement of nursing from vocation to profession, or more specifically, how the search for nursing

Previous authors: Martha Raile Alligood, Elizabeth Chong Choi, Juanita Fogel Keck, and Ann Marriner Tomey.

substance led to this outstanding time in nursing history and how the theory era affected nursing as an academic discipline and practice profession. Although there were sustained efforts toward the development of nursing as a profession, it was not until the last half of the twentieth century that nursing leaders came to understand the need for conceptual and theoretical approaches in nursing research to develop the knowledge base essential for professional nursing practice (Batey, 1977; Hardy, 1978). Nursing knowledge development was a driving force during this period as the baccalaureate degree became accepted as the first educational level for professional nursing and nursing began to be recognized as an academic discipline in higher education. Nurses worked to develop and clarify a substantive body of nursing knowledge with the goals of being recognized as a profession, raising the quality of patient care, and providing a professional style of practice. Thus the history of nursing provides the context needed to understand the nursing theory era and recognize the essential nature of theory for professional nursing practice.

The history and significance of nursing theory leads logically into analysis, the final section of this chapter. Analysis of nursing theoretical works and its role in knowledge development is presented as an essential process of critical reflection required for knowledge development. The criteria for analysis of each theorist's work are presented along with a brief discussion of how each criterion contributes to our understanding of theory use in education, research, administration, and practice (Chinn & Kramer, 2004).

HISTORY OF NURSING THEORY

The history of professional nursing begins with Florence Nightingale. It was Nightingale who envisioned nurses as a body of educated women at a time when women were neither educated nor employed in public service. Following her years of service organizing and caring for the wounded in Scutari during the Crimean War, her vision and her establishment of a school of nursing at St. Thomas' Hospital in London marked the birth of modern nursing. Nightingale's pioneering activities in nursing practice and her subsequent writings about nursing served as a guide for establishing nursing schools in the United States at the beginning of the twentieth century (Kalisch & Kalisch, 2003; Nightingale, 1859/1969). In the past century, nursing began with a strong emphasis on practice. Throughout that century, nurses worked toward the development of the profession in what has been described as successive historical eras (Alligood, 2002a).

The curriculum era addressed the question of what prospective nurses should study in order to learn how to nurse. In this era the emphasis was on what courses nursing students needed to take, with the goal of arriving at a standardized curriculum. By the mid-1930s a standardized curriculum was published. However, it was also in this era that the idea of moving nursing education from hospital-based diploma programs into colleges and universities emerged. Even so, it was the middle of the century before this goal began to be acted upon in many states (Kalisch & Kalisch, 2003).

As more and more nurses sought degrees in higher education, the research era, as it is deemed, began to emerge. This era came about as more and more nurses embraced higher education and arrived at a common understanding of the scientific age: that research was the path to new nursing knowledge. Nurses began to participate in research, and research courses began to be included in nursing curricula of the many developing graduate programs (Alligood, 2002a).

Thus the research era was followed closely by the graduate education era. Master's degree programs in nursing emerged to meet the public need for nurses with specialized nursing education. Many of these programs included a nursing research course. It was also in this era that most master's nursing programs began to include a course in concept development or nursing theory that introduced students to one or more of the early nursing theorists and the knowledge development process (Alligood, 2002a).

The theory era was a natural outgrowth of the research and graduate education eras. With an increased understanding of research and knowledge development, it soon became obvious that research without theory produced isolated information, and it was research and theory together that produced nursing science. In the early years of the theory era, doctoral education in nursing flourished and the emphasis was on theory development more than use of theory in nursing practice. However, within the contemporary phase of the theory era, an emphasis on the use of theory at the middle range level has emerged for theory-based nursing practice, as well as continued theory development (Alligood & Tomey, 1997, 2002; Batey, 1977; Chinn & Kramer, 2004; Fawcett, 2000; Tomey & Alligood, 2002). Each of the eras addressed nursing knowledge in a unique way that contributed and can be recognized in the history of nursing. They addressed the pervading question of the century: What is the nature of the knowledge that is needed for the practice of nursing? In addition, each era addressed that question according to the level of understanding at the time (Alligood, 2002a).

Nightingale's (1859/1969) vision of nursing has been practiced for more than a century, and theory development in nursing has evolved rapidly over the past 4 decades, leading to the recognition of nursing as an academic discipline with a substantive body of knowledge (Alligood, 2002a, 2002b; Alligood & Tomey, 2002; Chinn & Kramer, 2004; Fawcett, 2000; Tomey & Alligood, 2002; Walker & Avant, 2004). In the mid-1800s, Nightingale expressed with firm conviction that nursing knowledge was distinct from medical knowledge. She described a nurse's proper function as putting the patient in the best condition for nature (God) to act upon him or her. She put forth the idea that care of the sick is based on knowledge of persons and their surroundings, which was a different knowledge base than that physicians used for their practice. Despite this early edict from Nightingale in the 1850s, it was 100 years later during the 1950s before members of the nursing profession began serious discussion about the need to develop, articulate, and test nursing theory (Alligood, 2002d; Alligood, 2004; Chinn & Kramer, 2004; Meleis, 2004; Walker & Avant, 2004). Until the emergence of nursing as a science in the 1950s, nursing practice was based primarily on principles and traditions passed on through an ap-

prenticeship model of education and hospital-kept procedure manuals or handbooks that came from years of experience and use (Alligood, 2002a; Kalisch & Kalisch, 2003).

Although some nursing leaders aspired for nursing to develop as a profession and an academic discipline, nursing practice continued to reflect a vocational heritage more than a professional vision. The transition from vocation to profession included successive eras of history as nurses searched for a body of substantive knowledge on which to base nursing practice. The curriculum era, which emphasized course selection and content for nursing programs, gave way to the research era, with a focus on the research process and the goal of developing new knowledge.

In the mid-1970s, evaluation of 25 years of nursing research revealed that nursing lacked conceptual connections and theoretical frameworks (Batey, 1977). An awareness of the need for concept and theory development coincided with two other significant milestones in the evolution of nursing theory. One was the standardization of curricula for nursing master's education through the National League for Nursing accreditation criteria for baccalaureate and higher degree programs, and the second was the decision that doctoral education for nurses should be in nursing (Alligood, 2002a). The nursing theory era, coupled with a new awareness of nursing as a profession and an academic discipline in its own right, emerged from debates and discussions in the 1960s regarding the proper direction and appropriate discipline for nursing knowledge development. The awareness of the need for nursing doctorates and nursing science is evidenced by an explosive proliferation of nursing doctoral programs and nursing theory literature that was collected and reprinted by Nicoll (1986, 1992, 1997). The transition in the 1970s from vocation to profession was a major turning point for nursing because nurses asked the question, "Will nursing be other-discipline based or be nursing based?" The history records the answer, "Nursing practice will be based on nursing science" (Alligood, 2002a; Fawcett, 1978). According to Meleis (2004), this progress in nursing theory is a most significant aspect of the scholarly evolution and a cornerstone of the nursing discipline.

The 1980s was a period of major developments in nursing theory characterized as a transition from the preparadigm period to the paradigm period (Fawcett, 1984; Hardy, 1978). The prevailing nursing paradigms (models) provided various perspectives for nursing practice, administration, education, research, and further theory development. In the 1980s, Fawcett's proposal that global nursing concepts represented a nursing metaparadigm introduced an organizing structure for the existing nursing frameworks in the nursing literature (Fawcett, 1978, 1984, 2000). Classifying the nursing models as paradigms within a metaparadigm of the concepts *person, environment, health,* and *nursing* united the nursing theoretical works into a systematic view. This view clarified and improved the comprehension of knowledge development process by embedding the theorists' works in a larger context and facilitating an understanding of the growth of nursing as a science within the paradigm perspectives (Alligood & Tomey, 2002; Fawcett, 2000).

The body of nursing science and research, education, administration, and practice continue to expand through nursing scholarship. Papers are presented at national and international conferences. Newsletters, journals, and books, written by the communities of scholars associated with each of the various nursing models and theories, describe the theoretical base of practice and research with a selected model or theory within their paradigm perspectives (Alligood, 2004; Fawcett, 2000).

These observations of nursing science development bring Kuhn's (1970) ideas of normal science to life. Clearly his philosophy of science furthers our understanding of the evolution of nursing theory through an understanding of paradigm science (Kuhn, 1970). It is important to remember that theory emerged through individual efforts of various nursing leaders across the country, and it is only in retrospect that they have been viewed collectively in a systematic structure of knowledge. Theory development emerged as a product of the professional scholarship and growth process of nurse leaders, administrators, educators, and practi-

tioners who sought higher education and saw the limitations of theory from other disciplines such as medicine to describe, explain, or predict nursing outcomes. These leaders labored to establish a scientific basis for nursing management, curricula, practice, and research. Theory's function to convey an organizing structure and the meaning in these processes caused a convergence of ideas resulting in the emergence of what is referred to today as the *nursing theory era* (Alligood, 2002b; Alligood & Tomey, 2002; Cody, 1997; Nicoll, 1986, 1992, 1997).

The accomplishment of normal science ushers in the utilization phase of the theory era; that is, an emphasis on theory use and application in nursing practice, education, administration, and research (Alligood, 2002c). For the discipline of nursing, this emphasis on utilization restores the centrality of practice and recognizes theory and research as tools of practice rather than ends in their own right. The reader is referred to the third edition of Alligood and Tomey's text, *Nursing Theory: Utilization Application* (2006, in press) for case presentations and a more thorough discussion of the utilization and application of nursing theoretical works in nursing practice.

This brief history provides a context for the study of the nursing theorists and their work. In this new century the theory era continues with an emphasis on the use of nursing knowledge to guide the critical thinking required for professional practice. Middle range theories guide the thought and action of nursing practice (Alligood, 2002c; Alligood & Tomey, 1997; Fawcett, 2000; Smith & Leihr, 2003). Preparation for professional nursing includes an introduction to the works of selected nursing theorists.

Four general kinds of theoretical works are brought together in this text. Box 1-1 lists the theorists included in this text, grouped according to type of theoretical work. The first type is nursing philosophy. Philosophy sets forth the meaning of nursing phenomena through analysis, reasoning, and logical argument or presentation. Early works that predate or introduce the nursing theory era have contributed to knowledge development by providing direction or forming a basis for subsequent developments. Later works reflect more recent expansion in the areas of human science and its methods

(Alligood, 2002b; Meleis, 2004). Selected works classified as nursing philosophies are presented in Unit II, Chapters 6 through 11.

A second type, nursing conceptual models, comprises the nursing works of the grand theorists or pioneers in nursing (Chinn & Kramer, 2004; Fawcett, 2000; Meleis, 2004). Fawcett (2000) explains, "A conceptual model provides a distinct frame of reference for its adherents . . . that tells them how to observe and interpret the phenomena of interest to the discipline" (p. 16). The nursing models of these grand theorists are comprehensive and include their perspectives on each of the meta-paradigm concepts: person, environment, health, and nursing (Fawcett, 2000; Tomey & Alligood, 2002). Most nursing conceptual models have grand theories that the theorists have derived from their own models. Nursing models have explicit or implicit grand theories within them. The grand theories differ from the models in that they propose direction or action for members of the profession (Alligood & Tomey, 2002). An excellent example of a grand theory derived from a nursing model may be observed in Roy's work, where a grand theory of the person as an adaptive system is derived from her Adaptation Model. The highly abstract level of grand theories facilitates the derivation of many middle range theories from them that are specific to nursing practice (Alligood 2002d). Works classified as nursing models are in Unit III, Chapters 12 through 19.

The third type, nursing theory, may have been derived from works in other disciplines and related to nursing from earlier nursing philosophies and theories, from nursing grand theories, or from nursing conceptual models (Alligood, 2002c; Fawcett, 2000). A work classified as a nursing theory is less abstract than a grand theory but not as specific as a middle range theory. Theories may be specific to a particular aspect of nursing practice. Orlando gives an excellent example because her theory is specific to a style of communication within the nurse-patient relationship and the nursing process. Nursing theories are presented in Unit IV, Chapters 20 through 26.

The fourth type, middle range theory, has a narrower focus yet and is much more concrete

$\mathcal{B}$ox **1-1**

Types of Nursing Theoretical Works

PHILOSOPHIES
Nightingale
Watson
Ray
Benner
Martinsen
Eriksson

CONCEPTUAL MODELS AND GRAND THEORIES
Levine
Rogers
Orem
King
Neuman
Roy
Johnson
Boykin and Schoenhofer

THEORIES
Orlando
Pender
Leininger
Newman
Parse
Erickson, Tomlin, and Swain
Husted and Husted

MIDDLE RANGE NURSING THEORIES
Mercer
Mishel
Reed
Wiener and Dodd
Eakes, Burke, and Hainsworth
Barker
Kolcaba
Beck
Swanson
Ruland and Moore

than grand theory or nursing theory in its level of abstraction (Alligood 2002b, 2002d; Chinn & Kramer, 2004; Fawcett, 2000). Therefore, middle range theories are more precise and focus on answering specific nursing practice questions. They specify such factors as the age group of the patient, the family situation, the health condition, the location of the patient and, most importantly, the action of the nurse (Alligood, 2002c). Middle range theories address the specifics of nursing situations within the perspective of the model or theory from which they are derived (Alligood, 2002b, 2002c, 2002d; Fawcett, 2000). There are examples of middle range theories in the nursing literature that have been developed inductively rather than deductively. Selected middle range theories are presented in Unit V, Chapters 27 through 36. Table 1-1 presents examples of theoretical knowledge at each level of abstraction.

Table **1-1**

Knowledge Structure Levels with Examples	
STRUCTURE LEVEL	**EXAMPLE**
Metaparadigm	Person, environment, health, and nursing
Philosophy	Nightingale
Conceptual models	Neuman's systems model
Grand theory	Neuman's theory of optimal client stability
Theory	Optimal client stability for healthy aging
Middle range theory	Optimal client stability for healthy aging by intervening to maintain patient activity with body recall in community settings

Modified from Alligood, M. R., & Tomey, A. M. (2006, in press). Nursing theory: Utilization & application (3rd ed.). St. Louis: Mosby; and Fawcett, J. (2000). Contemporary nursing knowledge: Conceptual models of nursing and nursing theories. Philadelphia: F. A. Davis.

SIGNIFICANCE OF NURSING THEORY

At the beginning of the twentieth century, nursing was neither an academic discipline nor a profession. However, the accomplishments of the past century have led to the recognition of nursing in both areas. Although some may use these two terms (*discipline* and *profession*) interchangeably, their meanings are not the same. Although the discipline and profession are definitely interrelated, they have specific meanings that are important to understand, as follows:

- A **discipline** is specific to academia and refers to a branch of education, a department of learning, or a domain of knowledge (Donaldson & Crowley, 1978; Orem, 2001; Styles, 1982).
- A **profession** refers to a specialized field of practice; this is founded upon the theoretical structure of the science or knowledge of that discipline and the accompanying practice abilities (Donaldson & Crowley, 1978; Orem, 2001; Styles, 1982).

The achievements of the profession in the past century were highly relevant to nursing science development, but they did not come easily. History shows that many nurses pioneered the various causes and challenged the status quo with creative ideas for both the health of people and the development of nursing. Their achievements have ushered in this exciting time when nursing is recognized as both an academic discipline and a profession (Fitzpatrick, 1983; Kalisch & Kalisch, 2003; Meleis, 2004). In this section the pertinent question is: What is the significance of the theoretical works for the discipline and the profession of nursing? The answer to that question is: Nursing theoretical works represent the most comprehensive ideas and systematic presentations of nursing knowledge; therefore nursing theoretical works are vital to the future of both the discipline and the profession of nursing.

Significance for the Discipline

As nurses entered academia in larger numbers during the last half of the twentieth century, the goal to develop knowledge as a basis for nursing practice began to be realized. University baccalaureate programs proliferated, master's programs in nursing were developed, and the standardization of curricula increased through the accreditation process. As mentioned earlier in this chapter, nursing passed through eras of gradual development (Alligood, 2002a). Nursing leaders presented several different perspectives for the development of nursing science. Some advocated nursing as an applied science and others proclaimed nursing as a basic science (Donaldson & Crowley, 1978; Johnson, 1959; Rogers, 1970). History provides the evidence of the consensus that was reached; nursing research became essential content in both master's and baccalaureate nursing curricula.

In 1977, after *Nursing Research* had been in existence for 25 years, studies were comprehensively reviewed and the strengths and weaknesses of the research noted. Batey (1977) called attention to the importance of nursing conceptualizations to the research process and the role of a conceptual framework in the design of research for the production of science. This emphasis on the importance of conceptualization for nursing research projects and the development of conceptual frameworks for nursing curricula were precursors to the theory development era that moved nursing toward the goal of developing nursing knowledge to guide nursing practice. At that time, nursing theoretical works began to be published (Johnson, 1968, 1974; King, 1971; Levine, 1969; Neuman, 1974; Orem, 1971; Rogers, 1970; Roy, 1970). Soon after that, Fawcett (1978) presented her double helix metaphor that clarified the interdependent relationship of theory and research and became a classic reference on the topic. It was also about this time that earlier nursing scholars such as Henderson, Nightingale, Orlando, Peplau, and Wiedenbach began to be recognized for the relevant nature of their theoretical writings. Educators developed many of these early works as frameworks to structure curriculum content or guide the teaching of nursing practice in nursing programs. For example, Orlando's (1961, 1972) theory was the outcome of a nationally funded research project designed to study nursing practice.

When the Nurse Educator Nursing Theory Conference was held in New York City in 1978, the major theorists were brought together on the same stage for the first time. Most of them began their presentations by stating that they did not view themselves as theorists. Although an understanding of the significance of these works for nursing was limited at the time, young master's and doctoral students in the audience seemed to be aware of the significance of the event. By the second or third time, the audience just laughed at the theorists' denials of being theorists and then became silent and listened carefully to what each of the theorists had to share.

Also noteworthy, Donaldson and Crowley (1978) presented the keynote address at the Western Commission of Higher Education in Nursing Conference in 1977 as new nursing doctoral programs were beginning to open. They reopened the discussion of the nature of nursing science. The published version of the keynote address has become a classic reference for students to learn about nursing as a discipline and to clarify the difference between the discipline and the profession. The authors called for both basic and applied research and asserted that the use of this knowledge was vital to nursing as both a discipline and a profession.

Another critical topic the authors addressed had to do with the nature of nursing knowledge. The authors noted that the discipline and profession were inextricably linked, but failure to recognize and separate them from each other anchored nursing in a vocational view rather than a professional view. They then raised the question of whether the discipline of nursing even existed. Soon after this, nursing conceptual frameworks began to be noted as frameworks for curricula in nursing programs and as nursing conceptual models that addressed the major and most abstract concepts (metaparadigm) of nursing. This creative conceptualization of a nursing metaparadigm and a conceptual-theoretical structure of nursing knowledge clarified the works of the major nursing theorists as conceptual frameworks and paradigms of nursing. This organization of nursing theoretical works introduced a cohesive, systematic view of the theoretical knowledge that had been developed by the theorists at different times and in different parts of the country. Each nursing conceptual model was classified as such based on its performance in relation to a set of criteria for analysis and evaluation (Fawcett, 1984). Viewing the separate nursing works collectively under the metaparadigm umbrella led to increased understanding of the nursing theoretical works as a body of knowledge. In short, the significance of theory for the discipline of nursing is that the discipline is dependent upon theory for its continued existence.

The theoretical works have taken nursing to a higher professional level. The emphasis has shifted from a focus on knowledge about how nurses function with concentration on the nursing process to a focus on what nurses know and how they use what they know to guide their thinking and decision making while concentrating on the patient.

Frameworks and theories are designed to provide nurses with a perspective of the patient, and that perspective is characteristic of a profession. Professionals provide public service with practice that is focused on those whom they serve. The nursing process continues to be used in practice, but it is no longer the primary focus. That colleges and schools of nursing in universities across the country award degrees in nursing verifies the existence of unique nursing knowledge. This knowledge forms the basis for recognition of nursing as a discipline, and that knowledge is passed on to those entering the profession. Every discipline or field of knowledge includes theoretical knowledge. Therefore, nursing as an academic discipline is dependent upon the existence of nursing knowledge. This knowledge is transmitted to those entering the profession as a basis for their practice in the profession. Kuhn (1970), the philosopher of science, has stated, "The study of paradigms . . . is what mainly prepares the student for membership in the particular scientific community with which he [or she] will later practice" (p. 11). This is important to all nurses, but it is particularly important to those entering the profession because "in the absence of a paradigm . . . all of the facts that could possibly pertain to the development of a given science are likely to seem equally relevant" (Kuhn, 1970, p. 15). Finally, with regard to the priority of paradigms, he states, "By studying them and by practicing with them, the members of their corresponding community learn their trade" (Kuhn, 1970, p. 43). Master's-level nurses and students apply and test theoretical knowledge in their practice and test nursing knowledge in their theses. Doctoral level students who study to become nurse scientists develop nursing theory, test theory, and contribute new nursing science through theory-based research studies.

Significance for the Profession

Not only is theory essential for the existence of nursing as an academic discipline, it is also vital to the practice of professional nursing. Although the topic of nursing as a profession became less urgent at the end of the twentieth century, it had been a primary topic throughout much of the century as nursing made consistent progress toward professional status. Clearly, nursing is recognized as a profession today. Throughout much of the twentieth century, the criteria for a profession were used as a guide for its development. Nursing was the subject of a number of sociological studies of professional development that used various sets of criteria. For example, Bixler and Bixler (1959) published a set of criteria tailored to nursing in the *American Journal of Nursing*. They said that a profession does the following:

1. Utilizes in its practice a well-defined and well-organized body of specialized knowledge [that] is on the intellectual level of the higher learning
2. Constantly enlarges the body of knowledge it uses and improves its techniques of education and service by the use of the scientific method
3. Entrusts the education of its practitioners to institutions of higher education
4. Applies its body of knowledge in practical services vital to human and social welfare
5. Functions autonomously in the formulation of professional policy and in the control of professional activity thereby
6. Attracts individuals of intellectual and personal qualities who exalt service above personal gain and who recognize their chosen occupation as a life work
7. Strives to compensate its practitioners by providing freedom of action, opportunity for continuous professional growth, and economic security (pp. 1142-1146)

These criteria have historical value because they facilitate an understanding of the developmental path that nursing has followed. For example, a knowledge base that is well defined, organized, and specific to the discipline was formalized during the last half of the twentieth century, but this knowledge is not static. Rather, it continues to grow in relation to the profession's goals for the human and social welfare of the society that nurses serve. That is, although the body of knowledge is important, the theories and research are vital to the discipline and the profession as new knowledge continues to be generated. The application of nursing knowledge in practice is a criterion that is currently at the forefront with an emphasis on accountability for nursing practice, theory-based nursing practice, and the growing recognition that middle range theory is specific to nursing practice (Alligood & Tomey, 2002).

During the last decades of the twentieth century and in anticipation of the new millennium, ideas to move nursing forward were published. For example, Styles (1982) developed a distinction between a collective nursing profession and the individual nurse as a professional and called for internal developments based on ideals and beliefs of nursing for a new endowment. Her premise was that the profession needed a new, positive approach for the future, devoid of past problems, to make progress in professional development. To a similar end, Fitzpatrick (1983) presented a historical chronicle of the twentieth century achievements of the century leading to the professional status of nursing. Each references a more detailed background and history specific to the development of nursing as a profession. In this text we recognize nursing as a profession and emphasize the relationship between nursing theoretical works and that achievement. There are similarities and differences in the sets of criteria used to evaluate the status of professions; however, they all require developing and using a body of knowledge that is foundational to the practice of the given profession (Styles, 1982).

As individual nurses grow in their professional status, the use of substantive knowledge for theory-based nursing is a quality that is characteristic of their practice. This commitment to theory-based practice is most beneficial to patients because it provides a systematic, knowledgeable approach to their care. It also serves the profession of nursing because nurses are recognized for the contribution they make to the health care of society. As noted previously in relation to the discipline of nursing, the development of knowledge is an important activity for nurse scholars to pursue. It is important that nursing continue to be recognized and respected as a scholarly discipline that contributes to the health of society. Finally, and most importantly, nursing theory is a useful tool for reasoning, critical thinking, and decision making in nursing practice, as follows:

> Nursing practice settings are complex, and the amount of data (information) confronting nurses is virtually endless. Nurses must analyze a vast amount of information about each patient and decide what to do. A theoretical approach helps practicing nurses not to be overwhelmed by the mass of information and to progress through the nursing process in an orderly manner. Theory enables them to organize and understand what happens in practice, to analyze patient situations critically; for clinical decision making; to plan care and propose appropriate nursing interventions; and to predict patient outcomes from the care and evaluate its effectiveness. (Alligood, 2004, p. 247)

Professional practice requires a systematic approach that is focused on the patient, and the theoretical works provide just such perspectives of the patient. The types of theoretical works presented in this text are examples of the various perspectives. Philosophies of nursing, conceptual models of nursing, grand theories, nursing theories, and middle range theories guide the thought and action of the nurse in the data processing and actions of nursing practice.

With the background of the history and significance of nursing theory for the discipline and profession considered thus far in this chapter and with the introduction to levels of abstraction in various types of theory in a structure of nursing knowledge, we now turn to the topic of analysis of theory, a systematic process employed for the critical review of nursing theoretical works.

ANALYSIS OF THEORY

Analysis is an important process that is a vital step in the preparation for using nursing theoretical works in education, research, administration, or practice. Critical review of the work prior to its use leads to a better understanding of the work. Analysis of theory is the process carried out to acquire the knowledge of the theoretical work. The criteria for analysis of each theoretical work included in this text are clarity, simplicity, generality, empirical precision, and derivable consequences (Chinn & Kramer, 2004). Analysis, critique, and evaluation are all methods of studying nursing theoretical works critically. The process is useful for learning about the works and is especially essential for nurse scientists who intend to test, expand, or extend the works. Areas in need of further development are often discovered through the process of critique or analysis. Therefore, analysis is an important process for learning, for developing research projects, and for expanding the science associated with the theoretical works of nursing in the future.

Clarity

> How clear is this theory? (Chinn & Kramer, 2004, p. 117)

Consistency and semantic and structural clarity are important. To assess these, the major concepts, subconcepts, and their definitions are identified. Words often have multiple meanings within and across disciplines; therefore, a word should be defined carefully and specifically to the framework (philosophy, conceptual model, or theory) from which it is derived. Diagrams and examples may facilitate clarity and should be consistent. The logical development should be clear, and assumptions should be consistent with the theory's goals (Chinn & Kramer, 2004; Reynolds, 1971; Walker & Avant, 2004).

Reynolds (1971) refers to intersubjectivity when he states, "There must be shared agreement of the definitions of concepts and relationships between concepts within a theory" (p. 13). Hardy (1978) refers to meaning and logical adequacy when she states, "Concepts and relationships between concepts must be clearly identified and valid" (p. 106). Ellis (1968) refers to "the criterion of terminology" to evaluate theory and addresses "the danger of lost meaning when terms are borrowed from other disciplines and used in a different context" (p. 221). Walker and Avant (2004) assert that the logical adequacy of a theory is determined by the logical structure of the concepts and statements as proposed in the theory.

Simplicity

> How simple is this theory? (Chinn & Kramer, 2004, p. 117)

Simplicity is valued in theory development. Chinn and Kramer (2004) suggest that nurses in practice need simple forms of theory, such as middle range, to guide practice. A theory should be sufficiently comprehensive and at a level of abstraction sufficient to provide guidance, but it should have as few concepts as possible with simplistic relations to aid clarity. Reynolds (1971) contends, "the most useful theory provides the greatest sense of understanding" (p. 135). Walker and Avant (2004) suggest that parsimony is elegant in its simplicity, yet broad in content.

Generality

> How general is this theory (Chinn & Kramer, 2004, p. 117)

To determine the generality of a theory, the scope of concepts and goals within the theory are examined. The more limited the concepts and goals, the less general is the theory. Chinn and Kramer (2004) believe that the situations the theory applies to should not be limited. Ellis (1968) states, "The broader the scope, the greater the significance of the theory" (p. 129). The significance of scope has become better understood in recent years as doctoral students have come to understand that the more abstract the work, the more middle range theories can be derived from the work. Rogers' (1986) Theory of Accelerating Change is an excellent example of an abstract theory from which numerous middle range theories have been derived.

Empirical Precision

> How accessible is this theory? (Chinn & Kramer, 2004, p. 118)

Empirical precision is linked to the testability and ultimate use of a theory, and it refers to the "extent that the defined concepts are grounded in observable reality" (Hardy, 1978, p. 144). She states, "How well the evidence supports the theory is indicative of empirical adequacy . . . should be a match between theoretical claims and the empirical evidence" (p. 105). Reynolds (1971) refers to empirical relevance and the trait that "anyone be able to examine the correspondence between a particular theory and the objective empirical data" (p. 18). He notes that other scientists should be able to evaluate and verify results by themselves. Walker and Avant (2004) clarify that theory must generate hypotheses and be useful to scientists to add to the body of knowledge. Ellis (1968) emphasizes the tentative nature of theories and that they are subject to change.

Derivable Consequences

> How important is this theory? (Chinn & Kramer, 2004, p. 118)

Chinn and Kramer (2004) propose that if research, theory, and practice are to be meaningfully related, then nursing theory should lend itself to research testing, and research testing should lead to knowledge that guides practice. Furthermore, they suggest that nursing theory guides research and practice, generates new ideas, and differentiates the focus of nursing from other professions. Ellis (1968) indicates that to be considered useful, "it is essential for theory to develop and guide practice . . . theories

should reveal what knowledge nurses must, and should, spend time pursuing" (p. 220).

You will see these five criteria for the analysis of theory—clarity, simplicity, generality, empirical precision, and derivable consequences—because they are used in the chapters for critical reflection of each theoretical work. They are sufficiently broad criteria for analysis of nursing philosophies, conceptual models and grand theories, theories, and middle range theories.

SUMMARY

This chapter has provided an introduction to nursing theory with discussions of its history, significance, and analysis. The nurse's professional power is increased when using theoretical knowledge, because systematically developed methods guide critical thinking and decision making. As nurses use theory to guide their practice, they are more likely to be successful because they more quickly sort patient data, decide what nursing action is needed, and deliver care with an outcome expectation. They are also able to explain the framework they use for practice to other health professionals. Therefore, theory contributes to the achievement of professional autonomy by guiding practice, education, and research within the profession. Finally, the study of theory develops analytical skills and critical thinking ability, clarifies values and assumptions, and guides the purposes of nursing practice, education, and research (Alligood & Tomey, 2002; Chinn & Kramer, 2004; Cody, 1997; Fawcett, 2000; Meleis, 2004; Tomey & Alligood, 2002).

Nurses are recognizing the rich heritage of the works of the nursing theorists; that is, the philosophies, conceptual models, theories, and middle range theories of nursing. The contributions represent the status of nursing as a discipline as further developments occur. Most importantly, models and theories guide the critical thinking of nurses and are more and more accepted by the nursing community (Cody, 1997). Debates about what each model represents have given way to embracing how each model represents the diverse values of nurses. Today we see further clarification of these theoretical works as they are used as frameworks for structuring practice with predictable outcomes. Most important, the philosophies, models, theories, and middle range theories are being used in nursing education, administration, research, and practice.

Recognition of normal science from the theoretical works has occurred in this era. The scholarship of the past 2 decades alone demonstrates this outcome, not only as nursing literature around the philosophies, models, theories, and middle range theories has expanded quantitatively, but also as nursing scholarship has improved qualitatively. As more nurses have acquired higher education, a greater understanding of nursing theoretical works has expanded. Use of theory by nurses has increased dramatically the capacity for knowledge development, and the benefits for nursing practice have emerged (Alligood, 2002a; Chinn & Kramer, 2004; George, 2002; Johnson & Webber, 2001; McEwen & Willis, 2002; Parker, 2001).

REFERENCES

Alligood, M. R. (2002a). The nature of knowledge needed for nursing practice. In M. R. Alligood & A. M. Tomey (Eds.), *Nursing theory: Utilization & application* (2nd ed., pp. 3-14). St. Louis: Mosby.

Alligood, M. R. (2002b). Models and theories in nursing practice. In M. R. Alligood & A. M. Tomey (Eds.), *Nursing theory: Utilization & application* (2nd ed., pp. 15-39). St. Louis: Mosby.

Alligood, M. R. (2002c). Models and theories: Critical thinking structures. In M. R. Alligood & A. M. Tomey (Eds.), *Nursing theory: Utilization & application* (2nd ed., pp. 41-61). St. Louis: Mosby.

Alligood, M. R. (2002d). Areas for further development of theory-based nursing practice. In M. R. Alligood & A. M. Tomey (Eds.), *Nursing theory: Utilization & application* (2nd ed., pp. 453-463). St. Louis: Mosby.

Alligood, M. R. (2004). Nursing theory: The basis for professional nursing practice. In K. K. Chitty (Ed.), *Professional nursing: Concepts and challenges* (4th ed., pp. 271-298). Philadelphia: W. B. Saunders.

Alligood, M. R., & Tomey, A. M. (Eds.). (1997). *Nursing theory: Utilization & application.* St. Louis: Mosby.

Alligood, M. R., & Tomey, A. M. (Eds.). (2002). *Nursing theory: Utilization & application* (2nd ed.). St. Louis: Mosby.

Alligood, M. R., & Tomey, A. M. (Eds.). (2006, in press). *Nursing theory: Utilization & application* (3rd ed.). St. Louis: Mosby.

Batey, M. V. (1977). Conceptualization: Knowledge and logic guiding empirical research. *Nursing Research, 26*(5), 324-329.

Bixler, G. K., & Bixler, R. W. (1959). The professional status of nursing. *American Journal of Nursing, 59*(8), 1142-1146.

Chinn, P. L., & Kramer, M. K. (2004). *Integrated knowledge development in nursing* (6th ed.). St. Louis: Mosby.

Cody, W. K. (1997). Of tombstones, milestones, and gemstones: A retrospective and prospective on nursing theory. *Nursing Science Quarterly, 10*(1), 3-5.

Donaldson, S. K., & Crowley, D. M. (1978). The discipline of nursing. *Nursing Outlook, 26*(2), 1113-1120.

Ellis, R. (1968). Characteristics of significant theories. *Nursing Research, 17*(5), 217-222.

Fawcett, J. (1978). The relationship between theory and research: A double helix. *ANS Advances in Nursing Science, 1*(1), 49-62.

Fawcett, J. (1984). The metaparadigm of nursing: Current status and future refinements. *Image: The Journal of Nursing Scholarship, 16*, 84-87.

Fawcett, J. (2000). *Contemporary nursing knowledge: Conceptual models of nursing and nursing theories.* Philadelphia: F. A. Davis.

Fitzpatrick, M. L. (1983). *Prologue to professionalism.* Bowie, MD: Robert J. Brady.

George, J. (2002). *Nursing theories* (5th ed.). Upper Saddle River, NJ: Prentice-Hall.

Hardy, M. E. (1978). Perspectives on nursing theory. *ANS Advances in Nursing Science, 1*(1), 27-48.

Johnson, B., & Webber, P. (2001). *An introduction to theory and reasoning in nursing.* Philadelphia: J. B. Lippincott.

Johnson, D. (1959). The nature of a science of nursing. *Nursing Outlook, 7*, 291-294.

Johnson, D. (1968). One conceptual model for nursing. Unpublished paper presented at Vanderbilt University. Nashville, TN.

Johnson, D. (1974, Sept/Oct). Development of the theory: A requisite for nursing as a primary health profession. *Research Nursing, 23*, 372-377.

Kalisch, P. A., & Kalisch, B. J. (2003). *The advance of American nursing* (4th ed.). Philadelphia: Lippincott Williams & Wilkins.

King, I. (1971). *Toward a theory of nursing.* New York: John Wiley.

Kuhn, T. S. (1970). *The structure of scientific revolutions.* Chicago: University of Chicago Press.

Levine, M. (1969). *Introduction to clinical nursing.* Philadelphia: F. A. Davis.

McEwen, M., & Wills, E. (2002). *Theoretical basis of nursing.* Philadelphia: Lippincott Williams & Wilkins.

Meleis, A. (2004). *Theoretical nursing: Development and progress* (4th ed.). Philadelphia: Lippincott Williams & Wilkins.

Neuman, B. (1974). The Betty Neuman health systems model: A total person approach to patient problems. In

J. P. Riehl & C. Roy (Eds.), *Conceptual models for nursing practice* (pp. 94-114). New York: Appleton-Century-Crofts.

Nicoll, L. (1986). *Perspectives on nursing theory.* Boston: Little, Brown.

Nicoll, L. (1992). *Perspectives on nursing theory* (2nd ed.). Philadelphia: J. B. Lippincott.

Nicoll, L. (1997). *Perspectives on nursing theory* (3rd ed.). Philadelphia: J. B. Lippincott.

Nightingale, F. (1969). *Notes on nursing: What it is and what it is not.* New York: Dover. (Originally published 1859.)

Orem, D. (1971). *Nursing: Concepts of practice.* St. Louis: Mosby.

Orem, D. (2001). *Nursing: Concepts of practice* (6th ed.). St. Louis: Mosby.

Orlando, I. (1961). *The dynamic nurse-patient relationship.* New York: G. P. Putnam's Sons.

Orlando, I. (1972). *The discipline and teaching of nursing process.* New York: G. P. Putnam's Sons.

Parker, M. (2001). *Nursing theory and nursing practice.* Philadelphia: F. A. Davis.

Reynolds, P. D. (1971). *A primer for theory construction.* Indianapolis: Bobbs-Merrill.

Rogers, M. E. (1970). *An introduction to the theoretical basis of nursing.* Philadelphia: F. A. Davis.

Rogers, M. E. (1986). Science of unitary human beings. In V. Malinski (Ed.), *Explorations on Martha Rogers' science of unitary human beings.* Norwalk, CT: Appleton-Century-Crofts.

Roy, C. (1970). Adaptation: A conceptual framework for nursing. *Nursing Outlook, 18,* 42-45.

Smith, M., & Leihr, P. (2003). *Middle range theory for nursing.* New York: Springer Publishing.

Styles, M. M. (1982). *On nursing: Toward a new endowment.* St. Louis: Mosby.

Tomey, A. M., & Alligood, M. R. (2002). *Nursing theorists and their work* (5th ed.). St. Louis: Mosby.

Walker, L. O., & Avant, K. C. (2004). *Strategies for theory construction in nursing* (4th ed.). Norwalk, CT: Appleton Lange.

History and Philosophy of Science

Sue Marquis Bishop and Sonya R. Hardin

$\mathcal{M}$odern science is a relatively new intellectual activity. Established 400 years ago, modern science has occupied only a short time in the history of humankind (Bronowski, 1979). Scientific activity has persisted because it has improved quality of life and has satisfied human needs for creative work, a sense of order, and the desire to understand the unknown (Bronowski, 1979; Gale, 1979; Piaget, 1970). The development of science requires formalizing given phenomena of interest and events concerning each science. The construction of nursing theories is the formalization of attempts to describe, explain, predict, or control states of affairs in nursing (nursing phenomena).

HISTORICAL VIEWS OF THE NATURE OF SCIENCE

To formalize the science of nursing, basic questions must be considered, such as: What is science, knowledge, and truth? What methods produce

Previous author: Sue Marquis Bishop.

scientific knowledge? These are philosophical questions. The term *epistemology* is concerned with the theory of knowledge in philosophical inquiry. The particular philosophical perspective selected to answer these questions will influence how scientists perform scientific activities, how they interpret outcomes, and even what they regard as science and knowledge (Brown, 1977). Although philosophy has been documented as an activity for 3000 years, formal science is a relatively new human pursuit (Brown, 1977; Foucault, 1973). Scientific activity has only recently become the object of investigation.

Two competing theories of science, rationalism and empiricism, have evolved in the era of modern science with several variations. Gale (1979) labeled these alternative epistemologies as centrally concerned with the power of reason and the power of sensory experience. Gale noted similarity in the divergent views of science in the time of the classical Greeks. For example, Aristotle believed advances in biological science would develop through systematic observation of objects and events in the natural world, whereas Pythagoras believed knowledge of the natural world would develop from mathematical reasoning (Brown, 1977; Gale, 1979).

Rationalism

Rationalist epistemology emphasizes the importance of *a priori* reasoning as the appropriate method for advancing knowledge. The scientist in this tradition approaches the task of scientific inquiry by developing a systematic explanation (theory) of a given phenomenon (Gale, 1979). This conceptual system is analyzed by addressing the logical structure of the theory and the logical reasoning involved in its development. Theoretical assertions derived by deductive reasoning are then subjected to experimental testing to corroborate the theory. Reynolds (1971) labeled this approach the *theory-then-research strategy.* If the research findings fail to correspond with the theoretical assertions, additional research is conducted or modifications are made in the theory and further tests are devised; otherwise, the theory is discarded in favor of an alternative explanation (Gale, 1979; Zetterberg, 1966). Popper (1962) argued that science would evolve more rapidly through the process of conjectures and refutations by devising research in an attempt to refute new ideas.

The rationalist view is most clearly evident in the work of Einstein, the theoretical physicist, who made extensive use of mathematical equations in developing his theories. The theories Einstein constructed offered an imaginative framework, which has directed research in numerous areas (Calder, 1979). As Reynolds (1971) noted, if someone believes that science is a process of inventing descriptions of phenomena, the appropriate strategy for theory construction is the theory-then-research strategy. In Reynolds' view, "As the continuous interplay between theory construction (invention) and testing with empirical research progresses, the theory becomes more precise and complete as a description of nature and, therefore, more useful for the goals of science" (Reynolds, 1971, p. 145).

Empiricism

The empiricist view is based on the central idea that scientific knowledge can be derived only from sensory experience. Francis Bacon (Gale, 1979) received credit for popularizing the basis for the empiricist approach to inquiry. Bacon believed that scientific truth was discovered through generalizing observed facts in the natural world. This approach, called the *inductive method,* is based on the idea that the collection of facts precedes attempts to formulate generalizations, or as Reynolds (1971) called it, the *research-then-theory strategy.*

The strict empiricist view is reflected in the work of the behaviorists Watson and Skinner. In a 1950 paper, Skinner asserted that advances in the science of psychology could be expected if scientists would focus on the collection of empirical data. He cautioned against drawing premature inferences and proposed a moratorium on theory building until further facts were collected. Skinner's (1950) approach to theory construction was clearly inductive. His view of science and the popularity of behaviorism have been credited with influencing psychology's shift in emphasis from the building of theories to the gathering of facts between the 1950s and 1970s (Snelbecker, 1974). The difficulty with the inductive mode of inquiry is that the world presents an infinite number of possible observations and, therefore, the scientist must bring ideas to her experiences to decide what to observe and what to exclude (Steiner, 1977). Although Skinner disclaimed to be developing a theory in his early writings, Bixenstine (1964, p. 465) noted, "Skinner is startlingly creative in applying the conceptual elements of his, let's be frank, theory to a wide variety of issues, ranging from training pigeons in the guidance of missiles, to developing teaching machines, to constructing a model society."

EARLY TWENTIETH CENTURY VIEWS OF SCIENCE AND THEORY

During the first half of this century, philosophers focused on the analysis of theory structure, whereas scientists focused on empirical research (Brown,

1977). There was minimal interest in the history of science, the nature of scientific discovery, or the similarities between the philosophical view of science and the scientific methods (Brown, 1977). *Positivism,* a term first used by Comte, emerged as the dominant view of modern science (Gale, 1979). Modern logical positivists believed empirical research and logical analysis were two approaches that would produce scientific knowledge. Logical positivists hailed the system of symbolic logic, published from 1910 to 1913 by Whitehead and Russell, as an appropriate approach to discovering truth (Brown, 1977).

The logical empiricists offered a more lenient view of logical positivism and argued that theoretical propositions must be tested through observation and experimentation (Brown, 1977). This perspective is rooted in the idea that empirical facts exist independently of theories and offer the only basis for objectivity in science (Brown, 1977). In this view, objective truth exists independently of the researcher, and the task of science is to discover it. The empiricist view shares similarities with Aristotle's view of biological science and Bacon's inductive method as the true method of scientific inquiry (Gale, 1979). This view of science is often presented in methods courses as the single orthodox view of the scientific enterprise, and is taught in the following manner: "The scientist first sets up an experiment; observes what occurs . . . ; reaches a preliminary hypothesis to describe the occurrence; runs further experiments to test the hypothesis [and] finally corrects or modifies the hypothesis in light of the results" (Gale, 1979, p. 13).

The increasing use of computers, which permit the analysis of large data sets, may have contributed to the acceptance of the positivist approach to modern science (Snelbecker, 1974). However, in the 1950s, the literature began to reflect an increasing challenge to the positivist view, thereby ushering in a new view of science (Brown, 1977).

EMERGENT VIEWS OF SCIENCE AND THEORY IN THE LATE TWENTIETH CENTURY

In the latter years of the twentieth century, several authors presented analyses challenging the positivist

position, thus offering the basis for a new perspective of science (Brown, 1977; Foucault, 1973; Hanson, 1958; Kuhn, 1962; Toulmin, 1961). Foucault (1973) published his analysis (first published in French in 1966) of the epistemology of human sciences from the seventeenth to the nineteenth century. His major thesis stated that empirical knowledge was arranged in different patterns at a given time and in a given culture. Over time, he found changes in the focus of inquiry in what was regarded by scholars as scientific knowledge and in how knowledge was organized. Further, he concluded that humans only recently emerged as objects of study. Schutz (1967), in his *Phenomenology of the Social World,* argued that scientists seeking to understand the social world cannot cognitively know an external world that is independent of their own life experiences.

In 1977, Brown argued that a new intellectual revolution in philosophy, which emphasized the history of science, was replacing formal logic as the major analytical tool in the philosophy of science. One of the major perspectives in the new philosophy was the focus on science as a process of continuing research rather than the emphasis on accepted findings. In this emergent epistemology, the emphasis was on understanding scientific discovery and understanding the processes involved in changes in theories over time.

Empiricists argue that for science to maintain objectivity, data collection and analysis must be independent of theory (Brown, 1977). This assertion is based on the position that objective truth exists in the world, just waiting to be discovered. Brown (1977) argues that the new epistemology challenged the empiricist view of perception by acknowledging that theories play a significant role in determining what the scientist will observe and how it will be interpreted. The following story, related to Marquis Bishop by her grandmother, illustrates Brown's thesis that observations are concept laden; that is, an observation is influenced by ideas in the mind of the observer:

A husband and wife are sitting by the fire silently watching their firstborn son asleep in the cradle. The mother looks at her infant son and imagines him learning to talk and then to walk. She continues her reverie by imagining him playing with friends, coming home from school, and then going to college. She ends her daydreaming by visualizing him elected president of the United States. She smiles and glances up at her husband, who also had been staring intently at their son. "What are you thinking, honey?" The husband replies, "I was just thinking that I can't imagine how anyone could build a fine cradle like this, sell it for $24.95, and still make a profit."

Brown (1977) presented the example of a chemist and a child walking together past a steel mill. The chemist perceived the odor of sulfur dioxide and the child smelled rotten eggs. The two observers in the two examples above responded to the same observable data with distinctly different cognitive interpretations. In studying to become family therapists, students may analyze videotapes of family therapy sessions to learn the different approaches to family therapy. Novice student therapists tend to focus on the content of family interaction (what one member says to another) or the behavior of individual family members. After studying the system's view of families, which focuses on patterned transactions among family members, students then can recognize and describe transactions among family members that they did not perceive during the first viewing of the videotapes. For example, the son withdraws when his parents argue, or the wife grits her teeth when her husband speaks. Concepts and theories create boundaries for selecting observable phenomena and for reasoning about specific patterns. For example, the social network concept may be more fruitful, in some instances, for studying social relations than the group concept, because it focuses attention on a more complex set of relationships that are beyond the boundaries of any one setting (Bishop, 1984; Irving, 1977).

If scientists perceive patterns in the empirical world based on their presupposed theories, however, how can new patterns ever be perceived or new discoveries become formulated? Gale (1979) answered this question by arguing that the scientist is able to perceive forceful intrusions from the environment that challenge his or her *a priori* mental set, thereby raising questions regarding the current theoretical perspective. Brown (1977) maintained that, although a presupposed theoretical framework influences perception, theories are not the single determining factor of the scientist's perception. He identified the following three different views of the relationship between theories and observation:

1. Scientists are merely passive observers of occurrences in the empirical world. Observable data are objective truth waiting to be discovered.
2. Theories structure what the scientist perceives in the empirical world.
3. Presupposed theories and observable data interact in the process of scientific investigation (Brown, 1977, p. 298).

Brown's argument for an interactionist's perspective coincides with the scientific consensus in the study of pattern recognition in how humans process information. The following distinct minitheories have directed research efforts in this area: (1) the data-driven, or bottom-up, theory and (2) the conceptually driven, or top-down, theory (Norman, 1976). In the former, cognitive expectations (what is known or ways of organizing meaning) are used to select input and process incoming information from the environment. The second theory asserts that incoming data are perceived as unlabeled input and analyzed as raw data with increasing levels of complexity until all the data are classified. Current research evidence suggests that human pattern recognition progresses through an interaction of both data-driven and conceptually driven processes, and it uses sources of information in both currently organized, cognitive categories and in stimuli from the sensory environment. The interactionist's perspective also is clearly reflected in Piaget's theory of human cognitive functioning:

Piagetian man actively selects and interprets environmental information in the construction of his own knowledge, rather than passively copying the information just as it is presented to his senses. While paying attention to and taking account of the structure of the environment during knowledge seeking, Piagetian man reconstrues and reinterprets that environment [according to] his own mental framework . . . The mind neither copies the world . . . nor does it ignore the world [by] creating a private mental conception of it out of whole cloth. The mind meets the environment in an extremely active, self-directed way. (Flavell, 1977, p. 6)

If the thesis is accepted that objective truth does not exist and science is an interactive process between invented theories and empirical observations, how are scientists to determine truth and scientific knowledge? In the new epistemology, science is viewed as an ongoing process. Much importance is given to the idea of consensus among scientists. As Brown (1977) concluded, it is a myth that science can establish final truths. Tentative consensus based on reasoned judgments about the available evidence is the most that can be expected. In this view, scientific knowledge is what the community of scientists in any given historical era regard as scientific knowledge. Current consensus among scientists determines the truth of a given theoretical statement by concluding whether or not it presents an adequate description of reality (Brown, 1977). This consensus is possible through the collaboration of many scientists as they make their work available for public review and debate and as they build upon previous inquiries (Randall, 1964). "The individual (scientist) introduces ideas, the scientific community appraises them" by its objective criteria (Randall, 1964, p. 59).

In any given era and in any given discipline, science is structured by an accepted set of presuppositions that define the phenomena for study and define the appropriate methods for data collection and interpretation (Brown, 1977; Foucault, 1973; Kuhn, 1962). These presuppositions set the boundaries for the scientific enterprise in a particular field. In Brown's view of the transactions between theory and empirical observation:

Theory determines what observations are worth making and how they are to be understood, and observation provides challenges to accepted theoretical structures. The continuing attempt to produce a coherently organized body of theory and observation is the driving force of research, and the prolonged failure of specific research projects leads to scientific revolutions. (1977, p. 167)

The presentation and acceptance of a revolutionary theory may alter the existing presuppositions and theories, thereby creating a different set of boundaries and procedures. The result is a new set of problems or a new way to interpret observations; that is, a new picture of the world (Kuhn, 1962). In this view of science, the emphasis must be placed on ongoing research rather than established findings.

INTERDEPENDENCE OF THEORY AND RESEARCH

Traditionally, theory building and research have been presented to students in separate courses. Often, this separation has caused problems for students in understanding the nature of theories and in comprehending the relevance of research efforts (Winston, 1974). The acceptance of the positivist view of science may have influenced the sharp distinction between theory and research methods (Gale, 1979). Although theory and research can be viewed as distinct operations, they are regarded more appropriately as interdependent components of the scientific process (Dubin, 1978). In constructing a theory, the theorist must be knowledgeable about available empirical findings and be able to take these into account because theory is, in part, concerned with organizing and formalizing available knowledge of a given phenomenon. The theory is subject to revision if the hypotheses fail to correspond with empirical findings, or the theory may be abandoned in favor of an alternative explanation that accounts for the new information (Brown, 1977; Dubin, 1978; Kuhn, 1962).

In contemporary theories of science, the scientific enterprise has been described as a series of phases with an emphasis on the discovery and verification (or acceptance) phases (Gale, 1979; Giere, 1979). According to Gale, these phases are concerned primarily with the presentation and testing of new ideas. New ways of thinking about phenomena or new data are introduced to the scientific community during the discovery phase. During this time, the focus is on presenting a persuasive argument to show that the new conceptions represent an improvement over previous conceptions (Gale, 1979). Verification is characterized by the scientific community's efforts to critically analyze and test the new conceptions in an attempt to refute them. The new views are then subjected to testing and analyses (Gale, 1979). However, Brown (1977) argued that discovery and verification could not be viewed as distinct phases, because the scientific community does not usually accept a new conception until it has been subjected to significant testing. Only then can it be accepted as a new discovery.

In any scientific discipline, it is not appropriate to judge a theory on the basis of authority, faith, or intuition; it should be judged on the basis of scientific consensus (Randall, 1964). For example, if a specific nursing theory is deemed acceptable, this judgment should not be made because a respected nursing leader advocates the theory. Personal feelings, such as "I like this theory" or "I don't like this theory," should not provide the basis for judgment, either. The theory should be judged acceptable only on the basis of logical and conceptual or empirical grounds. The scientific community makes these judgments (Gale, 1979).

The advancement of science is thus a collaborative endeavor in which many researchers evaluate and build on each others' work. Theories, procedures, and findings from empirical studies must be made available for critical review by scientists for evidence to be cumulative. The same procedures can be used to support or refute a given analysis or finding. A theory is accepted when scientists agree that it provides a description of reality that captures the phenomenon of available research findings (Brown, 1977). The acceptance of a scientific hypothesis depends on the appraisal of the coherence of theory, which involves questions of logic, and the correspondence of the theory, which involves efforts to relate the theory to observable phenomena through research (Steiner, 1978). Gale (1979) labeled these criteria as epistemological and metaphysical concerns.

The consensus regarding the correspondence of the theory is, therefore, not based on a single study.

Repeated testing is crucial. The study must be replicated under the same conditions, and the theoretical assertions must be explored under different conditions or with different measures. Consensus is, therefore, based on accumulated evidence (Giere, 1979). When the theory does not appear to be supported by research, the scientific community does not necessarily reject it. Rather than agreeing that a problem exists with the theory itself, the community may make judgments about the validity or the reliability of the measures used in testing the theory or about the appropriateness of the research design. These possibilities are considered in critically evaluating all attempts to test a given theory.

Scientific consensus is necessary in three key areas for any given theory as follows: (1) agreement on the boundaries of the theory; that is, the phenomenon it addresses and the phenomena it excludes (criterion of coherence), (2) agreement on the logic used in constructing the theory to further understanding from a similar perspective (criterion of coherence), and (3) agreement that the theory fits the data collected and analyzed through research (criterion of correspondence) (Brown, 1977; Dubin, 1978; Steiner, 1977; Steiner, 1978). Essentially, consensus in these three areas constitutes an agreement among scientists to "look at the same 'things,' to do so in the same way, and to have a level of confidence certified by an empirical test" (Dubin, 1978, p. 13). Therefore, the theory must be capable of being operationalized for testing to check it against reality. Retroductive, deductive, and inductive forms of reasoning may be used as science progresses by building theoretical descriptions and explanations of reality, attempting to account for available findings, deriving testable hypotheses, and evaluating theories from the perspective of new empirical data (Steiner, 1978).

Most research may be considered within the category that Kuhn (1962) called *normal science.* Scientific inquiry in normal science involves testing a given theory, developing new applications of a theory, or extending a given theory. Occasionally, a new theory with different assumptions is developed that could replace previous theories. Kuhn (1962) described this as revolutionary science and described the theory with different presuppositions as a revolutionary theory. A change in the accepted presuppositions creates a set of boundaries and procedures that suggest a new set of problems or a new way to interpret observations (Kuhn, 1962).

In the social and behavioral sciences, there is some challenge to the assumptions underlying the accepted methods of experimental design, measurement, and statistical analysis that emphasizes the search for universal laws and emphasizes the use of procedures for the random assignment of subjects across contexts. Mishler (1979) argued that, in studying behavior, scientists should develop methods and procedures that are dependent on context for meaning rather than eliminate context by searching for laws that hold across contexts. This critique of the methods and assumptions of research is emerging from phenomenological and ethnomethodological theorists who view the scientific process from a very different paradigm (Bowers, 1992; Hudson, 1972; Mishler, 1979; Pallikkathayil & Morgan, 1991).

The proper focus of research is not the attempt to prove a theory or hypothesis, but the attempt to set up research to refute a given hypothesis (Popper, 1962). Repeated failed attempts at refutation lend support to the theory and acceptance of the theory by the scientific community (Dubin, 1978). However, the emphasis is always placed on ongoing research rather than established findings (Brown, 1977). In the future, new information or a new, compelling way to view the same evidence may lead to a reappraisal of the theory. One previously accepted theory may be abandoned for another theory if it fails to correspond with empirical findings or if it does not present clear directions for further research. The scientific community judges the selected alternative theory to account for available data and to suggest further lines of inquiry (Brown, 1977).

Popper observed that refutations of a given theory frequently are viewed as a failure of the theorist or the theory. In his view, "Every refutation should be regarded as a great success; not merely as a success of the scientist who refuted the theory, but also of the scientist who created the refuted theory and who thus . . . suggested, if only indirectly, the refutation experiment" (1962, p. 243).

There is neither a single science nor a single scientific method. There are several sciences, each with unique phenomena and structure and methods for inquiry (Springagesh & Springagesh, 1986). However, the commonality among sciences concerns the scientists' efforts to separate truth from speculation to advance knowledge (Snelbecker, 1974). In questions regarding the structure of knowledge in a given science, the consensus of scientists in the discipline decide what is to be regarded as scientific knowledge and the methods of inquiry (Brown, 1977; Gale, 1979).

Consensus has emerged in the field of nursing that the knowledge base for nursing practice is incomplete, and the development of a scientific base for nursing practice is a high priority for the discipline. The postpositivist and interpretive paradigms have achieved a degree of acceptance in nursing as paradigms to guide knowledge development (Ford-Gilboe, Campbell, & Berman, 1995). Postpositivism focuses on discovering patterns that may describe, explain, and predict phenomena. It rejects the older, traditional positivist views of an ultimate objective knowledge that is observable only through the senses (Ford-Gilboe et al., 1995; Weiss, 1995). The interpretive paradigm tends to promote understanding by addressing the meanings of the participants' social interaction that emphasize situation, context, and the multiple cognitive constructions that individuals create from everyday events (Ford-Gilboe et al., 1995). A critical paradigm for knowledge development in nursing also has been described as an emergent, postmodern paradigm that provides the framework for inquiring about the interaction between social, political, economic, gender, and cultural factors and the experiences of health and illness (Ford-Gilboe et al., 1995). A broad conception of postmodernism includes the particular philosophies that challenge the "objectification of knowledge," such as phenomenology, hermeneutics, feminism, critical theory, and poststructuralism (Omery, Kasper, & Page, 1995).

The various sciences are at different stages of development. Physics, with the exception of mathematics, is considered the most exacting of the sciences; the life sciences, such as botany, are not as well developed scientifically; the social sciences are even less developed. Until the late 1950s, use of the term *nursing science* in the literature was uncommon. The philosophy of nursing has been developing over a 150-year period; however, Fry (1999) concluded that philosophical inquiry was only a recent development in nursing, and was not yet a well-defined field in nursing. She cited the following evidence of increasing interest and productivity in the philosophy of nursing as a field of inquiry: (1) establishment of the Institute for Philosophical Nursing Research at the University of Alberta in the 1980s, (2) increased publication of articles and books on nursing philosophy, and (3) establishment of the journal *The Philosophy of Nursing*. It has been argued that evolutionary changes associated with the information age are changing nurses' views of possible realities and are creating a philosophical shift in nursing (Silva, Sorrell, & Sorrell, 1995; Carper, 1978). This shift was viewed as transferring the focus from an exclusive, philosophical emphasis on epistemological questions about knowing to a focus on ontological questions about meaning, being, and reality (Silva et al., 1995).

Compared with other developing sciences, nursing science is in the early stages of scientific development. During the early twenty-first century, the evidence is that a greater number of nursing scholars are actively engaged in the advancement of knowledge for the discipline of nursing.

SCIENCE AS A SOCIAL ENTERPRISE

The process of scientific inquiry may be viewed as a social enterprise (Mishler, 1979). In Gale's words, "Human beings do science" (1979, p. 290). Therefore, it might be anticipated that social, economic, or political factors may influence the scientific enterprise (Brown, 1977). For example, the popularity of certain ideologies may influence how phenomena are viewed and what problems are selected for study (Hudson, 1972). In addition, the availability of funds for research in a specified area may increase research activity in that area. However,

science does not depend on the personal characteristics or persuasions of any given scientist or group of scientists, but it is powerfully self-correcting within the community of scientists (Randall, 1964). Science progresses by "reasoned judgments on the part of scientists and through debate within the scientific community" (Brown, 1977, p. 167).

REFERENCES

Bishop, S. M. (1984). Perspectives on individual-family-social network interrelations. *Interrelational Journal of Family Therapy, 6*(2), 124-135.

Bixenstine, E. (1964). Empiricism in latter-day behavioral science. *Science, 145,* 465.

Bowers, L. (1992). Ethnomethodology I: An approach to nursing research. *International Journal of Nursing Studies, 29*(1), 59-67.

Bronowski, J. (1979). *The visionary eye: Essays in the arts, literature and science.* Cambridge, MA: MIT Press.

Brown, H. (1977). *Perception, theory and commitment: The new philosophy of science.* Chicago: University of Chicago Press.

Calder, N. (1979). *Einstein's universe.* New York: Viking.

Carper, B. (1978). Fundamental patterns of knowing in nursing. *ANS Advances in Nursing Science, 1*(1), 13-23.

Dubin, R. (1978). *Theory building.* New York: Free Press.

Flavell, J. H. (1977). *Cognitive development.* Englewood Cliffs, NJ: Prentice-Hall.

Ford-Gilboe, M., Campbell, J., & Berman, H. (1995). Stories and numbers: Coexistence without compromise. *ANS Advances in Nursing Science, 18*(1), 14-26.

Foucault, M. (1973). *The order of things: An archaeology of the human sciences.* New York: Vintage Books.

Fry, S. (1999). The philosophy of nursing. *Scholarly Inquiry for Nursing Practice: An International Journal, 13*(1), 5-15.

Gale, G. (1979). *Theory of science: An introduction to the history, logic and philosophy of science.* New York: McGraw-Hill.

Giere, R. N. (1979). *Understanding scientific reasoning.* New York: Holt, Rhinehart, & Winston.

Hanson, N. R. (1958). *Patterns of discovery.* Cambridge, MA: Cambridge University Press.

Hudson, L. (1972). *The cult of the fact.* New York: Harper & Row.

Irving, H. W. (1977). Social networks in the modern city. *Social Forces, 55,* 867-880.

Kuhn, T. S. (1962). *The structure of scientific revolutions.* Chicago: University of Chicago Press.

Mishler, E. G. (1979). Meaning in context: Is there any other kind? *Harvard Educational Review, 49,* 1-19.

Norman, D. A. (1976). *Memory and attention: An introduction to human information processing.* New York: John Wiley & Sons.

Omery, A., Kasper, C. E., & Page, G. G. (1995). *In search of nursing science.* Thousand Oaks, CA: Sage Publications.

Pallikkathayil, L., & Morgan, S. (1991). Phenomenology as a method for conducting clinical research. *Applied Nursing Research, 4*(4), 195-200.

Piaget, J. (1970). *The place of the sciences of man in the system of sciences.* New York: Harper & Row.

Popper, K. (1962). *Conjectures and refutations.* New York: Basic Books.

Randall, J. H. (1964). *Philosophy: An introduction.* New York: Barnes & Noble.

Reynolds, P. (1971). *A primer in theory construction.* Indianapolis, IN: Bobbs-Merrill.

Schutz, A. (1967). *The phenomenology of the social world.* Evanston, IL: Northwestern University Press.

Silva, M. C., Sorrell, J. M., & Sorrell, C. D. (1995). From Carper's patterns of knowing to ways of being: An ontological philosophical shift in nursing. *ANS Advances in Nursing Science, 18*(1), 1-13.

Skinner, B. F. (1950). Are theories of learning necessary? *Psychological Review, 57,* 193-216.

Snelbecker, G. (1974). *Learning theory, instructional theory, and psychoeducational design.* New York: McGraw-Hill.

Springagesh, K., & Springagesh, S. (1986). Philosophy and scientific approach. *Contemporary Philosophy, 11*(6), 18-20.

Steiner, E. (1977). *Criteria for theory of art education.* Unpublished monograph presented at Seminar for Research in Art Education. Philadelphia.

Steiner, E. (1978). *Logical and conceptual analytic techniques for educational researchers.* Washington, DC: University Press.

Toulmin, S. (1961). *Foresight and understanding.* New York: Harper & Row.

Weiss, S. J. (1995). Contemporary empiricism. In A. Omery, C. E. Kasper, & G. G. Page (Eds.), *In search of nursing science.* Thousand Oaks, CA: Sage Publications.

Winston, C. (1974). *Theory and measurement in sociology.* New York: John Wiley & Sons.

Zetterberg, H. L. (1966). *On theory and verification in sociology.* Totowa, NJ: Bedminster Press.

*L*ogical Reasoning

Sue Marquis Bishop and Sonya R. Hardin

*L*ogic is a branch of philosophy concerned with the analysis of inferences and arguments. An inference involves forming a conclusion based on some evidence. Although the common meaning of argument implies a disagreement, in logic, an argument consists of a conclusion and its supportive evidence, such that the premises justify the conclusion. The evidence supporting a conclusion may involve one or more theoretical statements, or premises. The tools of logic permit the analysis of reasoning from the premises to the conclusion (Pospesel, 1974).

A theory may be developed through deductive, inductive, or retroductive forms of reasoning. The internal coherence of a theory may therefore be assessed by using the criterion of logical development. This analysis seeks to assess if the development of the series of theoretical statements in the theory follow a logical form of reasoning. Traditionally, deductive and retroductive approaches have been presented in the literature as systematic procedures for devising theory. An in-depth discussion of these forms is beyond the scope of this chapter. It is

Previous author: Sue Marquis Bishop.

important, however, to grasp the basic differences between these forms of reasoning in order to understand how a given theorist may choose to approach the task of theory building and to understand how to proceed in the process of the evaluation of the coherence of the theory.

DEDUCTION

Deduction is a form of logical reasoning in which specific conclusions are inferred from more general premises or assertions. Reasoning proceeds from the more general assertions to specific conclusions. A theory that is developed deductively usually has a lengthy sequence of theoretical statements that have been derived from a few broad axioms or general statements. Derived conclusions may offer predictions or hypotheses that can be tested empirically. The deductive argument usually takes the form of a syllogism with general premises and a conclusion. The deductive form of reasoning is defined as follows:

1. If A were true, then B would be true.
2. A is true.
3. Therefore B is true (Steiner, 1978).

In logical analysis, letters are often substituted for concepts because the emphasis on the analysis of the argument is focused on the form of the argument. Examples A and B are valid deductive arguments with letter notation.

EXAMPLE A

Premise 1: All victims of abuse have low self-esteem. (**All S are M**)
Premise 2: Jennifer and Tom are victims of abuse. (**All P are S**)
Conclusion: Therefore Jennifer and Tom have low self-esteem. (**Ergo, all P are M**)

EXAMPLE B

Premise 1: All patients with heart failure have low oxygen saturation, crackles in the lungs, shortness of breath, and peripheral edema. (**All S are M**)
Premise 2: Mrs. Morris, a 54-year-old female, is admitted to the telemetry unit with a diagnosis of heart failure. (**All P are S**)
Conclusion: The nurse can expect that Mrs. Morris will have low oxygen saturation, crackles in the lungs, shortness of breath, and peripheral edema. (**Ergo, all P are M**)

In Examples A and B, the conclusions follow from, or were deduced from, the general premises. These are therefore valid deductive arguments. In the above examples, no new information is presented in the conclusion that is not at least implied in the premises. There may be a lengthy number of premises in a given argument preceding the conclusion.

In the nursing literature, arguments are not often presented in the form demonstrated in Example A, with the premises and conclusions placed in order and clearly labeled. However, with practice, it is possible to sharpen skills in identifying the arguments and labeling the premises and conclusions from reading narrative text (Salmon, 1973). The conclusion may be presented at the beginning, end, or middle of an argument (Salmon, 1973). Salmon suggests that certain words or phrases are clues that indicate specific statements are presented as premises or conclusions. Examples of terms that often precede a premise include *since, for,* and *because.* Examples of terms that often precede a conclusion include *therefore, consequently, hence, so,* and *it follows that* (Salmon, 1973).

Arguments may be evaluated in two different ways as follows: (1) the validity of the argument may be assessed as to whether the conclusion logically follows the premises, and (2) the content of the premises may be assessed in terms of the truth or falsity of the statements (Pospesel, 1974).

The validity of a deductive argument refers to the logic involved in reasoning from the premises to the conclusion to ensure that, if the premises are true, the conclusion must be true (Pospesel, 1974; Salmon, 1973; Steiner, 1978). A deductive argument may contain all true statements, or one or more false statements, and it may be considered either valid or invalid. This judgment is made on the basis of whether the conclusion is supported by the premises.

EXAMPLE C

Premise: All victims of abuse have low self-esteem.
Premise: Justin has low self-esteem.
Conclusion: Therefore Justin is a victim of abuse.

Although Justin may be the victim of abuse, the truth or falsity of the conclusion or any of the statements is not an issue when evaluating the validity of an argument. In Example C, the premises do not present any supportive evidence that Justin is a victim of abuse. Further, the premises do not assert that only victims of abuse have low self-esteem. Justin's low self-esteem could be from other antecedents or causes, such as he may have significant physical deformities and poor social support that negatively influenced his social development. The conclusion therefore goes beyond the explicit and implicit information in the premises. This is not a valid argument. Compare the reasoning in Examples A and B with that of Example C. Whereas validity refers to the form of the deductive argument, truth refers to the content of a given theoretical statement. Therefore it is inappropriate to label a single theoretical statement as valid or label an argument as true (Salmon, 1973).

In a valid deductive argument, if the premises are true, the conclusion must be true. This combination is marked (R) in Figure 3-1. Therefore it is impossible for the conclusion to be false. This combination is marked (S) in Figure 3-1. However, if one or more of the premises is false, two outcomes are possible: the conclusion may be either true or false.

Example D presents a deductively valid argument that illustrates how false premises lead to a false conclusion. This combination is marked (X) in Figure 3-1.

EXAMPLE D

Premise: The golf ball is larger than the tennis ball. (**False**)
Premise: The tennis ball is larger than the basketball. (**False**)
Conclusion: Therefore the golf ball is larger than the basketball. (**False**)

As Figure 3-1 suggests and Example E illustrates, it is also possible that a valid argument can lead to one or more false premises and a true conclusion. This combination is marked (Y) in Figure 3-1.

The conclusion is:

		True	False
If the premises are:	All true	Necessary (R)	Impossible (S)
	Not all true	Possible (Y)	Possible (X)

(R) If the premises are true, it *necessarily follows* that the conclusion be true.
(S) If the premises are true, it is therefore *impossible* for the conclusion to be false.
(Y), (X) If one or more of the premises are false, it is *possible* the conclusion may be *either* true or false.

Figure **3-1** Potential outcomes of a valid deductive argument. (From Giere, R. N. [1979]. *Understanding scientific reasoning.* New York: Holt, Rinehart & Winston. Reprinted with permission of Wadsworth, an imprint of Wadsworth Group, a division of Thomson Learning.)

EXAMPLE E

Premise: The tennis ball is larger than the basketball. (**False**)
Premise: The basketball is larger than the golf ball. (**True**)
Conclusion: Therefore the tennis ball is larger than the golf ball. (**True**)

It may be helpful to study Examples D and E to understand how the conclusions are derived from the information given in the premises. In science, deductive arguments can be a powerful form of reasoning to derive new conclusions by making explicit implied information. Then these derived conclusions can be subjected as hypotheses to empirical testing to test their correspondence with research findings.

INDUCTION

Induction is a form of logical reasoning in which a generalization is induced from a number of specific, observed instances. Inductive reasoning has not been as well developed as deductive reasoning (Pospesel, 1974). The form of the inductive argument is as follows:
1. A is true of $b_1, b_2 \ldots b_n$.
2. $b_1, b_2 \ldots b_n$ are some members of class B.
3. Therefore A is true of all members of class B (Steiner, 1978).

The inductive form is based on the assumption that members of any given class share common characteristics. Therefore, what is true for any randomly selected members of the class is accepted as true for all members of the class (Steiner, 1978). Suppose a sample of abuse victims has been selected for study. Example F presents an argument in the inductive form that may be developed based on this hypothetical study.

EXAMPLE F

Premise: Every victim of abuse who has been observed has low self-esteem.
Conclusion: All victims of abuse have low self-esteem.

In another study, a sample of the population of fathers and their newborns has been selected for study. Fathers selected for the study live in the southern city of Charlotte, North Carolina, and are white-collar professionals and Asian. Example G presents an argument in the inductive form that may be developed based on a father-newborn pair study of bonding.

EXAMPLE G

Premise: Every father in the study developed a strong loving bond with his newborn within 2 weeks of birth.
Conclusion: All new fathers develop a strong loving bond with their newborns within 2 weeks of birth.

The premise in Example G states observations from a number of instances; that is, a limited number of subjects and limited to one ethnic, regional, and socioeconomic group. The conclusion states a generalization that extends beyond the observations to the entire class of fathers and their newborns.

The inductive generalization also may be stated in terms of a mathematical quantity (Salmon, 1973). For example, assume a researcher surveys a sample of 400 nurses to determine their opinions about whether nurses should establish independent private practices. Results indicate that 60% of nurses in the sample support independent private practice activities in nursing. The inductive statement may be stated as follows:

EXAMPLE H

Premise: Sixty percent of nurses in the sample support independent private practice activities in nursing.
Conclusion: Sixty percent of all nurses support independent private practice activities in nursing.

In a deductive argument, if the premises are true, the conclusion must be true. The inductive argument can have true premises and produce a false conclusion. An inductive conclusion based on limited or biased evidence can clearly lead to a fallacious argument and perhaps a false conclusion (Salmon, 1973). Suppose the argument in Example G was developed through one observational study with five middle-class Asian fathers from a Midwestern city. The conclusion that all fathers develop a strong and loving bond with their newborns within 2 weeks may or may not be true. In any case, this conclusion is not warranted based on the limited number of observed instances. There is insufficient evidence in this case to justify the conclusion about all fathers in America or the world, or even the middle-class, Midwest, or Asian families.

Even if the sample size is appropriately sufficient (or based on several studies), the sample may be biased. Assume that the sample of nurses in Example H was drawn from nursing faculty in large research universities. The opinions of this select group of nurses may be expected to differ in some respects from, and may not reflect the opinions of, all nurses or even of nursing faculty in all schools of nursing. Considering a number of factors in selecting representative samples can help avoid introducing bias into observations. This reasoning is the basis for the random selection of subjects in research projects. Descriptive and inferential statistics are used to characterize the sample of the population and help with decisions about the strength of the evidence (Giere, 1979). The inductive inference has been termed the *statistical inference* (Steiner, 1978; Weiner, 1958).

In inductive arguments, the inferred conclusion goes beyond the implicit and explicit information in the premises. In Example G, not all fathers and newborns have been observed. This conclusion is inferred on the basis of selected instances. In a deductive argument, the conclusion can be considered true if the argument is structured so implicit information in the premises is made explicit (Salmon, 1973). Conversely, the inductive argument goes beyond the information in the premises. The inductive argument expands upon the presented information. Giere (1979) has argued that this characteristic permits the justification of scientific conclusions that may not be justifiable by deductive reasoning, because they contain information beyond the premises. An example would be a scientific hypothesis about the future based on observations in the present (Giere, 1979).

Whereas deductive arguments are considered either valid or invalid, the concept of validity does not apply to inductive arguments. The correctness of inductive arguments is not viewed in either/or terms; it is viewed on degrees of strength and measured in terms of the probability with which the premises lead to a given conclusion (Salmon, 1973). Then the inferred conclusion can be determined to have low, medium, or high probability (Salmon, 1973). Statistical procedures can be used in making these judgments. In Example A, the conclusion can be false only if one or more of the premises are false; that is, if all victims of abuse do not have low self-esteem or if Jennifer and Tom are not victims of abuse. If these are true, the conclusion must be true. However, in Example F, the reasoning suggests that all victims of abuse have low self-esteem. The premises state that only selected victims of abuse have been observed. The premises may lend some support for the conclusion. That victims of abuse without low self-esteem were not observed may be considered some evidence, but it will not preclude the possibility that a victim with high self-esteem will not be observed in the future (Salmon, 1973). Factors from other studies such as severity of the abuse, age at abuse, length of time victim was abused, and subsequent environmental supports, for example, may theoretically change or further specify the assertions that can be made about abuse victims.

Deductive arguments are considered to preserve truth, whereas inductive arguments can be a source of new information (Giere, 1979; Salmon, 1973). Scientific generalizations about instances not observed in the present or projections about the future are examples. Although this form of reasoning is useful in advancing science, the very nature of induction may introduce error into the scientific process (Gramling, Lambert, & Pursley-Crotteau, 1998). Even if the premises were accurate, the accuracy of the conclusion cannot be certain. In Giere's view, if the premises are assumed to be true, then "the difference between a good inductive argument and a valid deductive argument is that the deductive argument guarantees the truth of its conclusion while the inductive argument guarantees only an appropriately high probability of its conclusion" (1979, pp. 37-38).

RETRODUCTION*

Whereas deduction and induction may explicate and evaluate ideas, retroduction originates ideas (Steiner, 1977). The retroductive form of reasoning is an approach to theoretical inquiry that uses analogy as a method for devising theory. In 1878, Pierce described three kinds of reasoning as comprising the major steps of inquiry: (1) retroduction, (2) deduction, and (3) induction as cited in Steiner (1978). According to Steiner (1978), Pierce viewed retroductive reasoning as the first stage in the search for understanding some surprising phenomenon in which a viewpoint offering a possible explanation is identified. Pierce stated that once a viewpoint was identified that held the promise of explaining an observed phenomenon, deductive reasoning was used to develop the explanation. Pierce considered the final stage of inquiry in terms of induction and focused on checking out the devised hypotheses in experience (Steiner, 1978). Steiner[†] further developed the theory models approach using retroductive inference as a method for devising theory. Following is the form of the retroductive inference:

1. The surprising fact, C, is observed.
2. If A were true, C would be a matter of course.
3. Therefore there is reason to suspect that A is true (Steiner, 1976b).

An analysis of the preceding form reveals that the theory models (or retroductive inference) approach does not establish truth. Its function is to originate ideas about selected phenomena that can be further developed and tested. The theory models approach is most useful as a strategy for devising theory in a field that has few available theories, and innovation is indicated to advance the knowledge in describing

---

*This discussion of retroduction has been adapted from the work of Elizabeth Steiner (Steiner, 1977; Steiner, 1978; Stevens, 1979; Tsai, 2003). Copyright Elizabeth Steiner. All rights reserved.

[†]Elizabeth Steiner's earlier work on theory models was published under her married name of Maccia (Maccia, Maccia, & Jewett, 1963; Norman, 1976).

and understanding selected observations (Steiner, 1978; Walker & Avant, 1995).

The retroductive theorist approaches the development of a wanted theory by identifying a source theory in another field that may have the potential for developing the wanted theory. The theory models approach is based on the use of analogy and metaphor between two sets of phenomena. This requires that the theorist possess considerable creativity and an intuitive knowledge of the phenomena of interest (Steiner, 1976b). The theory models approach is represented as follows (Steiner, 1977; Steiner, 1978):

Theory 1 $\longrightarrow$ Theory $\longrightarrow$ Theory 2
                        model
(Source theory)   (Wanted theory)

Therefore, theory models are not models of, but are models for, devising representations of selected phenomena (Steiner, 1976b). The theory model is essentially a metamodel, which serves as a model to develop theory (Steiner, 1977). To devise a theory using retroductive inference, the theorist seeks out a source theory to form a theory model. The wanted theory is devised from this theory model. The source theory is selected on the basis of a similarity in structure, form, or relationships between the two sets of phenomena (Steiner, 1978). The selected source theory is perceived to present ideas that may be useful for developing a theory about the observations of interest. These ideas are selected from theory 1 and formed into a point of view or theory model that will serve as the framework for developing theory 2. This approach is based on the assumption that new conjectures, or ideas, in a given field may be devised from other conjectures and theories in other fields (Maccia & Maccia, 1966; Maccia et al., 1963; Steiner, 1978). The ideas selected from theory 1 for the theory model may involve any combination of concepts, hypothesized relationships, or theory structures. The viewpoint presented by the theory model is used to develop theory 2 by adding content to the theory model and by altering concepts and relationships to fit the phenomenon of interest for theory 2. It should be clear that this

process of theory building is not simply borrowing a theory from one field and applying it unchanged to another (Steiner, 1976a). The retroductive inference theory-building process, then, can result in a new nursing theory.

The theory models approach cannot be considered reductive, because theory 1 is not equivalent to theory 2 (Maccia et al., 1963; Steiner, 1977; Steiner, 1978). To be reductive, the theorist would simply borrow concepts and hypotheses and use them, as formulated, in a new context. This approach cannot be considered deductive, either, because theory 2 was not developed by deduction from theory 1. The hypotheses in theory 2 cannot be derived from theory 1 (Steiner, 1977, 1978). A theory devised by this method must meet the criteria for adequacy of a theory (Steiner, 1977, 1978). The new theory can then be evaluated by its correspondence with available scientific nursing literature and hypotheses can be empirically tested through research.

The use of analogy to develop theory has been a common occurrence in the development of many scientific fields. In Sigmund Freud's time, the machine model was a popular advanced model. Freud used the notion of machine operations to develop his theoretical assertions about psychological tension-reduction relationships in his theory of psychosexual development. Three or more decades ago, basic texts in human anatomy and physiology used the telephone switchboard as an analogy for explaining brain function. The computer is used often as a model for contemplating the brain and for developing theories of human information processing (Norman, 1976; Shepherd, 1974). In nursing, general systems theory has been used as a model for developing nursing theory (Nursing Theories Conference Group, 1990).

Stevens (1979) argued that in many instances nursing research has had minimal impact on nursing practice, because the research was based on the categories and characteristics of borrowed theories. In this instance, the borrowed theory was utilized, unchanged, in the new context. Although theories in other fields may suggest a possible framework for addressing phenomena in the field of nursing, this framework needs to be contextualized within nursing. That is, aspects of the borrowed theory need to be altered to reflect the appropriate categories and characteristics within nursing. Steiner's development of the theory models approach provides guidelines for using this strategy in theory building.

Walker and Avant's (1995) derivation strategy for theory construction draws from the theory models approach that Steiner developed. Walker and Avant (1995) present examples of using the derivation strategy to use and reformulate concepts, theoretical statements, and theories from other fields to the nursing field. Villarruel, Bishop, Simpson, Jemmott, and Fawcett (2001) emphasized that more systematic analysis of borrowed theories needs to occur to contextualize the theory in nursing and examine whether it is adequate to describe, explain, or predict nursing phenomena.

Dalton (2003) used a modified version of theory derivation to develop a theory of triadic collaborative decision making in nursing practice. She selected aspects of Kim's dyadic theory of nurse-patient decision making and added additional key concepts and relationships from nursing practice (e.g., family caregiver) to expand the theory model to a triadic theory of decision making. The inclusion of the family caregiver concept introduced other elements into the model that required the addition of information from the literature about the family caregiver and the relationship of the caregiver with the patient and nurse (e.g., concepts about caregivers and coalition formation among participants in the model). The resulting theory of client-nurse-family caregiver collaborative decision making then was analyzed for its correspondence with the literature. Dalton (2003) has subjected aspects of the theory to initial testing in a field study.

In Gramling and colleagues' (1998) approach to theoretical retroduction, the goal was to develop a theoretical model of stressors and coping in young women. Aspects of the Lazarus and Folkman transactional theory of coping were selected and aspects of women's development from the literature were added to the model. The resulting framework guided a qualitative study with 26 women. Findings were incorporated within the new model of coping for young women. Tsai (2003) utilized the Roy Adaptation Model to devise a middle range theory of caregiver stress by selecting concepts and relationships and adding information within the context of caregivers and the chronically ill.

In contrast to the reasoning based on traditional logical assumptions presented in this chapter, scholarly work is also ongoing with other unconventional approaches to logic. For example, Bosque (1995) used fuzzy logic in nursing to devise a theoretical perspective of nurse and machine symbiosis in the design of a new neonatal pulse oximeter alarm. Their approach used fuzzy set theory and fuzzy logic theory, which provides a model for modes of reasoning that are approximate rather than exact.

The theory models approach (retroductive inference) permits the translation and expansion of ideas within the milieu of nursing and may result in the development of a new nursing theory. This approach may be useful in the development of a mid-range nursing theory. A nursing theory devised by this method can be developed further through the use of deductive strategies. The new theory can be subjected to rigorous analysis for congruence with the existing research literature, and hypotheses can be subjected to rigorous testing in empirical studies. Table 3-1 (see pp. 32-33) presents a summary of deductive, inductive, and retroductive forms of reasoning.

Table **3-1**

Deduction, Induction, and Retroduction Summary		
TYPE	**QUESTION**	**TECHNIQUES**
DEDUCTION	Given that the premises are true, what other propositions may be inferred as necessary conclusions from the premises?[a]	Logical and conceptual analysis[a]
INDUCTION	Given that the premises are true, what is the strength of the link between them and the conclusion?[a]	Logical and conceptual analysis based on statistical analysis[c,d]
RETRODUCTION	Given a surprising observation, what explanation would result in the expectation that the observation would be a matter of course?[a]	Logical and conceptual analysis[c]

[a]Steiner, 1976b.
[b]Steiner, 1978.
[c]Steiner, 1976a.
[d]Stevens, 1979.
[e]Giere, 1979.
[f]Maccia et al., 1963.

DEFINITION	EXAMPLE	QUESTION
	Premises	*Explicates and derives further truths*
(1) If A were true, then B would be true (2) A is true (3) Therefore B is true[b]	All victims of abuse have low self-esteem. Mary and Tom are victims of abuse. *Conclusion* Mary and Tom have low self-esteem.	If premises are true, establishes truth of something else by derivation[c]
(1) A is true of $b_1, b_2 \ldots b_n$ (2) $b_1, b_2 \ldots b_n$ are some members of class B (3) Therefore A is true of all members of class B[b]	*Premise* $b_1, b_2 \ldots b_n$ victims of abuse who have been observed have low self-esteem. *Conclusion* All victims of abuse have low self-esteem.	*Evaluates and expands information* Based on probability of observed cases Does not establish truth Establishes probability of certainty, strength of evidence New data may change conclusion[c,e]
(1) The surprising fact, C, is observed. (2) But if A were true, C would be a matter of course. (3) Therefore there is reason to expect that A is true[b].	*Proposition 1* The role of expecting reward determines a relation between student and teacher that establishes a path for influence of the teacher on the student[f]. *Proposition 2* The role of expecting care and comfort determines a relation between patient and nurse that establishes a path for influence of the nurse on the patient.	*Originates ideas* Does not establish truth. Suggests lines of thought worthy of exploration and testing[c]

REFERENCES

Bosque, E. M. (1995). Symbiosis of nurse and machine through fuzzy logic: Improved specificity of neonatal pulse oximeter alarm. *ANS Advances in Nursing Science, 18*(2), 67-75.

Dalton, J. M. (2003). Development and testing of the theory of collaborative decision-making in nursing practice for triads. *Journal of Advanced Nursing, 41*(1), 22-33.

Giere, R. N. (1979). *Understanding scientific reasoning.* New York: Holt, Rinehart, & Winston.

Gramling, L. F., Lambert, V. A., & Pursley-Crotteau, S. (1998). Coping in young women: Theoretical retroduction. *Journal of Advanced Nursing, 28*(5), 1082-1091.

Kim, H. S. (1983). Collaborative decision making in nursing practice: A theoretical framework. In P. L. Chin (Ed.), *Advances in nursing theory development,* Rockville, MD: Aspen.

Maccia, E. S., & Maccia, G. (1966). *Construction of educational theory derived from three educational theory models* (Project No. 5-0638). Washington, DC: U.S. Department of Health, Education, and Welfare.

Maccia, E. S., Maccia, G., & Jewett, R. (1963). *Construction of educational theory models* (Cooperative Research Project No. 1632). Washington, DC: Office of Education, U.S. Department of Health, Education, and Welfare.

Norman, D. A. (1976). *Memory and attention: An introduction to human information processing.* New York: John Wiley & Sons.

Nursing Theories Conference Group. (1990). *Nursing theories: The base for professional nursing practice* (3rd ed.). Norwalk, CT: Appleton & Lange.

Pospesel, H. (1974). *Propositional logic.* Englewood Cliffs, NJ: Prentice Hall.

Salmon, W. C. (1973). *Logic.* Englewood Cliffs, NJ: Prentice Hall.

Shepherd, G. M. (1974). *The synaptic organization of the brain.* New York: Oxford University Press.

Steiner, E. (1976a). *Logical and conceptual analytic techniques for educational researchers.* Unpublished paper presented at the American Educational Research Association, San Francisco.

Steiner, E. (1976b): *The complete act of educational inquiry.* Unpublished paper.

Steiner, E. (1977). *Criteria for theory of art education.* Unpublished paper presented at the Seminar for Research in Art Education, Philadelphia.

Steiner, E. (1978). *Logical and conceptual analytic techniques for educational researchers.* Washington, DC: University Press.

Stevens, B. (1979). *Nursing theory: Analysis, application, evaluation.* Boston: Little, Brown.

Tsai, P. (2003). A middle-range theory of caregiver stress. *Nursing Science Quarterly, 16*(2), 137-145.

Villarruel, A. M., Bishop, T. L., Simpson, E. M., Jemmott, L. S., & Fawcett, J. (2001). Borrowed theories, shared theories, and the advancement of nursing knowledge. *Nursing Science Quarterly, 14*(2), 158-163.

Walker, L. O., & Avant, K. C. (1995). *Strategies for theory construction in nursing.* Norwalk, CT: Appleton & Lange.

Weiner, P. (1958). *Values in universe of chance.* New York: Doubleday.

Theory Development Process

Sue Marquis Bishop and Sonya R. Hardin

heory development in nursing is an essential component in nursing scholarship to advance the knowledge of the discipline. Nursing theories that are clearly set forth promote understanding and analysis of nursing phenomena and guide the scholarly development of the science of nursing practice through research. Once a nursing theory has been identified that fits an area or phenomenon of interest, several issues must be considered, such as the completeness of the theory, any missing components or relationships, the theory's internal consistency, the theory's correspondence with available empirical findings, and whether it is operationally defined for testing. Analyses of this nature logically lead to the consideration of the next steps in the development of the theory. The goal is to continue to direct attention and energies to the critical analysis of existing incomplete theories in terms of their potential for further development. Scientific evidence can accumulate to support or refute theoretical assertions or provide the basis for suggesting modifications in a nursing theory only through repeated and rigorous research.

Previous author: Sue Marquis Bishop.

Nursing theory development is not a mysterious, magical activity, but a scholarly activity that is pursued systematically. The availability of more systematically developed theories would provide a clearer understanding of nursing and would enable the exploration of whether this understanding corresponds with activities in nursing practice. Rigorous development of nursing theories, then, is a high priority for the development of the nursing profession.

It is important to grasp the concept of *systematic development*. Approaches to the construction of theory differ. However, one aspect they have in common is the agreement among scientists to approach theory development in a precise and systematic fashion, making the stages in the development of the theory explicit. The nurse who systematically devises a theory of nursing and presents it to the nursing community for public review and scholarly debate by nursing scholars is engaging in the process essential to advancing theory development. When this scholarly work is published in the literature, nurse theoreticians and researchers can review and critique the adequacy of the logical processes used in the development of the theory and

Table 4-1

Theory Components and Their Contributions to the Theory	
THEORY COMPONENTS	**CONTRIBUTIONS TO THE THEORY**
CONCEPTS AND DEFINITIONS	
Concepts	Describe and classify phenomena
Theoretical definitions of concept	Establish meaning
Operational definitions of concept	Provide measurement
RELATIONAL STATEMENTS	
Theoretical statements	Relate concepts to one another; permit analysis
Operational statements	Relate concepts to measurements
LINKAGES AND ORDERING	
Linkages of theoretical statements	Provide rationale of why theoretical statements are linked; add plausibility
Linkages of operational statements	Provide rationale for how measurement variables are linked; permit testability
Organization of concepts and definitions into primitive and derived terms	Eliminates overlap (tautology)
Organization of statements and linkages into premises and derived hypotheses and equations	Eliminates inconsistency

Modified from Hage, J. (1972). *Techniques and problems in theory construction in sociology.* New York: John Wiley & Sons.

correspondence of the theoretical assertions to available research findings. They can then proceed to empirically test the presented hypotheses through research. The ultimate goal is, of course, to advance nursing knowledge through the systematic development of theory.

THEORY COMPONENTS*

In the metatheoretical arena concerned with the study of how theories are developed, there is some agreement in the scientific community on selected scholarly terms, definitions, and understandings (e.g., meaning of theoretical and operational concepts, conditional statements) so that scholarly

*Discussion of the three categories of theory components modified from Hage's six theory components: Hage, J. (1972). *Techniques and problems of theory construction in sociology.* New York: John Wiley & Sons.

review and analysis can occur. It is important to grasp the essential terms and agreed-upon meanings in order to understand the theory development process.

Hage (1972) identified components of a complete theory and specified the contribution each makes to the whole theory (Table 4-1). He argued that failure to include one or more of the components resulted in the elimination of that particular contribution to the total theory. These aspects of a theory are discussed as a basis for understanding the function of each element in the theory-building process.

Concepts and Definitions

Concepts, the building blocks of theories, classify the phenomena of interest (Kaplan, 1964). In any separate discussion of concepts, it is crucial to recognize that concepts must not be considered separately from the theoretical system in which they are embedded and from which they derive their meaning. Concepts may have completely different meanings in different theoretical systems. Scientific progress is based on the critical review and testing of a researcher's work by the scientific community. It is, therefore, important that there be agreement as to the meaning of scientific concepts.

Concepts may be abstract or concrete. Abstract concepts are independent of a specific time or place, whereas concrete concepts relate to a particular time or place (Hage, 1972; Reynolds, 1971).

ABSTRACT CONCEPTS	CONCRETE CONCEPTS
Social system	The Marquis family
	2 South Surgery Floor, Memorial Hospital
	Nurse-patient-family caregiver
Debate	Bush-Kerry debate
Telemetry	Electrocardiogram, Holter monitor

The Marquis family, the surgery unit, and the nurse-patient-family caregiver triad are specific examples of the more general, abstract concept of social system. In a given theoretical system, then, the definition, characteristics, and functioning of a social system can be theorized to operate in the more specific instances, such as the nurse-patient-family caregiver social system.

Concepts may be classified as *discrete* or *continuous concepts*. This system of labels differentiates the concepts that vary along a continuum from the concepts that specify categories of phenomena. A discrete concept identifies categories or classes of phenomena, such as patient, nurse, or environment. A student can become a nurse or choose another profession, but he or she cannot become a partial nurse. Therefore, phenomena are identified as either belonging to, or not belonging to, a given class or category. For that reason, discrete concepts have been called *nonvariable concepts*. Sorting phenomena into nonvariable, discrete categories carries the

assumption that the reality associated with the given phenomenon is captured by the classification (Hage, 1972). The amount or degree of the variable is not an issue. Many years ago, Max Weber devised the discrete concept of bureaucracy as an ideal type to characterize organizations (Merton, 1967). Organizations were then classified as *bureaucratic* or *nonbureaucratic*. The definition of the discrete concept is critical in knowing how to classify the phenomenon.

Theories may be developed using a series of nonvariable discrete concepts (and subconcepts) to build typologies. Blegen and Tripp-Reimer (1997) argued that the development of taxonomies of nursing diagnoses, nursing interventions, and nursing outcomes can facilitate theory building for nursing practice. Typologies consist of a systematic arrangement of the concepts. For example, a typology on marital status could be partitioned into marital statuses in which a population could be classified, such as married, divorced, widowed, or single. These discrete categories could be partitioned further to permit the classification of an additional variable in this typology, for example, gender. In Table 4-2, an either/or decision is made for each of the 270 subjects in a hypothetical study. The subjects either fall in the category or they do not; there is no in-between or degree of how much they can be in the category (e.g., it is not possible to be partly widowed or highly single). The typology could be partitioned further by adding the discrete concept of children, so that subjects could be classified further for each of the gender and marital status categories as *have children* and *no children*.

A continuous concept, on the other hand, permits the classification of dimensions or gradations of a phenomenon across a continuum, such as degree of marital conflict. For example, marital couples may be classified across a range representing the degree of marital conflict in their relationships according to some measure.

Degree of Marital Conflict

0 ←——————→ 120

Low   High

Table 4-2

Typology of Marital Status and Gender

| | MARITAL STATUS | | | |
PARTICIPANTS	SINGLE	MARRIED	DIVORCED	WIDOWED
Male	15	75	23	6
Female	25	72	41	13
TOTAL	40	147	64	19

Other continuous concepts that may be used to classify couples could include amount of communication, number of shared activities, or number of children. Examples of continuous concepts that may be used to classify patients could be degree of temperature, level of anxiety, or age. Nurses are conceptualizing pain as a continuous concept when they ask patients to rate their pain on a scale from 0 to 10 to classify pain threshold or painful events.

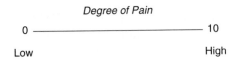

Note that continuous concepts are not expressed in either/or terms, but are conceptualized in *degrees on a continuum.* The use of variable concepts based on a range or a continuum tends to be focused on one dimension, without assuming that a single dimension captures all the reality connected with the phenomenon. Additional dimensions may be devised to measure further aspects of the phenomenon. In contrast to the nonvariable term *bureaucracy,* variable concepts, such as rate of conflict, ratio of professional to nonprofessional staff, communication flow, or ratio of registered nurses to patients, may be used to characterize health care organizations. Although nonvariable concepts are useful in classifying phenomena in theory development,

Hage (1972) argued that major breakthroughs have occurred in several disciplines when the focus shifted from nonvariable to variable concepts, because variable concepts permit the scoring of the phenomenon's full range on a continuum.

The development of concepts, then, permits the description and classification of phenomena (Hage, 1972). The labeled concept suggests boundaries for selecting phenomena to observe and for reasoning about the phenomena of interest. New concepts may focus attention on new phenomena or they may facilitate thinking about and classifying phenomena in a different way (Hage, 1972).

Concept analysis has received attention by nursing scholars, as well as in nursing education programs (Walker & Avant, 1983). Scholarly analysis of the concepts in nursing theories is a critical step in the process of theoretical inquiry. Some recent examples in the literature include: analysis of the concept of parent-infant attachment focused on enhancing clarification of this concept (Goulet, Bell, St-Cyr Tribble, Paul, & Lang, 1998), Keenan's analysis of the concept of autonomy as relevant to nursing practice (1999), concept analysis of facilitation in relation to nursing practice (Harvey, et al., 2002), analysis of the concept of equity and its relationship to health visiting services in Britain (Almond, 2002), and Schilling, Grey, and Knafl's (2002) analysis of the concept of self-management of child and adolescent type I diabetes.

Concept analysis must necessarily involve concept definitions. The development of science is a collaborative endeavor, in which the community of scientists review, critique, test, and build upon each others' work. Therefore, it is crucial that the concepts are as clearly defined as possible to reduce any ambiguity in understanding the given concept or set of concepts. Although it is not possible to eliminate perceived differences in meaning entirely, offering explicit definitions can minimize these differences. In the development of a complete theory, both theoretical and operational definitions provide meaning for the concept and a basis for seeking empirical indicators. Theoretical definitions also permit consideration of the relationship between a given concept and other theoretical ideas. For example, Haas (1999) analyzed concepts similar to the concept of quality of life with the goal of enhancing clarity and integration in research with related concepts.

Yet a clear meaning for concepts is not enough. If theories are to be tested against reality, then concepts must be measurable. Operational definitions relate the concepts to observable phenomena by specifying empirical indicators. The concept name and the theoretical and operational definitions (Table 4-3) establish reference points for locating the concept; that is, viewing the concept as it is related to the theoretical systems and the observable environment (Hage, 1972).

Relational Statements

Statements in a theory that can be classified as definitions relate to specific concepts. Whereas definitions provide descriptions of the concept, relational statements assert relationships between the properties of two or more concepts or variables. If concepts

Table 4-3

Examples of Theoretical and Operational Definitions

CONCEPT	THEORETICAL DEFINITION	OPERATIONAL DEFINITION
Body temperature	Homeothermic range of one's internal environment maintained by the thermoregulatory system of the human body	Degree of temperature measured by oral thermometer taken for 1 minute under the tongue
Heart failure	Inadequate cardiac function to meet the circulatory demands*	Stage of heart failure is measured by the NYHA classification[†]
Spirituality	A pandimensional awareness of the mutual human/environmental field process (integrality) as a manifestation of higher frequency patterning (resonance) associated with innovative, increasingly creative and diverse (helicy) experiences[‡]	Score on the Spiritual Inventory Belief Scale (SIBS), an instrument that measures a person's spirituality as the search for meaning and purpose[§] The SIBS has four subscales: 1) Internal/fluid 2) Humility/personal application 3) External/meditative 4) External/ritual[¶]

*Hussey & Hardin, 2003.
[†]AHA, 2004.
[‡]Malinski, 1994.
[§]Hatch, Burg, Naberhaus, & Hellmich, 1998.
[¶]Hardin, Hussey, & Steele, 2003.

can be considered the building blocks of theory, theoretical statements can be thought of as the chains that link the concepts. Concepts, therefore, must be connected with one another in a series of theoretical statements to devise a nursing theory. The development of a theoretical hypothesis asserting a connection between two or more concepts introduces the possibility of analysis (Hage, 1972).

In the connections between variables, one variable may be assumed to influence a second. In this instance, the first variable may be labeled an antecedent (or determinant) variable and the second a consequent (or resultant) variable. In this case, the first variable may be viewed as the independent and the second as the dependent variable (Giere, 1997). The complexity of nursing presents a situation in which multiple antecedents and consequences may be involved in studying a selected phenomenon. However, Zetterberg (1966) concluded that the development of two-variate theoretical statements could be an important intermediate step in the development of a theory. These statements can be reformulated later as the theory evolves or as new information becomes available.

Theoretical assertions may be expressed as either a necessary or sufficient condition, or both. These labels characterize the conditions that help explain the nature of the relationship between the two variables in the theoretical statements. For example, a relational statement expressed as a sufficient condition could be: If nurses react with approval of patients' self-care behaviors (*NA*), patients increase their efforts in self-care activities (*PSC*). This is a type of compound statement linking antecedent and consequent variables. The statement does not assert the truth of the antecedent. Rather, the assertion is made that if the antecedent is true, then the consequent is true (Giere, 1979). In addition, no assertion appears in the statement explaining why the antecedent is related to the consequent. In symbolic notation form, the above statements can be expressed as:

$$NA \longrightarrow PSC$$
(Antecedent/determinant $\longrightarrow$
Consequent/resultant)

A sufficient condition asserts that one variable can result in the occurrence of another variable. It does not claim it is the only variable that can result in the occurrence of the other variable. This statement asserts that nurse approval of a patient's self-care behaviors is sufficient for the occurrence of the patient's self-care activities. However, patient assumption of self-care activities resulting from other factors, such as the patient's health status and personality variables, is not ruled out. There could be other antecedents that are sufficient conditions for the patient's assumption of self-care activities.

A statement in the form of a necessary condition asserts that one variable is required for the occurrence of another variable. For example:

If patients are motivated to get well (WM = wellness motivation), then they will adhere to their prescribed treatment regimen (AR).

$$WM \longrightarrow AR$$

This means that adherence to a treatment regimen (*AR*) never occurs when wellness motivation (*WM*) does not occur. It is not asserted that the patients' adherence to the treatment regimen stems from their wellness motivation. However, it is asserted that if the wellness motivation is absent, patients will not assume strict adherence to their treatment regimens. The wellness motivation is a necessary, but not a sufficient, condition for the occurrence of this consequent.

The term *if* is generally used to introduce a sufficient condition, whereas *only if* and *if . . . then* are used to introduce necessary conditions (Giere, 1979). In most instances, conditional statements are not both necessary and sufficient. However, it is possible for a statement to express both conditions. In such instances, the term *if and only if* is used to imply that the conditions are both necessary and sufficient for one another. In this case, (1) the consequent never occurs in the absence of the antecedent and (2) the consequent always occurs when the antecedent occurs (Giere, 1979). It should be noted, however, that not all conditional statements are causal. For example, the following statement, "If this month is November, then the next month is December," does not assert that November causes December to occur. Rather, the sequence of months suggests that December follows November (Dubin, 1978; Giere, 1979).

Giere (1997) differentiated between deterministic models and probabilistic models in his discussion of causal statements. Theoretical statements from a deterministic model assert that the presence or absence of one variable determines the presence or absence of a second variable. The probabilistic model is another approach derived from the view that humans and other complex social and environmental phenomena are thus best conceptualized from a probability framework. Probabilistic statements generally are based on statistical data and assert relationships between variables that do not occur in every instance, but are likely to occur based on some estimate of probability. As an example, it has been asserted that a routine lack of exercise may likely lead to obesity, a growing national health problem. It is clear that a routine lack of exercise (*LE*) does not always lead to obesity, because not all couch potatoes become medically obese (*MO*). However, the probability of developing medical obesity (*P MO*) may be increased for persons who routinely avoid exercise at least to some degree of probability. In symbolic notation:

$$\text{IF } LE \longrightarrow P\,MO$$

The development of relational statements that assert connections between variables provides for analysis and establishes the basis for explanation and prediction (Hage, 1972).

Linkages and Ordering

Specification of linkages is an important part of the development of theory (Hage, 1972). Although the theoretical statements assert connections between concepts, the rationale for the stated connections must be developed. Development of theoretical linkages offers an explanation of why the variables in the theory may be connected in some manner; that is, the theoretical reasons for asserting particular interrelationships (Hage, 1972). Hage suggested that this rationale added plausibility to the theory. Operational linkages, on the other hand, contribute the element of testability to the theory by specifying how measurement variables are connected (Hage, 1972). Although operational definitions provide for the measurability of the concepts, operational linkages provide for the testability of the assertions. The operational linkage contributes a perspective for understanding the nature of the relationship between concepts, such as whether the relationship between the concepts is negative or positive, linear or curvilinear (Hage, 1972).

A theory may be considered fairly complete if it presents the elements of concepts, definitions, statements, and linkages. Complete development of the theory, however, requires organizing the concepts and definitions into primitive and derived terms and organizing the statements and linkages into premises and hypotheses and equations (Hage, 1972). As the theory evolves, concepts and theoretical statements multiply and it is necessary to establish some logical organization of all the theory components. This process of ordering may identify any existing overlap between concepts and definitions (Hage, 1972). The conceptual arrangement of statements and linkages into premises and equations may reveal areas of inconsistency (Hage, 1972). Premises (or axioms) are regarded as the more general assertions from which the hypotheses are derived in the form of equations. It is generally agreed that conceptual ordering of theoretical statements and their linkages is indicated when the theory contains a large number of theoretical statements.

A formal theory is a systematically developed, conceptual system that addresses a given set of phenomena. There are different ideas about how this conceptual system should be organized to constitute a theory. Reynolds (1971) described three forms for organizing theory: *set-of-laws, axiomatic,* and

Set-of-Laws Form
Laws (overwhelming empirical support) 1. 2. 3. Empirical generalizations (some empirical support) 1. 2. 3. 4. Hypotheses (no empirical support) 1. 2. 3. 4. 5.

Figure **4-1 Set-of-laws form.** (From Reynolds, P. [1971]. *A primer in theory construction.* Indianapolis, IN: Bobbs-Merrill. Used with permission from Allyn & Bacon, a division of Pearson Education.)

causal process.* Each is a different conceptual approach to organization with different limitations.

The set-of-laws approach attempts to organize findings from empirical research. Empirical findings from available research, in an area of particular interest, are identified from the literature for evaluation. Findings are evaluated and sorted into the categories of laws, empirical generalizations, and hypotheses based on the degree of research evidence supporting each assertion (Reynolds, 1971). Reynolds (1971) discussed limitations to the set-of-laws approach to theory building.

First, the nature of research requires focusing on the relationships between a limited set of variables, which are often two variables. Attempts to develop a set-of-laws theory from statements of findings, therefore, may result in a lengthy number of statements that assert the relationships between two or more variables. This lengthy set of generalizations may be difficult to organize and interrelate. Second,

for research to be conducted, concepts must be operationally defined so they can be measurable. Therefore, in the statements of empirical findings, the more highly abstract or theoretical concepts that might be useful in developing an understanding of the phenomenon of interest may be eliminated (Foster, 1997).

Reynolds (1971) concluded that although the set-of-laws form may provide for the classification of phenomena or the predictions of relationships between selected variables, it does not permit understanding, which is crucial for the advancement of science. Finally, Reynolds (1971) noted that each statement in the set-of-laws form is considered to be independent, because the various statements have not been interrelated into a system of description and explanation (Figure 4-1). Therefore, each statement must be tested. The statements are not interrelated; therefore, research support for one statement does not provide support for any other statement. Research efforts must be more extensive.

The set-of-laws approach to theory building is consistent with the view that scientific knowledge consists of empirical findings and science is

*Set of laws, axiomatic, and causal theory forms discussion based largely on arguments advanced by Reynolds, P. (1971). *A primer in theory construction.* Indianapolis, IN: Bobbs-Merrill.

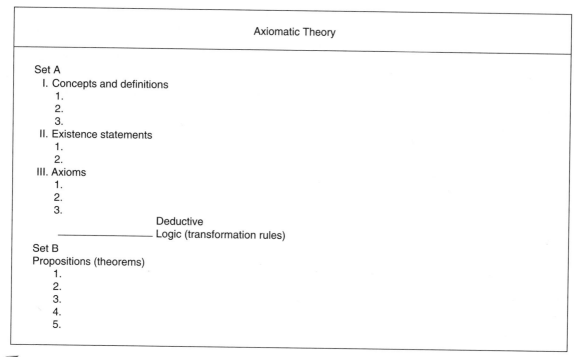

Figure **4-2 Axiomatic theory represented in schematic form.** (Developed from Werkmeister, W. [1959]. Theory construction and the problem of objectivity. In L. Gross [Ed.], *Symposium of sociological theory.* Evanston, IL: Row, Peterson, & Co. [schemata]; and Reynolds, P. [1971]. *A primer in theory construction.* Indianapolis, IN: Bobbs-Merrill [terminology].)

advanced by conducting research and searching for patterns in the data (Meleis, 1985). Patterns do not arise from empirical data of their own accord, and the theorist must bring ideas to experience to conceptualize and order theoretical relationships (Steiner, 1978). Reynolds (1971) stated that this might be difficult to do with a lengthy list of empirical findings in the set-of-laws form.

In contrast to the set-of-laws forms, the axiomatic form of theory organization is an interrelated, logical system. Specifically, an axiomatic theory consists of explicit definitions, a set of concepts, a set of existence statements, and a set of relationship statements arranged in hierarchical order (Reynolds, 1971). The concepts include highly abstract concepts, intermediate concepts, and more concrete concepts. The set-of-existence statements describe situations in which the theory is applicable.

Statements helping to delineate the boundaries of the theory are referred to as describing the scope conditions of the theory (Dubin, 1978; Hage, 1972; Reynolds, 1971). The relational statements consist of axioms and propositions. The highly abstract, theoretical statements, or axioms, are organized at the top of the hierarchy. All other propositions are developed through logical deduction from the axioms (Gross, 1959) or from other more abstract propositions (Figure 4-2). This results in a highly interrelated, explanatory system.

In the axiomatic form, the theoretical statements may not be contradictory (Werkmeister, 1959), because a basic principle of logic asserts that when two statements are contradictory, one or both of the statements must be false (Salmon, 1973). Axiomatic theorists seek to avoid this problem by developing a conceptual system with a few broad axioms from which a set of propositions can be derived. As science progresses and new empirical data become known, the general axioms may be modified or extended. However, if these additions to the logical system produce contradictions in the theory, the theory must be rejected for a theory without contradictions (Schlotfeldt, 1992). New theories often subsume portions of previous theories as special cases (Brown, 1977). For example, Einstein's theory of relativity incorporated Newton's law of gravitation as a special case within the theory. Axiomatic theories are not common in the social and behavioral sciences, but they are clearly evident in the fields of physics and mathematics. For example, Euclidean geometry is an axiomatic theory (Werkmeister, 1959; Zetterberg, 1966).

Developing theories in axiomatic form has several advantages (Reynolds, 1971; Salmon, 1973). First, because theory is a highly interrelated set of statements in which some statements are derived from others, all concepts do not need to be operationally defined (Reynolds, 1971). This allows the theorist to incorporate some highly abstract concepts that may not be measurable, but provide explanation. The interrelated axiomatic system may also be more efficient for explanation than the lengthy number of theoretical statements in the set-of-laws form. In addition, empirical support for one theoretical statement may be judged to provide support for the theory, thereby permitting less extensive research than the requirement to test each statement in the set-of-laws form. In certain instances, the axiomatic theory may be organized in a causal process form to increase understanding.

The distinguishing feature of the causal process form of theory is the development of theoretical statements that specify causal mechanisms between independent and dependent variables. This form of theory organization consists of a set of concepts, a set of definitions, a set of existence statements, and a set of theoretical statements specifying causal process (Reynolds, 1971). Concepts include abstract and concrete ideas. Existence statements function as they do in axiomatic theories to describe the scope

conditions of the theory; that is, the situations to which the theory applies (Dubin, 1978; Hage, 1972; Reynolds, 1971). In contrast to the hierarchical arrangement in the axiomatic theory, causal process theories contain a set of statements describing the causal mechanisms or effects of one variable upon one or more other variables. Causal process theories may be limited to a few variables or they may be quite complex, with several variables. Figure 4-3 displays a causal model for active coping. The broken lines show direction of expected linkage based upon the researchers' hypotheses. The dotted lines indicate new links given the data that have been analyzed. The numbers along the lines refer to the following four studies that were conducted and analyzed in the proposed causal model:

1. Informal caregivers of psychiatrically ill
2. Informal caregivers of demented relatives
3. Professional caregivers of elderly patients
4. Elderly spouses (Ducharme, & Rowat, 1992)

The causal statements specify the hypothesized effects of one variable upon one or more other variables. In complex causal process theories, feedback loops and paths of influence through several variables may be hypothesized in the set of interrelated causal statements (Mullins, 1971; Nowak, 1975). Reynolds (1971) concluded that the causal process form of theory provides for an explanation of the process of how events happen. He identified several advantages of the causal process form of organization. First, like axiomatic theory, it provides for highly abstract, theoretical concepts. Second, like axiomatic theory, this form permits more efficient research testing with its interrelated theoretical statements. Finally, the causal process statements provide a sense of understanding in the phenomenon of interest that is not possible with other forms. However, Turner (1978) observed that causal process theories might not include highly abstract concepts, because a number of available theories simply contain descriptions of causal connections among events. This approach does permit the development of a causal explanation of the sequence of events that may affect the phenomenon of interest (Turner, 1978).

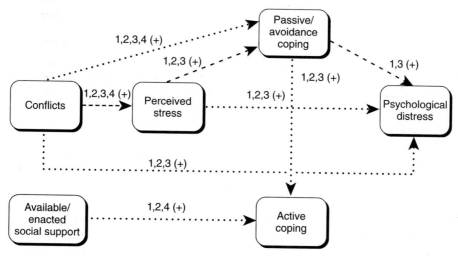

Figure **4-3 Causal model of active coping.** (From Ducharme, F., Ricard, N., Duquette, A., Lévesque, L., & Lachance, L. [1998]. Empirical testing of a longitudinal model derived from the Roy Adaptation Model. *Nursing Science Quarterly, 11*[4], 149-159.)

CONTEMPORARY ISSUES IN NURSING THEORY DEVELOPMENT

Theoretical Boundaries and Levels to Advance Nursing Science

Since Fawcett's (1984) discussion of four metaparadigm concepts in nursing, of person, environment, health, and nursing, general agreement emerged among nursing scholars that this framework was fruitful to pursue the development of nursing science. In general, a metaparadigm should specify the broad boundaries of the domain of interest in a discipline, for example, to set apart the domain of nursing from other disciplines, such as medicine, clinical exercise physiology, or sociology. Fawcett (2000) argued that a metaparadigm also should define the totality of all phenomena inherent in the discipline in a parsimonious way, as well as be perspective-neutral and international in scope. Her definition of perspective-neutral was that the metaparadigm concepts do not reflect any particular conceptual model or paradigm. Yet, in the nursing literature, these concepts have been defined in distinctly different ways that reflect a specific conceptual theory or paradigm, such as different conceptions of health. Thorne and colleagues (1998) proposed that it was not productive to continue the "metaparadigm debates" about which conceptual system should define these concepts and proposed the adoption of a "middle ground" definition that would allow different philosophical perspectives. Scholarly debates can be expected to continue as the community of nursing scholars engages in scholarship and inquiry to reach consensus about the boundaries of the nursing discipline and approaches to advance nursing knowledge (e.g., Monti & Tingen, 1999), such as the level of theories to develop to advance the discipline.

In the development of theories in a variety of disciplines, theories have been categorized at different levels of abstraction from metatheory (theory about theories) to grand theory (broad and general theories) to middle range theory and microrange theory. In the discipline of nursing, the earlier focus on the development and refinement of grand nursing theories has evolved to increasing emphasis on the development of middle range theories and focused situation-specific theories (e.g., Acton, Irvin, Jensen,

Hopkins, & Miller, 1997; Good, 1998; Im & Meleis, 1999; Lawson, 2003; Liehr & Smith, 1999; Smith, et al., 2002).

Middle range theories described by Merton (1967) focus on a specific phenomena (rather than attempt to address a broader range of phenomena) and are comprised of hypotheses with two or more concepts that are linked together in a conceptual system. A middle range theory can be thought of as in the middle of a continuum between a broad and general conception of nursing phenomena (grand theories) and a narrow and specific focus of a very limited nursing phenomenon (situation-based theories). It has been argued that middle range theories facilitate the conceptions of relationships between theory, nursing practice, and patient outcomes in focused areas.

In 1996, Lenz (in Liehr & Smith, 1999) identified the following six approaches for devising middle range theories:

1. Inductive approach through research
2. Deductive approach from grand nursing theories
3. Integration of nursing and nonnursing theories
4. Derivative (retroductive) approach from non-nursing theories
5. Theories devised from guidelines for clinical practice
6. Synthesis approach from research findings

In Liehr and Smith's (1999) review of 10 years of nursing literature on developing middle range theories in the late 1980s and 1990s, they found 22 middle range theories that could be categorized in five of the six Lenz approaches to theory building. They did not find any theories that reportedly were devised by synthesizing research findings. Examples in nursing literature of the range of different approaches to middle range theory building include using a standard of care to develop a middle range theory of the peaceful end of life for terminally ill patients (Ruland & Moore, 1998), using clinical guidelines to develop a mid-range theory of acute pain management (Good, 1998), using grounded theory to devise a mid-range theory of intervention for boys who have molested children (Lawson, 2003), and analyzing pooled empirical data from several research studies based on Roy's Theory of Adaptation in nursing to verify if the same pattern of relationships exists with different populations (Ducharme, Ricard, Duquette, Lévesque, & Lachance, 1998).

There is some difference of opinion among nursing scholars currently as to the definition of a middle range theory and whether some nursing theories should be classified as grand theories or middle range theories. The recent nursing literature emphasizes the importance of relating middle range theories to broader nursing theories and paradigms and continuing to pursue empirical testing and the replication of studies to advance nursing knowledge. Fahs, Morgan, and Kalman (2003) argued that greater attention needs to be focused on the replication of research studies to ensure that nursing scholars can provide "a (reliable) research-to-practice link" . . . that (provides) "safe, effective, quality care to consumers" (p. 70).

As the nursing discipline develops, it is critical that scholarly efforts to synthesize nursing knowledge continue, as the integration of knowledge establishes the linkages that can advance the science of nursing and the practice of nursing. The nursing literature reflects a call from nursing scholars to focus increased attention on developing methodologies to synthesize nursing knowledge (e.g., Copnell, 1998).

Nursing Theory, Practice, and Research

Theory-testing research may lead to the decision to abandon one nursing theory in favor of another theory that explains available research data more adequately. It is therefore critical that theory-testing research in nursing continues to receive emphasis if nursing science is to advance. Several nursing scholars have presented criteria for evaluating theory-testing research in nursing (e.g., Silva, 1986 and Acton, Irvin, & Hopkins, 1991). These criteria emphasize the importance of using a nursing theory to design the purpose and focus of the study, to derive hypotheses, and to relate the significance of the findings back to the nursing theory.

In addition to the call for more rigorous theory-testing research in nursing, both nursing scholars and practitioners are arguing for the need for increased attention to the relationships among theory, research, and practice. Their recommendations include the following:

- Continued development of nursing theories that are relevant to nurses' specialty practice
- Increased collaboration between scientists and practitioners (Lorentzon, 1998)
- Increased encouragement of nurse researchers' efforts to communicate research findings to relevant practitioners
- Increased efforts to relate middle range theories to nursing paradigms
- Increased emphasis on clinical research
- Increased use of nursing theories in clinical decision making

(See Chinn and Kramer, 2004; Cody, 1999; Hoffman and Bertus, 1991; Liehr and Smith, 1999; Lutz, Jones, and Kendall, 1997; Reed, 2000; and Sparacino, 1991.) Malinski (2000) and others have urged increased attention to nursing theory–based research and to strengthening nursing theory–based curricula, especially in master's and doctoral programs.

Regarding the use of nursing knowledge in clinical practice, Cody asserted, "It is a professional nurse's ethical responsibility to utilize the knowledge base of her or his discipline" (1997, p. 4). In 1992, in the first issue of the journal *Clinical Nursing Research,* Schlotfeldt stated the following:

> It will be nursing's clinical scholars . . . that will identify the human phenomena that are central to nurses' practice . . . and that provoke consideration of the practice problems about which knowledge is needed but is not yet available. It is nursing's clinical scholarship that must be depended on to generate promising theories for testing that will advance nursing knowledge and ensure nursing's continued essential services to humankind. (1992, p. 9)

In summary, contemporary nursing scholars are emphasizing the following in the theory-building process:

- Continued development of theoretical inquiry in nursing
- Continued scholarship with middle range theories and situation-specific theories, including efforts to relate to nursing theories and paradigms
- Greater attention to synthesizing nursing knowledge
- Development of stronger nursing theory-research-practice linkages

CREATIVITY IN THEORY BUILDING

A number of strategies for developing theory have been presented in the literature. The theorist who attempts to approach theory construction in a mechanical way by applying structured procedures, however, may have limited success. Theory building involves discovery and creativity. A scientific theory is clearly an invention of the human brain. Bronowski (1979) has written about similarities in the processes of constructing theories and in designing works of art, and he believed that each required a high level of imagination. In his view, "There is no difference in the use of such words as 'beauty' and 'truth' in the poem and such symbols as 'energy' and 'mass' in the equation" (Bronowski, 1979, p. 21).

Although it is possible to teach specific techniques and content, it is not known how to facilitate creativity and originality in students. Rosenberg (1978, p. 2) stated, "You can teach someone how to look, but not how to see, how to search, but not how to find." Rosenberg asserted that although creativity cannot be taught, it can be nurtured.

Bronowski (1979, p. 22) suggests that a sense of "imagination, playfulness, and participation" is essential for the theorist and for the reader who seeks to understand theories. According to Bronowski (1979, pp. 22-23), "If science is a form of imagination, if all experiment is a form of play, then science cannot be dry as dust. Science, or art, every creative activity is fun. If a theorem in science seems dull to you, that is because you are not reading it with the same active sense of participation (and imagination) which you bring to the reading of a poem."

In addition to imagination, developing and presenting theories requires personal discipline. As Mills (1959) emphasized long ago, innovative ideas tend to occur in an unconnected, ambiguous form. Self-discipline is required to work with, develop, and express the idea in written form for others to review (Hoffman & Bertus, 1991).

REFERENCES

Acton, G., Irvin, B., & Hopkins, B. (1991). Theory-testing research: Building the science. *ANS Advances in Nursing Science, 14*(1), 52-61.

Acton, G., Irvin, B., Jensen, B., Hopkins, B., & Miller, E. (1997). Explicating middle-range theory through methodological diversity. *ANS Advances in Nursing Science, 19*(3), 78-85.

Almond, P. (2002). An analysis of the concept of equity and its application to health visiting. *Journal of Advanced Nursing, 37*(6), 598-606.

American Heart Association (AHA). (2004). Diagnosing heart disease. Dallas: AHA. Retrieved April 26, 2004, from *http://www.americanheart.org/presenter.jhtml?identifier=330*

Blegen, M., & Tripp-Reimer, T. (1997). Implications of nursing taxonomies for middle-range theory development. *ANS Advances in Nursing Science, 19*(3), 37-49.

Bronowski, J. (1979). *The visionary age: Essay with arts, literature, and science.* Cambridge, MA: MIT Press.

Brown, H. (1977). *Perception, theory and commitment: The new philosophy of science.* Chicago: University of Chicago Press.

Chinn, P., & Kramer, M. (1991). *Theory and nursing: A systematic approach* (3rd ed.). St. Louis: Mosby.

Cody, W. (1997). Of tombstones, milestones, and gemstones: A retrospective and prospective on nursing theory. *Nursing Science Quarterly, 10*(1), 3-5.

Cody, W. (1999). Middle range theories: Do they foster the development of nursing science? *Nursing Science Quarterly, 12*(1), 9-14.

Copnell, B. (1998). Synthesis in nursing knowledge: An analysis of two approaches. *Journal of Advanced Nursing, 27,* 870-874.

Dubin, R. (1978). *Theory building.* New York: Free Press.

Ducharme, F., Ricard, N., Duquette, A., Lévesque, L., & Lachance, L. (1998). Empirical testing of a longitudinal model derived from the Roy Adaptation Model, *Nursing Science Quarterly, 11*(2), 149-159.

Ducharme, F., & Rowat, K. (1992). Conjugul supports family coping behaviors and the well-being of elderly couples. *Can. J. Res. 24*(1), 5-22.

Fahs, P. S., Morgan, L. L., & Kalman, M. (2003). A call for replication. *Journal of Nursing Scholarship, 35*(1), 67-72.

Fawcett, J. (1984). The metaparadigm of nursing: Present status and future refinements. *Image: The Journal of Nursing Scholarship, 16*(3), 84-87.

Fawcett, J. (2000). *Analysis and evaluation of contemporary nursing knowledge: Nursing models and theories.* Philadelphia: F. A. Davis.

Foster, L. (1997). Addressing epistemologic and practical issues in multimethod research: A procedure for conceptual triangulation. *ANS Advances in Nursing Science, 20*(2), 1-12.

Giere, R. N. (1979). *Understanding scientific reasoning.* New York: Holt, Rhinehart, & Winston.

Giere, R. N. (1997). *Understanding scientific reasoning* (4th ed.). Fort Worth, TX: Harcourt, Brace College Publishers.

Good, M. (1998). Middle range theory of acute pain management: Use in research. *Nursing Outlook, 46,*120-124.

Goulet, C., Bell, L., St-Cyr Tribble, D., Paul, D., & Lang, A. (1998). A concept analysis of parent-infant attachment. *Journal of Advanced Nursing, 28*(5), 1071-1081.

Gross, L. (1959). *Symposium on sociological theory.* Evanston, IL: Row, Peterson & Co.

Haas, B. K. (1999). Clarification and integration of similar quality of life concepts. *Image: The Journal of Nursing Scholarship, 31*(3), 215-220.

Hage, J. (1972). *Techniques and problems of theory construction in sociology.* New York: John Wiley & Sons.

Hardin, S. R., Hussey, L.C., & Steele, L. (2003). Spirituality as integrality among chronic heart failure patients: A pilot study. *Visions: The Journal of Rogerian Nursing Science, 11,* 1, 43-53.

Harvey, G., Loftus-Hills, A., Rycroft-Malone, J., Titchen, A., Kitson, A., McCormack, B., et al. (2002). Getting evidence into practice: The role and function of facilitation. *Journal of Advanced Nursing, 37*(6), 577-588.

Hatch, R. L., Burg, M. A., Naberhaus, D. S., & Hellmich, L. K. (1998). The Spiritual Involvement and Beliefs Scale: Development and testing of a new instrument. *Journal of Family Practice, 46,* 6.

Hoffman, A., & Bertus, P. (1991). Theory and practice: Bridging scientists' and practitioners' roles. *Archives of Psychiatric Nursing, 7*(1), 2-9.

Hussey, L.C., & Hardin, S. R. (2003). Sex-related differences in heart failure. *Heart & Lung, 32*(4), 215-225.

Im, E., & Meleis, A. (1999). Situation-specific theories: Philosophical roots, properties and approach. *ANS Advances in Nursing Science, 22*(2), 11-24.

Kaplan, A. (1964). *The conduct of inquiry: Methodology for behavioral science.* New York: Chandler.

Keenan, J. (1999). A concept analysis of autonomy. *Journal of Advanced Nursing, 29*(3), 556-562.

Lawson, L. (2003). Becoming a success story: How boys who have molested children talk about treatment. *Journal of Psychiatric and Mental Health Nursing, 10,* 259-268.

Liehr, P., & Smith, M. J. (1999). Middle range theory: Spinning research and practice to create knowledge for the new millennium. *ANS Advances in Nursing Science, 21*(4), 81-91.

Lorentzon, M. (1998). The way forward: Nursing research or collaborative health care research? *Journal of Advanced Nursing, 27,* 675-676.

Lutz, K., Jones, K., & Kendall, J. (1997). Expanding the praxis debate: Contributions to clinical inquiry. *ANS Advances in Nursing Science, 20*(2), 13-22.

Malinski, V. (1994). Spirituality: A pattern manifestation of the human/environment mutual process. *Visions: The Journal of Rogerian Science, 2*(1), 12-18.

Malinski, V. (2000). Research-based evaluation of conceptual models of nursing. *Nursing Science Quarterly, 13*(2), 103-110.

Meleis, A. (1985). *Theoretical nursing: Development and progress.* Philadelphia: J. B. Lippincott.

Merton, R. K. (1967). *On theoretical sociology.* New York: Free Press.

Mills, C. W. (1959). On intellectual craftsmanship. In L. Gross (Ed.), *Symposium on sociological theory.* Evanston, IL: Row, Peterson, & Co.

Monti, E., & Tingen, M. (1999). Multiple paradigms of nursing science. *ANS Advances in Nursing Science, 21*(4) 64-80.

Mullins, N. (1971). *The art of theory: Construction and use.* New York: Harper & Row.

Nowak, S. (1975). Causal interpretations of statistical relationships in social research. In H. Blalock (Ed.), *Quantitative sociology: International perspectives on mathematical and statistical modeling.* New York: Academic Press.

Reed, P. (2000). Nursing reformation: Historical reflections and philosophic foundations. *Nursing Science Quarterly, 13*(2), 129-136.

Reynolds, P. (1971). *A primer in theory construction.* Indianapolis, IN: Bobbs-Merrill.

Rosenberg, J. (1978). *The practice of philosophy.* Englewood Cliffs, NJ: Prentice Hall.

Ruland, C. M., & Moore, S. M. (1998). Theory construction based on standards of care: A proposed theory of the peaceful end of life. *Nursing Outlook, 46,* 169-175.

Salmon, W. D. (1973). *Logic.* Englewood Cliffs, NJ: Prentice Hall.

Schilling, L. S., Grey, M., & Knafl, K. A. (2002). The concept of self-management of type I diabetes in children and adolescents: An evolutionary concept analysis. *Journal of Advanced Nursing, 37*(1), 87-99.

Schlotfeldt, R. (1992). Why promote clinical nursing scholarship? *Clinical Nursing Research, 1*(1), 5-8.

Silva, M. (1986). Research testing nursing theory: State of the art. *ANS Advances in Nursing Science, 9*(10), 1-11.

Smith, C. E., Pace, K., Kochinda, C., Kleinbeck, S. V., Koehler, J., & Popkess-Vawter, S. (2002). Caregiving Effectiveness Model evolution to a midrange theory of home care: A process for critique and replication. *ANS Advances in Nursing Science, 25,* 50-64.

Sparacino, P. (1991). The reciprocal relationship between practice and theory. *Clinical Nurse Specialist, 5*(3), 138.

Steiner, E. (1978). *Logical and conceptual analytic techniques for educational researchers.* Washington, DC: University Press.

Thorne, S., Canam, C., Dahinten, S., Hall, W., Henderson, A., & Kirkham, S. R. (1998). Nursing's metaparadigm concepts: Disimpacting the debates. *Journal of Advanced Nursing, 27,* 1257-1268.

Turner, J. (1978). *The structure of sociological theory.* Homewood, IL: Dorsey Press.

Walker, L., & Avant, K. (1983). *Strategies for theory construction in nursing.* Norwalk, CT: Appleton-Century-Crofts.

Werkmeister, W. (1959). Theory construction and the problem of objectivity. In L. Gross (Ed.), *Symposium of sociological theory.* Evanston, IL: Row, Peterson, & Co.

Zetterberg, H. L. (1966). *On theory and verification in sociology.* New York: John Wiley & Sons.

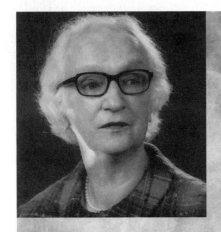

$\mathcal{H}$ildegard E. Peplau
1909-1999

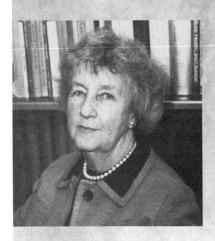

$\mathcal{V}$irginia Henderson
1897-1996

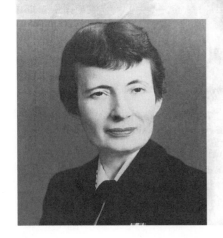

$\mathcal{F}$aye Glenn Abdellah
1919-present

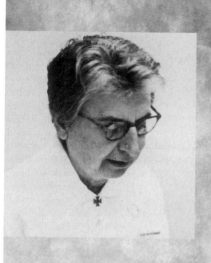

Ernestine Wiedenbach
1900-1996

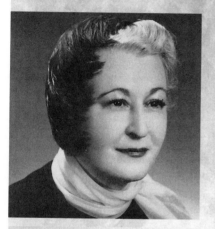

Lydia Hall
1906-1969

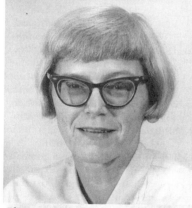

Joyce Travelbee
1926-1973

Photo Credit: Louisiana State
University Health Sciences Center,
School of Nursing, New Orleans, LA.

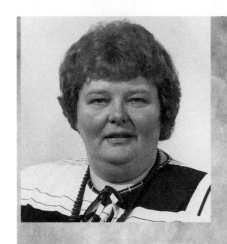

Kathryn E. Barnard
1938-present

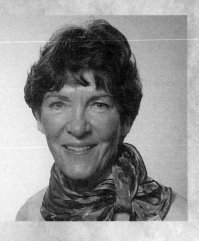

Evelyn Adam
1929-present

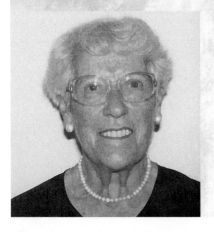

Nancy Roper
1918-2004

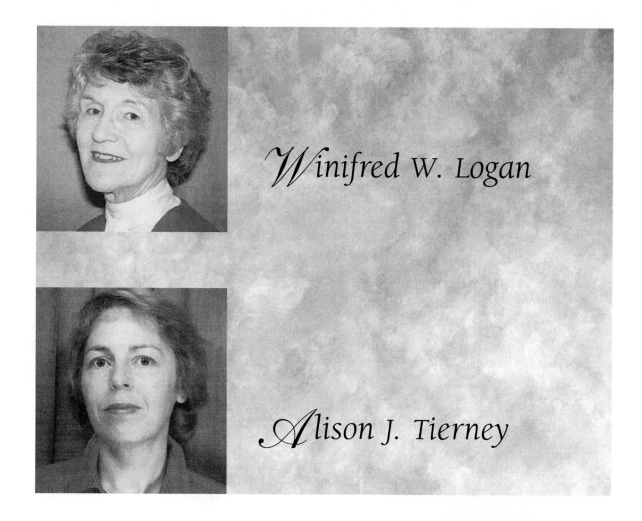

Winifred W. Logan

Alison J. Tierney

Nursing Theorists of Historical Significance

Ann Marriner Tomey

HILDEGARD E. PEPLAU
Theory of Interpersonal Relations

Hildegard E. Peplau's contributions to nursing in general and to the specialty of psychiatric nursing in particular have been enormous. She is considered the mother of psychiatric nursing, but her contribution to the professionalization of nursing transcends what she gave to psychiatric nursing. She promoted professional standards and regulation through credentialing. She introduced the concept of advanced nursing practice. Starting in the early 1950s she published many texts, beginning with *Interpersonal Relations in Nursing* (1952). She taught psychodynamic nursing and stressed the importance of the nurse's ability to understand his or her own behavior to help others identify perceived difficulties. She identified the following four phases of the nurse-patient relationship (Figure 5-1):

1. Orientation
2. Identification
3. Exploitation
4. Resolution

Peplau diagramed changing aspects of nurse-patient relationships (Figure 5-2) and proposed and described the following six nursing roles (Figure 5-3):

1. Stranger
2. Resource person
3. Teacher
4. Leader
5. Surrogate
6. Counselor

In addition, she discussed four psychobiological experiences that compel destructive or constructive responses, as follows:

1. Needs
2. Frustrations
3. Conflicts
4. Anxieties

Peplau was influenced by Freud, by Maslow, by Sullivan's interpersonal relationship theories, and by the contemporaneous psychoanalytical model. She was the first nurse author to borrow theory from other scientific fields and synthesize a theory for nursing. She used the psychological model to develop her Theory of Interpersonal Relations. Peplau's work is categorized as a theory for the practice of nursing.

VIRGINIA HENDERSON
Definition of Nursing

Virginia Henderson viewed the patient as an individual requiring help toward achieving independence. She envisioned the practice of nursing as independent from the practice of physicians and acknowledged her interpretation of the nurse's function as a synthesis of many influences. Her philosophy is based on work by Thorndike (an American psychologist), her experience in rehabilitation nursing, and Orlando's work regarding the conceptualization of deliberate nursing action (Orlando, 1961). Henderson emphasized the art of nursing and identified the 14 basic human needs on which nursing care is based. Her contributions include defining nursing, delineating autonomous nursing functions, stressing goals of interdependence for the patient, and creating self-help concepts. Her self-help concepts influenced the works of Abdellah and Adam (Abdellah, Beland, Martin, & Matheney, 1960; Adam, 1980, 1991).

Henderson made enormous contributions to nursing during more than 60 years of service as a nurse, teacher, author, and researcher, and she published extensively throughout those years. She directed the Yale-sponsored Nursing Studies Index Project that resulted in a four-volume annotated index to nursing's biographical, analytical, and historical literature from 1900 to 1959. Her definition of nursing first appeared in 1955 in the fifth edition of *Textbook of the Principles and Practice of Nursing* by Harmer and Henderson. Henderson stated the following:

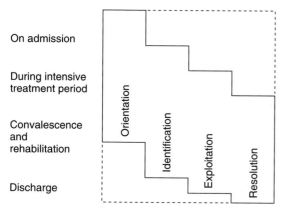

Figure **5-1 Overlapping phases in nurse-patient relationships.** (From Peplau, H. E. [1952]. *Interpersonal relations in nursing.* New York: G. P. Putnam's Sons.)

> The unique function of the nurse is to assist the individual, sick or well, in the performance of those activities contributing to health or its recovery (or to peaceful death) that he would perform unaided if he had the necessary strength, will, or knowledge and to do this in such a way as to help him gain independence as rapidly as possible. (1955, p. 7)

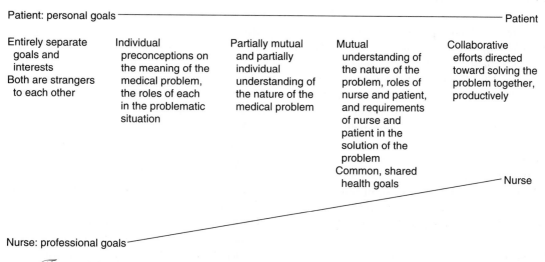

Figure **5-2 Continuum showing changing aspects of nurse-patient relationships.** (From Peplau, H. E. [1952]. *Interpersonal relations in nursing.* New York: G. P. Putnam's Sons.)

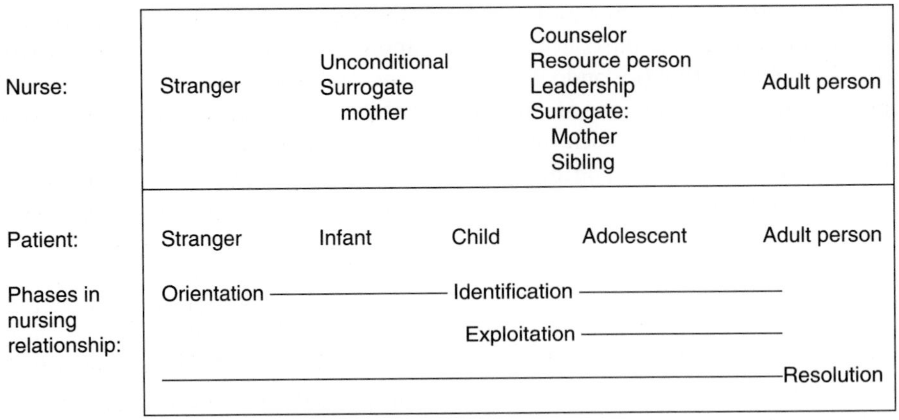

Nurse:	Stranger	Unconditional Surrogate mother	Counselor Resource person Leadership Surrogate: Mother Sibling	Adult person
Patient:	Stranger	Infant	Child Adolescent	Adult person

Phases in nursing relationship:

Orientation ———————— Identification ————————

Exploitation ————————

————————————————————————Resolution

Figure **5-3 Phases and changing roles in nurse-patient relationships.** (From Peplau, H. E. [1952]. *Interpersonal relations in nursing.* New York: G. P. Putnam's Sons.)

In *The Nature of Nursing: A Definition and Its Implications for Practice, Research, and Education,* Henderson (1966) identified 14 basic needs upon which nursing care is based (Box 5-1). She identified the following three levels of nurse-patient relationships in which the nurse acts as the following:

1. A substitute for the patient
2. A helper to the patient
3. A partner with the patient

She supported empathetic understanding and stated that the nurse must "get inside the skin of each of her patients in order to know what he needs" (Henderson, 1964, p. 63). Although she believed that the functions of nurses and physicians overlap, Henderson asserted that the nurse works in interdependence with other health professionals and with the patient, and used wedges of a pie graph to represent their relative contributions. The sizes of pieces vary, depending upon the patient's needs, but the goal is for the patient to represent the majority of the pie as he or she gains independence. In *The Nature of Nursing: Reflections After 25 Years,* Henderson (1991) added addenda to each chapter of the 1966 edition to present changes in her views and to explain her opinions. Henderson's work may be viewed as a philosophy of nursing.

FAYE GLENN ABDELLAH
Twenty-One Nursing Problems

Faye Glenn Abdellah is recognized as one of the country's leading researchers in health and public policy and an international expert on health problems. Among her numerous positions, she was Chief Nurse Officer of the United States Public Health Service for 17 years (1970–1987) and the first woman and first nurse to be Deputy Surgeon General (1982–1989). Her work is based on the problem-solving method and has had a great impact on nursing curriculum development. Problem solving is the vehicle for delineating nursing (patient) problems as the patient moves toward a healthy outcome.

Abdellah views nursing as both an art and a science that molds the attitude, intellectual competencies, and technical skills of the individual nurse into the desire and ability to help people cope with their health needs, whether they are ill or well. Although she believes that nursing actions are carried out under general or specific medical direction, she has formulated 21 nursing problems based on a review of nursing research studies (Box 5-2). She used Henderson's 14 basic human needs (see Box 5-1) and nursing

Box 5-1

Henderson's 14 Needs

1. Breathe normally.
2. Eat and drink adequately.
3. Eliminate body wastes.
4. Move and maintain desirable postures.
5. Sleep and rest.
6. Select suitable clothes; dress and undress.
7. Maintain body temperature within a normal range by adjusting clothing and modifying the environment.
8. Keep the body clean and well groomed and protect the integument.
9. Avoid dangers in the environment and avoid injuring others.
10. Communicate with others in expressing emotions, needs, fears, or opinions.
11. Worship according to one's faith.
12. Work in such a way that there is a sense of accomplishment.
13. Play or participate in various forms of recreation.
14. Learn, discover, or satisfy the curiosity that leads to normal development and health and use the available health facilities.

From Henderson, V. A. (1991). *The nature of nursing: Reflections after 25 years* (pp. 22-23). New York: National League for Nursing Press.

research to establish the classification of nursing problems.

Her work differs from that of Henderson; Abdellah's problems are formulated in terms of nursing-centered services, which are used to determine the patient's needs. Her contribution to nursing theory development consists of a systematic analysis of research reports to formulate the 21 nursing problems that served as an early guide for comprehensive nursing care. The typology of her 21 nursing problems first appeared in the 1960 edition of *Patient-Centered Approaches to Nursing*

(Abdellah et al., 1960). It evolved in *Preparing for Nursing Research in the 21st Century: Evolution, Methodologies, and Challenges* (Abdellah & Levine, 1994). The 21 nursing problems have progressed to a second-generation development of patient problems and patient outcomes, instead of nursing problems and nursing outcomes. Abdellah's work is considered a philosophy of nursing.

ERNESTINE WIEDENBACH
The Helping Art of Clinical Nursing

Ernestine Wiedenbach concentrated on the art of nursing and focused on the needs of the patient. Wiedenbach's work grew from 40 years of experience, primarily in maternity nursing. Her definition of nursing reflects her background. She stated the following: "People may differ in their concept of nursing, but few would disagree that nursing is nurturing or caring for someone in a motherly fashion" (Wiedenbach, 1964, p. 1).

Wiedenbach's orientation is a philosophy of nursing, which guides the nurse's action in the art of nursing. Wiedenbach specified the following four elements:
1. Philosophy
2. Purpose
3. Practice
4. Art

She postulated that clinical nursing is directed toward meeting the patient's perceived need-for-help. Her vision of nursing reflected the period when considerable emphasis was placed on the art of nursing. She followed Orlando's theory of deliberate rather than automatic nursing and incorporated the steps of the nursing process.

In her book (1964), *Clinical Nursing: A Helping Art*, the concepts and subconcepts (Figure 5-4) include the following:
I. Patient
   A. Need-for-help
II. Nurse
   A. Purpose
   B. Philosophy
   C. Practice

Box 5-2

Abdellah's Typology of 21 Nursing Problems

1. To maintain good hygiene and physical comfort
2. To promote optimal activity: exercise, rest, sleep
3. To promote safety through prevention of accident, injury, or other trauma and through the prevention of the spread of infection
4. To maintain good body mechanics and prevent and correct deformity
5. To facilitate the maintenance of a supply of oxygen to all body cells
6. To facilitate the maintenance of nutrition of all body cells
7. To facilitate the maintenance of elimination
8. To facilitate the maintenance of fluid and electrolyte balance
9. To recognize the physiological responses of the body to disease conditions—pathological, physiological, and compensatory
10. To facilitate the maintenance of regulatory mechanisms and functions
11. To facilitate the maintenance of sensory function

12. To identify and accept positive and negative expressions, feelings, and reactions
13. To identify and accept interrelatedness of emotions and organic illness
14. To facilitate the maintenance of effective verbal and nonverbal communication
15. To promote the development of productive interpersonal relationships
16. To facilitate progress toward achievement and personal spiritual goals
17. To create or maintain a therapeutic environment
18. To facilitate awareness of self as an individual with varying physical, emotional, and developmental needs
19. To accept the optimum possible goals in the light of limitations, physical and emotional
20. To use community resources as an aid in resolving problems arising from illness
21. To understand the role of social problems as influencing factors in the cause of illness

---

From Abdellah, F. G., Beland, I. L., Martin, A., & Matheney, R. V. (1960). *Patient-centered approaches to nursing.* New York: Macmillan. Reprinted with the permission of Scribner, a division of Simon & Schuster.

   1. Knowledge
   2. Judgment
   3. Skills
 D. Ministration
 E. Validation
 F. Coordination
   1. Reporting
   2. Consulting
   3. Conferring
 G. Art
   1. Stimulus
   2. Preconception

   3. Interpretation
   4. Actions
     a. Rational
     b. Reactionary
     c. Deliberative

She proposed that nurses identify patients' need-for-help through the following (Figure 5-5):

1. Observing behaviors consistent or inconsistent with their comfort
2. Exploring the meaning of their behavior
3. Determining the cause of their discomfort or incapability

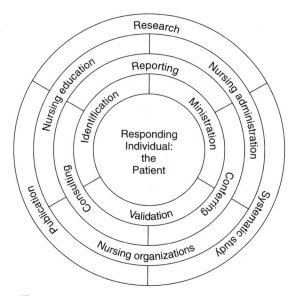

Figure **5-4** Clinical nursing: the relationship between its focus and its constituents. (From Wiedenbach, E. [1964]. *Clinical nursing: A helping art* [p. 108]. New York: Springer.)

4. Determining whether they can resolve their problems or have a need-for-help

Following that, the nurse administers the help needed (Figure 5-6) and validates that the need-for-help was met (Figure 5-7) (Wiedenbach, 1964). Wiedenbach's work may be considered a philosophy of nursing.

LYDIA HALL
Core, Care, and Cure Model

Lydia Hall used her philosophy of nursing to design and develop the Loeb Center for Nursing at Montefiore Hospital in New York. She served as administrative director of the Loeb Center from its opening in 1963 until her death in 1969. Most of her work was published in the 1960s. In 1964, her work was presented in "Nursing: What Is It?" in *The Canadian Nurse.* In 1969, it was discussed in "The Loeb

Center for Nursing and Rehabilitation" in the *International Journal of Nursing Studies.*

She proposed that nursing functions differ, using three interlocking circles to represent aspects of the patient. She labeled the circles as the body (the care), the disease (the cure), and the person (the core) (Figure 5-8). Nurses function in all three circles but to different degrees. They also share the circles with other providers. Hall believed that professional nursing care hastened recovery and that as less medical care was needed, more professional nursing care and teaching were necessary. Hall stressed the autonomous function of nursing. Her conceptualization encompasses adult patients who have passed the acute stage of illness. The goal for the patient was rehabilitation and success in self-actualization and self-love. Her contribution to nursing theory was the development and use of her philosophy of nursing care at the Loeb Center in New York. She also recognized professional nurses and encouraged them to make a contribution to patient outcomes. Hall's work may be viewed as a philosophy of nursing.

JOYCE TRAVELBEE
Human-to-Human Relationship Model

Joyce Travelbee published predominantly in the mid-1960s. She died in 1973 at a relatively young age. Travelbee (1966, 1971) proposed her Human-to-Human Relationship Theory in her book, *Interpersonal Aspects of Nursing.* She wrote about illness, suffering, pain, hope, communication, interaction, empathy, sympathy, rapport, and therapeutic use of self. She proposed that nursing was accomplished through human-to-human relationships that began with (1) the original encounter, which progressed through stages of (2) emerging identities, (3) developing feelings of empathy and, later, (4) sympathy, until (5) the nurse and patient attained rapport in the final stage (Figure 5-9). Travelbee's theory extended the interpersonal relationship theories of Peplau and Orlando, but her unique synthesis of their ideas differentiated her work in terms of

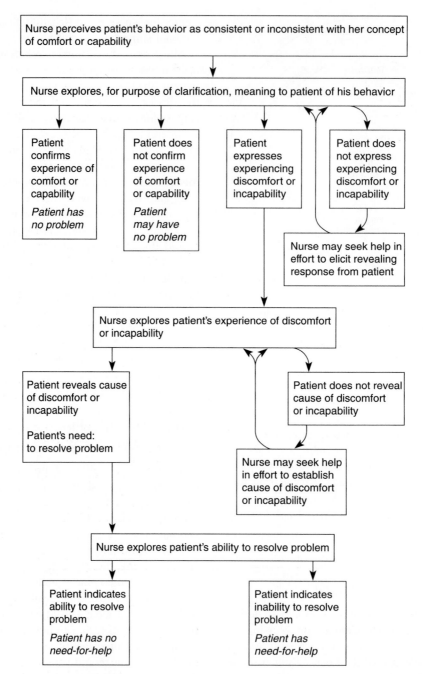

Figure **5-5 Identification of a need-for-help.** (From Wiedenbach, E. [1964]. *Clinical nursing: A helping art* [p. 60]. New York: Springer.)

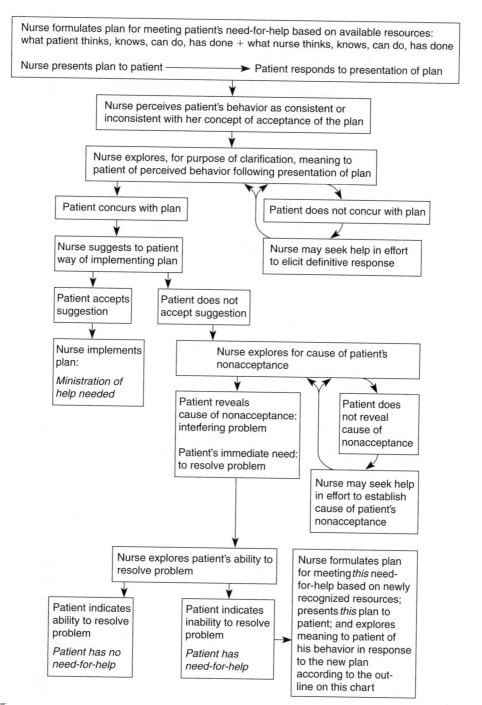

Figure **5-6 Ministration of help.** (From Wiedenbach, E. [1964]. *Clinical nursing: A helping art* [p. 61]. New York: Springer.)

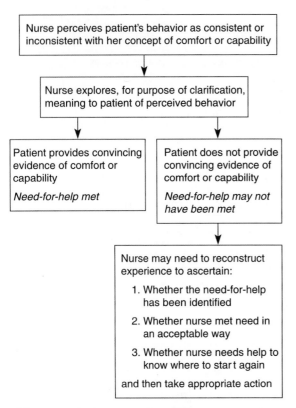

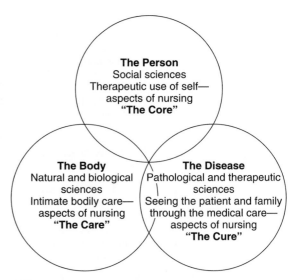

Figure **5-8 Core, Care, and Cure Model.** (From Hall, L. [1964, Feb.]. Nursing: What is it? *The Canadian Nurse, 60*[2], 151.)

Figure **5-7 Validation that need-for-help was met.** (From Wiedenbach, E. [1964]. *Clinical nursing: A helping art* [p. 62]. New York: Springer.)

the therapeutic human relationship between nurse and patient. Travelbee's emphasis on caring stressed empathy, sympathy, rapport, and the emotional aspects of nursing. The work is categorized as a nursing theory.

KATHRYN E. BARNARD
Child Health Assessment Interaction Model

Kathryn E. Barnard is an active researcher who has published extensively about infants and children since the mid-1960s. She began by studying mentally and physically handicapped children and adults, moved into studying the activities of the well child, and then expanded her work to include methods of evaluating the growth and development of children and mother-infant relationships. (Barnard, 1978) She was also concerned about disseminating research and, consequently, developed the Nursing Child Assessment Satellite Training Project.

Although Barnard never intended to develop theory, the longitudinal nursing-child assessment study provided the basis for her Child Health Assessment Interaction Theory (Figure 5-10). Barnard proposes that the individual characteristics of each member influence the parent-infant system and that adaptive behavior modifies those characteristics to meet the needs of the system. Barnard's theory borrows from psychology and human development and focuses on mother-infant interaction with the environment. Her theory is based on scales developed to measure the effects of feeding, teaching, and environment. With continuous research, she has refined the theory and provided a close link to

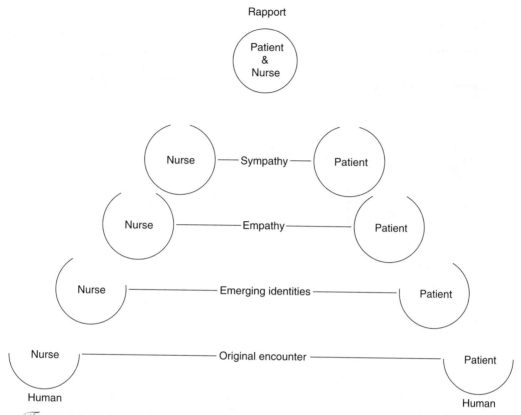

Figure **5-9 Human-to-human relationship.** (Conceptualized by William Hobble and Theresa Lansinger based on Joyce Travelbee's writings.)

practice. She models the role of researcher in clinical practice as she engages in theory development in practice for the advancement of nursing science. Barnard's work is a theory of nursing.

EVELYN ADAM
Conceptual Model for Nursing

Evelyn Adam is a Canadian nurse who started publishing in the mid-1970s. Much of her work focuses on development models and theories on the concept of nursing. She uses a model she learned from Dorothy Johnson. In her book, *To Be a Nurse* (1980),

she applies Virginia Henderson's definition of nursing to Johnson's model and identifies the assumptions, beliefs and values, and major units. In the latter category, she includes the goal of the profession, the beneficiary of the professional service, the role of the professional, the source of the beneficiary's difficulty, the intervention of the professional, and the consequences. She expanded her work in the 1991 second edition. Adam's work is a good example of using a unique basis of nursing for further expansion. She has contributed to theory development by clarification and explication of earlier work. Adam's work is a theory of nursing.

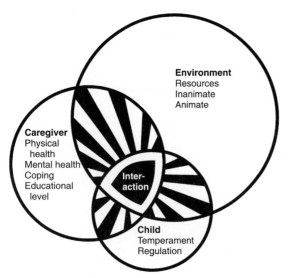

Figure **5-10** Child Health Assessment Model. (From Sumner, G., & Spietz, A. [Eds.]. [1994]. *NCAST caregiver/parent-child interaction teaching manual* [p. 3]. Seattle: NCAST Publications, University of Washington School of Nursing.)

NANCY ROPER, WINIFRED W. LOGAN, AND ALISON J. TIERNEY
A Model for Nursing Based on a Model of Living

After 15 years as a principal tutor in a school of nursing, Nancy Roper began her career as a full-time writer during the 1960s. Her MPhil research study, published in a monograph as *Clinical Experience in Nurse Education* (1976), provided the base for her later work with Winifred Logan and Alison Tierney. She, along with theorists Logan and Tierney, authored *The Elements of Nursing* in 1980, 1985, and 1990. The trio again collaborated in the fourth and most recent edition of *The Elements of Nursing Based on a Model of Living* (1996). During the 1970s Roper conducted research to discover the core of nursing, based on a Model of Living (Figure 5-11). This was in response to the use of qualifiers for naming nursing practice according to the ideas of

Table **5-1**

Comparison of the Main Concepts in the Model of Living and the Model for Nursing

MODEL OF LIVING	MODEL FOR NURSING
12 ALs	12 ALs
Life span	Life span
Dependence-independence continuum	Dependence-independence continuum
Factors influencing the ALs	Factors influencing the ALs
Individuality in living	Individualizing nursing

From Roper, N., Logan, W. W., & Tierney, A. J. (1996). *The elements of nursing: A model for nursing based on a model of living* (4th ed., p. 33). Edinburgh: Churchill Livingstone. *ALs*, Activities of living.

medical practice. Three decades of study of the elements of nursing by Roper evolved into a Model for Nursing with five main factors that influenced the ALs (Figure 5-12 and Table 5-1).

Rather than revise the fourth edition of their textbook, the theorists prepared a monograph (Roper, Logan, & Tierney, 2000) about the model, *The Roper-Logan-Tierney Model of Nursing: Based on Activities of Living*, without the application of the model. Holland, Jenkins, and Solomon (2003) explored the use of the Roper-Logan-Tierney Model of Nursing. They used case studies and exercises about adult patients with a variety of health problems in acute-care and community-based settings to help students develop problem-solving skills.

In the Model of Nursing, the 12 activities of living (ALs) include maintaining a safe environment, communicating, breathing, eating and drinking, eliminating, personal cleansing and dressing, controlling body temperature, mobilizing, working and playing, expressing sexuality, sleeping, and dying. Life span ranges from birth to death, and the dependence-independence continuum ranges from total depen-

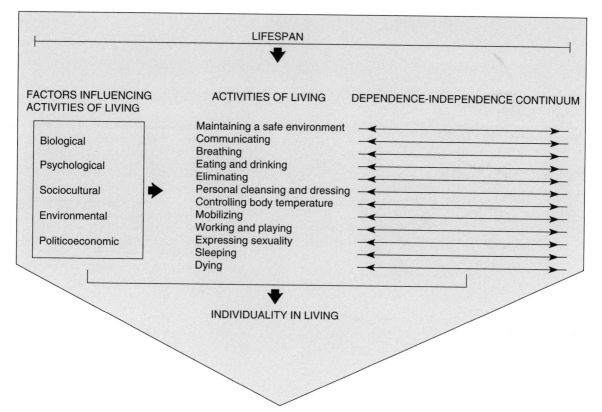

LIFESPAN

**FACTORS INFLUENCING
ACTIVITIES OF LIVING**

Biological

Psychological

Sociocultural

Environmental

Politicoeconomic

ACTIVITIES OF LIVING

Maintaining a safe environment
Communicating
Breathing
Eating and drinking
Eliminating
Personal cleansing and dressing
Controlling body temperature
Mobilizing
Working and playing
Expressing sexuality
Sleeping
Dying

DEPENDENCE-INDEPENDENCE CONTINUUM

INDIVIDUALITY IN LIVING

Figure **5-11 Diagram of the Model of Living.** (From Roper, N., Logan W. W., & Tierney, A. J. [1996]. *The elements of nursing: A model for nursing based on a model of living* [4th ed., p. 20]. Edinburgh: Churchill Livingstone.)

dence to total independence. The five groups of factors influencing the ALs are biological, psychological, sociocultural, environmental, and politicoeconomic (see Figure 5-12). Individuality of living is the way in which the individual attends to the ALs in regard to the individual's place on the life span, on the dependence-independence continuum, and as influenced by biological, psychological, sociocultural environmental, and politicoeconomic factors.

In the Model of Nursing, the five components can be used to describe the individual in relation to maintaining health, preventing disease, coping

during periods of sickness and rehabilitation, coping positively during periods of chronic ill health, or coping when dying. Individualizing nursing is accomplished by using the process of nursing, which involves four phases: (1) assessing, (2) planning, (3) implementing, and (4) evaluating (see Figure 5-12). The process is simply a method of logical thinking, and it needs to be used with an explicit nursing model. The patient's individuality in living (see Figure 5-11) must be borne in mind in all four phases of the process. This model has been used as a guide for nursing practice, research, and education.

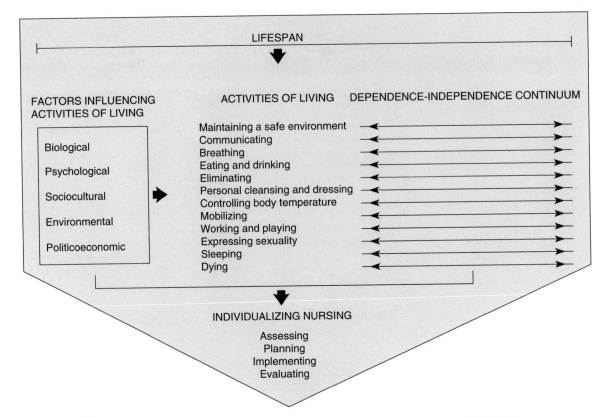

Figure **5-12 Diagram of the Model for Nursing.** (From Roper, N., Logan, W. W., & Tierney, A. J. [1996]. *The elements of nursing: A model for nursing based on a model of living* [4th ed, p. 34]. Edinburgh: Churchill Livingstone.)

REFERENCES

Abdellah, F. G., Beland, I. L., Martin, A., & Matheney, R. V. (1960). *Patient-centered approaches to nursing.* New York: Macmillan.

Abdellah, F. G., & Levine, E. (1994). *Preparing for nursing research in the 21st century: Evolution, methodologies, challenges.* New York: Springer.

Adam, E. (1980). *To be a nurse.* Philadelphia: W. B. Saunders.

Adam, E. (1991). *To be a nurse* (2nd ed.). Montreal: W. B. Saunders Company Canada.

Barnard, K. E. (1978). *Nursing child assessment and training: Learning resource manual.* Seattle: University of Washington.

Hall, L. E. (1964, Feb.). Nursing: What is it? *The Canadian Nurse, 60,* 150-154.

Hall, L. E. (1969). The Loeb Center for nursing and rehabilitation. *International Journal of Nursing Studies, 6,* 81-95.

Harmer, B., & Henderson, V. (1955). *Textbook of the principles and practice of nursing.* New York: Macmillan.

Henderson, V. (1964, Aug.). The nature of nursing. *American Journal of Nursing, 64,* 62-68.

Henderson, V. (1966). *The nature of nursing: A definition and its implications for practice, research, and education.* New York: Macmillan.

Henderson, V. A. (1991). *The nature of nursing: Reflections after 25 years.* New York: National League for Nursing Press.

Holland, K., Jenkins, J., & Solomon, J. (2003). *Applying the Roper-Logan-Tierney Model in practice.* Edinburgh: Churhill Livingstone.

Orlando, I. (1961). *The dynamic nurse-patient relationship.* New York: G. P. Putnam's Sons.

Peplau, H. (1952). *Interpersonal relations in nursing.* New York: G. P. Putnam's Sons.

Roper, N. (1976). *Clinical experience in nurse education* (Research monograph). Edinburgh: Churchill Livingstone.

Roper, N. (1980). *The elements of nursing: A model for nursing.* Edinburgh: Churchill Livingstone.

Roper, N. (1985). *The elements of nursing: A model for nursing* (2nd ed.). Edinburgh: Churchill Livingstone.

Roper, N. (1990). *The elements of nursing: A model for nursing based on a model of living* (3rd ed.). Edinburgh: Churchill Livingstone.

Roper, N., Logan, W., & Tierney, A. J. (2000). *The Roper-Logan-Tierney model of nursing: Based on activities of living.* Edinburgh: Churchill Livingstone.

Roper, N., Logan, W. W., & Tierney, A. J. (1996). *The elements of nursing: A model for nursing based on a model for living* (4th ed.). Edinburgh: Churchill Livingstone.

Travelbee, J. (1966). *Interpersonal aspects of nursing.* Philadelphia: F. A. Davis.

Travelbee, J. (1971). *Interpersonal aspects of nursing* (2nd ed.). Philadelphia: F. A. Davis.

Wiedenbach, E. (1964). *Clinical nursing: A helping art.* New York: Springer.

Philosophies

- Nursing philosophy sets forth the meaning of nursing phenomena through analysis, reasoning, and logical argument.

- Philosophies contribute to nursing knowledge by providing direction for the discipline and forming a basis for professional scholarship, which leads to new theoretical understanding.

- Nursing philosophies represent early works that predate the theory era and later works of a philosophical nature.

- Philosophies are works that provide a broad understanding, which are used to further the discipline in its professional application.

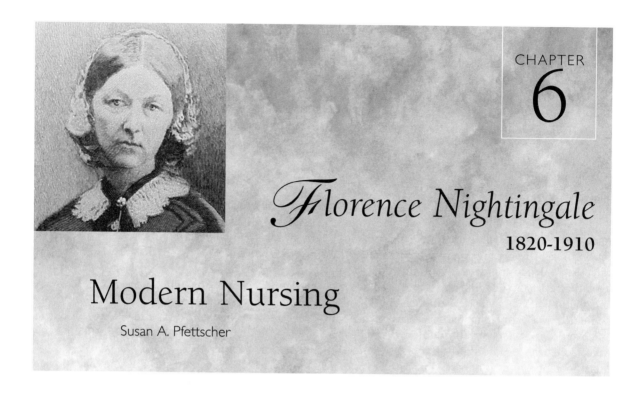

Florence Nightingale
1820-1910

Modern Nursing

Susan A. Pfettscher

CREDENTIALS AND BACKGROUND OF THE THEORIST

Florence Nightingale, the founder of modern nursing, was born on May 12, 1820. At the time of her birth, her parents were on an extended European tour. Her parents, Edward and Frances Nightingale, named their daughter after her birthplace—Florence, Italy. The Nightingales were a well-educated, affluent, aristocratic Victorian family that maintained residences in Derbyshire (with Lea Hurst as their original home) and in Hampshire (Embley Park). This latter residence was near London, which allowed the family to participate in London's spring and autumn social seasons.

Although the extended Nightingale family was large, the immediate family included only Florence

Previous authors: Susan A. Pfettscher, Karen R. de Graff, Ann Marriner Tomey, Cynthia L. Mossman, and Maribeth Slebodnik.

Nightingale and her elder sister, Parthenope. During her childhood, Nightingale's father educated her much more broadly and rigorously than other young women of her time. Nightingale was tutored by her father and others in mathematics, languages, religion, and philosophy (all subjects that later influenced her work). Although she participated in the usual Victorian aristocratic activities and social events during her adolescence, Nightingale developed the sense that her life should become more useful.

In 1837, Nightingale wrote about her calling in her diary: "God spoke to me and called me to his service" (Holliday & Parker, 1997, p. 41). The nature of her service and calling was unclear to her for some time. After she understood that she was called to become a nurse, she was finally able to complete her training in 1851 when she was accepted for training at Kaiserwerth, Germany, a Protestant religious community with a hospital facility. She stayed there for approximately 3 months and, at the end, her teachers declared her trained as a nurse.

Following her return to England, Nightingale began to examine hospital facilities, reformatories, and charitable institutions. Only 2 years after completing her training (in 1853), she became the superintendent of the Hospital for Invalid Gentlewomen in London.

During the Crimean War, Nightingale received a request from Sidney Herbert (a family friend and Secretary of War) to go to Scutari, Turkey, to provide trained nurses to care for wounded British soldiers. She arrived there in November of 1854, accompanied by 34 newly recruited nurses who met her criteria for professional nursing; these were young middle-class women with some basic general education. To achieve her mission of providing nursing care, she needed to address the environmental problems that existed, including the lack of sanitation and the presence of filth (few chamber pots, contaminated water, contaminated sheets and blankets, and overflowing cesspools). In addition, the soldiers were faced with exposure, frostbite, louse infestations, and opportunistic diseases during their recovery from battle wounds (Thomas, 1993).

Nightingale's work in improving these deplorable conditions made her a popular and revered person to the soldiers, but the support of physicians and military officers was less than enthusiastic. She was called The Lady of the Lamp, as immortalized in the poem "Santa Filomena" by Henry Wadsworth Longfellow (Longfellow, 1857), because she made ward rounds during the night providing emotional comfort to those soldiers. In Scutari Nightingale became critically ill with Crimean fever, which might actually have been typhus or brucellosis and which may have affected her physical condition years later.

After the war Nightingale returned to England to great accolades, particularly from the royal family (Queen Victoria), the soldiers who had served in and survived the Crimean War, their families, and the families of those who died at Scutari. She was awarded funds in recognition of this work, which she used to establish a teaching institution for nurses at St. Thomas' Hospital and King's College Hospital in London. Within a few years after it was founded, the Nightingale School began receiving requests to establish new schools at hospitals worldwide. Florence Nightingale's reputation as the founder of modern nursing was established (Lobo, 1995).

Nightingale devoted her energies not just to the development of nursing as a vocation (profession), but even more to local, national, and international societal issues and causes in an attempt to improve the living environments of the poor and to create social change (Isler, 1970). She continued to concentrate on army sanitation reform, the functions of army hospitals, sanitation in India, and sanitation and health care for the poor in England. Her writings, *Notes on Matters Affecting the Health, Efficiency, and Hospital Administration of the British Army Founded Chiefly on the Experience of the Late War* (Nightingale, 1858a), *Notes on Hospitals* (Nightingale, 1858b), and *Report on Measures Adopted for Sanitary Improvements in India from June 1869 to June 1870* (Nightingale, 1870), reflect her continuing concerns about these issues, particularly for the military.

Shortly after her return to England, Nightingale confined herself to her residence in London, citing her continued ill health and relapses. Until age 80, she wrote between 15,000 and 20,000 letters to friends, acquaintances, allies, and opponents. Her written word was strong and clear and conveyed her beliefs, observations, and desire for changes in health care and society. Through these writings, she was able to influence the issues and the world that concerned her. When necessary and when her health allowed, she received powerful visitors in her home to maintain her dialogue with them, plot strategies to support causes, and carry out her work.

During her lifetime, Nightingale's work was recognized through the many awards she received from her own country and from many other countries. She was able to work into her 80s until she lost her vision; she died in her sleep on August 13, 1910, at age 90.

Modern biographers and essayists have attempted to analyze Nightingale's lifework through her family relationships, notably with her parents and sister. Film dramatizations have focused frequently and inaccurately on her personal relationships with her family and friends. Although her personal and public life holds great intrigue for many, these retrospective analyses are often either very negative and harshly critical or overly positive in their descriptions of this Victorian leader and founder of modern nursing. Many biographies have been written describing Nightingale's life and work. Cook (1913) wrote the first original and comprehensive biography of Nightingale, which was based on her written papers but may have been biased by her family's involvement in and oversight of this project. It remains the most positive biography written. Shortly thereafter, Strachey (1918) was the first to describe her in negative terms; in his book, *Eminent Victorians*, he referred to her as arrogant and manipulative. O'Malley (1931) wrote a more positive biography focusing on her life from 1820 to 1856; however, the second volume which would have described the rest of her life and activities was never published. Woodham-Smith's book (1951) chronicles her entire life and was drawn primarily from original documents made available by her family. This is the biography with which most Americans are familiar and which has endured as the definitive biography of Nightingale's life; although more balanced, it maintains a positive tone. In 1982, F. B. Smith (1982) wrote *Florence Nightingale: Reputation and Power*, which was critical of both Nightingale's character and her work. Most recently, Small (1998) published yet another biography entitled *Florence Nightingale: Avenging Angel*. Again, he is critical of specific aspects of her character and work but is more balanced in his presentation. In an Internet-published paper originally presented in 2000, Small notes that Nightingale's life "is better documented than perhaps any previous life in history" because of the vast amount of family and personal papers that remain available today (Small, 2000). Small also advises that any biography is subject to the "prejudices" and interpretations of its author. His concerns and disagreements with other biographers, notably F. B. Smith, have been documented on his Web site (*http://www.florence-nightingale-avenging-angel.co.uk*). This controversy and intrigue has been made even more complicated by a recent analysis of Nightingale's behavior, leading an American physician to diagnose her as manic-depressive and songwriter/singer Country

Joe McDonald to speculate that she suffered from toxic poisoning associated with factories near her home (McDonald, n.d.).

In addition, a plethora of children's books have been written by American and English authors about Nightingale's life and work. Internet searches reveal thousands of sites that provide various articles, resources, and commentaries, both positive and negative, about Nightingale.

During their professional careers, Kalisch and Kalisch (1983a, 1983b, 1987) provided a critique of media portrayals that may assist the reader in better understanding the many histories of Florence Nightingale; their techniques may provide methods of analyzing more recent publications and events to persons interested in studying Nightingale's life and work. Dossey's (2000) comprehensive book, *Florence Nightingale: Mystic, Visionary, Healer*, provides the reader with another in-depth history and interpretation of Nightingale's personal life and her work. Using quotes from Nightingale's own writings (her diaries and letters) and from those of people with whom she interacted and corresponded during her lifetime, Dossey focused on interpreting the spiritual nature of her being and her lifework, creating yet another way of looking at her. Macrae (2001) explored Nightingale's personal spirituality as she interprets it from review of writings and documents and as an introduction/prelude to her descriptions of spirituality for nurses' lives based on Nightingale's writings.

Finally, all of Nightingale's surviving writings are in the process of being published as the *Collected Works of Florence Nightingale*. To date, five of the sixteen volumes have been published under the leadership of sociologist Lynn McDonald (McDonald, 2001-present). This large project will likely spawn an increasing number of articles and books that will further explore, interpret, and speculate on her life and work.

THEORETICAL SOURCES FOR THEORY DEVELOPMENT

Many factors influenced the development of Nightingale's philosophy of nursing. Her personal, societal, and professional values and concerns were all integral to the development of her beliefs. She combined her individual resources and concerns with the societal and professional resources available to her to produce change.

As noted, Nightingale's education was an unusual one for a Victorian girl. Her tutelage in subjects such as mathematics and philosophy by her well-educated, intellectual father provided her with knowledge and conceptual thinking abilities that were unique for women of her time. Although her parents initially opposed her desire to continue to study mathematics, they relented and allowed her to receive additional tutoring from well-respected mathematicians. Her aunt, Mai, a devoted relative and companion, described her as having a great mind; this was a description not used at the time for Victorian women, but one that was accepted for Nightingale. It remains unknown whether or not Nightingale was a genius who would have become a great leader and thinker under any circumstance, or whether her unique, formal education and social status were necessary for this to occur at the time. Would Nightingale become such a leader if born today? What would nursing be today if she had not been born at that time and in that place?

The Nightingale family's aristocratic social status provided her with easy access to people of power and influence. Many were family friends such as Stanley Herbert, who remained an ally and staunch supporter until his death. Nightingale learned to understand the political process of Victorian England through the experiences of her father during his short-lived political foray and through his continuing role as an aristocrat involved in the political and social activities of his community. She most likely relied on this foundation and her own experiences as she waged political battles for her causes.

Nightingale also recognized the societal changes of her time and their impact on the health status of individuals. The industrial age had descended upon England, creating new social classes, new diseases, and new social problems. Dickens' social commentaries and novels provided English society with scathing commentaries on health care and the need for health and social reform in England. In his novel,

Martin Chuzzlewit (Dickens, 1987), his portrayal of Sairey Gamp as a drunken, untrained nurse provided society with an image of the horrors of Victorian nursing practice. Nightingale's alliance with Dickens undoubtedly influenced her definitions of nursing and health care and her theory for nursing; that relationship also provided her with a forum to express her views about social and health care issues (Dossey, 2000; Kalisch & Kalisch, 1983a; Woodham-Smith, 1951).

Similar dialogues with many political leaders, intellectuals, and social reformers of the day (John Stuart Mill, Benjamin Jowett, Edwin Chadwick, and Harriet Marineau) developed Nightingale's philosophical and logical thinking, which is evident in her philosophy and theory of nursing (Dossey, 2000; Kalisch & Kalisch, 1983a; Woodham-Smith, 1951). Most likely these dialogues inspired her to continue to strive to change the things she viewed as unacceptable in the society in which she lived. No other nursing leader could better exemplify Chinn and Jacobs' statement that "when individual or professional values are in conflict with and challenge societal values, there is potential for creating change in society" (1983, p. 46).

Finally, Nightingale's religious affiliation and beliefs were especially strong sources for her nursing theory. Reared as a Unitarian, her belief that action for the benefit of others is a primary way of serving God was the foundation for defining her nursing work as a religious calling. In addition, the Unitarian community strongly supported education as a means of developing divine potential and helping people move toward perfection in their lives and in their service to God. Nightingale's faith provided her with personal strength throughout her life and provided her with the belief that education was a critical factor in establishing the profession of nursing. Also, religious conflicts of the time, particularly between the Angelican and Catholic Churches in the British Empire, may have provided her with the strongly held belief that nursing could and should be a secular profession (Dossey, 2000; Helmstadter, 1997; Nelson, 1997; Woodham-Smith, 1951). Despite her strong religious beliefs and her acknowledgment of her calling, this was not a requirement for her nurses. Indeed, her opposition to the work of the nuns in Crimea (she reported that they were proselytizing) escalated the conflict to the level of the Vatican's involvement (Dossey, 2000; Woodham-Smith, 1951). As parish nursing has seen a resur-gence in the United States and missionary work by nurses continues throughout the world, Nelson's review of pastoral care in the nineteenth century provides an interesting historical view of the role of religious service in nursing (Nelson, 1997).

MAJOR CONCEPTS *&* DEFINITIONS

Nightingale's theory focused on the environment. Murray and Zentner (1975) define environment as "all the external conditions and influences affecting the life and development of an organism and capable of preventing, suppressing, or contributing to disease, accidents, or death" (p. 149). Although Nightingale never used the term *environment* in her writing, she did define and describe in detail the concepts of ventilation, warmth, light, diet, cleanliness, and noise, which are components of the environment.

Although Nightingale often defined concepts precisely, she did not separate the patient's environment specifically into physical, emotional, or social aspects; she apparently assumed that all of these aspects were included in the environment. When reading *Notes on Nursing* (Nightingale, 1969) and her other writings, it is easy to identify her emphasis on the physical environment. In the context of the specific issues that she had identified and struggled to improve and correct in various settings (war-torn environment and workhouses) and in the context of the time, this emphasis appears to be most appropriate (Gropper, 1990). Her concern about healthy surroundings included not only the hospital settings in both Crimea and England, it also extended to the private homes of patients and to the physical living conditions of the poor. She believed that healthy surroundings were necessary for proper nursing care. Her theory of the five essential components of environmental health (pure air, pure water, efficient drainage, cleanliness, and light) is as essential today as it was 150 years ago.

Proper ventilation for the patient seemed to be of greatest concern to Nightingale; her charge to nurses was to "keep the air he breathes as pure as the external air, without chilling him" (Nightingale, 1969, p. 12). Notwithstanding her rejection of the germ theory (newly developed at the time), Nightingale's emphasis on proper ventilation indicates that she seemed to recognize this environmental component as a source of disease and recovery.

The concept of light was also of importance in Nightingale's theory. In particular, she identified direct sunlight as a particular need of patients. She noted that "light has quite as real and tangible effects upon the human body. . . . Who has not observed the purifying effect of light, and especially of direct sunlight, upon the air of a room?" (Nightingale, 1969, pp. 84-85). To achieve the beneficial effects of sunlight, nurses were instructed to move and position patients to expose them to sunlight.

Cleanliness as a concept is another critical component of Nightingale's environmental theory (Nightingale, 1969). In this regard, she specifically addressed the patient, the nurse, and the physical environment. She noted that a dirty environment (floors, carpets, walls, and bed linens) was a source of infection through the organic matter it contained. Even if the environment was well ventilated, the presence of organic material created a dirty area; therefore, the appropriate handling and disposal of bodily excretions and sewage was required to prevent contamination of the environment. Finally, Nightingale advocated bathing patients on a frequent, even daily, basis at a time

Continued

MAJOR CONCEPTS & DEFINITIONS—cont'd

when this practice was not the norm. In addition, she required that nurses also bathe daily, that their clothing be clean, and that they wash their hands frequently (Nightingale, 1969). This concept held special significance not only for individual patient care, it was also critically important in improving the health status of the poor living in crowded, environmentally inferior conditions with inadequate sewage and limited access to pure water (Nightingale, 1969).

Nightingale included the concepts of warmth, quiet, and diet in her environmental theory. In addition to discussing the ventilation in the room or home, Nightingale provided a description for measuring the patient's body temperature through palpation of extremities to assess for heat loss (Nightingale, 1969). The nurse was instructed to manipulate the environment continually to maintain both ventilation and patient warmth by using a good fire, opening windows, and properly positioning the patient in the room.

The need for quiet was also a concept that required assessment and intervention by the nurse (Nightingale, 1969). Noise created by physical activities in the environment (room) was to be avoided because it could harm the patient.

Nightingale was also concerned with the patient's diet (Nightingale, 1969). She instructed nurses not only to assess dietary intake, but also to assess both the meal schedule and its effect on the patient. She believed that patients with chronic illnesses could be starved to death and that intelligent nurses were those who were successful in meeting their patients' nutritional needs.

Another component of Nightingale's theory was that of a definition or description of *petty management* (Nightingale, 1969). The nurse was in control of the environment both physically and administratively. The nurse had to control the environment to protect the patient from both physical and psychological harm; for example, the nurse protected the patient from receiving upsetting news, from seeing visitors who could negatively affect recovery, and from experiencing sudden disruptions of sleep. In addition, Nightingale recognized that pet visits (small animals) might be of comfort to the patient. Nightingale also believed that the nurse remained in charge of the environment even when she was not physically present, because she was to oversee others who worked in her absence.

USE OF EMPIRICAL EVIDENCE

Nightingale's reports describing health and sanitary conditions in the Crimea and in England identify her as an outstanding scientist and empirical researcher. Her expertise as a statistician is also evident in the reports that she generated throughout her lifetime on the varied subjects of health care, nursing, and social reform.

Nightingale's carefully collected information that illustrated the efficacy of her hospital nursing system and organization during the Crimean War is perhaps her best-known work. Her report of her experiences and collected data in *Notes on Matters Affecting the Health, Efficiency, and Hospital*

Administration of the British Army Founded Chiefly on the Experience of the Late War (Nightingale, 1858a) was submitted to the British Royal Sanitary Commission. This commission had been organized in response to Nightingale's charges of poor sanitary conditions. The data in this report provided a strong argument in favor of her proposed reforms in the Crimean hospital barracks. According to Cohen (1984), she invented the polar-area diagram to represent dramatically the extent of needless death in the British military hospitals in the Crimea. In this article, Cohen summarized the work of Nightingale as both a researcher and a statistician by noting that "she helped to pioneer the revolutionary notion that social phenomena could be objectively measured and subjected to mathematical analysis" (1984, p. 128). Palmer (1977) described Nightingale's research skills as including recording, communicating, ordering, coding, conceptualizing, inferring, analyzing, and synthesizing. The observation of social phenomena at both an individual and a systems level was especially important to Nightingale and served as the basis of her writings. Nightingale emphasized the concurrent use of observation and the performance of tasks in the education of nurses and expected them to continue to use these concurrent activities in their work.

MAJOR ASSUMPTIONS
Nursing

Nightingale believed that every woman, at one time in her life, would be a nurse in the sense that nursing is having the responsibility for someone else's health. Nightingale's book *Notes on Nursing* was originally published in 1859 to provide women with guidelines for caring for their loved ones at home and to give advice on how to "think like a nurse" (Nightingale, 1969, p. 4). Trained nurses, however, learned and applied additional scientific principles to their work and were more skilled in observation and reporting of patients' health status while performing interventions that would allow the patient to recover.

Person

In most of her writings, Nightingale referred to the person as a *patient*. Nurses performed tasks to and for the patient and controlled the patient's environment to enhance recovery. For the most part, Nightingale described a passive patient in this relationship. However, there are specific references to the patient performing self-care when possible and, in particular, being involved in the timing and substance of meals; thus, the patient was not a totally passive individual. The nurse was instructed to ask the patient about his or her preferences, which reveals the belief that Nightingale saw each patient as an individual. However, Nightingale (1969) emphasized that the nurse was in control of and responsible for the patient's environment and, by default, in control of some personal choices and behaviors. One can also infer from her writings, particularly those about soldiers in the Crimea, that Nightingale had respect for persons of various backgrounds and was not judgmental about social worth. Indeed, her conviction about the need for secular nurses supports respect for, persons without judgment of their religious beliefs or lack thereof.

Health

Nightingale defined health as being well and using every power (resource) that the person has to the fullest extent in living his or her life. Additionally, she saw disease and illness as a reparative process that nature instituted when a person did not attend to health concerns. Nightingale envisioned the maintenance of health through the prevention of disease via environmental control and social responsibility; what she described is modern public health nursing and the more modern concept of health promotion. She distinguished the concept of health nursing as different from nursing a sick patient to enhance recovery or from living better until death. This concept of health nursing exists today in the role of the district nurse and health worker in England and in other countries where lay health care workers are used to maintain health and teach people how to prevent disease and illness. It is also a model that is employed by many public health agencies and departments in the United States with minor alterations.

Environment

Fitzpatrick and Whall describe Nightingale's concept of environment as "those elements external to and which affect the health of the sick and healthy person" and included "everything from the patient's food and flowers to the patient's verbal and non-verbal interactions" (1983, pp. 16-17). Little, if anything, in the patient's world is excluded from her definition of environment. Her admonition to nurses, both those providing care in the home and trained nurses in hospitals, was to create and maintain a therapeutic environment that would enhance the comfort and recovery of the patient. Her treatise on rural hygiene is an incredibly specific description of environmental problems and their results and includes practical solutions to these problems for households and communities (Halsall, 1997).

Nightingale's assumptions and understanding about the environmental conditions of the day were most relevant to her philosophy. She believed that sick poor people would benefit from environmental improvements that affected both their bodies and minds. She believed that nurses could be instrumental in changing the social status of the poor by improving their physical and psychological living conditions.

Many aristocrats of the time were unaware of the living conditions of the poor, not unlike current societal behaviors. Nightingale's mother, however, had visited and provided care to poor families in the communities surrounding their estates; Nightingale accompanied her on these visits as a child and continued them on her own when she was older. Thus Nightingale's understanding of physical environments and their effect on health status was acquired through firsthand observation and experience beyond her own comfortable living situation.

THEORETICAL ASSERTIONS

Nightingale believed that disease was a reparative process; disease was nature's effort to remedy a process of poisoning or decay, or a reaction against the conditions in which a person was placed. Although these concepts seem ridiculous today, they were more scientific than the prevailing ones of the time (e.g., disease as punishment). Nightingale did not provide a definition of nature. She often capitalized the word nature in her writings, thereby suggesting that it was synonymous with God. Her Unitarian religious beliefs would support this view of God as nature. However, when she used the word nature without capitalization, it is unclear whether or not the intended meaning is different and

perhaps synonymous with an organic pathological process. Nightingale believed that nursing's role was to prevent an interruption of the reparative process and to provide optimal conditions for its enhancement, thus ensuring the patient's recovery.

Nightingale was totally committed to nursing education (training). Although she wrote *Notes on Nursing* (1969) for all women, her primary treatise was that women were to be specifically trained to provide care for the sick person and that nurses providing preventive health care (public health nursing) required even more training. Nightingale (1969) also felt that nurses needed to be excellent observers of their patients and the environment; observation was an ongoing activity for trained nurses. In addition, she believed that nurses needed to use common sense in their nursing practice, coupled with observation, perseverance, and ingenuity. Finally, Nightingale believed that people desired good health, that they would cooperate with the nurse and nature to allow the reparative process to occur, and that they would also alter their environment to prevent disease.

Although Nightingale has often been maligned or ridiculed for not embracing the germ theory, she very clearly understood the concept of contagion and contamination through organic materials from the patient and the environment. Many of her observations are consistent with the concepts of infection and the germ theory; for example, she embraced the concept of vaccination against various diseases. Small (2004) argues that Nightingale did indeed believe in a germ theory but not in the one that suggests that that there are disease germs causing inevitable infections. Such a theory was antithetical to her belief that sanitation and good hygiene could prevent infection. Her belief that appropriate manipulation of the environment would prevent disease underlies modern sanitation activities.

Nightingale did not explicitly discuss the caring behaviors of nurses. She wrote very little about interpersonal relationships except as they influenced the patient's reparative processes. She did describe the phenomenon of being called to nursing and the need for commitment to nursing work. From the perspectives of Victorian England and her religious beliefs, these descriptions may describe a caring component of her nursing theory. Her own example of nursing practice in the Crimea provides evidence of caring behaviors. These include her commitment to observing her patients at night, a new concept and practice; sitting with them during the dying process; standing beside them during surgical procedures; writing letters for them; and providing reading materials, including a reading room, during their recuperation. Finally, she wrote letters to their families following soldiers' deaths.

Nightingale believed that nurses should be moral agents. She addressed their professional relationship with their patients; she instructed them on the principle of confidentiality and advocated for care to the poor to improve their health and social situations. In addition, she commented on patient decision making, a component of a relevant modern ethical concept. Nightingale (1969) called for concise and clear decision making by the nurse and physician regarding the patient, noting that indecision (irresolution) or changing the mind is more harmful to the patient than the patient having to make a decision.

LOGICAL FORM

Nightingale used inductive reasoning to extract laws of health, disease, and nursing from her observations and experiences. Her childhood education, particularly in philosophy and mathematics, may have contributed to her logical thinking and inductive reasoning abilities. For example, her observations of the conditions in the Scutari hospital led her to conclude that the contaminated, dirty, dark environment led to disease. Not only could she prevent disease from flourishing in such an environment, but she also recognized that disease prevention would be achieved through environmental controls. From her own nursing training, her brief experience as a superintendent in London, and her experiences in the Crimea, she was able to make observations and form the principles for nursing training and patient care (Nightingale, 1969).

ACCEPTANCE BY THE NURSING COMMUNITY
Practice

Nightingale's nursing principles remain applicable today. The environmental aspects of her theory (ventilation, warmth, quiet, diet, and cleanliness) remain integral components of nursing care. As nurses begin practice in the twenty-first century, these concepts continue to be relevant; in fact, they have increased relevance as the global society faces new issues of disease control. While modern sanitation and water treatment have controlled traditional sources of disease fairly successfully in the United States, contaminated water remains a health issue in many communities, due to environmental changes or to the introduction of less common contaminants. Global travel has dramatically altered the actual and potential spread of diseases more rapidly than previously anticipated. In addition, modern sanitation, adequate water treatment, and recognition and control of other methods of disease transmission remain challenges for nurses worldwide.

New environmental concerns are created by modern architecture (e.g., sick-building syndrome); nurses need to ask whether modern, environmentally controlled buildings meet Nightingale's principle of good ventilation. On the other hand, controlled environments increasingly protect the public from second-hand cigarette smoke, toxic gases, auto emissions, and other environmental hazards. Disposal of these wastes, including toxic waste, and the use of chemicals in this modern society also challenge professional nurses and other health care professionals to reassess the concept of a healthy environment (Butterfield, 1999; Gropper, 1990; MNA, 1999; Sessler, 1999; Shaner, 1998).

In health care facilities, the ability to control room temperature for an individual patient is often increasingly difficult. That same environment may create great noise through activities and the technology (equipment) used to assist the patient's reparative process. Nurses are looking in a scholarly way at these problems as they continue to affect patients and the health care system (McCarthy, Ouimet, &

Daun, 1991; McLaughlin, McLaughlin, Elliott, & Campalani, 1996; MNA, 1999; Pope, 1995).

Monteiro (1985) provided the American public health community with a comprehensive review of Nightingale's work as a sanitarian and social reformer, again reminding them of the extent of her impact on health care in various settings and her concern about poverty and sanitation issues. Although other disciplines in the United States have increasingly addressed such issues, it is clear that there is an active role for nurses and nursing both in providing direct patient care and in the social and political arena to ensure healthy environments for all citizens.

Although some of Nightingale's rationales have been modified or disproved by medical advances and scientific discovery, many of her concepts and portions of her theory have endured both the tests of time and technological advances. In reading and interpreting Nightingale's Victorian writings, remembering the uniqueness of her early life and considering the sociopolitical nature of the era, it is clear that much of her theory remains relevant for nursing today. Concepts from Nightingale's writings continue to be cited in the nursing literature, from political commentary to scholarly research. Several authors have recently analyzed Nightingale's petty management concepts and actions, again identifying some of the timelessness and universality of her management style (Decker & Farley, 1991; Henry, Woods, & Nagelkerk, 1990; Monteiro, 1985; Nightingale, 1969; Ulrich, 1992).

Finally, several writers have analyzed Nightingale's role in the suffrage movement, especially in the context of feminist theory development. Although she has been criticized for not actively participating in this movement, Nightingale indicated in a letter to John Stuart Mill that she could do work for women in other ways (Woodham-Smith, 1951). Although she supported the principle of political power for women, she did not feel she had time to participate actively in this movement. Her essay entitled *Cassandra* (1852) appears to reflect a great support for the concept that is now known as *feminism*. Nightingale's other writings also support her belief that upper social class women should be useful, contributing members of society

and should not be engaged only in idle, social roles (Woodham-Smith, 1951). Scholars continue to assess and analyze her role and position in the feminist movement of this modern era (Dossey, 2000; Hektor, 1994; Holliday & Parker, 1997; Welch, 1990).

Education

Nightingale's principles of nursing training (instruction in scientific principles and practical experience for the mastery of skills) provided a universal template for early nurse training schools, beginning with St. Thomas' Hospital and King's College Hospital in London. Using the Nightingale model of nurse training, the following three experimental schools were established in the United States in 1873 (Ashley, 1976):

1. Bellevue Hospital in New York
2. New Haven Hospital in Connecticut
3. Massachusetts Hospital in Boston

The influence of this training system and many of its principles is still evident in today's nursing programs.

Although Nightingale advocated the nursing school's independence from a hospital to ensure that students would not be involved in the hospital's labor pool as part of their training, American nursing schools were unable to achieve such independence for many years (Ashley, 1976). Nightingale (Decker & Farley, 1991) believed that the art of nursing could not be measured by licensing examinations, but she used testing methods, including case studies (notes), for nursing probationers at St. Thomas' Hospital.

Clearly Nightingale understood that good practice could result only from good education. This message resounds throughout her writings on nursing. Nightingale historian Joanne Farley responded to a modern nursing student by noting that "Training is to teach a nurse to know her business. . . . Training is to enable the nurse to act for the best . . . like an intelligent and responsible being" (Decker & Farley, 1991, pp. 12-13). It is difficult to imagine what the care of sick human beings would be like if Nightingale had not defined the educational needs of nurses and established these first schools.

Research

Nightingale's interest in scientific inquiry and statistics continues to define the scientific inquiry used in nursing research. She was exceptionally efficient and resourceful in her ability to gather and analyze data; her ability to represent data graphically was first identified in the polar diagrams, the graphic illustration style that she invented (Agnew, 1958; Cohen, 1984). Her empirical approach to solving problems of health care delivery is obvious in the data she often included in her numerous letters.

If Nightingale's writings are defined and analyzed as theory, they lack the complexity and testability found in modern nursing theories. Therefore, her theory cannot generate the nursing research that is employed to test modern theories. However, concepts that Nightingale identified have served as the basis for current research, which adds to modern nursing science and practice. A review of the current nursing literature suggests that controversy regarding Nightingale's place as the matriarch or icon of nursing has escalated throughout the international nursing community. This controversy continues in the twenty-first century. However, her concepts still serve as the basis of continued analysis and nursing research throughout the world; they are also frequently cited to support current nursing practices.

Finally, it is interesting to note that Nightingale used brief case studies, possible exemplars, to illustrate a number of the concepts she discussed in *Notes on Nursing* (1969). Scholarly nurses have refined this technique for inclusion in texts and research studies; such a style thus had an auspicious beginning in nursing education and literature.

FURTHER DEVELOPMENT

Nightingale's philosophy and theory of nursing is stated clearly and concisely in *Notes on Nursing* (1969), Nightingale's most widely known work. The text's content seems most amenable to theory analysis. Nightingale organized the chapters of this text by concept; however, continued discussion of other concepts may appear in a specific chapter as it relates

to the discussion. Fitzpatrick and Whall (1983) refer to this approach as a *set-of-laws theory*. They define laws as theoretical statements with overwhelming empirical support.

Hardy (1978) proposed that Nightingale formulated a grand theory, which explains the totality of behavior. Grand theories tend to be somewhat vague, without specific definition of terms and concepts and without full development of relationships between concepts. They often provide formulations that cannot be tested. This type of theory is an early development that relies on anecdotal situations to illustrate its meaning and support its claims. Although her work might also be classified as lower level theory, Nightingale provided the foundation for the development of both nursing practice and current nursing theories.

CRITIQUE
Simplicity

Nightingale's theory contains the following three major relationships:
1. Environment to patient
2. Nurse to environment
3. Nurse to patient

She believed that the environment was the main factor creating illness in a patient; she regarded disease as "the reactions of kindly nature against the conditions in which we have placed ourselves" (Nightingale, 1969, p. 56). Nightingale recognized not only the harmfulness of an environment, she also emphasized the benefit of good environments in preventing disease.

The nurse's practice includes manipulation of the environment in a number of ways to enhance patient recovery. Elimination of contamination and contagion and the exposure to fresh air, light, warmth, and quiet were all identified as elements to be controlled or manipulated in the environment. Nightingale began to develop relationships between some of these elements in her discussions of contamination and ventilation, light and patient position in the room, cleanliness and darkness, and noise and patient stimulation. She also described the relationship between the sickroom and the rest of the house and the relationship between the house and the surrounding neighborhood. In addition, Nightingale recognized the need to manipulate the environment to prevent disease, as evidenced by her discussion of the homes of the poor, the workhouses, and preventing exposure of children to measles.

The nurse-patient relationship may be the least well defined in Nightingale's writings. Yet there are suggestions of cooperation and collaboration between the nurse and patient in her discussions of a patient's eating patterns and preferences, the comfort of a beloved pet to the patient, the protection of the patient from emotional distress, and the conservation of energy while allowing the patient to participate in self-care. Finally, it is interesting to note that Nightingale discussed the concept of observation extensively, including its use to guide the care of patients and to measure improvement or lack of response to nursing interventions. This aspect of training and practice would suggest the origins of the nursing process (Ulrich, 1992). Combining the concepts that Nightingale identified does not aid in increasing their simplicity; her original statements are expressed in an economical form. Diagrams of these concepts and their relationships have been proposed, thereby supporting their logic and simplicity (Fitzpatrick & Whall, 1983).

Nightingale provided a descriptive, explanatory theory rather than one of prediction. Its environmental focus with its epidemiological components had predictive potential, but Nightingale never tested the theory in that manner. It is unclear whether Nightingale intended to develop a theory of nursing. She did intend to define the science and art of nursing and provide general rules with explanations that would result in good nursing care for patients. Thus her objective of setting forth general rules for the practice and development of nursing was met through this simple theory.

Generality

Nightingale's theory has been used to provide general guidelines for all nurses since she introduced it more than 150 years ago. Although some activities that she described are no longer relevant, the universality and timelessness of her concepts remain pertinent. The relation concepts (nurse, patient, and environment) are applicable in all nursing settings today. To address her audience of women who may provide care to another (not only professional nurses), the theory she proposed remains relevant. Therefore it meets the criterion of generality.

Empirical Precision

Concepts and relationships within Nightingale's theory frequently are stated implicitly and are presented as truths rather than tentative, testable statements. In contrast to her quantitative research on mortality performed in the Crimea, Nightingale advised nurses that their practice should be based on their observations and experiences rather than systematic, empirical research. If she were addressing the development of the art of nursing, her admonitions would be amenable to study via qualitative or phenomenological research methodology.

Derivable Consequences

To an extraordinary degree, Nightingale's writings direct the nurse to action on behalf of the patient and the nurse. These directives encompass the areas of practice, research, and education. Her principles that attempt to shape nursing practice are the most specific. She urges nurses to provide physicians with "not your opinion, however respectfully given, but your facts" (Nightingale, 1969, p. 122). Similarly, she advised that "if you cannot get the habit of observation one way or other, you had better give up the being a nurse, for it is not your calling, however kind and anxious you may be" (Nightingale, 1969, p. 113). Her encouragement for a measure of independence and precision previously unknown in nursing may still guide and motivate nurses today as the profession continues to evolve.

Nightingale's view of humanity was consistent with her theories of nursing. She believed in a creative, universal humanity with the potential and ability for growth and change (Dossey, 2000; Hektor, 1994; Palmer, 1977). Deeply religious, she viewed nursing as a means of doing the will of her God. Perhaps it is because she viewed nursing as a divine calling that she relegated the patient to a relatively passive role with his or her wants and needs provided by the nurse. The zeal and self-righteousness that comes from being a reformer might explain some of her beliefs and the practices that she advocated. Finally, the period and place in which she lived, Victorian England, must be considered and understood to better understand her views.

Nightingale's basic principles of environmental manipulation and psychological care of the patient can be applied in contemporary nursing settings. Although her rejection of the germ theory and her inability to recognize a unified body of nursing knowledge that is testable (rather than relying only on personal observation and experience) have subjected her to some criticism or ridicule, other parts of her theory and her activities are relevant to nursing's professional identity and practice.

SUMMARY

Florence Nightingale is a unique figure in the history of the world. No other woman has been and is still revered as an icon by so many people in so many diverse geographical locations around the globe. Few others figures still stimulate such interest in, controversy about, and interpretation of their lives and work. The nursing profession continues to embrace her as the founder of modern nursing, although controversy still reigns about her current influences on its work.

Nightingale defined the professional skills, behaviors, and knowledge required for nursing and the nurses who were trained for this work. Remnants of those descriptions serve the nursing profession well today, although their origins are probably not known or remembered by most of today's nurses.

Based on scientific and social changes in the world, some of her observations have been rejected.

However, close analysis reveals that the underlying beliefs, philosophy, and observations continue to be valid. Nightingale did not consciously attempt to develop what is considered a theory of nursing; she provided the first definitions from which nurses can develop theory and conceptual models and frameworks that inform professional nursing today. Her lifework (professional career) embodies the current definition of all nurses as clinicians, researchers, educators, and leaders. Other professionals increasingly identify her as their matriarch—mathematicians revere her for her work as an outstanding statistician while epidemiologists, public health professionals, and lay health care workers trace the origins of their disciplines to her descriptions of people who perform health promotion and disease prevention; sociologists are recognizing her leadership role in defining communities, their social ills, and in working to correct societal problems as a way to improve the health of its members.

Nurses, both students and practitioners, would be wise to become familiar with her original writings and review the many books and documents that are increasingly available. If you have read *Notes on Nursing* before, rereading it can reveal new and inspirational ideas as well as a brief look at her wry sense of humor. The logic and common sense that are embodied in her writings can serve to stimulate productive thinking for the individual nurse and the nursing profession. Nightingale's philosophy gives food for thought that continues to nourish the profession nearly 150 years later. Reading the work that is now becoming available can expand our thinking and horizons beyond the narrow aspects of our nursing careers and professions. To emulate the life of Nightingale is to become good citizens and leaders in our communities, our country, and our world. It is only right that Nightingale should continue to be recognized as the brilliant and creative founder of modern nursing and its first nursing theorist. What would Nightingale say about nursing today? Whatever she would say, she would probably objectively and logically provide an incredible analysis and critique.

Case Study

You are caring for an 82-year-old woman who has been hospitalized for several weeks for burns that she sustained on her lower legs during a cooking accident. Prior to her admission, she had lived alone in a small apartment. She reported on admission that she has no surviving family. Her support system appears to be other elders who live in her neighborhood. Due to transportation difficulties, most of them are unable to visit frequently. One of her neighbors has reported that she is caring for the patient's dog, a Yorkshire terrier. As you care for this lady, she begs you to let her friend bring her dog to the hospital. She says that none of the other nurses have listened to her about such a visit. As she asks you about this, she begins to cry and tells you that they have never been separated. You recall that the staff indicated their concern about this woman's well-being during report that morning. They said that she has been eating very little and seems to be depressed. Based on Nightingale's work, identify specific interventions that you would take in caring for this patient.

1. Describe what action, if any, you would take regarding her request to see her dog. Discuss the theoretical basis of your decision and action based on your understanding of Nightingale's work.
2. Describe and discuss what nursing diagnoses you would make and interventions you would initiate to address her nutritional status and emotional well-being.
3. As this patient's primary nurse, identify and discuss the planning that you would undertake regarding her discharge from the hospital. Identify members of the discharge team and their roles in this process. Describe how you would advocate for this patient based on Nightingale's observations and descriptions of the role of the nurse.

CRITICAL THINKING *Activities*

1. Using Nightingale's concepts of ventilation, light, noise, and cleanliness, analyze the setting in which you are practicing nursing, working as an employee or student.

2. Using Nightingale's theory, evaluate the nursing interventions you have identified for an individual patient in your facility or practice.

3. Your community has reported an outbreak of an airborne infection (e.g., *Legionella* infection [Legionnaire's disease], histoplasmosis, or coccidioidomycosis [valley fever]). Identify Nightingale's theories and commentaries that apply to this situation in regard to infection, the work required by health care professionals, and its societal influences on the health of citizens. Analyze the similarities between her theories and current practices.

REFERENCES

Agnew, L. R. (1958, May). Florence Nightingale, statistician. *American Journal of Nursing, 58,* 644.

Ashley, J. A. (1976). *Hospitals, paternalism, and the role of the nurse.* New York: Teachers College Press.

Butterfield, P. (1999). Integrating environmental health into clinical nursing. *Journal of the New York State Nurses Association, 30*(1), 24-27.

Chinn, P., & Jacobs, M. (1983). *Theory and nursing: A systematic approach.* St. Louis: Mosby.

Cohen, I. B. (1984, March). Florence Nightingale. *Scientific American, 250*(3), 128-137.

Cook, E. T. (1913). *The life of Florence Nightingale.* London: Macmillan.

Decker, B., & Farley, J. K. (1991, May/June). What would Nightingale say? *Nurse Educator, 16*(3), 12-13.

Dickens, C. (1987). *Life and adventures of Martin Chuzzlewit.* London: New Oxford Press.

Dossey, B. M. (2000). *Florence Nightingale: Mystic, visionary, healer.* Springhouse, PA: Springhouse Corporation.

Fitzpatrick, J., & Whall, A. (1983). *Conceptual models of nursing.* Bowie, MD: Prentice Hall.

Gropper, E. I. (1990). Florence Nightingale: Nursing's first environmental theorist. *Nursing Forum, 25*(3), 30-33.

Halsall, P. (1997). *Modern history sourcebook: Florence Nightingale: Rural hygiene.* New York: Paul Halsall.

Retrieved January 25, 2004, from *http://www. fordham.edu/halsall/mod/nightingale-rural.html.*

Hardy, M. (1978). Perspectives on nursing theory. *ANS Advances in Nursing Science, 1*, 37-48.

Hektor, M. (1994, Nov.). Florence Nightingale and the women's movement: Friend or foe? *Nursing Inquiry, 1*(1), 38-45.

Helmstadter, C. (1997). Doctors and nurses in the London teaching hospitals: Class, gender, religion, and professional expertise, 1850-1890. *Nursing History Review, 5*, 161-167.

Henry, B., Woods, S., & Nagelkerk, J. (1990). Nightingale's perspective of nursing administration. *Nursing and Health Care, 11*(4), 200-206.

Holliday, M. E., & Parker, D. L. (1997). Florence Nightingale, feminism and nursing. *Journal of Advanced Nursing, 28*, 483-488.

Isler, C. (1970). *Florence Nightingale: Rebel with a cause.* Oradell, NY: Medical Economics.

Kalisch, B. J., & Kalisch, P. A. (1983a, April). Heroine out of focus: Media images of Florence Nightingale. Part I: Popular biographies and stage productions. *Nursing and Health Care, 4*(4), 181-187.

Kalisch, B. J., & Kalisch, P. A. (1983b, May). Heroine out of focus: Media images of Florence Nightingale. Part II: Film, radio, and television dramatizations. *Nursing and Health Care, 4*(5), 270-278.

Kalisch, P. A., & Kalisch B. J. (1987). *The changing image of the nurse.* Menlo Park, CA: Addison-Wesley.

Lobo, M. L. (1995). Florence Nightingale. In J. B. George (Ed.), *Nursing theories: The base for professional nursing practice.* Norwalk, CT: Appleton & Lange.

Longfellow, H. W. (1857). Santa Filomena. *Atlantic Monthly, 1*(1), 22-23.

Macrae, J. A. (2001). *Nursing as a spiritual practice: A contemporary application of Florence Nightingale's views.* New York: Springer Publishing.

McCarthy, D. O., Ouimet, M. E., & Daun, J. M. (1991, May). Shades of Florence Nightingale: Potential impact of noise stress on wound healing. *Holistic Nursing Practice, 5*(4), 39-48.

McDonald, C. J. (n.d.). *Country Joe McDonald's tribute to Florence Nightingale.* Berkeley, CA: Country Joe McDonald. Retrieved January 25, 2004, from *http:// www.countryjoe.com/nightingale.*

McDonald, L. (Ed.). (2001-present). *The collected works of Florence Nightingale.* Ontario, Canada: Wilfred Laurier University Press. Retrieved January 25, 2004, from *http://www.sociology.uoguelph.ca/fnightingale.*

McLaughlin, A., McLaughlin, B., Elliott, J., & Campalani, G. (1996). Noise levels in a cardiac surgical intensive care unit: A preliminary study conducted in secret. *Intensive and Critical Care Nursing, 12*(4), 226-230.

Michigan Nurses Association (MNA). (1999). Nursing practice: Moving toward environmentally responsible health care. *Michigan Nurse, 72*(1), 8-9.

Monteiro, L. A. (1985, Feb.). Florence Nightingale on public health nursing. *American Journal of Public Health, 75*, 181-186.

Murray, R., & Zentner, J. (1975). *Nursing concepts in health promotion.* Englewood Cliffs, NJ: Prentice Hall.

Nelson, S. (1997). Pastoral care and moral government: Early nineteenth century nursing and solutions to the Irish question. *Journal of Advanced Nursing, 26*, 6-14.

Nightingale, F. (1852). *Cassandra.* Unpublished essay.

Nightingale, F. (1858a). *Notes on matters affecting the health, efficiency, and hospital administration of the British army founded chiefly on the experience of the late war. Presented by request to the Secretary of State for War.* London: Harrison & Sons.

Nightingale, F. (1858b). *Notes on hospitals: Being two papers read before the National Association for the Promotion of Social Science, at Liverpool, in October 1858. With evidence given to the Royal Commissioner on the state of the army in 1857.* London: John W. Park and Son.

Nightingale, F. (1870). *Report on measures adopted for sanitary improvements in India from June 1869 to June 1870: Together with abstracts.* London.

Nightingale, F. (1969). *Notes on nursing: What it is and what it is not.* New York: Dover.

O'Malley, I. B. (1931). *Life of Florence Nightingale, 1820-1856.* London: Butterworth.

Palmer, I. S. (1977, March/April). Florence Nightingale: Reformer, reactionary, researcher. *Nursing Research, 26*, 84-89.

Pope, D. S. (1995, Winter). Music, noise, and the human voice in the nurse-patient environment. *Image: The Journal of Nursing Scholarship, 27*, 291-295.

Sessler, A. (1999). Doing more than doing no harm: Nursing professionals turn their attention to the environment. *On-Call, 2*(4), 20-23.

Shaner, H. (1998). Pollution prevention for nurses: Minimizing the adverse environmental impact of healthcare delivery. *Vermont Registered Nurse, 64*(4), 9-11.

Small, H. (1998). *Avenging angel.* New York: St. Martin's Press.

Small, H. (2000, Sept. 7). *Florence Nightingale's 20th century biographies.* Paper originally presented to the Friends of Florence Nightingale Museum, London. Retrieved January 25, 2004, from *http://www.florence-nightingale-avenging-angel.co.uk/biograph.htm.*

Small, H. (2004). *Florence Nightingale, Avenging Angel.* London: Hugh Small. Retrieved December 20, 2004 from *http://www.florence-nightingale-avenging-angel. co.uk.*

Smith, F. B. (1982). *Florence Nightingale: Reputation and power.* New York: St. Martin.

Strachey, L. (1918). *Eminent Victorians.* London: Chatto & Windus.

Thomas, S. P. (1993, April/June). The view from Scutari: A look at contemporary nursing. *Nursing Forum, 28*(2), 19-24.

Ulrich, B. T. (1992). *Leadership and management according to Florence Nightingale.* Norwalk, CT: Appleton & Lange.

Welch, M. (1990, June). Florence Nightingale: The social construction of a Victorian feminist. *Western Journal of Nursing Research, 12,* 404-407.

Woodham-Smith, C. (1951). *Florence Nightingale.* New York: McGraw-Hill.

BIBLIOGRAPHY
Primary Sources
Books

Nightingale, F. (1911). *Letters from Miss Florence Nightingale on health visiting in rural districts.* London: King.

Nightingale, F. (1954). *Selected writings* (Compiled by Lucy R. Seymer). New York: Macmillan.

Nightingale, F. (1957). *Notes on nursing.* Philadelphia: J. B. Lippincott. (Originally published 1859.)

Nightingale, F. (1969). *Notes on nursing: What it is and what it is not.* New York: Dover.

Nightingale, F. (1974). *Letters of Florence Nightingale in the history of nursing archive.* Boston: Boston University Press.

Nightingale, F. (1976). *Notes on hospitals.* New York: Gordon.

Nightingale, F. (1978). *Notes on nursing.* London: Duckworth.

Nightingale, F. (1992). *Notes on nursing.* Philadelphia: J. B. Lippincott. (Commemorative edition with commentaries by contemporary nursing leaders.)

Journal Articles*

Nightingale, F. (1930, July). Trained nursing for the sick poor. *International Nursing Review, 5,* 426-433.

Nightingale, F. (1954, May). Maternity hospital and midwifery school. *Nursing Mirror, 99,* ix-xi, 369.

Nightingale, F. (1954). The training of nurses. *Nursing Mirror, 99,* iv-xi.

Secondary Sources
Reviews

[Review of the article *Selected writings*]. (1955, April). *Royal Sanitary Institute Journal, 75,* 75-276.

[Review of the article *Selected writings*]. (1955, May). *American Journal of Nursing, 55,* 162.

[Review of the article *Selected writings*]. (1955, May). *Nursing Times, 52,* 502-503, 507.

*All published posthumously.

[Review of the book *Cassandra: An essay*]. (1981, May). *American Journal of Nursing, 81,* 1059-1061.

[Review of the book *Florence Nightingale*]. (1950, Nov.). *Nursing Mirror, 92,* 31.

[Review of the book *Florence Nightingale*]. (1950, Dec.). *Nursing Times, 46,* 1285, 16.

[Review of the book *Florence Nightingale*]. (1951, June). *Journal of the American Medical Association, 146,* 605.

[Review of the book *Florence Nightingale*]. (1951, Aug.). *Public Health Nursing, 43,* 459.

[Review of the book *Notes on nursing: What it is and what it is not*]. (1970, June). *Nursing Times, 66,* 828.

[Review of the book *Notes on nursing: What it is and what it is not*]. (1970, Oct.). *Nursing Mirror, 131,* 47.

[Review of the book *What it is and what it is not, the science and art*]. (1980, Oct.). *Nursing Times, 76,* 187.

[Review of the book *What it is and what it is not, the science and art*]. (1980, Dec.). *Nursing Mirror, 151,* 41.

[Review of the book *What it is and what it is not, the science and art*]. (1981, Feb.) *Australian Nurses Journal, 10,* 29.

Books

Aiken, C. A. (1915). *Lessons from the life of Florence Nightingale.* New York: Lakeside.

Aldis, M. (1914). *Florence Nightingale.* New York: National Organization for Public Health Nursing.

Andrews, M. R. (1929). *A lost commander.* Garden City, NY: Doubleday.

Baly, M. E. (1986). *Florence Nightingale: The nursing legacy.* New York: Methuen.

Barth, R. J. (1945). *Fiery angel: The story of Florence Nightingale.* Coral Gables, FL: Glade House.

Bishop, W. J. (1962). *A bio-bibliography of Florence Nightingale.* London: Dawson's of Pall Mall.

Boyd, N. (1982). *Three Victorian women who changed their world.* New York: Oxford.

Bull, A. (1985). *Florence Nightingale.* North Pomfret, VT: David and Charles.

Bullough, V. L., Bullough, B., & Stanton, M. P. (Eds.). (1990). *Florence Nightingale and her era: A collection of new scholarship.* New York: Garland.

Calabria, M., & Macrae, J. (Eds.). (1994). *Suggestions for thought by Florence Nightingale: Selections and commentaries.* Philadelphia: University of Pennsylvania Press.

Collins, D. (1985). *Florence Nightingale.* Milford, MI: Mott Media.

Columbia University Faculty of Medicine and Department of Nursing. (1937). *Catalogue of the Florence Nightingale collection.* New York: Author.

Cook, E. T. (1913). *The life of Florence Nightingale.* London: Macmillan.

Cook, E. T. (1941). *A short life of Florence Nightingale.* New York: Macmillan.

Cope, Z. (1958). *Florence Nightingale and the doctors.* Philadelphia: J. B. Lippincott.

Cope, Z. (1961). *Six disciples of Florence Nightingale.* New York: Pitman.

Davies, C. (1980). *Rewriting nursing history.* London: Croom Helm.

Dossey, B. M. (2000). *Florence Nightingale: Mystic, visionary, healer.* Springhouse, PA: Springhouse.

Editors of *RN.* (1970). *Florence Nightingale: Rebel with a cause.* Oradell, NJ: Medical Economics.

French, Y. (1953). *Six great Englishwomen.* London: H. Hamilton.

Goldie, S. (1987). *I have done my duty: Florence Nightingale in the Crimea War, 1854-1856.* London: Manchester University Press.

Goldsmith, M. L. (1937). *Florence Nightingale: The woman and the legend.* London: Hodder and Stoughton.

Gordon, R. (1979). *The private life of Florence Nightingale.* New York: Atheneum.

Hall, E. F. (1920). *Florence Nightingale.* New York: Macmillan.

Hallock, G. T., & Turner, C. E. (1928). *Florence Nightingale.* New York: Metropolitan Life Insurance Co.

Herbert, R. G. (1981). *Florence Nightingale: Saint, reformer, or rebel?* Melbourne, FL: Krieger.

Holmes, M. (n.d.). *Florence Nightingale: A cameo life-sketch.* London: Woman's Freedom League.

Huxley, E. J. (1975). *Florence Nightingale.* London: Putnam.

Hyndman, J. A. (1969). *Florence Nightingale: Nurse to the world.* Cleveland, OH: World Publishing.

Keele, J. (Ed.). (1981). *Florence Nightingale in Rome.* Philadelphia: American Philosophical Society.

Lammond, D. (1935). *Florence Nightingale.* London: Duckworth.

Macrae, J. A. (2001). *Nursing as a spiritual practice: A contemporary application of Florence Nightingale's views.* New York: Springer Publishing.

Miller, B. W. (1947). *Florence Nightingale: The lady with the lamp.* Grand Rapids, MI: Zondervan.

Miller, M. (1987). *Florence Nightingale.* Minneapolis: Bethany House.

Mosby, C. V. (1938). *Little journey to the home of Florence Nightingale.* New York: C. V. Mosby.

Muir, D. E. (1946). *Florence Nightingale.* Glasgow: Blackie and Son.

Nash, R. (1937). *A sketch for the life of Florence Nightingale.* London: Society for Promoting Christian Knowledge.

O'Malley, I. B. (1931). *Life of Florence Nightingale, 1820-1856.* London: Butterworth.

Pollard, E. (1902). *Florence Nightingale: The wounded soldiers' friend.* London: Partridge.

Presbyterian Hospital School of Nursing. (1937). *Catalogue of the Florence Nightingale collection.* New York: Author.

Quiller-Couch, A. T. (1927). *Victor of peace.* New York: Nelson.

Quinn, V., & Prest, J. (Eds.). (1987). *Dear Miss Nightingale: A selection of Benjamin Jowett's letters to Florence Nightingale, 1860-1893.* Oxford: Clarendon Press.

Rappe, E. C. (1977). *God bless you, my dear Miss Nightingale.* Stockholm: Almqvist och Wiksell.

Sabatini, R. (1934). *Heroic lives.* Boston: Houghton.

Saint Thomas's Hospital. (1960). *The Nightingale training school: St. Thomas's Hospital, 1860-1960.* London: Author.

Selanders, L. C. (1993). *Florence Nightingale: An environmental adaptation theory.* Newbury Park, CA: Sage Publications.

Seymer, L. R. (1951). *Florence Nightingale.* New York: Macmillan.

Shor, D. (1987). *Florence Nightingale.* Lexington, NH: Silver.

Small, H. (1998). *Avenging angel.* New York: St. Martin's Press.

Smith, F. B. (1982). *Florence Nightingale: Reputation and power.* New York: St. Martin's Press.

Stark, M. (1979). *Introduction to Cassandra: An essay by Florence Nightingale.* Old Westbury, NY: Feminist Press.

Stephenson, G. E. (1924). *Some pioneers in the medical and nursing world.* Shanghai: Nurses's Association of China.

Strachey, L. (1918). *Eminent Victorians.* London: Chatto & Windus.

Tooley, S. A. (1905). *The life of Florence Nightingale.* New York: Macmillan.

Turner, D. (1986). *Florence Nightingale.* New York: Watts.

Vicinus, M., & Nergaard, B. (1990). *Ever yours, Florence Nightingale.* Cambridge, MA: Harvard University Press.

Wilson, W. G. (1940). *Soldier's heroine.* Edinburgh: Missionary Education Movement.

Woodman-Smith, C. (1983). *Florence Nightingale.* New York: Atheneum.

Woodham-Smith, C. B. (1951). *Florence Nightingale, 1820-1910.* New York: McGraw-Hill.

Woodham-Smith, C. B. (1951). *Lonely crusader: The life of Florence Nightingale, 1820-1910.* New York: Whittlesey House.

Woodham-Smith, C. B. (1956). *Lady-in-chief.* London: Methven.

Woodham-Smith, C. B. (1977). *Florence Nightingale, 1820-1910.* London: Collins.

Book Chapters

Reed, P. G., & Zurakowski, T. L. (1989). Nightingale: A visionary model for nursing. In J. Fitzpatrick & A. Whall (Eds.), *Conceptual models of nursing: Analysis and application.* Bowie, MD: Robert J. Brady.

Torres, G. C. (1990). Florence Nightingale. In Nursing Theories Conference Group, J. B. George (Chairperson), *Nursing theories: The base for profes-*

sional nursing practice. Englewood Cliffs, NJ: Prentice Hall.

Unpublished Dissertations

Hektor, L. M. (1992). *Nursing, science, and gender: Florence Nightingale and Martha E. Rogers.* Unpublished doctoral dissertation, University of Miami, Miami.

Newton, M. E. (1949). *Florence Nightingale's philosophy of life and education.* Unpublished doctoral dissertation, Stanford University, Stanford, CA.

Parker, E. (1994). *Of writing and nursing: A study of. . . .* Unpublished doctoral dissertation, University of Nevada, Reno.

Selanders, L. C. (1992). *An analysis of the utilization of power by Florence Nightingale.* Unpublished doctoral dissertation, Western Michigan University, Kalamazoo, MI.

Tschirch, P. (1992). *The caring tradition: Nursing ethics in the United States, 1890-1915.* Unpublished doctoral dissertation, The University of Texas at Galveston, Graduate School of Biomedical Science, Galveston, TX.

Journal Articles

A criticism of Miss Florence Nightingale. (1907, Feb.). *Nursing Times, 3,* 89.

Address by the Archbishop of York. (1970, May). Florence Nightingale. *Nursing Times, 66,* 670.

Address given at fiftieth anniversary of founding by Florence Nightingale of first training school for nurses at St. Thomas's Hospital, London, England. (1911, Feb.). *American Journal of Nursing, 11,* 331-361.

A passionate statistician. (1931, May). *American Journal of Nursing, 31,* 566.

Attewell, A. (1998). Florence Nightingale's relevance to nurses. *Journal of Holistic Nursing, 16,* 281-291.

Baly, M. (1986, June). Shattering the Nightingale myth. *Nursing Times, 82*(24), 16-18.

Baly, M. E. (1969, Jan.). Florence Nightingale's influence on nursing today. *Nursing Times, 65*(Suppl.), 1-4.

Barber, E. M. (1935, July). A culinary campaign. *Journal of the American Dietetic Association, 11,* 89-98.

Barber, J. A. (1999). Concerning our national honour: Florence Nightingale and the welfare of Aboriginal Australians. *Collegian: Journal of the Royal College of Nursing Australia, 6*(1), 36-39.

Barker, E. R. (1989, Oct.). Caregivers as casualties . . . war experiences and the postwar consequences for both Nightingale- and Vietnam-era nurses. *Western Journal of Nursing Research, 11,* 628-631.

Barritt, E. R. (1973). Florence Nightingale's values and modern nursing education. *Nursing Forum, 12,* 7-47.

Berentson, L. (1982, April/May). Florence Nightingale: Change agent. *Registered Nurse, 6*(2), 3, 7.

Bishop, W. J. (1957, May). Florence Nightingale's letters. *American Journal of Nursing, 57,* 607.

Bishop, W. J. (1960, May). Florence Nightingale's message for today. *Nursing Outlook, 8,* 246.

Blanc, E. (1980, May). Nightingale remembered: Reflections on times past. *California Nurse, 75*(10), 7.

Blanchard, J. R. (1939, June). Florence Nightingale: A study in vocation. *New Zealand Nursing Journal, 32,* 193-197.

Boylen, J. O. (1974, April). The Florence Nightingale-Mary Stanley controversy: Some unpublished letters. *Medical History, 18*(2), 186-193.

Bridges, D. C. (1954, April). Florence Nightingale centenary. *International Nurses Review, 1,* 3.

Brow, E. J. (1954, April). Florence Nightingale and her international influence. *International Nursing Review, 1,* 17-19.

Brown, E. (2000). Nightingale's values live on. *Kai Tiaki: Nursing New Zealand, 6*(3), 31.

Carlisle, D. (1989, Dec.). A nightingale sings . . . Florence Nightingale . . . unknown details of her life story. *Nursing Times, 85*(50), 38-39.

Charatan, F. B. (1990, Feb.). Florence Nightingale: The most famous nurse in the world. *Today's OR Nurse, 12*(2), 25-30.

Cherescavich, G. (1971, June). Florence, where are you? *Nursing Clinics of North America, 6,* 217-223.

Choa, G. H. (1971, May). Speech by Dr. the Hon. G. H. Choa at the Florence Nightingale Day Celebration on Wednesday, 12th May, 1971, at City Hall, Hong Kong. *Nursing Journal, 10,* 33-34.

Clayton, R. E. (1974, April). How men may live and not die in India: Florence Nightingale. *Australian Nurses Journal, 2,* 10-11.

Coakley, M. L. (1989, Winter). Florence Nightingale: A one-woman revolution. *Journal of Christian Nursing, 6,* 20-25.

Cohen, S. (1997). Miss Loane, Florence Nightingale, and district nursing in late Victorian Britain. *Nursing History Review, 5,* 83-103.

de Guzman, G. (1935, July). Florence Nightingale. *Filipino Nurse, 10,* 10-14.

Dennis, K. E., & Prescott, P. A. (1985, Jan.). Florence Nightingale: Yesterday, today, and tomorrow. *ANS Advances in Nursing Science, 7*(2), 66-81.

de Tornayay, R. (1976, Nov./Dec.). Past is prologue: Florence Nightingale, *Pulse, 12*(6), 9-11.

Dwyer, B. A. (1937, Jan.). The mother of our modern nursing system. *Filipino Nurse, 12,* 8-10.

Florence Nightingale: Rebel with a cause. (1970, May). *Registered Nurse, 33,* 39-55.

Florence Nightingale: The original geriatric nurse. (1980, May). *Oklahoma Nurse, 25*(4), 6.

Gibbon, C. (1997). The influence of Florence Nightingale's image on Liverpool nurses 1945-1995. *International History of Nursing Journal, 2*(3), 17-26.

Gordon, J. E. (1972, Oct.). Nurses and nursing in Britain. 21. The work of Florence Nightingale. I. For the health of the army. *Midwife Health Visitor and Community Nurse, 8*, 351-359.

Gordon, J. E. (1972, Nov.). Nurses and nursing in Britain. 22. The work of Florence Nightingale. II. The establishment of nurse training in Britain. *Midwife Health Visitor and Community Nurse, 8*, 391-396.

Gordon, J. E. (1973, Jan.). Nurses and nursing in Britain. 23. The work of Florence Nightingale. III. Her influence throughout the world. *Midwife Health Visitor and Community Nurse, 9*, 17-22.

Hoole, L. (2000). Florence Nightingale must remain as nursing's icon. *British Journal of Nursing, 4*, 189.

Ifemesia, C. C. (1976, July/Sept.). Florence Nightingale (1820-1910). *Nigerian Nurse, 8*(3), 26-34.

Kelly, L. Y. (1976, Oct.). Our nursing heritage: Have we renounced it? (Florence Nightingale). *Image: The Journal of Nursing Scholarship, 8*(3), 43-48.

Large, J. T. (1985, May). Florence Nightingale: A multifaceted personality. *Nursing Journal of India, 76*(5), 110, 114.

LeVasseur, J. (1998). Student scholarship: Plato, Nightingale, and contemporary nursing. *Image: The Journal of Nursing Scholarship, 30*, 281-285.

Light, K. M. (1997). Florence Nightingale and holistic philosophy. *Journal of Holistic Nursing, 15*(1), 25-40.

Macmillan, K. (1994, April/May). Brilliant mind gave Florence her edge . . . Florence Nightingale. *Registered Nurse, 6*(2), 29-30.

Macrae, J. (1995, Spring). Nightingale's spiritual philosophy and its significance for modern nursing. *Image: The Journal of Nursing Scholarship, 27*, 8-10.

McDonald, L. (1998). Florence Nightingale: Passionate statistician. *Journal of Holistic Nursing, 16*, 267-277.

Monteiro, L. A. (1985, Nov.). Response in anger: Florence Nightingale on the importance of training for nurses. *Journal of Nursing History, 1*(1), 11-18.

Rabstein, C. (2000). Patron saint or has-been? . . . Role models: Is Florence Nightingale holding us back? *Nursing, 30*(1), 8.

Selanders, L. C. (1998). Florence Nightingale: The evolution and social impact of feminist values in nursing. *Journal of Holistic Nursing, 16*(2), 227-243.

Selanders, L. C. (1998). The power of environmental adaptation: Florence Nightingale's original theory for nursing practice. *Journal of Holistic Nursing, 16*, 247-263.

Sparacino, P. S. A. (1994, March). Clinical practice: Florence Nightingale: A CNS role model. *Clinical Nurse Specialist, 8*(2), 64.

Stronk, K. (1997). Florence Nightingale: Mother of all nurses. *Journal of Nursing Jocularity, 7*(2), 14.

Ulrich, B. T. (1999). Continuing education. Still so much to do: The legacy of Florence Nightingale. *Nurse Week, 12*(25), 10-12.

Watson, J. (1998). Reflections: Florence Nightingale and the enduring legacy of transpersonal human caring. *Journal of Holistic Nursing, 16*, 292-294.

Welch, M. (1986, April). Nineteenth-century philosophic influences on Nightingale's concept of the person. *Journal of Nursing History, 1*(2), 3-11.

Wheeler, W., & Walker, M. (1999, May). Florence: Death of an icon . . . Florence Nightingale. *Nursing Times, 95*(19), 24-26.

Widerquist, J. G. (1992, Jan./Feb.). The spirituality of Florence Nightingale. *Nursing Research, 41*, 49-55.

Widerquist, J. G. (1997). Sanitary reform and nursing: Edwin Chadwick and Florence Nightingale. *Nursing History Review, 5*, 149-160.

Williams, B. (2000). Florence Nightingale: A relevant heroine for nurses today? *California Nurse, 96*(1), 9, 27.

Videotape

The Helene Fuld Health Trust (Producer). (1990). *Florence Nightingale. The nurse theorists. Portraits of excellence* (Videotape). Athens, OH: Studio Three Productions, a division of Samuel Merritt College, Oakland, CA.

Web Sites*

About.com Women's History: Quotes by Women—Women's Voices. Retrieved December 20, 2004, from: *http://womenshistory.about.com/cs/quotes/a/qu_nightingale*

BBC archives for Florence Nightingale. Retrieved December 20, 2004, from: *http://www.bbc.co.uk* (Type "Florence Nightingale" into the search function.)

*Author's note: Several thousand Web sites about Florence Nightingale are available via Internet search engines. It appears that many of these sites are linked to closed sources (e.g., libraries), which do not allow access by direct Web addresses. A wealth of information is available through the use of these links from search engines, which also access archived information that is no longer available via a Web address. The user should review these sites carefully and attempt to identify the source of the information posted to determine its validity. Various university mathematics departments also feature wonderful essays about the statistical work done by Nightingale; these sites may provide links to data that are not found easily and, therefore, can be exciting for students who are interested in this aspect of her work. Two such sites include York University in Canada and Agnes Scott College in Decatur, Georgia, where many of the library holdings describe and post Nightingale letters owned by that institution—documents not easily accessible elsewhere. Enjoy visiting these Web sites!

Country Joe McDonald's Tribute to Florence Nightingale. Retrieved December 20, 2004, from: *http://www.countryjoe.com/nightingale*

Florence Nightingale, Avenging Angel. Retrieved December 20, 2004, from: *http://www.florence-nightingale-avenging-angel.co.uk*

Internet Modern History Sourcebook—Florence Nightingale: Rural Hygiene. Retrieved December 20, 2004, from: *http://www.fordham.edu/halsall/mod/nightingale-rural.html*

The Collected Works of Florence Nightingale. Retrieved December 20, 2004, from: *http://www.sociology.uoguelph.ca/fnightingale/*

The Florence Nightingale Museum. Retrieved December 20, 2004, from: *http://www.florence-nightingale.co.uk*

VSU College of Nursing Florence Nightingale Page. Retrieved December 20, 2004, from: *http://www.valdosta.edu/nursing/history_theory/florence*

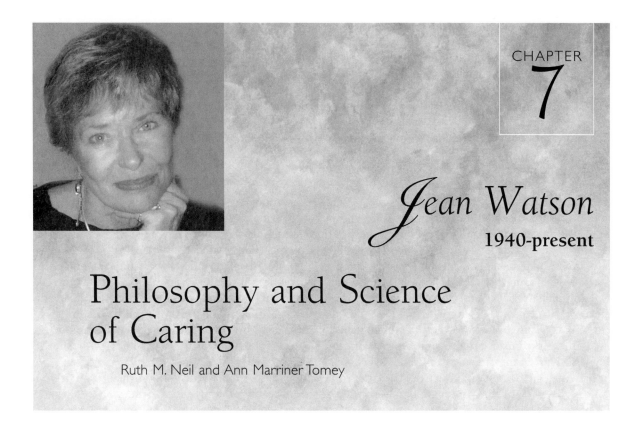

Jean Watson
1940-present

Philosophy and Science of Caring

Ruth M. Neil and Ann Marriner Tomey

CREDENTIALS AND BACKGROUND OF THE THEORIST

Margaret Jean Harman Watson was born in southern West Virginia and grew up during the 1940s and 1950s in the small town of Welch, West Virginia, in the Appalachian Mountains. As the youngest of eight children, she was surrounded by an extended family–community environment.

Previous authors: Tracey J. F. Patton, Deborah A. Barnhart, Patricia M. Bennett, Beverly D. Porter, and Rebecca S. Sloan. In addition, Ruth Neil updated the chapter in 1990. The authors wish to thank Dr. Jean Watson for her ongoing inspiration and support, along with her review of the content of this chapter for accuracy and her assistance in updating the references and bibliography.

Watson attended high school in West Virginia and then the Lewis Gale School of Nursing in Roanoke, Virginia. After graduation in 1961, she married her husband, Douglas, and moved west to his native state of Colorado. Douglas, whom Watson describes not only as her physical and spiritual partner, but also as her best friend, died in 1998. She has two grown daughters, Jennifer (born in 1963) and Julie (born in 1967), and five grandchildren. She continues to live in Boulder, Colorado.

After moving to Colorado, Watson continued her nursing education and graduate studies at the University of Colorado. She earned a baccalaureate degree in nursing in 1964 at the Boulder campus, a master's degree in psychiatric-mental health nursing in 1966 at the Health Sciences campus, and a doctorate in educational psychology and counseling in 1973 at the Graduate School, Boulder campus. After Watson completed her doctoral degree, she joined the School of Nursing faculty of the University of Colorado Health Sciences Center in Denver, where she has served in both faculty and administrative positions. She has served as chairperson and assistant dean of the undergraduate program, and she was involved in early planning and implementation of the nursing Ph.D. program in Colorado, which was initiated in 1978. She was coordinator and director of the Ph.D. program between 1978 and 1981. In 1981 and 1982, she pursued international sabbatical studies and diverse learning experiences in New Zealand, Australia, India, Thailand, and Taiwan. Upon her return, she was appointed dean of the University of Colorado School of Nursing and Associate Director, Nursing Practice at University Hospital from 1983 to 1990. She is currently a Distinguished Professor of Nursing and holds the Murchinson-Scoville Endowed Chair in Caring Science at the University of Colorado School of Nursing. She continues to offer her basic theory courses as part of the International Certificate Program in Caring-Healing, which can be taken for credit twice a year. Information about these courses and other selected in-resident studies with Dr. Watson can be obtained by contacting her at the Web site *http://www2.uchsc.edu/son/caring/content.*

During her deanship, she was instrumental in the development of a postbaccalaureate nursing curriculum in human caring, health, and healing, which leads to a career professional clinical doctoral degree (ND). This pilot ND program was selected as a national demonstration program by the Helene Fuld Health Trust in New York and was funded by the Trust and Colorado clinical health care agencies. The program was implemented in 1990 as a partnership between nursing education and practice, whereby clinical and academic agencies in Colorado and beyond work jointly to restructure simultaneously nursing education and nursing practice for the future.

The Center for Human Caring was established in the 1980s by Watson and colleagues at the University of Colorado; it was the nation's first interdisciplinary center with an overall commitment to develop and use knowledge of human caring and healing as the moral and scientific basis of clinical practice and nursing scholarship and as the foundation for efforts to transform the current health care system (Watson, 1986). During its existence, the center developed and sponsored numerous clinical, educational, and community scholarship activities and projects in human caring, including participation of national and international scholars in residence.

During her career, Watson has been active in community programs, having served as an earlier founder and member of the Board of Boulder County Hospice, and she has initiated numerous collaborations with area health care facilities. The recipient of several research and advanced education federal grants and awards, Watson has also received numerous university and private grants and extramural funding for her faculty and administrative projects and scholarships in human caring.

Other honors include honorary doctoral degrees from at least six universities in the United States and abroad including Assumption College in Worcester, Massachusetts, the University of Akron, Ohio, the University of West Virginia, Göteborg University in Sweden, Luton University in London, and the University of Montreal in Quebec, Canada. Watson also received the high honor of Distinguished Professor of Nursing at the University of Colorado in 1992. In 1993, she was the recipient of the National League for Nursing (NLN) Martha E. Rogers Award, which recognizes a nurse scholar who has made significant contributions to nursing knowledge that advance the science of caring in nursing and health sciences. Between 1993 and 1996, Watson served as a member of the Executive Committee, the Governing Board, and as an officer for the NLN. She was president from 1995 to 1996. In 1997, she was given an honorary lifetime certification as a holistic nurse.

In 1998, she was recognized as a Distinguished Nurse Scholar by New York University and in 1999, she was honored with the national Norman Cousins Award by the Fetzer Institute in recognition of her commitment to developing, maintaining, and exemplifying relationship-centered care practices (Watson, personal communication, August 14, 2000).

Watson's national and international work includes distinguished lectureships throughout the United States at well-known universities including Boston College, Catholic University, Adelphi University, Columbia University–Teachers College, State University of New York, and at universities and scholarly meetings in numerous foreign countries including Canada, England, Finland, Sweden, Germany, Australia, Nova Scotia, Micronesia, Portugal, Scotland, Korea, Israel, Japan, Spain, New Zealand, Thailand, Taiwan, Denmark, Brazil, and Venezuela.

Her international activities also include an International Kellogg Fellowship in Australia (1982), a Fulbright Research and Lecture Award to Sweden and other parts of Scandinavia (1991), and a lecture tour in the United Kingdom (1993). She has also been involved in international projects and received invitations in New Zealand, India, Thailand, Taiwan, Israel, Japan, Venezuela, Korea, and others.

Watson is featured in several nationally distributed videotapes on nursing theory. These include "Circles of Knowledge" and "Conversations on Caring with Jean Watson and Janet Quinn" from the NLN, "Portraits of Excellence: Nursing Theorists and Their Work" from the Helene Fuld Health Trust, and "Theory in Practice" from the NLN. The latter features the Denver Nursing Project in Human Caring, a nurse-directed caring center for persons with acquired immunodeficiency syndrome (AIDS) (Watson, personal correspondence, August 14, 2000). The Denver Nursing Project in Human Caring was a clinical (caring-theory based) demonstration project of the University of Colorado Center for Human Caring and School of Nursing and served patients from 1988 to 1996.

More recent media productions include the NLN-produced videotape, "Applying the Art and Science of Human Caring, Parts I and II"; "A Meta-Reflection on Nursing's Present," an audiotape produced by the American Holistic Nurses Association; and "Private Psalm: A Mantra and Meditation for Healing," a compact disc set. (See the complete listing of audiovisual productions at the end of this chapter and on the Web.)

Watson's publications reflect the evolution of her theory of caring. Her writings have been geared toward educating nursing students and providing them with the ontological, ethical, and epistemological basis for their praxis and research directions. Much of her current work began with the 1979 publication that was reprinted in 1985 and has been translated into Korean and French, *Nursing: The Philosophy and Science of Caring*, which she says began as class notes for a course she was developing. She says the book "emerged from her quest to bring new meaning and dignity to the world of nursing and patient care—care that seemed too limited in its scope at the time, largely defined by medicine's paradigm and traditional biomedical science models" (Watson, 1997, p. 49).

Nursing: Human Science and Human Care—A Theory of Nursing, published in 1985 and reprinted in 1988 and 1999, was her second major work. The purpose of this book was to address some of the conceptual and philosophical problems that still existed in nursing. She hoped that others would join her as she sought to "elucidate the human care process in nursing, preserve the concept of the person in our science, and better our contribution to society" (Watson, 1988, p. ix). This book has been translated into Chinese, German, Japanese, Korean, Swedish, Norwegian, Danish, and probably, by now, other languages (Watson, personal communication, August 14, 2000).

Postmodern Nursing and Beyond was published in 1999 and is Watson's most recent work. This work projects nursing and health care into the mid–twenty-first century. It seeks to illuminate ". . . a model of caring and healing practices that take medicine, nursing, and the public beyond traditional Western medicine, beyond the 'cure at all costs' approach" (Watson, 1999, p. xii) and embeds caring and healing practices in a new paradigm that acknowledges the symbiotic relationship between humankind-technology-nature and the larger, expanding universe. "It offers a search for the spiritual aspects of our being and our approaches to health and healing" (Watson, 1999, p. xiv).

In the dedication section of *Postmodern Nursing and Beyond* (Watson, 1999), which has been translated into Portuguese and Japanese, Watson described recent traumatic personal experiences that contributed to her insights as expressed in the book. One of these was an accidental injury in 1997 that resulted in the loss of her left eye despite many months of trying to save it. The other was her husband's death in 1998. Watson states that she is now "attempting to integrate these wounds into my life and work. One of the gifts through the suffering was the privilege of experiencing and receiving my own theory through the care from my husband and loving nurse friends and colleagues" (Watson, personal communication, August 31, 2000).

In Watson's (1979) original *Nursing: The Philosophy and Science of Caring*, she referred to caring as "central to nursing" (p. 9). Caring is a moral ideal rather than a task-oriented behavior and includes such characteristics as the actual caring occasion and the transpersonal caring moment, phenomena that occur when an authentic caring relationship exists between the nurse and the patient. One of her earliest written treatises on the caring model was presented at an American Nurses Association Division of Practice Meeting in 1979 (Watson, Burckhardt, Brown, Block, & Hester, 1979). As her work evolved, Watson posited that caring is intrinsically related to healing: "Such an ethic and ethos of caring, healing, and health comprises nursing's professional context and mission—its *raison d'être* to society" (Watson, 1997, p. 50).

THEORETICAL SOURCES

In addition to traditional nursing knowledge and the works of Nightingale and Henderson, Watson acknowledges the work of Leininger, Gadow, and Peplau as background for hers (Watson, 1985a, 1997). In her more recent work, Watson refers to that of others such as Maslow, Heidegger, Erickson, Selye, Lazarus, Whitehead, de Chardin, and Sartre. In addition, she acknowledges philosophical and intellectual guidance from feminist theory, quantum physics, wisdom traditions, and perennial philosophy (Watson, 1995, 1997, 1999). To develop her framework, Watson drew heavily on the sciences and the humanities, providing a phenomenological, existential, and spiritual orientation.

Watson explains that the concepts she defined to bring new meaning to nursing's paradigm were "derived from clinically inducted, empirical experiences, combined with my philosophical, intellectual and experiential background; thus my early work emerged from my own values, beliefs, and perceptions about personhood, life, health, and healing . . ." (Watson, 1997, p. 49).

Watson attributes her emphasis on the interpersonal and transpersonal qualities of congruence, empathy, and warmth to the views of Carl Rogers and more recent writers of transpersonal psychology. Rogers described several incidents that led to the formulation of his thoughts on human behavior. One of these involved learning that "it is the client who knows what hurts and that the facilitator should allow the direction of the therapeutic process to come from the client" (Rogers, 1961, pp. 11-12). Rogers believed that "through understanding" the patient would come to accept himself, an initial step toward a positive outcome (Rogers, 1961, pp. 18-19). The therapist, motivated by a warm interest in the patient, helps by clarifying and stating feelings about which the patient has been unclear. Together, the therapist and the patient understand the meaning of the patient's experience. Another crucial concept of Rogerian theory is that the therapist-patient relationship is more important to the outcome than adherence to traditional methods. Rogers states:

> In my early professional years I was asking the question, "How can I treat, or cure, or change this person?" Now I phrase the question in this way: "How can I provide a relationship which this person may use for his own personal growth?" (Rogers, 1961, p. 33)

(For additional information about Rogers, see Betz and Whitehorn [1956] and Seeman [1954]).

Watson points out that Rogers' phenomenological approach, with his view that nurses are not here to manipulate and control others, but rather to understand, was profoundly influential at a time when "clinicalization" (therapeutic control and manipulation of the patient) was considered the norm (Watson, personal communication, August 31, 2000).

Watson believes a strong liberal arts background is also essential to the process of holistic care for patients. She believes the study of the humanities expands the mind and increases thinking skills and personal growth. Watson compares the current status of nursing with the mythological Danaides, who attempted to fill a broken jar with water, only to see water flow through the cracks. Until nursing merges theory and practice through the combined study of the sciences and the humanities, she believes similar cracks will be evident in the scientific basis of nursing knowledge (Watson, 1981, 1997).

Yalom's 11 curative factors stimulated Watson's thinking about the psychodynamic and human components that could apply to nursing and caring and, consequently, to her 10 carative factors in nursing (Watson, 1979). Although Watson still says the 10 carative factors continue to embrace the core of nursing, she is emerging toward more fluid and evolutionary language: caritas, making explicit connections between caring and love (Watson, personal correspondence, 2004).

Watson's work has been called a treatise, a conceptual model, a framework, and a theory. This chapter uses the terms *theory* and *framework* interchangeably. In addition, Watson states that, both retrospectively and prospectively, her work "can be read as philosophy, ethic, or even paradigm or worldview" (Watson, 1997, p. 50).

MAJOR CONCEPTS *&* DEFINITIONS

Watson bases her theory for nursing practice on the following 10 carative factors. Each has a dynamic phenomenological component that is relative to the individuals involved in the relationship as encompassed by nursing. The first three interdependent factors serve as the "philosophical foundation for the science of caring" (Watson, 1979, pp. 9-10). As Watson's ideas and values have evolved, she translated the 10 carative factors into caritas processes. In caritas processes, there is a decidedly spiritual dimension and overt evocation of love and caring (*http://www2.uchsc.edu/son/caring/content/wct.asp*). (See Table 7-1 [p. 104] for the original carative factors and the caritas process interpretation.)

I. FORMATION OF A HUMANISTIC-ALTRUISTIC SYSTEM OF VALUES

Humanistic and altruistic values are learned early in life but can be influenced greatly by nurse educators. This factor can be defined as satisfaction through giving and extension of the sense of self (Watson, 1979).

2. INSTILLATION OF FAITH-HOPE

This factor, incorporating humanistic and altruistic values, facilitates the promotion of holistic nursing care and positive health within the patient population. It also describes the nurse's role in developing effective nurse-patient interrelationships and in promoting wellness by helping the patient adopt health-seeking behaviors (Watson, 1979).

3. CULTIVATION OF SENSITIVITY TO SELF AND TO OTHERS

The recognition of feelings leads to self-actualization through self-acceptance for both the nurse and the patient. As nurses acknowledge their sensitivity and feelings, they become more genuine, authentic, and sensitive to others (Watson, 1979).

4. DEVELOPMENT OF A HELPING-TRUST RELATIONSHIP

The development of a helping-trust relationship between the nurse and patient is crucial for trans-

Continued

MAJOR CONCEPTS & DEFINITIONS—cont'd

personal caring. A trusting relationship promotes and accepts the expression of both positive and negative feelings. It involves congruence, empathy, nonpossessive warmth, and effective communication. Congruence involves being real, honest, genuine, and authentic. Empathy is the ability to experience and, thereby, understand the other person's perceptions and feelings and to communicate those understandings. Nonpossessive warmth is demonstrated by a moderate speaking volume, a relaxed, open posture, and facial expressions that are congruent with other communications. Effective communication has cognitive, affective, and behavior response components (Watson, 1979).

5. PROMOTION AND ACCEPTANCE OF THE EXPRESSION OF POSITIVE AND NEGATIVE FEELINGS

The sharing of feelings is a risk-taking experience for both nurse and patient. The nurse must be prepared for either positive or negative feelings. The nurse must recognize that intellectual and emotional understandings of a situation differ (Watson, 1979).

6. SYSTEMATIC USE OF THE SCIENTIFIC PROBLEM-SOLVING METHOD FOR DECISION MAKING

Use of the nursing process brings a scientific problem-solving approach to nursing care, dispelling the traditional image of a nurse as the doctor's handmaiden. The nursing process is similar to the research process in that it is systematic and organized (Watson, 1979).

7. PROMOTION OF INTERPERSONAL TEACHING-LEARNING

This factor is an important concept for nursing in that it separates caring from curing. It allows the patient to be informed and shifts the responsibility for wellness and health to the patient. The nurse facilitates this process with teaching-learning techniques that are designed to enable patients to provide self-care, determine personal needs, and provide opportunities for their personal growth (Watson, 1979).

8. PROVISION FOR SUPPORTIVE, PROTECTIVE, AND CORRECTIVE MENTAL, PHYSICAL, SOCIOCULTURAL, AND SPIRITUAL ENVIRONMENT

Nurses must recognize the influence that internal and external environments have on the health and illness of individuals. Concepts relevant to the internal environment include the mental and spiritual well-being and sociocultural beliefs of an individual. In addition to epidemiological variables, other external variables include comfort, privacy, safety, and clean, aesthetic surroundings (Watson, 1979).

9. ASSISTANCE WITH GRATIFICATION OF HUMAN NEEDS

The nurse recognizes the biophysical, psychophysical, psychosocial, and intrapersonal needs of self and patient. Patients must satisfy lower-order needs before attempting to attain higher-order needs. Food, elimination, and ventilation are examples of lower-order biophysical needs, whereas activity, inactivity, and sexuality are considered lower-order psychophysical needs. Achievement and affiliation are higher-order psychosocial needs. Self-actualization is a higher-order intrapersonal-interpersonal need (Watson, 1979).

10. ALLOWANCE FOR EXISTENTIAL-PHENOMENOLOGICAL FORCES

Phenomenology describes data of the immediate situation that help people understand the phenomena in question. Existential psychology is a science of human existence that uses phenomenological analysis. Watson considers this factor difficult to understand. It is included to provide a thought-provoking experience leading to a better understanding of the self and others.

Watson believes that nurses have the responsibility to go beyond the 10 carative factors and to facilitate patients' development in the area of health promotion through preventive health actions. This goal is accomplished by teaching patients personal changes to promote health, providing situational support, teaching problem-solving methods, and recognizing coping skills and adaptation to loss (Watson, 1979).

USE OF EMPIRICAL EVIDENCE

Watson and her colleagues have attempted to study the concept of caring by collecting data to use in classifying caring behaviors, to describe the similarities and differences between what nurses consider care and what patients consider care, and to generate testable hypotheses around the concept of nursing care. They studied responses from registered nurses, nursing students, and patients to the same open-ended questionnaire covering a variety of aspects of (1) taking care of and (2) caring about patients. Their findings revealed a discrepancy in the values considered most important by patients, nursing students, and registered nurses. They stressed the need for further study to clarify what behaviors and values are important from each viewpoint. The study also raised a question about differences in values for persons in various situations and the question of meeting minimum care needs before the quality of care can be evaluated (Watson, 1981).

Watson's research into caring incorporates empiricism, but it emphasizes methodologies that begin with nursing phenomena rather than the natural sciences (Leininger, 1979). She has used human science, empirical phenomenology, and transcendent phenomenology in her work. She has also investigated new language, such as metaphor and poetry, to communicate, convey, and elucidate human caring and healing (Watson, 1987). In her inquiry and writing, she increasingly incorporates her conviction that there is a sacred relationship between humankind and the universe (Watson, 1997). *Instruments for Assessing and Measuring Caring in Nursing and Health Sciences* was published in 2002 to facilitate the collection of evidence and received the American Journal of Nursing Book of the Year Award.

MAJOR ASSUMPTIONS

In her first book, *Nursing: The Philosophy and Science of Caring* (1979), Watson states the major assumptions of the science of caring in nursing as follows:

1. Caring can only be effectively demonstrated and practiced interpersonally.
2. Caring consists of carative factors that result in the satisfaction of certain human needs.
3. Effective caring promotes health and individual or family growth.
4. Caring responses accept a person not only as he or she is now but as what he or she may become.
5. A caring environment offers the development of potential while allowing the person to choose the best action for himself or herself at a given time.
6. Caring is more "healthogenic" than is curing. The practice of caring integrates biophysical knowledge with knowledge of human behavior to generate or promote health and to provide ministrations to those who are ill. A science of caring is therefore complementary to the science of curing.
7. The practice of caring is central to nursing (Watson, 1979, pp. 8-9).

Gaut identified three conditions necessary for caring. These include "(1) an awareness and knowledge about one's need for care; (2) an intention to act, and actions based on knowledge; (3) a positive change as a result of caring, judged solely on the basis of welfare of others" (Gaut, 1983, pp. 313-324). Watson expanded Gaut's work by adding two additional conditions, "an underlying value and moral commitment to care; and a will to care" (Watson, personal communication, August 3, 1997).

In her second book, *Nursing: Human Science and Human Care—A Theory of Nursing*, Watson states, "both nursing education and the healthcare delivery system must be based on human values and concern for the welfare of others" (Watson, 1985a, p. 33). To further define the social and ethical responsibilities of nursing and to explicate the human care concepts in nursing, Watson proposes the following 11 assumptions related to human care values:

1. Care and love comprise the primal and universal psychic energy.
2. Care and love, often overlooked, are the cornerstones of humanness; nourishment of these needs fulfills humanity.
3. The ability to sustain the caring ideal and ideology in practice will affect the development of civilization and determine nursing's contribution to society.
4. Caring for the self is a prerequisite to caring for others.
5. Historically, nursing has held a human care and caring stance in regard to people with health-illness concerns.
6. Caring is the central unifying focus of nursing practice—the essence of nursing.
7. Caring, at the human level, has been increasingly deemphasized in the health care system.
8. Technological advancements and institutional constraints have sublimated nursing's caring foundation.
9. A significant issue for nursing today and in the future is the preservation and advancement of human care.
10. Only through interpersonal relationships can human care be effectively demonstrated and practiced.
11. Nursing's social, moral, and scientific contributions to humankind and society lie in its commitments to human care ideals in theory, practice, and research (Watson, 1988).

In *Postmodern Nursing and Beyond*, Watson (1999) seeks to describe a more fundamental ontological shift in human consciousness that evokes a return to the sacred core of humankind and its relation with the universe, connecting with a sense of the divine and inviting awe and mystery back into life and work. Such thinking holds a sense of reverence and openness for the infinite possibilities contained within an individual's inner and outer space. It offers a search for the spiritual aspects of being and approaches to health and healing.

This ontological shift invites practitioners to embark upon the following paths:

- Path of awareness, of awakening to the sacred feminine archetype-cosmology to rebalance the disorder of conventional modern medicine and the modern, cultural mindset.
- Path of cultivation of higher/deeper self and a higher consciousness: transpersonal self.
- Path of honoring the sacred within and without; open to deeper explorations of the mystery of the human body and life-healing processes: postmodern-transpersonal body.
- Path of acknowledging the metaphysical-spiritual level, attending to the nonphysical, spiritual dimensions of existence.
- Path of acknowledging quantum concepts and phenomena such as caring-healing energy, intentionality and consciousness, as paths toward expanding human existence and the evolving human consciousness.
- Path of honoring the connectedness of all; unitary consciousness; the eternal "caring moment"; "transpersonal caring-healing".
- Path of honoring the unity of mindbodyspirit; both immanence and transcendence of the human being and becoming.
- Path of reintegrating the caring-healing arts, as an artistry of being into healing practices: ontological competencies.
- Path of creating healing space: healing architecture.
- Path of a relational ontology, open to new epistemologies of existence.
- Path of moving beyond the modern-postmodern into the open, transpersonal space and the new thinking required for the next millennium (Watson, 1999, p. xv)

THEORETICAL ASSERTIONS

According to Watson, nurses are interested in understanding health, illness, and the human experience. Within the philosophy and science of caring, she tries to define an outcome of scientific activity with regard to the humanistic aspects of life. She attempts to make nursing an interrelationship of quality of life, including death, and the prolongation of life (Watson, 1979).

Watson believes nursing is concerned with health promotion, restoration, and illness prevention. Health, more than the absence of illness, is an elusive concept because it has a subjective nature (Watson, 1979). Health refers to "unity and harmony within the mind, body, and soul" and is associated with the "degree of congruence between the self as perceived and the self as experienced" (Watson, 1988, p. 48).

According to Watson, *caring* is a nursing term representing the factors nurses use to deliver health care to patients. She states that by responding to others as unique individuals, the caring person perceives the feelings of the other and recognizes the uniqueness of the other (Watson, 1985a).

Using the 10 carative factors, the nurse provides care to various patients. Each carative factor describes the caring process of how a patient attains, or maintains, health or dies a peaceful death. Conversely, Watson describes *curing* as a medical term referring to the elimination of disease (Watson, 1979). In her initial work, *Nursing: The Philosophy and Science of Caring*, Watson (1979) describes the following basic premises of a science for nursing:

1. Caring (and nursing) has existed in every society. Every society has had some people who have cared for others. A caring attitude is transmitted by the culture of the profession as a unique way of coping with its environment. The opportunities for nurses to obtain advanced education and engage in higher-level analyses of problems and concerns in their education and practice have allowed nursing to combine its humanistic orientation with the relevant science.
2. There is often a discrepancy between theory and practice or between the scientific and artistic aspects of caring, partly because of the disjunction between scientific values and humanistic values.

Expanding on her previous work, Watson (1985a) added the following components for the context of human science theory development:

1. A philosophy of human freedom, choice, and responsibility
2. A biology and psychology of holism (nonreducible persons interconnected with others and nature)
3. An epistemology that allows not only for empirics but also for advancement of esthetics, ethical values, intuition, and process discovery
4. An ontology of time and space
5. A context of interhuman events, processes, and relationships
6. A scientific world view that is open

As Watson's work evolved, she continued to focus more on the human care process and the transpersonal aspects of caring-healing. The basic premises Watson stated in *Nursing: Human Science and Human Care—A Theory of Nursing* are a reflection of the interpersonal-transpersonal-spiritual aspects of her work (Watson, 1985a). These aspects represent an integration of her beliefs and values about human life and provide the foundation for further development of her theory, as follows:

1. A person's mind and emotions are windows to the soul . . .
2. A person's body is confined in time and space, but the mind and soul are not confined to the physical universe . . .
3. A nurse may have access to a person's mind, emotions, and inner self indirectly through any sphere—mind, body or soul—provided the physical body is not perceived or treated as separate from the mind and emotions and higher sense of self (soul) . . .
4. The spirit, inner self, or soul (geist) of a person exists in and for itself . . .
5. People need each other in a caring, loving way . . .
6. To find solutions, it is necessary to find meanings . . .
7. The totality of experience at any given moment constitutes a phenomenal field . . . (Watson, 1985a, pp. 50-51).

Watson's evolving work continues to make it explicit that humans cannot be treated as objects and humans cannot be separated from self, other, nature, and the larger universe. The caring-healing paradigm is located within a cosmology that is both metaphysical and transcendent with the co-evolving human in the universe. The context calls for a sense of reverence and sacredness with regard to life and all living things. It incorporates both art and science, as they are also being redefined, acknowledging a convergence between the two (Watson, 1997).

LOGICAL FORM

The framework is presented in a logical form. It contains broad ideas and addresses many situations on the health-illness continuum. Watson's definition of caring as opposed to curing delineates nursing from medicine. This concept is helpful in classifying the body of nursing knowledge as a separate science.

Since 1979 the development of the theory has been toward clarifying the person of the nurse and the person of the patient. Another emphasis has been on existential-phenomenological and spiritual factors.

Watson's theory has foundational support from theorists in other disciplines, such as Rogers, Erikson, and Maslow. She is adamant in her support for nursing education that incorporates holistic knowledge from many disciplines and integrates the humanities, arts, and sciences. She believes the increasingly complex requirements of the health care system and patient needs require nurses to have a broad, liberal education. The ideals, content, and theory of liberal education must be integrated into professional nursing education (Sakalys & Watson, 1986).

Watson has recently incorporated dimensions of a postmodern paradigm shift throughout her theory of transpersonal caring. Modern theoretical underpinnings have been associated with concepts such as steady-state maintenance, adaptation, linear interactions, and problem-based nursing practice. The postmodern approach moves beyond this point; the redefining of such a nursing paradigm leads to a more holistic, humanistic, open system wherein harmony, interpretation, and self-transcendence are the emerging directions reflected in this epistemological shift. Watson (1999) believes that nursing must be challenged to construct and co-construct ancient and new knowledge toward an ever-evolving humanity of possibilities to further clarify nursing for a new era. "The theory evolution has tended to place greater emphasis on transpersonal caring, intentionality, caring consciousness, and the caring field" (Watson, personal communication, August 21, 2000).

ACCEPTANCE BY THE NURSING COMMUNITY

Practice

Institutions that are seeking a holistic approach to nursing care are integrating many aspects of Watson's theoretical commitment to caring. For example, nursing journals concerned with the delivery of nursing care contain increasing numbers of articles that refer to Watson and incorporate the importance of caring as an essential domain of nursing (Brenner, Boyd, Thompson, Cervantez, Buerhaus, & Leininger, 1986).

Watson's theory is being validated clinically in a variety of settings and with various populations. With the nursing shortage, the emergence of magnet hospital initiatives has generated more recent interest in the use of Watson's caring theory as context and framework for transforming nursing practice from the inside out. The clinical settings have included critical care units, neonatal intensive care units, and pediatric and gerontological care units (Byrd, 1988; Cronin & Harrison, 1988; Miller, 1987; Ray, 1987; Sithichoke-Rattan, 1989; Swanson, 1991). (See Watson's Web site [*http://www2uchsc.edu/son/caring/content/*] for more information about clinical agencies using this work—for example, Miami Baptist Hospital, Resurrection Health System [Chicago], Denver Veteran's

Administration Hospital, and Children's Hospital [Denver], Inova Health System [Virginia], Baptist Central Hospital [Kentucky], Elmhurst Hospital [New York] Pascak Valley Hospital [New Jersey], Sarasota Memorial Hospital and Tampa Memorial Hospital [Florida], and Scripps Memorial Hospital [California], among others.)

The systems and populations have included women who have miscarried, women who have had newborns in intensive care units, and women who have been identified as socially at risk (Swanson, 1990, 1991 & 2000); patients who have had myocardial infarction (Cronin & Harrison, 1988); oncology patients (Larson, 1987); people with acquired immunodeficiency syndrome (Neil, 1990); and the elderly (Clayton, 1989). Montgomery (1993) studied healing through communication. The relationship of caring to nursing administration has also been examined (Miller, 1987; Nyberg, 1989, 1998; Ray, 1987, 1989). In 2002 Watson's book, *Instruments for Assessing and Measuring Caring in Nursing and Health Science*, was published.

The acuity level of hospitalized individuals, the short length of hospital stays, and the increasing complexity of technology have been identified as possibly interfering with the implementation of the caring theory. However, more recently this caring theory focus is considered one of the solutions needed to address health care reform and system reform at a deep, ethical level, enabling nurses to follow their own professional practice model. New initiatives for this model are emerging under Watson's leadership as "Nightingale units," where caring-healing excellence is manifested within current institutions seeking major nursing reform at individual and environmental levels.

Education

Watson has been active in curriculum planning at the University of Colorado. Her framework has been taught in numerous baccalaureate nursing curricula, including Bellarmine College in Louisville, Kentucky; Assumption College in Worcester, Massachusetts; Indiana State University in Terre Haute; and Florida Atlantic University in Boca Raton. In addition, these concepts are now used widely in nursing programs in Australia, Sweden, Finland, and the United Kingdom.

Critics of Watson's work have concentrated on the use of undefined terms, incomplete treatment of subject matter when describing the 10 carative factors, and a lack of attention to the pathophysiological aspect of nursing. Watson (1985a) addresses these aspects in both her first book, *Nursing: The Philosophy and Science of Caring* (1979, 1988), and the preface of her second book, *Nursing: Human Science and Human Care—A Theory of Nursing* (1985), where she defines her intent to describe the core of nursing (those aspects of the nurse-patient relationship resulting in a therapeutic outcome) rather than the trim of nursing (the procedures, tasks, and techniques used in practice settings). With this focus, the framework is not limited to any nursing specialty. Although she emphasizes that both the core and the trim are necessary, she believes that the trim cannot be the center of a professional model of "nursing qua nursing" (Watson, 1997, p. 50). Watson (1985a) hopes her work will help nurses develop a meaningful moral and philosophical base for practice. A study of Watson's framework leads the reader through a thought-provoking experience by emphasizing deep inner reflection and personal growth, communication skills, use of self-transpersonal growth, attention to both nurse and patient, and the human caring process that potentiates human health and healing.

Research

Watson and colleagues are attempting to research the caring framework and to arrive at empirical data amenable to research techniques (Hester & Ray, 1987; Morse, Bottorff, Neander, & Solberg, 1991; Morse, Solberg, Neander, Bottorff, & Johnson, 1990; Watson, 1985b; Watson & Lea, 1997). However, this abstract framework is difficult to study concretely. Watson believes that a chasm often exists between the essential qualities and subject matter of nursing and the methods used for research. As with her concern for uniting the liberal arts with nursing education, she hopes that nursing research will incorporate and explore esthetic, metaphysical, empirical, and contextual methodologies (Leininger, 1979; Watson, 1987).

Morse and colleagues (1990, 1991) have analyzed the caring literature for themes related to conceptual and theoretical development. They conclude that the abstractness of the concept and the clinical reality in some situations (e.g., the brief interactions with patients afforded by outpatient or office visits) has limited the development of a knowledge base in Watson's caring theory, whether caring exists in nursing situations that have yet to develop interpersonally and whether caring is unique to nursing.

Patient outcomes in caring transactions need further study.

Research and practice must focus on both subjective and objective patient outcomes in determining whether caring is the essence of nursing. The development of behaviors and predictors of change is critical to further development of this work. (See Box 7-1 for information on the use of caring instruments.)

FURTHER DEVELOPMENT

Early nursing research traditionally followed the received view format in which single-factor methodology is compared with rigorous standards of truth,

Box **7-1**

Survey of Use of Caring Instruments in Current Literature

CARING ASSESSMENT INSTRUMENT (CARE-Q)

Greenhalgh, Vanhanen, & Kyngas, 1998

Holroyd, Yue-kuen, Fung-shan, & Waiwan, 1998

Larsson, Peterson, Lampic, von Essen, & Sjoden, 1998

Smith, 1997

CARING ATTRIBUTES PROFESSIONAL SELF-CONCEPT-TECHNOLOGICAL INFLUENCE (CAPSTI)

Arthur, D., Pang, S., Wong, T., Alexander, M. F., Drury, J., Eastwood, et al., 1999

CARING BEHAVIORS ASSESSMENT (CBA)

Gay, 1999

Manogin, Bechtel, & Rami, 2000

Marini, 1999

Mullins, 1996

Schultz, Bridgham, Smith, & Higgins, 1998.

CARING BEHAVIOR INVENTORY (CBI)

Wolf, 1998

CARING DIMENSIONS INVENTORY (CDI)

Watson & Lea, 1997

CARING EFFICACY SCALE

Coates, 1997

CARING PROFESSIONAL SCALE (CPS)

Swanson, 2000

HOLISTIC CARING INTERVENTION

Lathem, 1996

PROFESSIONAL CARING BEHAVIOR

Harrison, 1995

NOTE: For more extensive information, including instruments and author contact information, see Watson, J. (2002). *Assessing and measuring caring in nursing and health science.* New York: Springer.

operational definitions, and observational criteria (Seeman, 1954; Watson, 1981). Watson writes about the inadequacy of this methodology for studying the multidimensional phenomena of nursing care. She proposes that as nursing advances in its doctoral programs, the process of scientific development will be used on itself. Nursing research will adopt the received view, reject it, and synthesize new ideas, which will result in a new nursing model for the next century.

Watson has identified some critical issues for future research conditions that foster the person as an end and not a means in a highly technological society and has also identified conditions that promote caring when humanity is threatened (Watson, 1985a). This theory lends itself to creative research methodologies that assist nursing in formulating a philosophical base for professional human care concepts.

CRITIQUE
Clarity

Watson's theory uses nontechnical, yet sophisticated, language. At times, lengthy phrases (e.g., "symbiotic relationship between humankind-technology-nature") (Watson, 1999 p. xiv) and sentences need to be read more than once to gain meaning. Her increasing inclusion of metaphor, personal reflections, artwork, and poetry make her complex concepts more tangible and more aesthetically appealing. She continues to refine her theory and has recently revised the original carative factors which she now describes as caritas processes. The word *caritas* comes from a Greek word meaning "to cherish, to appreciate, to give special attention to—even loving attention to." Table 7-1 outlines an evolution of Watson's thinking.

Simplicity

Watson draws on a number of disciplines to formulate her theory. To understand the theory as it is presented, the reader does best by being familiar with broad subject matter. It is viewed as complex when considering the existential-phenomenological nature of her work, which is partly because many nurses have a limited liberal arts background and baccalaureate nursing curricula have limited integration of liberal arts.

Generality

The theory seeks to provide a moral and philosophical basis for nursing. The scope of the framework encompasses all aspects of the health-illness continuum. In addition, the theory addresses aspects of preventing illness and experiencing a peaceful death, thereby increasing its generality. The carative factors that Watson described have provided important guidelines for nurse-patient interactions; however, some critics have stated that the generality is limited by the emphasis placed on the psychosocial aspects rather than the physiological aspects of caring.

Another characteristic of the theory is that it does not furnish explicit directions about what to do to achieve authentic caring-healing relationships. It is more about being than about doing and it must be internalized thoroughly by the nurse to be actualized in practice. Nurses who want concrete guidelines may not feel secure when trying to rely on this theory alone.

Empirical Precision

Although the framework is difficult to study empirically, Watson draws heavily on widely accepted work from other disciplines. This solid foundation strengthens her views. Watson describes her theory as descriptive and she acknowledges the evolving nature of the theory and welcomes input by others. The theory does not lend itself to research conducted with traditional scientific methodologies. In her second book, *Nursing: Human Science and Human Care—A Theory of Nursing*, Watson (1985a) addresses the issue of methodology. The methodologies relevant to studying transpersonal caring and developing nursing as a human science and art can be classified as qualitative, naturalistic, or phenomenological. Watson does acknowledge that a

Table 7-1

Carative Factors and Caritas Process	
CARATIVE FACTORS	**CARITAS PROCESS**
1. "The formation of a humanistic-altruistic system of values"	"Practice of loving-kindness and equanimity within the context of caring consciousness"
2. "The instillation of faith-hope"	"Being authentically present and enabling and sustaining the deep belief system and subjective life-world of self and one being cared for"
3. "The cultivation of sensitivity to one's self and to others"	"Cultivation of one's own spiritual practices and transpersonal self going beyond the ego self"
4. "Development of a helping-trust relationship" became "development of a helping-trusting, human caring relation" (in 2004 Watson Web site)	"Developing and sustaining a helping trusting authentic caring relationship"
5. "The promotion and acceptance of the expression of positive and negative feelings"	"Being present to, and supportive of, the expression of positive and negative feelings as a connection with deeper spirit and self and the one-being-cared for"
6. "The systematic use of the scientific problem-solving method for decision making" became "systematic use of a creative problem-solving caring process" (in 2004 Watson Web site)	"Creative use of self and all ways of knowing as part of the caring process; to engage in the artistry of caring-healing practices"
7. "The promotion of transpersonal teaching-learning"	"Engaging in genuine teaching-learning experience that attends to unity of being and meaning attempting to stay within other's frame of reference"
8. "The provision of supportive, protective, and (or) corrective mental, physical, societal and spiritual environment"	"Creating healing environment at all levels (physical as well as nonphysical, subtle environment of energy and consciousness, whereby wholeness, beauty, comfort, dignity and peace are potentiated)"
9. "The assistance with gratification of human needs"	"Assisting with basic needs, with an intentional caring consciousness, administering 'human care essentials', which potentiate alignment of mindbodyspirit, wholeness, and unity of being in all aspects of care"
10. "The allowance for existential-phenomenological forces" became "allowance for existential-phenomenological-spiritual forces" (in 2004 Watson Web site)	"Opening and attending to spiritual-mysterious, and existential dimensions of one's own life-death; soul care for self and the one-being-cared for"

From Watson, J. (1979). *Nursing: The philosophy and science of caring* (pp. 9-10). Boston: Little, Brown & Co. (for original carative factors); and Watson, J. (2004). *Theory of human caring* (Web site). Denver, CO: Jean Watson/University of Colorado School of Nursing. Retrieved June 3, 2004, from *http://www2.uchsc.edu/son/caring/content/wct.asp* (for caritas processes and revised carative factors).

combination of qualitative-quantitative inquiry may also be useful.

Derivable Consequences

Watson's theory continues to provide a useful and important metaphysical orientation for the delivery of nursing care. Watson's theoretical concepts, such as use of self, patient-identified needs, the caring process, and the spiritual sense of being human, may help nurses and their patients find meaning and harmony in a period of increasing complexity. Watson's rich and varied knowledge of philosophy, the arts, the human sciences, and traditional science and traditions, joined with her prolific ability to communicate, has enabled professionals in many disciplines to share and recognize her work.

SUMMARY

Jean Watson began developing her theory while assistant dean of the undergraduate program and it evolved in the early planning and implementation of the nursing Ph.D. program at the University of Colorado. Her first book started as class notes that emerged from teaching in an innovative, integrated curriculum. She became coordinator and director of the Ph.D. program when it was initiated in 1978 and served until 1981. While serving as Dean of the University of Colorado School of Nursing, she was instrumental in the development of a postbaccalaureate nursing curriculum in human caring that leads to a career professional clinical doctoral degree (ND) that was implemented in 1990 and has been a national demonstration program. She initiated the Center for Human Caring that was the nation's first interdisciplinary center with a commitment to develop and use knowledge of human caring for practice and scholarship. She worked from Yalom's 11 curative factors to formulate her 10 carative factors. She modified the 10 factors slightly over time and developed the caritas processes that have a spiritual dimension and use a more fluid and evolutionary language. She added spiritual aspects. She believes that the core of nursing is those nurse-patient relationships that result in a therapeutic outcome.

Case Study

A young woman has prematurely delivered her second infant. The infant had considerable difficulty and expired shortly after birth. Her husband is with her. Some friends are taking care of their 2-year-old child. The parents of the couple live a great distance away and are working. What caring practices can the nurse implement?

CRITICAL THINKING *Activities*

Critical thinking with Watson's philosophy and science of caring offers a holistic and humanistic approach in the assessment, diagnosis, planning, implementation, and evaluation phases of the nursing process. On the basis of 10 carative assumptions, Watson's theory provides a framework on which nurses can establish a precedent of collaboration to assist the patient in gaining control, knowledge, and health. The following exercises demonstrate critical and reflective thinking from the perspective of Watson's theory:

1. Examine your own values and beliefs to ascertain how each of Watson's 10 carative assumptions would fit with your own personal philosophy of caring in relation to the patient, environment, health, and nursing.

2. Develop a mission statement with your teammates, integrating your shared beliefs about basing your practice on caring. Revisit this periodically and discuss how your values and beliefs are evolving.

3. Think of a time in your life when you felt someone truly cared for you. Then think of a time when you demonstrated care for another person. (These can be either health care–related or not.) Then identify the major characteristics of those interactions.

4. Make a list of caring behaviors from your own thoughts. Then look at *Instruments for Assessing and Measuring Caring in Nursing and Health Science* (Watson, 2002) and make a list of caring behaviors from the instruments. Compare and contrast the lists.

5. In her third book, *Postmodern Nursing and Beyond*, Watson (1999) included a chapter entitled "Exercises for Experiencing the Transpersonal Body." Her hope for the continued evolution of transpersonal caring-healing depends so strongly on the continuing spiritual evolution of each individual; therefore, a brief description of her own approach to personal meditation follows.

   She suggests that participants close their eyes, breathe deeply, and find a quiet place inside themselves. "Then allow yourself to be quiet and still . . . try to dwell there . . . feel the lovely sensation of just being still and quiet . . . and access a sense of inner peace" (Watson, 1999, p. 171). She continues the discussion by describing how the meditation can lead to a reconnection for the participant between mind and body. Watson advises, "Feel yourself in your body; explore your body and gently note points of tension" (Watson, 1999, p. 173). "Once you have explored the body and experienced the sensations, you can move to more focused breathing, concentrating on a given word, or a visual image that comforts and soothes you" (Watson, 1999, p. 174).

   The concluding words of the chapter are like a benediction. "In cultivating one's transpersonal self, one experiences the 'at-one-ment' of all. May you be graced on your spiritual journey and deepened through your contemplative practices, whatever they may be" (Watson, 1999, p. 175).

REFERENCES

Arthur, D., Pang, S., Wong, T., Alexander, M. F., Drury, J., Eastwood, et al. (1999). Caring attributes, professional self-concepts and technological, influences in a sample of registered nurses in eleven countries. *International Journal of Nursing Studies, 36*, 387-396.

Betz, B. J., & Whitehorn, J. C. (1956). *The relationship of the therapist to the outcome of therapy in schizophrenia. Research techniques in schizophrenia. Psychiatric research reports #5*. Washington, DC: American Psychiatric Association.

Brenner, P., Boyd, C., Thompson, T., Cervantez, M., Buerhaus, P., & Leininger, M. (1986, Jan.). The care symposium: Considerations for nursing administrators. *Journal of Nursing Administration, 16*(1), 25-26.

Byrd, R. (1988). Positive therapeutic effects of intercessory prayer in a coronary care unit population. *Southern Medical Journal, 81*(7), 826-829.

Clayton, G. (1989). Research testing Watson's theory. In J. Riehl-Siska (Ed.), *Conceptual models for nursing practice* (pp. 245-252). Norwalk, CT: Appleton & Lange.

Coates, C. (1997). The caring efficacy scale: Nurses' self reports of caring in practice settings. *Advanced Practice Nursing Quarterly, 3*(1), 53-59.

Cronin, S., & Harrison, B. (1988). Importance of nursing care behaviors as perceived by patient after myocardial infarction. *Heart and Lung, 17*(4), 374-380.

Gaut, D. (1983). Development of a theoretically adequate description of caring. *Western Journal of Nursing Research, 5*(4), 313-324.

Gay, S. (1999). Meeting cardiac patients' expectations of caring. *Dimensions of Critical Care Nursing, 18*(4), 46–50.

Greenhalgh, J., Vanhanen, L., & Kyngas, H. (1998). Nurse caring behaviors. *Journal of Advanced Nursing, 27*, 927-932.

Harrison, E. (1995). Nurse caring: The new health care paradigm. *Journal of Nursing Care Quality, 9*(4), 14-23.

Hester, N. O., & Ray, M. A. (1987). *Assessment of Watson's carative factors: A qualitative research study*. Paper presented at the International Nursing Research Congress, Edinburgh, Scotland.

Holroyd, E., Yue-kuen, C., Fung-shan, L., & Waiwan, W. (1998). *Journal of Advance Nursing, 28*(6), 1289-1294.

Larson, P. (1987). Comparison of cancer patients' and professional nurses' perceptions of important nurse caring behaviors. *Heart and Lung, 16*(2), 187-193.

Larsson, G., Peterson, V. W., Lampic, C., von Essen, L., & Sjoden, P. (1998). Cancer patient and staff ratings of the importance of caring behaviors and their relation to patient anxiety and depression, *Journal of Advanced Nursing, 27*, 855-864.

Lathem, C. P. (1996). Predictors of patient outcomes following interactions with nurses. *Western Journal of Nursing Research, 15*(5), 548-564.

Leininger, M. (1979). Preface. In J. Watson (Ed.), *Nursing: The philosophy and science of caring.* Boston: Little, Brown.

Manogin, T. W., Bechtel, G., & Rami, J. S. (2000). Caring behaviors by nurses: Women's perceptions during childbirth. *JOGNN, 29*(2), 153-157.

Marini, B. (1999). Institutionalized older adults' perceptions of nurse caring behaviors. *Journal of Gerontological Nursing, 25*(5), 11-16.

Miller, K. (1987). The human care perspective in nursing administration. *Journal of Nursing Administration, 17*(2), 10-12.

Montgomery, C. (1993). *Healing through communication: The practice of caring.* Newbury Park, CA: Sage.

Morse, J., Bottorff, J., Neander, W., & Solberg, S. (1991). Comparative analysis of conceptualizations and theories of caring. *Image: The Journal of Nursing Scholarship, 23*(2), 119-126.

Morse, J., Solberg, S., Neander, W., Bottorff, J., & Johnson, J. (1990). Concepts of caring and caring as a concept. *ANS Advances in Nursing Science, 13*(1), 1-14.

Mullins, I. L. (1996). Nurse caring behaviors for persons with AIDS/HIV. *Applied Nursing Research, 9*(1), 18-23.

Neil, R. (1990). Watson's theory of caring in nursing: The rainbow of and for people living with AIDS. In M. E. Parker (Ed.), *Nursing theories in practice* (pp. 289-301). New York: National League for Nursing.

Nyberg, J. (1989). The element of caring in nursing administration. *Nursing Administration Quarterly, 13*(3), 9-16.

Nyberg, J. (1998). *A caring approach in nursing administration.* Boulder, CO: University of Colorado Press.

Ray, M. (1987). Technological caring: A new model in critical care. *Dimensions of Critical Care Nursing, 6,* 166-173.

Ray, M. (1989). The theory of bureaucratic caring in nursing practice in the organizational culture. *Nursing Administration Quarterly, 13*(2), 31-42.

Rogers, C. R. (1961). *On becoming a person: A therapist's view of psychology.* Boston: Houghton Mifflin.

Sakalys, J. A., & Watson, J. (1986). Professional education: Post-baccalaureate education for professional nursing. *Journal of Professional Nursing, 2*(2), 91-97.

Schultz, A. A., Bridgham, C., Smith, M. E., & Higgins, D. (1998). Perceptions of caring: Comparison of antepartum and postpartum patients. *Clinical Nursing Research, 7,* 363-378.

Seeman, J. (1954). Counselor judgments of therapeutic process and outcome. In C. R. Rogers & R. F. Dymond (Eds.), *Psychotherapy and personality change* (pp. 272-299). Chicago: University of Chicago Press.

Sithichoke-Rattan, N. (1989). A clinical application of Watson's theory. *Pediatric Nursing, 15*(5), 458-462.

Smith, M. (1997). Nurses' and patients' perceptions of most important caring behaviors in a long-term care setting. *Geriatric Nursing, 18*(2), 70-73.

Swanson, K. (1990). Providing care in the NICU: Sometimes an act of love. *ANS Advances in Nursing Science, 13*(1), 60-73.

Swanson, K. (1991). Empirical development of a middle range theory of caring. *Nursing Research, 40*(3), 161-166.

Swanson, K. (2000). Predicting depressive symptoms after miscarriage: A path analysis based on the Lazarus Paradigm. *Journal of Women's Health & Gender Based Medicine, 9*(2), 191-206.

Watson, J. (1979). *Nursing: The philosophy and science of caring.* Boston: Little, Brown.

Watson, J. (1981, July). Nursing's scientific quest. *Nursing Outlook, 29,* 413-416.

Watson, J. (1985a). *Nursing: Human science and human care—A theory of nursing.* Norwalk, CT: Appleton-Century-Crofts.

Watson, J. (1985b). Reflections on new methodologies for study of human care. In M. Leininger (Ed.), *Qualitative research methods in nursing* (pp. 343-349). Orlando, FL: Grune & Stratton.

Watson, J. (1986, Dec.). The dean speaks out: Center for human caring established. *The University of Colorado School of Nursing News,* 1-6.

Watson, J. (1987). Nursing on the caring edge: Metaphorical vignettes. *ANS Advances in Nursing Science, 10*(1), 10-18.

Watson, J. (1988). *Nursing: Human science and human care—A theory of nursing.* New York: National League for Nursing.

Watson, J. (1995). Post modernism and knowledge development in nursing. *Nursing Science Quarterly, 8*(2), 60-64.

Watson, J. (1997). The theory of human caring: Retrospective and prospective. *Nursing Science Quarterly, 10*(1), 49-52.

Watson, J. (1999). *Postmodern nursing and beyond.* Edinburgh: Churchill Livingstone.

Watson, J. (2002). *Instruments for assessing and measuring caring in nursing and health sciences.* New York: Springer. (AJN Book of the Year Award, 2002; Japanese translation in print.)

Watson, J., Burckhardt, C., Brown, L., Block, D., & Hester, N. (1979). A model of caring: An alternative health care model for nursing practice and research. In *Clinical and scientific sessions: Division of practice* (pp. 32-44, Order No. NP-59 3W8179190), Kansas City, MO: American Nurses Association.

Watson, R., & Lea, A. (1997). The caring dimensions inventory (CDI): Content validity, reliability and scaling. *Journal of Advanced Nursing, 25,* 87-94.

Wolf, Z. R., Miller, P. D., & Devine, M. (1998). Relationship between nurse caring and patient satisfaction, *MEDSURG Nursing, 7*(2), 99-105.

BIBLIOGRAPHY
Primary Sources
Publications

A continually updated list of caring theory publications is available through the University of Colorado School of Nursing Web site at *http://www.uchsc.edu/nursing/watsoncaring.html*. Accessed June 3, 2004.

Books

Bevis, E. O., & Watson, J. (1989, reprinted in 2000). *Toward a caring curriculum: A new pedagogy for nursing.* New York: National League for Nursing.

Chinn, P., & Watson, J. (Eds.). (1994). *Art and aesthetics of nursing.* New York: National League for Nursing.

Leininger, M., & Watson, J. (Eds.). (1990). *The caring imperative in education.* New York: National League for Nursing.

Taylor, R., & Watson, J. (Eds.). (1989). *They shall not hurt: Human suffering and human caring.* Boulder, CO: University Press of Colorado.

Watson, J. (1979, reprinted 1985 by University Press of Colorado). *Nursing: The philosophy and science of caring.* Boston: Little, Brown. [Translated into French.]

Watson, J. (1985, reprinted 1988, reprinted by NLN & Bartlett, 1999). *Nursing: Human science and human care.* Norwalk, CT: Appleton-Century-Crofts. [Translated into Japanese, Swedish, Chinese, Korean, German, Norwegian, and Danish.]

Watson, J. (1985). *Nursing: The philosophy and science of caring* [2nd printing]. Boulder, CO: University Press of Colorado.

Watson, J. (1988). *Nursing: Human science and human care* [2nd printing]. New York: National League for Nursing. [Translated into Japanese, 1990.]

Watson, J. (1999). *Postmodern nursing and beyond.* Edinburgh, Scotland: Churchill Livingstone/W. B. Saunders. [Translated into Japanese, 2001.]

Watson, J. (2002). *Instruments for assessing and measuring caring in nursing and health sciences.* New York: Springer. [AJN Book of the Year Award, 2002; Japanese translation in print.]

Watson, J. (2005). *Caring science as sacred science.* Philadelphia: F. A. Davis.

Watson, J. (Ed.). (1994). *Applying the art and science of human caring.* New York: National League for Nursing.

Watson, J., Jones, W., & Levin, J. (Eds.). (1999). *Essentials of complementary alternative medicine.* Philadelphia: Lippincott Williams & Wilkins.

Watson, J., & Ray, M. (Eds.). (1988). *The ethics of care and the ethics of cure: Synthesis in chronicity.* New York: National League for Nursing.

Chapters, Monographs, and Forewords

Watson, J. (1980). Self losses. In F. Bower (Ed.), *Nursing and the concept of loss* (pp. 51-84). New York: Wiley.

Watson, J. (1981). Some issues related to a science of caring for nursing practice. In M. Leininger (Ed.), *Caring: An essential human need* (pp. 61-67). Proceedings from National Caring Conference, University of Utah. Thorofare, NJ: Charles B. Slack.

Watson, J. (1982). The nurse-client relationship. In L. Sonstegard, K. Kowalski, & B. Jennings (Eds.), *Women's health care* (pp. 45-56). New York: Grune & Stratton.

Watson, J. (1983). Delivery and assurance of quality health care: A rights based foundation. In R. Luke, J. Krueger, & R. Madrow (Eds.), *Organization and change in health care quality assurance* (pp. 13-19). Rockville, MD: Aspen Systems.

Watson, J. (1985). Reflection on different methodologies for the future of nursing. In M. Leininger (Ed.), *Qualitative research methods in nursing* (pp. 343-349). Orlando, FL: Grune & Stratton.

Watson, J. (1987). The dream curriculum. In National League for Nursing (Ed.), *Patterns in nursing: Strategic planning for nursing education* (pp. 91-104). New York: Author.

Watson, J. (1988). A case study: Curriculum in transition. In National League for Nursing (Ed.), *Curriculum revolution: Mandate for change* (pp. 1-8). New York: Author.

Watson, J. (1988). Introduction. In J. Watson & M. Ray (Eds.), *The ethics of care and the ethics of cure: Synthesis in chronicity* (pp. 1-3). New York: National League for Nursing.

Watson, J. (1988). The professional doctorate as an entry level into practice. In National League for Nursing (Ed.), *Perspectives* (pp. 41-47). New York: Author.

Watson, J. (1989). Human caring and suffering: A subjective model for health sciences. In R. Taylor & J. Watson (Eds.), *They shall not hurt* (pp. 125-135). Boulder, CO: University Press of Colorado.

Watson, J. (1989). Preface and introduction. In M. Krysl (Ed.), *Midwife and other poems on caring* (pp. v, vii-viii). New York: National League for Nursing.

Watson, J. (1989). Watson's philosophy and theory of human caring in nursing. In J. Riehl-Sisca (Ed.), *Conceptual models for nursing practice* (3rd ed.) (pp. 219-236). Norwalk, CT: Appleton & Lange.

Watson, J. (1990). Foreword. In L. Hill & N. Smith (Eds.), *Self care nursing: Promotion of health* (pp. xi-xii). Norwalk, CT: Appleton & Lange.

Watson, J. (1990). Human caring: A public agenda. From revolution to renaissance. In J. Stevenson & T. Tripp-Reiner (Eds.), *Knowledge about care and caring: State of the art and future developments* (pp. 41-48).

Proceedings of a Wingspread Conference, Racine, WI, Feb. 1-3, 1989. St. Louis: American Academy of Nursing.

Watson, J. (1990). Informed moral passion. In *Proceedings for the 1989 National Forum of Doctoral Education in Nursing*, Indianapolis: Indiana University School of Nursing.

Watson, J. (1990). Preface. In G. Gaut & M. Leininger (Eds.), *Caring: The compassionate healer*. New York: National League for Nursing.

Watson, J. (1990). Preface. In M. Leininger & J. Watson (Eds.), *The caring imperative in education* (pp. xiii-xiv). New York: National League for Nursing.

Watson, J. (1990). Transformation in nursing: Bring care back to health care. In National League for Nursing (Ed.), *Curriculum revolution: Redefining the student-teacher relationship* (pp. 15-20). New York: National League for Nursing.

Watson, J. (1990). Transpersonal caring: A transcendent view of person, health, and healing. In M. Parker (Ed.), *Nursing theories in practice* (pp. 277-288). New York: National League for Nursing.

Watson, J. (1991). Foreword. In A. Pearson & R. McMahon (Eds.), *Nursing as therapy*. London & New York: Chapman and Hall.

Watson, J. (1991). Introduction. In M. Leininger (Ed.), *Theory of transcultural nursing*. New York: National League for Nursing.

Watson, J. (1991). Preface: The caring imperative on education. In R. Neil & R. Watts (Eds.), *Caring and nursing: Explorations in feminist perspectives* (pp. ix-x). New York: National League for Nursing.

Watson, J. (1992). Notes on nursing: Guidelines for caring then and now. In F. Nightingale (Ed.), *Notes on nursing*. Philadelphia: J. B. Lippincott.

Watson, J. (1992). Prelude. In E. Gee (Ed.), *The light around the dark*. New York: National League for Nursing.

Watson, J. (1994). A frog, a rock, a ritual: An eco-caring cosmology. In E. Schuster & C. Brown (Eds.), *Caring and environmental connection*. New York: National League for Nursing.

Watson, J. (1994). Anthology on art and esthetics. In J. Watson & P. Chinn (Eds.), *Art and aesthetics as passage between centuries*. New York: National League for Nursing.

Watson, J. (1994). Foreword/chapter. In C. Johns (Ed.), *The Burford NDU model. Caring in practice*. Oxford: Blackwell Scientific.

Watson, J. (1994). Introduction. In J. Watson (Ed.), *Applying the art and science of human caring* (pp. 1-10). New York: National League for Nursing.

Watson, J. (1994). Overview of caring theory. In J. Watson (Ed.), *Applying the art and science of human caring*. New York: National League for Nursing.

Watson, J. (1994). Poeticizing as truth through language. In P. L. Chinn & J. Watson (Eds.), *Art and aesthetics in nursing* (pp. 3-17). New York: National League for Nursing.

Watson, J. (1995). Into the future. In O. Slevin & L. Basford (Eds.), *Theory and practice of nursing: An integrated approach to patient care* (2nd ed.). Cheltenham, UK: Nelson Thornes.

Watson, J. (1996). Art, caring, spirituality, and humanity. In E. Farmer (Ed.), *Exploring the spiritual dimension of care* (pp. 29-40). Wiltshire, England: Mark Allen.

Watson, J. (1996). Artistry and caring: Heart and soul of nursing. In D. Marks-Maran & P. Rose (Eds.), *Reconstructing nursing: Beyond art and science* (pp. 54-63). London: Bailliere Tindall Ltd (Division of Harcourt Brace).

Watson, J. (1996). Beyond art and science. In D. Marks-Maran & P. Rose (Eds.), *Reconstructing nursing: Beyond art and science*. London: Bailliere Tindall.

Watson, J. (1996). Foreword. In A. Pearson & R. McMahon (Eds.), *Nursing as therapy* (2nd printing, 1998). Cheltenham, UK: Stanley Thomas.

Watson, J. (1996). Nursing, caring-healing paradigm. In D. Pesat (Ed.), *Capsules of comments in psychiatric nursing*. St. Louis: Mosby.

Watson, J. (1996). Poeticizing as truth on nursing inquiry. In J. Kikuchi, H. Simmons, & D. Romyn (Eds.), *Truth on nursing inquiry* (pp. 125-138). Thousand Oaks, CA: Sage.

Watson, J. (1996). Watson's theory of transpersonal caring. In P. J. Walker & B. Neuman (Eds.), *Blueprint for use of nursing models: Education, research, practice and administration* (pp. 141-184). New York: National League for Nursing Press.

Watson, J. (1997). A meta-reflection of reflective practice. In C. Johns (Ed.), *Reflective practice*. Oxford, UK: Blackwell Science.

Watson, J. (1997). Window on theory of human caring (special contributor). In M. T. O'Toole (Ed.), *Miller-Keane encyclopedia & dictionary of medicine, nursing, & allied health*. Philadelphia: W. B. Saunders.

Watson, J. (1999). Alternative therapies and nursing practice. In J. Watson (Ed.), *Nurse's handbook of alternative and complementary therapies*. Springhouse, PA: Springhouse.

Watson, J. (1999). Foreword. In B. M. Dossey, L. Keegan, & C. Guzzetta (Eds.), *Holistic nursing: A handbook for practice* (3rd ed.). Gaithersburg, MD: Aspen Publishers.

Watson, J. (1999). Postmodern nursing and beyond. In N. Chaska (Ed.), *The nursing profession: Nursing theories and nursing practice* (pp. 343-354). Philadelphia: F. A. Davis.

Watson, J. (1999). Postscript. In C. Johns (Ed.), *Becoming a reflective practitioner*. Oxford, UK: Blackwell Science.

Watson, J. (2000). Foreword. In M. Knapp & M. Knapp, *Souls that are linked*, Britan Della Cor Publisher.

Watson, J. (2000). *Monograph of instruments for measuring and assessing caring*. New York: Springer Publishing.

Watson, J. (2000). Postmodern nursing and beyond. In N. L. Chaska (Ed.), *The nursing profession: Tomorrow's vision and beyond* (pp. 299-308). Thousand Oaks, CA: Sage.

Watson, J. (2000). Reconsidering caring in the home. In R. Rice (Ed.), *Home care nursing practice: Concepts, applications* (3rd ed.). St. Louis: Mosby.

Watson, J. (2000). Theory of human caring. In J. M. Parker (Ed.), *Nursing theories in practice*. Philadelphia: F. A. Davis.

Watson, J. (2001). Foreword. In M. A. Anderson, *Nursing leadership: Management and professional practice* (pp. v-vi). Philadelphia: F. A. Davis.

Watson, J. (2001). Foreword. In R. Locsin (Ed.), *Advancing technology, caring, nursing*. Westport, CT: Auburn House.

Watson, J. (2001). Jean Watson: Theory of human caring. In M. E. Parker (Ed.), *Nursing theories and nursing practice* (pp. 343-354). Philadelphia: F. A. Davis.

Watson, J. (2002). Illuminating the spiritual journey. Jean Watson tells her story. In P. Burkhardt & M. G. Nagai-Jackson (Eds.), *Spirituality: Living our connectedness* (pp. 181-186). New York: Delmar.

Watson, J. (2003). Meditation: Contemplative practice. In K. Wren & C. Norred, *Real-world nursing survival guide*. Philadelphia: Harcourt.

Watson, J. (2004). Epilogue on home health nursing. In R. Rice (Ed.), *Home care nursing: Practice and concepts* (4th ed.). St. Louis: Elsevier.

Watson, J. (2004). Foreword. In M. Koloroutis (Ed.), *Creative health care management. Relationship-based care delivery: A model for transforming care*. Minneapolis: Creative Health Care Management.

Watson, J. (2004). Foreword. In K. Sitz, *Understanding nursing theory: A creative beginning*. Sudbury, MA: Jones and Bartlett.

Watson, J. (2004, in press). Foreword. In L. Wright, *Spirituality, suffering, and illness*. Philadelphia: F. A. Davis.

Watson, J. (1998, 2005). Meta-reflection of reflective practice and where it leads. In C. Johns & D. Freshwater (Eds.), *Tranforming nursing through reflective practice* Oxford UK: Blackwell Science Oxford, UK: Blackwell.

Watson, J. (2001, 2005). Jean Watson's Theory of Human Caring. In M. Parker (Ed.), *Nursing theories and nursing practice*. Philadelphia: F. A. Davis.

Watson, J., & Bevis, E. (1990). Coming of age for a new age. In N. L. Chaska (Ed.), *The nursing profession: Turning points* (pp. 100-105). St. Louis: Mosby.

Watson, J., Burckhardt, C., Brown, L., Block, D., & Hester, N. (1979). Model of caring: An alternative health care model for nursing and research. *Clinical and Scientific Sessions* (pp. 32-44). Kansas City, MO: American Nurses Association.

Watson, J., & Chinn, P. L. (1994). Art and esthetics as passage between centuries. In J. Watson & P. L. Chinn (Eds.), *Art and esthetics nursing* (pp. xiii-xviii). New York: National League for Nursing.

Watson, J., & Chinn, P. L. (1994). Introduction to esthetics and art of nursing. In P. L. Chinn & J. Watson (Eds.), *Anthology on art and esthetics in nursing*. New York: National League for Nursing.

Watson, J., Jackson, R., & Borbasi, S. (2004, in press). Constructing caring. In S. Borbasi (Ed.), *Caring and the discipline of nursing*. Melbourne, Australia: Blackwell.

Watson, J., & Ray, M. (Eds) (1988). *The ethics of care and the ethics of cure synthesis in chronicity*. New York: National League for Nursing.

Journal Articles

Carozza, V., Congdon, J. A., & Watson, J. (1978, Nov.). An experimental educationally sponsored pilot internship program. *Journal of Nursing Education, 17*, 14-20.

Fawcett, J., Watson, J., Neuman, B., & Hinton-Walker, P. (2001). On missing theories and evidence. *Journal of Nursing Scholarship, 33*(2), 115-119.

Krysl, M., & Watson, J. (1988, Jan.). Poetry on caring and addendum on center for human caring. *ANS Advances in Nursing Science, 10*(2), 12-17.

Quinn, J., Smith, M., Swanson, K., Ritenbaugh, C., & Watson, J. (2003). The healing relationship in clinical nursing: Guidelines for research. *Journal of Alternative Therapies, 9*(3), A65-A79.

Sakalys, J., & Watson, J. (1985, Sept./Oct.). New directions in higher education: A review of trends. *Journal of Professional Nursing, 1*(5), 293-299.

Sakalys, J., & Watson, J. (1986, Mar./Apr.). Professional education: Post-baccalaureate education for professional nursing. *Journal of Professional Nursing, 2*(2), 91-97.

Watson, J. (1968, Feb.). Death—A necessary concern for nurses. *Nursing Outlook, 15*(1), 448. [Reprinted as Watson, J. (1972). Death—A necessary concern for nurses. In *The dying patient: A nursing perspective* (Contemporary Nursing Series, pp. 196-200). New York: American Journal of Nursing Publication Co.]

Watson, J. (1976). Research and literature on children's responses to injections: Some general nursing implications. *Pediatric Nursing, 2*(1), 7-8.

Watson, J. (1976). Research: Question-answer. Creative approach to researchable questions. *Nursing Research, 25*(6), 439.

Watson, J. (1976, Jan./Feb.). The quasi-rational element in conflict: A review of selected conflict literature. *Nursing Research, 25,* 19-23.

Watson, J. (1977). Follow-up study of University of Colorado undergraduate nursing program. *Colorado Nurse, 77*(1), 6-19.

Watson, J. (1978). Conceptual systems of undergraduate nursing students compared with college students at large and practicing nurses. *Nursing Research, 27*(3), 151-155.

Watson, J. (1979). Research answer. Content analysis. *Western Journal of Nursing Research, 1*(3), 214-219.

Watson, J. (1980). [Response to review of *Nursing: Philosophy and science of caring*]. *Western Journal of Nursing Research, 2*(2), 514-515.

Watson, J. (1980). [Review of the book *Nursing: Philosophy and science of caring*]. *Western Journal of Nursing Research, 2*(2), 514-515.

Watson, J. (1980). [Review of the book *Starting point: An introduction to the dialectic of existence*]. *Western Journal of Nursing Research, 2*(3), 637-638.

Watson, J. (1981). Conceptual systems of students and practicing nurses. *Western Journal of Nursing Research, 3*(2), 172-192.

Watson, J. (1981). Nursing's scientific quest. *Nursing Outlook, 29*(7), 413-416.

Watson, J. (1981, Aug.). Professional identity crisis— Is nursing finally growing up? *American Journal of Nursing, 81,* 1488-1490.

Watson, J. (1981). Response to Conceptual systems, students, practitioner. *Western Journal of Nursing Research, 3*(2), 197-198.

Watson, J. (1981, reprinted 1983). The lost art of nursing. *Nursing Forum, 20*(3), 244-249.

Watson, J. (1982, Aug.). Traditional v. tertiary: Ideological shifts in nursing education. *The Australian Nurses Journal, 12*(2), 44-46.

Watson, J. (1983, Fall). Commentary on instructor directed research model. *Western Journal of Nursing Research, 5*(4), 310-311.

Watson, J. (1987, Oct.). Nursing on the caring edge: Metaphorical vignettes. *ANS Advances in Nursing Science, X*(1), 10-18.

Watson, J. (1987). [Review of the book *Health as expanding consciousness*]. *Journal of Professional Nursing, 3*(5), 315.

Watson, J. (1987). [Review of the book *Practical psychotherapy*]. *Journal of Psychosocial Nursing and Mental Health Services, 25*(3), 42.

Watson, J. (1988). Human caring as moral context for nursing education. *Nursing and Health Care, 9*(8), 422-425.

Watson, J. (1988). New dimensions of human caring theory. *Nursing Science Quarterly, 1*(4), 175-181.

Watson, J. (1988). Of nurses, women and the devaluation of caring. [Review of the book *Images of Nurses: Perspectives for history, art, and literature*]. *Medical Humanities Review, 2*(2), 60-62.

Watson, J. (1988). Response to caring and practice. Construction of the nurses' world. *Scholarly Inquiry for Nursing Practice: An International Journal, 2*(3), 217-221.

Watson, J. (1989). Caring theory. *Journal of Japan Academy of Nursing Science, 9*(2), 29-37.

Watson, J. (1989, Oct.). Keynote address: Caring theory. *Journal of Japan Academy of Nursing Science, 9*(2), 9-37.

Watson, J. (1990). Caring knowledge and informed moral passion. *ANS Advances in Nursing Science, 13*(1), 15-24.

Watson, J. (1990). Caring knowledge and informed moral passion. *ANS Advances in Nursing Science, 15*(1), 13-24.

Watson, J. (1990). Reconceptualizing nursing ethics: A response. *Scholarly Inquiry for Nursing Practice: An International Journal, 4*(3), 219-221.

Watson, J. (1990). The moral failure of the patriarchy. *Nursing Outlook, 28*(2), 62-66.

Watson, J. (1991). From revolution to renaissance. *Revolution: Journal of Nurse Empowerment, 1*(1), 94-100.

Watson, J. (1991). Robb, Dock, and Nutting: I wish I'd been there. *Nursing and Health Care, 12*(4), 210.

Watson, J. (1992). Response to caring, virtue, theory, and a foundation for nursing ethics. *Scholarly Inquiry for Nursing Practice: An International Journal, 6*(2), 169-171.

Watson, J. (1992, Summer). Response to caring, virtue through a foundation for nursing ethics. A response to Pamela Salsberry. *Scholarly Inquiry for Nursing Practice: An International Journal, 6*(2), 169-171.

Watson, J., & Phillips, S. (1992). A call for educational reform: Colorado nursing doctorate model as exemplar. *Nursing Outlook, 40,* 20-26.

Watson, J. (1993). Dr. Jean Watson with E. Henderson— An interview. *Alberta Association of Registered Nurses Newsletter, 49*(6), 10-12.

Watson, J. (1993). Should NPs, CNMs, and CNAs, etc., add graduate credentials? *Open Mind, 2*(3), 2.

Watson, J. (1994). Guest editorial. *Nursing Praxis in New Zealand, 9*(1), 2-5.

Watson, J. (1994). Have we arrived or are we on our way out? Promises, possibilities, and paradigms. (Invited editorial). *Image: The Journal of Nursing Scholarship, 26*(2), 86.

Watson, J. (1995). Advanced nursing practice and what might be. *Journal of Nursing and Health Care, 16*(2), 78-83.

Watson, J. (1995). A Fulbright in Sweden: Runes, academics, archetypal motifs, and other things. *Image: The Journal of Nursing Scholarship, 27*(1), 71-75.

Watson, J. (1995). A yearning for new debates. *NLN Update, 1*(3), 6-8.

Watson, J. (1995). Nursing's caring-healing model as an exemplar for alternative medicine. *Journal of Alternative Therapies in Health and Medicine, 1*(3), 64-69.

Watson, J. (1995). Postmodernism and knowledge development in nursing. *Nursing Science Quarterly, 8*(2), 60-64.

Watson, J. (1995). President's message: Challenges and summons from within and without. *Journal of Nursing and Health Care, 16*(6), 340.

Watson, J. (1995). President's message: Visioning on: Toward action transformation. *Journal of Nursing and Health Care, 16*(5), 290.

Watson, J. (1995). [Review of the book *Healing power of aromatherapy*]. *Journal of Alternative Therapies in Health and Medicine, 1*(3), 64-69.

Watson, J. (1996). President's message: From discipline specific to "inter" to "multi" to "transdisciplinary" health care education and practice. *Journal of Nursing and Health Care, 17*(2), 90-91.

Watson, J. (1996, May). [Review of the book *Healing nutrition*]. *Journal of Alternative Therapies in Health and Medicine, 2*(3), 91.

Watson, J. (1996, May). The wait, the wonder, the watch: Caring in a transplant unit. *Journal of Clinical Nursing, 5*(3), 199-200.

Watson, J. (1996). United States of America: Can nursing theory and practice survive? *International Journal of Nursing Practice, 2*(4), 241-243.

Watson, J. (1997). Dancing for life. New questions for nursing: To dance or not to dance? *Scholarly Inquiry for Nursing Practice*, ••.

Watson, J. (1997). From the mountaintop to the marsh/fens: Punting on the River Cam. (Guest editorial). *Journal of Clinical Nursing, 6*(1), 3-4.

Watson, J. (1997). [Review of the book *Kitchen table wisdom*].

Watson, J. (1997). The future of nursing-scholarship. *Image: The Journal of Nursing Scholarship, 29*(2), 117.

Watson, J. (1997). The theory of human caring: Retrospective and prospective. *Nursing Science Quarterly, 10*(1), 49-52.

Watson, J. (1998). Nightingale and the enduring legacy of transpersonal human caring. *Journal of Holistic Nursing, 16*(2), 292.

Watson, J. (1999, Spring). Aesthetic expressions of caring: Private psalms—Surrendering to the sacred. Personal professional reflections on caring and healing. *International Journal of Human Caring, 3*(3), 34.

Watson, J. (2000). Leading via caring-healing: The fourfold way toward transformative leadership. *Nursing Administration Quarterly, 25*(1), 1-6.

Watson, J. (2000). Philosophical perspectives in home care: Reconsidering caring. *Journal of Geriatric Nursing, 21*(6), 330-331.

Watson, J. (2000). Reconsidering caring in the home. *Journal of Geriatric Nursing, 21*(6), 330-333.

Watson, J. (2000). Via negative: Considering caring by way of non-caring. *Australian Journal of Holistic Nursing, 7*(1), 4-8.

Watson, J. (2001). Post-hospital nursing: Shortages, shifts, and script. *Nursing Administration Quarterly, 25*(3), 77-82.

Watson, J. (2002). Caring and healing our living and dying. *The International Nurse, 14*(2), 4-5.

Watson, J. (2002). Holistic nursing and caring: A values-based approach. *Journal of Japan Academy of Nursing Science, 22*(2), 69-74.

Watson, J. (2002). Intentionality and caring-healing consciousness: A theory of transpersonal nursing. *Holistic Nursing Journal, 16*(4), 12-19.

Watson, J. (2002). Metaphysics of virtual caring communities. *International Journal of Human Caring, 6*(1).

Watson, J. (2002, Spring). Nursing: Seeking its source and survival [Guest editorial]. *ICU Nursing Web Journal, Spring*(9), 1-7. Retrieved June, 7, 2004, from http://www.nursing.gr/J.W.editorial.pdf.

Watson, J. (2003). Love and caring: Ethics of face and hand. *Nursing Administration Quarterly, 27*(3), 197-202.

Watson, J. (2004). Caritas and communitas: An ethic for caring science. *Journal Japan Academy of Nursing Science, 24*(3), 66-67.

Watson, J. (2004). The relational core of nursing practice as partnership [Invited commentary]. *Journal of Advanced Nursing, 47*(3).

Watson, J. Bauer, R., & Biley, F. (2002). Bavarian nursing secret: An inside view. *Reflections on Nursing Leadership: Sigma Theta Tau International Magazine, 28*(1), 26-28.

Watson, J., Biley, F. C., & Biley, A. M. (2001). Aesthetics, postmodern nursing, complementary therapies and more: An Internet dialogue. *Theoria: Journal of Nursing Theory, 10*(3), 13-16.

Watson, J., Biley, F. C., & Biley, A. M. (2002). Aesthetics, postmodern nursing, complementary therapies, and more: An Internet dialogue. *Complementary Therapies in Nursing and Midwifery, 8*, 81-83.

Watson, J., & Foster, R. (2003). The Attending Nurse Caring Model: Integrating theory, evidence, and advanced caring-healing therapeutics for transforming professional practice. *Journal of Clinical Nursing, 12*, 360-365.

Watson, J., & Smith, M. C. (2002). Caring science and the science of unitary human beings: A trans-theoretical discourse for nursing knowledge development. *Journal of Advanced Nursing, 7*(5), 452-461.

Abstracts, Proceedings, and Other Publications

Bevis, E., & Watson, J. (1989). *Coming of age for a new age* (Abstract). International Council of Nurses, 19th Quadrennial Congress. Seoul, Korea.

Watson, J. (1975, Dec.). Invitational farewell address to graduating class of 1975. *CU School of Nursing Commencement Exercise Bulletin.* Denver, CO.

Watson, J. (1977, Feb.). Preparation of faculty for nurse practitioner role. The future of nurse practitioners. *Proceedings of WICHE Conference,* Boulder, CO: Western Interstate Commission for Higher Education.

Watson, J. (1978, Jan.). Integration of practitioner skills in an undergraduate nursing curriculum. *Proceedings of HEW, Division of Nursing Conference,* Denver.

Watson, J. (1979, Dec.). *Terminal progress report, HEW research project, division of nursing research, conceptual systems, students, practitioners.* (Health, Education, and Welfare Report No. NU-000590). Washington, DC.

Watson, J. (1981, Apr.). The need to clarify faculty governance. (University of Colorado publication). *Silver and Gold Record,* 2.

Watson, J. (1982). A hospice home care program. *Kellogg Publication* (No. 2). Centre for Advanced Studies in Health Sciences, Western Australian Institute of Technology. Based on presentation at international conference. Care of Dying in Australia and Third World, Perth, Western Australia.

Watson, J. (1982). Changing demands and perspectives in nursing education. *Kellogg Publication* (No. 4). Centre for Advanced Studies in Health Sciences, Australia Institute of Technology, Perth: Western Australia.

Watson, J. (1982). Ethical issues in nursing and health sciences. *Kellogg Publication* (No. 6). Centre for Advanced Studies in Health Sciences, West Australia Institute of Technology, Perth: Western Australia.

Watson, J. (1982). *Final Report.* Visiting Kellogg Fellow Centre for Advanced Studies Division of Health Sciences. West Australia Institute of Technology, Bentley, Western Australia.

Watson, J. (1982). Ideological shifts between traditional hospital training and tertiary nursing education. *Kellogg Publication* (No.7). Centre for Advanced Studies in Health Sciences, West Australia Institute of Technology, Perth: Western Australia.

Watson, J. (1982). Issues of interdisciplinary health education and practice. *Kellogg Publication* (No. 3). Centre for Advanced Studies in Health Sciences, West Australia Institute of Technology, Perth: Western Australia.

Watson, J. (1982). Nursing's "new" art and "new" science. *Kellogg Publication* (No. 5). Centre for Advanced Studies in Health Sciences, West Australia Institute of Technology, Perth: Western Australia.

Watson, J. (1982). Review of the misguided cell. *Kellogg Publication* (No. 8). Centre for Advanced Studies in Health Sciences, Sunderland, MA: Sinauer Associates.

Watson, J. (1982). Understanding loss and grief. *Kellogg Publication* (No. 1). Centre for Advanced Studies in Health Sciences, Western Australia Institute of Tech-

nology, Perth: Western Australia. Based on presentation at international conference. Care of Dying in Australia and Third World, Perth, Perth: Western Australia.

Watson, J. (1983-1984). University of Colorado planning directions for year 2000. *University of Colorado School of Nursing Newsletter,* 1 Denver, CO.

Watson, J. (1984-1990). The Dean speaks out. *University of Colorado School of Nursing Newsletter.* Denver, CO.

Watson, J. (1985, Jan.). *Nursing education and current trends—Needs and supply data.* Report to Colorado Commission on Higher Education. Denver, CO.

Watson, J. (1987). *Academic and clinical collaboration: Advancing the art and science of human caring* (Communicating nursing research, vol. 20; Collaboration in nursing research: Advancing the science of human care, pp. 1-16). Proceedings of the Western Society for Research in Nursing Conference, Western Institute of Nursing, Tempe, AZ.

Watson, J. (1989). *Humanitarian-human caring paradigm for nursing education* (Abstract). International Council of Nurses, 19th Quadrennial Congress, Seoul, Korea.

Watson, J. (1993). *Poeticizing as truth.* Proceedings of 1993 Institute for Philosophical Nursing, University of Alberta, Canada.

Watson, J. (1994). *Postmodern crisis in science and method.* Proceedings of National Institutes of Health-Office of Alternative Medicine Conference, Bethesda, MD.

Watson, J. (2000). *Importance of story and health care.* Second National Gathering on Relationship-Centered Caring, Fetzer Institute Conference, Scottsdale, AZ.

Watson, J. (2001). *Reconnecting spirit: Caring and healing our living and dying.* International Parish Nursing Conference, Westberg Symposium, St. Louis, MO.

Unpublished Manuscript

Watson, J. (1973). *The effect of feelings and various forms of feedback upon conflict in a political group problem-solving situation.* Unpublished doctoral dissertation, University of Colorado, Denver.

Audiovisual or Media Productions

Watson, J. (1974). *Interview of patient with progressive-permanent threat to steady state maintenance—Mr. J.* (Audiotape). Denver: University of Colorado School of Nursing Learning Resource Laboratory.

Watson, J. (1981, Fall). *A phenomenological approach to person* (Videotape). Denver: University of Colorado Health Sciences Center Educational Resources Production.

Watson, J. (1987, Feb.). *The balance between objectivity and caring* (Audiotape). Denver: The Value of Many Voices Conference, Rose Medical Center, The Center for Applied Biomedical Ethics.

Watson, J. (1988). *It's nice to be loved* (Videotape about the Denver Nursing Project in Human Caring). Denver: Raven Films.

Watson, J. (1988). *The power of caring: the power to make a difference* (Videotape). Denver: Center for Human Caring, University of Colorado Health Sciences Center, School of Nursing.

Watson, J. (1989). *The nurse theorists: portraits of excellence* (Videotape). New York: Helene Fuld Health Trust.

Watson, J. (1989). *Theories at work* (Videotape). New York: National League for Nursing.

Watson, J. (1994). *A guide to applying the art and science of human caring* (Videotape). Denver: University of Colorado, Center for Human Caring.

Watson, J. (1994). *Applying the art and science of human caring. Parts I and II* (Videotape). New York: National League for Nursing, in conjunction with Denver: University of Colorado, Center for Human Caring.

Watson, J. (1996). *Nursing perspectives.* In Alternative medicine: Implications for clinical practice (Video conference; David Eisenberg, M. D., director). Boston: Harvard Medical School Department of Continuing Education and Beth Israel Hospital Department of Medicine.

Watson, J. (1999). *Private psalms. A mantra and meditation for healing* (CD-ROM). Denver: University of Colorado Health Sciences Center Bookstore. (Music by Dallas Smith and Susan Mazer). (Available from traci.mathis@uchsc.edu.)

Watson, J., Chinn, P., & Schroeder, C. (1992). *A dialogue with nursing theorists* (Videotape). Denver: University of Colorado Health Sciences Center Production.

Watson, J., Peterson, C., & Walsh, K. (1974, Nov.). *Surgical preparation of hospitalized child* (Videotape). Denver: University of Colorado Medical Center Educational Resources Production.

SECONDARY SOURCES
Book

Brencick, J., & Webster, G. (1999). *Philosophy of nursing.* Albany, NY: State University of New York.

Chapters and Monographs

Burns, P. (1991). Elements of spirituality and Watson's theory of transpersonal caring. Expansion of focus. In P. L. Chinn (Ed.), *Anthology of caring* (pp. 141-153). New York: National League for Nursing.

Duffy, J. R. (1992). The impact of nursing caring on patient outcomes. In D. Gaut (Ed.), *The presence of caring in nursing* (pp. 113-136). New York: National League for Nursing.

Fawcett, J. (2000). Watson's theory of human caring. In J. Fawcett (Ed.), *Analysis and evaluation of contemporary nursing knowledge: Nursing models and theories* (pp. 657-687). Philadelphia: F. A. Davis.

Morris, D. L. (1998). Watson's human care model. In J. J. Fitzpatrick (Ed.), *Encyclopedia of Nursing Research* (pp. 593-595). New York: Springer.

Neil, R. M. (1990). Watson's theory of caring in nursing. The rainbow of and for people living with AIDS. In M. E. Parker (Ed.), *Nursing theories in practice* (pp. 289-301). New York: National League for Nursing.

Neil, R. M. (1995). Evidence in support of basing a nursing center on nursing theory: The Denver nursing project in human caring. In B. Murphy (Ed.), *Nursing centers: The time is now* (pp. 33-46). New York: National League for Nursing.

Nyberg, J. (1994). Implementing Watson's theory of caring. In J. Watson (Ed.), *Applying the art and science of human caring* (pp. 53-61). New York: National League for Nursing.

Journal Articles

Bent, K. N. (1999). The ecologies of community caring. *ANS Advances in Nursing Science, 21,* 29-36.

Biley, A. (2000). [Review of the book *Postmodern nursing and beyond*]. *Journal of Clinical Nursing, 9,* 649-653.

Burchiel, R. N. (1995). The Watson theory of human care applied to ASPO/Lamaze perinatal education. *Journal of Perinatal Education, 6,* 1, 43-47.

Coates, C. J. (1997). The caring efficacy scale: Nurses' self-reports of caring in practice settings. *Advanced Practice Nursing Quarterly, 3*(1), 53-59.

Eddins, B. B., & Riley-Eddins, E. A. (1997). Watson's theory of human caring: The twentieth century and beyond. *Journal of Multicultural Nursing and Health, 3,* 30-35.

Falk, R., & Adeline, R. (2000). Watson's philosophy, science and theory of human caring as a conceptual framework for guiding community health nursing practice. *ANS Advances in Nursing Science, 23*(2), 34-50.

Fawcett, J. (2002). The nurse theorists: 21st century updates—Jean Watson. *Nursing Science Quarterly, 15*(3), 214-219.

From, M. A. (1995). Utilizing the home setting to teach Watson's theory of human caring. *Nursing Forum, 30,* 5-11.

Horrigan, B. (2000). Regions hospital opens holistic nursing unit. *Alternative Therapies, 6*(4), 92-93.

Jensen, K. P., Back-Pettersson, S. R., & Segesten, K. M. (1993). The caring moment and the green-thumb phenomenon among Swedish nurses. *Nursing Science Quarterly, 6,* 98-104.

Kilby, J. W. (1997). Case study: Transpersonal caring theory in perinatal loss. *Journal of Perinatal Education, 6*(2), 45-50.

Marck, B. B. (1995). Watson's theory of caring: A model for implementation in practice. *Journal of Nursing Care Quality, 9*(4), 43-54.

McNamara, S. A. (1995). Perioperative nurses' perceptions of caring practices. *AORN Journal, 61,* 377, 380-385.

Mullaney, J. A. (2000, June). The lived experience of using Watson's actual caring occasion to treat depressed women. *Journal of Holistic Nursing, 18*(2), 129-142.

Nelson-Marten, P., Hecomovich, K., & Pangle, M. (1998). Caring theory: A framework for advanced practice nursing. *Advanced Practice Nursing Quarterly, 4,* 70-77.

Norred, C. (2000). Minimizing preoperative anxiety with alternative caring-healing therapies. *AORN Journal, 72*(3), 1-4.

Nyman, C. S., & Lutzen, K. (1999). Caring needs of patients with rheumatoid arthritis. *Nursing Science Quarterly, 12*(2), 164-169.

Perry, B. (1997). Beliefs of eight exemplary nurses related to Watson's nursing theory. *Canadian Oncology Nursing Journal, 8*(2), 97-101.

Ray, M. A. (1997). Consciousness and the moral ideal: A transcultural analysis of Watson's theory of transpersonal caring. *Advanced Practice Nursing Quarterly, 3,* 25-31.

Saewyc, E. (2000, June). Nursing theories of caring. *Journal of Holistic Nursing, 18*(2), 109-113.

Schindel-Martin, L. (1991). Using Watson's theory to explore the dimensions of adult polycystic kidney disease. *American Nephrology Nurses' Association Journal, 18,* 493-496.

Schroeder, C. (1993). Nursing's response to the crisis of access, costs, and quality in health care. *ANS Advances in Nursing Science, 16*(1), 1-20.

Schroeder, C., & Maeve, M. K. (1992). Nursing care partnerships at the Denver nursing project in human caring: An application and extension of caring theory in practice. *ANS Advances in Nursing Science, 15*(2), 25-38.

Smith, M. C. (1997). Nursing theory-guided practice: Practice guided by Watson's theory. The Denver nursing project in human caring. *Nursing Science Quarterly, 10,* 56-58.

Swanson, K. M. (1991). Empirical development of a middle range theory of caring. *Nursing Research, 40,* 161-166.

Updike, P., Cleveland, M. J., & Nyberg, J. (2000). Complementary caring-healing practices of nurses caring for children with life-challenging illnesses and their families: A pilot project with case reports. *Alternative Therapies, 6*(4), 108-112.

Walker, C. A. (1996). Coalescing the theories of two nurse visionaries: Parse and Watson. *Journal of Advanced Nursing, 24,* 988-996.

Ward, S. (1998). Caring and healing in the 21st century. *MCN Journal, 23*(4), 210-215.

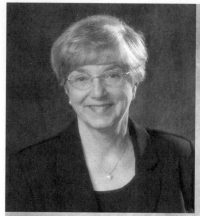

Photo credit: M. Dauley, Artistic
Images, Littleton, CO.

Marilyn Anne Ray

1938-present

Theory of Bureaucratic Caring

Sherrilyn Coffman

CREDENTIALS OF THE THEORIST

Marilyn Anne (Dee) Ray was born in Hamilton, Ontario, Canada, and grew up in a family of six children. When Ray was 15, her father became seriously ill, was hospitalized, and almost died. A nurse saved his life. Marilyn decided that she would become a nurse so that she could help others and perhaps save their lives, too.

In 1958, Marilyn Ray graduated from St. Joseph Hospital School of Nursing, Hamilton, and left for Los Angeles, California. She worked at the University of California, Los Angeles Medical Center on a number of units, including obstetrics and gynecology, emergency department, and cardiac and critical care with adults and children. In Southern California she enjoyed meeting new friends from different cultures and cared for children from vulnerable populations. While working with people of diverse cultures, particularly African-Americans and Latinos, Ray began to see how important cultures were in the development of people's views about nursing and the world.

In 1965, Ray returned to school for her BSN and MSN in Maternal-Child Nursing at the University of Colorado, School of Nursing. This is where she met Dr. Madeleine Leininger, who was the first nurse anthropologist and the Director of the Federal Nurse-Scientist program. Through her mentorship, Leininger profoundly influenced Ray's life. Ray took a special interest in her first courses on nursing and anthropology, including childhood and culture. She studied organizations as small cultures, and her research project in graduate school involved the study of a children's hospital as a small culture. While being educated at University of Colorado, she worked in organizations and practiced in critical care with children and adults, renal dialysis, and occupational health nursing with family-centered care.

In the mid-1960s, Ray became a citizen of the United States. Shortly afterward, in 1967, she joined and was commissioned as an officer in the United States Air Force Reserve, Nurse Corps (and Air National Guard). She graduated as a flight nurse from the School of Aerospace Medicine at Brooks Air Force Base, Texas, and served as an aeromedical evacuation nurse. She cared for combat casualties and other patients onboard different types of aircraft during the Viet Nam conflict. Since that time, Ray has served more than 30 years in different positions in the Air Force—flight nurse, clinician, administrator, educator, and researcher—and held the rank of colonel for more than 10 years. Her interest in space nursing stimulated her to attend the program for educators at Marshall Space Flight Center in Huntsville, Alabama. She remains a charter member of the Space Nursing Society. In 1990 she was the first nurse to go to the Soviet Union with the Aerospace Medical Association when the former USSR opened its space operations to American space engineers and physicians. Ray was called to active duty during the First Persian Gulf War in 1991, at which time she was assigned to Eglin Air Force Base, Florida, where she orchestrated discharge planning and later conducted research in the emergency department.

Ray is the recipient of a number of medals, including Air Force commendation medals for nursing education and research developments received during her Air Force career. Most notably, in 2000 she received the Federal Nursing Services Essay Award from the Association of Military Surgeons of the United States for their research on the impact of TRICARE/Managed Care on Total Force Readiness. This award recognized her accomplishments as part of a research program on economics and the nurse-patient relationship that received

nearly $1 million in funding from the TriService Military Nursing Research Council. Ray remains a mentor and consultant for funded research on the study titled *Air Force Combat Casualty Aeromedical Nursing Post-9-11* Major Mona Ternus at Old Dominion University, School of Nursing, leads the study.

Ray's first teaching positions were at the University of California San Francisco and the University of San Francisco in undergraduate nursing education. At that time, she was privileged to be on the faculty of nursing at the University of California San Francisco with Drs. Barney Glaser and Anselm Strauss, authors of the grounded theory method. This association intensified her interest in qualitative research methods. She continued to be intrigued by the study of nursing as a culture and had opportunities to teach students from various American and Asian cultures. During the summer of 1971, she traveled to Mexico with colleagues to study anthropology and health. She acknowledges how much she learned about aboriginal peoples and their fascinating life ways from the people of a small village.

During the years 1973 to 1977, Ray returned to Canada to be with her family. She joined the nursing faculty at McMaster University in Hamilton, Ontario, and taught in the family nurse practitioner program. In this position, Ray again had the opportunity to integrate culture and health into the curriculum. This was an exciting time, because the McMaster University Health Sciences Center was initiating evidence-based teaching, education, and practice. Ray completed a Master of Arts in Cultural Anthropology at McMaster University and studied human relationships, decision making and conflict, and the hospital as an organizational culture. Her clinical work at that time was in the area of neonatal intensive care at McMaster University Health Sciences Center.

Ray was thrilled when she received a letter from Leininger asking if she would be interested in applying for the first transcultural nursing doctoral program in the United States. At the University of Utah, where she studied with her mentor Dr. Leininger, Ray met wonderful colleagues who have taken their places in the history of nursing by their research and scholarly work, especially, Drs. Joyceen Boyle, Joan Uhl-Pierce, Kathryn McCance, and Janice Morse. Ray's doctoral dissertation (1981a) was related to the study of caring in the complex hospital organizational culture. From this research, the Theory of Bureaucratic Caring emerged, which is the focus of this chapter.

During her doctoral studies, Ray married James L. Droesbeke, whom she credits as her inspiration, friend, and love of her life. He was a constant support and help to her over the course of her career until his untimely death from cancer in 2001. Today, Jim remains a significant spiritual influence in her personal and professional life. After completing her doctorate in 1984 and as she began her married life in Denver, Colorado, Ray was able to rejoin the University of Colorado School of Nursing. She designed and taught the first qualitative nursing research course to graduate students at the University of Colorado and continued teaching the course while a full-time faculty member. After leaving her full-time position, she returned each summer to teach in the doctoral program an advanced interpretive qualitative course. Ray continues to be a visiting professor, serving on several doctoral dissertation committees, with access to the research skills of Dr. Carol Vojir in the Center for Nursing Research.

At the University of Colorado, Ray had the good fortune to work with Dr. Jean Watson, who was and continues to be a nursing leader, advancing the theory and practice of human caring in nursing. With Watson and several other scholars, Ray founded the International Association for Human Caring. At that time, Dr. Max van Manen from the University of Alberta was her mentor in phenomenology and hermeneutic human science research methods. Through the University of Colorado, Ray continued her study and teaching of phenomenology and other qualitative research approaches with Dr. Francelyn Reeder and directed the dissertation work of Dr. Alice Davidson, focusing on the new sciences of complexity.

In 1989, Ray accepted the appointment as the Christine E. Lynn Eminent Scholar at Florida Atlantic University, College of Nursing, a position she held until 1994. Her appointment as the first in-residence eminent scholar was made through the efforts of Dr. Anne Boykin, Dean of the College of Nursing, who has been advancing nursing as caring in the curriculum and research. Florida Atlantic University has developed the Center for Caring, which houses many of the caring memorabilia since the inception of the International Association for Human Caring in 1977. Ray also held the position of Yingling Visiting Scholar Chair at Virginia Commonwealth University, School of Nursing, from 1994 to 1995. Ray has been a visiting professor at universities in Australia and New Zealand, promoting and advancing the teaching and research of human caring. Ray has written several theoretical and research publications in transcultural caring, transcultural ethics, and caring inquiry while serving as an eminent scholar and visiting professor.

Ray continues in a teaching role as a full professor at Florida Atlantic University, Christine E. Lynn College of Nursing, Boca Raton, Florida, where she is a faculty member in both the Master of Science and Doctor of Nursing Science programs. Ray's interest in transcultural nursing remains a common theme in her research, teaching, and practice. With Dr. Sherrilyn Coffman she completed a grounded theory research study of high-risk pregnant African-American women (Coffman & Ray, 1999, 2002). Learning more about vulnerable populations gave Ray a deeper understanding of the needs of these populations, particularly related to equal access to health care and the importance of caring communities. Ray held the position of vice president of Floridians for Health Care (universal health care) from 1998 to 2000. She has been a Certified Transcultural Nurse since 1988 and is a member of the International Transcultural Nursing Society. She has made international presentations on transcultural caring and ethics in countries ranging from China to Saudi Arabia and England. In 1984, Ray was awarded the Leininger Transcultural Nursing Award given for excellence in transcultural nursing. Ray serves on the review boards of the *Journal of Transcultural Nursing* and *Qualitative Health Research,* and has written a book on transcultural caring in nursing and health (Ray, in press).

Ray's research interests continue to focus on nurses, nurse administrators and patients in critical care and intermediate care, and in nursing administration in the complex hospital organizational cultures. She has developed a program of research with Dr. Marian Turkel with federal funding from the TriService Nursing Research Program, studying the nurse-patient relationship as an economic resource (Turkel & Ray, 2000, 2001, 2003). These studies have focused on the impact of caring relationships on patient and economic outcomes in complex organizations. With Turkel, Ray has published in the areas of complex caring relational theory, organizational transformation through caring and ethical choice making, instrument development on organizational caring, economic and political caring, and caring organization creation. Teaching in the new doctoral program at Florida Atlantic University gives Ray opportunities to continue to influence complex organizations and create caring organizations and environments in local, national, and global contexts.

THEORETICAL SOURCES

Ray's interest in caring as a topic of nursing scholarship was stimulated by her work with Leininger, beginning in 1968, focusing on transcultural nursing and ethnographic-ethnonursing research methods. She used ethnographic methodology in combination with phenomenology to generate substantive and formal grounded theories, resulting in the overarching Theory of Bureaucratic Caring (Ray, 1981a, 1984, 1989). The formal theory focuses on nursing in complex organizations, such as hospitals. What distinguishes organizations as cultures is the foundation in anthropology, or the study of how people behave in communities and the significance or meaning of work life (Louis, 1985). Organizational cultures are viewed as social constructions, symbolically formed through meaning in interaction (Smircich, 1985).

Ray's earlier work (1989) was influenced by the philosophy of Hegel, who posited the interrelationship between thesis, antithesis, and synthesis (Moccia, 1986). In Ray's theory the thesis of caring (humanistic, spiritual, ethical) and the

antithesis of bureaucracy (technological, economic, political, legal) were synthesized as bureaucratic caring.

As she revisited and continued to develop her formal theory, Ray (2001) discovered that her study findings fit well with explanations from chaos theory, quantum physics' contribution to the science of complexity. Chaos theory describes simultaneous order and disorder, and order within disorder (the edge of chaos). An underlying order or interconnectedness exists in apparently random events. (Briggs & Peat, 1984). Mathematical studies, from which chaos theory originated, have shown that what may seem random is actually part of a larger pattern. Application of this theory to organizations demonstrates that within a state of chaos, the system is held within boundaries that are well ordered (Wheatley, 1999). Furthermore, chaos is necessary to new creative ordering. The creative process, as conceptualized in chaos theory, is described by Briggs and Peat as follows:

> ... when we enter the vital turbulence of life, we realize that, at bottom, everything is always new. Often we have simply failed to notice this fact. When we're being creative, we take notice. (1999, p. 30)

Ray compares change in complex organizations with this creative process and challenges nurses to step back and renew their perceptions of everyday events, to discover the embedded meanings. This is particularly important during organizational change.

Complexity is a more general concept than chaos and focuses on wholeness or holonomy (the whole is in the part and the part in the whole). Complex systems, such as organizations, have a great many agents interacting with each other in multiple ways. As a result, these systems are dynamic and always changing. Systems behave in nonlinear fashion because they do not react proportionately to inputs. Small inputs can have large effects and may create different effects at different times. For example, a simple intervention such as asking a colleague for help with a procedure may be accommodated easily or may be seen as unreasonable on a busy day. This makes the behavior of complex systems impossible to predict (Vicenzi, White, & Begun, 1997). Nevertheless, this chaos exists only because the entire system is holistic. Briggs and Peat (1999, pp. 156-157) describe this "chaotic wholeness" as "full of particulars, active and interactive, animated by nonlinear feedback and capable of producing everything from self-organized systems to fractal self-similarity to unpredictable chaotic disorder." These ideas are influential in Ray's ongoing development of bureaucratic caring theory, which suggests that multiple system inputs are interconnected with caring in the whole of the organizational culture. Nurses involved in small group work can apply these ideas by broadening the scope of information utilized in decision making, considering all possible relevant factors.

Ray's reflection on the Theory of Bureaucratic Caring as holographic was influenced by the historic revolution taking place in science based on the new holographic world view (Ray, 2001). The discovery of interconnectedness between apparently unrelated subatomic events has intrigued scientists. In experiments, electrons were found to lose their individual properties as they spun, charged, and changed from matter to energy to meet the requirements of the whole. In this process, the electrons did not remain as parts; they were drawn together by a process of internal connectedness. Scientists concluded that systems possess the capacity to self-organize; therefore, attention is shifting away from describing parts and instead focusing on the totality as an actual process (Wheatley, 1999). The conceptualization of the hologram portrays how every structure interpenetrates and is interpenetrated by other structures—so the part is the whole, and the whole is reflected in every part (Talbot, 1991).

The hologram has provided scientists with a new way of understanding order. Bohm conceptualized the universe as a kind of giant, flowing hologram (Talbot, 1991). He asserted that our day-to-day reality is really an illusion, like a holographic image. Bohm termed our conscious level of existence as the *explicate* (which means unfolded) order and the deeper layer of reality of which humans are usually unaware the *implicate,* or enfolded, order. In the Theory of Bureaucratic Caring, Ray compares the health care structures of political, legal, economic, educational, physiological, social-cultural, and technological with the explicate order and spiritual-ethical caring with the implicate order. An example related to health care might focus on a case manager's decisions about obtaining resources for a client's care in the home. At first glance, explicate structures such as the legal managed care contract or the physical needs of the client might appear to be enough information. However, through the case manager's caring relationship with the client, more implicate issues may emerge, such as the client's values and desires. In truth, each nursing situation involves countless enfoldings and unfoldings between the explicate and implicate orders, and both are important in the decision-making process.

Ray (2001) states that the Theory of Bureaucratic Caring fits with numerous paradigms in nursing. Synthesis of the concept of caring and the organizational context draws from theoretical work in each of these paradigms. The theory fits within the totality paradigm because the components of nursing, person, health, and environment characterize the nature of nursing practice. The simultaneity paradigm, which illuminates the human-environmental connection in nursing, is consistent with dynamic relationships within Ray's theory. The emphasis on wholeness in Ray's theory is also consistent with ideas from the unitary-transformative paradigm, that the human being is an evolving energy field identified by pattern and interaction with the larger whole.

USE OF EMPIRICAL EVIDENCE

The Theory of Bureaucratic Caring was generated from qualitative research involving health professionals and clients in the hospital setting. The research focused on caring in the organizational culture and first appeared in the doctoral dissertation in 1981, and in other literature in 1984 and

MAJOR CONCEPTS & DEFINITIONS

The theoretical processes of awareness of viewing truth or seeing the good of things (caring), and of communication, are central to the theory. The dialectic of spiritual-ethical caring (the implicate order) in relation to the surrounding structures of political, legal, economic, educational, physiological, social-cultural, and technological (the explicate order) illustrates that everything is interconnected with caring and the system within a macrocosm of the whole culture. In the model (see Figure 8-2), everything is infused with spiritual-ethical caring (the center) by its integrative and relational connection to the structures of organizational life. Spiritual-ethical caring is involved with qualitatively different processes, such as political, economic, and technological ones.

This interconnectedness of concepts led Ray to reflect upon the Theory of Bureaucratic Caring as a holographic theory (Ray, 2001). Holography means that everything is a whole in one context and a part in another—each part being in the whole and the whole being in the part (Talbot, 1991). Spiritual-ethical caring is both a part and a whole. Likewise, every part secures its meaning from each of the parts, which can also be considered wholes. The theory is holographic, because every structure interpenetrates and is interpenetrated by everything else—so the part is the whole, and the whole is reflected in every part.

Definitions of major concepts in the Theory of Bureaucratic Caring are listed in the following sections.

CARING

Caring is defined as a complex, transcultural, relational process, grounded in an ethical, spiritual context. As such, caring is the relationship between charity and right action, between love as compassion in response to suffering and need, and justice or fairness in terms of what ought to be done. Caring occurs within a culture or society, in-cluding personal culture, hospital organizational culture, or society and global culture (M. Ray, personal communication, March 27, 2002).

SPIRITUAL-ETHICAL CARING

Spirituality involves creativity and choice and is revealed in attachment, love, and community. The ethical imperatives of caring that join with the spiritual relate to our moral obligations to others. This means never treating people simply as a means to an end or as an end in itself, but rather as beings who have the capacity to make choices. Spiritual-ethical caring for nursing focuses on how the facilitation of choices for the good of others can or should be accomplished (Ray, 1989, 1997a).

EDUCATIONAL

Formal and informal educational programs, use of audiovisual media to convey information, and other forms of teaching and sharing information are examples of educational factors related to the meaning of caring (Ray, 1981a, 1989).

PHYSICAL

Physical factors relate to the physical state of being, including biological and mental patterns. Because the mind and body are interrelated, each pattern influences the other (Ray, 2001).

SOCIAL-CULTURAL

Examples of social and cultural factors are ethnicity and family structures; intimacy with friends and family; communication; social interaction and support; understanding interrelationships, involvement, and intimacy; and structures of cultural groups, community, and society (Ray, 1981a, 1989, 2001).

LEGAL

Legal factors related to the meaning of caring include responsibility and accountability; rules

---

MAJOR CONCEPTS & DEFINITIONS—cont'd

and principles to guide behaviors, such as policies and procedures; informed consent; rights to privacy; malpractice and liability issues; client, family, and professional rights; and the practice of defensive medicine and nursing (Ray, 1981a, 1989).

TECHNOLOGICAL

Technological factors include nonhuman resources, such as the use of machinery to maintain the physiological well-being of the patient, diagnostic tests, pharmaceutical agents, and the knowledge and skill needed to utilize these resources (Ray, 1987, 1989). Also included with technology are computer-assisted practice and documentation (M. Ray, personal communication, June 16, 2004).

ECONOMIC

Factors related to the meaning of caring include money, budget, insurance systems, limitations,

and guidelines imposed by managed care organizations and, in general, allocation of scarce human and material resources to maintain the economic viability of the organization (Ray, 1981a, 1989). Caring as an interpersonal resource should be considered, as well as goods, money, and services (Turkel & Ray, 2000, 2001, 2003).

POLITICAL

Political factors and the power structure within health care administration influence how nursing is viewed in health care and include patterns of communication and decision making in the organization; role and gender stratification among nurses, physicians, and administrators; union activities, including negotiation and confrontation; government and insurance company influences; uses of power, prestige, and privilege; and in general, competition for scarce human and material resources (Ray, 1989).

1989. The purpose of the dissertation study was to generate a theory of the dynamic structure of caring in a complex organization. The methodologies used were grounded theory mixed with phenomenology (meaning of experience) and ethnography (the patterns of organizational culture) to elicit the meaning of caring to study participants.

The grounded theory approach is a qualitative research method that uses a systematic set of procedures to develop an inductive grounded theory about a phenomenon. The aim of the researcher is to construct what the participants see as their social reality (Strauss & Corbin, 1990). This process results in the evolution of substantive theory (caring data generated from experience) and formal theory (integrated synthesis of caring and bureaucratic structures).

Ray spent more than 7 months in the field studying caring in all areas of a hospital, from nursing to

materials management to administration, including nursing administration. More than 200 respondents participated in the purposive and convenience sample. The principal question asked of participants was "What is the meaning of caring to you?" A process of dialogue and exploration of caring evolved from in-depth interviews, participant observation, caregiving, and documentation by field notes (Ray, 1989).

The discovery of bureaucratic caring began as a substantive theory and evolved to a formal theory. The substantive theory emerged as Differential Caring and revealed that the meaning of caring differentiates itself by its context. Dominant caring dimensions vary by areas of practice or hospital units. For example, an intensive care unit has a dominant value of technological caring (i.e., monitors, ventilators, treatments, and pharmacotherapeutics) and an oncology unit has a value of a more intimate, spiritual caring (i.e., family focused, comforting, compassionate). Staff nurses valued caring in terms of its relation to patients, while administrators valued caring as more system related, such as safeguarding the economic well-being of the hospital.

The formal Theory of Bureaucratic Caring symbolized a dynamic structure of caring. This structure emerges from the dialectic between the thesis of caring as humanistic (social, education, ethical, and religious-spiritual structures) and the antithesis of caring as bureaucratic (economic, political, legal, and technological structures). The dialectic of caring in relation to the various structures illustrates that everything is interconnected with caring, and the organizational system in a macrocosm of the whole of culture.

The evolution of Ray's theory development is illustrated in Figure 8-1, which contains diagrams of

the bureaucratic caring structure published in 1981 and 1989. In the original grounded theory (see Figure 8-1, *A*), the political and economic structures each occupied a larger dimension to illustrate their increasing influence on the nature of institutional caring (Ray, 1981a). Subsequent research conducted in intensive care and intermediate care units (Ray, 1989) emphasized the differential nature of caring, through its competing structures of political, legal, economic, technological-physiological, spiritual-religious, ethical, and educational-social elements (see Figure 8-1, *B*). Ray was one of the first nurse researchers to focus on caring in the high-technology area of critical care, where her work was truly innovative. In her 1987 article on technological caring, she noted that "critical care nursing is intensely human, moral, and technocratic" (p. 172). Ray encouraged other researchers to study this area

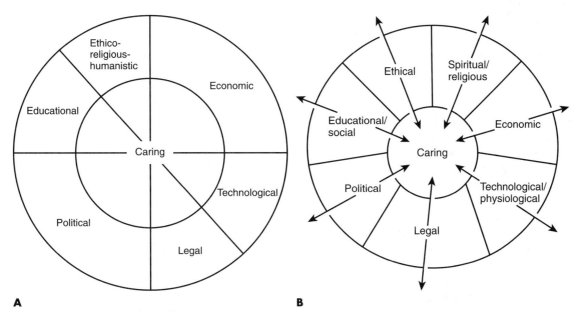

*F*igure 8-1 **A,** The original grounded Theory of Bureaucratic Caring. (From Ray, M. A. [1981a]. A study of caring within an institutional culture. *Dissertation Abstracts International, 42*[06]. [University Microfilm No. 8127787]) **B,** Subsequent grounded theory revealing differential caring. (From Parker, M. E. [2001]. *Nursing theories and nursing practice.* Philadelphia, F. A. Davis. Graphics redrawn from originals by J. Castle and B. Jensen, Nevada State College, Henderson, NV.)

to enhance nursing's understanding of both the advantages and limitations of technology in critical care. The *Dimensions of Critical Care Nursing* journal presented Ray with the researcher of the year award for this groundbreaking work.

With continued reflection and analysis of her work, combined with research on the economics of the nurse-patient relationship, Ray began to illuminate the more ethical-spiritual realm of nursing (Figure 8-2) (Ray, 2001). Spiritual-ethical caring became a dominant modality because of discoveries that focused on the nurse-patient relationship. The qualitatively different systems, such as political, economic, social-cultural, and physiological, when presented as open and interactive, are a whole and operate by the choice-making of nursing (Davidson & Ray, 1991; Ray, 1994a). Spiritual-ethical caring in nursing suggests how choice making for the good of others can or should be accomplished.

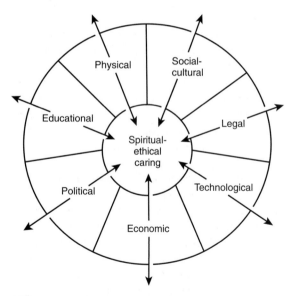

Figure 8-2 **The holographic Theory of Bureaucratic Caring.** (From Parker, M. E. [2001]. *Nursing theories and nursing practice.* Philadelphia: F. A. Davis. Graphics redrawn from originals by J. Castle and B. Jensen, Nevada State College, Henderson, NV.)

Ray's research reveals that nursing (caring) is practiced and lived out at the margin between the humanistic-spiritual dimension and the system dimension in complex organizations. These findings are consistent with world views from the new science of complexity, which proposes that phenomena that are antithetical actually coexist (Briggs & Peat, 1999; Ray, 1998). Thus, both technological and humanistic systems exist together. Complexity theory helps to explain why there is a resolution of the paradox between differing systems (thesis and antithesis), represented in the synthesis, or the Theory of Bureaucratic Caring.

In summary, the Theory of Bureaucratic Caring emerged from grounded theory methodology, blended with phenomenology and ethnography. The initial theory was examined using the philosophy of Hegel. The theory was revisited in 2001 after continuing research, and findings were examined in light of complexity science and chaos theory, resulting in the holographic Theory of Bureaucratic Caring (see Figure 8-2).

MAJOR ASSUMPTIONS
Nursing

Nursing is holistic, relational, spiritual, and ethical caring that seeks the good of self and others in complex community, organizational, and bureaucratic cultures. Dwelling more deeply with the nature of caring reveals that the foundation of spiritual caring is love. By knowledge of the inner mystery of the inspirational life within, love calls forth a responsible ethical life that enables the expression of concrete actions of caring in the lives of nurses. As such, caring is cultural and social. Transcultural caring encompasses beliefs and values of compassion or love and justice or fairness, which find significance in the social realm where relationships are formed and transformed. Transcultural caring is a unique lens through which human choices can occur and where understanding in health and healing can emerge. Thus, through compassion and justice, nursing strives toward excellence in the activities of caring in the dynamics of complex cultural contexts of relationships, organizations, and communities (M. Ray, personal communication, May 25, 2004).

Person

A person is a spiritual and cultural being. Persons are created by God, the Mystery of Being, and engage co-creatively in human organizational and transcultural relationships to find meaning and value (M. Ray, personal communication, May 25, 2004).

Health

Health is a pattern of meaning for individuals, families, and communities. In all human societies, beliefs and caring practices about illness and health are central features of culture. Health is not simply the consequence of a physical state of being. People construct their reality of health in terms of biology, mental patterns, characteristics of their image of the body, mind and soul, ethnicity and family structures, structures of society and community (political, economic, legal and technological), and experiences of caring that give meaning to lives in complex ways. The social organization of health and illness in the society (the health care system) determines the way people are recognized as sick or well, the way health or illness is presented to health care professionals, and the way health or illness is interpreted by the individual. Thus, health is intimately connected to the way people (including nurses) in a culture group, an organizational culture, or a bureaucratic system construct reality and give and find meaning (Helman, 1997; M. Ray, personal communication, May 25, 2004).

Environment

Environment is a complex spiritual, ethical, ecological, and cultural phenomenon. This conceptualization of environment embodies knowledge and conscience about the beauty of life forms and symbolic (representational) systems or patterns of meaning. These patterns are transmitted historically, preserved, or changed through caring values, attitudes, and communication. Functional forms identified in the social structure or bureaucracy (i.e., political, legal, technological, and economic) play a role in understanding the meaning of caring, cooperation, and conflict in human cultural groups and complex organizational environments. Nursing practice in environments embodies the elements of the social structure and spiritual and ethical caring patterns of meaning (M. Ray, personal communication, May 25, 2004).

THEORETICAL ASSERTIONS

Person, nursing, environment, and health are integrated into the structure of the Theory of Bureaucratic Caring. The theory implies that there is a dialectical relationship (thesis, antithesis, synthesis) between the human (person and nurse) dimension of spiritual-ethical caring and the structural (nursing, environment) dimensions of the bureaucracy or organizational culture (technological, economic, political, legal, and social). For Ray, the dialectic of caring and bureaucracy is synthesized into a theory of bureaucratic caring. Bureaucratic caring, the synthetic margin between the human and structural dimensions, is where nurses, patients, and administrators integrate person, nursing, health, and environment.

The theoretical assertions within the Theory of Bureaucratic Caring are as follows:

1. *The meaning of caring is highly differential depending on its structures* (social-cultural, educational, political, economic, physical, technological, legal). The substantive theory of Differential Caring discovered that caring in nursing is contextual and is influenced by the organizational structure or culture. The meaning of caring varied in the emergency department, intensive care unit, oncology unit, and other areas of the hospital. The meaning of caring was further influenced by the role and position a person

held. For example, patients primarily expressed the need for human care, while physicians' descriptions were predominantly in the technical sphere. The meaning of caring emerged as differential because no clear definition or meaning of caring was identified (Ray, 1989). The theoretical statement that describes the substantive theory of Differential Caring is formulated as follows:

> In a hospital, differential caring is a dynamic social process that emerges as a result of the various values, beliefs, and behaviors expressed about the meaning of caring. Differential Caring relates to competing [cooperating] educational, social, humanistic, religious/spiritual, and ethical forces as well as political, economic, legal, and technological forces within the organizational culture that are influenced by the social forces within the dominant American [world] culture (Ray, 1989, p. 37).

2. *Caring is bureaucratic,* given the extent to which its meaning can be understood in relation to the organizational structure (Ray, 1989, 2001). In the theoretical model (see Figure 8-2) everything is infused with spiritual-ethical caring by its integrative and relational connection to the structures of organizational life (e.g., political, educational). Spiritual-ethical caring is both a part and a whole, just as each of the organizational structures is both part and whole. Every part secures its purpose and meaning from the other parts.
3. *Caring is the primordial construct and consciousness of nursing.* Spiritual-ethical caring and the organizational structures in Figure 8-2, when integrated, open, and interactive, are a whole and must operate by conscious choice. Nurses' choice making occurs with the interest of humanity at heart, utilizing ethical principles as the compass in deliberations. Ray (2001) states, "Spiritual-ethical caring for nursing does not question whether or not to care in complex systems, but intimates how sincere deliberations and ultimately the facilitation of choices for the good of others can or should be accomplished" (p. 429).

LOGICAL FORM

The formal Theory of Bureaucratic Caring was induced primarily by comparative analysis and insight into the whole of the experience. Review of the literature on nursing, philosophy, social processes, and organizations was combined with the substantive theory titled Differential Caring that Ray discovered through ethnography, phenomenology, and grounded theory research. These ideas were integrated and analyzed through a process that was both inductive and logical. It was inductive in building on the data from the substantive theory and the literature. At the same time, it was logical in drawing upon the philosophical argument of Hegel's dialectic (Moccia, 1986) and complexity science to synthesize caring and bureaucracy to a new theoretical formulation (Ray, 2001).

ACCEPTANCE BY THE NURSING COMMUNITY
Practice

The Theory of Bureaucratic Caring has direct implications for clinical and administrative nursing. In the clinical setting, staff nurses are challenged to integrate knowledge, skills, and caring all at once (Turkel, 2001). Given economic constraints, nurses cannot practice the art of caring in isolation from meeting the physiological needs of the patient. This synthesis of behaviors and knowledge reflects the holistic nature of the Theory of Bureaucratic Caring. At the edge of chaos, contemporary issues such as inflation of health care costs serve as the catalyst for change within corporate health care organizations.

The ethical component, embedded in spiritual-ethical caring (see Figure 8-2), addresses nurses' moral obligations to others. Ray (2001) emphasizes that "transformation can occur even in the businesslike atmosphere of today if nurses reintroduce the spiritual and ethical dimensions of caring. The deep values that underlie choice to do good for the many will be felt both inside and outside organizations" (p. 429).

Results of Ray's research, based on bureaucratic caring theory, have been disseminated to practice settings. Miller (1995) summarized the work of Ray and other theorists and encouraged nurse executives to examine their daily caring skills and to use these skills in administrative practice. Nyberg studied with Ray and acknowledged the impact of Ray's ideas in her own book, *A Caring Approach in Nursing Administration* (Nyberg, 1998). In her book, Nyberg urged nurse administrators to create a more caring and compassionate system, while still being accountable for organizational management, costs, and economic forces. Turkel and Ray's (2003) study with United States Air Force personnel resulted in dissemination of findings and increased awareness of issues among civilian and military policy makers.

Ray has addressed the impact of diverse cultures on the health care system. The Transcultural Communicative Caring Tool provides guidelines to help nurses understand the needs, adversity, problems, and questions of people that arise in culturally dynamic health care situations (Ray & Turkel, 2000). The dimensions of the tool are as follows:

1. Compassion
2. Advocacy
3. Respect
4. Interaction
5. Negotiation
6. Guidance

To assist nurses with transcultural assessment, Ray developed an instrument for assessing older adults (Ray, 2000).

Ray's research has shown that nurses, patients, and administrators value the caring intentionality that is co-created in the nurse-patient or administrator-nurse relationship. By creating ethical caring relationships, administrators and staff can transform the work environment (Ray, Turkel, & Marino, 2002). The Theory of Bureaucratic Caring suggests that organizations fostering ethical choices, respect, and trust will become the successful organizations of the future.

Education

The theory is useful to nursing education because of its broad focus on caring in nursing and its conceptualization of the health care system. The holographic theory combines differentiation of structures within a holistic framework. Discussion of the structures or forces within complex organizations (e.g., legal, economic, social-cultural) provides an overview of factors involved in nursing situations. Infusion of these structures with spiritual-ethical caring emphasizes the moral imperatives and choice-making of nurses.

When developing a new baccalaureate nursing program at Nevada State College, the faculty was particularly drawn to the theory because of its description of the dimensions relevant to nursing within a philosophy of caring. The conceptual framework of the new nursing program combined Ray's Theory of Bureaucratic Caring with theoretical ideas from Watson (1985) and Johns (2000). Figure 8-3 depicts the ways in which nurses and clients interact in the health care system and how reflection on practice influences this process.

The description of the conceptual framework, as illustrated in Figure 8-3, is as follows:

> . . . the holographic theory of caring recognizes the interconnectedness of all things, and that everything is a whole in one context and a part of the whole in another context. Spiritual-ethical caring, the focus for communication, infuses all nursing phenomena, including physical, social-cultural, legal, technological, economic, political, and educational forces. The arrows reflect the dynamic nature of spiritual-ethical caring by the nurse and the forces that influence the changing structure of the health care system. These forces impact both the client/patient and the nurse. (Nevada State College, 2003, p. 2)

While in the health care system, the client-patient and nurse come together in a dynamic transpersonal caring relationship (Watson, 1985). This means that the nurse, through communication, views the person as having the capacity to make choices. Through reflection on experience, the nurse assesses which force(s) has the most influence on the nursing situation (Johns, 2000). The nurse draws upon empirical, ethical, and personal knowledge to inform and influence the aesthetic response to the

Nevada State College
Nursing Organizing Framework

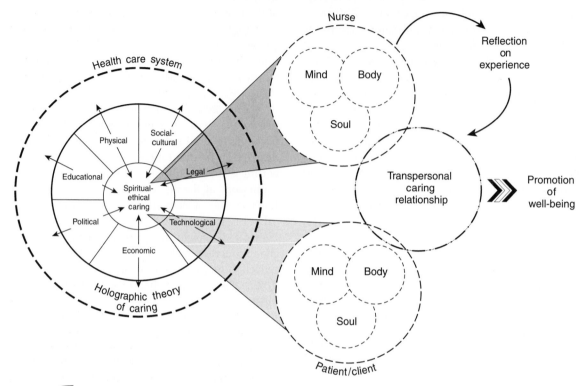

$\mathscr{F}$igure 8-3 Nevada State College Nursing Organizing Framework. (Reprinted with permission of Nevada State College, Department of Nursing, Henderson, NV, 2003. Graphics redrawn from original by J. Castle, Nevada State College, Henderson, NV.)

patient. Through the nurse's caring activities within the transpersonal relationship, the goal of nursing can be achieved—the promotion of well-being through caring (Nevada State College, 2003).

The Theory of Bureaucratic Caring is being used to guide curriculum development in the master's of science program in nursing administration at Florida Atlantic University (Turkel, 2001). Structures from the theory, including ethical, spiritual, economic, technological, legal, political, and social, serve as a framework to explore current health care issues. Students are challenged to analyze the contemporary economic structure of health care from the perspective of a caring lens. Caring within the

health care delivery system is a key concept in nursing courses.

Research

From Ray's research resulting in the Theory of Bureaucratic Caring, she developed a phenomenological-hermeneutic approach that guides her current studies (Ray, 1985, 1991, 1994b). This research methodology is particularly significant for nurse researchers, because it is grounded in the philosophy of humanism and caring and encourages nurses to utilize phenomenological hermeneutics through the lens of caring. The evolution of Ray's research methods began with ethnography-ethnonursing, grounded theory, and phenomenology, culminating in Caring Inquiry and Complex Caring Dynamics approaches. These approaches consist of generation of data by inquiring into the meaning of participants' life-world and relational experiences. Interviews and narrative discourse are the primary methods of data generation in the ethnography and ethnonursing, grounded theory, and phenomenological approaches. In Caring Inquiry the ontology of caring is a part of the approach to data generation. Complex Caring Dynamics includes not only qualitative data generation and analysis but also complex quantitative research data collection and analysis techniques. Through reflection, the researcher dwells on the essential meanings of phenomena. Further reflection facilitates the interpretation of the interview data, with the purpose of transforming data into interpretative themes and metathemes. The goal of the research approach is to capture the unity of meaning and synthesize meanings into a theory or conceptual model.

Based on the Theory of Bureaucratic Caring, Ray and Turkel have developed a program of research focusing on nursing in complex organizations. These studies have further explored the meaning of caring and the nature of nursing among hospital nurses, administrators, and clients-patients. A TriService Nursing Research Program grant supported extensive research on nursing as an economic resource. Table 8-1 outlines publications that describe this ongoing program.

FURTHER DEVELOPMENT

Ray's development of the Theory of Bureaucratic Caring is ongoing in her program of research and scholarship. Her work is a synthesis of nursing science, ethics, philosophy, complexity science, anthropology, economics, and organizational management. Ray described her most recent program of research sponsored by the TriService Nursing Research Program in *Nursing Science Quarterly* (Turkel & Ray, 2001). It included instrument development and psychometric testing of the Nurse-Patient Relationship Resource Analysis, now referred to as the *Organizational Caring Tool.* The tool consists of two Likert-type questionnaires, one for health care professionals and one for patients, which measure the nurse-patient relationship as an economic resource. This tool will help researchers link the noneconomic resources of caring, professional status, and patient education to the traditional economic resources of money, goods, and services. This type of research is at the cutting edge in nursing and will lead to further understanding of the concepts and relationships in the Theory of Bureaucratic Caring.

CRITIQUE
Clarity

The major structures, spiritual-religious, ethical, technological-physiological, social, legal, economic, political, and educational, are defined in Ray's 1989 publication. These definitions have semantic clarity and are consistent with definitions commonly used by practicing nurses. The definitions also have semantic consistency, meaning that the concepts of the theory are used in ways that are consistent with their definition (Chinn & Kramer, 2004). Although most terms did not change from the 1989 article to the 2001 publication, some concepts were combined or separated as Ray's development of the theory evolved. For purposes of this manuscript, all currently used terms were clarified with the theorist. The formal definitions of terms *spiritual-ethical caring, social-cultural, physical,* and *technological,* as they relate to the theory, are published for the first time in this chapter.

The diagram presented in Figure 8-2 enhances clarity. The interrelationship of spiritual-ethical caring with all other structures and the openness of the system are depicted by the organization of concepts and the dynamic arrows. The holographic nature of the diagram cannot be depicted in a one-dimensional drawing but must be left to the imagination of the reader. Ray's description (2001, pp. 428-429) of the theory assists the reader in imaging the theory relationships as holographic.

Table 8-1

Research Publications Related to the Theory of Bureaucratic Caring

YEAR	CITATION	RESEARCH FOCUS AND FINDINGS
1981	Ray, M. A. Study of caring within an institutional culture. *Dissertation Abstracts International, 42*(06). (University Microfilms No. 8127787)	The dissertation analyzed the meaning of caring expressions and behavior among 192 participants in a hospital culture. The substantive theory of Differential Caring and the formal Theory of Bureaucratic Caring were abstracted.
1984	Ray, M. The development of a classification system of institutional caring. In M. Leininger (Ed.), *Care: The essence of nursing and health.* Thorofare NJ: Slack.	The discussion examines the construct of caring within the cultural context of the hospital. The classification system included cultural caring symbols of psychological, practical, interactional, and philosophical factors.
1987	Ray, M. Technological caring: A new model in critical care. *Dimensions in Critical Care Nursing, 6*(3), 166-173.	This phenomenological study examined the meaning of caring to critical care unit nurses. The study showed that ethical decisions, moral reasoning, and choice undergo a process of growth and maturation.
1989	Ray, M. A. The theory of bureaucratic caring for nursing practice in the organizational culture. *Nursing Administration Quarterly, 13*(2), 31-42.	Caring within the organizational culture was the focus of the study. It describes the substantive theory of Differential Caring and the formal Theory of Bureaucratic Caring. With caring at the center of the model, the study included ethical, spiritual-religious, economic, technological-physiological, legal, political, and educational-social structures.
1989	Valentine, K. Caring is more than kindness: Modeling its complexities. *Journal of Nursing Administration, 19*(11), 28-34.	Nurses, patients, and corporate health managers provided quantitative and qualitative data to define caring. Data were organized using the categorization schema developed by Ray (1984).
1993	Ray, M. A. A study of care processes using total quality management as a framework in a USAF regional hospital emergency service and related services. *Military Medicine, 158*(6), 396-403.	This descriptive study investigated access to care processes in a military regional hospital emergency service using a total quality management framework. The study lends support to the need for a decentralized, coordinated health care system with more authority and control given to local commands.

Table 8-1

Research Publications Related to the Theory of Bureaucratic Caring—cont'd

YEAR	CITATION	RESEARCH FOCUS AND FINDINGS
1997	Ray, M. The ethical theory of existential authenticity: The lived experience of the art of caring in nursing administration. *Canadian Journal of Nursing Research, 29*(1), 111-126.	Existential authenticity was uncovered as the unity of meaning of caring by nurse administrators. This was described as an ethic of living and caring for the good of nursing staff members and the good of the organization.
1998	Ray, M. A. A phenomenologic study of the interface of caring and technology in intermediate care: Toward a reflexive ethics for clinical practice. *Holistic Nursing Practice, 12*(4), 69-77.	This phenomenological study examined the meaning of caring for technologically dependent patients. Results revealed that vulnerability, suffering, and the ethical situations of moral blurring and moral blindness were the dynamics of caring for these patients.
2000	Turkel, M., & Ray, M. Relational complexity: A theory of the nurse-patient relationship within an economic context. *Nursing Science Quarterly, 13*(4), 307-313.	The formal theory of Relational Complexity illuminated that the caring relationship is complex and dynamic, is both process and outcome, and is a function of both economic and caring variables; that, as a mutual process, is lived all at once as relational and system self-organization.
2001	Ray, M., & Turkel, M. Impact of TRICARE/Managed Care on Total Force Readiness. *Military Medicine, 166*(4), 281-289.	A phenomenological study was conducted to illuminate the life world descriptions of experiences of USAF active duty and reserve personnel with managed care in the military and civilian health care systems. The research illuminated the need for policy change to better meet the health care needs of these USAF personnel and their families.
2001	Turkel, M., & Ray, M. Relational complexity: From grounded theory to instrument theoretical testing. *Nursing Science Quarterly, 14*(4), 281-287.	The article describes a series of studies to examine the relationship development and among caring, economics, cost, quality, and the nurse-patient relationship. Results of theory testing showed that relational caring as a process was the strongest predictor of the outcome—relational self-organization that is aimed at well-being.

Continued

Table 8-1

RESEARCH PUBLICATIONS RELATED TO THE THEORY OF BUREAUCRATIC CARING—cont'd	
YEAR CITATION	**RESEARCH FOCUS AND FINDINGS**
2002 Ray, M., Turkel, M., & Marino, F. The transformative process for nursing in workforce redevelopment. *Nursing Administration Quarterly, 26*(2), 1-14.	Relational self-organization is a shared, creative response to a continuously changing and interconnected work environment. Strategies of respecting, communicating, maintaining visibility, and engaging in participative decision making are the transformative processes leading to growth and transformation.
2003 Turkel, M. A journey into caring as experienced by nurse managers. *International Journal for Human Caring, 7*(1), 20-26.	The purpose of this phenomenological study was to capture the meaning of caring as experienced by nurse managers. Essential themes that emerged were growth, listening, support, intuition, receiving gifts, and frustration.
2003 Turkel, M., & Ray, M. A process model for policy analysis within the context of political caring. *International Journal for Human Caring, 7*(3), 17-25.	This phenomenological study illuminated the experiences of USAF personnel with managed care in the military and civilian health care systems. A model outlining the process of policy analysis was generated.

USAF, United States Air Force.

Simplicity

The theory helps to simplify the dynamics of complex bureaucratic organizations. From the numerous descriptions of the inductive grounded theory study, Ray derived the integrative concept of spiritual-ethical caring and the seven interrelated concepts of physical, social-cultural, legal, technological, economic, political, and educational structures. When the complexity of the bureaucratic organization is appreciated, the number of concepts is minimal.

Generality

The Theory of Bureaucratic Caring is a philosophy that addresses the nature of nursing as caring. Alligood and Tomey (2002) note that philosophies set forth the general meaning of nursing and nursing phenomena. Ray's theory addresses questions such as, "What is the nature of caring in nursing?" and "What is the nature of nursing practice as caring?" Philosophies are broad and propose general ideas about how the profession of nursing fulfills its moral obligation to society. The Theory of Bureaucratic Caring proposes that nurses are choice makers guided by spiritual-ethical caring, in relation to legal, economic, technological, and other structures.

The Theory of Bureaucratic Caring provides a unique view of health care organizations and how nursing phenomena interrelate as wholes and parts of the system. Concepts or phenomena were derived logically from inductive research. Ray's analysis incorporated ideas from complexity science. The conceptualization of the health care system as holographic emphasizes the holistic nature of concepts and relationships. As nurses in all areas of nursing practice study these new conceptualizations, they may question older, linear ideas about cause and effect. Therefore the Theory of Bureaucratic Caring has the potential to change the paradigm or way of thinking of all practicing nurses.

Empirical Precision

Because the Theory of Bureaucratic Caring is generated by grounded theory, and continued revisions to the theory are based largely on research, empirical precision is high. This means that the defined concepts are grounded in observable reality. The theory corresponds directly to the research data that are summarized in published reports (Ray, 1981a, 1981b, 1984, 1987, 1989, 1997b, 1998).

The theory is being used by Dr. Ray, Dr. Marian Turkel, and colleagues to generate a program of research on the nurse-patient relationship as an economic resource (Ray, 1998; Ray, et al., 2002; Turkel, 2003; Turkel & Ray, 2000, 2001, 2003). These studies are generating models that provide guidance for nursing practice and increase nurses' understanding of the dynamics of health care organizations. Ray (2001) proposes that bureaucratic caring theory culminates "in a vision for understanding the deeper reality of nursing life" (p. 426).

Derivable Consequences

The issues that confront nurses today include economic constraints in the managed care environment and the effects of these constraints (e.g., staffing ratios) on the nurse-patient relationship. These are the very issues that the Theory of Bureaucratic Caring addresses. Nurses in administrative, research, and clinical roles can use the political and economic dimensions of the theory as a framework to inform their practice. The theory is very relevant to the contemporary world in which nurses work.

Ray and Turkel have generated middle range theories from their program of research based on the Theory of Bureaucratic Caring. Existential authenticity was uncovered by Ray (1997b) as the unity of

meaning of nurse administrator caring art. Nurse administrators described an ethic of living caring for the good of their staff nurses and for the good of the organization. Relational complexity is a theory focusing on the nurse-patient relationship within an economic context (Turkel & Ray, 2000, 2001). Study data showed that relational caring between administrators, nurses, and patients was the strongest predictor of the outcome, relational self-organization, which is aimed at well-being. Relational self-organization is a shared, creative response involving growth and transformation (Ray, et al., 2002). Transformative processes that can lead to relational self-organization include respecting, communicating, maintaining visibility, and engaging in participative decision making in the workplace. Ray's work has also identified the need for a new reflexive ethics for clinical practice, to increase understanding of how deep values and moral interactions shape ethical decisions (Ray, 1998).

SUMMARY

The Theory of Bureaucratic Caring challenges all participants in nursing to think beyond their usual paradigms, to envision the world more holistically and to consider the universe as a hologram. Appreciation of the interrelatedness of all persons, environments, and events is key to understanding this theory. The theory provides a unique view of health care organizations and how nursing phenomena interrelate as wholes and parts of the system. One of the unique constructs within Ray's theory is technological caring.

The theory was derived inductively from research and synthesized through further reflection and analysis. Ray acknowledges the influences of the philosophy of Hegel, chaos theory, complexity science, and the holographic world view. Theory development continues through Ray's current research and scholarship. Ray challenges nurses to envision the spiritual and ethical dimensions of caring, in order to build the profession that nurses want. Ray states that insights from the Theory of Bureaucratic Caring will inform nurses to use their creativity and imagination to transform the work world.

Case Study

Mrs. Smith was a 73-year-old widow who lived alone with no significant social support. She had been suffering from emphysema for several years and had had frequent hospitalizations for respiratory problems. On the last hospital admission her pneumonia quickly progressed to organ failure. Death appeared to be imminent, as she went in and out of consciousness, alone in her hospital room. The medical-surgical nursing staff and the Nursing Director focused on making her end-of-life period as comfortable as possible. Based on discussions with unit staff, the Nursing Director reorganized patient assignments. Over the next few hours, a staff member who had volunteered her assistance provided personal care for Mrs. Smith. With help from her team, the nurse turned, bathed, and suctioned Mrs. Smith. She quietly sang hymns in her room, creating a peaceful environment that expressed caring for her and calmed the nursing unit staff. Mrs. Smith died with caring persons at her bedside, and the unit staff felt comforted that she had not died alone.

1. What caring behaviors prompted the nursing staff to approach the Nursing Director for help with this situation?
2. What issues from the structure of the Theory of Bureaucratic Caring impacted this situation (ethical, spiritual, legal, social-cultural, economic)?
3. How did the Nursing Director balance these issues? What considerations went into her decision making?
4. What were the interrelationships between persons in this environment; that is, how were staff, patient, and administrators connected in this situation?

CRITICAL THINKING *Activities*

1. Read the book, *The Spirit Catches You and You Fall Down* by Anne Fadiman (1998). This is the story of a 3-month-old infant diagnosed with epilepsy and the cultural differences experienced by her Laotian refugee parents and American health care personnel. Although social-cultural forces were predominant in this situation, what other structures or forces were important in this story (see Figure 8-2)? What were the meanings of this child's seizure disorder to the family and to the professional staff? Using insights gained from the Theory of Bureaucratic Caring, describe alternative approaches to transcultural care in this situation.

2. Think back on a problem that you encountered in a clinical practice situation. What structures within the health care system were involved (social-cultural, legal, political, physical, educational, economic, technological)? How were these structures or issues interrelated? Would envisioning these structures holographically (each as a whole and as a part of a whole) change your perception of the situation and your nursing approaches?

3. How does the Theory of Bureaucratic Caring enlarge your views about a complex organization where you work? Describe how staff members' interactions with each other reflect caring. Is caring described differently by staff in different clinical roles and work areas? What decisions and choices reflecting spiritual-ethical caring occur regularly in each setting?

REFERENCES

Alligood, M. R., & Tomey, A. M. (2002). *Nursing theory: Utilization & application.* St. Louis: Mosby.

Briggs, J., & Peat, F. D. (1984). *Looking glass universe: The emerging science of wholeness.* New York: Simon & Schuster.

Briggs, J., & Peat, F. D. (1999). *Seven life lessons of chaos: Spiritual wisdom from the science of change.* New York: Harper Collins.

Chinn, P. L., & Kramer, M. K. (2004). *Integrated knowledge development in nursing.* St. Louis: Mosby.

Coffman, S., & Ray, M. A. (1999). Mutual intentionality: A theory of support processes in pregnant African American women. *Qualitative Health Research, 9*(4), 479-492.

Coffman, S., & Ray, M. A. (2002). African American women describe support processes during high-risk pregnancy and postpartum. *Journal of Obstetric, Gynecologic, and Neonatal Nursing, 31*(5), 536-544.

Davidson, A., & Ray, M. (1991). Studying the human-environment phenomenon using the science of complexity. *ANS Advances in Nursing Science, 14*(2):73-87.

Fadiman, A. (1998). *The spirit catches you and you fall down.* New York: Farrar, Straus, & Giroux.

Helman, C. (1997). *Culture, health and illness* (3rd ed.). Oxford, UK: Butterworth-Heinemann.

Johns, C. (2000). *Becoming a reflective practitioner.* Oxford, UK: Blackwell Science.

Louis, M. (1985). An investigator's guide to workplace culture. In P. Frost, L. Moore, M. Louis, L. C. Lundberg, & J. Martin (Eds.), *Organizational culture* (pp. 73-93). Beverly Hills, CA: Sage.

Miller, K. (1995). Keeping the care in nursing care: Our biggest challenge. *Journal of Nursing Administration, 25*(11), 29-32.

Moccia, P. (1986). *New approaches to theory development* (Pub. No. 15-1992). New York: National League for Nursing.

Nevada State College. (2003, August 19). *Nursing organizing framework.* Henderson, NV: Author.

Nyberg, J. J. (1998). *A caring approach in nursing administration.* Niwot, CO: University Press of Colorado.

Ray, M. (1981a). A study of caring within an institutional culture. *Dissertation Abstracts International, 42*(06). (University Microfilms No. 8127787)

Ray, M. (1981b). A philosophical analysis of caring within nursing. In M. Leininger (Ed.), *Caring: An essential human need* (pp. 25-360). Thorofare, NJ: Slack.

Ray, M. (1984). The development of a classification system of institutional caring. In M. Leininger (Ed.), *Care: The essence of nursing and health* (pp. 95-112). Thorofare, NJ: Slack.

Ray, M. (1987). Technological caring: A new model in critical care. *Dimensions in Critical Care Nursing, 6*(3), 166-173.

Ray, M. (1989). The Theory of Bureaucratic Caring for nursing practice in the organizational culture. *Nursing Administration Quarterly, 13*(2), 31-42.

Ray, M. A. (1985). A philosophical method to study nursing phenomena. In M. Leininger (Ed.), *Qualitative research methods in nursing* (pp. 81-92). New York: Grune & Stratton.

Ray, M. A. (1991). Caring inquiry: The esthetic process in the way of compassion. In D. Gaut & M. Leininger (Eds.), *Caring: The compassionate healer* (pp. 181-189). New York: National League for Nursing Press.

Ray, M. A. (1994a). Complex caring dynamics: A unifying model for nursing inquiry. *Theoretic and Applied Chaos in Nursing, 1*(1), 23-32. (Journal renamed *Complexity and Chaos in Nursing.*)

Ray, M. A. (1994b). The richness of phenomenology: Philosophic, theoretic, and methodologic concerns. In J. Morse (Ed.), *Critical issues in qualitative research methods* (pp. 116-135). Newbury Park, CA: Sage.

Ray, M. A. (1997a). Consciousness and the moral ideal: A transcultural analysis of Watson's theory of transpersonal caring. *Advanced Practice Nursing Quarterly, 3*(1):25-31.

Ray, M. A. (1997b). The ethical theory of existential authenticity: The lived experience of the art of caring in nursing administration. *Canadian Journal of Nursing Research, 29*(1), 111-126.

Ray, M. A. (1998). A phenomenologic study of the interface of caring and technology: A new reflexive ethics in intermediate care. *Holistic Nursing Practice, 12*(4), 71-79.

Ray, M. A. (2000). Transcultural assessment of older adults. In S. Garratt & S. Koch (Eds.), *Assessing older people: A practical guide for health professionals.* Sydney, Australia: MacLennan & Petty.

Ray, M. A. (2001). The Theory of Bureaucratic Caring. In M. Parker (Ed.), *Nursing theories and nursing practice* (pp. 422-431). Philadelphia: F. A. Davis.

Ray, M. A. (in press). *Transcultural awareness and caring in nursing and health care.* Philadelphia: F. A. Davis.

Ray, M. A., & Turkel, M. C. (2000). Culturally based caring. In L. Dunphy & J. Winland-Brown (Eds.), *Advanced practice nursing: A holistic approach* (pp. 43-55). Philadelphia: F. A. Davis.

Ray, M., Turkel, M., & Marino, F. (2002). The transformative process for nursing in workforce redevelopment. *Nursing Administration Quarterly, 26*(2), 1-14.

Smircich, L. (1985). Is the concept of culture a paradigm for understanding organizations and ourselves? In P. Frost, L. Moore, M. Louis, L. C. Lundberg, & J. Martin (Eds.), *Organizational culture* (pp. 55-72). Beverly Hills, CA: Sage.

Strauss, A., & Corbin, J. (1990). *Basics of qualitative research: Grounded theory procedures and techniques.* Newbury Park, CA: Sage.

Talbot, M. (1991). *The holographic universe.* New York: Harper Collins.

Turkel, M. (2001). Applicability of bureaucratic caring theory to contemporary nursing practice: The political and economic dimensions. In M. Parker (Ed.), *Nursing theories and nursing practice* (pp. 433-444). Philadelphia: F. A. Davis.

Turkel, M. (2003). A journey into caring as experienced by nurse managers. *International Journal for Human Caring, 7*(1), 20-26.

Turkel, M., & Ray, M. (2000). Relational complexity: A theory of the nurse-patient relationship within an economic context. *Nursing Science Quarterly, 13*(4), 307-313.

Turkel, M., & Ray, M. (2001). Relational complexity: From grounded theory to instrument development and theoretical testing. *Nursing Science Quarterly, 14*(4), 281-287.

Turkel, M., & Ray, M. (2003). A process model for policy analysis within the context of political caring. *International Journal for Human Caring, 7*(3), 17-25.

Vicenzi, A. E., White, K. R., & Begun, J. W. (1997). Chaos in nursing: Make it work for you. *American Journal of Nursing, 97*(10), 26-31.

Watson, J. (1985). *Nursing: Human science and human care.* Norwalk, CT: Appleton-Century-Crofts.

Wheatley, M. J. (1999). *Leadership and the new science: Discovering order in a chaotic world.* San Francisco: Berrett-Koehler.

BIBLIOGRAPHY

Primary Sources

Books

Ray, M. (in press). *Transcultural awareness and caring in nursing and health care.* Philadelphia: F. A. Davis.

Watson, J., & Ray, M. (Eds.). (1988). *The ethics of care and the ethics of cure: Synthesis in chronicity.* New York: National League for Nursing. (Released, 1989; translated into Swedish.)

Book Chapters

Ray, M. A. (1979). Discussion of "An ethnoscientific approach to selected aspects of illness behavior among an urban American Indian population." In M. Leininger (Ed.), *Transcultural nursing* (pp. 723-725). New York: Masson International Nursing Publications.

Ray, M. A. (1981). A philosophical analysis of caring within nursing. In M. Leininger (Ed.), *Caring: An essential human need* (pp. 25-36). Thorofare, NJ: Charles B. Slack.

Ray, M. A. (1984). The development of a nursing classification system of institutional caring. In M. Leininger (Ed.), *Care: The essence of nursing: and health* (pp. 95-112). Thorofare, NJ: Charles B. Slack.

Ray, M. A. (1985). A philosophical method to study nursing phenomena. In M. Leininger (Ed.), *Qualitative research methods in nursing* (pp. 81-92). New York: Grune & Stratton.

Ray, M. A. (1988). Ethical dilemmas in the clinical setting—Time constraints, conflicts in interprofessional decision-making. In J. Watson & M. Ray (Eds.), *The ethics of care and the ethics of cure: Synthesis in chronicity* (pp. 37-39). New York: National League for Nursing.

Ray, M. A. (1990). Phenomenological method in nursing research. In N. Chaska (Ed.), *The nursing profession: Turning points* (pp. 173-179). New York: McGraw-Hill.

Ray, M. A. (1991). Caring inquiry: The esthetic process in the way of compassion. In D. Gaut & M. Leininger (Eds.), *Caring: The compassionate healer* (pp. 181-189). New York: National League for Nursing Press.

Ray, M. A. (1992). Phenomenological method for nursing research. In J. Poindexter (Ed.), *Nursing theory. Research & Practice Summer Research Conference monograph* (pp. 163-174). Detroit: Wayne State University.

Ray, M. A. (1994). Environmental encountering through interiority. In E. Schuster & C. Brown (Eds.), *Exploring our environmental connections* (pp. 113-118). New York: National League for Nursing Press.

Ray, M. A. (1994). The quality of authentic presence: Transcultural caring inquiry in primary care. In J. Wang & P. Simoni (Eds.), *Proceedings of First International and Interdisciplinary Health Research Symposium* (pp. 69-72). At Peking Union Medical College Hospital, Beijing, China, and Zhejiang Medical University, Hangzhou, China (Chinese translation). Morgantown, WV: West Virginia University.

Ray, M. A. (1994). The richness of phenomenology: Philosophic, theoretic, and methodologic concerns. In J. Morse (Ed.), *Critical issues in qualitative research methods* (pp. 116-135). Newbury Park, CA: Sage. (Translated into Spanish, 2004.)

Ray, M. A. (1995). Transcultural health care ethics: Pathways to progress. In J. Wang (Ed.), *Health care and culture* (pp. 3-9). Morgantown, WV: West Virginia University.

Ray, M. A. (1997). Illuminating the meaning of caring: Unfolding the sacred art of divine love. In M. S. Roach (Ed.), *Caring from the heart: The convergence between caring and spirituality* (pp. 163-178). New York: Paulist Press.

Ray, M. A. (1999). Caring foundations of deacony. In T. Ryokas & K. Keissling (Eds.), *Spiritus-Lux-Caritas* (pp. 225-236). Lahti, Finland: Deaconal Institution of Lahti. (Translated into German, 1999, University of Heidelberg, Germany.)

Ray, M. A. (1999). Critical theory as a framework to enhance nursing science. In E. Polifroni & M. Welch (Eds.), *Perspectives on philosophy of science in nursing* (pp. 382-386). Philadelphia: Lippincott.

Ray, M. A. (2000). Transcultural assessment of older adults. In S. Koch & S. Garratt (Eds.), *Assessing older people: A practical guide for health professionals.* Sydney, Australia: MacLennan & Petty.

Ray, M. A. (2001). Complex culture and technology: Toward a global caring communitarian ethics of nursing. In R. Locsin (Ed.), *Concerning technology and caring* (pp. 41-52). Westport, CT: Greenwood Publishing Group.

Ray, M. A. (2001). The Theory of Bureaucratic Caring. In M. Parker (Ed.), *Nursing theories and nursing practice* (pp. 421-444). Philadelphia: F. A. Davis.

Ray, M. A., & Turkel, M. C. (2000). Culturally based caring. In L. Dunphy & J. Winland-Brown (Eds.), *Advanced practice nursing: A holistic approach* (pp. 43-55). Philadelphia: F. A. Davis.

Journal Articles

Coffman, S., & Ray, M. A. (1999). Mutual intentionality: A theory of support processes in pregnant African American women. *Qualitative Health Research, 9*(4), 479-492.

Coffman, S., & Ray, M. A. (2002). African American women describe support processes during high-risk pregnancy and postpartum. *Journal of Obstetric, Gynecologic, and Neonatal Nursing, 31*(5), 536-544.

Davidson, A., & Ray, M. (1991). Studying the human-environment relationship using the science of complexity. *ANS Advances in Nursing Science, 14*(2), 73-87.

Ray, M. A. (1978). Toward a concept of caring and a model of health anthropology. *Anthropology at McMaster, 14*(1), 25-29.

Ray, M. A. (1987). Health care economics and human caring in nursing: Why the moral conflict must be resolved. *Journal of Family and Community Health, 10*(1), 35-43.

Ray, M. A. (1987). Technological caring: A new model in critical care. *Dimensions of Critical Care Nursing, 2*(3), 166-173.

Ray, M. A. (1989). An analysis of caring within nursing research and practice. *Woman of Power, 11*(2), 42-43.

Ray, M. A. (1989). A theory of bureaucratic caring for nursing practice in the organizational culture. *Nursing Administration Quarterly, 13*(2), 31-42. (Also translated and published in Japanese.)

Ray, M. A. (1989). Gloomy outlook for world health. *The International Nurse, 2*(3), 6.

Ray, M. A. (1989). Transcultural caring: Political and economic caring visions. *Journal of Transcultural Nursing, 1*(1), 17-21.

Ray, M. A. (1990). Critical reflective analysis of Parse's and Newman's research methodologies. *Nursing Science Quarterly, 3*(1), 44-46.

Ray, M. A. (1991). Nurses caring for America: An Air Force Reserve nurse's experience. *The Florida Nurse, 39*(9), 6-7.

Ray, M. A. (1992). Critical theory as a framework to enhance nursing science. *Nursing Science Quarterly, 5*(3), 98-101.

Ray, M. A. (1992). What does critical theory have to do with nursing inquiry? *The Florida Nurse, 40*(2), 11.

Ray, M. A. (1993). A study of care processes using Total Quality Management as a framework in a USAF regional hospital emergency service and related services. *Military Medicine, l58*(6), 396-403.

Ray, M. A. (1993). A theory of bureaucratic caring for nursing practice in the organizational culture. *The Japanese Journal of Nursing Research, 1*, 14-24.

Ray, M. A. (1994). Communal moral experience as the research starting point for health care ethics. *Nursing Outlook, 42*(3), 104-109.

Ray, M. A. (1994). Complex caring dynamics: A unifying model for nursing inquiry. *Theoretic and Applied Chaos in Nursing, 1*(1), 23-32. (Journal renamed *Complexity and Chaos in Nursing.*)

Ray, M. A. (1994). Interpretive analysis of Olson's book, *The Life of Illness: One Woman's Journey. Qualitative Health Research, 2*(2), 250-253.

Ray, M. A. (1994). Transcultural nursing ethics: A framework and model for transcultural ethical analysis. *Journal of Holistic Nursing, 12*(3), 251-264.

Ray, M. A. (1997). Consciousness and the moral ideal: Transcultural analysis of Watson's Transpersonal Caring Theory. *Advanced Nursing Practice Journal, 3*(1), 25-31.

Ray, M. A. (1997). The ethical theory of Existential Authenticity: The lived experience of the art of caring in nursing administration. *Canadian Journal of Nursing Research, 22*(1), 111-126. (Abstract also published in French.)

Ray, M. A. (1998). Complexity and nursing science. *Nursing Science Quarterly, 11*(3), 91-93.

Ray, M. A. (1998). The interface of caring and technology: A new reflexive ethics in intermediate care. *Holistic Nursing Practice, 12*(4), 71-79.

Ray, M. A. (1999). The future of caring in the challenging health care environment. *International Journal for Human Caring, 3*(1), 7-11.

Ray, M. (1999). Transcultural caring in primary care. *National Academies of Practice Forum, 1*(1), 177-182.

Ray, M. A., Didominic, V. A., Dittman, P. W., Hurst, P. A., Seaver, J. B., Sorbello, B. C., et al. (1995). The edge of chaos: Caring and the bottom line. *Nursing Management, 9*, 48-50.

Ray, M., & Turkel, M. (2001). Impact of TRICARE/Managed Care on Total Force Readiness. *Military Medicine, 166*(4), 281-289.

Ray, M., Turkel, M., & Marino, F. (2002). The transformative process for nursing in workforce redevelopment. *Nursing Administration Quarterly, 26*(2), 1-14.

Turkel, M., & Ray, M. (2000). Relational complexity: A theory of the nurse-patient relationship within an economic context. *Nursing Science Quarterly, 13*(4), 307-313.

Turkel, M., & Ray, M. (2001). Relational complexity: From grounded theory to instrument development and theoretical testing. *Nursing Science Quarterly, 14*(4), 281-287.

Turkel, M., & Ray, M. (2003). A process model for policy analysis within the context of political caring. *International Journal for Human Caring, 7*(3), 17-25.

Dissertation

Ray, M. (1981a). A study of caring within an institutional culture. *Dissertation Abstracts International, 42*(06). (University Microfilm No. 8127787)

Secondary Sources
Books

Johns, C. (2000). *Becoming a reflective practitioner.* Oxford, England: Blackwell Science.
Nyberg, J. J. (1998). *A caring approach in nursing administration.* Niwot, CO: University Press of Colorado.

Book Chapters

Tappen, R., Turkel, M., & Hall, R. (1997). Nursing in transition: A response to the changing health care system. In A. Moorehead & P. Huber (Eds.), *Nursing roles: Evolving or recycled?* Thousand Oaks, CA: Sage.
Turkel M. (2000). Applicability of bureaucratic caring theory to contemporary nursing practice: The political and economic dimensions. In M. Parker (Ed.), *Nursing theories and nursing practice.* Philadelphia: F. A. Davis.
Turkel, M. (2000). Directing and organizing patient care. In M. Tappen (Ed.), *Leadership and management,* (4th ed.). Philadelphia: F. A. Davis.
Turkel, M. (2001). Applicability of bureaucratic caring theory to contemporary nursing practice: The political and economic dimensions. In M. Parker (Ed.), *Nursing theories and nursing practice* (pp. 433-444). Philadelphia: F. A. Davis.
Turkel, M. (2001). Challenging contemporary practices in critical care settings. In N. Locsin (Ed.), *Advancing technology, caring and nursing.* Westport, CT: Auburn House.

Journal Articles

Barry, C. D. (2001). Creating a quilt: An aesthetic expression of caring for nursing students. *International Journal for Human Caring, 6*(1), 25-29.
Beckerman, A. (1995). Cardiac catheterization: The patients' perspective. *Heart & Lung, 24*(3), 213-219.
Chiu, W. (1996). Resolving the ethical dilemma of nurse managers over chemically-dependent colleagues. *Nursing Ethics, 3*(4), 285-293.
Cody, W. K. (1998). Critical theory and nursing science: Freedom in theory and practice. *Nursing Science Quarterly, 11*(2), 44-46.
Davidhizar, R. (1995). Dilemma for the nurse manager: The stress of caring "too much." *Today's OR Nurse, 17*(2), 36-38.

Davidhizar, R. (2002). Management toolbox: Strategies for effective confrontation. *Radiologic Technology, 73*(5), 476-478.
Davis, R. (1997). Community caring: An ethnographic study within an organizational culture. *Public Health Nursing, 14*(2), 92-100.
Davis, R. (2000). Holographic community: Reconceptualizing the meaning of community in an era of health care reform. *Nursing Outlook, 48*(6), 294-301.
DeMarco, R. F. (1998). Caring to confront in the workplace: An ethical perspective for nurses. *Nursing Outlook, 46*(3), 130-135.
Dyson, J. (1996). Nurses' conceptualizations of caring attitudes and behaviors. *Journal of Advanced Nursing, 23*(6), 1263-1269.
Elliott, R. L. (1997). Cultural patterns in rural Russia. *Journal of Multicultural Nursing and Health, 3*(1), 22-28.
Ford, K. (1997). Promoting independence in people with Alzheimer's disease. *Elderly Care, 9*(3), 12-16.
Fulbrook, P. (1999). On the receiving end: Experiences of being a relative in critical care. Part 2. *Nursing in Critical Care, 4*(4), 179-185.
Gaydos, H. L. (2001). On calling and character: Caring as archetypal act. *International Journal for Human Caring, 5*(1), 8-13.
Goldberg, B. (1998). Connection: An exploration of spirituality in nursing care. *Journal of Advanced Nursing, 27*(4), 836-842.
Huffman, C. (1997). The nurse-technology relationship: The case of ultrasonography. *Journal of Obstetric, Gynecologic and Neonatal Nursing, 26*(6), 673-682.
Jakobsson, L. (1997). Met and unmet nursing care needs in men with prostate cancer. An explorative study. Part II. *European Journal of Cancer Care, 6*(2), 117-123.
Jenny, J. (1996). Caring and comfort metaphors used by patients in critical care. *Image: The Journal of Nursing Scholarship, 28*(4), 349-352.
Jones, J. (1997). Your experiences. The guiding light of a good yarn: How stories from the past provide a link to the future of emergency nursing practice. *Australian Emergency Nursing Journal, 1*(2), 42-46.
Käppeli, S. (2001). Compassion—A forgotten tradition of nursing? *Pflege, 14*(5), 293-306.
King, S. J. (2000). Caring for adolescent females with anorexia nervosa: Registered nurses' perspective. *Journal of Advanced Nursing, 32*(1), 139-147.
Korniewicz, D. M. (1997). The preferable future for nursing. *Nursing Outlook, 45*(3), 108-113.
Locsin, R. C. (1995). Machine technologies and caring in nursing. *Image: The Journal of Nursing Scholarship, 27*(3), 201-203.
Miller, K. (1995). Keeping the care in nursing care: Our biggest challenge. *Journal of Nursing Administration, 25*(11), 29-32.

Milne, H. A. (1996). Considering nursing resource as "caring time." *Journal of Advanced Nursing, 23*(4), 810-819.

Palo-Bengtsson, L. (1997). Social dancing in the care of persons with dementia in a nursing home setting . . . including commentary by Watson J. *Scholarly Inquiry for Nursing Practice, 11*(2), 101-123.

Pelletier, D. (1997). The cardiac nurse's role: An Australian Delphi study perspective. *Clinical Nurse Specialist, 11*(6), 255-263.

Pelletier, D. (2000). Australian clinicians and educators identify gaps in specialist cardiac nursing practice. *Australian Journal of Advanced Nursing, 17*(3), 24-30.

Rickard, M. (1996). Caring and justice: A study of two approaches to health care ethics. *Nursing Ethics, 3*(3), 212-223.

Schoenhofer, S. O. (1998). Giving of oneself on another's behalf: The phenomenology of everyday caring. *International Journal for Human Caring, 2*(2), 23-29.

Scholes, J. (1996). Therapeutic use of self: How the critical care nurse uses self to the patient's therapeutic benefit. *Nursing in Critical Care, 1*(2), 60-66.

Seedhouse, D. (1997). The importance of care. *Lamp, 54*(3), 35, 37-38.

Turkel, M. (2001). Struggling to find a balance: The paradox between caring and economics. *Nursing Administration Quarterly, 26*(1), 67-82.

Turkel, M. (2003). A journey into caring as experienced by nurse managers. *International Journal for Human Caring, 7*(1), 20-26.

Turkel, M., Tappen, R., & Hall, R. (1999). Moments of excellence. *Journal of Gerontological Nursing, 25*(1), 7-12.

Turkel, M. C. (2000). Relational complexity: A theory of the nurse-patient relationship within an economic context. *Nursing Science Quarterly, 13*(4), 307-313.

Turkel, M. J. (1999). Moments of excellence: Nurses' response to role redesign in long-term care. *Journal of Gerontological Nursing, 25*(1), 7-12.

Valentine, K. (1989). Caring is more than kindness: Modeling its complexities. *Journal of Nursing Administration, 19*(11), 28-34.

Wallace, C. L. (1995). Nursing as the promotion of well-being: The client's experience. *Journal of Advanced Nursing, 22*(2), 285-289.

Walsh, M. (2000). Chaos, complexity and nursing. *Nursing Standard, 14*(32), 39-42.

Wuest, J. (1997). Fraying connections of caring women: An exemplar of including difference in the development of explanatory frameworks. *Canadian Journal of Nursing Research, 29*(2), 99-116.

Wuest, J. (2001). Precarious ordering: Toward a formal theory of women's caring. *Journal of Health Care for Women International, 22*(1/2), 167-193.

Other Publication

Gaut, D. A. (1993). *A global agenda for caring* (Pub No. 15-2518). New York: National League for Nursing Press.

Theses and Dissertations

Didominic, V. (1996). Ethical evaluation by nephrology nurse administrators: An exploratory-descriptive study. *Dissertation Abstracts International, 34*(02). (University Microfilms No. 1376812)

Dittman, P. W. (1996). The work-life views of the nurse manager during transition from primary care to patient-focused care. *Dissertation Abstracts International, 34*(02). (University Microfilms No. 1376813)

Herp, C. A. (1996). Meanings of folk and professional health care experienced by Guatemalan Mayans in Southeast Florida. *Dissertation Abstracts International, 34*(06). (University Microfilms No. 1380713)

Quinn, C. M. (2000). The lived experience of caring and the nurse executive: A phenomenological study. *Dissertation Abstracts International, 38*(04). (University Microfilms No. 1398084)

Ross, M. A. (1996). The nurses' experience of being assisted in practice by multiskilled personnel. *Dissertation Abstracts International, 35*(02). (University Microfilms No. 1382401)

Swinderman, T. D. (1997). Caring in nurse managers as described by staff nurses. *Dissertation Abstracts International, 35*(06). (University Microfilms No. 1385321)

Turkel, M. J. (1997). Struggling to find a balance: A grounded theory study of the nurse-patient relationship within an economic context. *Dissertation Abstracts International, 58*(08). (University Microfilms No. 9805958)

Wright, C. A. (2001). Public health nurse managers' perception of Total Quality Management initiatives. *Dissertation Abstracts International, 39*(02). (University Microfilms No. 1401204)

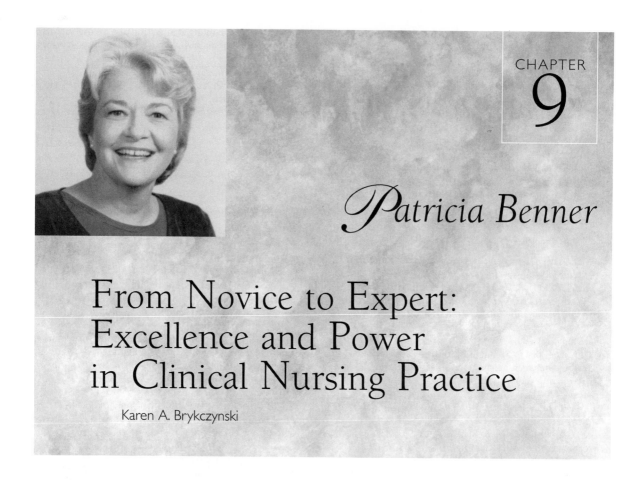

Patricia Benner

From Novice to Expert: Excellence and Power in Clinical Nursing Practice

Karen A. Brykczynski

CREDENTIALS AND BACKGROUND OF THE THEORIST

Patricia Benner was born in Hampton, Virginia, and spent her childhood in California, where she received her early and professional education. Majoring in nursing, she obtained a bachelor of arts degree from Pasadena College in 1964. In 1970, she earned a master's degree in nursing, with her major emphasis in medical-surgical nursing, from the University of California, San Francisco (UCSF) School of Nursing. Her Ph.D. in stress, coping, and health was conferred in 1982 by the University of California, Berkeley, and her dissertation was

Previous authors: Jullette C. Mitre, Sr. Judith E. Alexander, and Susan L. Keller. The author wishes to express appreciation to Patricia Benner for critiquing this chapter.

published in 1984 (Benner, 1984b). Benner has a wide range of clinical experience including acute medical-surgical, critical care, and home health care. She has held staff and head nurse positions.

Benner has a rich background in research and began this part of her career in 1970 as a postgraduate nurse researcher in the School of Nursing at UCSF. Upon completion of her doctorate in 1982, Benner achieved the position of associate professor in the Department of Physiological Nursing at UCSF and became a tenured professor in 1989. In 2002, she moved to the Department of Social and Behavioral Sciences at UCSF, where she is a professor and first occupant of the Thelma Shobe Cook Endowed Chair in Ethics and Spirituality. She continues to teach at the doctoral and master's levels and serves on 8 to 10 dissertation committees per year.

Benner acknowledges that her thinking in nursing has been influenced greatly by Virginia Henderson. Henderson (1989) commented that because of the nature and scope of Benner's *From Novice to Expert: Excellence and Power in Clinical Nursing Practice* (1984a), it had the potential to materially affect practice and preparation of nurses for practice. The Institute for Nursing Healthcare Leadership commemorated the impact of this book on nursing practice with a celebration of the 20 years since its publication at its conference Charting the Course: The Power of Expert Nurses to Define the Future in Boston in September 2003, and they presented Benner with an award for 20 years of collecting and extending clinical wisdom, experiential learning, and caring practices. In the foreword to Benner's work, *The Primacy of Caring: Stress and Coping in Health and Illness* (Benner & Wrubel, 1989), Henderson commented the following regarding the publication:

. . . a wide-ranging and scholarly work that demonstrates familiarity with an impressive body of literature, dating back to ancient Greece, that bears on the argument underlying their central themes of caring, stress and coping. (p. ix)

The research described in the book by Benner, Tanner, and Chesla (1996), *Expertise in Nursing Practice: Caring, Clinical Judgment, and Ethics,* is a continuation and expansion of the research described in *From Novice to Expert.* In the foreword to the 1996 book, Barbara Stevens Barnum wrote the following:

This work continues to challenge our traditional understanding of what it means to know, to be, and to act skillfully and ethically in nursing practice. Equally important, the book enables the reader to see how we might begin to shape our systems to better accommodate expert caring work. One of the truths of learning made clear by this work is that clinical learning is a dialogue between principles and practice. (pp. vii-viii)

Clinical Wisdom in Critical Care: A Thinking-in-Action Approach by Benner, Hooper-Kyriakidis, and

Stannard (1999) constitutes phase two of the articulation research of critical care nursing practice begun in *Expertise in Nursing Practice: Caring, Clinical Judgment, and Ethics.* Articulation refers to "describing, illustrating, and giving language to taken-for-granted areas of practical wisdom, skilled know-how, and notions of good practice" (Benner et al., 1999, p. 5). In the first foreword to this book, Joan Lynaugh wrote the following:

Perhaps the most important accomplishment of this text is its insistence on incorporating all the elements of critical care: clinical thinking and thinking ahead, caregiving to patients and families, ethical and moral issues, dealing with breakdown and technological hazard, communication and negotiation among all participants, teaching and coaching, and understanding the linkages between the larger systems and the individual patient. (Benner et al., 1999, p. vi)

In the second foreword, Joyce Clifford wrote the following of the work:

. . . provides the nurse administrator a wonderful understanding of the way organizational design can facilitate the caregiving process of clinical experts . . . [and] also provides guidance to those entrusted with the development of practice environments that promote the clinical learning and advancement of those just entering the profession. (Benner et al., 1999, p. vii)

Benner has published extensively and has been the recipient of numerous honors and awards, including the 1984, 1989, 1996, and 1999 *American Journal of Nursing (AJN)* Book of the Year awards for *From Novice to Expert: Excellence and Power in Clinical Nursing Practice* (1984a), *The Primacy of Caring: Stress and Coping in Health and Illness* (1989, with Wrubel), *Expertise in Nursing Practice: Caring, Clinical Judgment, and Ethics* (1996, with Tanner and Chesla), and *Clinical Wisdom in Critical Care: A Thinking-in-Action Approach* (1999, with Hooper-Kyriakidis & Stannard), respectively. *The Crisis of Care: Affirming and Restoring Caring Practices in the Helping Professions* (1994), edited by Susan S.

Phillips and Patricia Benner, was selected for the CHOICE list of Outstanding Academic Books for 1995. Benner's books have been translated into 10 languages. Several of her articles have also been translated and read worldwide. Benner received the AJN media CD-ROM of the year award for *Clinical Wisdom and Interventions in Critical Care: A Thinking-in-Action Approach* (2001, with Hooper-Kyriakidis and Stannard).

In 1985, Benner was inducted into the American Academy of Nurses; in 1989, she received the National League for Nursing's Linda Richards Award for leadership in education. In 1990, she received the Excellence in Nursing Research and Excellence in Nursing Education Award from the Organization of Nurse Executives—California. She also received the Alumnus of the Year Award from Point Loma Nazarene College (formerly Pasadena College) in 1993. In 1994, Benner became an Honorary Fellow in the Royal College of Nursing, United Kingdom. In 1995, she received the Helen Nahm Research Lecture Award from the faculty at UCSF in recognition of her contribution to nursing science and research.

Benner received an award for outstanding contributions to the profession by the National Council of State Boards of Nursing in 2002 for her work on developing an instrument to capture the sources and nature of nursing errors. The instrument is entitled Taxonomy of Error, Root Cause and Practice (TERCAP) analysis audit tool. She received the American Association of Colleges of Nursing Pioneering Spirit Award in May 2004 for her work on skill acquisition and articulating nursing knowledge in critical care. She is invited worldwide to lecture and lead workshops on health, stress and coping, skill acquisition, and ethics. Benner and her husband and colleague, Richard Benner, consult with nurses in hospitals around the world regarding their approach to clinical practice development models (CPDMs) (Benner & Benner, 1999).

Benner was appointed Nursing Education Study Director for the Carnegie Foundation's Preparation for the Professions Program (PPP) in March 2004. This is a nationwide study that will be integrated with a study of other professions, particularly medical education. The project focuses on the role of nursing schools in preparing nurses by addressing issues of teaching and learning, instruction, curriculum assessment, and institutional context.

THEORETICAL SOURCES

Benner studies clinical nursing practice in an attempt to discover and describe the knowledge embedded in nursing practice; that is, knowledge accrues over time in a practice discipline and is developed through dialogue in relationship and in situational context. She refers to this work as *articulation research,* as noted earlier. One of the first philosophical distinctions that Benner made was to differentiate between practical and theoretical knowledge. Benner stated that knowledge development in a practice discipline "consists of extending practical knowledge (know-how) through theory-based scientific investigations and through the charting of the existent 'know-how' developed through clinical experience in the practice of that discipline" (1984a, p. 3). She believes that nurses have been delinquent in documenting their clinical learning and "this lack of charting of our practices and clinical observations deprives nursing theory of the uniqueness and richness of the knowledge embedded in expert clinical practice" (Benner, 1983, p. 36). Benner has contributed extensively to the description of the know-how of nursing practice.

Scientists have long distinguished interactional causal relationships as "knowing that" from "knowing how." Citing Kuhn (1970) and Polanyi (1958), philosophers of science, Benner (1984a) emphasizes the difference in knowing how, a practical knowledge that may elude precise abstract formulations, and knowing that, which lends itself to theoretical explanations. Knowing that is the way an individual comes to know by establishing causal relationships between events. Knowing how is skill acquisition that may defy knowing that; that is, an individual may know how before the development of a theoretical explanation. Benner (1984a) maintains that practical knowledge may extend theory or be developed before scientific formulas. Clinical situations are always more varied and complicated than theoretical accounts; therefore, clinical practice is an area of inquiry and a source of knowledge development. Clinical practice embodies the notion of excellence. By studying practice, nurses can uncover new knowledge. Nursing must develop the knowledge base of its practice (know-how) and, through scientific investigation and observation, it must begin to record and develop the know-how of clinical expertise. Ideally, practice and theory set up a dialogue that creates new possibilities. Theory is derived from practice and practice is altered or extended by theory.

Hubert Dreyfus introduced Benner to phenomenology. Stuart Dreyfus, in operations research, and Herbert Dreyfus, in philosophy, both professors at the University of California at Berkeley, developed the Dreyfus Model of Skill Acquisition (Dreyfus & Dreyfus, 1980; Dreyfus & Dreyfus, 1986), which Benner applied in her work, *From Novice to Expert*. She credits Jane Rubin's (1984) scholarship, teaching, and colleagueship as sources of inspiration and influence, especially in relation to the works of Heidegger (1962) and Kierkegaard (1962). Richard Lazarus (Lazarus & Folkman, 1984; Lazarus, 1985) has mentored her in the field of stress and coping. Judith Wrubel has been a participant and co-author with Benner for years, collaborating on the ontology of caring and caring practices (Benner & Wrubel, 1989). Additional philosophical and ethical influences on Benner's work include Joseph Dunne (1993), Knud Løgstrup (1995a, 1995b, 1997), Alistair MacIntyre (1981, 1999), (Alvsvåg, 2006), Maurice Merleau-Ponty (1962), Onora O'Neill (1996), and Charles Taylor (1971, 1982, 1989, 1991, 1993, 1994).

Benner (1984a) adapted the Dreyfus model to clinical nursing practice. The Dreyfus brothers developed the skill acquisition model by studying the performance of chess masters and pilots in emergency situations (Dreyfus & Dreyfus, 1980; Dreyfus & Dreyfus, 1986). The model is situational and describes five levels of skill acquisition and

development: (1) novice, (2) advanced beginner, (3) competent, (4) proficient, and (5) expert. The model posits that changes in four aspects of performance occur in movement through the levels of skill acquisition as follows: (1) movement from a reliance on abstract principles and rules to use of past, concrete experience, (2) shift from reliance on analytical, rule-based thinking to intuition, (3) change in the learner's perception of the situation from viewing it as a compilation of equally relevant bits to viewing it as an increasingly complex whole in which certain parts stand out as more or less relevant, and (4) passage from a detached observer, standing outside the situation, to one of a position of involvement, fully engaged in the situation (Benner, Tanner, & Chesla, 1992).

The performance level can be determined only by consensual validation of expert judges and the assessment of the outcomes of the situation (Benner, 1984a). In applying the model to nursing, Benner noted "experience-based skill acquisition is safer and quicker when it rests upon a sound educational base" (1984a, p. xix). Benner (1984a) defines skill and skilled practice to mean implementing skilled nursing interventions and clinical judgment skills in actual clinical situations. In no case does this refer to context-free psychomotor skills or other demonstrable enabling skills outside the context of nursing practice.

In subsequent research further explicating the Dreyfus model, Benner identified two interrelated aspects of practice that also distinguish the levels of practice from advanced beginner to expert (Benner et al., 1992, 1996). First, clinicians at different levels of practice live in different clinical worlds, recognizing and responding to different situated needs for action. Second, clinicians develop what Benner terms *agency*, or the sense of responsibility toward the patient, and evolve into fully participating members of the health care team.

Benner attempted to highlight the growing edges of clinical knowledge rather than to describe a typical nurse's day. Benner's explanation of nursing practice goes beyond the rigid application of rules and theories and is based on "reasonable behavior that responds to the demands of a given situation" (1984a, p. xx). The skills acquired through nursing experience and the perceptual awareness that expert nurses develop as decision makers from the "gestalt of the situation" lead them to follow their hunches as they search for evidence to confirm the subtle changes they observe in patients (1984a, p. xviii).

The concept that experience is defined as the outcome when preconceived notions are challenged, refined, or refuted in actual situations is based on Heidegger's (1962) and Gadamer's (1970) work. As the nurse gains experience, clinical knowledge becomes a blend of practical and theoretical knowledge. Expertise develops as the clinician tests and modifies principle-based expectations in the actual situation. Heidegger's influence is evident in this and in Benner's subsequent writings on the primacy of caring. Benner refutes the dualistic Cartesian descriptions of mind-body person and espouses Heidegger's phenomenological description of person as a self-interpreting being who is defined by concerns, practices, and life experiences. Persons are always situated; that is, they are engaged meaningfully in the context of where they are. Persons come to situations with an understanding of the self in the world. Heidegger (1962) termed *practical knowledge* as the kind of knowing that occurs when an individual is involved in the situation. Persons share background meanings, skills, and habits derived from their cultural practices.

By virtue of being humans we have embodied intelligence, meaning that we come to know things through being in situations. When a familiar situation is encountered, there is embodied recognition of its meaning. For example, once having witnessed someone develop a pulmonary embolus, a nurse notices qualitative nuances and has recognition ability for observing it prior to others who have never seen it before. Benner and Wrubel (1989) stated, "Skilled activity, which is made possible by our embodied intelligence, has been long regarded as 'lower' than intellectual, reflective activity" but argue that intellectual, reflective capacities are dependent on embodied knowing (p. 43). Embodied knowing and the meaning of being are premises for the capac-

ity to care; things matter and "cause us to be involved in and defined by our concerns" (p. 42).

While doing her doctoral studies at Berkeley, Benner was a research assistant to Richard S. Lazarus (Lazarus, 1985; Lazarus & Folkman, 1984), who is known for his development of stress and coping theory. As part of Lazarus' larger study, Benner conducted a study of midcareer males' meaning of work and coping, which was published as *Stress and Satisfaction on the Job: Work Meanings and Coping of Mid-Career Men* (1984b). In this study, coping is defined as a form of practical knowledge, and it was determined that work meanings influence what is experienced as stress and what coping options are available to the individual. Lazarus' Theory of Stress and Coping is described as phenomenological; that is, the person is understood to constitute and be constituted by meanings. Stress is described as the disruption of meanings, and coping is what the person does about the disruption. Both doing something and refraining from doing something about the stressful situation are ways of coping. Coping is bound by the meanings inherent in what the person interprets as stressful. The person must be understood as a "participant self" in a situation that is shaped by reflective and nonreflective meanings and concerns (Benner & Wrubel, 1989, p. 63). Different possibilities arise from the way the person is in the situation. Benner uses this key concept to describe clinical nursing practice in terms of nurses making a positive difference by being in the situation in a caring way.

Benner's approach to knowledge development that began with *From Novice to Expert* (1984a) constitutes the commencement of a growing, living tradition for learning from clinical nursing practice through collection and interpretation of exemplars (Benner, 1994; Benner & Benner, 1999; Benner, et al., 1996; Benner, et al., 1999). Benner and Benner stated the following:

Effective delivery of patient/family care requires collective attentiveness and mutual support of good practice embedded in a moral community of practitioners seeking to create and sustain good practice. . . . This vision of practice is taken from the Aristotelian tradition in ethics (Aristotle, 1985) and the more recent articulation of this tradition by Alasdair MacIntyre (1981), where practice is defined as a collective endeavor that has notions of good internal to the practice .... However, such collective endeavors must be comprised of individual practitioners who have skilled know how, craft, science, and moral imagination, who continue to create and instantiate good practice. (Benner & Benner, 1999, pp. 23-24)

Benner expresses that nursing is a cultural paradox in a highly technical society, which is slow to value and articulate caring practices. She feels that the value of extreme individualism makes it difficult to perceive the brilliance of caring in expert nursing practice. Benner (2003) calls for a relational ethic that is based on practice to balance the dominant focus on rights and justice.

MAJOR CONCEPTS *&* DEFINITIONS

NOVICE

In the novice stage of skill acquisition in the Dreyfus model, the person has no background experience of the situation in which he or she is involved. Context-free rules and objective attributes must be given to guide performance. There is difficulty discerning between relevant and irrelevant aspects of a situation. Generally, this level applies to students of nursing, but Benner has suggested that nurses at higher levels of skill in one area of practice could be classified at the novice level if placed in an area or situation unfamiliar to them (Benner, 1984a).

ADVANCED BEGINNER

The advanced beginner stage in the Dreyfus model develops when the person can demonstrate marginally acceptable performance having coped with enough real situations to note, or to have pointed out by a mentor, the recurring meaningful components of the situation. The advanced beginner has enough experience to grasp aspects of the situation (Benner, 1984a). Unlike attributes and features, aspects cannot be objectified completely because they require experience based on recognition in the context of the situation.

Nurses functioning at this level are guided by rules and are oriented by task completion. They have difficulty grasping the current patient situation in terms of the larger perspective. However, Dreyfus and Dreyfus (1996) state the following:

Through practical experience in concrete situations with meaningful elements which neither the instructor nor student can define in terms of objective features, the advanced beginner starts intuitively to recognize these elements when they are present. We call these newly recognized elements 'situational' to distinguish them from the objective elements of the skill domain that the beginner can recognize prior to seeing concrete examples. (p. 38)

Clinical situations are viewed by nurses at the advanced beginner stage as a test of their abilities and the demands of the situation placed on them rather than in terms of the patient needs and responses (Benner et al., 1992). Advanced beginners feel highly responsible for managing patient care, yet they still rely on the help of those more experienced (Benner et al., 1992). Benner places most newly graduated nurses at this level.

COMPETENT

Through learning from actual practice situations and by following the actions of others, the advanced beginner moves to the competent level (Benner et al., 1992). The competent stage of the Dreyfus model is typified by considerable conscious and deliberate planning that determines which aspects of the current and future situations are important and which can be ignored (Benner, 1984a).

Consistency, predictability, and time management are important in competent performance. A

Continued

MAJOR CONCEPTS *&* DEFINITIONS—cont'd

sense of mastery is acquired through planning and predictability (Benner et al., 1992). There is an increased level of efficiency, but "the focus is on time management and the nurse's organization of the task world rather than on timing in relation to the patient's needs" (Benner et al., 1992, p. 20). The competent nurse may display hyperresponsibility for the patient, often more than is realistic, and may exhibit an ever-present and critical view of the self (Benner et al., 1992).

The competent stage is most pivotal in clinical learning, because the learner must begin to recognize patterns and determine which elements of the situation warrant attention and which can be ignored. The competent nurse devises new rules and reasoning procedures for a plan while applying learned rules for action on the basis of the relevant facts of that situation. To become proficient, the competent performer must allow the situation to guide responses (Dreyfus & Dreyfus, 1996). Studies point to the importance of active teaching and learning in the competent stage to coach nurses making the transition from competency to proficiency (Benner et al., 1996; Benner et al., 1999).

PROFICIENT

At the proficient stage of the Dreyfus model, the performer perceives the situation as a whole (the total picture) rather than in terms of aspects, and the performance is guided by maxims. The proficient level is a qualitative leap beyond the competent. Now the performer recognizes the most salient aspects and has an intuitive grasp of the situation based on background understanding (Benner, 1984a).

Nurses at this level demonstrate a new ability to see changing relevance in a situation, including the recognition and the implementation of skilled responses to the situation as it evolves. They no longer rely on preset goals for organization, and

they demonstrate an increased confidence in their knowledge and abilities (Benner et al., 1992). At the proficient stage, there is much more involvement with the patient and family. (See the Case Study.) The proficient stage is a transition into expertise (Benner et al., 1996).

EXPERT

The fifth stage of the Dreyfus model is achieved when "the expert performer no longer relies on analytical principle (rule, guideline, maxim) to connect her or his understanding of the situation to an appropriate action" (Benner, 1984a, p. 31). Benner described the expert nurse as having an intuitive grasp of the situation and as being able to identify the region of the problem without losing time considering a range of alternative diagnoses and solutions. There is a qualitative change as the expert performer "knows the patient," meaning knowing typical patterns of responses and knowing the patient as a person. Key aspects of the expert nurse's practice are as follows (Benner et al., 1996):

- Demonstrating a clinical grasp and resource-based practice
- Possessing embodied know-how
- Seeing the big picture
- Seeing the unexpected

The expert nurse has this ability to recognize patterns on the basis of deep experiential background. For the expert nurse, meeting the patient's actual concerns and needs is of utmost importance, even if it means planning and negotiating for a change in the plan of care. There is almost a transparent view of the self (Benner et al., 1992).

ASPECTS OF A SITUATION

The aspects are the recurring meaningful situational components recognized and understood in context because the nurse has previous experience (Benner, 1984a).

MAJOR CONCEPTS *&* DEFINITIONS—cont'd

ATTRIBUTES OF A SITUATION

The attributes are measurable properties of a situation that can be explained without previous experience in the situation (Benner, 1984a).

COMPETENCY

Competency is "an interpretively defined area of skilled performance identified and described by its intent, functions, and meanings" (Benner, 1984a, p. 292). This term is unrelated to the competent stage of the Dreyfus model.

DOMAIN

This is an area of practice having a number of competencies with similar intents, functions, and meanings (Benner, 1984a).

EXEMPLAR

An exemplar is an example of a clinical situation that conveys one or more intents, meanings, functions, or outcomes easily translated to other clinical situations (Benner, 1984a).

EXPERIENCE

Experience is not a mere passage of time, but an active process of refining and changing preconceived theories, notions, and ideas when confronted with actual situations; it implies there is a dialogue between what is found in practice and what is expected (Benner & Wrubel, 1982).

MAXIM

This is a cryptic description of skilled performance that requires a certain level of experience to recognize the implications of the instructions (Benner, 1984a).

PARADIGM CASE

A paradigm case is a clinical experience that stands out and alters the way the nurse will perceive and understand future clinical situations (Benner, 1984a). Paradigm cases create new clinical understanding and open new clinical perspectives and alternatives.

SALIENCE

Salience describes a perceptual stance or embodied knowledge whereby aspects of a situation stand out as more or less important (Benner, 1984a).

COMPORTMENT

Comportment refers to style and manner of acting and interacting, which includes gestures, posture, and stance (Benner et al., 1999).

HERMENEUTICS

Hermeneutics means interpretive. The term derives from biblical and judicial exegesis. As used in research, *hermeneutics* refers to describing and studying "meaningful human phenomena in a careful and detailed manner as free as possible from prior theoretical assumptions, based instead on practical understanding" (Packer, 1985, pp. 1081-1082).

USE OF EMPIRICAL EVIDENCE

Benner's early work focused on the anticipatory socialization of nurses. Benner and Kramer (1972) studied the differences between nurses who worked in special care units and those who worked in regular hospital units. Benner was a research consultant for a nursing activity study to determine the use and productivity of nursing personnel in 1974 and 1975. Concurrently, she was a consultant on a study of new nurse work-entry. Benner and Benner (1979) conducted a systematic evaluation of the competencies, the job finding, and the work-entry problems of new graduate nurses. Benner also studied methods of increasing teacher competencies through the use of a mobile microteaching laboratory.

From 1978 to 1981, Benner was the author and project director of a federally funded grant, Achieving Methods of Intraprofessional Consensus, Assessment and Evaluation, known as the AMICAE project. This research led to the publication of *From Novice to Expert* (1984a) and numerous articles. Benner directed the AMICAE project to develop evaluation methods for participating schools of nursing and hospitals in the San Francisco area. It was an interpretive, descriptive study that led to the use of Dreyfus' five levels of competency to describe skill acquisition in clinical nursing practice. In describing the interpretive approach, Benner (1984a) explains that it seeks a rich description of nursing practice from observation and narrative accounts of actual nursing practice to provide the text for interpretation (hermeneutics).

The nurses' descriptions of patient care situations in which they made a positive difference "present the uniqueness of nursing as a discipline and an art" (Benner, 1984a, p. xxvi). More than 1200 nurse participants completed questionnaires and interviews as part of the AMICAE project. Paired interviews with preceptors and preceptees were "aimed at discovering if there were distinguishable, characteristic differences in the novice's and expert's descriptions of the same clinical incident" (Benner, 1984a, p. 14). Further interviews and participant observations were conducted with 51 nurse-clinicians and other newly graduated nurses and senior nursing students to "describe characteristics of nurse performance at different stages of skill acquisition" (Benner, 1984a, p. 15). The purpose "of the inquiry has been to uncover meanings and knowledge embedded in skilled practice. By bringing these meanings, skills, and knowledge into public discourse, new knowledge and understandings are constituted" (Benner, 1984a, p. 218).

Thirty-one competencies emerged from the analysis of the transcripts of interviews about nurses' detailed descriptions of patient care episodes that included their intentions and interpretations of the events. From these competencies identified from actual practice situations, the following seven domains were inductively derived on the basis of similarity of function and intent (Benner, 1984):

1. The helping role
2. The teaching-coaching function
3. The diagnostic and patient-monitoring function
4. Effective management of rapidly changing situations
5. Administering and monitoring therapeutic interventions and regimens
6. Monitoring and ensuring the quality of health care practices
7. Organizational work-role competencies

Each of these domains was described with the related competencies from the actual practice situations describing nursing practice. Benner presented the domains and competencies of nursing practice as an open-ended interpretive framework for enhancing the understanding of the knowledge embedded in nursing practice. As a result of the socially embedded, relational, and dialogical nature of clinical knowledge, the domains and competencies need to be adapted for use in each institution through the study of clinical practice at each specific locale (Benner & Benner, 1999). Such adaptations have been implemented in many institutions for nursing staff in hospitals around the world (Alberti, 1991; Balasco & Black, 1988; Brykczynski, 1998; Dolan, 1984; Gaston, 1989; Gordon, 1986; Hamric, Whitworth, & Greenfield, 1993; Lock & Gordon, 1989; Nuccio, et al., 1996; Silver, 1986a, 1986b). The domains and competencies have also been useful for ongoing articulation of the knowledge embedded in advanced practice nursing (Brykczynski, 1999; Fenton, 1985; Fenton & Brykczynski, 1993; Lindeke, Canedy, & Kay, 1997; Martin, 1996).

Benner and Wrubel (1989) have further explained and developed the background to their ongoing study of the knowledge embedded in nursing practice in *The Primacy of Caring: Stress and Coping in Health and Illness.* They note that the primacy of caring is three-pronged "as the producer of both stress and coping in the lived experience of health and illness, . . . as the enabling condition of nursing practice (indeed any practice), and the ways that nursing practice based in such caring can positively affect the outcome of an illness" (1989, p. 7).

Benner extended the research presented in 1984 *From Novice to Expert* and features this work in 1996 *Expertise in Nursing Practice*. This later book is based on a 6-year study of 130 hospital nurses, primarily critical care nurses, examining the acquisition of clinical expertise and the nature of clinical knowledge, clinical inquiry, clinical judgment, and expert ethical comportment. The key aims of the extension of this research were as follows:

- Delineate the practical knowledge embedded in expert practice.
- Describe the nature of skill acquisition in critical care nursing practice.
- Identify institutional impediments and resources for the development of expertise in nursing practice.
- Begin to identify educational strategies that encourage the development of expertise.

In the introduction to the 1996 work, Benner stated, "In the study we found that examining the nature of the nurse's agency, by which we mean the sense and possibilities for acting in particular clinical situations, gave new insights about how perception and action are both shaped by a practice community" (Benner et al., 1996, p. xiii). As a result of the study, there was a clearer understanding of the distinctions between engagement with a problem or situation and the requisite nursing skills of interpersonal involvement. It appears that these nursing skills are learned over time experientially. The skill of involvement seems central in gaining nursing expertise. Understanding of the interlinkage of clinical and ethical decision making (i.e., how an individual's notions of good and poor outcomes and visions of excellence shape clinical judgments and actions) was enhanced by this research. This study represents phase one of the articulation project to describe the nature of critical care nursing practice.

Phase two took place from 1996 to 1997 and included 76 nurses (32 of them advanced practice nurses) from six different hospitals. This work is presented in the book published in 1999 by Benner and colleagues, *Clinical Wisdom in Critical Care*. The following nine domains of critical care nursing practice were identified as broad themes in phase two of this work:

1. Diagnosing and managing life-sustaining physiological functions in unstable patients
2. Using the skilled know-how of managing a crisis
3. Providing comfort measures for the critically ill
4. Caring for patients' families
5. Preventing hazards in a technological environment
6. Facing death: end-of-life care and decision making
7. Communicating and negotiating multiple perspectives
8. Monitoring quality and managing breakdown
9. Using the skilled know-how of clinical leadership and the coaching and mentoring of others

The nine domains of critical care nursing practice were used as broad themes to interpret the data, with the incorporation of the descriptions of the following six aspects of clinical judgment and skillful comportment:

1. Reasoning-in-transition
2. Skilled know-how
3. Response-based practice
4. Agency
5. Perceptual acuity and the skill of involvement
6. Links between clinical and ethical reasoning

Identification of clinical grasp and clinical forethought (two pervasive habits of thought linked with action in nursing practice in phase two of this articulation project) enriched the understanding of clinical judgment (Benner et al., 1999). Benner explained that clinical grasp is as follows:

> . . . clinical inquiry in action that includes problem identification and clinical judgment across time about the particular transitions of particular patients and families. It has four components: making qualitative distinctions, engaging in detective work, recognizing changing clinical relevance, and developing clinical knowledge in specific patient populations. (Benner et al., 1999, p. 317)

She added that clinical forethought, although playing a role in clinical grasp, "also plays an essential role in structuring the practical logic of clinicians. Clinical forethought refers to at least four habits of thought and action: future think, clinical forethought about specific diagnoses and injuries, anticipation of risks for particular patients, and seeing the unexpected" (Benner et al., 1999, p. 317).

MAJOR ASSUMPTIONS

Benner incorporates the following assumptions (as delineated in Brykczynski's 1985 dissertation; see also Benner 1984a) in her ongoing articulation research:

- There are no interpretation-free data. This abandons the assumption from natural science that there is an independent reality whose meaning can be represented by abstract terms or concepts (Taylor, 1982).
- There are no nonreactive data. This abandons the false belief from natural science that one can neutrally observe brute data (Taylor, 1982).
- Meanings are embedded in skills, practices, intentions, expectations, and outcomes. They are taken for granted and often are not recognized as knowledge. According to Polanyi (1958), a context possesses existential meaning, and this distinguishes it from "denotative or more generally, representative meaning" (p. 58). He claims that transposing a significant whole into terms of its constituent parts deprives it of any purpose or meaning.
- People sharing a common cultural and language history have a background of common meanings that allows for understanding and interpretation. Heidegger (1962) refers to this as *primordial understanding,* after the writings of Dilthey (1976) in the late 1800s and early 1900s, asserting that cultural organization and meanings precede and influence individual understanding.
- The meanings embedded in skills, practices, intentions, expectations, and outcomes cannot be made completely explicit; however, they can be interpreted by someone who shares a similar language and cultural background and can be consensually validated by the participants and relevant practitioners. Humans are self-interpreting beings (Heidegger, 1962). Hermeneutics is the interpretation of cultural contexts and meaningful human action.
- Humans are integrated, holistic beings. The mind-body split is abandoned. Embodied intelligence enables skilled activity that is transformed through experience and mastery (Dreyfus & Dreyfus, 1980; Dreyfus & Dreyfus, 1986). Benner stated, "This model assumes that all practical situations are far more complex than can be described by formal models, theories and textbook descriptions" (1984a, p. 178). The hierarchical elevation of intellectual, reflective activity above embodied skilled activity ignores the point that skilled action is a way of knowing and that the skilled body may be essential for the more highly esteemed levels of human intelligence (Dreyfus, 1979).

Benner and her collaborators explicated the themes of nursing, person, situation, and health in their publications.

Nursing

Nursing is described as a caring relationship, an "enabling condition of connection and concern" (Benner & Wrubel, 1989, p. 4). "Caring is primary because caring sets up the possibility of giving help and receiving help" (Benner & Wrubel, 1989, p. 4). "Nursing is viewed as a caring practice whose science is guided by the moral art and ethics of care and responsibility" (Benner & Wrubel, 1989, p. xi). Benner and Wrubel (1989) understand nursing practice as the care and study of the lived experience of health, illness, and disease and the relationships among these three elements.

Person

Benner and Wrubel (1989) use Heidegger's phenomenological description of person, which they describe as "A person is a self-interpreting being, that is, the person does not come into the world predefined but gets defined in the course of living a life. A person also has . . . an effortless and nonreflective understanding of the self in the world" (p. 41). "The person is viewed as a participant in common meanings" (Benner & Wrubel, 1989, p. 23).

Finally, the person is embodied Benner and Wrubel (1989) have conceptualized the following four major aspects of understanding that the person must deal with:

1. The role of the situation
2. The role of the body
3. The role of personal concerns
4. The role of temporality

Together, these aspects of the person make up the person in the world. This view of the person is based on the works of Heidegger (1962), Merleau-Ponty (1962), and Dreyfus (1979, 1991). Their goal is to overcome Cartesian dualism, the view that the mind and body are distinct, separate entities (Visintainer, 1988).

Benner and Wrubel (1989) define embodiment as the capacity of the body to respond to meaningful situations. On the basis of the work of Merleau-Ponty (1962), Dreyfus (1979, 1991), and Dreyfus and Dreyfus (1986), they outline the following five dimensions of the body (Benner & Wrubel, 1989):

1. The unborn complex, unacculturated body of the fetus and newborn baby
2. The habitual skilled body complete with socially learned postures, gestures, customs, and skills evident in bodily skills such as sense perception and "body language" that are "learned over time through identification, imitation, and trial and error" (Benner & Wrubel, 1989, p. 71)
3. The projective body that is set (predisposed) to act in specific situations (for example, opening a door or walking)
4. The actual projected body indicating an individual's current bodily orientation or projection in a situation that is flexible and varied to fit the situation, such as when an individual is skillful in using a computer
5. The phenomenal body, the body aware of itself with the ability to imagine and describe kinesthetic sensations

They point out that nurses attend to all of these dimensions of the body and seek to understand the role of embodiment in particular situations of health, illness, and recovery.

Health

On the basis of the work of Heidegger (1962) and Merleau-Ponty (1962), Benner and Wrubel focus "on the lived experience of being healthy and being ill" (1989, p. 7). Health is defined as what can be assessed, whereas well-being is the human experience of health or wholeness. Well-being and being ill are understood as distinct ways of being in the world. Health is described as not just the absence of disease and illness. Also, on the basis of the work of Kleinman, Eisenberg, and Good (1978) a person may have a disease and not experience illness, because illness is the human experience of loss or dysfunction, whereas disease is what can be assessed at the physical level (Benner & Wrubel, 1989).

Situation

Benner and Wrubel (1989) use the term *situation* rather than *environment,* because situation conveys a social environment with social definition and meaningfulness. They use the phenomenological terms *being situated* and *situated meaning,* which are defined by the person's engaged interaction, interpretation, and understanding of the situation. "Personal interpretation of the situation is bounded by the way the individual is in it" (Benner & Wrubel, 1989, p. 84). This means that each person's past, present, and future, which include their own personal meanings, habits, and perspectives, influence the current situation.

THEORETICAL ASSERTIONS

Benner (1984a) stated that there is always more to any situation than theory predicts. The skilled practice of nursing exceeds the bounds of formal theory. Concrete experience provides learning about the exceptions and shades of meaning in a situation. The knowledge embedded in practice can lead to discovering and interpreting theory, precedes and extends theory, and synthesizes and adapts theory in caring nursing practice. Some of the relationship statements included in Benner's work follow:

- "Discovering assumptions, expectations, and sets can uncover an unexamined area of practical knowledge that can then be systematically studied and extended or refuted" (Benner, 1984a, p. 8).
- Clinical knowledge is embedded in perceptions rather than precepts.
- "Perceptual awareness is central to good nursing judgment and . . . [for the expert] begins with vague hunches and global assessments that initially bypass critical analysis; conceptual clarity follows more often than it precedes" (Benner, 1984a, p. xviii).
- Formal rules are limited and discretionary judgment is needed in actual clinical situations.
- Clinical knowledge develops over time, and each clinician develops a personal repertoire of practice knowledge that can be shared in dialogue with other clinicians.
- "Expertise develops when the clinician tests and refines propositions, hypotheses, and principle-based expectations in actual practice situations" (Benner, 1984a, p. 3).

LOGICAL FORM

Through qualitative descriptive research, Benner applied the Dreyfus Model of Skill Acquisition to clinical nursing practice. By following the model's logical sequence, Benner was able to identify the performance characteristics and teaching-learning needs inherent at each level of skill. In reporting her research, Benner used exemplars taken directly from interviews and observation of expert practice to help the reader form a clear picture of such practice. The goal of Benner's research is to bring meanings and knowledge embedded in skilled practice into public discourse. Benner (1984a) claims that new knowledge and understanding are constituted by articulating meanings, skills, and knowledge that were previously taken for granted and embedded in clinical practice.

ACCEPTANCE BY THE NURSING COMMUNITY
Practice

Benner describes clinical nursing practice by using an interpretive phenomenological approach. *From Novice to Expert* (1984a) includes several examples of the application of her work in practice settings (Dolan, 1984; Huntsman, Lederer, & Peterman, 1984; Ullery, 1984). As noted earlier, Benner's approach has been used to aid in the development of clinical promotion ladders, new graduate orientation programs, and clinical knowledge development seminars. Symposia focusing on excellence in nursing practice have been held for staff development, recognition, and reward and as a way to demonstrate clinical knowledge development in practice (Dolan, 1984). Fenton (1984) reported the use of Benner's approach in an ethnographic study of the performance of clinical nurse-specialists. Her findings included identification and description of competencies of nurses functioning at an advanced level of preparation. Balasco and Black (1988) and Silver (1986a, 1986b) used Benner's work as a basis for differentiating clinical knowledge development and career progression in nursing.

Neverveld (1990) used Benner's rationale and format in her development of basic and advanced preceptor workshops. Farrell and Bramadat (1990) used Benner's paradigm case analysis in a collaborative educational project between a university school of nursing and a tertiary care teaching hospital to better understand the development of clinical reasoning skills in actual practice situations. Crissman and Jelsma (1990) applied Benner's findings in developing a cross-training program to address staffing imbalances. They delineated specific cross-training performance objectives for novice nurses, but also provided support for the experiential judgment needed to function in unfamiliar settings by designating a preceptor in the clinical area. The aim is for the novice to be able to perform more like an advanced beginner with an experienced nurse available as a resource.

Benner has been cited extensively in nursing literature regarding nursing practice concerns and the role of caring in such practice. She continues to advance understanding of the knowledge embedded in clinical situations through publications (Benner 1985a, 1985b, 1987; Benner & Tanner, 1987; Benner, et al., 1996; Benner et al., 1999). Benner edited a clinical exemplar series in the *American Journal of Nursing* during the 1980s. (See this chapter in the fifth edition of this book [2002].) In 2001, she began editing a series called Current Controversies in Critical Care in the *American Journal of Critical Care*. (See the *Journals* listing in this chapter's bibliography.)

Education

Benner (1982) has critiqued the concept of competency-based testing by contrasting it with the complexity of the proficiency and expert stages described in the Dreyfus Model of Skill Acquisition and the 31 competencies described in the AMICAE project (Benner, 1984a). In summary, she stated, "Competency-based testing seems limited to the less situational, less interactional areas of patient care where the behavior can be well defined and patient and nurse variations do not alter the performance criteria" (1982, p. 309).

Fenton (1984, 1985) described the application of the domains of clinical nursing practice as the basis for studying the skilled performance of clinical nurse specialists (CNSs). Her analysis validated that the CNSs studied demonstrated competencies in common with those skills of expert nurses reported in the AMICAE project. She also identified additional areas of skilled performance for the CNSs including the consulting role, and she delineated five preliminary categories relevant for curriculum evaluation in the graduate program. Ethical, clinical, and political dilemmas, positions or stances that promote success or failure, and new knowledge that blends the empirical and theoretical were among these categories.

According to Barnum (1990), it was not Benner's development of the seven domains of nursing practice that has had the greatest impact on nursing education, but the "appreciation of the utility of the Dreyfus model in describing learning and thinking

in our discipline" (p. 170). As a result of Benner's application of the Dreyfus model, nursing educators have realized that learning needs at the early stages of clinical knowledge development are different from those required at later stages. These differences need to be acknowledged and valued in developing nursing education programs appropriate for the background experience of the students. Some in nursing have come to appreciate that knowledge does develop in practice and that practice is more complex than any one theory can encompass, but the platonic quest for application of abstract theories continues to be a strong thrust in academia.

In *Expertise in Nursing Practice,* Benner and colleagues (1996) emphasized the importance of learning the skill of involvement and caring through practical experience, the articulation of knowledge with practice, and the use of narratives in undergraduate education. This work provides further support for the thesis that it may be better to place a new graduate with a competent nurse preceptor who can explain nursing practice in ways that the beginner comprehends than with the expert, whose intuitive knowledge may elude beginners who do not have the experienced know-how to grasp the situation.

In *Clinical Wisdom in Critical Care,* Benner and colleagues (1999) urged greater attention to experiential learning and presented the work as a guide to teaching. They designed a highly interactive CD-ROM to accompany the book (Benner et al., 2001).

Research

The preceding example by Fenton (1984, 1985) presented an application of educational research. Lock and Gordon (1989), medical anthropologists who had been research assistants on the AMICAE project, extended the inquiry to study the formal models used in nursing practice and medicine. They concluded that formal models may serve as maps that direct care, substitute knowledge, and result in conformity. Gordon (1984) cautions that a misuse of formal models occurs when nurses apply models without using judgment, when they use models to exert control, when they use language from models that may cover up meanings, or when they do not understand the meaning of the models. And finally, "formal models should be used with discretion" as tools and should not eclipse the relational, holistic, intuitive aspects of nursing (p. 242).

FURTHER DEVELOPMENT

Benner's philosophy of nursing practice provides concept definitions and in-depth descriptions of each from nursing practice. From these situated descriptions, competencies in seven domains have been derived from actual nursing practice (Benner, 1984a). Additionally, nine domains have been described for critical care nursing practice (Benner et al., 1999), and the domains and competencies have been modified to reflect advanced practice nursing (Brykczynski, 1999; Fenton, 1984, 1985; Fenton & Brykczynski, 1993). These descriptions of nursing practice follow Benner's approach to maintaining the context of the clinical situations so that the descriptions are holistic or synthetic and not procedural and elemental.

The competencies within each domain are in no way intended as an exhaustive list. Instead, the situation-based interpretive approach to describing nursing practice seeks to overcome some of the problems of reductionism and the problem of global and overly general descriptions based on nursing process categories (Benner, 1984a). In a further description this approach, Benner (1992) examined the role of narrative accounts in understanding the notion of good or ethical caring in expert clinical nursing practice. "The narrative memory of the actual concrete event is taken up in embodied know-how and comportment, complete with emotional responses to situations. The narrative memory can evoke perceptual or sensory memories that enhance pattern recognition" (p. 16).

Dunlop (1986) explored the nursing literature related to the science of caring. She drew a distinction between a science for caring and a science of caring. She stated, "A science of caring implies that caring can be operationalized in some way as a set of behaviors, which can be observed, counted or measured" (p. 666). Benner has taken a hermeneutical form to uncover the knowledge embedded in clinical nursing practice. Dunlop stated, "As she does this, she is also uncovering the nursing-caring with which it is deeply intertwined" (p. 668). Dunlop noted that "it does not provide us with any universal truths about caring in general or about nursing-caring in particular—indeed it does not make any such pretension" (p. 668).

CRITIQUE
Simplicity

Benner has developed an interpretive descriptive account of clinical nursing practice. The concepts are the levels of skilled practice from the Dreyfus model, including novice, advanced beginner, competent, proficient, and expert. She used these five concepts to describe nursing practice from interviews, observations, and the analysis of transcripts of exemplars that nurses provided. From these descriptions, competencies were identified and these were grouped inductively into seven domains of nursing practice on the basis of common intentions and meanings (Benner, 1984a). Benner and colleagues' (1996) study of critical care nursing practice explored the differentiation of levels of practice in depth and suggested, as noted earlier, that nurses at different levels live in different worlds in the Heideggerian sense. Benner's ongoing articulation research project has also produced nine domains of critical care nursing practice (Benner et al., 1999). The model is relatively simple in regard to the five stages of skill acquisition, and it provides a comparative guide for identifying levels of nursing practice from individual nurse descriptions and observations of actual nursing practice. The interpretations are validated by consensus.

A degree of complexity is encountered in the subconcepts for differentiation among the levels of competency and the need to identify meanings and intentions. This interpretive approach is designed to overcome the constraints of the rational-technical approach to the study and description of practice.

Although a decontextualized (object) description of the novice level of performance is possible, such a description of expert performance would be difficult, if not impossible, and of limited usefulness because of the limits of objectification. In other words, the philosophical problem of infinite regress would be encountered in attempting to specify all the aspects of expert practice objectively. Instead, a holistic understanding of the particular situation is required for expert performance.

Generality

The novice to expert skill acquisition model has universal characteristics; that is, it is not restricted by age, illness, health, or location of nursing practice. However, the characteristics of theoretical universality imply properties of operationalization for prediction that are not a part of this perspective. Indeed, this phenomenological perspective critiques the limits of universality in studies of human practices. The interpretive model of nursing practice has the potential for universal application as a framework, but the descriptions are limited by dependence on the actual clinical nursing situations from which they must be derived. Its use depends on the understanding of the five levels of competency and the ability to identify the characteristic intentions and meanings inherent at each level of practice.

Although clinical knowledge is relational and contextual and involves local, specific, historical issues, it is generalizable in terms of the translation of meanings to similar situations (Guba & Lincoln, 1982). To capture the contextual and relational aspects of practice, Benner uses narrative accounts of actual clinical situations and maintains that this approach enables the reader to recognize similar intents and meanings, although the objective circumstances may be quite different. An example of generalizability or transferability as used here follows: upon reading or hearing a narrative about a nurse connecting with a family whose child is dying, other nurses can relate the knowledge and meanings conveyed to experiences they may have

had with families of patients of any age who were dying.

Empirical Precision

The model was empirically tested using qualitative methodologies; 31 competencies, 7 domains of nursing practice, and 9 domains of critical care nursing practice were derived inductively. Subsequent research suggests that the framework is applicable and useful for continued development of knowledge embedded in nursing practice. This approach to knowledge development honors the primacy of caring and the central ethic of care and responsibility embedded in expert nursing practice that don't show up if we use only scientific, technical, and organizational strategies for legitimizing expert nursing care (Benner, 1999).

It is precisely the use of an alternative qualitative process of discovering nursing knowledge that makes it difficult to address the body of Benner's work within a rational-empirical framework for critique. Positivistic science seeks formulas and theories to apply in practice. Using the quantitative scientific approach, the nurse would look for lawlike relational statements to predict practice. Instead, using the qualitative interpretive approach, Benner describes expert nursing practice in many exemplars. Her work can be considered as hypothesis generating rather than hypothesis testing. Benner provides no universal "how to" for nursing practice, but instead provides a methodology for uncovering and entering into the situated meaning of expert nursing care.

Derivable Consequences

Although clinical nurses around the world enthusiastically received *From Novice to Expert* (1984a), some academicians and administrators initially interpreted it as promoting traditionalism and devaluing education and theory for nursing practice (Christman, 1985). Benner's qualitative interpretive approach to interpretation of the meaning and level of nursing practice creates doubt among objective researchers who seek precision and control. An ongoing debate has developed over cognitive interpretations of Benner's concepts of expertise and intuition (Benner, 1996b; Cash, 1995; Darbyshire, 1994; English, 1993; Paley, 1996). Yet these phenomenological concepts were never intended to be operationalized and objectified.

Benner's perspective is phenomenological, not cognitive. She stated, "Clinical judgment and caring practices require attendance to the particular patient across time, taking into account changes and what has been learned. In this vision of clinical judgment, skilled know-how and action are linked" (Benner, 1999, p. 316). The strength of the Benner model is that data-based research contributes to the science of nursing as a practice discipline (Darbyshire, 1994). The significance of Benner's research findings lies in her conclusion that "a nurse's clinical knowledge is relevant to the extent to which its manifestation in nursing skills makes a difference in patient care and patient outcomes" (Benner & Wrubel, 1982, p. 11).

The approach to generalization is through understanding common meanings, skills, practices, and embodied capacities rather than through general abstract laws that explain and predict. Such common meanings, skills, and practices are socially embedded in nurse schooling and in the practice and tradition of nursing. The knowledge embedded in clinical nursing practice should be brought forth as public knowledge to further a greater understanding of nursing practice. Benner (1984a) believes the scope and complexity of nursing practice are too extensive to rely on idealized, decontextualized views of practice or experiments. Benner (1992) stated, "The platonic quest to get to the general so that we can get beyond the vagaries of experience was a misguided turn . . . . We can redeem the turn if we subject our theories to our unedited, concrete, moral experience and acknowledge that skillful ethical comportment calls us not to be beyond experience but tempered and taught by it" (p. 19).

The generalizations possible with the interpretive approach are depicted through exemplars that demonstrate relational and contextually relevant intents and aspects of clinical knowledge. The applicability and relevance of the common approaches used for universality or generalization in physics and the natural sciences are questioned by the interpretive approach that claims that the basis for generalization in clinical knowledge cannot be structural or mechanistic, but must be based on common meanings and practices. Preferred strategies for generalization in clinical practice are not based on abstraction through removing the situation or context (objectification), but by showing how the skilled knowledge, intent, content, and notion of good in clinical knowledge can be depicted by exemplars that illustrate the role of the situation.

Benner claims that this is not a privativistic or subjectivistic approach, but an attempt to overcome the limits of subject-object descriptions. Her call is to "increase public storytelling" to validate nursing as an ethical caring practice and "to extend, alter, and preserve ethical distinctions and concerns" (Benner, 1992, pp. 19-20). Benner (1996a) stated, "We have overlooked practitioner stories that demonstrate that compassion can be wise and, in the long run, less costly than 'defensive' adversarial commodified technocures" (pp. 35-36). Benner's work is useful in that it frames nursing practice in the context of what nursing actually is and does rather than from idealized theoretical descriptors that are context free.

SUMMARY

Benner seeks to affirm and restore nurses' caring practices during a time when nurses are rewarded more for efficiency, technical skills, and measurable outcomes. She maintains that caring practices are imbued with knowledge and skill about everyday human needs and that in order to be experienced as caring, these practices must be attuned to the particular person being cared for and to the particular situation as it unfolds. Benner's philosophy of nursing practice is a dynamic, emerging holistic perspective that holds that philosophy, practice, research, and theory are interdependent, interrelated, and hermeneutic. Her hope voiced in the preface to *From Novice to Expert* (1984a) that the domains and competencies would not be deified by system builders seems to have been largely realized, as those who have sought to apply these concepts have honored the contextual background on which they are based.

Benner maintains that there is excellence and power in clinical nursing practice that can be made visible through what she describes as *articulation research*. Intricate nuanced descriptions of situational contexts are the essence of this research approach that dictates that data be collected through situation-based dialogue and observation of actual practice. The situational context guides interpretation of meanings such that there can be agreement among interpreters. This is a holistic approach that emphasizes identification and description of meanings embedded in clinical practice. The holistic approach is maintained throughout the research process from beginning to end. The situational context is maintained as narratives are interpreted through dialogue among researchers and clinicians.

Case Study

A case study from the peer-identified nurse expert project that this author (Brykczynski, 1993-1995, 1998) conducted as part of a nursing service clinical ladder enhancement process is selected here to illustrate how to apply Benner's approach to knowledge development in clinical nursing practice. This project was undertaken to identify and describe expert staff nursing practices at our institution. Exemplars were obtained and participant observations were conducted to yield narrative text that was then interpreted using Benner's multiphase interpretive phenomenological process (Benner, 1984a, 1994). In the final phase of data analysis, Benner's domains and competencies of nursing practice (Benner, 1984a) were incorporated as an interpretive framework. A critical aspect of using Benner's approach is to realize that the domains and competencies form a dynamic evolving interpretive framework that is used in interpreting the narrative and observational data collected. They are not used initially as a prescriptive abstract theoretical framework that might circumscribe the study.

The nurse who described this situation had approximately 8 years of experience in critical care, and she noted that it was significant to her practice because it taught her how to integrate taking care of a family in crisis along with taking care of a critically ill patient. This was a paradigm case for the nurse, who learned many things from it that impacted her future practice. Mrs. Walsh is a pseudonym for a woman in her 70s who was in critical condition following repeat coronary artery bypass graft (CABG) surgery. Her family had lived nearby when Mrs. Walsh had her first CABG surgery. They had moved out of town but returned to our institution where the first surgery had been performed successfully. Mrs. Walsh remained critically ill and unstable for several weeks prior to her death. Her family was very anxious because of Mrs. Walsh's unstable and deteriorating condition, and for the first few weeks there was always a family member with her, 24 hours a day.

The nurse became involved with this family while Mrs. Walsh was still in surgery, because they were very anxious that the procedure was taking longer than it had the first time and made repeated calls to the critical care unit asking about the patient. The nurse met with the family and offered to go into the operating room to talk with the cardiac surgeon so as to better inform the family of their mother's status.

One of the helpful things the nurse did to assist this family was to establish a consistent group of nurses to work with Mrs. Walsh, so that the family members could establish trust and feel more confident about the care their mother was receiving. This eventually enabled the family members to leave the hospital for intervals to get some rest. The nurse related that this was a family whose members were affluent, educated, and well-informed, and they came in prepared with lists of questions. A consistent group of nurses who were familiar with Mrs. Walsh's particular situation helped both the family members and the nurses to be more satisfied and less anxious. The family developed a close relationship with the three nurses who consistently cared for Mrs. Walsh and shared details about Mrs. Walsh and her life with them.

The nurse related that there was a tradition in this particular critical care unit not to involve family members in care. She broke that tradition when she responded to the son's and daughter's helpless feelings by teaching them some simple things that they could do for their mother. They learned to give some basic care, such as bathing her. The nurse acknowledged that involving family members in direct patient care with a critically ill patient is complex and requires knowledge and sensitivity. She believes that a developmental process is involved in working with families.

She noted that after lots of experience and a high degree of comfort with highly technological skills, it becomes okay for family members to be in the room when care is provided. She pointed out that direct observation by anxious family members can be disconcerting to those insecure with their skills when family members ask things like: "Why are you doing this? Nurse 'So and So' does it differently." She commented that nurses need to learn to be flexible and to reset priorities. They should be able to let some things wait that don't need to be done right away to give the family some time with the patient. One of the things the nurse did to coordinate was to meet with the family to see what times worked best for them, and then she posted family time on the patient's activity schedule outside her cubicle to communicate the plan to others involved in Mrs. Walsh's care.

When Mrs. Walsh died the son and daughter wanted to participate in preparing her body. This had never been done in this unit, but after checking to see that there was no policy forbidding it, the nurse invited them to participate. They turned down the lights, closed the doors, put music on, and the nurse, patient's daughter, and son all cried together while they prepared Mrs. Walsh to be taken to the morgue. The nurse took care of all the intravenous lines and tubes while the children bathed her. The nurse gives evidence of how finely tuned her skill of involvement was with this family when she explained that she felt uncomfortable at first because she thought that the son and

daughter should be sharing this time alone with their mother. Then she realized that they really wanted her to be there with them. This situation taught her that families of critically ill patients need care as well. The nurse explained that this was a paradigm case for motivating her to move into a CNS role, with expansion of her sphere of influence from her patients during her shift to other shifts, other patients and their families, and other disciplines.

Domain: The Helping Role of the Nurse

This narrative exemplifies the meaning and intent of several competencies in this domain, in particular creating a climate for healing and providing emotional and informational support to patients' families (Benner, 1984a). Incorporating the family as participants in the care of a critically ill patient requires a high level of skill that cannot be developed until the nurse feels competent and confident in technical critical care skills. This nurse had many years of experience in this unit, and she felt that providing care for their mother was so important to these children that she broke tradition in her unit and taught them how to do some basic comfort and hygiene measures. The nurse related that the other nurses in this critical care unit held the belief that active family involvement in care was intrusive and totally out of line. A belief such as this is based on concerns for patient safety and efficiency of care, yet it cuts the family off from being fully involved in the caring relationship. This nurse demonstrated moral courage, commitment to care, and advocacy in going against the tradition in her unit of excluding family members from direct care. She had 8 years of experience in this unit and her peers respected her, so she was able to change practice by starting with this one patient-family situation and involving the other two nurses working with them.

Chesla's (1996) research points to a gap between theory and practice with respect to including families in patient care. Eckle (1996) studied family presence with children in emergency situations and concluded that in times of crisis the needs of families must be addressed to provide effective and compassionate care. The skilled practice of including the family in care emerged as significantly meaningful in the narrative text from the peer-identified nurse expert study. It was defined as an additional competency in the domain called the *helping role of the nurse* and was named *maximizing the family's role in care* (Brykczynski, 1998). The intent of this competency is to assess each situation as it arises and develops over time, so that family involvement in care can adequately address specific patient-family needs and they are neither excluded from involvement nor do they have participation thrust upon them.

This narrative illustrates how Benner's approach is dynamic and specific for each institution. The belief that being attuned to family involvement in care is in part a developmental process is supported by Nuccio and colleagues' (1996) description of this aspect of care in the CPDM at their institution. They observed that novice nurses begin by recognizing their feelings associated with family-centered care, while expert nurses develop creative approaches to include patients and families in care. The intricate process of finely tuning the nurse's collaboration with families in critical care is further delineated by Levy (2004) in her interpretive phenomenological study articulating the practices of nurses with critically burned children and their families. Other domains of nursing practice are also relevant to this narrative, but they will not be discussed due to space limitations.

CRITICAL THINKING *Activities*

1. Describe clinical situations from your own experience or those of colleagues that you have observed that illustrate how nurses at various levels of skill development from novice to expert involve patients and families in care.

2. Discuss the clinical narrative provided here in terms of the rights and justice approach to ethical decision making, and then describe what the care and responsibility approach to relational ethics would add to this perspective. You may want to refer to Benner's (2003) chapter, "Finding the Good Behind the Right" to assist you in responding to this challenge.

3. Describe and give examples of what is meant by the statement that the caring practices, intervention skills, clinical judgment, and collaboration skills articulated with Benner's approach can increase the visibility of nursing practice in the following three senses: (1) to the individual nurse, (2) to nursing colleagues, and (3) to the health care system.

4. Obtain a videotape of the movie "At First Sight" produced by MGM in 1999. View it and identify examples from the movie to illustrate the phenomenology of how the massage therapist, played by Val Kilmer, constructed his world as a blind person, and contrast this with how his architect love interest, played by Mira Sorvino, constructed her world as a sighted person. Articulate how the massage therapist was like a novice when his sight was restored and relate insights gained from this exercise to skill development in nursing practice.

REFERENCES

Alberti, A. M. (1991). Advancing the scope of primary nurses in the NICU. *Journal of Perinatal and Neonatal Nursing, 5*(3), 44-50.

Alvsvåg, H. (2006). Kari Martinsen: Philosophy of caring. In A. M. Tomey & M. R. Alligood (Eds.), *Nursing theorists and their work* (6th ed.) St. Louis: Mosby.

Aristotle (1985). *Nicomachean ethics* (T. Irwin, Trans.). Indianapolis: Hackett.

Balasco, E. M., & Black, A. S. (1988). Advancing nursing practice: Description, recognition, and reward. *Nursing Administration Quarterly, 12*(2), 52-62.

Barnum, B. (1996). Foreword. In P. Benner, C. Tanner, & C. Chesla (Eds.), *Expertise in nursing practice: Caring, clinical judgment, and ethics.* New York: Springer.

Barnum, B. J. (1990). *Nursing theory: Analysis, application, evaluation.* Glenview, IL: Scott, Foresman.

Benner, P. (1982, May). Issues in competency-based training. *Nursing Outlook, 20*(5), 303-309.

Benner, P. (1983). Uncovering the knowledge embedded in clinical practice. *Image: The Journal of Nursing Scholarship, 15*(2), 36-41.

Benner, P. (1984a). *From novice to expert: Excellence and power in clinical nursing practice.* Menlo Park, CA: Addison-Wesley.

Benner, P. (1984b). *Stress and satisfaction on the job: Work meanings and coping of mid-career men.* New York: Praeger.

Benner, P. (1985a). The oncology clinical nurse specialist: An expert coach. *Oncology Nursing Forum, 12*(2), 40-44.

Benner, P. (1985b). Quality of life: A phenomenological perspective on explanation, prediction, and understanding in nursing science. *ANS Advances in Nursing Science, 8*(1), 1-14.

Benner, P. (1987, Sept.). A dialogue with excellence. *American Journal of Nursing, 87*(9), 1170-1172.

Benner, P. (1992). The role of narrative experience and community in ethical comportment. *ANS Advances in Nursing Science, 14*(2), 1-21.

Benner, P. (1994). The tradition and skill of interpretive phenomenology in studying health, illness, and caring practices. In P. Benner (Ed.), *Interpretive phenomenology: Embodiment, caring, and ethics in health and illness* (pp. 99-126). Thousand Oaks, CA: Sage.

Benner, P. (1996a). Embodiment, caring and ethics: A nursing perspective: The 1995 Helen Nahm lecture. *The Science of Caring, 8*(2), 30-36.

Benner, P. (1996b). A response by P. Benner to K. Cash. Benner and expertise in nursing: A critique. *International Journal of Nursing Studies, 33*(6), 669-674.

Benner, P. (1999). Claiming the wisdom and worth of clinical practice. *Nursing and Health Care Perspectives, 20*(6), 312-319.

Benner, P. (2003). Finding the good behind the right: A dialogue between nursing and bioethics. In F. G. Miller, J. C. Fletcher, &. J. M. Humber (Eds.), *The nature and prospect of bioethics: Interdisciplinary perspectives* (pp. 113-139). Totowa, NJ: Humana Press.

Benner, P., & Benner, R. V. (1979). *The new nurses' work entry: A troubled sponsorship.* New York: Tiresias.

Benner, P., & Benner, R. V. (1999). The clinical practice development model: Making the clinical judgment, caring and collaborative work of nurses visible. In B. Haag-Heitman (Ed.), *Clinical practice development: Using novice to expert theory* (pp. 17-42). Gaithersburg, MD: Aspen.

Benner, P., Hooper-Kyriakidis, P., & Stannard, D. (1999). *Clinical wisdom in critical care: A thinking-in-action approach.* Philadelphia: W. B. Saunders.

Benner, P., & Kramer, M. (1972, Jan.). Role conceptions and integrative role behavior of nurses in special care and regular hospital nursing units. *Nursing Research, 21*(1), 20-29.

Benner, P., Stannard, D., & Hooper-Kyriakidis, P. (2001). *Clinical wisdom and interventions in critical care: A thinking-in-action approach* (CD-ROM). Philadelphia: W. B. Saunders.

Benner, P., & Tanner, C. (1987, Jan.). Clinical judgment: How expert nurses use intuition. *American Journal of Nursing, 87*(1), 23-31.

Benner, P., Tanner, C., & Chesla, C. (1992). From beginner to expert: Gaining a differentiated clinical world in critical care nursing. *ANS Advances in Nursing Science, 14*(3), 13-28.

Benner, P., Tanner, C., & Chesla, C. (1996). *Expertise in nursing practice: Caring, clinical judgment, and ethics.* New York: Springer.

Benner, P., & Wrubel, J. (1982). Skilled clinical knowledge: The value of perceptual awareness. *Nurse Educator, 7*(3), 11-17.

Benner, P., & Wrubel, J. (1989). *The primacy of caring: Stress and coping in health and illness.* Menlo Park, CA: Addison-Wesley.

Brykczynski, K. A. (1985). Exploring the clinical practice of nurse practitioners (Doctoral dissertation, University of California, San Francisco). *Dissertation Abstracts International, 46,* 3789B. (University Microfilms No. DA8600592)

Brykczynski, K. A. (1993-1995). Principal investigator. Developing a profile of expert nursing practice. Project of the UTMB Nursing Service Task Force studying expert nursing practice, supported by UTMB Joint Ventures. Galveston, TX: University of Texas Medical Branch.

Brykczynski, K. A. (1998). Clinical exemplars describing expert staff nursing practice. *Journal of Nursing Management, 6,* 351-359.

Brykczynski, K. A. (1999). An interpretive study describing the clinical judgment of nurse practitioners. *Scholarly Inquiry for Nursing Practice: An International Journal, 13*(2), 141-166.

Cash, K. (1995). Benner and expertise in nursing: A critique. *International Journal of Nursing Studies, 32*(6), 527-534.

Chesla, C. A. (1996). Reconciling technologic and family care in critical-care nursing. *Image: The Journal of Nursing Scholarship, 28*(3), 199-203.

Christman, L. (1985). [Review of *From Novice to Expert* (1984) by Patricia Benner]. *Nursing Administration Quarterly, 9*(4), 87-89.

Clifford, J. (1999). Foreword. In P. Benner, P. Hooper-Kyriakidis, & D. Stannard (Eds.), *Clinical wisdom in critical care: A thinking-in-action approach.* Philadelphia: W. B. Saunders.

Crissman, S., & Jelsma, N. (1990). Cross-training: Practicing effectively on two levels. *Nursing Management, 21*(3), 64a-64h.

Darbyshire, P. (1994). Skilled expert practice: Is it "all in the mind"? A response to English's critique of Benner's novice to expert model. *Journal of Advanced Nursing, 19*, 755-761.

Dilthey, W. (1976). *Selected writings* (H. P. Rickman, Trans. & Ed.). London: Cambridge University Press. (Original work published 1833-1911.)

Dolan, K. (1984). Building bridges between education and practice. In P. Benner (Ed.), *From novice to expert: Excellence and power in clinical nursing practice* (pp. 275-284). Menlo Park, CA: Addison-Wesley.

Dreyfus, H. L. (1979). *What computers can't do.* New York: Harper & Row.

Dreyfus, H. L. (1991). *Being-in-the-world: A commentary on being and time dimension. I.* Cambridge, MA: M. I. T. Press.

Dreyfus, H. L., & Dreyfus, S. E. (1986). *Mind over machine.* New York: The Free Press.

Dreyfus, H. L., & Dreyfus, S. E. (1996). The relationship of theory and practice in the acquisition of skill. In P. Benner, C. Tanner, & C. Chesla (Eds.), *Expertise in nursing practice: Caring, clinical judgment, and ethics* (pp. 29-47). New York: Springer.

Dreyfus, S. E., & Dreyfus, H. L. (1980, Feb.). *A five-stage model of the mental activities involved in directed skill acquisition.* Unpublished report supported by the Air Force Office of Scientific Research, USAF (Contract F49620-79-c-0063). Berkeley, CA: University of California, Berkeley.

Dunlop, M. J. (1986). Is a science of caring possible? *Journal of Advanced Nursing, 11*, 661-670.

Dunne, J. (1993). *Back to the rough ground: Practical judgment and the lure of technique.* Notre Dame, IN: Indiana University Press.

Eckle, N. J. (1996). Family presence—Where would you want to be? *Critical Care Nurse, 16*(1), 102.

English, I. (1993). Intuition as a function of the expert nurse: A critique of Benner's novice to expert model. *Journal of Advanced Nursing, 18*, 387-393.

Farrell, P., & Bramadat, I. J. (1990). Paradigm case analysis and stimulated recall: Strategies for developing clinical reasoning skills. *Clinical Nurse Specialist, 4*(3), 153-157.

Fenton, M. V. (1984). Identification of the skilled performance of master's prepared nurses as a method of curriculum planning and evaluation. In P. Benner (Ed.), *From novice to expert: Excellence and power in clinical nursing practice* (pp. 262-274). Menlo Park, CA: Addison-Wesley.

Fenton, M. V. (1985). Identifying competencies of clinical nurse specialists. *Journal of Nursing Administration, 15*(12), 31-37.

Fenton, M. V., & Brykczynski, K. A. (1993). Qualitative distinctions and similarities in the practice of clinical nurse specialists and nurse practitioners. *Journal of Professional Nursing, 9*(6), 313-326.

Gadamer, G. (1970). *Truth and method.* London: Sheer & Ward.

Gaston, C. (1989). Inservice education: Career development for South Australian nurses. *Australian Journal of Advanced Nursing, 6*(4), 5-9.

Gordon, D. R. (1984). Research application: Identifying the use and misuse of formal nursing models in nursing practice. In P. Benner (Ed.), *From novice to expert: Excellence and power in clinical nursing practice* (pp. 225-243). Menlo Park, CA: Addison-Wesley.

Gordon, D. R. (1986). Models of clinical expertise in American nursing practice. *Social Science and Medicine, 22*(9), 953-961.

Guba, E. G., & Lincoln, Y. S. (1982). Epistemological and methodological bases of naturalistic inquiry. *Educational Communications and Technology Journal, 30*, 233-252.

Hamric, A. B., Whitworth, T. R., & Greenfield, A. S. (1993). Implementing a clinically focused advancement system. *Journal of Nursing Administration, 23*(9), 20-28.

Heidegger, M. (1962). *Being and time* (J. MacQuarrie & E. Robinson, Trans.). New York: Harper & Row.

Henderson, V. (1989). Foreword. In P. Benner & J. Wrubel (Eds.), *The primacy of caring: Stress and coping in health and illness.* Menlo Park, CA: Addison-Wesley.

Huntsman, A., Lederer, J. R., & Peterman, E. M. (1984). Implementation of staff nurse III at El Camino Hospital. In P. Benner (Ed.), *From novice to expert: Excellence and power in clinical nursing practice* (pp. 244-257). Menlo Park, CA: Addison-Wesley.

Kierkegaard, S. (1962). *The present age* (A. Dur, Trans.). New York: Harper & Row.

Kleinman, A., Eisenberg, L., & Good, B. (1978). Culture, illness, and care. Clinical lessons from anthropologic and cross-cultural research. *Annals of Internal Medicine, 88*, 251-258.

Kuhn, T. S. (1970). *The structure of scientific revolutions* (2nd ed.). Chicago: University of Chicago Press.

Lazarus, R. S. (1985). The trivialization of distress. In J. C. Rosen & L. J. Solomon (Eds.), *Preventing health risk behaviors and promoting coping with illness* (Vol. 8, pp. 279-298). Hanover, NH: University Press of New England.

Lazarus, R. S., & Folkman, S. (1984). *Stress appraisals and coping.* New York: Springer.

Levy, K. (2004). Practices that facilitate critically burned children's healing. *Qualitative Health Research, 13*(10), 1-21.

Lindeke, L. L., Canedy, B. H., & Kay, M. M. (1997). A comparison of practice domains of clinical nurse specialists and nurse practitioners. *Journal of Professional Nursing, 13*(5), 281-287.

Lock, M., & Gordon, D. R. (Eds.). (1989). *Biomedicine examined.* Boston, MA: Kluwer Academic.

Løgstrup, K. E. (1995a). *Metaphysics* (Vol. I; R. L. Dees, Trans.). Milwaukee, WI: Marquette University Press.

Løgstrup, K. E. (1995b). *Metaphysics* (Vol. II; R. L. Dees, Trans.). Milwaukee, WI: Marquette University Press.

Løgstrup, K. E. (1997). *The ethical demand* (with introduction by A. MacIntyre & H. Fink). Notre Dame, IN: University of Notre Dame Press.

Lynaugh, J. (1999). Foreword. In P. Benner, P. Hooper-Kyriakidis, & D. Stannard (Eds.), *Clinical wisdom in critical care: A thinking-in-action approach.* Philadelphia: W. B. Saunders.

MacIntyre, A. (1981). *After virtue: a study in moral theory.* Notre Dame, IN: University of Notre Dame.

MacIntyre, A. (1999). *Dependent rational animals: Why human beings need the virtues.* Chicago: Open Court.

Martin, L. L. (1996). *Factors affecting performance of advanced nursing practice.* Doctoral dissertation, Virginia Commonwealth University, School of Nursing. (University Microfilms No. 9627443)

Merleau-Ponty, M. (1962). *Phenomenology of perception* (C. Smith, Trans.) London: Routledge and Kegan Paul.

Neverveld, M. E. (1990, July/Aug.). Preceptorship: One step beyond. *Journal of Nursing Staff Development, 6*(4), 186-189, 194.

Nuccio, S. A., Lingen, D., Burke, L. J., Kramer, A., Ladewig, N., Raum, J., et al. (1996). The clinical practice developmental model: The transition process. *Journal of Nursing Administration, 26,* 29-37.

O'Neill, O. (1996). *Towards justice and virtue. A constructive account of practical reasoning.* Cambridge, MA: Cambridge University Press.

Packer, M. J. (1985). Hermeneutic inquiry in the study of human conduct. *American Psychologist, 40*(10), 1081-1093.

Paley, J. (1996). Intuition and expertise: Comments on the Benner debate. *Journal of Advanced Nursing, 23*(4), 665-671.

Phillips, S., & Benner, P. (Eds.). (1994). *The crisis of care: Affirming and restoring caring practices in the helping professions.* Washington, DC: Georgetown University Press.

Polanyi, M. (1958). *Personal knowledge.* Chicago: University of Chicago Press.

Rubin, J. (1984). *Too much of nothing: Modern culture, the self and salvation in Kierkegaard's thought* (Unpublished doctoral dissertation). Berkeley, CA: University of California, Berkeley.

Silver, M. (1986a). A program for career structure: A vision becomes a reality. *The Australian Nurse, 16*(2), 44-47.

Silver, M. (1986b). A program for career structure: From neophyte to expert. *The Australian Nurse, 16*(2), 38-41.

Taylor, C. (1971). Interpretation and the sciences of man. *The Review of Metaphysics, 25,* 3-34.

Taylor, C. (1982). Theories of meaning. Dawes Hicks Lecture. Read November 6, 1980. *Proceedings of the British Academy* (pp. 283-327). Oxford, UK: University Press.

Taylor, C. (1989). *Sources of the self: The making of modern identity.* Cambridge, MA: Harvard.

Taylor, C. (1991). *Ethics of authenticity.* Cambridge, MA: Harvard.

Taylor, C. (1993). Explanation and practical reason. In M. Nussbaum & A. Sen (Eds.). *The quality of life* (pp. 208-231). Oxford, UK: Clarendon.

Taylor, C. (1994). Philosophical reflections on caring practices. In S. S. Phillips & P. Benner (Eds.), *The crisis of care: Affirming and restoring caring practices in the helping professions* (pp. 174-187). Washington, DC: Georgetown University Press.

Ullery, J. (1984). Focus on excellence. In P. Benner (Ed.), *From novice to expert: Excellence and power in clinical nursing practice* (pp. 258-261). Menlo Park, CA: Addison-Wesley.

Visintainer, M. (1988). [Review of the book *The Primacy of Caring: Stress and Coping in Health and Illness*]. *Image: The Journal of Nursing Scholarship, 20*(2), 113-114.

BIBLIOGRAPHY*
Primary Sources
Books

Benner, P. (2001). *From novice to expert.* Upper Saddle River, NJ: Prentice Hall.

Benner, P., Hooper-Kyriakidis, P., & Stannard, D. (1999). *Clinical wisdom in critical care: A thinking-in-action approach.* Philadelphia: W. B. Saunders.

Benner, P., Tanner, C., & Chesla, C. (1996). *Expertise in nursing practice: Caring, clinical judgment, and ethics.* New York: Springer.

Gordon, S., Benner, P., & Noddings, N. (Eds.). (1996). *Caregiving readings in knowledge, practice, ethics, and politics.* Philadelphia: University of Pennsylvania Press.

Book Chapters

Benner, P. (1997). A dialogue between virtue ethics and care ethics. In D. Thomasma (Ed.), *The moral philosophy of Edmund Pellegrino* (pp. 47-61). Dordrecht, Netherlands: Kluwer.

*For references prior to 1995, please refer to Tomey, A. M., & Alligood, M. R. (2002). *Nursing theorists and their work* (5th ed.). St. Louis: Mosby.

Benner, P. (1998). When health care becomes a commodity: The need for compassionate strangers. In J. F. Kilner, R. D. Orr, & J. A. Shelly (Eds.), *The changing face of health care* (pp.119-135). Grand Rapids, MI: William B. Eerdmans.

Benner, P. (2000). The quest for control and the possibilities of care. In M. A. Wrathall & J. Malpas (Eds.), *Heidegger, coping and cognitive science: Essays in honor of Hubert L. Dreyfus* (Vol. 2, pp. 293-383). Cambridge, MA: M. I. T. Press.

Benner, P. (2001). The phenomenon of care. In S. K. Tombs (Ed.), *Handbook of phenomenology and medicine* (pp. 351-369). Dordrecht, Netherlands: Kluwer Academic Publishers.

Benner, P. (2002). Learning through experience and expression: Skillful ethical comportment in nursing practice. In E. D. Pellegrino, D. C. Thomasma, & J. L. Kissel (Eds.), *The healthcare professional as friend and healer; building on the work of Edmund Pellegrino* (pp. 49-64). Washington, DC: Georgetown University Press.

Benner, P. (2003). Clinical practice development. In *Clinical practice development* (pp. 90-98). Tokyo, Japan: Shoshina.

Benner, P. (2003). Clinical reasoning articulating experiential learning in nursing practice. In O. Slevin & L. Basford (Eds.), *Theory and practice of nursing* (2nd ed., pp. 176-186). London, UK: Nelson Thornes Ltd.

Benner, P. (2003). Finding the good behind the right: A dialogue between nursing and bioethics. In F. G. Miller, J. C. Fletcher, &. J. M. Humber (Eds.), *The nature and prospect of bioethics: Interdisciplinary perspectives* (pp. 113-139). Totowa, NJ: Humana Press.

Benner, P. (2003). The role of narrative in reflecting on practice and experiential learning. In *Clinical practice development* (pp. 76-88). Tokyo, Japan: Shoshina.

Benner, P., & Benner, R. V. (1999). The clinical practice development model: Making the clinical judgment, caring and collaborative work of nurses visible. In B. Haag-Heitman (Ed.), *Clinical practice development, using novice to expert theory* (pp. 17-42). Gaithersburg, MD: Aspen.

Benner, P., & Gordon, S. (1996). Caring practice. In S. Gordon, P. Benner, & N. Noddings (Eds.), *Caregiving, readings in knowledge, practice, ethics and politics* (pp. 40-55). Philadelphia: University of Pennsylvania Press.

Journal Articles

Benner, P. (1996). A dialogue between virtue ethics and care ethics. *Theoretical Medicine, 23,* 1-15.

Benner, P. (1996). A response by P. Benner to K. Cash, Benner expertise in nursing: A critique. *International Journal of Nursing Studies, 33*(6), 669-674.

Benner, P. (1996). Embodiment, caring and ethics: A nursing perspective. The 1995 Helen Nahm Lecture. *Science of Caring, 8*(2), 30-36.

Benner, P. (1999). Claiming the wisdom and worth of clinical practice. *Nursing and Health Care Perspectives, 20*(6), 312-319.

Benner, P. (2000). Seeing the person beyond the disease, current controversies in critical care. *American Journal of Critical Care, 10*(2), 60-62.

Benner, P. (2000). The roles of embodiment, emotion and lifeworld for rationality and agency in nursing practice. *Nursing Philosophy, 1,* 5-19.

Benner, P. (2000). The wisdom of our practice. *AJN, 100*(10), 99-101, 103, 105.

Benner, P. (2001). Breathing new life into practice communities. *American Journal of Critical Care, 10*(3), 188-190.

Benner, P. (2001). Creating a culture of safety and improvement: A key to reducing medical error. *American Journal of Critical Care, 10*(4), 281-284.

Benner, P. (2001). Curing, caring, and healing in medicine: Symbiosis and synergy or syncretism? *Park Ridge Center Bulletin, 23,* 11-12.

Benner, P. (2001). Death as a human passage: Compassionate care for persons dying in critical care units. *American Journal of Critical Care, 10*(5), 355-359.

Benner, P. (2001). Seeing the person beyond the disease. Current controversies in critical care. *American Journal of Critical Care, 10*(2), 121-124.

Benner, P. (2001). Taking a stand on experiential learning and good practice. *American Journal of Critical Care, 10*(1), 60-62.

Benner, P. (2002). Caring for the silent patient. *American Journal of Critical Care, 11*(5), 480-481.

Benner, P. (2002). Creating compassionate institutions that foster agency and respect. *American Journal of Critical Care, 11*(2), 164-166.

Benner, P. (2002). Developing clinical expertise in undergraduate education (in Japanese). *Expert Nurse, 12*(15), 107-113.

Benner, P. (2002). Living organ donors: Respecting the risks involved in the "gift of life." *American Journal of Critical Care, 11*(3), 266-268.

Benner, P. (2002). One year after September 11: Revisiting our ethical visions of freedom and justice. *American Journal of Critical Care, 11*(6), 572-573.

Benner, P. (2003). Avoiding ethical emergencies. *American Journal of Critical Care, 12*(1), 71-72.

Benner, P. (2003). Beware of technological imperatives and commercial interests that prevent best practices! *American Journal of Critical Care, 12*(5), 469-471.

Benner, P. (2003). [Book review for *From detached concern to empathy: Humanizing medical practice,* J. Halpern, Ed.] *The Cambridge Quarterly for Health Care Ethics, 12*(1), 134-136.

Benner, P. (2003). Creating a more responsible public dialogue about the social, ethical, and legal aspects of genomics. *American Journal of Critical Care, 12*(3), 259-261.

Benner, P. (2003). Enhancing patient advocacy and social ethics. Current controversies in critical care. *American Journal of Critical Care, 12*(4), 374-375.

Benner, P. (2003). Reflecting on what we care about. Current controversies in critical care. *American Journal of Critical Care, 12*(2), 165-166.

Benner, P. (2004). Seeing the person beyond the disease. Current controversies in critical care. *American Journal of Critical Care, 13*(1), 75-78.

Benner, P., Brennan, Sr. M. R., Kessenich, C. R., & Letvak, S. A. (1996). Critique of Silva's philosophy, science and theory: Interrelationships and implications for nursing research. *Image: The Journal of Nursing Scholarship, 29*(3), 214-215.

Benner, P., Ekegren, K., Nelson, G., Tsolinas, T., & Ferguson-Dietz, L. (1997). The nurse as a wise, skillful and compassionate stranger. *American Journal of Nursing, 97*(11), 27-34.

Benner, P., Kerchner, S., Corless, I. B., & Davies, B. (2003). Current controversies in critical care. Attending death as a human passage: Core nursing principles for end-of-life care. *American Journal of Critical Care, 12*(6), 558-561.

Benner, P., Sheets, V., Uris, P., Malloch, K., Schwed, K., & Jamison, D. (2002). Individual, practice, and system causes of errors in nursing: A taxonomy. *Journal of Nursing Administration, 32*(10), 509-523.

Benner, P., Stannard, D., & Hooper, P. L. (1996). "Thinking-in-action" approach to teaching clinical judgment: A classroom innovation for acute care advanced practice nurses. *Advanced Practice Nursing Quarterly, 1*, 70-77.

Benner, P., Tanner, C. A., & Chesla, C. A. (1996). Nurse practitioner extra. Becoming an expert nurse. (Adapted with permission from Benner, Tanner, & Chesla [Eds.]. *Expertise in nursing practice: caring, clinical judgment, and ethics.* NY: Springer Publishing.) *AJN, 97*(6), Contin Care Extra Ed, 16BBB, 16DDD.

Benner, P., Tanner, C. A., & Chesla, C. A. (1996). The social fabric of nursing knowledge. (Adapted with permission from Benner, Tanner, & Chesla [Eds.]. *Expertise in nursing practice: Caring, clinical judgment, and ethics.* New York: Springer Publishing). *AJN, 97*(7), Nurse Pract Extra Ed, 16BBB.

Brant, M., Rosen, L., & Benner, P. (1998, Nov.). Nurses as skilled samaritans. "The nurse as wise, skillful, and compassionate stranger." *AJN, 98*(4), Contin Care Extra Ed, 22-23.

Cohen H., & Benner, P. (2002). Errors in nursing. Individual, practice, and system causes of errors in nursing: A taxonomy. *JONA, 32*(10), 509-523.

Day, L., & Benner, P. (2002). Ethics, ethical comportment, and etiquette. *American Journal of Critical Care, 11*(1), 76-79.

Ekegren, K., Nelson, G., Tsolinas, A., Ferguson-Dietz, L., & Benner, P. (1997). The nurse as wise, skillful, and compassionate stranger. *AJN, 97*, 26-34.

Emami, A., Benner, P., Ekman, S. L. (2001). A sociocultural health model for late-in-life immigrants. *Journal of Transcultural Nursing, 12*(1), 15-24.

Emami, A., Benner, P., Lipson, J. G., Ekman, S. L. (2000). Health as continuity and balance in life. *Western Journal of Nursing Research, 22*, 812-825.

Fowler, M., & Benner, P. (2001). The new code of ethics for nurses: A dialogue with Marsha Fowler. *American Journal of Critical Care, 10*(6), 434-437.

Benner, P., et al. (1996). Survey reactions of nursing leaders: A grim prognosis for health care? *AJN, 96*(11), 43.

Puntillo, K. A., Benner, P., Drought, T., Drew, B., Stotts, N., Stannard, D., Rushton, C., et al. (2001). White, C. End-of-life issues in intensive care units: A national random survey of nurses knowledge and beliefs. *American Journal of Critical Care, 10*(4), 216-229.

Weiss, S. M., Malone, R. E., Merighi, J. R., & Benner, P. (2002). Economism, efficiency, and the moral ecology of good nursing practice. *Canadian Journal of Nursing Research, 34*(2), 95-119.

Videotape

Benner, P., Tanner, C., & Chesla, C. (1992). *From beginner to expert: Clinical knowledge in critical care nursing* (Videotape). Helene Fuld Trust Fund. Athens, OH: Studio Three Productions, FITNE.

CD-ROM

Benner, P., Stannard, D., & Hooper-Kyriakidis, P. (2001). *Clinical wisdom and interventions in critical care: A thinking-in-action approach* (CD-ROM). Philadelphia: W. B. Saunders.

Secondary Sources
Doctoral Dissertations

The following doctoral dissertations were supervised by Patricia Benner:

Boller, J. E. (2001). The ecology of exercise: An interpretive phenomenological account of exercise in the lifeworld of persons on maintenance hemodialysis (Doctoral dissertation, University of California, San Francisco). *Dissertation Abstracts International,* B62/12, 5638. (University Microfilms No. 3034743)

Brykczynski, K. A. (1985). Exploring the clinical practice of nurse practitioners (Doctoral dissertation, University of California, San Francisco). *Dissertation Abstracts International,* 46, 3789B. (University Microfilms No. DA8600592)

Chesla, C. A. (1988). Parents' caring practices and coping with schizophrenic offspring, an interpretive study

(Doctoral dissertation, University of California, San Francisco). Dissertation Abstracts International 49-B, 2563. (University Microfilms No. AAD88-13331)

Cho, A. (2001). Understanding the lived experience of heart transplant recipients in North America and South Korea: An interpretive phenomenological cross-cultural study (Doctoral dissertation, University of California, San Francisco). *Dissertation Abstracts International*, B62/12, 5639. (University Microfilms No. 3034721)

Day, L. J. (1999). Nursing care of potential organ donors. An articulation of ethics, etiquette and practice (Doctoral dissertation, University of California, San Francisco). *Dissertation Abstracts International*, 60-B, 5431. (University Microfilms No. AADAA-19951464)

Doolittle, N. (1990). Life after stroke (Doctoral dissertation, University of California, San Francisco). *Dissertation Abstracts International*, 51-B, 1742. (University Microfilms No. AAD90-24963)

Dunlop, M. (1990). Shaping nursing knowledge: An interpretive analysis of curriculum documents from NSW Australia (Doctoral dissertation, University of California, San Francisco). *Dissertation Abstracts International*, 51-B, 659. (University Microfilms No. AAD90-16380)

Gordon, D. (1984). Expertise, formalism, and change in American nursing practice: A case study. Medical anthropology program (Doctoral dissertation, University of California, San Francisco). *Dissertation Abstracts International*, 46-A, 738. (University Microfilms No. AAD85-09101)

Hartfield, M. (1985). Appraisal of anger situations and subsequent coping responses in hypertensive and normotensive adults: A comparison (Doctoral dissertation, University of California, San Francisco). *Dissertation Abstracts International*, 46-B, 4452. (University Microfilms No. AAD85-24005)

Hooper, P. L. (1995). Expert titration of multiple vasoactive drugs in post-cardiac surgical patients: An interpretive study of clinical judgment and perceptual acuity (Doctoral dissertation, University of California, San Francisco). *Dissertation Abstracts International*, 57-B, 238. (University Microfilms No. AAD85-19614338)

Kesselring, A. (1990). The experienced body, when taken-for-grantedness falters: A phenomenological study of living with breast cancer (Doctoral dissertation, University of California, San Francisco). *Dissertation Abstracts International*, 52-B, 1955. (University Microfilms No. AAD91-19579)

Leonard, V. W. (1993). Stress and coping in the transition to parenthood of first time mothers with career commitments: An interpretive study (Doctoral dissertation, University of California, San Francisco). *Dissertation Abstracts International*, 54-A, 3221. (University Microfilms No. AAD94-02354)

Lionberger, H. (1986). Phenomenological study of therapeutic touch in nursing practice: An interpretive study of nurses' practice of therapeutic touch (Doctoral dissertation, University of California, San Francisco). *Dissertation Abstracts International*, 46-B, 2624. (University Microfilms No. AAD85-24008)

MacIntyre, R. (1993). Sex, drugs, and T-cell counts in the gay community: Symbolic meanings among gay men with asymptomatic HIV infections (immune deficiency) (Doctoral dissertation, University of California, San Francisco). *Dissertation Abstracts International*, 54-B, 4601. (University Microfilms No. AAD94-06617)

Mahrer-Imhof, R. (2003). Couples' daily experiences after the onset of cardiac disease: An interpretive phenomenological study (Doctoral dissertation, University of California, San Francisco).

Malone, R. (1995). The almshouse revisited: Heavy users of emergency services (Doctoral dissertation, University of California, San Francisco). *Dissertation Abstracts International*, 56-B, 6036. (University Microfilms No. AADAA-19606591)

McKeever, L. C. (1988). Menopause: An uncertain passage. An interpretive study (Doctoral dissertation, University of California, San Francisco). *Dissertation Abstracts International*, 49-B, 3677. (University Microfilms No. AAD88-24678)

Plager, K. A. (1995). Practical well-being in families with school-age children: An interpretive study (Doctoral dissertation, University of California, San Francisco). *Dissertation Abstracts International*, 56-B, 6039. (University Microfilms No. AADAA-16906593)

Popell, C. L. (1983). An interpretive study of stress and coping among parents of school-age developmentally disabled children (Doctoral dissertation, Wright Institute of Graduate Psychology). *Dissertation Abstracts International*, 44-B, 1604. (University Microfilms No. AAD83-20854)

Raingruber, B. J. (1998). Moving in a climate of care: Styles and patterns of interaction between nurse-therapists and clients: An interpretive study (Doctoral dissertation, University of California, San Francisco). *Dissertation Abstracts International*, 58-B, 6482. (University Microfilms No. AAD98-18661)

Schilder, E. (1986). The use of physical restraints in an acute care medical ward (immobilization) (Doctoral dissertation, University of California, San Francisco). *Dissertation Abstracts International*, 47-B, 4826. (University Microfilms No. AAD87-08453)

SmithBattle, L. (1992). Caring for teenage mothers and their children: Narratives of self and ethics of intergenerational caregiving (Doctoral dissertation, University of California, San Francisco). *Dissertation Abstracts International*, 53-B, 4594. (University Microfilms No. AAD93-03555)

Stainton, M. C. (1985). Origins of attachment: Culture and cue sensitivity (Doctoral dissertation, University of California, San Francisco). *Dissertation Abstracts International, 46-B,* 3786. (University Microfilms No. AAD86-00606)

Stannard, P. (1997). Reclaiming the house: An interpretive study of nurse-family interactions and activities in critical care (Doctoral dissertation, University of California, San Francisco). *Dissertation Abstracts International, 58-B,* 4147. (University Microfilms No. AAD98-06902)

Stevens, M. (1984). Adolescents coping with hospitalization for surgery (Doctoral dissertation, University of California, San Francisco). *Dissertation Abstracts International, 45-B,* 3977. (University Microfilms No. AAD85-03742)

Stuhlmiller, C. (1991). An interpretive study of appraisal and coping of rescue workers in an earthquake disaster: The Cypress collapse (Doctoral dissertation, University of California, San Francisco). *Dissertation Abstracts International, 52-B,* 4671. (University Microfilms No. AAD92-05240)

Warnian, L. (1987). *A hermeneutical study of group psychotherapy* (Unpublished doctoral dissertation). Berkeley, CA: University of California, Berkeley.

Weiss, S. M. (1996). Possibility or despair: Biographies of aging (Doctoral dissertation, University of California, San Francisco). *Dissertation Abstracts International, 57-B,* 3662. (University Microfilms No. AAD96-34295)

Moccia, P. (1987). *Nursing theory: A circle of knowledge* (Videotape). New York: National League for Nursing.

Web Sites

Home Page of Patricia Benner. Accessed December 20, 2004: *http://www.bennerassociates.com*

Home Page for Hubert Dreyfus. Accessed December 20, 2004: *http://ist-socrates.berkeley.edu/~hdreyfus*

CHAPTER 10

*K*ari Martinsen

1943-present

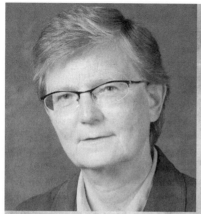

Photo credit: Lars Jakob Løtvedt,
Bergen Norway.

Philosophy of Caring

Herdis Alvsvåg

Translators: Bjørn Follevåg and Kirsten Costain Schou

CREDENTIALS AND BACKGROUND OF THE THEORIST

Kari Marie Martinsen is a nurse and philosopher, born and raised in Oslo, the capital city of Norway. She was born in 1943 during the German occupation of Norway during the second World War (1940-1945). Her parents were both in the Resistance and her father worked illegally. After the war, moral and sociopolitical discussions dominated home life, a home consisting of three generations: a younger sister, parents, and a grandmother. Both parents were economists educated at the University of Oslo, and her mother worked all of her adult life outside the home.

After high school, Martinsen began studies at Ulleval College of Nursing in Oslo and became a nurse in 1964. She worked in clinical practice at the hospital for 1 year while doing preparatory studies

for acceptance to the university. But before embarking upon a university degree, she gained further education in nursing and became a psychiatric nurse in 1966. She worked for 2 years at Dikemark Psychiatric Hospital near Oslo and was engaged there for several years in psychiatric care of outpatients.

Both as a nurse and a psychiatric nurse, she became concerned over social inequalities and inequalities in the health service. Health, illness, care, and treatment were unequally distributed. Some patients received help, support, and care while others waited, often without getting the help they needed. Further, she became aware that there were discrepancies between health care theories, ideals, and goals on the one hand, and the practical and concrete results of nursing, medicine, and the health service on the other. She began to pose questions about how a society and a profession must be constituted in order to support and aid the ill and those

167

who fall outside the employment market. One question she posed to the nursing profession was, How must it operate if it is not to let down its weakest patients and those that need care the most? What then followed was the question of how the nurse can care for the person who is ill, when medical science relates foremost to physical illnesses. In other words, Martinsen asked how we in the health services can care adequately for the subjects of our care when we are so closely allied with a science that objectifies the patient. She posed questions about whether that same objectification will occur with the increasing emphasis on a scientific base for the discipline of nursing.

These foundational questions brought Martinsen to further study, this time a bachelor's degree in psychology at the University of Oslo in 1968. At this point, she planned to take a master's degree in psychology. In order to qualify, she had to take an intermediate examination in physiology and another free credit at the intermediate level. She took the physiology examination in 1969. She chose philosophy as her other intermediate subject and took that examination in 1971. Both examinations were taken at the University of Oslo. Her encounter with philosophy and phenomenology changed her plans. She realized that philosophy could contribute more to the existential questions with which she was concerned than could psychology. It was phenomenology that brought her to the University of Bergen, Norway's next-largest city.

From 1972 to 1974, she was a student at the of Institute of Philosophy at the University of Bergen. In her graduate degree in philosophy thesis (Magister artium) printed in 1975, she grappled philosophically with questions that disturbed her as a citizen, professional, and health care worker. The title of the dissertation is *Philosophy and Nursing: A Marxist and Phenomenological Contribution* (Martinsen, 1975). The work created debate and received much critical attention. The dissertation directed a critical gaze toward the nursing profession for its refusal to take up or take seriously the consequences for the discipline of nursing of uncritically adopting the characteristics of a profession, and the consequences of uncritically embracing a scientific base

for nursing. Such a development could contribute to distancing nurses from the patients who need them most. This first dissertation written by a nurse in Norway analyzed the discipline of nursing from a critical philosophical and social perspective.

During the mid-1970s in Norway there was a great lack of nursing teachers for the nursing colleges, and this was also the situation in Bergen. The rectors of the three nursing colleges in Bergen took the initiative to establish a temporary nursing teacher–training course in order to address this problem. The course was jointly established by the University of Bergen, the three nursing colleges in Bergen, and the county. A nurse with university-level qualifications was needed to head the program. Martinsen was asked to be Dean of the Faculty of Nursing Teachers' Training in Bergen, which she did from 1976 to 1977.

Through her philosophical studies and the sociological issues she encountered in nursing and nursing education, Martinsen developed an interest in nursing history. How did the education of nurses in Norway begin, who was responsible for its inception, and what did they wish to achieve? In order to look more closely at some of these issues, Martinsen applied for and received a grant from the Norwegian Nurses' Association in 1976. She was affiliated with the Institute for Hygiene and Social Medicine at the University of Bergen, and she lectured there to medical students in social medicine while lecturing in nursing at the nursing teachers' training program of which she was dean.

At that time, an intense debate was underway about nursing education in Norway. A public committee proposed the retention of the traditional 3-year degree but eventually agreed to alter this to a system of stage-based qualification. That is to say that after completion of 1 year, a student was a qualified care assistant, and with a further 2 years, a qualified nurse. This meant the end of the principle of a comprehensive 3-year degree. Nurses throughout the country, with the Norwegian Nurses' Association at the forefront, marched in protest to save the 3-year nursing degree. Sides in this debate remained rigidly opposed, and the tone of the political discourse on the issue of nursing education was heated.

Martinsen threw herself into this debate. She suggested that nursing education be changed to a 4-year program but gave her approval to the principle of stage-based education. She sketched an educational model in which one is qualified as a care assistant after 2 years and a nurse after 4 years (Martinsen, 1976). With the comprehensive 3-year degree as the stated goal for the nursing association, her suggestion was viewed as a provocation.

In 1978, she received a grant from Norway's General Science Research Council. She was now attached to the historical institute at the University of Oslo. There she worked on her recently begun project on the social history of nursing while lecturing master's degree students in sociopolitical history. From 1981 to 1985 she was a scientific assistant at the Historical Institute at the University of Bergen. In addition to her own research, Martinsen lectured and supervised master's degree students in feminist history and developed a database of Norwegian feminist history.

The period from 1976 to 1986 can be described as a historical phase in Martinsen's work (Kirkevold, 2000). She published several historical articles (Martinsen, 1977, 1978, 1979a, 1979b). Close collaborators during this phase were professor of social history Anne Lise Seip, professor of feminist history Ida Blom, and professor of sociology Kari Wærness. In 1979, Martinsen and Wærness published a "lit torch" of a book with the provocative title, *Caring Without Care?* (Martinsen & Wærness, 1979). The questions posed by the authors concern whether nursing was moving away from the sickbed, whether caring for the ill and infirm was disappearing with the advent of increasingly technical care and treatment, and whether nurses were becoming administrators and researchers who increasingly relinquish the concrete and executive work of care to other occupational groups.

To aid ill and care-dependent people as women's work has long historical roots. However, the existence of the professionally trained nurse is not very old in Norway, originating in the late 1800s. The deaconesses (Christian lay sisters) were the first trained health workers in Norway, educated at the different deaconess houses in Germany. Martinsen described how these first trained nurses built up nursing education in Norway and how they expanded, wrote textbooks, and practiced nursing both in institutions and the home. They were the forerunners of Norway's public health system. This pioneer period was described by Martinsen in her book, *Nursing History: Frank and Engaged Deaconesses: A Caring Profession Emerges 1860-1905* (Martinsen, 1984). Based on this work, Martinsen became a doctor of philosophy in 1984 at the University of Bergen.

In connection with her defense, she prepared two lectures: Health Policy Problems and Health Policy Thinking Behind the Hospital Law of 1969 (Martinsen, 1989a) and The Doctors' Interest in Pregnancy—Part of Perinatal Care: The Period ca. 1890-1940 (Martinsen, 1989b). During the 10-year historical phase of her work, beginning in the middle of 1970, she wrote about nursing's social history and feminist history, and on the social history of medicine.

From 1986, she worked for 2 years as Associate Professor at the Institute for Health and Social Medicine at the University of Bergen. She lectured and supervised master's degree students and occupied herself with publishing a series of philosophical and historical papers. The book was published in 1989, *Caring, Nursing and Medicine. Historical-Philosophical Essays* (Martinsen, 1989c). It was divided into three parts: the philosophy of caring and caring in nursing, essays on nursing history, and medicine and the history of the health service. This book drew together the threads of Martinsen's historical phase and marked the beginning of a more philosophical period (Kirkevold, 2000) in her work. The book has several editions. The 2003 publication included a lengthy interview with the author (Karlsson & Martinsen, 2003). Fundamental problems in caring and interpretations of the meaning of discernment are what preoccupy her from 1985 to 1990. In a collection of articles published in Denmark in 1990 she contributed a paper entitled "Moral Practice and Documentation in Practical Nursing." In it, she wrote:

> Moral practice is based upon *caring*. Caring does not merely form the value foundation of nursing;

it is a fundamental precondition of our life.... Discretion demands emotional involvement and the capacity for situational analysis in order to assess alternatives for action.... To learn moral practice in nursing is to learn how the moral is founded in concrete situations. It is accounted for through experiential objectivity or through discretion, in action or in speech. In both cases what is concerned is learning good nursing. (Martinsen, 1990, pp. 60, 64-65)

In 1990, Martinsen moved to Denmark. She was employed at the University of Århus to establish master's degree and Ph.D. programs in nursing. She remained there for 5 years. Her philosophical foundation was further developed during these years through encounters with Danish life-philosophy (Martinsen, 2002a) and theological tradition. In *Caring, Nursing and Medicine: Historical-Philosophical Essays,* Martinsen (1989c, 2003b) connected the concept of caring to the German philosopher Martin Heidegger (1889-1976). While she was living in Denmark, Heidegger's role as a Nazi sympathizer during the second World War became clearer to her. At that time, a series of academic articles was published which prove that Heidegger was a member of the national Socialist Party in Germany, and that he betrayed his Jewish colleagues and friends such as Emund Husserl (1859-1938) and Hannah Arendt (1906-1975). Heidegger was banned from teaching for several years after the war because of his involvement with the Nazis (Lubcke, 1983).

Martinsen confronts Heidegger and her own thinking about his philosophy in *From Marx to Løgstrup: On Morality, Social Criticism and Sensuousness in Nursing* (Martinsen, 1993b). Knud E. Løgstrup (1905-1985) was a Danish theologian and philosopher. Precisely because life and learning cannot be separated, it became important for Martinsen to go to sources other than Heidegger in order to illustrate the fundamental aspects of caring. K. E. Løgstrup represented an alternative source. K. E. Løgstrup died in 1985. Martison knows him through his books. Rosemarie Løgstrup, Løgstrup's wife, was originally German. She met her husband in Germany, while both were studying philosophy, and later translated his books into German. While Martinsen lived and worked in Denmark, she visited Rosemarie Løgstrup several times. Their friendship and scholarly conversations were continued after Martinsen moved back to Norway.

While Martinsen lived and worked in Denmark, she met Patricia Benner on several occasions in public dialogues in Norway and Denmark, and again in 1996 in California. One of these dialogues took place at a conference at the University of Tromsø. Martinsen published it with the title "Ethics and Vocation, Culture and the Body" (Martinsen, 1997b). She also continued dialogues with Katie Eriksson, a Finnish professor of nursing.

Eriksson and Martinsen met in Norway, Denmark, Sweden, and Finland. In the beginning, the discussions with Eriksson were tense and strained, but they developed over time to include good and enlightening conversations. Martinsen (1996) published these conversations in a book with the title, *Phenomenology and Caring: Three Dialogues.* Eriksson wrote an afterword for the book. Martinsen's first chapter in this book is entitled "Caring and Metaphysics—Has Nursing Science Got Room for This?," the second, "The Body and Spirit in Practical Nursing," and the third, "The Phenomenology of Creation—Ethics and Power: Løgstrup's Philosophy of Religion Meets Nursing Practice." This is impressive language, similar to that of the dialogues Martinsen conducted with Benner, and in her preface to the book she wrote the following:

> The dialogues between the Finnish nurse researcher Katie Eriksson and myself deal with the "big words" in nursing. The words about which we speak and write are compassion, hope, suffering, pain, sacrifice, shame, violation, doubt. These are big words. But they are no bigger than their location in life, our everyday nursing situation. Mercy, writes the Danish theologian and philosopher Løgstrup, is the renewal of life, it is to afford others life.... What else is nursing but to release the patients possibilities for living within the life cycle we inhabit between life and death? We must venture into life amongst our fellow persons in order to experience the meaning of these big words. (Martinsen, 1996, p. 7)

While Martinsen taught in Århus, she was also Professor II beginning in 1994 at the Department of

Nursing Science at the University of Tromsø. In 1997, she moved north and was subsequently made professor full time. She remained for only 1 year in this position. She experienced a lack of time for her research and writing, and became a freelancer in 1998.

The period from 1990 is characterized by philosophical research. The foundational philosophical and ontological questions and their meaning for nursing dominated her thought. She worked during this period with disparate projects and published in several journals and article collections in addition to her own books. Two books from this period are already mentioned (Martinsen, 1993b, 1996). In 2000, *The Eye and the Call* (Martinsen, 2000b) was published. The titles of the chapters in this book ring more poetically than before: "To See With the Eye of the Heart," "Ethics, Culture and the Vulnerability of the Flesh," "The Call—Can We Be Without It?," and "The Act of Love and the Call." Martinsen also worked with ideas about space and architecture. Space and architecture can maintain human dignity. This she wrote about first in an article with the poetic title, "The House and the Song, the Tears and the Shame: Space and Architecture as Caretakers of Human Dignity" (Martinsen, 2001). In 2004, she was working on a book project about space and architecture in the health service.

Martinsen has held positions at two nursing colleges, one deaconal (Christian) college in Bergen and one in Oslo. From 1989 to 1990 she was employed as researcher at Bergen Deaconess University College, Bergen. From 1999 to autumn 2004 she was Professor II part time at the Lovisenberg Deconal University College, Oslo. Ideas and academic ventures sprouted and flourished easily around her, and she drew others into academic projects. While she was employed in Bergen she edited a collection of articles to which several nursing college teachers contributed, *The Thoughtful Nurse* (Martinsen, 1993a). Lovisenberg Deconal University College in Oslo, with Martinsen's assistance, took the initiative to publish a new edition of the first nursing textbook published in Norway, originally in 1877 (Nissen, 2000). Martinsen (2000a) wrote an afterword that places the text within a context of academic nursing. With a colleague in Oslo who is Professor II in theology, Martinsen edited another collection of articles. In addition to the editors, the college lecturers again contributed articles to the book, this time with the title *Ethics, Discipline, and Refinement: Elizabeth Hagemann's Ethics Book—New Readings* (Martinsen & Wyller, 2003). The book provided an analysis of a text on ethics for nurses published in 1930 and used as a textbook right up to 1965. When the ethics text was republished in 2003, it was interpreted in the light of two French philosophers, Pierre Bourdieu (1930-2002) and Michel Foucault (1926-1984), as well as the German sociologist Max Weber (1864-1920).

With these last publications, Martinsen returned to her roots in history. The historical and philosophical threads seem to merge. They are both present in the different phases of her thought but color her work differently during the different periods.

In 2002, Martinsen made her way back to the University of Bergen, where she was hired as professor at the Department of Public Health and Primary Health Care, section for nursing science. Teaching and supervision of master's and doctoral students is central now. She arranges doctoral courses and is much in demand as supervisor and lecturer in the Nordic countries.

THEORETICAL SOURCES

In her analysis of the profession of nursing in the early 1970s, Martinsen looked to three philosophers in particular. These are the German philosopher, politician, and social theorist Karl Marx (1818-1883), the German philosopher and founder of phenomenology Edmund Husserl (1859-1938), and the French philosopher and phenomenologist of the body Merleau-Ponty (1908-1961). Later on, she broadened her theoretical sources to include other philosophers, theologians, and sociologists.

Karl Marx: Critical Analysis— A Transformative Practice

Marxist philosophy gave Martinsen some analytical tools with which to describe the reality of the discipline of nursing and the social crisis in which it found itself. This crisis consisted of the failure of the discipline to examine its nature as fragmented, specialized, and technically calculating, at the same time as it pretended to hold a holistic perspective on care. She found that the discipline was part of positivism and the capitalist system, without a praxis of liberation. A "reversed care–law" governs such that those who need care most receive the least. Marx criticized individualism and the satisfaction of the needs of the rich at the expense of the poor. Martinsen's view is that it is important to expose this phenomenon as it occurred in the health service. Such revelation can be a force for change of this reality. She writes that we must question the nature of nursing, its content and inner structure, its historical origins, and the genesis of the profession. This can result in a critical nursing practice in which the practitioner views her occupation and profession in a historical and social context. Her historical interest has a critical and transformative intention.

Edmund Husserl: Phenomenology as the Natural Attitude

Husserl's phenomenology is important to Martinsen's critiques of science and positivism. Positivism's view of the self lies in its attitude of objectification and its dehumanizing (in the sense of reduction to the nature of the "thing"), calculating attitude toward the person. Husserl viewed phenomenology as a strict science. The strict methodological processes of phenomenology produce an attitude of composed reflection over our scientific reality such that we can uncover structures and contexts within which we otherwise perform taken-for-granted and unconscious work. This practice is about making the taken-for-granted problematic. By problematizing the security of a taken-for-granted self-understanding, we find opportunities to grasp "the thing itself," which will always reveal itself to be contradictory and perspective. Phenomenology works with the prescientific, that which we encounter in the natural attitude, when we are directed toward something with the intent to recognize and understand it meaningfully. Phenomenology insists upon context, wholeness, involvement, engagement, the body, and the lived life. We live in contexts, in time and space, and we live historically. The body cannot be divided up into body and soul; it is whole and relates to other bodies, to things in the world, and to nature.

Merleau-Ponty: The Body as the Natural Attitude

Merleau-Ponty builds upon Husserl's thought, but focuses more than any other thinker on the human body in the world. Both Husserl and Merleau-Ponty criticized Descartes (1596-1650), who separates the person from the world in which one lives with other persons. The body is the natural attitude in the world. The nursing profession is related to the body in all aspects. We use the body in the work of care and we relate to other bodies in need of nursing, treatment, and care. Our bodies and those of our patients express themselves through actions, attitudes, words, tone of voice, and gestures. Phenomenology involves the acts of interpretation, description, and recognition of the lived life, the everyday life that people live together with others in a mutual natural world, including the professional contexts in which caring is enacted.

Martin Heidegger: Existential Being as Caring

Martin Heidegger (1889-1976) was a German phenomenologist and a student of Husserl, among others. He investigated existential Being, that is to say that which is and how it is. Martinsen connects the concept of caring to Heidegger because he "has caring as a central concept in his thought. . . . The point is to try to elicit the fundamental qualities of caring, or what caring is and encompasses" (Martinsen, 1989c, p. 68). She wrote further, "An analysis of our practical life and an analysis of what caring is are inseparable. To investigate the one is at the same time to investigate the other. Together they form an inseparable unit. Caring is a foundational concept in understanding the person" (Martinsen, 1989c, p. 69). With phenomenology and Heidegger as a backdrop, Martinsen gave content to caring:

caring will always have at least two parts as a precondition. One has concern and anxiety for the other. Caring involves how we relate to each other, how we show concern for each other in our daily life. Caring is the most natural and the most fundamental aspect of human existence.

As mentioned earlier, Martinsen revised her perspective on Heidegger (Martinsen, 1993b). Precisely because life and philosophy cannot be separated, it is important for Martinsen to go to other sources besides Heidegger in order to describe the fundamental aspects of caring. At the same time she did not reject "Heidegger's original and acute thought" (Martinsen, 1993b, p. 17). She turned back to Heidegger when she wrote about what it is to dwell. Heidegger had examined exactly this concept termed *to dwell*. To dwell is always, first and foremost, to live amongst things (Martinsen, 2001). Here we see that Heidegger underscores something of what Merleau-Ponty is also concerned with when he states that the things we surround ourselves with are not merely things for us, objectively speaking, but participate in shaping our lives. We leave something of ourselves within these things with which we reside when we dwell. It is the body that dwells, surrounded by an environment.

Knud Eiler Løgstrup: Ethics as a Primary Condition of Human Existence

K. E. Løgstrup (1905-1981) was a Danish philosopher and theologian who built his thought on the work of two other Danish writers, Nikolaj Frederik Severin Grundtvig (1783-1872) and Søren Aaby Kierkegaard (1813-1855). Løgstrup used Grundtvig's writings to think with, while with Kierkegaard he had an enduring struggle. These two are, like Løgstrup, also philosophers and theologians. In the "void" after Heidegger, Løgstrup's work became important for Martinsen. Human perception and lived experience was central (Martinsen, 1993b). Løgstrup can be summarized through two intellectual strands: phenomenology and creation theology, the latter containing his philosophy of religion. As a phenomenologist he sought to reveal and analyze the essential phenomena of human existence. Through his phenomenological investigations, Løgstrup arrived at what he termed *sovereign* or *spontaneous life utterances:* trust, hope, compassion, and the openness of speech. That these are essential is to say that they are precultural characteristics of our existence. As characteristics they provide conditions for our culture, conditions for our existence; they make human community possible (Lubcke, 1983). With Heidegger, caring is such a characteristic. Caring must be present if existence is to prevail, because existence is characterized by our constant relationship with that which is different from ourselves. With Løgstrup, the sovereign life utterances were the necessary characteristics for human coexistence.

Martinsen wrote that for Løgstrup, metaphysics and ethics are interwoven in the concept of creation:

> They are characteristic phenomena which carry us, such that caring for the other arises out of the condition of our having been created. Caring for the other reveals itself in human relationship through trust, open speech, hope and compassion. These phenomena, which Løgstrup also calls sovereign life utterances, are "born ethical." By that is meant that they are essentially ethical. Trust, open speech, hope and compassion are fundamentally good without requiring our justification. If we try to gain dominion over them, they are destroyed. Metaphysics and ethics, or rather metaphysical ethics, is practical. It is linked to questions of life in which the person is stripped of omnipotence. (Martinsen, 1993b, pp. 17-18)

We must care for existence, not seek to control it: "Western culture is singular in its need to understand and control. It has moved away from the cradle of our culture and our religion in the narrative of creation from the Old Testament. In it 'guarding,' 'watching,' and care on one side, and cultivation and use on the other formed a unified opposition" (Martinsen, 1996, p. 79). That these are unified opposites is to say that they singularly and in themselves are opposites which separate and are insurmountable, but when they are adjusted to one another they enter into an opposition which unifies and which creates a sound whole. To care for, guide and guard, cultivate and make use of, that is to say cultivate and use in a caring manner as a unified opposition, means that we do not become domineering and exploitative, but restrained and thoughtful in our dealings with one another and with nature.

The ethical question is how a society combats suffering and takes care of those who need help. In a nursing context, Martinsen formulates the question in this way, "How do we as nurses take care of the person's eternal meaning, the individual's unending worth—independent of what the individual is good for, can be used for or can achieve? Can I bear to see the other as the other, and yet not as fundamentally different from myself?" (Martinsen, 1993b, p. 18).

Max Weber: Vocation as the Duty to Serve One's Neighbor Through One's Work

Max Weber (1864-1920) was a German sociologist and had great significance in the philosophy of social science. Weber sought to understand the meaning of human action, and he was a critic of the society he saw emerging with the advent of industrialization. Martinsen found in Weber a new alliance in addition to Marx in the criticism of both capitalism and science. While Løgstrup was a philosopher of religion, Weber was a sociologist of religion. Weber also criticized the West for its boundless intervention and its boundless consumption. Science disenchants the created world precisely because it relates to that which was created as objects in its objectification of all that is (Martinsen, 2000b, 2001, 2002b).

Martinsen was particularly concerned with joining Weber in her explication of vocation (Martinsen, 2000b). Weber looked to Martin Luther (1483-1546) who discussed vocation in the secular sense, as follows:

> Vocation is work in the sense of a life's occupation or a restricted field of work, in which the individual will endow his fellow person. . . . The

young Luther linked vocation to work, and understood it as an act of neighbourly love. Vocation is understood on the basis of the notion of creation, that we are created in order to care for one another through work. (Martinsen 2000b, pp. 94-95)

In other words, vocation is in the service of creation. With reference to the young Luther, Martinsen wrote that vocation "means that we are placed in life contexts which demand something of us. It is a challenge that I, in this my vocation, meet and attend to my neighbour. It lies in existence as a law of life" (Martinsen, 1996, p. 91).

Michel Foucault: The Effect of His Method Intensifying Phenomenologists' Phenomenology

Phenomenologists underscore the importance of history to our experience. Martinsen (1975) referred to Foucault in her dissertation in philosophy but was most concerned with this philosopher in connection with her historical works from 1976 on (Martinsen 1978, 1989a, 2001, 2002b, 2003a). Foucault (1926-1984) was a French philosopher and historian of ideas. He was concerned with fracture and difference, not continuity and context. He claimed that within each historical epoch and within the different cultures there reside some common structures, systems of terms and forms of thought that shape societies. In this way, Foucault confronted subjective philosophy that emphasizes the person as a private and independent individual. For example, Foucault asked about which fundamental conditions were present during the historical epoch in which institutions for the insane were created, and in later epochs he began to define the insane as mentally ill. Something new had happened; on what did it depend? Why did it happen and what was to be achieved in society? What actions were undertaken; were there alliances of power and did it involve establishing discipline? To question in this way is to dig away several layers of understanding such that we come past the general conception in order to understand the meaning of history in a different way. Foucault elicits the basal social distinctions that make it possible to characterize people. They are dug out of tacit preconditions (Lubcke, 1983). In this way Foucault's method intensified the phenomenological process. He asked us to think differently from the manner of thinking within the epoch and within the contexts in which we live. The gaze became not only descriptive, but also critical.

Martinsen stated that, in caring for the other, we related to the other in a different way and looked for different things than those looked for within natural science and objectifying medicine with their "classification gaze" and "examining gaze" (Martinsen, 1989b, pp. 142-168; Martinsen, 2000a). Such gazes require special space; caring requires different types of space for the development of different types of knowledge. The question we must take with us into caring in the health service is: which disciplinary characteristics or structures are to be found in our practice today, in nursing practice and its spatial arrangements? What will it mean to think differently from those of our particular epoch? Is it here we find a critical nursing, and what will a critical nursing practice mean today to the health service and to research?

Paul Ricoeur: The Bridge-Builder

Ricoeur (1913-present) is a French philosopher. His position is often termed *critical hermeneutics* or *hermeneutic phenomenology*. He seeks to build a bridge between natural science and human science, between phenomenology and structuralism and other divided positions. He writes for example about time and narrative, language and history, discernment and science. Ricoeur is concerned with communication between people, on what it is to understand one another. He is concerned with everyday language and its many meanings, in contrast to the language of science. Martinsen wrote the following:

> The culture of medicine is dominated by an abstract conceptual language in which words are embedded in different classifications, and in which they are not always tested in connection with the concrete situation. . . . In the everyday language of the caring tradition on the other hand, words are followed by the manner in which they unfold in the different contexts of meaning they enter into in concrete caring—in company with the patient and the professional community. As spoken in everyday language, the words are distinguished by their power of expression, where they strike a tone. (Martinsen, 1996, p. 103)

Martinsen referred to several parallels in the philosophy of language of Løgstrup and Ricoeur.

Major Concepts & Definitions

Martinsen is reluctant to provide definitions of terms. Definitions have a tendency to close off concepts. She writes to the contrary that the content of concepts should be given and that it is important to circumscribe the meaningful content of a term, explain what the term means, but avoid having terms lodged fast in definitions.

CARE

Care "forms not only the value base of nursing, but is a fundamental precondition for our lives. Care is the positive development of the person through the Good" (Martinsen, 1990, p. 60). Care is a trinity: relational, practical, and moral simultaneously (Alvsvåg, 2003; Martinsen, 2003b). Caring is directed outward toward the situation of the other. In professional contexts, caring requires education and training. "Without professional knowledge, concern for the patient becomes mere sentimentality" (Martinsen, 1990, p. 63). Neither guardianship, negligence, nor sentimentality is an expression of care.

Continued

MAJOR CONCEPTS *&* DEFINITIONS—cont'd

PROFESSIONAL JUDGMENT AND DISCERNMENT

These qualities are linked to the concrete. It is through the exercise of professional judgment in practical, living contexts that we learn clinical observation. It is "training not only to see, listen and touch clinically, but to see, listen and touch clinically in a good way" (Martinsen, 1993b, p. 147). The patient makes an impression on us, we are moved bodily, the impression is sensuous. "Because perception has an analogue character it evokes variation and context in the situation" (Martinsen, 1993b, p. 146), one thing is reminiscent of another and this recollection creates a connection between the impressions in the situation, professional knowledge, and previous experience. Discretion expresses professional knowledge through the natural senses and everyday language.

MORAL PRACTICE IS FOUNDED ON CARE

"Moral practice is when empathy and reflection work together such that caring can be expressed in nursing" (Martinsen, 1990, p. 60). The moral is present in concrete situations, which must be accounted for. Our actions need to be accounted for; they are learned and justified through the objectivity of empathy, which consists of empathy and reflection. This means in concrete terms to discover how the other will be best helped, and the basic conditions are recognition and empathy (Martinsen, 1990). Sincerity and judgment enter into moral practice (Martinsen, 1990).

PERSON-ORIENTED PROFESSIONALISM

Person-oriented professionalism is "to demand professional knowledge which affords the view of the patient as a suffering person, and which protects his integrity. It challenges professional competence and humanity in a benevolent reciprocation, gathered in a communal basic experience of the protection and care for life. . . . It demands an engagement in what we do, that one wants to invest something of oneself in encounters with the other, and that one is obligated to do one's best for the person one is to care for, watch or nurse. It is about having an understanding of one's position within a life context that demands something from one, and about placing the other at the centre, about the caring encounter's orientation toward the other" (Martinsen, 2000b, pp. 12, 14).

SOVEREIGN LIFE UTTERANCES

Sovereign life utterances are phenomena that accompany the creation itself. They exist as precultural phenomena in all societies; they are present as potentials. They are beyond human control and influence, and are therefore sovereign. Those over which we do have power are the conditions for the realization of the sovereign life utterances in our lives. Sovereign life utterances are openness, mercy, trust, hope, and love. These are phenomena we can receive in the same way that we receive time, space, air, water, and food (Alvsvåg, 2003). Unless we receive them, life disintegrates. Life is self-preservation through reception (Martinsen, 2000b). Sovereign life utterances are preconditions for care, simultaneously as caring actions are necessary conditions for the realization of the sovereign life utterances in the concrete life. We can act in such a way that openness, trust, hope, mercy, and love are realized through our interactions, or we can shut them out. Without them, caring cannot be realized. At the same time, caring actions clear the way for the realization of the sovereign life utterances in our personal and our professional lives. Care can bring the patient to experience the meaning of love and mercy; caring can light hope or give it sustenance, and caring can be that which makes trust and openness foremost in relations with the nurse. In the same way, lack of care can block the other's experience of mercy;

MAJOR CONCEPTS & DEFINITIONS

it can create mistrust and an attitude of restraint in relation to the health service.

THE UNTOUCHABLE ZONE

This term refers to a zone we must not interfere with in encounters with the other and encounters with nature. It refers to boundaries for which we must have respect. The untouchable zone creates a certain protective distance in the relation; it ensures impartiality and demands argumentation, theory, and professionalism. In caring, the untouchable zone is united with its opposite which is openness, in which closeness, vulnerability, and motive have their correct place. Openness and the untouchable zone constitute a unifying contradiction in caring (Martinsen, 1990).

VOCATION

Vocation "is a demand life makes to me in a completely human way to encounter and care for one's fellow person. Vocation is given as a law of life concerning neighborly love which is foundationally human" (Martinsen, 2000b, p. 87). It is an ethical demand to take care of one's neighbor. For this reason, nursing requires a personal refinement in addition to professional knowledge (Malchau, 2000).

THE EYE OF THE HEART

This concept stems from the parable of the Good Samaritan. The heart says something about the existence of the whole person, about being accosted by the suffering of the other and the situation the other is in. In sensuous and perception, we are moved before we understand, but we are also challenged by the afterthought of understanding. To see and be seen with the eye of the heart is a form of participatory attention based on a reciprocation which unifies perception and understanding, in which the eye's understanding is led by senses (Martinsen, 2000b).

THE REGISTERING EYE

The registering eye is objectifying and the perspective is that of the observer. It is concerned with finding connections, systematizing, ranking, classifying, and placing in a system. The registering eye represents an alliance between modern natural science, technology, and industrialization. If one as a patient is exposed to, or if one as a professional employs this gaze in a one-sided manner, compassion is lifted out of the situation, and the will to life is reduced (Martinsen, 2000b).

USE OF EMPIRICAL EVIDENCE

In Martinsen's philosophy of caring, language and the reflection involved in professional judgment and narrative are ways of accounting convincingly for case conditions, situations, and phenomena (Martinsen, 1997a, 2002c, 2003c, 2004a, 2004b). She writes that obvious perceptions must be accounted for convincingly. With reference to Husserl she points to different forms of evidence: the undoubtable (apodictic), the exhaustive, and the partial. Each type represents different evidential requirements. Facts, themes, and situations provide different forms of evidence. For example, we cannot accept mathematical evidence that is undoubtable and transfer this to physical objects and persons. This is because here the partial or perspective evidence is at the level of that for which it must be convincingly accounted. In this field it is discernment and narrative that can clarify the empirical facts of a case in an evidentiary, enlightening, or convincing manner (Martinsen 2003c, 2004a, 2004b). To exercise discretion is to interpret those impressions we get of the patient. The professional knowledge and experience one has built up give one a horizon of understanding that is flexible in encounters with the patient's situation (Martinsen, 1990, 2002c). The narrative can both describe and prescribe action (Kjær, 2000; Martinsen, 1997a). "A good narrative tells existential morality into being, and makes practical action unavoidable" (Martinsen, 1993b, p. 161).

MAJOR ASSUMPTIONS
Nursing

Although care goes beyond nursing, caring is fundamental to nursing and to other work of a caring nature. Caring involves having consideration for, taking care of, and being concerned about the other. When we speak about caring, three things must be simultaneously present; we could call them the triumvirate of caring: caring must be relational, practical, and moral (Alvsvåg, 2003). That it is relational means that caring requires at least two people. Martinsen describes it thus:

> The one has concern and anxiety for the other. When the one suffers, the other will "grieve" (in the sense of suffer with) and *provide for* the alleviation of pain. . . . Caring is the most natural and the most fundamental aspect of the person's existence. In caring the relationship between people is the most essential element. . . . The essence of the person is that one is created for the sake of others— for one's own sake. . . . The point here is that caring always presupposes others. Further, that I can never understand myself or realise myself alone or independent of others. (Martinsen 1989e, p. 69)

Caring is practical. It is about concrete and practical action. Caring is trained and learned through its practice. Caring is also moral: "If caring is to be genuine, I must relate to the other from an *attitude* (mood, 'befindlichkeit') which acknowledges the other in light of *his* situation . . . [We must] neither overestimate nor underestimate his ability to help himself" (Martinsen, 1989c, p. 71). Caring requires a correct understanding of the situation and this presupposes a good evaluation of which goals lie in the caring situation: "Caring work in nursing is essentially directed towards persons not capable

of self-help who are ill and in need of care. To encounter the ill person with caring through the work of care involves a set of preconditions such as knowledge, skills, and organization" (Martinsen, 1989c, p. 75). We need training in all types of caring work. We must practice and reflect alone and with others in order to develop professional judgment. Caring and professional judgment are integrated in nursing (Martinsen, 1990, 1997a, 2003c, 2004b).

Person

It is the meaning-bearing, fellowship of tradition which turns the individual into the person. The person cannot be torn away from the social milieu and the community of persons (Martinsen, 1975). In one way there is a parallel between the person and the body. It is as bodies that we relate to ourselves, to others, and to the world (Alvsvåg, 2000; Martinsen, 1997a). The body is a unit of soul and flesh, or spirit and flesh. The person is bodily, and as bodies we both perceive and understand.

Health

Health is discussed from a sociohistorical perspective. Two rival historical health ideals, the classical Greek and the modern one of intervention and expansion, form the background when she writes, "Health does not only reflect the condition of the organism, it is also an expression of the current level of competence in medicine. To put it pointedly, the tendencies of the modern concept of health are such that if one has an unnecessary 'defect' or an organ which 'could' be better, one is not completely healthy" (Martinsen, 1989c, p. 146). The modern reductionistic health ideal upon which modern medicine is built is both analytic and individualistic; it is oriented toward all that is not "good enough." Combined with medicine's autonomy and resources it has yielded success in terms of treatment. Martinsen is concerned with the point that this ideology does not withstand critical examination. Medicine's damaging effects and insufficient service for people with chronic diseases and illnesses bring Martinsen to turn toward the conservative, classical health ideal. What is important is to cure sometimes, help often, and comfort always. This requires society to give people the opportunity to live the best life possible and the individual to live sensibly; both requirements have environmental implications. We must not change the environment at such a speed and to such an extent that the change exceeds our knowledge base; restraint and caution are required (Martinsen, 1989c, 2003b).

Environment: Space and Situation

The person is always in a particular situation in one place and in a particular space. In space are found time, ambience, and power (Martinsen, 2001, 2002b, 2002c). Martinsen asks what time, architecture, and knowledge do to the ambience of a space. Architecture, our intercourse with each other, use of objects, words, knowledge, our being-in-the-room—all set the tone and color the situation and the space. The person enters into the universal space, the natural space, but through dwelling creates cultural space. We build houses with rooms, and the activities of the health service take place in different rooms. "The sick-room is important as a physical, material and constructed place, but it is also a place we share with other people. . . . The room with its interior and objects make visible the patient's and the nurse's interpretation of it" (Martinsen, 2001, pp. 175-176). Our challenge is to give patients and each other dignity in these spaces. What is needed then is deliberate knowledge gathered in slowed down, deliberate spaces, "space in which to perceive—smell, listen, see and care" (Martinsen, 2001, p. 176).

THEORETICAL ASSERTIONS

People are created dependent and relational. Care is fundamental to human life. As humans we live not merely in fellowship with one another, but also enter into relationship with animals and with nature, and we relate to a creative force that sustains the whole. The person is fundamentally dependent upon community and the creation. To the created belong the sovereign life utterances, "These are firstly *given to* us, and secondly they are *sovereign*.

That is to say it is impossible for the person to avoid their power. . . . These are phenomena which are present in the service of life. They create life, they release life's possibilities" (Martinsen, 1996, p. 80).

The body is created whole. That is to say that need and spirit, or body and spirit, enter into a benevolent interaction, in which sensing cannot be avoided. Martinsen (1996) wrote the following:

> Sensing initiates interaction and maintains it. Care of the body becomes central. In this respect, nursing is secular vocational work which through professional care of the body protects and provides space for the life possibilities of the patient. The vocation is seen as a demand life makes on us to care for our neighbour, in this case the patient, through our work. It is work in the service of life processes. Vocation, the body and work are seen as a counterweight to the new (bodiless) spirituality in nursing. (p. 72)

Love of one's neighbor is coupled with a concrete, practical, professional, and moral discernment.

Sensuous and experience-based knowledge is the most fundamental and essential for the practice of nursing. Caring is learned through practical experience in concrete situations under the supervision of expert and experienced nurses (Martinsen, 1993b, 2003b).

Metaphysics is not speculation about that of which we cannot know anything. It is an interpretation of phenomena we all recognize through senses and can experience. These phenomena are prescientific and foundational.

LOGICAL FORM

Martinsen's logical form can be described as inductive and analogous. The inductive aspect of her thought has its source in that the experiences in life and in the health service are the starting point for her theoretical works. She turns toward philosophy and history in the hope of greater insight and understanding of the concrete work of nursing and the lived life. In her meeting with the philosophy of life and the phenomenology of creation she encounters the ontological and metaphysical in a different way than that of traditional philosophy. Life utterances, the creation, time, and space are ontological and metaphysical facts. Analogy would say that we can think these facts and recognize them in our concrete experiences in our practical life. They come to expression in meetings between persons, in narratives, and in the exercise of discernment. In this way metaphysics pries at the empirical, writes Martinsen with reference to Løgstrup (Martinsen, 1996). Further, she states "The narrative takes time, it is slow. It provides context through analogous forms of recognition, that is to say, it is relevant to us when we can recognize ourselves in the life phenomena it relates" (Martinsen, 2002b, p. 267).

Kirkevold (1998) writes the following:

> Martinsen does not mean to present a logically constructed theory. On the contrary, she distances herself from that view of knowledge that insists theory have a logical structure of terms, principles and rules. Martinsen's theory is an interpretive analysis of caring, upon which the author tries to shed light from several perspectives. Her treatment of this phenomenon must be said to be both extensive and thorough. (p. 180)

ACCEPTANCE BY THE NURSING COMMUNITY

Practice

Martinsen, herself, is reluctant to provide concrete directions for nursing work. She recommends instead that nurses "think with" and assess what she writes and speaks about in their own lives, own practice, and experience, and against this background imagine their way to alternatives of action. This is followed up by Kirkevold (1998):

> Martinsen's theory of caring is practically relevant as an overarching/general philosophy of nursing. It is clearly articulated and encompasses a precise formulation of how (one ought) to understand and approach patients and nursing. Its strength is the ability to promote reflection upon nursing practice in different contexts, in that it gives a clear picture of what the author believes must be present in

order for nursing to be considered caring or moral practice. (p. 181)

Many of these texts have, she further writes:

> . . . a normative character, and are intended to mobilize a counter-culture in nursing, which does not only revolutionize the discipline of nursing and its practice, but which also stands as a resisting force against the societal tendency to opposition of the concept of care. . . . In recent years the personal, inspiring and poetic style has become more pronounced. It communicates Martinsen's normatively founded philosophy of caring in a gripping way, and has therefore had great impact on nurses and students. (Kirkevold, 1998, p. 204)

Martinsen herself addresses practicing nurses through their professional journal, *Sykepleien*. Kirkevold writes, "In choosing the journal *Nursing* as a main vehicle for communicating her academic work, she has underscored her roots in practical nursing rather than in science" (Kirkevold, 1998, p. 203).

Education

Most nursing colleges in Norway and Denmark use Martinsen's texts, and her works form part of the curriculum at a variety of educational levels. The books are reprinted regularly and have had great impact, even though they have not been written as textbooks or as required course reading. Several prescribed texts for nursing education have dealt with her thought (Alvsvåg, 2003; Kirkevold 1998; Kristoffersen, 2002; Mekki & Tollefsen, 2000; Nielsen, 2003). In addition, other books have been written for nursing education in which the aim is to make Martinsen's thinking relevant for both nursing generally and for specific professional issues. For example, several college lecturers in Norway and Denmark produced an article compilation in 2000, which gives an introduction to Martinsen's thought and for which the target group is students (Alvsvåg & Gjengedal, 2000). In 2002 the book *The Philosophy of Caring in Practice: Thinking with Kari*

Martinsen in Nursing, was published (Austgard, 2002). The book takes concrete situations of caring and shows how philosophy can contribute to affect caring work in practice. It is written for teaching and clinical supervision. The book was translated into Danish in 2004 (Austgard, 2004). In 2003, a Danish nurse wrote a textbook of spiritual care. Central to the book is Martinsen's thinking, in addition to that of Katie Eriksson and Joyce Travelbee (Overgaard, 2003).

Research

In the same way as one in practical nursing can "think with" and assess what she writes, her writings can be applied in research. Countless dissertations based on practical, concrete, and more theoretical issues discuss the relationship between empirical experience and the case in light of Martinsen's terminology and philosophy. In 1993, on the occasion of Martinsen's 50th year the book, *Wisdom and Skill,* was published (Kirkevold, Nortvedt, & Alvsvåg, 1993). Kirkevold writes that Martinsen's thought and works have created a critical and constructive role model for research and professional development (Kirkevold, 1993). Ruth Olsen writes about the reflective practitioner (Olsen, 1993), a work she builds upon in her doctoral dissertation, later published under the title *Wise With Experience? On Sensation and Attention, Knowledge and Reflection in Practical Nursing* (Olsen, 1998).

FURTHER DEVELOPMENT

Caring can be understood on several levels: ontological, concrete, and practical, or at the level of the system or organization. In nursing we are encouraged to act in a professional and moral manner such that caring and the life utterances receive the space they need to emerge in nurse-patient encounters. We are challenged time after time to reflect critically over whether this happens or not. This involves the manifestation of a person-oriented professionalism, the manifestation of loving deeds in the profession again and again (Martinsen, 1993b, 2000b).

It is important, moreover, to develop a mode of thinking about caring in nursing research. Science in nursing will then face certain boundaries. The challenge is to develop a type of research which does not impoverish practice but which upgrades the available knowledge and wisdom and which is developed in practice, that is to say a practice-oriented research, a cooperation between researcher and practitioner (Martinsen, 1989c, 1993b). Kirkevold writes the following:

> Martinsen's theory is especially important because it is one of the few existing Norwegian nursing theories, and because it is one of the first Nordic nursing theories that gives expression for a new understanding of reality and the need for new nursing theories based upon this. (Kirkevold, 1998, p. 182)

At the organizational and social levels the concept of care is also relevant. It is important to develop social systems and organizations, such as the health service, so that a person-oriented professionalism can be facilitated. Martinsen writes about both a merciful and a political Samaritan (Martinsen, 1993b, 2000b, 2003b). At both the organizational and social levels what is important is how the political Samaritans facilitate the work of the merciful Samaritans.

CRITIQUE
Simplicity

At first glance, Martinsen's theory seems complex. At the same time, the question must be raised about whether this is because she turns so many of our familiar assumptions on their heads, as for example, that we as human beings are free, independent, and boundless in our capacity for activity and interference with the creation. Western societies live in a culture of individualism. Her view of humanity can be described as *collectivist.* She uses a poetic and philosophical rather than a scientific mode of speaking, which can also seem alien in a scientized society. She writes about general phenomena that affect us all and that we can easily recognize in our personal lives, either occupational or daily life. Seen this way, theory of caring is not hard to understand. Martinsen asks that we read slowly and imagine our own experiences in light of what she writes (Martinsen, 2000b).

Generality

Because Martinsen's nursing theory deals with the essential phenomena of life and nursing, those phenomena present in all human situations, it can be seen as relevant to patients in general. Her theory of care "seems to be relevant for all patients who, because of illness or other reasons need help and assistance" (Kirkevold, 1998, p. 181).

Empirical Precision

The patient's and the nurse's worlds of experience are diverse, nuanced, and multifaceted. A nuanced and varied language is required to deal with a multifaceted reality, one that is on par with that which is to be described. This language is close to philosophy and everyday language; it is a poetic language. We can say that the poetic language is most precise in relation to description of the manifold and situations open to interpretation. Reflection on professional judgment and professional narratives creates the contexts of a community of nursing and the tradition of nursing; we recognize situations and thus find professional and moral insight. This enables us to perform situation-dependent, good nursing, a professional moral practice.

Derivable Consequences

Martinsen's theory of caring is· a critique of the system, which at the same time imparts inspiration to the individual in concrete caring situations (Gjengedal, 2000). Gjengedal writes that Martinsen's motivation for theoretical work "has precisely a practical point of departure, a wish to understand and protect against devaluation of the aspect of care in nursing" (Gjengedal, 2000, p. 38). Devaluation of caring can occur if one uncritically accepts "a scientific perspective blind to the lived life and

all that gives meaning to being" (Gjengedal, 2000, p. 54).

The lived life is built on basic structures; being has meaning and this meaning exists from the beginning of life. As people and as nurses we are challenged to live such that positive meaning can be expressed in our human relations, for example in relations between patients and family members. How we express this in a concrete way in a nursing context is up to us as professionals to decide, but the philosophy on which Martinsen bases her thinking can provide ideas with which to reflect in specific situations.

Specific situations present themselves with both possibilities and limitations. Socially created structural arrangements such as lack of personnel, financial resources, and lack of institutional beds present many limitations on a daily basis. Opportunities for caring become more accessible within a caring state and this must be shaped by politically aware people:

> Because if society is to be such that all are to have the same opportunities to live their best life, we must ourselves be involved in turning the Welfare State into a State of Care. A caring state is not dictatorial, nor is it society's passive extended arm. The caring state exists only to the extent that we struggle for its existence. We must form it ourselves: through solidarity, through morally responsible action, through the fight for greater equality and for community and social integration. Caring is an active and radical concept. (Martinsen, 1989c, p. 62)

It is important to create conditions for good and equal health care and living standard for all, but in the fight over crowns or dollars to take as our starting point those who are weakest, who most need help, it is about turning the inverted law of care around such that those who have least receive most.

SUMMARY

Martinsen has both a personal and sociopolitical interest in the ill and in those who, for other reasons, fall outside of society. Her theoretical stance can be called critical and phenomenological. She takes as her starting point the idea that human beings are created and placed within a fundamentally good created order for which we have administrative responsibility. We are relational and dependent on each other and on the Creation. Therefore, caring, solidarity, and moral practice are unavoidable realities for us.

In her thought on the subject of caring, Martinsen challenges society, the politics of health care, and health care workers themselves to realize the values inherent in caring through concrete policies and practical nursing. She deliberately gives few directives for action. Rather, she asks us to think ourselves into the situations of patients and family members and to arrive at the best choices for action based on a rich situational understanding, professional insight, and caring.

Martinsen's thought has provoked, engaged, and created debate and professional development in nursing in the Nordic countries over the past 30 years. Her thought challenges us to both think and act well and correctly, critically, and differently in nursing, in education, and in research. Martinsen's "caring thought" contributes to the enlightenment of nursing and nursing research through its perspectives, concepts, and insights based on historical and philosophical scholarship and research.

Case Study

As nurses, we meet patients and family members in many different life situations. They are of all age groups, are acutely or chronically ill, will return to life and health, or are coming to the end of their lives and must face death as a reality in their own lives. Nurses meet patients and family members in their homes, at the hospital or the nursing home, in the school health service, at the local clinic, and so forth. Some meetings with patients and family members make a greater impression on us than others and most meetings represent situations of learning in one or more ways. Write a brief case study from your personal experience or make one up and discuss how caring is expressed in the situation.

CRITICAL THINKING *Activities*

Take as a starting point a concrete situation with which you have personal experience, either as an active participant, or in which you had a more observational role.

1. Discuss how caring and professional judgment and discretion are expressed in the situation.

2. Reflect over how the sovereign life utterances get space or lack of space in the situation.

3. From the starting point of the situation, discuss what is meant by person-oriented professionalism and moral practice.

REFERENCES*

Alvsvåg, H. (2000). Menneskesynet—Fra kroppsfenomenologi til skapelsesfenomenologi. I H. Alvsvåg & E. Gjengedal (red.), *Omsorgstenkning. En innføring i Kari Martinsens forfatterskap.* Bergen: Fagbokforlaget. [The view of the person—From the phenomenology of the body to creation phenomenology. In H. Alvsvåg & E. Gjengedal (Eds.), *Caring thought: An introduction to the writings of Kari Martinsen.* Bergen: Fagbokforlaget.]

Alvsvåg, H. (2003). Omsorg—Med utgangspunkt i Kari Martinsens omsorgstenkning. I B. K. Nielsen (red.), *Sygeplejebogen 2, 1. del Teoretisk-metodisk grundlag for klinisk sygepleje.* København: Gads Forlag. [Caring—From the starting point of Kari Martinsen's philosophy. In B. K. Nielsen (Ed.), *Nursing textbook 2, part 1. Theoretical-methodologic basis of clinical nursing.* Copenhagen: Gads Forlag.]

Alvsvåg, H., & Gjengedal, E. (red.) (2000). *Omsorgstenkning. En innføring i Kari Martinsens forfatterskap.* Bergen: Fagbokforlaget. [*Caring thought: An introduction to the writings of Kari Martinsen.* Bergen: Fagbokforlaget.]

Austgard, K. (2002). *Omsorgsfilosofi i praksis. Å tenke med Kari Martinsen i sykepleien.* Oslo: Cappelen Akademisk Forlag. [*Philosophy of caring in practice. Thinking with Kari Martinsen in nursing.* Oslo: Cappelen Akademisk Forlag.]

Austgard, K. (2004). *Omsorgsfilosofi i praksis. At tænke med Kari Martinsen i sygeplejen.* København: Akademisk Forlag. [*Philosophy of Caring in Practice: Thinking with*

*Norwegian titles are provided with approximate translation into English.

Kari Martinsen in Nursing. Copenhagen: Akademisk Forlag.]

Gjengedal, E. (2000). Omsorg og sykepleie. I H. Alvsvåg & E. Gjengedal (red.), *Omsorgstenkning: En innføring i Kari Martinsens forfatterskap.* Bergen: Fagbokforlaget. [Caring and nursing. In H. Alvsvåg & E. Gjengedal (Eds.), *Caring thought: An introduction to the writings of Kari Martinsen.* Bergen: Fagbokforlaget.]

Karlsson, B., & Martinsen, K. (2003). Prolog. I K. Martinsen, *Omsorg, sykepleie og medisin.* 2. utgave. Oslo: Universitetsforlaget. [Prologue. In K. Martinsen. *Caring, nursing and medicine: Historical-philosophical essays* (2nd ed.). Oslo: Universitetsforlaget.]

Kirkevold, M. (1993). Innledning. I M. Kirkevold, F. Nortvedt, & H. Alvsvåg (red.), *Klokskap og kyndighet. Kari Martinsens innflytelse på norsk og dansk sykepleie.* Oslo: ad Notam Gyldendal. [Introduction. In M. Kirkevold, F. Nortvedt, & H. Alvsvåg (Eds.), *Wisdom and skill: Kari Martinsen's influence on Norwegian and Danish nursing.* Oslo: ad Notam Gyldendal.]

Kirkevold, M. (1998). *Sykepleieteorier—Analyse og evaluering.* Oslo: ad Notam Gyldendal. 2. utgave. [*Nursing theories—Analysis and evaluation* (2nd ed.). Oslo: ad Notam Gyldendal.]

Kirkevold, M. (2000). Utviklingstrekk i Kari Martinsens forfatterskap. I H. Alvsvåg & E. Gjengedal (red.), *Omsorgstenkning—En innføring i Kari Martinsens forfatterskap.* Bergen: Fagbokforlaget. [Developmental characteristics in the writings of Kari Martinsen. In H. Alvsvåg & E. Gjengedal (Eds.), *Caring thought: An introduction to the writings of Kari Martinsen.* Bergen: Fagbokforlaget.]

Kirkevold, M., Nortvedt, F., & Alvsvåg, H. (red.) (1993). *Klokskap og kyndighet. Kari Martinsens innflytelse på norsk og dansk sykepleie.* Oslo: Gyldendal Academisk. [*Wisdom and skill. Kari Martinsen's influence on Norwegian and Danish nursing.* Oslo: Gyldendal Academisk.]

Kjær, T. (2000). Fænomenologi, etikk og fortælling: I H. Alvsvåg & E. Gjengedal (red.), *Omsorgstenkning—En innføring i Kari Martinsens forfatterskap.* Bergen: Fagbokforlaget. [Phenomenology, ethics and narrative. In H. Alvsvåg & E. Gjengedal (Eds.), *Caring thought: An introduction to the writings of Kari Martinsen.* Bergen: Fagbokforlaget.]

Kristoffersen, N. J. (2002). *Generell sykepleie.* Oslo: Universitetsforlaget. [*Fundamental nursing.* Oslo: Universitetsforlaget.]

Lubcke, P. (red.) (1983). *Politikens filosofiske leksikon.* København: Politikens Forlag. [*Politiken's philosophical lexicon.* Copenhagen: Politikens Forlag.]

Malchau, S. (2000). Kaldet. I H. Alvsvåg & E. Gjengedal (red.), *Omsorgstenkning—En innføring i Kari Martinsens forfatterskap.* Bergen: Fagbokforlaget. [The call. In H. Alvsvåg & E. Gjengedal (Eds.), *Caring thought: An introduction to the writings of Kari Martinsen.* Bergen: Fagbokforlaget.]

Martinsen K. (1975). *Filosofi og sykepleie. Et marxistisk og fenomenologisk bidrag.* Filosofisk institutts stensilserie nr. 34. Bergen: Universitetet i Bergen. [*Philosophy and nursing: A Marxist and phenomenological contribution* (Philosophical institute's stencil series no. 34). Bergen: University of Bergen.]

Martinsen, K. (1976). Historie og sykepleie—Momenter til en utdanningsdebatt. *Kontrast, 7,* 430-446. [History and nursing—Elements of an educational debate. *Contrast, 7,* 430-446.]

Martinsen, K. (1977). Nightingale—Ingen opprører bak myten. *Sykepleien 18*(65), 1022-1025. [Nightingale—No rebel behind the myth. *Nursing, 18*(65), 1022-1025.]

Martinsen, K. (1978). Det 'kliniske blikk' i medisinen og i sykepleien. *Sykepleien, 20*(66), 1271-1272. [The 'clinical gaze' in medicine and in nursing. *Nursing, 20*(66), 1271-1272.]

Martinsen, K. (1979a). Den engelske sanitation—Bevegelsen, hygiene og synet på sykdom. I Ø. Larsen (red.), *Synet på sykdom.* Oslo: Seksjon for medisinsk historie, Universitetet i Oslo. [The English sanitation movement, hygiene and the view of illness. In Ø. Larsen (Ed.), *The view of illness.* Oslo: University of Oslo (Section for medical history).]

Martinsen, K. (1979b). Diakonissesykepleiens framvekst. Fra vekkelser og kvinneforeninger til moderhus og fattigomsorg. I NAVF's sekretariat for kvinneforskning (red.), *Lønnet og ulønnet omsorg. En seminarrapport.* Arbeidsnotat nr. 5/79. Oslo: NAVF. [Development of the professional trained Christian nurses. From revival and woman's charitable groups to the mother house and care of the poor. In NAVF's Secretariat for Feminist Research (Ed.), *Paid and unpaid care: A seminar report.* Working paper no. 5/79. Oslo: NAVF.]

Martinsen, K. (1984). *Sykepleiens historie. Freidige og uforsagte diakonisser. Et omsorgsyrke vokser fram 1860-1905.* Oslo: Aschehoug/Tanum-Norli. [*History of nursing: Frank and engaged deaconesses: A caring profession emerges 1860-1905.* Oslo: Aschehoug/Tanum-Norli.]

Martinsen, K. (1989a). Helsepolitiske problemer og helsepolitisk tenkning bak sykehusloven av 1969. I K. Martinsen, *Omsorg, sykepleie og medisin. Historisk-filosofiske essays.* Oslo: Tano Forlag. [Health policy problems and health policy thinking behind the hospital law of 1969. In K. Martinsen, *Caring, nursing and medicine: Historical-philosophical essays.* Oslo: Tano Forlag.]

Martinsen, K. (1989b). Legers interesse for svangerskapet—En del av den perinatale omsorg. Tidsrommet ca. 1890-1940. I K. Martinsen, *Omsorg, sykepleie og medisin. Historisk-filosofiske essays.* Oslo: Tano Forlag. [The doctor's interest in pregnancy—Part of perinatal care: The period ca. 1890-1940. In K. Martinsen, *Caring, nursing and medicine: Historical-philosophical essays*. Oslo: Tano Forlag.]

Martinsen, K. (1989c). *Omsorg, sykepleie og medisin. Historisk-filosofiske essays*. Oslo: Tano Forlag. [*Caring, nursing and medicine: Historical-philosophical essays*. Oslo: Tano Forlag.]

Martinsen, K. (1990). Moralsk praksis og dokumentasjon i praktisk sykepleie. I T. Jensen, L. U. Jensen, & W. C. Kim (red.), *Grundlagsproblemer i sygeplejen. Etik, viden-skabsteori,ledelse & samfunn*. Aarhus: Philosophia. [Practice and documentation in practical nursing. In T. Jensen, L. U. Jensen, & W. C. Kim (Eds.), *Foundational problems in nursing: Ethics, theories of science, leadership and society*. Aarhus: Philosophia.]

Martinsen, K. (red.) (1993a). *Den omtenksomme syke-pleier*. Oslo: Tano. [*The thoughtful nurse*. Oslo: Tano.]

Martinsen, K. (1993b). *Fra Marx til Løgstrup. Om moral, samfunnskritikk og sanselighet i sykepleien*. Oslo: Tano Forlag. [*From Marx to Løgstrup: On morality, social criticism and sensuousness in nursing*. Oslo: Tano Forlag.]

Martinsen, K. (1996). *Fenomenologi og omsorg. Tre dialoger*. Oslo: Tano-Aschehoug. [*Phenomenology and caring: Three dialogues*. Oslo: Tano-Aschehoug.]

Martinsen, K. (1997a). De etiske fortellingene. *Omsorg, 1*(14), 58-63. [The ethical narratives. *Caring, 1*(14), 58-63.]

Martinsen, K. (1997b). Etikk og kall, kultur og kropp—En dialog med Patricia Benner. I M. Sæther (red.), *Syke-pleiekonferanse på Nordkalottens tak*. Tromsø: Univer-sitetet i Tromsø. [Ethics and vocation, culture and the body—A dialogue with Patricia Benner. In M. Sæther (Ed.), *Nursing conference on the roof of Nordkalotten*. Tromsø: University of Tromsø.]

Martinsen, K. (2000a). Kjærlighetsgjerningen og kallet. Betraktninger omkring Rikke Nissens "Lærebog i Syge-pleie for diakonisser". I R. Nissen, *Lærebog i Sygepleie. Med etterord av Kari Martinsen*. Oslo: Gyldendal Akademisk. [The loving act and the call. Reflections on Rikke Nissen's *textbook of nursing for deaconesses*. In R. Nissen, *Textbook of nursing. With afterword by Kari Martinsen*. Oslo: Gyldendal Akademisk.]

Martinsen, K. (2000b). *Øyet og kallet*. Bergen: Fagbokfor-laget. [*The eye and the call*. Bergen: Fagbokforlaget.]

Martinsen, K. (2001). Huset og sangen, gråten og skammen. Rom og arkitektur som ivaretaker av men-neskets verdighet. I T. Wyller (red.), *Skam. Perspektiver på skam, ære og skamløshet i det moderne*. Bergen: Fag-bokforlaget. [The house and the song, the tears and the shame: Space and architecture as caretakers of human dignity. In T. Wyller (Ed.), *Shame. Perspectives on shame, honor and shamelessness in modernity*. Bergen: Fagbokforlaget.]

Martinsen, K. (2002a). Livsfilosofiske betraktninger. *Diakoninytt, 3*(118), 8-12. [Reflections on the philoso-phy of life. *Deaconry News, 3*(118), 8-12.]

Martinsen, K. (2002b). Rommets tid, den sykes tid, pleiens tid. I I. T. Bjørk, S. Helseth, & F. Nortvedt (red.), *Møte mellom pasient og sykepleier*. Oslo: Gyldendal Akademisk. [The room's time, the ill person's time, nursing time. In I. T. Bjørk, S. Helseth, & F. Nortvedt (Eds.), *The meeting between patient and nurse*. Oslo: Gyldendal Akademisk.]

Martinsen, K. (2002c). Samtalen, kommunikasjonen og sakligheten i omsorgsyrkene. *Omsorg, 1*(19), 14-22. [Conversation, communication and professionality in the caring professions. *Caring, 1*(19), 14-22.]

Martinsen, K. (2003a). Disiplin og rommelighet. I K. Martinsen & T. Wyller (red.), *Etikk, disiplin og dannelse. Elisabeth Hagemanns etikkbok—Nye lesinger*. Oslo: Gyldendal Akademisk. [Discipline and spaciousness. In K. Martinsen & T. Wyller (Eds.), *Ethics, discipline and refinement: Elizabeth Hagemann's ethics book—New readings*. Oslo: Gyldendal Akademisk.]

Martinsen, K. (2003b). *Omsorg, sykepleie og medisin. Historisk-filosofiske essays*. 2. utgave. Oslo: Univer-sitetsforlaget. [*Caring, nursing and medicine: Historical-philosophical essays* (2nd ed.). Oslo: University Press.]

Martinsen, K. (2003c). Talens åpenhet og evidens—Dialog med Jens Bydam. *Klinisk Sygepleie, 4*(17), 36-46. [The openness of speech and evidence—Dialogue with Jens Bydam. *Clinical Nursing, 4*(17), 36-46.]

Martinsen, K. (2004a). *Samtalen, skjønnet og evidensen*. Oslo: Akribe. [*Dialog, Discernment and the Evidence*. Oslo: Akribe.]

Martinsen, K. (2004b). Skjønn—Språk og distanse—Dialog med Jens Bydam. *Klinisk Sygepleie, 2*(18), 50-56. [Discernment—Language and distance—Dialogue with Jens Bydam. *Clinical Nursing, 2*(18), 50-56.]

Martinsen, K., & Wærness, K. (1979). *Pleie uten omsorg?* Oslo: Pax Forlag A/S. [*Caring without care?* Oslo: Pax Forlag.]

Martinsen, K., & Wyller, T. (red.) (2003). *Etikk, disiplin og dannelse. Elisabeth Hagemanns etikkbok—Nye lesinger*. Oslo: Gyldendal Akademisk. [*Ethics, discipline and refinement: Elizabeth Hagemann's ethics book—New readings*. Oslo: Gyldendal Akademisk.]

Mekki, T. E., & Tollefsen, S. (2000). *På terskelen. Introduk-sjon til sykepleie som fag og yrke*. Oslo: Akribe. [*On the threshold: Introduction to nursing as discipline and profession*. Oslo: Akribe.]

Nielsen, B.K. (red.) (2003). *Sygeplejenbogen 2, 1. del. Teoretisk-metodisk grundlag for klinisk sygepleje*. Køben-havn: Gads Forlag. [*Nursing textbook 2, part 1. Theoretical-methodic basis of clinical nursing*. Copen-hagen: Gads Forlag.]

Nissen, R. (2000). *Lærebog i Sygepleie. Med etterord av Kari Martinsen*. Oslo: Gyldendal Akademisk. [*Textbook of* nursing. With an afterword by Kari Martinsen. Oslo: Gyldendal Akademisk.]

Olsen, R. (1993). Den reflekterte praktiker—Rapport fra et sykehjem. I Kirkevold, M., Nortvedt, F., & Alvsvåg, H. (red.), *Klokskap og kyndighet. Kari Martinsens innflytelse på norsk og dansk sykepleie*. Oslo: ad Notam Gyldendal (s. 200-208). [The reflective practitioner—Report from a nursing home. In M. Kirkevold, F. Nortvedt, & H. Alvsvåg (Eds.), *Wisdom and skill. Kari Martinsen's influence on Norwegian and Danish nursing* (pp. 200-208). Oslo: ad Notam Gyldendal.]

Olsen, R. H. (1998). *Klok av erfaring? Om sansing og oppmerksomhet, kunnskap og refleksjon i praktisk sykepleie.* Oslo: Tano Aschehoug. [*Wise with experience? On Sensation and Attention, Knowledge and Reflection in practical nursing.* Oslo: Tano Aschehoug.]

Overgaard, A. E. (2003). *Åndelig omsorg—En lærebog.* København: Nytt Nordisk Forlag Arnold Busck. [*Spiritual care—Textbook.* Copenhagen: Nyt Nordisk Forlag Arnold Busck.]

BIBLIOGRAPHY*
Primary Sources
Books

Martinsen K. (1975). *Filosofi og sykepleie. Et marxistisk og fenomenologisk bidrag.* Filosofisk institutts stensilserie nr. 34. Bergen: Universitetet i Bergen. [*Philosophy and nursing: A Marxist and phenomenological contribution.* Philosophical Institute's stencil series no. 34. Bergen: University of Bergen.]

Martinsen, K. (1979). *Medisin og sykepleie, historie og samfunn.* Oslo: Norsk Sykepleierforbund. [*Medicine and nursing, history and society.* Oslo: The Norwegian Nursing Association.]

Martinsen, K. (1984). *Sykepleiens historie. Freidige og uforsagte diakonisser. Et omsorgsyrke vokser fram 1860-1905.* Oslo: Aschehoug/Tanum-Norli. [*History of nursing: Frank and engaged deaconesses. A caring profession emerges 1860-1905.* Oslo: Aschehoug/Tanum-Norli.]

Martinsen, K. (1989). *Omsorg, sykepleie og medisin. Historisk-filosofiske essays.* Oslo: Tano Forlag. [*Caring, nursing and medicine. Historical-philosophical essays.* Oslo: Tano Forlag.]

Martinsen, K. (red.) (1993). *Den omtenksomme sykepleier.* Oslo: Tano. [*The thoughtful nurse.* Oslo: Tano.]

Martinsen, K. (1993). *Fra Marx til Løgstrup. Om moral, samfunnskritikk og sanselighet i sykepleien.* Oslo: Tano Forlag. [*From Marx to Løgstrup. On morality, social criticism and sensuousness in nursing.* Oslo: Tano Forlag.]

Martinsen, K. (1996). *Fenomenologi og omsorg. Tre*

*Norwegian titles are provided with approximate translation into English.

dialoger.* Oslo: Tano-Aschehoug. [*Phenomenology and caring. Three dialogues.* Oslo: Tano-Aschehoug.]

Martinsen, K. (2000). *Øyet og kallet.* Bergen: Fagbokforlaget. [*The eye and the call.* Bergen: Fagbokforlaget.]

Martinsen, K., & Wærness, K. (1979). *Pleie uten omsorg?* Oslo: Pax Forlag A/S. [*Caring without care?* Oslo: Pax Forlag.]

Martinsen, K., & Wyller, T. (red.) (2003). *Etikk, disiplin og dannelse. Elisabeth Hagemanns etikkbok—Nye lesinger.* Oslo: Gyldendal Akademisk. [*Ethics, discipline and refinement. Elizabeth Hagemann's ethics book—New readings.* Oslo: Gyldendal Akademisk.]

Martinsen, K. (2005). *Samtalen, skjønnet og evidensen.* Oslo: Akribe. *Dialog, discernment and evidence.* Oslo: Akribe.

Martinsen, K. (2006). *Rom og rommelighet.* Bergen: Fagbokforlaget. *Room and spaciousness.* Bergen: Fagbokforlaget.

Book Chapters

Martinsen, K. (1972). Samfunnets krise og sykepleiernes oppgave. I I. K. Haugen, T. Malmin, S. Midtgaard, & K. Nicolaysen (red.), *Pedialogen* (s. 3-14). Oslo: Norsk Sykepleierforbund. [The crises of society and the nursing objectives. In I. K. Haugen, T. Malmin, S. Midtgaard, & K. Nicolaysen (Eds.), *Pedialog* (pp. 3-14). Oslo: Norwegian Nursing Association.]

Martinsen, K. (1972). Sykepleie som sosial-moralsk praksis. I I. K. Haugen, T. Malmin, S. Midtgaard, & K. Nicolaysen (red.), *Pedialogen* (s. 15-36). Oslo: Norsk Sykepleierforbund. [Nursing as social and moral practice. In I. K. Haugen, T. Malmin, S. Midtgaard, & K. Nicolaysen (Eds.), *Pedialog* (pp. 15-36). Oslo: Norwegian Nursing Association.]

Martinsen, K. (1978). Fra ufaglært fattigsykepleie til profesjonelt yrke—Konsekvenser for omsorg. I B. Persson, K. Ravn, & R. Truelsen (red.), *Fokus på sygeplejen-79. Årbok* (s. 128-157). København: Munksgaard. [From unskilled nursing the poor to professional occupation—Consequences for nursing. In B. Persson, K. Ravn, & R. Truelsen (Eds.), *Focus on nursing* (Annual 79, pp. 128-157). Copenhagen: Munksgaard.]

Martinsen, K. (1979). Den engelske sanitation-bevegelsen, hygiene og synet på sykdom. I Ø. Larsen (red.), *Synet på sykdom* (s. 78-87). Oslo: Seksjon for medisinsk historie, Universitetet i Oslo. [The English sanitation movement: Hygiene and the view of illness. In Ø. Larsen (Ed.), *The view of illness* (pp. 78-87). Oslo: University of Oslo, Section for Medical History.]

Martinsen, K. (1979). Diakonissesykepleiens framvekst. Fra vekkelser og kvinneforeninger til moderhus og fattigomsorg. I NAVF's sekretariat for kvinneforskning (red.), *Lønnet og ulønnet omsorg. En seminarrapport* (Arbeidsnotat nr. 5, s.135-170). Oslo: NAVF. [Development of the professional trained Christian nurses: From revival and woman's charitable groups to the mother house and care of the poor. In NAVF's Secretariat for Feminist Research (Ed.), *Paid and unpaid care: A seminar report* (Working paper no. 5, pp. 135-170). Oslo: NAVF.]

Martinsen, K. (1979). Diakonissene. I E. Mehlum (red.), *Bak maskinene, under fanene.* Utgitt i forbindelse med "Kristiania-utstillingen" om arbeidsfolk i byen for 100 år siden (s. 54-56). Oslo: Tiden. [Deconesses. In E. Mehlum (Ed.), *Behind the machines and the banners* (pp. 54-56). Oslo: Tiden.] (Published in connection with "The Christiania (Oslo) exhibition" on the condition of workers 100 years ago.)

Martinsen, K. (1979). Sykepleien, historien og den omvendte omsorgen. I R. Wendt (red.), *Utveckling av omvårdnadsarbete* (s. 90-102). Lund: Studentlitteratur. [Nursing, history and the converse caring. In R. Wendt (Ed.), *Development of health care* (pp. 90-102). Lund: Studentlitteratur.]

Martinsen, K. (1979). Sykepleien i historisk perspektiv: Fra omsorg mot egenomsorg. I M. S. Fagermoen & R. Nord (red.), *Sykepleie: Teori/praksis* (s. 5-23). Oslo: Norwegian Nursing Association. [Nursing in a historical perspective: From care to self caring. In M. S. Fagermoen & R. Nord (Eds.), *Nursing: Theory/practice* (pp. 5-23). Oslo: Norwegian Nursing Association.]

Martinsen, K. (1981). Diakonisser. I H. F. Dahl, J. Elster, I. Iversen, S. Nørve, T. I. Romøren, R. Slagstad, m.fl. (red.), *Pax leksikon.* Oslo: Pax Forlag (s. 89-90). [Deaconsses. In H. F. Dahl, J. Elster, I. Iversen, S. Nørve, T. I. Romøren, R. Slagstad, et al. (Eds.), *Pax lexicon* (pp. 89-90). Oslo: Pax Forlag.]

Martinsen, K. (1981). Guldberg, Cathinka. I H. F. Dahl, J. Elster, I. Iversen, S. Nørve, T. I. Romøren, R. Slagstad, m.fl. (red.), *Pax leksikon* (s. 553-554). Oslo: Pax forlag. [Guldberg, Cathinka. In H. F. Dahl, J. Elster, I. Iversen, S. Nørve, T. I. Romøren, R. Slagstad, et al. (Eds.), *Pax lexicon* (pp. 553-554). Oslo: Pax Forlag.]

Martinsen, K. (1981). Nightingale, Florence. I H. F. Dahl, J. Elster, I. Iversen, S. Nørve, T. I. Romøren, R. Slagstad, m.fl. (red.), *Pax leksikon* (s. 448-449). [Nightingale, Florence. In H. F. Dahl, J. Elster, I. Iversen, S. Nørve, T. I. Romøren, R. Slagstad, et al. (Eds.), *Pax lexicon* (pp. 448-449). Oslo: Pax Forlag.]

Martinsen, K. (1981). Omsorg i sykepleie. I E. Barnes & S. Solbak (red.), *Sykepleielære 1. Lærebok for hjelpepleiere* (Kap. 3). Oslo: Aschehoug. [Care in nursing. In E. Barnes & S. Solbak (Eds.), *Nursing textbook 1. Textbook for licensed practical nurses* (Chapter 3). Oslo: Aschehoug.]

Martinsen, K. (1981). Sykepleier. I H. F. Dahl, J. Elster, I. Iversen, S. Nørve, T. I. Romøren, R. Slagstad, m.fl. (red.), *Pax leksikon* (s. 179-180). [Nurse. In H. F. Dahl, J. Elster, I. Iversen, S. Nørve, T. I. Romøren, R. Slagstad, et al. (Eds.), *Pax lexicon* (pp. 179-180). Oslo: Pax Forlag.]

Martinsen, K. (1981). Sykepleieraksjonen 1972. I H. F. Dahl, J. Elster, I. Iversen, S. Nørve, T. I. Romøren, R. Slagstad, m.fl. (red.), *Pax leksikon* (s. 180-181). Oslo: Pax forlag. [Nurses on strike 1972. In H. F. Dahl, J. Elster, I. Iversen, S. Nørve, T. I. Romøren, R. Slagstad, et al. (Eds.), *Pax lexicon* (pp. 180-181). Oslo: Pax Forlag.]

Martinsen, K. (1981). Sykepleierforbund, Norsk (NSF). I H. F. Dahl, J. Elster, I. Iversen, S. Nørve, T. I. Romøren, R. Slagstad, m.fl. (red.), *Pax leksikon* (s. 181-183). Oslo: Pax forlag. [Nursing association. In H. F. Dahl, J. Elster, I. Iversen, S. Nørve, T. I. Romøren, R. Slagstad, et al. (Eds.), *Pax lexicon* (pp. 181-183). Oslo: Pax Forlag.]

Martinsen, K. (1981). Trekk av hjelpepleiernes historie. I E. Barnes & S. Solbak (red.), *Sykepleielære 1. Lærebok for hjelpepleiere.* (Kap. 2). Oslo: Aschehoug. [Aspects of licensed practical nurse history. In E. Barnes & S. Solbak (Eds.), *Nursing textbook 1. Textbook for licensed practical nurses* (Chapter 2). Oslo: Aschehoug.]

Martinsen, K. (1985). Organisering av omsorg: diakonisser i Norge. I J. Bjørgum, K. Gundersen, S. Lie, & K. Vogt (red.), *Kvinnenes kulturhistorie* (s.131-134). Oslo: Universitetsforlaget. [Organization of care: deaconesses in Norway. In J. Bjørgum, K. Gundersen, S. Lie, & K. Vogt (Eds.), *Woman's cultural history* (pp. 131-134). Oslo: Universitetsforlaget.]

Martinsen, K. (1986). Sykepleierne—Helsemisjonerer, oppdragere og profesjonelle yrkeskvinner. I. Fredriksen & H. Rømer (red.), I *Kvinder, Mentalitet og arbejde. Kvindehistorisk forskning i Norden* (s.151-156). Aarhus: Aarhus universitetsforlag. [Nurses—Health missionaries, educators and professional working woman. In I. Fredriksen & H. Rømer (Eds.), *Woman, mentality and work: Research on feminist history in Nordic countries* (pp. 151-156). Aarhus: Aarhus universitetsforlag.]

Martinsen, K. (1987). Ledelse og omsorgsrasjonalitet—Gir patriarkatbegrepet innsikt? I NAVFs sekretariat for kvinneforskning (red.), *Kjønn og makt: teoretiske perspektiver* (s. 18-26). Arbeidsnotat nr. 2. Oslo: NAVF. [Leadership and rationality of care—Does the concept of patriarchy yield insight? In *Gender and power: theoretical perspectives* (Working paper no. 2, pp. 18-26). Oslo: NAVF.]

Martinsen K. (1989). Omsorg i sykepleien—In moralsk utfordring. I B. Persson, J. Petersen, & R. Truelsen (red.), *Fokus på sygeplejen-90* (s. 181-200). København: Munksgaard. [Caring in nursing—A moral challenge. In B. Persson, J. Petersen, & R. Truelsen (Eds.), *Focus on Nursing—90* (pp. 181-200). Copenhagen: Munksgaard.]

Martinsen, K. (1990). Fra resultater til situasjoner: Omsorg, makt og solidaritet. I Samkvind (Center for samfundsvidenskabelig kvindeforskning). *Kvinder og kommuner i Norden* (s. 61-82). København: Samkvind. [From results to situations: Care, power and solidarity. In Samkvind (Center for Feminist Research), *Woman* and municipals in Nordic country (pp. 61-82). Copenhagen: Samkvind.]

Martinsen, K. (1990). Moralsk praksis og dokumentasjon i praktisk sykepleie. I T. Jensen, L. U. Jensen, & W. C. Kim (red.), *Grundlagsproblemer i sygeplejen. Etik, vitenskabsteori, ledelse & samfunn* (s. 60-84). Aarhus: Philosophia. [Moral practice and documentation in practical nursing. In T. Jensen, L. U. Jensen, & W. C. Kim, *Foundational problems in nursing: Ethics, theories of science, leadership and society* (pp. 60-84). Aarhus: Philosophia.]

Martinsen, K. (1993). Etikk og diakoni. I P. Frølich, J. Midtbø, & A. Tang, *Bergen Diakonissehjem 75 år* (s. 22-26). Bergen: Bergen Diakonissehjem. [Etichs and Diaconi. In P. Frølich, J. Midtbø, & A. Tang, *Bergen Diakonissehjem 75 years* (pp. 22-26). Bergen: Bergen Diakonissehjem.]

Martinsen, K. (1993). Omsorgens filosofi og dens praksis. I H. M. Dahl (red.), *Omsorg og kjærlighet i velfærdsstaten* (Samfundsvidenskabelig kvindeforskning/Cekvina (s. 7-23). Århus: Universitetet i Århus. [Caring philosophy and its practice. In H. M. Dahl (Ed.), *Care and love in the welfare state* (Social scientifically woman studies, pp. 7-23). Århus: The University of Århus.]

Martinsen, K. (1995). Omsorgsfeltet i den kliniske sygepleje. I I. Andersen & M. G. Erikstrup (red.), *Statens sundhedsvidenskabelige forskningsråds sygeplejeforskningsinitiativ. Betydning for sygeplejepraksis* (s. 31-43). Århus: Århus Universitet. [Area for care in clinical nursing. In I. Andersen & M. G. Erikstrup (Eds.), *The state's initiative in nursing science. The significance for nursing practice* (pp. 31-43). Århus: Århus University.]

Martinsen, K. (1997). Etikk og kall, kultur og kropp—En dialog med Patricia Benner. I M. Sæther (red.), *Sykepleiekonferanse på Nordkalottens tak* (s. 111-157). Tromsø: Universitetet i Tromsø. [Ethics and vocation, culture and the body—A dialogue with Patricia Benner. In M. Sæther (Ed.), *Nursing conference on the roof of Nordkalotten* (pp. 111-157). Tromsø: University of Tromsø.]

Martinsen, K. (1999). Etikken og kulturen, og kroppens sårbarhet. I K. Christensen & L. J. Syltevik (red.), *Omsorgens forvitring? En antologi om utfordringer i velferdsstaten—Tilegnet Kari Wærness* (s. 241-269). Bergen: Fagbokforlaget. [Ethics and culture, and vulnerability of the body. In K. Christensen & L. J. Syltevik (Eds.), *Weathering of caring? An anthology about challenges in the welfare state—Dedicate Kari Wærness* (pp. 241-269). Bergen: Fagbokforlaget.]

Martinsen, K. (2000). Kjærlighetsgjerningen og kallet. Betraktninger omkring Rikke Nissens "Lærebog i Sygepleie for diakonisser". I R. Nissen, *Lærebog i Sygepleie. Med etterord av Kari Martinsen* (s. 245-300). Oslo: Gyldendal Akademisk. [The loving act and the call. Reflections on Rikke Nissen's *Textbook of nursing for deaconesses*. In R. Nissen, *Textbook of nursing. With afterword by Kari Martinsen* (pp. 245-300). Oslo: Gyldendal Akademisk.]

Martinsen, K. (2001). Huset og sangen, gråten og skammen. Rom og arkitektur som ivaretaker av menneskets verdighet. I T. Wyller (red.), *Skam: Perspektiver på skam, ære og skamløshet i det moderne* (s. 167-190). Bergen: Fagbokforlaget. [The house and the song, the tears and the shame: Space and architecture as caretakers of human dignity. In T. Wyller (Ed.), *Shame: Perspectives on shame, honor and shamelessness in modernity* (pp. 167-190). Bergen: Fagbokforlaget.]

Martinsen, K. (2002). Rikke Nissen. Kjærlighetsgjerningen og sykestuen. I R. Birkelund (red.), *Omsorg, kald og kamp. Personer og ideer i sygeplejens historie* (s. 305-328). København: Munksgaard forlag. [The loving act and the room for the sick. In R. Birkelund (Ed.), *Care, vocation and love in action and the sick-room. Persons and ideas in nursing history* (pp. 305-328). Copenhagen: Munksgaard.]

Martinsen, K. (2002). Rommets tid, den sykes tid, pleiens tid. I I. T. Bjørk, S. Helseth, & F. Nortvedt (red.), *Møte mellom pasient og sykepleier* (s. 250-271). Oslo: Gyldendal Akademisk. [The room's time, the ill person's time, nursing time. In I. T. Bjørk, S. Helseth, & F. Nortvedt (Eds.), *The meeting between patient and nurse* (pp. 250-271). Oslo: Gyldendal Akademisk.]

Martinsen, K. (2003). Disiplin og rommelighet. I K. Martinsen & T. Wyller (red.), *Etikk, disiplin og dannelse. Elisabeth Hagemanns etikkbok—Nye lesinger* (s. 51-85). Oslo: Gyldendal Akademisk. [Discipline and spaciousness. In K. Martinsen & T. Wyller (Eds.), *Ethics, discipline and refinement. Elizabeth Hagemann's ethics book—New readings* (pp. 51-85). Oslo: Gyldendal Akademisk.]

Martinsen, K. (2005). Å bo på sykehuset og erfare arkitektur. I K. Larsen (red.), *Arkitektur, kropp og læring*. København: Reitzels forlag. To dwell in hospitals and experience architecture. In K. Larsen (Ed.), *Architecture, body and learning*. København: Reitzels forlag.

Journal Articles

Martinsen, K. (1976). Historie og sykepleie—Momenter til en utdanningsdebatt. *Kontrast, 7*(12), 430-446. [History and nursing—Elements of an educational debate. *Contrast, 7*(12), 430-446.]

Martinsen, K. (1977). Nightingale—Ingen opprører bak myten. *Sykepleien, 18*(65), 1022-1025. [Nightingale—No rebel behind the myth. *Nursing, 18*(65), 1022-1025.]

Martinsen, K. (1978). Det 'kliniske blikk' i medisinen og i sykepleien. *Sykepleien, 20*(66), 1271-1272. [The "clinical gaze" in medicine and in nursing. *Nursing, 20*(66), 1271-1272.]

Martinsen, K. (1981). Omsorgens filosofi og omsorg i

praksis. *Sykepleien, 8*(69), 4-10. [The philosophy of caring—And the practice. *Nursing, 8*(69), 4-10.]

Martinsen, K. (1982). Den tvetydige veldedigheten. *Sosiologi i dag*, temanummer *Kvinner og omsorgsarbeid, 1*(12), 29-41. [The ambiguity of charity. *Sociology, 1*(12), 29-41.]

Martinsen, K. (1982). Diakonissene—De første faglærte sykepleiere. *Sykepleien, 7*(70), 6-9. [The deaconesses—The first professionally trained nurses. *Nursing, 7*(70), 6-9.]

Martinsen, K. (1985). Kallsarbeidere og yrkeskvinner: Diakonissene—Våre første sykepleiere. *Forskningsnytt*, temanummer: *Kvinner og arbeid, 1*, 18-23. [Woman with a calling and a profession: The deaconesses—Our first nurses. *News in Science, 1*, 18-23.]

Martinsen, K. (1985). Sykepleiertradisjonen—Et nødvendig korrektiv til dagens sykepleieforskning. *Sykepleien, 15*(73), 6-14. [The nursing tradition—A necessary corrective to today's nursing science. *Nursing, 15*(73), 6-14.]

Martinsen, K. (1986). Omsorg og profesjonalisering—Med fagutviklingen i sykepleien som eksempel. *Nytt om kvinneforskning, 2*(10), 21-32. [Care and professionalism—An example from the development in nursing. *News in Woman Science, 2*(10), 21-32.]

Martinsen, K. (1987). Arbeidsdeling—Kjønn og makt. *Sykepleien, 1*(74), 18-23. [Division of labor—Gender and power. *Nursing, 1*(74), 18-23.]

Martinsen, K. (1987). Endret kunnskapsideal og to pleiegrupper. *Sykepleien, 4*(74), 20-25. [A changing paradigm and two types of nurses. *Nursing, 4*(74), 20-25.]

Martinsen, K. (1987). Helsepolitiske problemer og helsepolitisk tenkning bak sykehusloven av 1969. *Historisk tidsskrift, 3*(66), 357-372. [Health policy problems and health policy thinking underlying the new hospital law. *History, 3*(66), 357-372.]

Martinsen, K. (1987). Ledelse og omsorgsrasjonalitet—Gir patriarkatbegrepet innsikt? *Sykepleien, 1*(74), 18-23. [Management and caring rationality—Does the concept of patriarchate give insight? *Nursing, 1*(74), 18-23.]

Martinsen, K. (1987). Legers interesse for svangerskapet—En del av den perinatale omsorg. Tidsrommet ca. 1890-1940. *Historisk tidsskrift, 3*(66), 373-390. [Doctors' interests in pregnancy—A part of perinatal care. *History, 3*(66), 373-390.]

Martinsen, K. (1987). Norsk Sykepleierskeforbund på barrikadene for utdanning fra første stund. *Sykepleien, 3*(74), 6-12. [The Norwegian Nursing Association on the barricades from day one. *Nursing, 3*(74), 6-12.]

Martinsen, K. (1988). Ansvar og solidaritet. En moralfilosofisk og sosialpolitisk forståelse av omsorg. *Sykepleien, 12*(75), 17-21. [Responsibility and solidarity. A moral-philosophical and sociopolitical understanding of caring. *Nursing, 12*(75) 17-21.]

Martinsen, K. (1988). Etikk og omsorgsmoral. *Sykepleien, 13*(75), 16-20. [Ethics and the moral practice of caring. *Nursing, 13*(75), 16-20.]

Martinsen, K. (1990). Diakoni er fellesskap og samhørighet. *Under Ulriken, 5*(30), 6-10. [Diaconi is community and fellowship. *Under Ulrikken, 5*(30), 6-10.]

Martinsen, K. (1991). Omsorg og makt, ord og kropp i sykepleien. *Sykepleien, 2*(78), 2-11, 29. [Caring and power, word and body in nursing profession. *Nursing, 2*(78), 2-11, 29.]

Martinsen, K. (1991). Under kjærlig forskning. Fenomenologiens åpning for den levde erfaring i sykepleien. *Perspektiv—Sygeplejersken, 36*(91), 4-15. [Compassionate research. Phenomenology opening up for lived experience in nursing. *Perspective—Nursing* (Danish), *36*(91), 4-15.]

Martinsen, K. (1993). Grunnforskning—Trofast og troløs forskning—Noen fenomenologiske overveielser. *Tidsskrift for Sygeplejeforskning, 1*(9), 7-28. [Basic research—Faithful and faithless research—Some phenomenological considerations. *Nursing Research* (Danish), *1*(9), 7-28.]

Martinsen, K. (1997). De etiske fortellinger. *Omsorg, 1*(14), 58-63. [The ethical narratives. *Caring, 1*(14), 58-63.]

Martinsen, K. (1997). Kallet—Kan vi være det foruten? *Tidsskrift for sygeplejeforskning, 2*(13), 9-41. [The vocation—Can we do without it? *Nursing Science, 2*(13), 9-41.]

Martinsen, K. (1998). Det fremmede og vedkommende (I). *Klinisk Sygepleje, 1*(12), 13-19. [Strangeness and relevant (I). *Clinical Nursing, 1*(12), 13-19.]

Martinsen, K. (1998). Det fremmede og vedkommende (II). *Klinisk Sygepleje, 1-2*(12), 78-84. [Strangeness and relevans (II). *Clinical Nursing, 2*(12), 78-84.]

Martinsen, K. (2001). Er det mørketid for filosofien? Et svar til Marit Kirkevold. *Tidsskrift for sygeplejeforskning* (dansk), *1*(17), 19-23. [Is Philosophy in shadow? A replay to Marit Kirkevold. *Nursing Science* (Danish), *1*(17), 19-23.]

Martinsen, K. (2002). Livsfilosofiske betraktninger. I *Diakoninytt, 3*(118), 8-12. [Reflections on the philosophy of life. *Deaconry News, 3*(118), 8-12.]

Martinsen, K. (2002). Samtalen, kommunikasjonen og sakligheten i omsorgsyrkene. *Omsorg, 1*(19), 14-22. [Conversation, communication and professionality in the caring professions. *Caring, 1*(19), 14-22.]

Martinsen, K. (2003). Talens åpenhet og evidens—Dialog med Jens Bydam. *Klinisk Sygepleje, 4*(17), 36-46. [The openness of speech and evidence—Dialogue with Jens Bydam. *Clinical Nursing, 4*(17), 36-46.]

Martinsen, K. (2004). Skjønn—Språk og distanse: dialog med Jens Bydam. *Klinisk Sygepleje, 2*(18), 50-56. [Discernment—Language and distance: Dialogue with Jens Bydam. *Clinical Nursing, 2*(18), 50-56.]

Martinsen, K., & Wærness, K. (1976). Sykepleierrollen— En undertrykt kvinnerolle i helsesektoren (I). *Sykepleien, 4*(64), 220-224. [The nursing role—An oppressed female role in National Health Service. *Nursing, 4*(64), 220-224.]

Martinsen, K., & Wærness, K. (1976). Sykepleierrollen— En undertrykt kvinnerolle i Helsesektoren (II). *Sykepleien, 5*(64), 274-275, 281-282. [The nursing role—An oppressed female role in National Health Service. *Nursing, 5*(64), 274-275, 281-282.]

Martinsen, K., & Wærness, K. (1980). Klientomsorg og profesjonalisering. *Sykepleien, 4*(68), 12-14. [Client care and the professionalization. *Nursing, 4*(68), 12-14.]

Publications in Press

Martinsen, K. (2005). *Samtalen, skjønnet og evidensen.* Oslo: Akribe. *[Dialog, Discernment and the Evidence.* Oslo: Akribe.]

Martinsen, K. (2005). Å bo på sykehuset og erfare arkitektur. I K. Larsen (red.), *Om hus og arkitektur* (premiliminær tittel). København: Reitzels Forlag. [To dwell in hospitals and experience architecture. In K. Larsen (Ed.), *About houses and architecture* (preliminary title). København: DPU's Forlag.]

Martinsen, K. (2005). *Rom og rommelighet.* Bergen: Fagbokforlaget. *[Room and spaciousness.* Bergen: Fagbokforlaget.]

Secondary Sources

Alvsvåg, H., & Gjengedal, E. (red.) (2000). *Omsorgstenkning. En innføring i Kari Martinsens forfatterskap.* Bergen: Fagbokforlaget. *[Caring thought: An introduction to the writings of Kari Martinsen.* Bergen: Fagbokforlaget.]

Austgard, K. (2002). *Omsorgsfilosofi i praksis. Å tenke med filosofen Kari Martinsen i sykepleien.* Oslo: Cappelen Akademisk Forlag. *[Philosophy of caring in practice: Thinking with philosopher Kari Martinsen in nursing.* Oslo: Cappelen Akademisk Forlag.]

Kirkevold, M., Nortvedt, F., & Alvsvåg, H. (red.) (1993). *Klokskap og kyndighet. Kari Martinsens innflytelse på norsk og dansk sykepleie.* Oslo: Gyldendal Academisk. *[Wisdom and skill: Kari Martinsen's influence on Norwegian and Danish nursing.* Oslo: Gyldendal Academisk.]

Mekki, T. E., & Tollefsen, S. (2000). *På terskelen. Introduksjon til sykepleie som fag og yrke.* Oslo: Akribe. *[On the threshold: An introduction to nursing as discipline and profession.* Oslo: Akribe.]

Olsen, R. (1998). *Klok av erfaring? Om sansing og oppmerksomhet, kunnskap og refleksjon i praktisk sykepleie.* Oslo: Tano Aschehoug. *[Wise with experience? On sensation and attention, knowledge and reflection in practical nursing.* Oslo: Tano Aschehoug.]

Overgaard, A. E. (2003). *Åndelig omsorg—En lærebog. Kari Martinsen, Katie Eriksson og Joyce Travelbee i nytt lys.* København: Nyt Nordisk Forlag Arnold Busck. *[Spiritual care—A textbook. Kari Martinsen, Katie Eriksson and Joyce Travelbee in a new light.* Copenhagen: Nyt Nordisk Forlag Arnold Busck.]

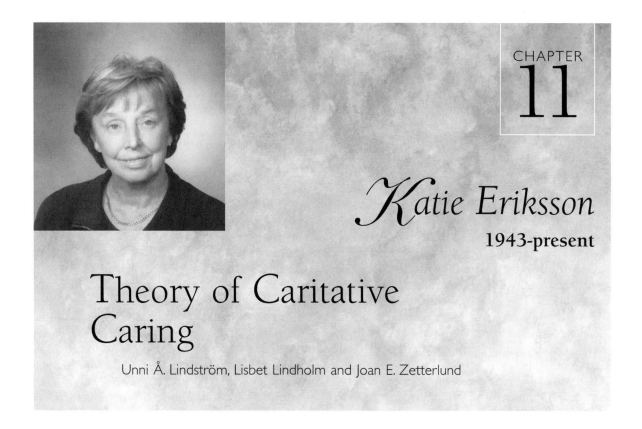

Katie Eriksson

1943-present

Theory of Caritative Caring

Unni Å. Lindström, Lisbet Lindholm and Joan E. Zetterlund

CREDENTIALS OF THE THEORIST

Katie Eriksson is one of the pioneers of caring science in the Nordic countries. When she started her career 30 years ago, she had to open the way for a new science. We who have followed her work and progress in Finland have noticed her excellent ability from the very beginning to have designed caring science as a discipline, while at the same time with her excellent pedagogical skill bringing to life the abstract substance of caring.

Eriksson was born on November 18, 1943, in Jakobstad, Finland. She belongs to the Finland-Swedish minority in Finland, and her native language is Swedish. She is a 1965 graduate of the Helsinki Swedish School of Nursing, and in 1967 she completed her public health nursing specialty education at the same institution. She graduated in 1970

from the nursing teacher education program at Helsinki Finnish School of Nursing. She continued her academic studies at University of Helsinki, where she received her M.A. degree in philosophy in 1974, her licentiate degree in 1976, and she defended her doctoral dissertation in pedagogy *(The Patient Care Process—An Approach to Curriculum Construction within Nursing Education. The Development of a Model for the Patient Care Process and an Approach for Curriculum Development Based on the Process of Patient Care)* in 1982 (Eriksson, 1974, 1976, 1981). In 1984, she was appointed Docent of Caring Science (part time) at University of Kuopio, the first docentship in caring science in the Nordic countries. She was appointed Professor of Caring Science at Åbo Akademi University in 1992. Between 1993 and 1999 she also held a professorship in caring science at University of Helsinki, Faculty of Medicine, where she has been a docent since 2001. Since January 1, 1996, she has served as Director of Nursing at Helsinki University Central Hospital, with responsibilities for research and development of caring science in connection with her professorship at Åbo Akademi University.

At the end of the 1960s and beginning of the 1970s, Eriksson worked in various fields of nursing practice, but she continued her studies at the same time. Her main area of work, however, has been in teaching and research. Since the beginning of the 1970s, Eriksson has systematically deepened her thoughts about caring, partly through the development of an ideal model for caring which has formed the basis for the caritative caring theory, and partly through the development of an autonomous humanistically oriented caring science. Eriksson is one of the few caring science researchers in the Nordic countries who has developed a caring theory, and she has been a forerunner of basic research in caring science.

Eriksson's scientific career and her professional experience comprise two periods: the years 1970 to 1986 at Helsinki Swedish School of Nursing, and the period from 1986 when she was invited to found the Department of Caring Science at Åbo Akademi University, which she has directed since 1987.

In 1972, after teaching for 2 years at the nursing education unit at Helsinki Swedish School of Nursing, she was assigned to start and develop an educational program to prepare nurse educators at that institution. Such a program taught in the Swedish language had not existed in Finland. This education program, with initial collaboration with University of Helsinki, was the beginning of caring science didactics. Under Eriksson's leadership, Helsinki Swedish School of Nursing developed one of the leading educational programs in caring science and nursing in the Nordic countries. It became the forerunner of education based on caring science and also of integration of research in the education. Eriksson was in charge of the program for 2 years, until she became dean at Helsinki Swedish School of Nursing in January 1974. She

remained the dean until September 1986, when she was nominated to plan and start academic education and research at Åbo Akademi University.

Toward the end of the 1980s, nursing science became a university subject in Finland, and professorial chairs were established at four Finnish universities and at the Finland-Swedish university, Åbo Akademi University. In 1986, Eriksson was called to plan an education and research program within the subject of caring science at Åbo Akademi University's Faculty of Education in Vaasa, Finland. A fully developed education program for health care, with three focus areas or options and a research education program for caring science, was created. The result of her planning was the establishment of the Department of Caring Science in 1987. It became an autonomous department within the Faculty of Education of Åbo Akademi University until 1992, when a new faculty, the Faculty of Social and Caring Sciences, was founded. A result of her work was that the education program for the M.A. in health and the caring science didactic education program were developed.

In 1987 a doctoral program was started under Eriksson's direction, and 23 doctoral dissertations have been published at the department. At her own department Eriksson, with her staff and researchers, has further developed the caritative theory of caring and caring science as an academic discipline. The department today has a leading position in the Nordic countries with students and researchers from those countries.

In addition to her work with teaching, research, and supervision, Eriksson is also the dean of the Department of Caring Science. One of her central tasks has been to develop Nordic and other international contacts within caring science.

Since the middle of the 1970s, Eriksson has been a very popular guest and keynote speaker, not only in Finland, but in all the Nordic countries and at various international congresses. In 1977, she was a guest speaker at Symposium of Medical and Nursing Education in Istanbul, Turkey; in 1978, she participated in the foundation of medical care teacher education in Reykjavik, Iceland; in 1982, she presented her nursing care didactic model at the First Open Conference of the Workgroup of European Nurse-Researchers in Uppsala, Sweden; and for several years she participated in education and advanced further education of nurses at the Statens Utdanningscenter for Helsopersonell (Federal Education Center for Nursing Staff) in Oslo, Norway. In 1988, she taught a course titled Basic Research in Nursing Care Science at the University in Bergen, Norway, and a course called Nursing Care Science's Theory of Science and Research at Umeå University in Sweden. She has worked as consultant at many educational institutions in Sweden; since 1975, she has been a regular lecturer at Nordiska Hälsovårdsskolan (The Nordic School of Public Health) in Gothenburg, Sweden. In 1991, she was a guest speaker at the 13th International Association for Human Caring (IAHC) Conference in Rochester, New York; in 1992, she presented her theory at the 14th IAHC Conference in Melbourne, Australia; and in 1993 she was the keynote speaker at the 15th IAHC Conference, Caring as Healing: Renewal Through Hope in Portland, Oregon (Eriksson, 1994b).

Since 1985, she has been a yearly keynote speaker at the annual congresses for nurse managers and, since 1996, at the annual caring science symposia in Helsinki, Finland. In many public dialogues with Professor Kari Martinsen from Norway, Eriksson has discussed basic questions about caring and caring science. Some of the dialogues have been published (Martinsen, 1996).

Eriksson has worked as a leader of many symposia: in 1975, for The Nordic Symposium about the Nursing Care Process (the first Nordic Nursing Care Science Symposium in Finland); in 1982, for The Symposium in Basic Research in Nursing Care Science; in 1985, for The Nordic Symposium in Nursing Care Science; in 1989 for the Nordic symposium titled Humanistic Caring; in 1991, for Nordic Caring Science Conference: Caritas & Passio in Vaasa, Finland; and in 1993, for the Nordic Caring Science Conference: To Care or Not to Care—The Key Question in Nursing in Vaasa, Finland.

Eriksson's caritative theory of caring came into clearer focus internationally in 1997 when the IAHC for the first time arranged its research conference in a European country. The Department of Caring Science had the honor of serving as the host of this conference, which was arranged in Helsinki, Finland, 1997, with the topic, "Human Caring: The Primacy of Love and Existential Suffering."

Eriksson is a member of several editorial committees for international journals in nursing and caring science. She has been invited to many universities in Finland and other Nordic countries as a faculty opponent for doctoral students and an expert consultant in her field. She is not only an adviser for her own research students, she is also a supervisor for research students at Kuopio and Helsinki universities, where she is an associate professor (docent). Eriksson also has served as chairperson of the Nordic Academy of Caring Science from 1999 to 2002.

Eriksson has produced an extensive list of textbooks, scientific reports, professional journal articles, and short papers. Her publications started at the beginning of the 1970s and include a total of about 400 titles. Some of her publications have been translated into other languages, mainly into Finnish. *Vårdandets Idé [The Idea of Caring]* has been published in Braille.

Eriksson has received many awards and honors for her professional and academic accomplishments, of which we want to mention several. In 1975, Eriksson was nominated by Finland to receive the 3M–ICN (International Council of Nurses) Nursing Fellowship award; in 1987, she was awarded the Sophie Mannerheim Medal of the Swedish Nursing Association in Finland; and in 1998, she received the Caring Science Gold Mark for academic nursing care, Helsinki University Central Hospital. Also in 1998, she received an Honorary Doctorate in Public Health from the Nordic School of Public Health, in Gothenburg, Sweden. Other awards include the 2001 Åland Islands medal for caring science activity in the province and the 2003 Topelius medal instituted by Åbo Akademi University in acknowledgement of good research. In 2003, she was honored nationally as a Knight, First Class, of the Order of the White Rose of Finland.

THEORETICAL SOURCES

Ever since the middle of the 1970s, Eriksson's leading thoughts have been not only to develop the substance of caring, but also to develop caring science as an independent discipline (Eriksson, 1988). From the beginning Eriksson wanted to go back to the great Greek classics by Plato, Socrates, and Aristotle, from whom she found her inspiration for the development of both the substance and the discipline of caring science (Eriksson, 1987a). From her basic idea of caring science as a humanistic science, she developed a meta-theory which she refers to as "the theory of science for caring science" (Eriksson, 1988, 2001).

When developing caring science as an academic discipline, her most important sources of inspiration besides Plato and Aristotle were Swedish theologian Anders Nygren (1972) and Hans-Georg Gadamer (1960/1994). Nygren and later Tage Kurtén (1987) have provided her with support for her division of caring science into systematic and clinical caring science. Eriksson introduces Nygren's concepts of motive research, context of meaning, and basic motive, which give the discipline a structure. The aim of motive research is to find the essential context, the leading idea of caring. The idea of motive research applied to caring science is, in an objective way, to show the characteristics of caring (Eriksson, 1992c).

The basic motive in caring science and caring is caritas, which constitutes the leading idea and keeps the various elements together. It gives both the substance and the discipline of caring science a distinctive character. In the development of the basic motive, St. Augustine (1957) and Søren Kierkegaard (1843/1943) also become important sources. In the further development of the discipline, Eriksson's thinking has been influenced by sources of theory of science such as Tomas Kuhn (1971) and Karl Popper (1997), and later by the American philosopher Susan Langer (1942) and the Finnish philosophers Eino Kaila (1939) and Georg von Wright (1986), who all

support the human science idea that science cannot exist without values.

For many years Eriksson collaborated with Håkan Törnebohm (1978), who had the first Nordic professorial chair in theory of science at the University of Gothenburg, Sweden. It is especially Törnebohm's research in and development of paradigms related to the development of various scientific cultures that have inspired Eriksson (Eriksson, 1989; Lindström, 1992).

The thought that concepts have both meaning and substance has been prominent in Eriksson's scientific work. This appears through a systematic analysis of fundamental concepts with the help of a semantic method of analysis rooted in the idea of hermeneutics, which professor in education Peep Koort (1975) developed. Koort, who was Eriksson's mentor, was also unmistakably her most important source of inspiration in her scientific work. Building on the foundation of his methodology, Eriksson has subsequently developed a model for concept development that has been of great importance to many researchers in their scientific work.

In her formulation of the caritative caring ethic, which Eriksson conceives as an ontological ethic, Emmanuel Lévinas' (1988) idea that ethics precedes ontology has been a guiding principle. Eriksson agrees especially with Lévinas' thought that the call to serve precedes dialogue, that ethics is always more important in relations with other human beings. The fundamental substance of ethics—caritas, love, and charity—is further supported by Aristotle's (1993), Nygren's (1972), Kierkegaard's (1843/1943), and St. Augustine's (1957) ideas. In the formulation of caritative ethics Eriksson has been inspired by Kierkegaard's ideas of the innermost spirit of a human being as a synthesis of the eternal and temporal; acting ethically is to will absolutely or to will the eternal (Kierkegaard, 1843/1943). In her stress on the importance of the knowledge of history of ideas for the preservation of the whole of spiritual culture, she finds support in Nikolaj Berdâev (1990), the Russian philosopher and historian. In intensifying the basic conception of the human being as body, soul, and spirit, Eriksson carries on an interesting dialogue with several theologians like Gustaf

Wingren (1960/1996), António Barbosa da Silva (1993), and Tage Kurtén (1987), while developing the subdiscipline she refers to as *caring theology*.

Perhaps the most prominent feature of Eriksson's thinking has been her clear formulation of the ontological, epistemological, and ethical basic assumptions with regard to the discipline of caring science. In the field of caring science the historical sources like Plato, Aristotle, and Socrates have served as guides for Eriksson whenever she has been looking for a basis for the substance of caring in its original historical form.

MAJOR CONCEPTS & DEFINITIONS

CARITAS

Caritas means love and charity. In caritas eros and agape are united, and caritas is by nature unconditional love. Caritas, which is the fundamental motive of caring science, also constitutes the motive for all caring. It means that caring is an endeavor to mediate faith, hope, and love through tending, playing, and learning.

CARING COMMUNION

Caring communion constitutes the context of meaning of caring and is the structure which determines caring reality. Caring gets its distinctive character through caring communion (Eriksson, 1990). It is a form of intimate connection which characterizes caring. Caring communion requires meeting in time and space, an absolute, lasting presence (Eriksson, 1992c). Caring communion is characterized by intensity and vitality, warmth, closeness, rest, respect, honesty, and tolerance. It cannot be taken for granted but presupposes a conscious effort to be with the other. Caring communion is seen as the source of strength and meaning in caring. Eriksson (1990) writes in *Pro Caritate*, referring to Lévinas:

> Entering into communion implies creating opportunities for the other—to be able to step out of the enclosure of his/her own identity, out of that which belongs to one towards that which does not belong to one and is nevertheless one's own—it is one of the deepest forms of communion. (pp. 28-29)

Joining in a communion means creating possibilities for the other. Lévinas suggests that considering someone as one's own son implies a relationship "beyond the possible" (1985, p. 71; 1988). In this relationship, the individual perceives the other person's possibilities as if they were his or her own. This requires the ability to move toward something which is no longer just one's own, but which belongs to oneself. It is one of the deepest forms of communion (Eriksson, 1992b). Caring communion is what unites and ties together and gives caring its significance (Eriksson, 1992a).

THE ACT OF CARING

The act of caring contains the caring elements (faith, hope, love, tending, playing, and learning) and involves the categories of infinity and eternity, and invites to deep communion. The act of caring is the art of making something very special out of something less special.

CARITATIVE CARING ETHICS

Caritative caring ethics comprises the ethics of caring, the core of which is determined by the caritas motive. Eriksson makes a distinction between caring ethics and nursing ethics. She also defines the foundations of ethics in care and its essential substance. Caring ethics deals with the basic relation between the patient and the nurse, the way in which the nurse meets the patient in an ethical sense. It is about the approach we have toward the patient. Nursing ethics deals with the

Continued

MAJOR CONCEPTS *&* DEFINITIONS—cont'd

ethical principles and rules which guide my work or my decisions. Caring ethics is the core of nursing ethics. The foundations of caritative ethics can be found not only in history, but also in the dividing line between theological and human ethics in general. Eriksson has been influenced by Nygren's (1966) human ethics and Lévinas' (1988) "face ethics," among others. Ethical caring is what we actually make explicit through our approach and the things we do for the patient in practice. An approach based on ethics in care means that we, without prejudice, see the human being with respect and that we confirm his or her absolute dignity. It also means that we are willing to sacrifice something of ourselves. The ethical categories which emerge as basic in caritative caring ethics are human dignity, the caring communion, invitation, responsibility, good and evil, and virtue and obligation. In an ethical act the good is brought out through ethical actions (Eriksson, 1995, 2003).

DIGNITY

Dignity constitutes one of the basic concepts of caritative caring ethics. Human dignity is partly absolute dignity, partly relative dignity. Absolute dignity is granted the human being through creation, while relative dignity is influenced and formed through culture and external contexts. A human being's absolute dignity involves the right to be confirmed as a unique human being (Eriksson, 1988, 1995, 1997a).

INVITATION

Invitation refers to the act that occurs when the carer welcomes the patient to the caring communion. The concept of invitation finds room for a place where the human being is allowed to rest, a place that breathes genuine hospitality, and where the patient's appeal for charity meets with a response (Eriksson, 1995; Eriksson & Lindström, 2000).

SUFFERING

Suffering is an ontological concept, described as a human being's struggle between good and evil in a state of becoming. Suffering implies in some sense dying away from something, and through reconciliation the wholeness of body, soul, and spirit is recreated, where the human being's holiness and dignity appear. Suffering is a unique, isolated total experience and is not synonymous with pain (Eriksson, 1984, 1993).

SUFFERING RELATED TO ILLNESS, TO CARE, AND TO LIFE

These are three different forms of suffering. Suffering related to illness is experienced in connection with illness and treatment. When the patient is exposed to suffering caused by care or absence of caring, the patient experiences suffering related to care, which is always a violation of the patient's dignity. Not to be taken seriously, not to be welcome, being blamed, or being subjected to exercise of power are various forms of suffering related to care. In the situation of being a patient, the entire life of a human being may be experienced as a suffering related to life (Eriksson, 1993, 1994a; Lindholm & Eriksson, 1993).

THE SUFFERING HUMAN BEING

The suffering human being is the concept that Eriksson uses to describe the patient. The patient refers to the concept of *patiens* (Latin), which means suffering. The patient is a suffering human being or a human being who suffers and patiently endures (Eriksson, 1994a; Eriksson & Herberts, 1992).

RECONCILIATION

Reconciliation refers to the drama of suffering. A human being who suffers wants to be confirmed in his or her suffering and be given time and space to suffer and reach reconciliation. Reconciliation implies a change through which a new wholeness is formed of the life the human being has lost in suffering. In reconciliation the importance of sacrifice emerges (Eriksson, 1994a). Having achieved reconciliation implies living with an imperfection with regard to oneself and others but seeing a way forward and a meaning in one's suffering. Reconciliation is a prerequisite of caritas (Eriksson, 1990).

CARING CULTURE

Caring culture is the concept that Eriksson (1987a) uses instead of environment. It characterizes the total caring reality and is based on cultural elements such as traditions, rituals, and basic values. Caring culture transmits an inner order of value preferences or ethos, and the different constructions of culture have their basis in the changes of value which ethos undergoes. If communion arises based on the ethos, the culture becomes inviting. Respect for the human being, his or her dignity and holiness, form the goal of the communion and the participation in a caring culture. The origin of the concept of culture is to be found in such dimensions as reverence, tending, cultivating, and caring and these dimensions are central to the basic motive of preserving and developing a caring culture (Eriksson, 1987a; Eriksson & Lindström, 2003).

USE OF EMPIRICAL EVIDENCE

From the beginning development of her theory, Eriksson has firmly established it in empiricism by systematically employing a hermeneutical and hypothetical deductive approach. Eriksson, in conformity with a humanistic scientific and hermeneutical way of thinking, has developed a caring science concept of evidence (Eriksson, Nordman, & Myllymäki, 1999). As her main argument for this, she points out that the natural scientific concept of evidence is too narrow to capture and reach the depth of the complex caring reality. Her concept of evidence is derived from Gadamer's concept of truth (Gadamer, 1960/1994), which encompasses the true, the beautiful, and the good. She points out, in accordance with Gadamer, that evidence cannot be connected solely with a method and empirical data. Evidence in a humanistic scientific perspective contains two aspects: a conceptual, logical one which she calls ontological, and an empirical one, each presupposing the other. The evidence concept developed by Eriksson has been shown to be empirically evident by having been tested in two comprehensive empirical studies, where the idea has been to develop evidence-based caring cultures in seven caring units in the Hospital District of Helsinki and Uusimaa (Eriksson & Nordman, 2004).

During the 1970s, Eriksson initially developed a nursing care process model (Eriksson, 1974), which later in her doctoral dissertation (1981) was formulated as a theory. Since then, Eriksson, step by step, has deepened her conceptual and logical understanding of the basic concepts and phenomena which have emerged from the theory. She has tested their validity in empirical contexts, where the concepts have assumed contextual and pragmatic attributes. This logical way of working, a constant movement between logical and empirical evidence, has been summarized by Eriksson in her model of concept development (Eriksson, 1997b). The validity of this model has been tested in several doctoral dissertations between the years 1995 and 2004 (Kasén, 2002; Lindwall, 2004; Nåden, 1998; Rundqvist, 2004; Sivonen, 2000; von Post, 1999). She started more comprehensive systematic as well as clinical research programs on caring when she was appointed director of the Department of Caring Science at Åbo Akademi University. All the 23 doctoral dissertations which have been written at the

Department of Caring Science between 1992 and 2004 are in different ways a test and validation of her ideas and theory.

MAJOR ASSUMPTIONS

Eriksson distinguishes between two kinds of major assumptions: axioms and theses. She regards the axioms as fundamental truths in relation to the conception of the world; the theses are fundamental statements concerning the general nature of caring science, and their validity is tested through basic research. The axioms and theses jointly constitute the ontology of caring science and are therefore also the foundation of epistemology (Eriksson, 1988, 2001). The caritative theory of caring is based on the following axioms and theses as modified and clarified from Eriksson's basic assumptions with her approval (Eriksson, 2002). The axioms are as follows:

- The human being is fundamentally an entity of body, soul, and spirit.
- The human being is fundamentally a religious being.
- The human being is fundamentally holy. Human dignity means accepting the human obligation of serving with love, of existing for the sake of others.
- Communion is the basis for all humanity. Human beings are fundamentally interrelated to an abstract and/or concrete other in a communion.
- Caring is something human by nature, a call to serve in love.
- Suffering is an inseparable part of life. Suffering and health are each other's prerequisites.
- Health is more than the absence of illness. Health implies wholeness and holiness.
- The human being lives in a reality which is characterized by mystery, infinity, and eternity.

The theses are as follows:

- Ethos confers the ultimate meaning on the caring context.
- The basic motive of caring is the caritas motive.
- The basic category of caring is suffering.
- Caring communion forms the context of meaning of caring and derives its origin from the ethos of love, responsibility, and sacrifice, namely caritative ethics.
- Health means a movement in becoming, being, and doing, striving for wholeness and holiness, which is compatible with endurable suffering.
- Caring implies alleviation of suffering in charity, love, faith, and hope. Natural basic caring is expressed through tending, playing, and learning in a sustained caring relationship, which is asymmetrical by nature.

The Human Being

The conception of the human being in Eriksson's theory is based on the axiom that the human being is an entity of body, soul, and spirit (Eriksson, 1987a, 1988). She emphasizes that the human being is fundamentally a religious being, but all human beings have not recognized this dimension. The human being is fundamentally holy, and this axiom is related to the idea of human dignity, which means accepting the human obligation of serving with love and existing for the sake of others. Eriksson stresses the necessity of understanding the human being in his ontological context. The human being is seen as in constant becoming; he is constantly in change and therefore never in a state of full completion. He is understood in terms of the dual tendencies that exist within him, engaged in a continued struggle and living in a tension between being and nonbeing. Eriksson sees the human being's conditional freedom as a dimension of becoming. She links her thinking with Kierkegaard's (1843/1943) ideas of free choice and the decision in the human being's various stages, the aesthetic, the ethical, and the religious stages, and she thinks that the human being's power of transcendency is the foundation of real freedom. The dual tendency of the human being also emerges in his effort to be unique, while he simultaneously longs for belonging in a larger communion.

The human being is fundamentally dependent on communion; he is dependent on another, and it is in the relationship between a concrete other (human being) and an abstract other (some form of God) that the human being constitutes himself and his being (Eriksson, 1987a). The human being seeks a communion where he can give and receive love, experience faith and hope, and be aware that his existence here and now has a meaning. According to Eriksson (1987b), the human being we meet in care is creative and imaginative, has desires and wishes, and is able to experience phenomena; therefore, a description of the human being only in terms of his needs is insufficient. When the human being is entering the caring context, he or she becomes a patient in the original sense of the concept, a suffering human being (Eriksson, 1994a).

Caritas

Love and charity, or caritas, as the basic motive of caring has been found in Eriksson (1987b, 1990, 2001) as a principal idea even in her early works. The caritas motive can be traced through semantics, anthropology, and the history of ideas (Eriksson, 1992c). According to Nygren (1966), caritas means human love and charity. Anthropologically, the essence of the human being is love. Giving love is a human characteristic (Lévinas, 1988). The history of ideas indicates that the foundation of the caring professions through the ages has been an inclination to help and minister to those suffering (Lanara, 1981).

Caritas constitutes the motive for caring, and it is through the caritas motive that caring gets its deepest formulation. This motive, according to Eriksson, is also the core of all teaching and fostering growth, and in all forms of human relations. In caritas, the two basic forms of love—eros and agape (Nygren, 1966)—are combined. When the two forms of love combine, generosity becomes a human being's attitude toward life, and joy its form of expression. The motive of caritas becomes visible in a special ethical attitude in caring, or what Eriksson calls a *caritative outlook,* and which she formulates and specifies in caritative caring ethics (Eriksson, 1995). Caritas constitutes the inner force which is connected with the mission to care. A carer who works in love also beams forth what Eriksson calls *claritas,* that is, the strength and light of beauty.

Caritas comprises love for one's neighbor and God, a human being's love for himself, a human being's love for everything created, and God's love for human beings. Eriksson sees the expressions of love as a development of the original virtues of mercy and the theological virtues of faith, hope, and love (Eriksson, 1987a, 1990). From the idea of caritas Eriksson has derived her whole caritative caring theory.

Caring

In accordance with the fundamental assumptions of caring science, Eriksson sees caring as an ontology and an expression of caritas (Eriksson, 1988). Caring is something natural and original. She thinks that the substance of caring can be understood only by a search for its origin. This origin is in the origin of the concept and in the idea of natural caring. The fundamentals of natural care are constituted by the idea of motherliness, which implies cleansing and nourishing, and spontaneous and unconditional love.

Natural basic caring is expressed through tending, playing, and learning in a spirit of love, faith, and hope. The characteristics of tending are warmth, closeness, and touch; playing is an expression of exercise, testing, creativity and imagination, and desires and wishes, while learning is aimed at growth and change. To tend, play, and learn implies sharing, and sharing, Eriksson (1987a) says, is "presence with the human being, life and God" (p. 38). True care is therefore "not a form of behavior, not a feeling or state. It is to be there—it is the way, the spirit in which it is done and this spirit is caritative" (Eriksson, 1998, p. 4). She brings out that caring through the ages can be seen as various expressions of love and charity, with a view to alleviating suffering and serving life and health. In her later texts she stresses that caring can also be seen as a search for truth, goodness, beauty and the eternal, and for what is permanent in caring and making it visible or evident (Eriksson, 2002). Her constant search has been centered on the question of what is care (the caring fundamentals) in caring. Eriksson emphasizes that caritative caring relates to the innermost core of nursing and she has distinguished between traditions that she calls *caring nursing* and *nursing care*. She means that nursing care is based on the nursing care process and that it represents good care only when it is based on the innermost core of caring. Caring nursing represents a kind of caring without prejudice that emphasizes the patient and his or her suffering and desires (Eriksson, 1994a).

Caritative caring arises in the encounter with the suffering human being in a caring relationship which involves fundamental communion (Eriksson, 1998). The core of the caring relationship between nurse and patient is described by Eriksson (1993) as an open invitation, and the invitation contains an affirmation that the other is always welcome. The constant open invitation is involved in what Eriksson (2003) today calls the *act of caring*. The act of caring expresses the innermost spirit of caring and recreates the basic motive of caritas. The caring act expresses the deepest holy element, the safeguarding of the individual patient's dignity. In the caring act the patient is invited to a genuine sharing, a communion, in order to make the caring fundamentals alive and active (Eriksson, 1987a) (i.e., appropriated to the patient). The appropriation has the consequence of somehow restoring the human being and making him or her more genuinely human. In an ontological sense, the ultimate goal of caring, according to Eriksson, cannot be only health, but it reaches further and includes human life in its entirety. Because the mission of the human being is to serve, to exist for the sake of others, the ultimate purpose of caring is to bring the human being back to this mission (Eriksson, 1994a).

Ethos

Eriksson uses the concept of ethos in accordance with Aristotle's (1935, 1997) idea that ethics is derived from ethos. In Eriksson's sense the ethos of caring science as well as that of caring consists of the idea of love and charity and the respect and honor of the holiness and dignity of the human being. Ethos is the sounding board of all caring. Ethos is ontology in which there is an "inner ought to," a target of caring "that has its own language and its

own key" (Eriksson, 2003, p. 23). Good caring and true knowledge become visible through ethos. Ethos originally refers to home or to the place where a human being feels at home. It symbolizes a human being's innermost space where he appears in his nakedness (Lévinas, 1989). Ethos and ethics belong together, and in the caring culture they become one (Eriksson, 2003). Eriksson thinks that ethos means that we feel called to serve a particular task. This ethos she sees as the core of caring culture. Ethos, which forms the basic force in caring culture, reflects the prevailing priority of values through which the basic foundations of ethics and ethical actions appear.

Suffering

At the beginning of the 1990s when Eriksson reintroduced the idea of suffering as a basic category of caring, she returned to the fundamental historical conditions of all caring, the idea of charity as the basis of alleviating suffering (Eriksson, 1984, 1993, 1994a, 1997a). That meant a change in the view of caring reality to a focus on the suffering human being. In an ontological sense she sees all suffering as a fight between evil and good. Her starting point is that suffering is an inseparable part of human life and that it has no distinct reason or definition. It has many faces and many characteristics, but it lacks an explicit language. Suffering as such has no meaning, but a human being can ascribe a meaning to it by becoming reconciled to it. Eriksson makes a distinction between endurable and unendurable suffering and thinks that an unendurable suffering paralyzes the human being, preventing him or her from growing, while endurable suffering is compatible with health. In its deepest meaning all suffering can be described in some sense as a form of dying, but it can also lead to renewal. Every human being's suffering is enacted in a drama of suffering. Alleviating a human being's suffering implies being a co-actor in the drama and confirming his or her suffering. A human being who suffers wants to have the suffering confirmed and be given time and space to become reconciled to it. The ultimate purpose of caring is to alleviate suffering. Eriksson has described three different forms: suffering related to illness, suffering related to care, and suffering related to life (Eriksson, 1993, 1994a, 1997a).

Health

Eriksson considers health in many of her earlier writings in accordance with an analysis of the concept in which she defines health as soundness, freshness, and well-being. The subjective dimension, or well-being, is emphasized strongly (Eriksson, 1976). In the current axiom of health she states that it is more than absence of illness; health implies being whole in body, soul, and spirit. Health means as a pure concept wholeness and holiness (Eriksson, 1984). In accordance with her view of the human being, Eriksson has developed various premises regarding the substance and laws of health, which have been summed up in an ontological health model. She sees health as both movement and integration. Health is a movement between actual and potential in a human being's active becoming, and it is an integrated part of human life. The health premise is a movement comprising various partial premises: health as movement implies a change; a human being is being formed or destroyed, but never completely; health is movement between actual and potential; health is movement in time and space; health as movement is dependent on vital force, vitality of body, soul, and spirit; the direction of the movement is determined by the human being's needs and desires; the will to find meaning, life, and love constitutes the source of energy of the movement; and health as movement strives toward a realization of one's potential (Eriksson, 1984).

In the ontological conception, health is conceived as a becoming, a movement toward a deeper wholeness and holiness. As a human being's inner health potential is touched, a movement occurs which becomes visible in the different dimensions of health as doing, being and becoming in a wholeness unique to human beings (Eriksson, Bondas-Salonen, Fagerström, Herberts, & Lindholm, 1990). In doing, the person's thoughts concerning health are focused on healthy life habits and avoiding illness; in being, the person strives for balance and harmony; in becoming, the human being becomes whole on a deeper level of integration.

Eriksson (1997a) sees that health and suffering belong together. Health becomes wholeness only through its combination with suffering. Health and suffering are two sides of the same movement, and they are integrated into each other and constantly present in a human being's life. In the health dimension of doing, human beings are unfamiliar with their suffering and want to explain it away. In the health dimension of being, they seek harmony and want to get away from suffering. In becoming, human beings are not unfamiliar with suffering; instead, they strive to reconcile themselves to the circumstances of life. Eriksson (1994a) thinks that suffering can give health a meaning by making the human being conscious of the contrasts of health and suffering.

THEORETICAL ASSERTIONS

Eriksson's fundamental idea when formulating theoretical assertions is that they connect four levels of knowledge: the meta-theoretical, the theoretical, the technological, and caring as art. The generation of theory takes place through dialectical movement between these levels, but here deduction constitutes the basic epistemological idea (Eriksson, 1981). The theory of science for caring science, which contains the fundamental epistemological, logical, and ethical standpoints, is formed on the meta-theoretical level. Eriksson (1988), in accordance with Nygren (1972), sees the basic motive as the element that permeates the formation of knowledge at all levels and gives scientific knowledge its unique characteristics. A common, clearly formulated ontology constitutes the foundation of both the caritative caring theory and caring science as a discipline. In accordance with Lévinas' (1988) thinking, Eriksson is of the opinion that ethics precedes ontology. The caritas motive, the ethos of love and charity, and the respect and reverence for human holiness and dignity, which determine the nature of caring, give the caritative caring theory its feature. This ethos, which encircles caring as science and as art, permeates caring culture and creates the preconditions for caring. The ethos is reflected in the process of nursing care, in the documentation, and in various care planning models.

Caring communion constitutes the context of meaning from which the various concepts in the theory are to be understood. Human suffering, which forms the basic category of caring, summons the carer to true caring (i.e., serving in love and charity). In the act of caring, the suffering human being, or patient, is invited and welcomed to the caring communion, where the patient's suffering can be alleviated through the act of caring in the drama of suffering that is unique to every human being. Alleviation of suffering implies that the carer is a co-actor in the drama and confirms the patient's suffering, and gives time and space to suffer until reconciliation is reached. Reconciliation is the ultimate aim of health or being and signifies a reestablishment of wholeness and holiness (Eriksson, 1997a).

The outer structure of caring is constituted by the nursing care process, structured as a hermeneutic course of events in which understanding is a necessary prerequisite of action. It creates a caring culture in which caritative caring is made possible.

LOGICAL FORM

Meta-theory has always had a fundamental place in Eriksson's thinking, and thought patterns in her epistemological work are anchored in Aristotle's theory of knowledge (Aristotle, 1935). Searching for knowledge, which is intrinsically hermeneutic and which has consistently taken place within the scope of an articulated theoretical perspective, is to be understood as a search for the original text in a historical-hermeneutic tradition, that which in the old hermeneutic sense represents truth (Gadamer, 1960/1994). In order to achieve the depth in the development of knowledge and theory which Eriksson has consistently striven for, she has used various logical models in which the hypothetical deductive method and hermeneutics have been guiding principles.

The logical form is constituted both in Eriksson's caritative theory of caring and in caring science as a discipline (Eriksson & Lindström, 1997). Eriksson stresses the importance of the logical form being created on the basis of the substance of caring (i.e., caritas), not on the basis of method. It is thus deduction combined with abduction that has formed the guiding logic. The language, words, and concepts are the carriers of the content of meaning, and Eriksson stresses the necessity of choosing words, concepts, and language which correspond to the tradition of human science.

In the dynamic change between the natural world and the world of science there has constantly occurred a striving toward the source of the true, the beautiful, and the good, that which is evident. Eriksson (1999) shapes her theory of scientific thought, in which reflection moves between patterns at different levels and the repertory of interpretation is subject to the theoretical perspective. The movement takes place distinctly between *dóxa* (empirical-perceptive knowledge) and *episteme* (rational-conceptual knowledge), and "the infinite." The movement thus takes place between the two basic epistemological categories of the theory of knowledge, perception, and conception. The infinite reaches beyond the rational concept-forming knowledge, of which epistemological categories mainly take the form of symbols and metaphors.

Eriksson has consistently applied three forms of inference—deduction, induction, and abduction or retroduction (Eriksson & Lindström, 1997)—that have given the theory a logical external structure. The substance of her caring theory has moved simultaneously by abductive leaps (Peirce, 1990; Eriksson & Lindström, 1997), which have sometimes created a new chaos but have carried Eriksson's thinking toward new discoveries. Through abduction the ideal model for caritative caring has been shaped, proceeding from historical and self-evident suppositions (Nygren, 1972). Eriksson has in this way made use of old original texts which testify to caritative caring as her research material. Through induction and deduction the validity of the theory has been tested continually.

Theory is conceived by Eriksson in accordance with the old Greek concept of theory, *theoria*, in the sense of seeing the beautiful and the good, participating in the common and dedicating it to others (Gadamer, 2000, p.49). Theory and practice are different aspects of the same core. The convincing force and potential of the whole theory are found in its innermost core, caritas, around which the generation of theory takes place. The caring substance is formed in a dialectical movement between the potential and actual, the abstract general and the concrete individual. With the help of logical abstract thinking combined with the logic of the heart (Pascal, 1971), the Theory of Caritative Caring becomes perceptible through the art of caring.

ACCEPTANCE BY THE NURSING COMMUNITY

Practice

A characteristic feature of Eriksson's manner of working is her way of structuring abstract thinking as a natural and obvious precondition of clinical activity and an evidence-based form of caring which opens up a deeper insight. Eriksson uses the concept of caring as art as an expression of a caring practice in which the abstract generality appears in a unique individual caritative act of caring.

Several nursing units in the Nordic countries have based their practice and caring philosophy on Eriksson's ideas and her caritative theory of caring. These include several clinics in the Hospital District of Helsinki and Uusimaa in Finland, Stiftelsen Hemmet in the Åland Islands of Finland, and Stora Sköndal in Sweden. Because Eriksson's thinking and process model of caring are general, the nursing care process model has proved to be applicable in all contexts of caring, from acute clinical caring and psychiatric care to health-promoting and preventive care.

Since the 1970s, Eriksson's nursing care process model has been systematically used, tested, and developed as a basis of nursing care and documentation at Helsinki University Central Hospital. From the beginning of the 1990s, Eriksson has served as the director of the clinical research program, "In the World of the Patient." This program comprises a number of empirical studies in various clinics within the whole district of university hospitals. In various studies, Eriksson's theory has been tested, and the results have been presented in doctoral and master's theses and published in professional and scientific journals. At present the study, In the Patient's World II: Alleviating the Patient's Suffering—Ethics and Evidence, which will lead to recommendations for the care of patients, is an ongoing research project that will become a handbook for clinical caring science.

The theoretical assumptions, the assertions, and the nursing care process model form the basis of the development of caring planning and documentation. Eriksson's model has been subjected to more comprehensive academic research (Fagerström, 1999; Kärkkäinen & Eriksson, 2003, 2004; Lukander, 1995; Turtiainen, 1999). Eriksson's thinking has been influential in nursing leadership and nursing administration, where the caritative theory of nursing forms the core of the development of nursing leadership at various levels of the nursing organization. That Eriksson's ideas about caring and her nursing care process model work in practice has been verified by everything from a multiplicity of essays and tests of learning in clinical practice to master's theses, licentiates' theses, and doctoral dissertations produced all over the Nordic countries.

Education

Since the 1970s Eriksson's theory has been integrated into the education of nurses at various levels and her books have been included continuously in the examination requirements in various forms of nursing education in the Nordic countries. The education for master's and doctoral degrees that started in 1986 at the Department of Caring Science, Åbo Akademi University, has been based entirely on Eriksson's ideas, and her caritative caring theory forms the core of the development of substance in education and research.

Eriksson started the first Finnish-Swedish education of caring science teachers in 1970. She subsequently for 15 years had the advantage of working with a team of teachers who have integrated her ideas and her caritative caring theory while at the same time developing caring didactics. Eriksson worked intensively to develop the caring science curriculum. In her book on didactics of caring (Eriksson, 1985), Eriksson further developed her curriculum theory and didactics. Her theory of caring didactics is based on a dialectic between a clearly articulated ontology, epistemology, and ethos which result in a didactics, an art of teaching, which is hermeneutical by nature. The caring science concepts and the theory run like a main thread through the whole education, independently of the level. Eriksson's build-up of caring science as a humanistic autonomous discipline, with its subdisciplines such as caring ethics, caring theology, and the history of ideas of caring (Eriksson, 1988, 2001), forms the basic structure of the organization of the curriculum and teaching on numerous levels (Eriksson, 1986).

Development of the caring science–centered curriculum and caring didactics continued in the educational and research program in caring science didactics. Development of teachers within the education of nurses forms a part of the master's degree program and has resulted in the first doctoral dissertation in the didactics of caring science (Ekebergh, 2001).

Eriksson realized at an early stage the importance of integrating academic courses in the education of nurses, and nowadays academic courses in caring science based on Eriksson's theory are offered as part of the continuing education of those who work in clinical practice. Approximately 200 nurses take part annually in these academic courses.

Because Eriksson sees caring science not as a profession-oriented but as a "pure" academic discipline, it has aroused interest among students in other disciplines and other occupational groups, such as teachers, social workers, psychologists, and theologians. Eriksson stresses that it is necessary for doctors, as well, to study caring science so that genuine interdisciplinary cooperation is to be achieved between caring science and medicine.

Research

Eriksson and her teaching and research colleagues at the Department of Caring Science have designed a research program based on her caring science tradition. The research program comprises systematic caring science, clinical caring science, the didactics of caring science, caring administration, and interdisciplinary research. Eriksson's caritative caring theory has been tested and further developed in various contexts with different methodological approaches both within the department's own research projects and in the 23 doctoral dissertations which so far have been published at the department.

Eriksson has always emphasized the importance of basic research as necessary for clinical research, and her main thesis is that substance should direct the choice of research method. In her book, *Pausen [The Pause]* (Eriksson, 1987b), she describes how the research object is structured, starting from the caritative theory of caring, and in her book, *Broar [Bridges]* (Eriksson, 1991), she describes the research paradigm and various methodological approaches based on a human science perspective. During the first few years, the emphasis lay on basic research with the focus on the development of the basic concepts and assumptions of the theory and on the fundamentals of history and the history of ideas. An especially strong point in Eriksson's research is the clearly formulated theoretical perspective that confers explicitness and greater depth to the generation of knowledge. The development of the theory and of research have always moved hand in hand with the focus on the various dimensions of the theory, and in this connection we wish to illustrate some central results of the research.

Eriksson has always emphasized the necessity of an exhaustive and systematic analysis of basic concepts, and she has developed her own model of concept development (Eriksson, 1991, 1997b), which has proved fruitful and is used by many researchers, including Nådén (1998) in his study of the art of caring, von Post (1999) in her study of the concept of natural care, Sivonen (2000) in studies of the concepts of soul and spirit, and Kasén (2002) in her study of the concept of caring relationship. Other studies have focused on the concept of dignity (Edlund, 2002), the concepts of power and authority (Rundqvist, 2004), and the concept of the body in a perioperative context (Lindwall, 2004).

A continued development of Eriksson's concept of health took place in the research project Den Mångdimensionella Hälsan [Multidimensional Health], which was in progress during the years 1987 to 1992 and resulted in the ontological health model (Eriksson, 1994a; Eriksson et al., 1990; Eriksson & Herberts, 1992). The project included several studies resulting in a number of master's theses. Of these, Lindholm's study of young people's conception of health (1998; Lindholm & Eriksson, 1998) and Bondas' study of women's health during their perinatal period (2000; Bondas & Eriksson, 2001) led to doctoral dissertations.

The ontological health model has subsequently formed the basis for several studies. Wärnå (2002), in her study concerning the worker's health, related Aristotle's theory of virtue to Eriksson's ontological health model. The result of the study opened quite a new line of thought in preventive health service in working environments, and continued research and development are now in progress in a number of factories in the wood-processing industry in Finland.

Since the mid-1980s, when suffering as the basic category in caring was made explicit in Eriksson's theory, examples of research related to suffering have been legion. One is Wiklund's (2000) study of suffering as struggle and drama, both among patients with heart disease and patients addicted to drugs. In several clinical studies, Råholm has focused on suffering and the alleviation of suffering in patients undergoing coronary bypass surgery (Råholm, Lindholm, & Eriksson, 2002; Råholm 2003). The manifestation of suffering in a psychiatric context has been studied by Fredriksson, who illustrates the possibilities of the caring conversation in the alleviation of suffering (Arman, 2003; Fredriksson, 2003; Fredriksson & Eriksson, 2003; Fredriksson & Lindström, 2002; Rehnsfeldt, 1999). In a Norwegian study, Nilsson (2004) studied suffering in patients in psychiatric noninstitutional care units with a high degree of ill health and found that the experience of loneliness is of basic importance. Caspari (2004) has in her study illustrated the importance of aesthetics for health and suffering.

In a cooperative project between researchers in Sweden and Finland, the suffering of women with breast cancer has been studied. The project comprises, among other things, intervention studies, in which the importance of different forms of care for the alleviation of suffering has been illustrated (Arman, Rehnsfeldt, Lindholm, & Hamrin, 2002; Arman-Rehnsfeldt & Rehnsfeldt 2003; Lindholm, Nieminen, Mäkelä, & Rantanen-Siljamäki, 2004). Arman-Rehnsfeldt has in her dissertation illustrated how the drama of suffering is formed among these women (Arman, 2003).

Continuous research has been carried out since the 1970s with a view toward developing caring science as an academic discipline, and a theory of science for caring science has been formulated (Eriksson, 1988, 2001; Eriksson & Lindström, 2000, 2003; Lindström, 1992). Eriksson has developed subdisciplines of caring science, which means that researchers of caring science and other scientific disciplines enter into dialogues with each other and constitute a research area. An example of this is the development of caritative caring ethics (Andersson, 1994; Eriksson, 1991, 1995; Fredriksson & Eriksson, 2001; Råholm & Lindholm, 1999; Råholm et al., 2002). Another interesting subdiscipline that Eriksson has developed is caring theology, within which she has articulated spiritual and doctrinal questions in caring with a scientific group of themes and in this respect has also cleared the way for new thinking. Caring theology, which has aroused great interest among caregivers in clinical practice, can nowadays be studied in academic courses.

Many researchers at universities, institutes of higher education, and clinics all over the Nordic countries make use of Eriksson's ideas and theory. This is evident in how frequently her literature is referenced. (Further discussion of this is not within the scope of this chapter.)

FURTHER DEVELOPMENT

Eriksson continues developing her thinking and the caritative caring theory with unabated energy and constantly finds new ways, while at the same time recreating and deepening what has been stated before. Systematic research and the development of caritative caring theory as well as the discipline of caring science take place chiefly within the scope of the research programs in her own department with her own staff and the postdoctoral group. The dissertation topics of the doctoral candidates are connected with the research programs and form an important contribution of knowledge to the ongoing development of Eriksson's thinking. During the last few years, Eriksson has emphasized the necessity of basic research in clinical caring science, where she has especially stressed the understanding of the research object, caring reality. She describes the object of research from three points of view: the experienced world, praxis as activity, and the real reality, which stretches beyond the empirical reality and constitutes the infinite. In the real reality, which carries the attributes of mystery, one finds something of the deepest potential of caring, and it is a reality that can be understood in Gadamer's sense, in the old Greek meaning of praxis, as a way of living, a mode of being, that is, an ontology (Gadamer, 2000). The development of knowledge in caring science becomes fundamentally different depending on what object of knowledge constitutes the focus of research (Eriksson & Lindström, 2003). Another central area of interest for Eriksson (2003) today is formed by the development of caritative caring ethics (i.e., the question of ethos, the basic values of caring, the ethical fundamentals of caring, and appropriation in the act of caring). A continued development of the caritative theory of caring also occurs, as has emerged before, through continued implementation and testing in various clinical contexts.

CRITIQUE
Clarity

The strong point of Eriksson's theory is the overall logical structure of the theory, in which every new concept becomes a part of an ever more comprehensive whole in which an element of internal logic can be seen clearly in the development of substance. Her main thesis has always been that a basic conceptual clarity will be needed before it becomes meaningful to develop the contextual features of the theory. Eriksson has used concept analysis and analysis of ideas as central methods, which has led to semantic and structural clarity. It has at the same time meant that the concepts may have assumed dimensions that have been regarded as strange to those who are not familiar with the theoretical perspective in which the development of the theory has taken place. We, who have for many years had the opportunity to follow Eriksson's work, have time and again been able to realize that her way of thinking forms a logical whole, where the abstract scientific reveals the concrete in a new understanding (i.e., provides an experience of evidence and verifies the convincing force of the theory).

Simplicity

The theoretical clarity of Eriksson's theory reflects the simplicity of the theory by showing the general in a clear and logical conceptual entirety. The hermeneutic approach has deepened the understanding of the substance and thus contributed to the simplicity of the theory (Gadamer, 1960/1994). The simplicity can also be understood as an expression of Gadamer's concept of theory by making it comprehensible that theory and practice belong together and reflect two sides of the same reality. Eriksson agrees with Gadamer's thought that understanding includes application, and the theory opens the way to deeper participation and communion. Eriksson (2003) formulates this process by the statement that "ideals reach reality and reality reaches the ideals" (p. 26).

Generality

Eriksson's theory is general in the sense that it aims at creating an ontological and ethical basis of caring, while at the same time it constitutes the core of the discipline and thus involves epistemology, as well. Eriksson's theory is also general as a result of the wide convincing force it receives through its theoretical core concepts and its theoretical axioms and theses. There may be a risk that a too-general theory becomes diffuse in relation to different caring contexts. Eriksson, however, has always stressed the importance of describing the core concepts on an optimal level of abstraction in order to include all of the complex caring reality while they simultaneously carry a wealth of signification which opens up understanding in various caring contexts.

Empirical Precision

Eriksson's thinking as a whole has reached an understanding that also extends to other disciplines and professions. She has developed a language and a rhetoric that can reach researchers as well as practitioners in the human scientific field. The empirical precision of Eriksson's theory is manifested through a combination of the clarity, simplicity, and generality of the theory combined with a rich substance and a clearly formulated ethos.

Derivable Consequences

Eriksson's work on developing her caritative caring theory for 30 years has been successful, and there is evidence to show that her thinking is of great importance to clinical practice, research, and education and also to the development of the discipline. By her development of the caritative theory of care, Eriksson has created her own caring science tradition, a tradition that has grown strong, and it is no exaggeration to say that it has set the tone in the Nordic countries.

SUMMARY

Eriksson has for many years been a guide and visionary who has gone before and "ploughed new furrows" in theory development. Eriksson's caritative theory and her whole caring science thinking have developed over the course of 30 years. Characteristic of her thinking is that while she is working at an abstract level developing concepts and theory, the theory is rooted in clinical reality and teaching. The whole caritative theory and the caring that are built up around the theoretical core get their distinctive character and deeper meaning through the ethos of caritas, love, and compassion that perme-

ates the whole. The ultimate goal of caring is to alleviate suffering and serve life and health. The conception of the human being as an entity of body, soul, and spirit, with a core of holiness and dignity, constitutes one of the basic axioms.

Knowledge formation, which Eriksson sees as a hermeneutic spiral, starts from the thought that ethics preceded ontology. In a concrete sense, this implies that the thought of human holiness and dignity is always kept alive in all phases of the search for knowledge. Ethics precedes ontology in theory as well as in practice.

Eriksson's caring science tradition and the academic discipline of caring science form the basis of the activity at the Department of Caring Science at Åbo Akademi University. Eriksson's caritative caring theory and the discipline of caring science have inspired many in the Nordic countries, and they are used as the basis for research, education, and clinical practice. Many of her original textbooks, published mainly in Swedish, have been translated into Finnish, Norwegian, and Danish.

Case Study

The following case study is presented in the form of an authentic description, by Ulf Donner, leader of the Foundation Home, a psychiatric nursing home in Finland that for 15 years has based its practice on Eriksson's caritative theory of caring.

Even at an early stage in our serving in caring science, we caregivers recognized ourselves in the caring science theory which stresses the healing force of love and compassion in the form of tending, playing, and learning in faith, hope, and charity. The caritative culture is made visible with the help of rituals, symbols, and traditions, for instance with the stone that burns with the light of the Trinity and the daily common time for spiritual reflection. In every meeting with the suffering human being, the attributes of love and charity are striven for, and the day involves discussions of reconciliation, forgiveness, and how we as caregivers can tend by nourishing and cleansing on the level of becoming, being, and doing. In the struggle in love and compassion to reach a fellow human being who because of suffering has withdrawn from the communion, to find common horizons, the sacrifice of the caregiver is constantly available.

We work with people who often have the feeling that they do not deserve the love they encounter and who in various ways try to convince us caregivers of this. We experience patients' disappointment in their destructive acts and we have constantly to remember that it may often be broken promises that produce such dynamics. Sometimes it may be difficult to recognize that suffering which is expressed in this way in an abstract sense seeks an embrace that does not give way but is strong enough to give shelter to this suffering in a way that makes a becoming movement possible. In recognizing what is bad and difficult, the horizons in the field of force are expanded and the possibility of bringing in a ray of light and hope is opened.

As caregivers we constantly ask ourselves whether the words, the language we use, bring promise and how we can create linguistic footholds in the void by means of images and symbols. In our effort to nourish and cleanse that which constitutes the basic movement of tending, we often recognize the importance of teaching the patient to be able to mourn disappointments and affirm the possibilities of forgiveness in the movement of reconciliation.

We also try to bring about the open invitation to the suffering human being to join a communion with the help of myths, legends, and tales concerned with human questions about evil–good, about questions of eternity and infinity. Reading aloud with common reflective periods often provides us caregivers with a possibility of getting closer to the patients without getting too close, and opens the door for the suffering the patient bears.

In the act of caring, we strive for openness with regard to the patient's face and a confirmative attitude that responds to the appeal that we can recognize that the patient directs to us. When we as caregivers respond to the patient's appeal for charity, we are faced with the task of confirming the holiness of the other as a human being. Our constant effort is to make it possible for the patient to reestablish his or her dignity, accomplish his or her human mission, and enter true communion.

CRITICAL THINKING *Activities*

1. Reflect on the meaning of caritas as the ethos of caring.
   a. How is caritas culture formed in a care setting?
   b. How do caritative elements appear in caring?
   c. Try to formulate an ethics based on caritas.

2. Health and suffering are each other's preconditions. Think about what this means in the care of a patient.

3. How have you recognized the elements of caring—faith, hope, love and tending, playing and learning—in a concrete caring situation? Give examples.

4. The most usual form of suffering related to care, suffering as a consequence of lack of caritative caring, is a violation of a human being's dignity. Think about a situation where this may occur and what can be done in order to prevent suffering related to care.

REFERENCES

Andersson, M. (1994). *Integritet som begrepp och princip. En studie av ett vårdetiskt ideal i utveckling.* Doktorsavhandling, Turku, Finland, Åbo Akademis Förlag, [*Integrity as a concept and as a principle in health care ethics.* Doctoral dissertation, Turku, Finland. Åbo Akademi University Press.]

Aristotle (1935). *Metaphysics, X-XIV oeconomica magna moralia.* (H. Tredennick & G. C. Armstrong, Trans.). Cambridge, MA: Harvard University Press.

Aristotle. (1993). *Den nikomachiska etiken.* Gothenburg, Sweden: Daidalos. [*The nicomachean ethics* (M. Ringbom, Trans. & Commentary). Gothenburg, Sweden: Daidalos.]

Aristotle. (1997). *Retoriikka.* Helsinki, Finland: Gaudeamus. [*Rhetoric* (P. Hohti, Trans.). Helsinki, Finland: Gaudeamus.]

Arman, M. (2003). *Lidande i existens i patientens värld—Kvinnors upplevelser av att leva med bröstcancer.* Doktorsavhandling, Turku, Finland, Åbo Akademis Förlag. [*Suffering and existence in the patient's world—Women's experiences of living with breast cancer.* Doctoral dissertation, Turku, Finland, Åbo Akademi University Press.]

Arman, M., Rehnsfeldt, A., Lindholm, L., & Hamrin, E. (2002). The face of suffering among women with breast cancer—Being in a field of forces. *Cancer Nursing, 25*(2), 96-103.

Arman-Rehnsfeldt, M., & Rehnsfeldt, A. (2003). Vittnesbördet som etisk grund i vårdandet. I K. Eriksson & U. Å. Lindström (red.), *Gryning II. Klinisk vårdvetenskap* (s. 109-121), Vaasa, Finland: Institutionen för vårdvetenskap, Åbo Akademi. ["Bearing witness as an ethical base in caring." In K. Eriksson & U. Å. Lindström (Eds.), *Dawn II. Clinical caring science* (pp. 109-121). Vaasa, Finland: Department of Caring Science, Åbo Akademi.]

Barbosa da Silva, A. (1993). *Vetenskap och männiksosyn i sjukvården: en introduktion till vetenskapsfilosofi och vårdetik.* Stockholm: Svenska hälso och sjukvårdens tjänstemannaförbund, (SHSTF). [*Science and view of human nature in nursing: an introduction to philosophy of science and caring ethics.* Stockholm: Svenska hälso och sjukvårdens tjänstemannaförbund, (SHSTF).]

Berdâev, N. A. (1990). *Historiens mening: ett försök till en filosofi om det mänskliga ödet.* Skellefteå, Sweden: Artos. [*The meaning of history: an attempt at philosophy of human fate.* Skellefteå, Sweden: Artos.]

Bondas, T. (2000). *Att vara med barn: en vårdvetenskaplig studie av kvinnors upplevelser under perinatal tid.* Doktorsavhandling, Turku, Finland, Åbo Akademis Förlag. [*To be with child: a study of women's lived experiences during the perinatal period from a caring science perspective.* Doctoral dissertation, Turku, Finland, Åbo Akademi University Press.]

Bondas, T., & Eriksson, K. (2001). Women's lived experiences of pregnancy: A tapestry of joy and suffering. *Qualitative Health Research, 11*(6), 824-840.

Caspari, S. (2004). *Det Gyldne snitt. Den estetiske dimensjon et etisk anliggende.* Doktorsavhandling, Turku, Finland: Åbo Academis Förlag. [*The golden section. The aesthetic dimension—A source of health.* Doctoral dissertation. Turku, Finland, Åbo Akademi University Press.]

Edlund, M. (2002). *Människans värdighet—Ett grundbegrepp inom vårdvetenskapen.* Doktorsavhandling, Turku, Finland, Åbo Akademis Förlag. [*Human dignity—A basic caring science concept.* Doctoral dissertation, Turku, Finland, Åbo Akademi University Press.]

Ekebergh, M. (2001). *Tillägnandet av vårdvetenskaplig kunskap. Reflexionens betydelse för lärandet.* Doktorsavhandling, Turku, Finland, Åbo Akademis Förlag. [*Acquiring caring science knowledge—The importance of reflection for learning.* Doctoral dissertation, Turku, Finland, Åbo Akademi University Press.]

Eriksson, K. (1974). *Vårdprocessen* (kompendium). Helsinki, Finland: Helsingfors svenska sjukvårdsinstitut. [*The nursing care process* (Compendium). Helsinki, Finland: Helsingfors svenska sjukvårdsinstitut.]

Eriksson, K. (1976). *Hälsa. En teoretisk och begreppsanalytisk studie om hälsan och dess natur som mål för hälsovårdsedukation.* Licentiatavhandling, Helsinki, Finland: Institutionen för pedagogik, Helsingfors universitet. [*Health. A conceptual analysis and theoretical study of health and its nature as a goal for health care education.* Unpublished Licentiate thesis, Helsinki, Finland: Department of Education, University of Helsinki.]

Eriksson, K. (1981). *Vårdprocessen—En utgångspunkt för läroplanstänkande inom vårdutbildningen. Utvecklande av en vårdprocessmodell samt ett läroplanstänkande utgående från vårdprocessen, n. 94.* Helsinki, Finland: Helsingfors universitet, Pedagogiska Institutionen. [*The nursing care process—An approach to curriculum construction within nursing education. The development of a model for the nursing care process and an approach for curriculum development based on the process of nursing care* (No. 94). Helsinki, Finland: Department of Education, University of Helsinki.]

Eriksson, K. (1984). *Hälsans idé.* Stockholm: Almqvist & Wiksell. [*The idea of health.* Stockholm: Almqvist & Wiksell.]

Eriksson, K. (1985). *Vårddidaktik.* Stockholm: Almqvist & Wiksell. [*Caring didactics.* Stockholm: Almqvist & Wiksell.]

Eriksson, K. (1986). *Annual report.* Helsingfors: Svenska Sjukvårdsinstitut.

Eriksson, K. (1987a). *Vårdandets idé.* Stockholm: Almqvist & Wiksell. [*The idea of caring.* Stockholm: Almqvist & Wiksell.]

Eriksson, K. (1987b). *Pausen. En beskrivning av vårdvetenskapens kunskapsobjekt.* Stockholm: Almqvist & Wiksell. [*The pause: A description of the knowledge object of caring science.* Stockholm: Almqvist & Wiksell.]

Eriksson, K. (1988). *Vårdvetenskap som disciplin, forknings-och tillämpningsområde* (Vårdforskninger 1/1988). Vaasa, Finland: Institutionen för vårdvetenskap, Åbo Akademi. [*Caring science as a discipline, field of research and application* (Caring research 1/1988). Vaasa, Finland: Department of Caring Science, Åbo Akademi.

Eriksson, K. (1989). Caring paradigms. A study of the origins and the development of caring paradigms among nursing students. *Scandinavian Journal of Caring Sciences, 3*(4), 169-176.

Eriksson, K. (1990). *Pro Caritate. En lägesbestämning av caritativ vård. Vårdforskninger 2/1990.* Vaasa, Finland: Institutionen för vårdvetenskap, Åbo Akademi. [*Cari-*

tative caring—A positional analysis. Vaasa, Finland: Department of Caring Science, Åbo Akademi.]

Eriksson, K. (1991). *Broar. Introduktion i vårdvetenskaplig metod.* Vaasa, Finland: Institutionen för vårdvetenskap, Åbo Akademi. [*Bridges. Introduction to the methods of caring science* (test ed.). Vaasa, Finland: Department of Caring Science, Åbo Akademi.]

Eriksson, K. (1992a). The alleviation of suffering—The idea of caring. *Scandinavian Journal of Caring Sciences, 6*(2), 119-123.

Eriksson, K. (1992b). Different forms of caring communion. *Nursing Science Quarterly, 5,* 93.

Eriksson, K. (1992c). Nursing: The caring practice "being there." In D. Gaut (Ed.), *The practice of caring in nursing* (pp. 201-210). New York: National League for Nursing Press.

Eriksson, K. (1993). Lidandets idé. I K. Eriksson (red.), *Möten med lidanden. Vårdforskning 4/1993* (s. 1-27). Vaasa, Finland: Institutionen för vårdvetenskap, Åbo Akademi. [The idea of suffering. In K. Eriksson (Ed.), *Encounters with suffering* (pp. 1-27). Vaasa, Finland: Department of Caring Science, Åbo Akademi.]

Eriksson, K. (1994a). *Den lidande människan.* Stockholm: Liber Förlag. [*The suffering human being.* Stockholm: Liber Förlag.] [English translation forthcoming from Nordic Studies Press, Chicago.]

Eriksson, K. (1994b). Theories of caring as health. In D. Gaut & A. Boykin (Eds.), *Caring as healing: Renewal through hope* (pp. 3-20). New York: National League for Nursing Press.

Eriksson, K., (Ed.). (1995). *Mot en caritativ vårdetik* (Vårdforskning 5/1995). Vaasa, Finland: Institutionen för vårdvetenskap, Åbo Akademi. [*Toward a caritative caring ethic* (Caring research 5/1995). Vaasa, Finland: Department of Caring Science, Åbo Akademi.]

Eriksson, K. (1997a). Caring, spirituality and suffering. In S. M. Roach (Ed.), *Caring from the heart: the convergence between caring and spirituality* (pp. 68-84). New York: Paulist Press.

Eriksson, K. (1997b). Perustutkimus ja käsiteanalyysi. I M. Paunonen & J. Vehvilänen-Julkunen, *Hoitotieteen tutkimusmetodiikka* (s. 50-75). Helsinki Porvoo, Finland: WSOY. [Basic research and concept analysis. In M. Paunonen & J. Vehvilänen-Julkunen, *The research methodology of caring science* (pp. 50-75). Helsinki Porvoo, Finland: WSOY.]

Eriksson, K. (1998). Understanding the world of the patient, the suffering human being: The new clinical paradigm from nursing to caring. In C. E. Guzzetta (Ed.), *Essential readings in holistic nursing* (pp. 3-9). Gaithersburg, MD: Aspen.

Eriksson, (1999, November). *Teoriutveckling inom vårdvetenskapen. Human vetenskaplig angreppspunkt.* Stockholm: Nordisk Akademi för Sykepleievitenskap, Kongress i Stockholm. [*Theory development in caring science. A humanistic approach.* Stockholm: Nordisk Akademi för Sykepleievitenskap, Kongress i Stockholm.]

Eriksson, K. (2001). *Vårdvetenskap som akademisk disciplin* (Vårdforskning 7/2001). Vaasa, Finland: Institutionen för vårdvetenskap, Åbo Akademi. [*Caring science as an academic discipline* (Caring research 7/2001). Vaasa, Finland: Department of Caring Science, Åbo Akademi.]

Eriksson, K. (2002). Caring science in a new key. *Nursing Science Quarterly, 15*(1), 61-65.

Eriksson, K. (2003). Ethos. I K. Eriksson & U. Å. Lindström (red.), *Gryning II. Klinisk vårdvetenskap* (s. 21-34). Vaasa, Finland: Institutionen för vårdvetenskap, Åbo Akademi. [Ethos, in K. Eriksson & U. Å. Lindström (Eds.), *Dawn II. Clinical caring science* (pp. 21-34). Vaasa, Finland: Department of Caring Science, Åbo Akademi.]

Eriksson, K., Bondas-Salonen, T., Fagerström, L., Herberts, S., & Lindholm, L. (1990). *Den mångdimensionella hälsan—En pilotstudie över uppfattningar bland patienter, skolungdomar och lärare* (Projektrapport). Vaasa, Finland: Vasa Sjukvårdsdistrikt kf. och Institutionen för vårdvetenskap, Åbo Akademi. [*Multidimensional health—A pilot study of how patients, school students, and teachers experience health* (Project Rep. 1). Vaasa, Finland: Vasa Sjukvårdsdistrikt kf. och Institutionen för vårdvetenskap, Åbo Akademi.]

Eriksson, K., & Herberts, S. (1992). *Den mångdimensionella hälsan. En studie av hälsobilden hos sjukvårdsledare och sjukvårdspersonal* (Projektrapport 2). Vaasa, Finland: Vasa sjukvårdsdistrikt kf. och Institutionen för vårdvetenskap, Åbo Akademi. [*The multidimensional health. A study of the view of health among health care leaders and health care personnel* (Project Rep. 2). Vaasa, Finland: Vasa sjukvårdsdistrikt kf. och Institutionen för vårdvetenskap, Åbo Akademi.]

Eriksson, K., & Lindström, U. Å. (1997). Abduction—A way to deeper understanding of the world of caring. *Scandinavian Journal of Caring Sciences, 11*(4), 195-198.

Eriksson, K., & Lindström, U. Å. (2000). Siktet, sökandet, slutandet—Om den vårdvetenskapliga kunskapen. I K. Eriksson & U. Å. Lindström (red.), *Gryning—En vårdvetenskaplig antologi* (s. 5-18). Vaasa, Finland: Institutionen för vårdvetenskap, Åbo Akademi. [In the prospect of, searching for, and ending of—The caring science knowledge. In K. Eriksson & U. Å. Lindström (Eds.), *Dawn. An anthology of caring science* (pp. 5-18). Vaasa, Finland: Department of Caring Science, Åbo Akademi.]

Eriksson, K., & Lindström, U. Å. (2003). Klinisk vårdvetenskap. I K. Eriksson & U. Å. Lindström (red.), *Gryning II. Klinisk vårdvetenskap* (s. 3-20). Vaasa, Finland: Institutionen för vårdvetenskap, Åbo

Akademi. [Clinical caring science. In K. Eriksson & U. Å. Lindström (Eds.), *Dawn II. Clinical caring science* (pp. 3-20). Vaasa, Finland: Department of Caring Science, Åbo Akademi.]

Eriksson, K., & Nordman, T. (2004). *Trojanska hästen II. Utvecklande av evidensbaserade vårdande kulturer.* Vaasa, Finland: Institutionen för vårdvetenskap, Åbo Akademi. [*Trojan Horse II. The development of evidence-based caring cultures.* Vaasa, Finland; The Department of Caring Science, Åbo Akademi University.]

Eriksson K., Nordman T., & Myllymäki, I., (1999). *Den trojanska hästen. Evidensbaserat vårdande och vårdarbete ur ett vårdvetenskapligt perspektiv* (Rapport 1). Institutionen för vårdvetenskap. Vaasa, Finland: Åbo Akademi; Helsingfors universitetscentralsjukhus & Vasa sjukvårdsdistrikt. [*The Trojan horse. Evidence-based caring and nursing care in a caring science perspective.* (Report). Department of Caring Science. Vaasa, Finland: Åbo Akademi; Helsingfors universitetscentralsjukhus & Vasa sjukvårdsdistrikt.]

Fagerström, L. (1999). *The patients' caring needs. To understand and measure the unmeasurable.* Doctoral dissertation. (Turku, Finland, Åbo Akademi University Press.)

Fredriksson, L. (2003). *Det vårdande samtalet.* Doktorsavhandling, Åbo Akademis Förlag, Turku, Finland. [*The caring conversation.* Doctoral dissertation, Turku, Finland, Åbo Akademi University Press.]

Fredriksson, L., & Eriksson, K. (2001). The patient's narrative of suffering—A path to health? An interpretetative research synthesis on narrative understanding. *Scandinavian Journal of Caring Sciences, 15*(1), 3-11.

Fredriksson, L., & Eriksson, K. (2003). The ethics of the caring conversation. *Nursing Ethics, 10*(2), 138-148.

Fredriksson, L., & Lindström, U. Å. (2002). Caring conversations—Psychiatric patients' narratives about suffering. *Journal of Advanced Nursing, 40*(4), 396-404.

Gadamer, H-G. (1994). *Truth and method* (2nd rev. ed., J. Weinsheimer & D. G. Marshall, Trans.). New York: Continuum. [Original work published 1960.]

Gadamer, H-G. (2000). *Teoriens lovprisning,* Århus: Systeme. [*Praise the theory.* New Haven: Yale University Press, 1998.] [German orig: *Lob der Theorie,* 3. Auflage, 1991.]

Kaila, E. (1939). *Den mänskliga kunskapen: vad den är och vad den icke är.* Helsinki, Finland: Söderström. [*Human knowledge: What it is and what it is not* (G. H. von Wright, Trans.). Helsinki, Finland: Söderström.]

Kasén, A. (2002). *Den vårdande relationen.* Doktorsavhandling, Turku, Finland, Åbo Akademis Förlag. [*The caring relationship.* Doctoral dissertation Turku, Finland, Åbo Akademi University Press.]

Kierkegaard, S. (1943). *Antingen—Eller* [Orig. 1843: *Enten—Eller.*]. Utgiver under pseudonymen Victor Eremita. Köpenhamn: Meyer. [*Either/or.* Princeton, N.

J.: Princeton University Press, 1987] [Original work published 1843.]

Koort, P. (1975). *Semantisk analys och konfigurationsanalys.* Lund, Sweden: Studentlitteratur. [*Semantic analysis and analysis of configuration.* Lund, Sweden: Studentlitteratur.]

Kuhn, T. (1971). *The structure of scientific revolutions.* Chicago: University of Chicago Press.

Kurtén, T. (1987). *Grunder för en kontextuell teologi: ett wittgensteinskt sätt att närma sig teologin I diskussion med Anders Jeffner.* Turku, Finland: Åbo Akademis Förlag. [*Bases for a contextual theology: a Wittgensteinian way of approaching theology in a discussion with Anders Jeffner.* Turku, Finland: Åbo Akademi University Press.]

Kärkkäinen, O., & Eriksson, K. (2003). Evaluation of patient records as a part of developing a nursing care classification. *Journal of Clinical Nursing, 12*(2), 198-205.

Kärkkäinen, O., & Eriksson, K. (2004). Structuring the documentation of nursing care on the basis of a theoretical process model. *Scandinavian Journal of Caring Sciences, 18*(2), 229-236.

Lanara, V. (1981). *Heroism as a nursing value.* Athens, Greece: Sisterhood Evniki.

Langer, S. K. (1942). *Filosofi i en ny tonart.* Stockholm: Geber. [*Philosophy in a new key.* Stockholm: Geber.]

Lévinas, E. (1985). *Ethics and infinity.* Pittsburgh: Duquesne University Press.

Lévinas, E. (1988). *Etik och oändlighet.* Stockholm-Lund: Symposion. [*Ethics and infinity.* Stockholm-Lund: Symposion.]

Lévinas, E. (1989). *The Lévinas reader* (S. Hand, Ed.). Oxford: Blackwell.

Lindholm, L. (1998). *Den unga människans hälsa och lidande.* Doktorsavhandling, Vaasa, Finland. Institutionen för vårdvetenskap, Åbo Akademi. [*The young person's health and suffering.* Doctoral dissertation, Vaasa, Finland. Åbo Akademi, Department of Caring Science.]

Lindholm, L., & Eriksson, K. (1993). To understand and to alleviate suffering in a caring culture. *Journal of Advanced Nursing, 18,* 1354-1361.

Lindholm, L., & Eriksson, K. (1998). The dialectic of health and suffering: An ontological perspective on young people's health. *Qualitative Health Research, 8*(4), 513-525.

Lindholm, L., Nieminen, A-L., Mäkelä, C., & Rantanen-Siljamäki, S. (2004). Significant others—A source of strength in the care of women with breast cancer. Manuscript submitted for publication.

Lindström, U. Å. (1992). *De psykiatriska specialsjukskötarnas yrkesparadigm.* Doktorsavhandling, Turku, Finland. Åbo Akademis Förlag. [*The professional paradigm of the qualified psychiatric nurses.* Doctoral dissertation, Turku, Finland, Åbo Akademi University Press.]

Lindwall, L. (2004). *Kroppen som bärare av hälsa och lidande.* Doktorsavhandling, Turku, Finland, Åbo Akademis Förlag. [*The body as a carrier of health and suffering.* Doctoral dissertation, Turku, Finland, Åbo Akademi University Press.]

Lukander, E. (1995). *Developing and testing a method: Nursing audit, for evaluation of nursing care.* Licentiate thesis, Kuopion yliopisto, Kuopio, Finland.

Martinsen, K., (Ed.). (1996). *Fenomenologi og omsorg.* Oslo, Norway: TANO. [*Phenomenology and care.* Oslo, Norway: TANO.]

Nilsson, B. (2004). *Savnets tone i ensomhetens melodi. Ensomhet hos aleneboende personer med alvorlig psykisk lidelse.* Doktorsavhandling, Turku, Finland, Åbo Akademis Förlag. [*The tune of want in the loneliness melody.* Doctoral dissertation, Turku, Finland, Åbo Akademi University Press.]

Nygren, A. (1966). *Eros och agape.* Stockholm: Aldus Bonniers. [*Eros and agape.* Stockholm: Aldus Bonniers.]

Nygren, A. (1972). *Meaning and method: prolegomena to a scientific philosophy of religion and a scientific theology.* London: Epworth Press.

Nåden, D. (1998). *Når sykepleie er kunstutøvelse. En undersøkelse av noen nødvendige forutsetninger for sykepleie som kunst.* Doktorsavhandling, Vaasa, Finland. Institutionen för vårdvetenskap, Åbo Akademi. [*When caring is an exercise of art. An examination of some necessary preconditions of nursing as art.* Doctoral dissertation, Department of Caring Science, Åbo Akademi, Vaasa, Finland.]

Pascal, B. (1971). *Tankar.* Uddevalla, Sweden: Bohusläningens AB. [*Thoughts.* Uddevalla, Sweden: Bohusläningens AB.]

Peirce, C. S. (1990). *Pragmatism och kosmologi. Valda uppsatser.* Gothenburg, Sweden: Daidalos. [*Pragmatism and cosmology* (Chosen essays). Gothenburg, Sweden: Daidalos.]

Popper, K. R. (1997). *Popper i urval av Miller. Kunskapsteori, vetenskapsteori.* Stockholm: Thales. [*Popper in selection of Miller. Theory of knowledge and theory of science.* Stockholm: Thales.]

Rehnsfeldt, A. (1999). *Mötet med patienten i ett livsavgörande skede.* Doktorsavhandling, Åbo Akademis Förlag, Turku, Finland. [*The encounter with the patient in a life-changing process.* Doctoral dissertation, Åbo Akademi University Press, Turku, Finland.]

Rundqvist, E. (2004). *Makt som fullmakt. Ett vårdvetenskapligt perspektiv.* Doktorsavhandling, Åbo Akademis Förlag, Turku, Finland. [*Power as authority. A caring science perspective.* Doctoral dissertation, Åbo Akademi University Press, Turku, Finland.]

Råholm, M-B. (2003). *I kampens och modets dialektik.* Doktorsavhandling, Åbo Akademis Förlag, Turku, Finland. [*In the dialectic of struggle and courage.* Dissertation, Åbo Akademi University Press, Turku, Finland.]

Råholm, M-B., & Lindholm, L. (1999). Being in the world of the suffering patient: A challenge to nursing ethics. *Nursing Ethics, 6,* 528-539.

Råholm, M-B., Lindholm, L., & Eriksson, K. (2002). Grasping the essence of the spiritual dimension reflected through the horizon of suffering—An interpretative research synthesis. *The Australian Journal of Holistic Nursing, 9,* 4-12.

Sivonen, K. (2000). *Vården och det andliga. En bestämning av begreppet 'andlig' ur ett vårdvetenskapligt perspektiv.* Doktorsavhandling, Turku, Finland, Åbo Akademis Förlag. [*Care and the spiritual dimension. A definition of the concept of "spiritual" in a caring science perspective.* Doctoral dissertation, Turku, Finland, Åbo Akademi University Press.]

St. Augustine, A. (1957). *Bekännelser.* Stockholm: Söderström. [*Confessions.* Stockholm: Söderström.]

Turtiainen, A-M. (1999). *Hoitotyön käytännön kuvaamisen yhtenäistäminen: Belgialaisen hoitotyön minimitiedoston (BeNMDS) kulttuurinen adaptio Suomeen.* Doktorsavhandling, Väitöskirja, Kuopion yliopisto, Kuopio, Finland. [*Methods to describe nursing with uniform language: The cross-cultural adaptation process of the Belgium Nursing Minimum Data Set in Finland.* Doctoral dissertation, Kuopio University, Kuopio, Finland.]

Törnebohm, H. (1978). *Paradigm i vetenskapsteorin* (Del 2. Rapport nr. 100). Gothenburg, Sweden: Institutionen för vetenskapsteori, Göteborgs universitet. [*Paradigms in the theory of science* (Part 2 Report nr. 100). Gothenburg, Sweden: Institutionen för vetenskapsteori, Göteborgs universitet.]

von Post, I. (1999). *Professionell naturlig vård ur anestesi och operationassjuksköterskors perspektiv.* Doktorsavhandling, Åbo Akademis Förlag, Turku, Finland. [*Professional natural care from the perspective of nurse anesthetists and operating room nurses.* Doctoral dissertation, Turku, Finland, Åbo Akademi University Press.]

von Wright, G. H. (1986). *Vetenskapen och förnuftet.* Helsinki, Finland: Söderström. [*Science and reason.* Helsinki, Finland: Söderström.]

Wiklund, L. (2000). *Lidandet som kamp och drama.* Doktorsavhandling, Turku, Finland, Åbo Akademis Förlag. [*Suffering as struggle and as drama.* Doctoral dissertation, Turku, Finland, Åbo Akademi University Press.]

Wingren, G. (1996). *Predikan: en principiell studie.* Lund, Sweden: Gleerup. [*The sermon: a study based on principles.* Lund, Sweden: Gleerup.] [Original work published 1960.]

Wärnå, C. (2002). *Dygd och hälsa.* Doktorsavhandling, Turku, Finland, Åbo Akademis Förlag. [*Virtue and health*. Doctoral dissertation, Turku, Finland, Åbo Akademi University Press.]

BIBLIOGRAPHY

Primary Sources

Articles in Scientific Journals With Referee Practice

Arman, M., Rehnsfeldt, A., Lindholm, L., Hamrin, E. & Eriksson, K. (2004). Suffering related to health care: A study of breast cancer patients' experiences. *International Journal of Nursing Practice, 10*(6), 248–256.

Bondas, T., & Eriksson, K. (2001). Women's lived experiences of pregnancy: A tapestry of joy and suffering. *Qualitative Health Research, 11*(6), 824-840.

Eriksson, K. (1976). Nursing—Skilled work or a profession. *International Nursing Review, 23*(4), 118-120.

Eriksson, K. (1979). Semantiska och kulturella aspekter på hälsobegreppet. *Finska Läkaresällskapets handlingar,* 74-81. [Semantic and cultural aspects of the concept of health. *Finska Läkaresällskapets handlingar,* 74-81.]

Eriksson, K. (1980). Hoitotieteen loogiset ja tieteenteoreettiset perusteet. *Sosiaalinen aikakauskirja, 14*(5), 6-10. [The theory of science and logical basics of caring science. *Sosiaalinen aikakauskirja, 14*(5), 6-10.]

Eriksson, K. (1980). Hoitotieteen teoreettisista malleista, käsitejärjestelmistä ja niiden merkityksestä alan kehittämisessä. *Sosiaalilääketieteellinen aikakauslehti, 17*(2), 66-70. [The importance of caring scientific theoretical models and concept systems for the development of the science. *Sosiaalilääketieteellinen aikakauslehti, 17*(2), 66-70.]

Eriksson, K. (1982). Sjukskötarnas strävan efter högskoleutbildning. *Kasvatus, 13*(3), 192-194. [The nurses strive for a university education. *Kasvatus, 13*(3), 192-194.]

Eriksson, K. (1982). Vad är vårdvetenskap? *Nordisk Medicin, 97,* 200-201. [What is caring science? *Nordisk Medicin, 97,* 200-201.]

Eriksson, K. (1982). Vård som teknologi och vetenskap. *Vård i Norden, 2,* 92-95. [Caring as technology and as a science. *Nordic Journal of Nursing Research and Clinical Studies, 2,* 92-95.]

Eriksson, K. (1984). Vårdvetenskapens och vårdforskningens nytta och giltighet. *Vård i Norden, 2*(4), 220-224. [The use and validity of caring science and caring research. *Nordic Journal of Nursing Research and Clinical Studies, 2*(4), 220-224.]

Eriksson, K. (1989). Caring paradigms. A study of the origins and the development of caring paradigms among nursing students. *Scandinavian Journal of Caring Sciences, 3*(4), 169-176.

Eriksson, K. (1989). Det finns en gemensam substans i allt vårdandet. *Vård i Norden, 15*(2), 27-28. [There is a common substance in all caring. *Nordic of Journal Nursing Research and Clinical Studies, 15*(2), 27-28.]

Eriksson, K. (1989). Motivforskning inom vårdvetenskapen. En beskrivning av vårdvetenskapens grundmotiv. *Hoitotiede, 1*(2), 61-67. [Motive research within caring science. A description of the basic motive in caring science. *Journal of Nursing Science, 1*(2), 61-67.]

Eriksson, K. (1990). Nursing science in a Nordic perspective. Systematic and contextual caring science. A study of the basic motive of caring and context. *Scandinavian Journal of Caring Sciences, 4*(1), 3-5.

Eriksson, K. (1992). Different forms of caring communion. *Nursing Science Quarterly, 5,* 93.

Eriksson, K. (1992). The alleviation of suffering—The idea of caring. *Scandinavian Journal of Caring Sciences, 6*(2), 119-123.

Eriksson, K. (1994). Hälsovårdskandidatutbildningen vid Helsingfors universitet—Historisk tillbakablick och visioner. *Hoitotiede, 3,* 122-126. [The bachelor's degree in health care at Helsinki University—A historical retrospect and visions. *Journal of Nursing Science, 3,* 122-126.]

Eriksson, K. (1995). Ars moriendi är ars vivendi. *Finsk tidskrift, 10,* 641-645. [Ars moriendi is ars vivendi. *Finsk tidskrift, 10,* 641-645.]

Eriksson, K. (1995). Teologi og bioetik. *Vård i Norden, 1,* 33. [Theology and bio-ethics. *Nordic Journal of Nursing Research and Clinical Studies, 1,* 33.]

Eriksson, K. (1997). Understanding the world of the patient, the suffering human being—The new clinical paradigm from nursing to caring. *Advanced Practice Nursing Quarterly, 3*(1), 8-13.

Eriksson, K. (1998). Hälsans tragedy. *Finsk tidskrift, 10,* 590-599. [The tragedy of health. *Finsk tidskrift, 10,* 590-599.]

Eriksson, K. (2002). Caring science in a new key. *Nursing Science Quarterly, 15*(1), 61-65.

Eriksson, K., Bondas, T., Lindholm, L., Kasén, A. & Matilainen, D. (2002). Den vårdvetenskapliga forskningstraditionen vid Institutionen för vårdvetenskap, Åbo Akademi. *Hoitotiede, 14*(6), 307-315. [The tradition of research at the Department of Caring Science, Åbo Akademi University. *Journal of Nursing Science, 14*(6), 307-315.]

Eriksson, K., Herberts, S., & Lindholm, L. (1994). Bilder av lidande—Lidande i belysning av aktuell vårdvetenskaplig forskning. *Hoitotiede, 4,* 155-162. [Views of suffering—Suffering in the light of current research within caring science. *Journal of Nursing Science, 4,* 155-162.]

Eriksson, K., & Lindström, U. Å. (1997). Abduction—A way to deeper understanding of the world of caring. *Scandinavian Journal of Caring Sciences, 11*(4), 195-198.

Eriksson, K., & Lindström, U. Å. (1999). Abduktion och pragmatism—Två vägar till framsteg inom vårdvetenskapen. *Hoitotiede, 11*(5), 292-299. [Abduction and pragmatism—Two ways to progress within caring science. *Journal of Nursing Science, 11*(5), 292-299.]

Eriksson, K., & Lindström, U. Å. (1999). En vetenskapsteori för vårdvetenskapen. *Hoitotiede, 11*(6), 358-364. [A theory of science for caring science. *Journal of Nursing Science, 11*(6), 358-364.]

Eriksson, K., & Lindström, U. Å. (1999). The fundamental idea of quality assurance. *International Journal for Human Caring, 3*(3), 21-27.

Eriksson, K., & von Post, I. (1999). A hermeneutic textual analysis of suffering and caring in the peri-operative context. *Journal of Advanced Nursing, 30*(4), 983-989.

Fagerström, L., Eriksson, K., & Bergbom Engberg, I. (1998). The patient's perceived caring needs as a message of suffering. *Journal of Advanced Nursing, 28*(5), 978-987.

Fagerström, L., Eriksson, K., & Bergbom Engberg, I. (1999). The patient's perceived caring needs—Measuring the unmeasurable. *International Journal of Nursing Practice, 5*(4), 199-208.

Fredriksson, L., & Eriksson, K. (2001). The patient's narrative of suffering—A path to health? An interpretetative research synthesis on narrative understanding. *Scandinavian Journal of Caring Sciences, 15*(1), 3-11.

Fredriksson, L., & Eriksson, K. (2003). The ethics of the caring conversation. *Nursing Ethics, 10*(2), 138-148.

Herberts, S., & Eriksson, K. (1995). Nursing leaders' and nurses' view of health. *Journal of Advanced Nursing, 22*, 868-878.

Kärkkäinen, O., & Eriksson, K. (2003). Evaluation of patient records as a part of developing a nursing care classification. *Journal of Clinical Nursing, 12*(2), 198-205.

Kärkkäinen, O., & Eriksson, K. (2004). A theoretical approach to documentation of care. *Nursing Science Quarterly, 17*(3), 2-6.

Lindholm, L., & Eriksson, K. (1993). To understand and to alleviate suffering in a caring culture. *Journal of Advanced Nursing, 18*, 1354-1361.

Lindholm, L., & Eriksson, K. (1998). The dialectic of health and suffering: An ontological perspective on young people's health. *Qualitative Health Research, 8*(4), 513-525.

Nåden, D., & Eriksson, K. (2000). The phenomenon of confirmation—An aspect of nursing as an art. *International Journal for Human Caring, 4*(3), 23-28.

Nåden, D., & Eriksson, K. (2002). Encounter: A fundamental category of nursing as an art. *International Journal for Human Caring, 6*(1), 34-40.

Nåden, D., & Eriksson, K. (2003). Semantisk begrepsanalyse—Et grunnleggende aspekt i en disiplins teoriutvikling. *Vård i Norden, 23*(1), 21-26. [Semantic concept analysis—A fundamental aspect in the theory development of a discipline. *Nordic Journal of Nursing Research and Clinical Studies, 23*(1), 21-26.]

Nåden, D., & Eriksson, K. (2004). Understanding the importance of values and moral attitudes in nursing care in preserving human dignity. *Nursing Science Quarterly, 17*(1), 86-91.

Nåden, D., & Eriksson, K. (2004). Values and moral attitudes in nursing care. Understanding the patient perspective. *Norsk Tidskrift for Sygepleieforskning, 6*(1), 3-17.

Rehnsfeldt, A. & Eriksson, K. (2004). The progression of suffering implies alleviated suffering. *Scandinavian Journal of Caring Sciences, 18*(3), 264–272.

Råholm, M-B., & Eriksson, K. (2001). Call to life: Exploring the spiritual dimension as a dialectic between suffering and desire experienced by coronary bypass patients. *International Journal for Human Caring, 5*(1), 14-20.

Råholm, M-B., Lindholm, L., & Eriksson, K. (2002). Grasping the essence of the spiritual dimension reflected through the horizon of suffering: An interpretative research synthesis. *The Australian Journal of Holistic Nursing, 9*(1), 4-13.

von Post, I., & Eriksson, K. (2000). The ideal and practice concepts of 'professional nursing care.' *International Journal for Human Caring, 4*(1), 14-22.

Wikström-Grotell, C., Lindholm, L., & Eriksson, K. (2002). Det mångdimensionella rörelsebegreppet i fysioterapin—En kontextuell analys. *Nordisk Fysioterapi, 6*, 146-184. [The multidimensional concept of movement in physiotherapy—A contextual analysis. *Nordisk Fysioterapi, 6*, 146-184.]

Articles in Compilation Works and Proceedings With Referee Practice
Compilation Works

Eriksson, K. (1971). En analys av sjuksköterskeutbildningen utgående från en utbildningsteknologisk model. I *Sairaanhoidon vuosikirja VIII* (s. 54-77). Helsinki, Finland: Sairaanhoitajien Koulutussäätiö. [An analysis of nursing education from an educational-technological model. In *Health care yearbook VIII* (pp. 54-77). Helsinki, Finland: Sairaanhoitajien Koulutussäätiö.]

Eriksson, K. (1974). Sairaanhoidon kehittäminen oppiaineena. I *Sairaanhoidon vuosikirja XI* (s. 9-21). Helsinki, Finland: Sairaanhoitajien Koulutussäätiö. [The development of health care as a subject. In *Health care yearbook XI* (pp. 9-21). Helsinki, Finland: Sairaanhoitajien Koulutussäätiö.]

Eriksson, K. (1977). Hälsa—En teoretisk och begreppsanalytisk studie om hälsa och dess nature. I *Sairaanhoidon vuosikirja XIV* (s. 55-195). [Health—A conceptual analysis and theoretical study of health and its nature. In *Health care yearbook XIV* (pp. 155-195). Helsinki, Finland: Sairaanhoitajien Koulutussäätiö.]

Eriksson, K. (1978). Modellen—Ett sätt att beskriva vårdskeendet. I *Sairaanhoidon vuosikirja XV* (s. 189-

225). Helsinki, Finland: Sairaanhoitajien Koulutussäätiö. [The model—A way of describing the act of nursing care. In *Health care yearbook XV* (pp. 189-225). Helsinki, Finland: Sairaanhoitajien Koulutussäätiö.]

Eriksson, K. (1982). Den vårdvetenskapscentrerade läroplanen—Ett alternativ för dagens vårdutbildning. I *Sairaanhoidon vuosikirja XIX* (s. 173-187). Helsinki, Finland: Sairaanhoitajien Koulutussäätiö. [The caring science centered curriculum—An alternative for health education today. In *Health care yearbook XIX* (pp. 173-187). Helsinki, Finland: Sairaanhoitajien Koulutussäätiö.]

Eriksson, K. (1983). Den fullvuxna insulindiabetikern i hälsovårdens vårdprocess. I *Sairaanhoidon vuosikirja XIX* (s. 428-430). Helsinki, Finland: Sairaanhoitajien Koulutussäätiö. [The adult insulin-dependent diabetic in the health care nursing process. In *Health care yearbook XIX* (pp. 428-430). Helsinki, Finland: Sairaanhoitajien Koulutussäätiö.]

Eriksson, K. (1983). Vårdområdet finner sin profil— Den vårdvetenskapliga eran har inlets. I *Epione, Jubileumsskrift 1898-1983* (s. 12-17). [The area of caring finds its profile—The caring science era has begun. In *Epione, Jubilee-script 1898-1983* (pp. 12-17). Helsinki, Finland: SSY-Sjuksköterskeföreningen i Finland.]

Eriksson, K. (1984). Ammatillisuus hoitamisessa. I Sairaanhoitajien Koulutussäätiö (red.), *Hoito-opin perusteet* (s. 125-129). Vaasa, Finland: Sairaanhoitajien Koulutussäätiö. [Professionalism in caring. In Sairaanhoitajien Koulutussäätiö (Ed.), *The basics of nursing science* (pp. 125-129). Vaasa, Finland: Sairaanhoitajien Koulutussäätiö.]

Eriksson, K. (1985). Vårdvetenskap—Aktuellt läge— Utvecklingens trender. I *Epione, SSY—Sjuksköterskeföreningen i Finland r.f:s rapport.* Helsinki, Finland: Sairaanhoitajien Koulutussäätiö. [Caring science— Current situation—Development trends. In *Epione, SSY—Sjuksköterskeföreningen in Finland* (r.f:s report) (pp. 7-17). Helsinki, Finland: Sairaanhoitajien Koulutussäätiö.]

Eriksson, K. (1986). Hoito, Caring—Hoitotyön primaari substanssi. Puheenvuoro 2. I T. Martikainen & K. Manninen (red.), *Hoitotyö ja koulutus* (s. 17-41). Hämeenlinna, Finland: Sairaanhoitajien Koulutussäätiö. [Caring—The primary substance of nursing. Speech 2. In T. Martikainen & K. Manninen (Eds.), *Nursing and education* (pp. 17-41). Hämeenlinna, Finland: Sairaanhoitajien Koulutussäätiö.]

Eriksson, K. (1987). Vårdvetenskapen som humanistisk vetenskap. I *Hoitotiede vuosikirja (s. 68-77)* [Caring science as a humanistic science. *Journal of Nursing Science Yearbook* 68-77.]

Eriksson, K. (1988). Vårdandets idé och ursprung. I *Panakeia. Vårdvetenskaplig årsbok* (s. 17-35). Stock-holm: Almqvist & Wiksell. [The origin and idea of caring. In *Panakeia. Caring science yearbook* (pp. 17-35). Stockholm: Almqvist & Wiksell.]

Eriksson, K. (1989). Ammatillisuus hoitamisessa. I *Hoito-opin perusteet* (2: 2 yppl., s. 125-129). Vaasa, Finland: Sairaanhoitajien Koulutussäätiö. [Professionalism in caring. In *The basics of nursing science* (2nd ed., pp. 125-129). Vaasa, Finland: Sairaanhoitajien Koulutussäätiö.]

Eriksson, K. (1990). Framtidsvisioner—om utvecklingen av sjukskötarens arbete. I *Epione, Jubileumsskrift 1898-1988* (s. 28-38). Helsinki, Finland: SSY-sjuksköterskeföreningen i Finland r.f. [Future visions of the development of the nurse's work. In *Epione, Jubilee-script 1898-1988* (pp. 28-38). Helsinki, Finland: SSY-sjuksköterske-föreningen i Finland r.f.]

Eriksson, K. (1991). Hälsa är mera än frånvaro av sjukdom. I *Centrum för vårdvetenskap, Vård—Utbildning—Utveckling—Forskning* (s. 1-2, 29-35). Stockholm: Karolinska Institutet. [Health is more than the absence of illness. In *Centrum för vårdvetenskap, Vård—Utbildning—Utveckling—Forskning* (pp. 1-2, 29-35). Stockholm: Karolinska Institutet.]

Eriksson, K. (1992). Nursing: The caring practice "being there." In D. Gaut (Ed.), *The Practice of caring in nursing* (pp. 201-210). New York: National League for Nursing Press.

Eriksson, K. (1993). De första åren—Några reflektioner kring den vårdvetenskapliga eran. I *Epione, Jubileumsskrift 1898-1993* (s. 7-15). Helsinki, Finland: SSY-Sjuksköterskeföreningen. [The first years— Reflections upon the era of caring science. In *Epione, Jubilee-script 1898-1993* (pp. 7-15). Helsinki, Finland: SSY-Sjuksköterskeföreningen.]

Eriksson, K. (1994). Theories of caring as health. In D. Gaut & A. Boykin (Eds.), *Caring as healing: Renewal through hope* (pp. 3-20). New York: National League for Nursing Press.

Eriksson, K. (1994). Vårdvetenskapen som autonom discipline. I H. Willman (red.), *Hygieia. Hoitotyön vuosikirja 1994* (s. 87-91).). Helsinki, Finland: Kirjayhtymä. [Caring science as an autonomous discipline. In H. Willman (Ed.), *Hygieia. Nursing yearbook 1994* (pp. 87-91). Helsinki, Finland: Kirjayhtymä.]

Eriksson, K. (1996). Efterskrift—Om vårdvetenskapens möjligheter och gränser. I K. Martinsen (red.), *Fenomenologi og omsorg* (s. 140-150). Oslo, Norway: TANO. [Postscript—About the possibilities and boundaries of caring science. In K. Martinsen (Ed.), *Phenomenology and caring* (pp. 140-150). Oslo, Norway: TANO.]

Eriksson, K. (1996). Om dokumentation—Vad den är och inte är. I K. Dahlberg (red.), *Konsten att dokumentera omvårdnad* (s. 9-13). Lund, Sweden: Studentlitteratur. [On documentation—What it is and what it is not. In

K. Dahlberg (ed.), *The art of documenting care* (pp. 9-13). Lund, Sweden: Studentlitteratur.]

Eriksson, K. (1996). Om människans värdighet. I T. Bjerkreim, J. Mathinsen, & R. Nord (red.), *Visjon, viten og virke. Festskrift till sykepleieren Kjellaug Lerheim, 70 år* (s. 79-86). Oslo, Norway: Universitetsförlaget. [On human dignity. In T. Bjerkreim, J. Mathinsen, & R. Nord (Eds.), *Vision, knowledge and influence. Jubilee-script for the nurse Kjellaug Lerheim, 70 years* (pp. 79-86). Oslo, Norway: Universitetsförlaget.]

Eriksson, K. (1997). Caring, spirituality and suffering. In S. M. Roach (Ed.), *Caring from the heart: The convergence between caring and spirituality* (pp. 68-84). New York: Paulist Press.

Eriksson, K. (1997). Mot en vårdetisk teori. I *Hoitotyön vuosikirja 1997. Pro Nursing RY:n vuosikirja, Hygieia* (s. 9-23). Helsinki, Finland: Kirjayhtymä. [Toward an ethical caring theory. In *Nursing yearbook 1997. Pro Nursing RY:s yearbook, Hygieia* (pp. 9-23). Helsinki, Finland: Kirjayhtymä.]

Eriksson, K. (1997). Perustutkimus ja käsiteanalyysi. I M. Paunonen & K. Vehviläinen-Julkunen (red.), *Hoitotieteen tutkimusmetodiikka* (s. 50-75). Helsinki, Finland: WSOY. [Basic research and conceptual analysis. In M. Paunonen & K. Vehviläinen-Julkunen (Eds.), *The research methodology of caring science* (pp. 50-75). Helsinki, Finland: WSOY.]

Eriksson, K. (1998). Epione—Vårdandets ethos. I *Epione, Jubileumsskrift 1898-1998* Helsinki, Finland: SSY-Sjuksköterskeföreningen. [Epione—The ethos of caring. In *Epione, Jubilee-script 1898-1998*. Helsinki, Finland: SSY-Sjuksköterskeföreningen.]

Eriksson, K. (1998). Människans värdighet, lidande och lidandets ethos. I *Suomen Mielenterveysseura, Tuhkaa ja linnunrata. Henkisyys mielenterveystyössä* (s. 67-82). Helsinki: Suomen Mielenterveysseura, SMS-julkaisut. [Human dignity, suffering and the ethos of suffering. In *Ashes and the Milky Way: Spirituality in mental health care nursing* (pp. 67-82). Helsinki: Suomen Mielenterveysseura, SMS-julkaisut.]

Eriksson, K. (1998). Understanding the world of the patient, the suffering human being: The new clinical paradigm from nursing to caring. In C. E. Guzzetta (Ed.), *Essential readings in holistic nursing* (pp. 3-9). Gaithersburg, MD: Aspen Publications.

Eriksson, K. (1999). Tillbaka till Popper och Kuhn—En evolutionär epistemologi för vårdvetenskapen. I J. Kinnunen, P. Meriläinen, K. Vehviläinen-Julkunen, & T. Nyberg (red.), *Terveystieteiden monialainen tutkimus ja yliopistokoulutus. Suunnistuspoluilta tiedon valtatielle. Professor Sirkka Sinkkoselle omistettu juhlakirja* (s. 21-35). Kuopio, Finland: Kuopion yliopiston julkaisuja E, Yhteiskuntatieteet 74. [Back to Popper and Kuhn—An evolutionary epistemology for caring science. In J. Kinnunen, P. Meriläinen, K. Vehviläinen-Julkunen, &

T. Nyberg (Eds.), *The multiscientific health science university education and research. Paths to the highway of science. A jubilee book dedicated to Professor Sirkka Sikkonen* (pp. 21-35). Kuopio, Finland: Kuopion yliopiston julkaisuja E, Yhteiskuntatieteet 74.]

Eriksson, K. (1999). Vårdvetenskapen—En akademisk disciplin. I S. Janhonen, I. Lepola, M. Nikkonen, & M. Toljamo (red.), *Suomalainen hoitotiede uudelle vuosituhannelle. Professori Maija Hentisen juhlakirja* (s. 59-64). Oulu, Finland: Oulun yliopiston hoitotieteen ja terveyshallinnon laitoksen julkaisuja 2. [Caring science—An academic discipline. In S. Janhonen, I. Lepola, M. Nikkonen, & M. Toljamo (Eds.), *The Finnish caring science in the new millennium. A jubilee-script dedicated to Professor Maija Hentinen* (pp. 59-64). Oulu, Finland: Oulun yliopiston hoitotieteen ja terveyshallinnon laitoksen julkaisuja 2.]

Eriksson, K. (2000). Caritas et passio—Liebe und leiden—Als grundkategorien der pflegewissenschaft. I T. Strom, *Diakonie an der Schwelle zum neuen Jahrtausend.* Heidelberg, Germany: Diakoniewissenschaftlichen Instituts, Universität Heidelberg. [Caritas et passio—Love and suffering as basic categories in caring science. In T. Strom, *The diaconate on the threshold of the new millennium.* Heidelberg, Germany: Diakoniewissenschaftlichen Instituts, Universität Heidelberg.]

Eriksson, K. (2002). Rakkaus—Diakoniatieteen ydin ja ethos? I M. Lahtinen & T. Toikkanen (red.), *Anno Domini. Diakoniatieteen vuosikirja 2002* (s. 155-164). Tampere, Finland: Tammerpaino. [Love—The core and ethos of deacony? In M. Lahtinen & T. Toikkanen (Eds.), *Anno Domini. Diakonic yearbook 2002* (pp. 155-164). Tampere, Finland: Tammerpaino.]

Eriksson, K. (2003). Diakonian erityisyys hoitotyössä. I M. Lahtinen & T. Toikkanen (red.), *Anno domini. Diakoniatieteen vuosikirja 2003* (s. 120-126). Tampere, Finland: Tammerpaino. [The uniqueness of deacony in nursing. In M. Lahtinen & T. Toikkanen (Eds.), *Anno Domini. Diakonic yearbook 2003* (pp. 120-126). Tampere, Finland: Tammerpaino.]

Eriksson, K., & Hamrin, E. (1988). Vårdvetenskapen formas—En tillbakablick och ett framtidsperspektiv. I *Panakeia, vårdvetenskaplig årsbok* (s. 9-16). Stockholm: Almqvist & Wiksell. [Caring science is formed—A historical and futuristic perspective. In *Panakeia, caring science yearbook* (pp. 9-16). Stockholm: Almqvist & Wiksell.]

Eriksson, K., Nordman, T., & Kasén, A. (1998). Reflective practice: A way to the patient's world and caring, the core of nursing. In C. Johns & D. Freshwater (Eds.), *Transforming nursing through reflective practice.* Oxford: Blackwell Science.

Eriksson, K., & Willman, H. (1972). Kohti parempaa ohjausta. I *Sairaanhoidon vuosikirja IX* (s. 131-139). Helsinki, Finland: Sairaanhoitajien Koulutussäätiö. [Toward a better counseling. In *Health care yearbook*

IX (pp. 131-139). Helsinki, Finland: Sairaanhoitajien Koulutussäätiö.]

Proceedings (Selected)

Eriksson, K. (1977). *A theoretical and principal framework on concepts in curricular planning in basic schools of nursing* (pp. 203-211). Istanbul, Turkey: Istanbul Medical Convention.

Eriksson, K. (1978). Sjukvårdsforskning: intentioner-områden-betingelser-problem. *Rapport fra SSN:s forskningsseminar Perspektiver på sykepleieforskning* (s. 30-43). Voksenåsen, Norway. Stockholm: SSN. [Health care research: Intentions—Areas—Conditions—Problems. *Report from SSN's research seminar perspectives on nursing care research* (pp. 30-43). Voksenåsen, Norway. Stockholm: SSN.]

Eriksson, K. (1982). Basforskning inom vård. *Kongressrapport* (s. 44-51). Stockholm: Högskolan för lärarutbildning. [Basic research within care. *Congress report* (pp. 44-51). Stockholm: Högskolan för lärarutbildning.]

Eriksson, K. (1982). *The patient care process—An approach to curriculum construction within nursing education.* 5th Work group meeting. First Open Conference (pp. 318-321). Uppsala, Sweden.

Eriksson, K. (1983). Vårdvetenskap. I L. Björkman (red.), *Rapport från Omvårdnads-konferens i Örebro* (s. 4-10). Sweden, Högskolan i Örebro. [Caring Science. In L. Björkman (Ed.), *Report from the nursing care conference in Örebro* (pp. 4-10). Sweden, Högskolan i Örebro.]

Eriksson, K. (1985). Bildning för yrke och framtid *SKUT-84. Dokumentation från Pedagogiska Fakulteten* (Nr, 21, s. 56-61). Vaasa, Finland: Åbo Akademi. [Education for profession and future (No. 21, pp. 56-61). *Documentation from the Faculty of Education,* Vaasa, Finland: Åbo Akademi.]

Eriksson, K. (1985). Utbildning—En kulturell metabolism. I H. Andersson & L. Finnäs (red.), *Finlandssvensk utbildningsforskning. Utbildningsforskning vid Jyväskylä universitet. Kasvatustieteiden Tutkimuslaitos. Selosteita ja Tiedotteita VIII* (s. 17-32). Jyväskylä, Finland: Jyväskylä University. [Education—A cultural metabolism. In H. Andersson & L. Finnäs (Eds.), *Finland-Swedish education research. Education research at the University of Jyväskylä. Faculty of education, department of research. Declarations and announcements VIII* (pp. 17-32). Jyväskylä, Finland: Jyväskylä University.]

Eriksson, K. (1986). Vårdvetenskapens utgångspunkt. *Studier för vårdutveckling. Rapport från Nordisk forskningskonferens. Mänskliga resurser—Omvårdnad och social omsorg* (No. 11, s. 29-33). Östersund, Sweden: Mitthögskolan i Östersund. [The starting point of caring science. *Studies for the development of care. Report from the Nordic Research Conference. Human Resources—Nursing Care And Social Caring* (No. 11, pp. 29-33). Östersund, Sweden: Mitthögskolan i Östersund.]

Eriksson, K. (1987). Livskvalitet i högteknologisk vård. Ett vårdvetenskapligt perspektiv. I Svensk Medicin, Hjärta och kärl. *Rapport från Svenska läkarstämman* (s. 6). Stockholm: SPRI. [The quality of life in high technological nursing. A caring science perspective. In *A report from Svenska läkarstämman* (p. 6). Stockholm: SPRI.]

Eriksson, K. (1987). Sykepleie—En kjærlighetsgjerning. I M. V. Hermansen (red.), *Sykepleie i tiden care* (s. 25-29). Oslo, Norway: Ullevål Sykehus. [Nursing care—An act of love. In M. V. Hermansen (Ed.), *A historical overview of nursing care* (pp. 25-29). Oslo, Norway: Ullevål Sykehus.]

Eriksson, K. (1991). Caritas-tanken. XIX Norditrans kongress. Helsingfors. Sammandrag av föreläsning. *Nordiatrans, 31,* 21-22. [The caritas thought. XIX Nordiatrans congress. Helsinki. A summary of the lecture. *Nordiatrans, 31,* 21-22.]

Eriksson, K. (1997). Introduction to the closing panel "Visions for the future" (Abstract). In 19th International Association for Human Caring Conference Proceedings, *Human Caring: The Primacy of Love and Existential Suffering* (p. 58). Helsinki, Finland.

Eriksson, K. (1998). På tröskeln till en andra generation inom vårdvetenskapen. I V nationella vårdvetenskapliga konferensen, *Vårdvetenskapens och vårdandets värld—Kunskaps-och värdegrund* (s. 17-20). Vaasa, Finland: Hoifofiede Seura [On the threshold of a second generation of caring science. In V nationella vårdvetenskapliga konferensen, *The world of caring and caring science—Knowledge and basic values* (pp. 17-20). Vaasa, Finland: Hoifofiede Seura.]

Eriksson, K., Bondas-Salonen, T., Herberts, S., Lindholm, L., & Matilainen, D. (1998). Multidimensional health—Toward an ontological health model (Abstract). In 4th International Multidisciplinary Qualitative Health Research Conference, *Book of abstracts* (p. 84). Vancouver, Canada: University of Alberta.

Books and Monographs

Eriksson, K. (1974). *Sjuksköterskeyrket—Hantverk eller profession.* Sjuksköterskors samarbete i Norden. Rapport från SSN:s expertgrupp för klargörande av vårdfunktionsområdet. Helsinki, Finland: SSN. [*The nursing profession—Skill or profession.* Collaboration of nurses in the Nordic countries. Report from SSN's expert group for the clarification of nursing. Helsinki, Finland: SSN.]

Eriksson, K. (1975). *Den teoretiska utgångspunkten för vårdprocessen.* Rapport från SSN:s symposium i Helsingfors. Helsinki, Finland: SSN. [*The theoretical starting point of the nursing care process.* A report from SSN:s symposium in Helsinki. Helsinki, Finland: SSN.]

Eriksson, K. (1976). Hoitotapahtuma. *Hoito-oppi 2.* Helsinki, Finland: Sairaanhoitajien Koulutussäätiö. [The nursing care process. *Nursing science 2.* Helsinki, Finland: Sairaanhoitajien Koulutussäätiö.]

Eriksson, K. (1976). *Hälsa. En teoretisk och begreppsanalytisk studie om hälsan och dess natur som mål för hälsovårdsedukation.* Licentiatavhandling, Helsinki, Finland: Institutionen för pedagogik, Helsingfors universitet. [*Health. A conceptual analysis and theoretical study of health and its nature as a goal for health care education.* Unpublished licentiate thesis, Helsinki, Finland: Department of Education University of Helsinki.]

Eriksson, K. (1979). *Vårdprocessen.* Stockholm: Almqvist & Wiksell. [*The nursing care process.* Stockholm: Almqvist & Wiksell.]

Eriksson, K. (1981). *Vårdprocessen—En utgångspunkt för läroplanstänkande inom vårdutbildningen. Utvecklande av en vårdprocessmodell samt ett läroplanstänkande utgående från vårdprocessen* (Nr. 94). Helsinki, Finland: Helsingfors universitet, Pedagogiska Institutionen. [*The nursing care process—An approach to curriculum construction within nursing education. The development of a model for the nursing care process and an approach for curriculum development based on the process of nursing care* (No. 94). Helsinki, Finland: Department of Education University of Helsinki.]

Eriksson, K. (1982). *Vårdprocessen.* (2:a uppl.). Stockholm: Almqvist & Wiksell. [*The nursing care process* (2nd ed.). Stockholm: Almqvist & Wiksell.]

Eriksson, K. (1983). *Introduktion till vårdvetenskap.* Stockholm: Almqvist & Wiksell. [*An introduction to caring science.* Stockholm: Almqvist & Wiksell.]

Eriksson, K. (1984). *Hälsans idé.* Stockholm: Almqvist & Wiksell. [*The idea of health.* Stockholm: Almqvist & Wiksell.]

Eriksson, K. (1985). *Hoitopedagogiikka I.* Helsinki, Finland: Sairaanhoitajien Koulutussäätiö. [*Caring pedagogy I.* Helsinki, Finland: Sairaanhoitajien Koulutussäätiö.]

Eriksson, K. (1985). *Hoitotapahtuma. Hoito-oppi 2* (Rev. uppl.). Helsinki, Finland: Sairaanhoitajien Koulutussäätiö. [*The nursing care process. nursing science 2* (Rev. ed.). Helsinki, Finland: Sairaanhoitajien Koulutussäätiö.]

Eriksson, K. (1985). *Johdatus hoitotieteeseen.* Helsinki, Finland: Sairaanhoitajien Koulutussäätiö. [*An introduction to caring science.* Helsinki, Finland: Sairaanhoitajien Koulutussäätiö.]

Eriksson, K. (1985). *Vårddidaktik.* Stockholm: Almqvist & Wiksell. [*Caring didactics.* Stockholm: Almqvist & Wiksell.]

Eriksson, K. (1985). *Vårdprocessen* (3: e uppl.). Stockholm: Almqvist & Wiksell. [*The nursing care process* (3rd ed.). Stockholm: Almqvist & Wiksell.]

Eriksson, K. (1986). *Hoito-opin didaktiikka.* Helsinki, Finland: Sairaanhoitajien Koulutussäätiö. [*The didactics of caring science.* Helsinki, Finland: Sairaanhoitajien Koulutussäätiö.]

Eriksson, K. (1986). *Introduktion till vårdvetenskap* (2: a uppl.). Stockholm: Almqvist & Wiksell. [*An introduction to caring science* (2nd ed.). Stockholm: Almqvist & Wiksell.]

Eriksson, K. (1987). *Hoitamisen idea.* Forssa, Sweden: Sairaanhoitajien Koulutussäätiö. [*The idea of health.* Forssa, Sweden: Sairaanhoitajien Koulutussäätiö.]

Eriksson, K. (1987). *Pausen. En beskrivning av vårdvetenskapens kunskapsobjekt.* Stockholm: Almqvist & Wiksell. [*The pause. A description of the knowledge object of caring science.* Stockholm: Almqvist & Wiksell.]

Eriksson, K. (1987). *Vårdandets idé.* Stockholm: Almqvist & Wiksell. [*The idea of caring.* Stockholm: Almqvist & Wiksell.]

Eriksson, K. (1988). *Hoito tieteenä.* Forssa, Sweden: Sairaanhoitajien Koulutussäätiö. [*Caring as a science.* Forssa, Sweden: Sairaanhoitajien Koulutussäätiö.]

Eriksson, K. (1988). *Vårdprocessen* (4: e uppl.). Stockholm: Almqvist & Wiksell. [*The nursing care process* (4th ed.). Stockholm: Almqvist & Wiksell.]

Eriksson, K. (1989). *Caritas-idea.* Helsinki, Finland: Sairaanhoitajien Koulutussäätiö. [*The idea of caritas.* Helsinki, Finland: Sairaanhoitajien Koulutussäätiö.]

Eriksson, K. (1989). *Hälsans idé health* (2:a uppl.). Stockholm: Almqvist & Wiksell. [*The idea of health* (2nd ed.). Stockholm: Almqvist & Wiksell.]

Eriksson, K. (1989). *Terveyden idea.* Helsinki, Finland: Sairaanhoitajien Koulutussäätiö. [*The idea of health.* Helsinki, Finland: Sairaanhoitajien Koulutussäätiö.]

Eriksson, K. (1991). *Broar. Introduktion i vårdvetenskaplig metod* (försöks uppl). Vaasa, Finland: Institutionen för vårdvetenskap, Åbo Akademi. [*Bridges. Introduction to the methods of caring science* (test ed.). Vaasa, Finland: Department of Caring Science, Åbo Akademi.]

Eriksson, K. (1992). *Broar. Introduktion i vårdvetenskaplig metod.* Vaasa, Finland: Institutionen för vårdvetenskap, Åbo Akademi. [*Bridges. Introduction to the methods of caring science.* Vaasa, Finland: Department of Caring Science, Åbo Akademi.]

Eriksson, K. (1994). *Det lidande människan.* Stockholm: Liber Förlag. [*The suffering human being.* Stockholm: Liber Förlag.] [English translation forthcoming from Nordic Studies Press, Chicago.]

Eriksson, K. (1995). *Det lidende menneske* (Danish translation). Copenhagen: Munksgaard. [*The suffering human being* (Danish translation). Copenhagen: Munksgaard.]

Eriksson, K. (1995). *Den lidende menneske* (Norwegian translation). Oslo: TANO. [*The suffering human being* (Norwegian translation). Oslo: TANO.]

Eriksson, K. (1996). *Omsorgens idé* (Danish translation). Copenhagen: Munksgaard. [*The idea of caring* (Danish translation). Copenhagen: Munksgaard.]

Eriksson, K. (1997). *Vårdandets idé* (Kassettband). Talboks- och punktskriftsbiblioteket. Stockholm: Almqvist & Wiksell. [*The idea of caring* (Audiotape). Talboks- och punktskriftsbiblioteket. Stockholm: Almqvist & Wiksell.]

Eriksson, K. (2001). *Gesundheit. Ein Schlüsselbegriff der Pflegetheorie.* (German translation). Bern, Germany: Verlag Hans Huber. [*The idea of health* (German translation). Bern, Germany: Verlag Hans Huber.]

Eriksson, K., & Barbosa da Silva, A. (Eds.). (1994). *Usko ja terveys—johdatus hoitoteologiaan.* (Finnish translation). Helsinki, Finland: Sairaanhoitajien Koulutussäätiö. [*Caring theology* (Finnish translation). Helsinki, Finland: Sairaanhoitajien Koulutussäätiö.]

Eriksson, K., Byfält, H., Leijonqvist, G-B., Nyberg, K., & Uuspää, B. (1986). *Hoitotaito.* Helsinki, Finland: Sairaanhoitajien Koulutussäätiö. [*The art of caring.* Helsinki, Finland: Sairaanhoitajien Koulutussäätiö.]

Eriksson, K., Byfält, H., Leijonqvist, G-B., Nyberg, K., & Uuspää, B. (1986). *Vårdteknologi.* Stockholm: Almqvist & Wiksell. [*Caring technology.* Stockholm: Almqvist & Wiksell.]

University and Department Publications

Eriksson, K. (1988). Fälthandledning—En filosofisk betraktelse. I A-L. Østern (red.), *Kvalitet i praktiken* (Nr. 35, s. 122-124). Vaasa, Finland: Pedagogiska Fakulteten, Åbo Akademi. [Field counseling—A philosophical contemplation. In A-L. Østern (Ed.), *Quality in practice* (No. 35, pp. 122-124). Vaasa, Finland: Faculty of Education, Åbo Akademi.]

Eriksson, K. (1988). *Vårdvetenskap som disciplin, forsknings-och tillämpningsområde. Vårdforskningar 1/1988.* Vaasa, Finland: Institutionen för vårdvetenskap, Åbo Akademi. [*Caring science as a discipline, field of research and application.* Vaasa, Finland: Department of Caring Science, Åbo Akademi.]

Eriksson, K. (1990). *Pro Caritate. En lägesbestämning av caritativ vård. Vårdforskningar 2/1990.* Vaasa, Finland: Institutionen för vårdvetenskap, Åbo Akademi. [*Pro Caritate. Caritative caring—A positional analysis.* Vaasa, Finland: Department of Caring Science, Åbo Akademi.]

Eriksson, K. (1991). Att lindra lidande. I K. Eriksson & A. Barbosa da Silva (red.), *Vårdteologi. Vårdforskningar 3/1991* (s. 204-221). Vaasa, Finland: Institutionen för vårdvetenskap, Åbo Akademi. [To alleviate suffering. In K. Eriksson & A. Barbosa da Silva (Eds.), *Caring theology* (pp. 204-221). Vaasa, Finland: Department of Caring Science, Åbo Akademi.]

Eriksson, K. (1991). *Pro Caritate. En lägesbestämning av caritativ vård. Vårdforskningar 2/1990* (2: a uppl.). Vaasa, Finland: Institutionen för vårdvetenskap, Åbo Akademi. [*Pro Caritate. Caritative caring—A positional analysis* (2nd ed.). Vaasa, Finland: Department of Caring Science, Åbo Akademi.]

Eriksson, K. (1991). Vårdteologins framväxt. I K. Eriksson & A. Barbosa da Silva (red.), *Vårdteologi. Vårdforskningar 3/1991* (s. 1-25). [The growth of caring theology. In K. Eriksson & A. Barbosa da Silva (Eds.), *Caring theology* (pp. 1-25). Vaasa, Finland: Department of Caring Science, Åbo Akademi.]

Eriksson, K. (1993). Lidandets idé. I K. Eriksson (red.), *Möten med lidanden. Vårdforskningar 4/1993* (s. 1-27). Vaasa, Finland: Institutionen för vårdvetenskap, Åbo Akademi. [The idea of suffering. In K. Eriksson (Ed.), *Encounters with suffering* (pp. 1-27). Vaasa, Finland: Department of Caring Science, Åbo Akademi.]

Eriksson, K. (1993). *Pro Caritate. En lägesbestämning av caritativ vård. Vårdforskningar 2/1990* (Red. 3). Vaasa, Finland: Institutionen för vårdvetenskap, Åbo Akademi. [*Pro Caritate. Caritative caring—A positional analysis* (3rd ed.). Vaasa, Finland: Department of Caring Science, Åbo Akademi.]

Eriksson, K. (red.). (1993). *Möten med lidanden. Vårdforskning 4/1993.* Vaasa, Finland: Institutionen för vårdvetenskap, Åbo Akademi. [*Encounters with suffering.* Vaasa, Finland: Department of Caring Science, Åbo Akademi.]

Eriksson, K. (red.). (1995). *Den mångdimensionella hälsan—Verklighet och visioner. Slutrapport.* Vaasa, Finland: Vasa sjukvårdsdistrikt kf. och Institutionen för vårdvetenskap, Åbo Akademi. [*Multidimensional health—Visions and reality. Final report.* Vaasa, Finland: Vasa sjukvårdsdistrikt kf. och Institutionen för vårdvetenskap, Åbo Akademi.]

Eriksson, K. (red.). (1995). *Mot en caritativ vårdetik. Vårdforskning 5/1995.* Vaasa, Finland: Institutionen för vårdvetenskap, Åbo Akademi. [*Toward a caritative caring ethic. Caring research 5/1995.* Vaasa, Finland: Department of Caring Science, Åbo Akademi.]

Eriksson, K. (1995). Mot en caritativ vårdetik. I K. Eriksson (red.), *Mot en caritativ vårdetik. Vårdforskning 5/1995* (s. 9-40). Vaasa, Finland: Institutionen för vårdvetenskap, Åbo Akademi. [Toward a caritative caring ethic. In K. Eriksson (Ed.), *Toward a caritative caring ethic. Caring research 5/1995.* (pp. 9-40). Vaasa, Finland: Department of Caring Science, Åbo Akademi.]

Eriksson, K. (1995). Vad är vårdetik? I K. Eriksson (red.), *Mot en caritativ vårdetik. Vårdforskning 5/1995* (s. 1-8). Vaasa, Finland: Institutionen för vårdvetenskap, Åbo Akademi. [What is caring ethic? In K. Eriksson (Ed.), *Toward a caritative caring ethic* (pp. 1-8). Vaasa, Finland: Department of Caring Science, Åbo Akademi.]. *Caring research 5/1995.*

Eriksson, K. (1997). Att insjukna i demens—Ett tungt lidande för patient och anhöriga. I B. Beck-Friis & G. Grahn (red.), *Leva med demenshandikapp.* Lund, Sweden: Lunds universitet: Stiftelsen Silviahemmet.

[Becoming ill with dementia—A burdensome suffering for the patient and his/her family. In B. Beck-Friis & G. Grahn (Eds.), *Living with the handicap of dementia* (Action in favor of people suffering from neurodegenerative diseases). Lund, Sweden: Lunds universitet, Stiftelsen Silviahemmet.]

Eriksson, K. (red.). (1998). *Jubileumsskrift 1987-1997.* Vaasa, Finland: Institutionen för vårdvetenskap, Åbo Akademi. [*Jubilee-script 1987-1997.* Vaasa, Finland: Department of Caring Science, Åbo Akademi.]

Eriksson, K. (1998). Vårdvetenskapens framväxt som akademisk disciplin—Ett finlandssvenskt perspektiv. I K. Eriksson (red.), *Jubileumsskrift 1987-1997* (s. 1-7). Vaasa, Finland: Institutionen för vårdvetenskap, Åbo Akademi. [The growth of caring science as an academic discipline—A Finland-Swedish perspective. In K. Eriksson (Ed.), *Jubilee-script 1987-1997* (pp. 1-7). Vaasa, Finland: Department of Caring Science, Åbo Akademi.]

Eriksson, K. (2001). *Vårdvetenskap som akademisk disciplin. Vårdforskning 7/2001.* Vaasa, Finland: Institutionen för vårdvetenskap, Åbo Akademi. [*Caring science as an academic discipline. Caring research 7/2001.* Vaasa, Finland: Department of Caring Science, Åbo Akademi.]

Eriksson, K. (2002). *Den trojanske hest. Evidensbasering og sygepleje.* (Danish translation). Copenhagen: Gads Förlag. [*The Trojan horse. Evidence-based nursing and caring through a caring science perspective* (Danish translation). Copenhagen: Gads Förlag.]

Eriksson, K. (2002). Idéhistoria som deldisciplin inom vårdvetenskapen. I K. Eriksson & D. Matilainen (red.), *Vårdandets och vårdvetenskapens idéhistoria. Strövtåg i spårandet av "caritas originalis." Vårdforskning 8/2002* (s. 1-14). Vaasa, Finland: Institutionen för vårdvetenskap, Åbo Akademi. [The history of ideas as a sub-discipline within caring science. In K. Eriksson & D. Matilainen (Eds.), *The history of ideas of caring and caring science. Wanderings in search of "caritas originalis." Caring research 8/2002* (pp. 1-14). Vaasa, Finland: Department of Caring Science, Åbo Akademi.]

Eriksson, K. (2002). Vårdandets idéhistoria. I K. Eriksson & D. Matilainen (red.), *Vårdandets och vårdvetenskapens idéhistoria. Strövtåg i spårandet av "caritas originalis." Vårdforskning 8/2002* (s. 15-34). Vaasa, Finland: Institutionen för vårdvetenskap, Åbo Akademi. [The history of ideas of caring. In K. Eriksson & D. Matilainen (Eds.), *The history of ideas of caring and caring science. Wanderings in search of "caritas originalis." Caring research 8/2002* (pp. 15-34). Vaasa, Finland: Department of Caring Science, Åbo Akademi.]

Eriksson, K. (2003). Ethos. I K. Eriksson & U. Å. Lindström (red.), *Gryning II. Klinisk vårdvetenskap* (s. 21-34). Vaasa, Finland: Institutionen för vårdvetenskap, Åbo Akademi. [Ethos. In K. Eriksson & U. Å. Lindström (Eds.), *Dawn II. Clinical caring science* (pp. 21-34).

Vaasa, Finland: Department of Caring Science, Åbo Akademi.]

Eriksson, K. (2003). Klinisk vårdvetenskap. I K. Eriksson & U. Å. Lindström (red.), *Gryning II. Klinisk vårdvetenskap* (s. 3-20). Vaasa, Finland: Institutionen för vårdvetenskap, Åbo Akademi. [Clinical caring science. In K. Eriksson & U. Å. Lindström (Eds.), *Dawn II. Clinical caring science* (pp. 3-20). Vaasa, Finland: Department of Caring Science, Åbo Akademi.

Eriksson, K., & Barbosa da Silva, A. (red.). (1991). *Vårdteologi. Vårdforskning 3/1991.* Vaasa, Finland: Institutionen för vårdvetenskap, Åbo Akademi. [*Caring theology. Caring research 3/1991.* Vaasa, Finland: Department of Caring Science, Åbo Akademi.

Eriksson, K., & Barbosa da Silva, A. (1991). Vårdteologi som vårdvetenskapens deldisciplin. I K. Eriksson & A. Barbosa da Silva (red.), *Vårdteologi. Vårdforskningar 3/1991* (s. 26-64). Vaasa, Finland: Institutionen för vårdvetenskap, Åbo Akademi. [Caring theology as a sub-discipline of caring science. In K. Eriksson & A. Barbosa da Silva (Eds.), *Caring theology. Caring research 3/1991* (pp. 26-64). Vaasa, Finland: Department of Caring Science, Åbo Akademi.]

Eriksson, K., Bondas-Salonen, T., Fagerström, L., Herberts, S., & Lindholm, L. (red.). (1990). *Den mångdimensionella hälsan. En pilotstudie över uppfattningar bland patienter, skolungdomar och lärare* (Projektrapport 1). Vaasa, Finland: Vasa sjukvårdsdistrikt kf. och Institutionen för vårdvetenskap, Åbo Akademi. [*Multidimensional health. A pilot study of understanding health among patients, students and teachers* (Project Rep. 1). Vaasa, Finland: Vasa sjukvårdsdistrikt kf. och Institutionen för vårdvetenskap, Åbo Akademi.]

Eriksson, K., Bondas-Salonen, T., Fagerström, L., Herberts, S., & Lindholm, L. (red.) (1990). *Moniulotteinen terveys. Esitutkimus potilaiden, koulunuorison ja opettajien keskuudessa vallitsevista käsityksistä* (Projektrapport 1). Vaasa, Finland: Vaasan sairaanhoitopiirin ja Institutionen för vårdvetenskap (Hoitotieteen laitos), Åbo Akademi. [*Multidimensional health. A pilot study of understanding health among patients, students and teachers* (Project Rep. 1). Vaasa, Finland: Vaasan sairaanhoitopiirin ja Institutionen för vårdvetenskap (Hoitotieteen laitos), Åbo Akademi.]

Eriksson, K., & Herberts, S. (1991). Tron i hälsans tjänst. I K. Eriksson & A. Barbosa da Silva (red.), *Vårdteologi. Vårdforskningar 3/1991* (s. 222-258). Vaasa Finland: Institutionen för vårdvetenskap, Åbo Akademi. [Faith in the service of health. In K. Eriksson & A. Barbosa da Silva (Eds.), *Caring theology. Caring research 3/1991* (pp. 222-258). Vaasa Finland: Department of Caring Science, Åbo Akademi.

Eriksson, K., & Herberts, S. (1992). *Den mångdimensionella hälsan. En studie av hälsobilden hos sjukvårdsledare och sjukvårdspersonal* (Projektrapport 2). Vaasa,

Finland: Vasa sjukvårdsdistrikt kf och Institutionen för vårdvetenskap, Åbo Akademi. [*Multidimensional health. A study of the views of health among health care leaders and health care personnel* (Project Rep. 2). Vaasa, Finland: Vasa sjukvårdsdistrikt kf och Institutionen för vårdvetenskap, Åbo Akademi.]

Eriksson, K., & Herberts, S. (1992). *Moniulotteinen terveys. Tutkimus sairaanhoitajien ja hoitohenkilökunnan terveyskuvasta* (Projektrapport 2). Vaasa, Finland: Vaasan sairaanhoitopiirin ja Institutionen för vårdvetenskap (Hoitotieteen laitos), Åbo Akademi. [*The multidimensional health. A study of the views of health among health care leaders and health care personnel* (Project Rep. 2). Vaasa, Finland: Vaasan sairaanhoitopiirin ja Institutionen för vårdvetenskap (Hoitotieteen laitos), Åbo Akademi.]

Eriksson, K., & Herberts, S. (1993). Lidande—En begreppsanalytisk studie. I K. Eriksson (red.), *Möten med lidanden. Vårdforskningar 4/1993* (s. 29-54). Vaasa, Finland: Institutionen för vårdvetenskap, Åbo Akademi. [A study of suffering—A concept analysis. In K. Eriksson (Ed.), *Encounters with suffering. Caring research 4/1993* (pp. 29-54). Vaasa, Finland: Department of Caring Science, Åbo Akademi.]

Eriksson, K., Herberts, S., & Lindholm, L. (1993). Bilder av lidande—Lidande i belysning av aktuell vårdvetenskaplig forskning. I K. Eriksson (red.), *Möten med lidanden. Vårdforskningar 4/1993 suffering* (s. 55-78). Vaasa, Finland: Institutionen för vårdvetenskap, Åbo Akademi. [Views of suffering—Suffering in the light of current caring science research. In K. Eriksson (Ed.), *Encounters with suffering. Caring research 4/1993* (pp. 55-78). Vaasa, Finland: Department of Caring Science, Åbo Akademi.]

Eriksson, K., & Koort, P. (1973). *Sjukvårdspedagogik* (Kompendium). Helsinki, Finland: Helsingfors svenska sjukvårdsinstitut. [*The pedagogy of nursing care* (Compendium). Helsinki, Finland: Helsingfors svenska sjukvårdsinstitut.]

Eriksson, K., & Lindholm, L. (1993). Lidande och kärlek ur ett psykiatriskt vårdperspektiv—En casestudie av mötet mellan mänskligt lidande och kärlek. I K. Eriksson (red.), *Möten med lidanden. Vårdforskningar 4/1993 suffering* (s. 79-137). Vaasa, Finland: Institutionen för vårdvetenskap, Åbo Akademi. [Love and suffering though a psychiatric caring perspective—A case study of the encounters with human love and suffering. In K. Eriksson (Ed.), *Encounters with suffering. Caring research 4/1993* (pp. 79-137). Vaasa, Finland: Department of Caring Science, Åbo Akademi.]

Eriksson, K., & Lindström, U. Å. (2000). *Gryning. En vårdvetenskaplig antologi.* Vaasa, Finland: Institutionen för vårdvetenskap, Åbo Akademi. [*Dawn. An anthology of caring science.* Vaasa, Finland: Department of Caring Science, Åbo Akademi.]

Eriksson, K., & Lindström, U. Å. (2000). Siktet, Sökandet, slutandet. I K. Eriksson & U. Å. Lindstöm, *Gryning. En vårdvetenskaplig antologi science* (s. 5-18). Vaasa, Finland: Institutionen för vårdvetenskap, Åbo Akademi. [Envisioning, seeking and ending. In K. Eriksson & U. Å. Lindström, *Dawn. An anthology of caring science* (pp. 5-18). Vaasa, Finland: Department of Caring Science, Åbo Akademi.]

Eriksson, K., & Lindström, U. Å. (red.). (2003). *Gryning II. Klinisk vårdvetenskap.* Vaasa, Finland: Institutionen för vårdvetenskap, Åbo Akademi. [*Dawn II. Clinical caring science.* Vaasa, Finland: Department of Caring Science, Åbo Akademi.]

Eriksson, K., & Matilainen, D. (red.). (2002). *Vårdandets och vårdvetenskapens idéhistoria. Strövtåg i spårandet av "caritas originalis". Vårdforskning 8/2002.* Vaasa, Finland: Institutionen för vårdvetenskap, Åbo Akademi. [Eriksson, K., & Matilainen, D. (eds.). *The history of ideas of caring and caring science. Wanderings in search of "caritas originalis." Caring research 8/2002.* Vaasa, Finland: Department of Caring Science, Åbo Akademi.]

Eriksson, K., & Nordman, T. (2004). *Den trojanska hästen II—Utvecklande av evidensbaserade vårdande kulturer.* Vaasa, Finland: Institutionen för vårdvetenskap, Åbo Akademi. [*The Trojan horse II—Development of evidence-based caring cultures.* Vaasa, Finland: Department of Caring Science, Åbo Akademi.]

Eriksson K., Nordman T., & Myllymäki I. (1999). *Den trojanska hästen. Evidensbaserat vårdande och vårdarbete ur ett vårdvetenskapligt perspektiv cultures* (Rap. 1). Vaasa, Finland: Institutionen för vårdvetenskap, Åbo Akademi; Helsingfors universitetscentralsjukhus & Vasa sjukvårdsdistrikt. [*The Trojan horse II—Development of evidence-based caring cultures* (Rep. 1). Vaasa, Finland: Institutionen för vårdvetenskap, Åbo Akademi; Helsingfors universitetscentralsjukhus & Vasa sjukvårdsdistrikt.

Eriksson, K., Nordman, T., & Myllymäki, I. (2000). *Troijan hevonen. Evidenssiin perustuva hoitaminen ja hoitotyö hoitotieteellisestä näkökulmasta.* Vaasa, Finland: Helsingin yliopistollinen keskussairaala: Institutionen för vårdvetenskap, Åbo Akademi & Vaasan sairaanhoitopiirin kuntayhtymä. [*The Trojan horse—Evidence-based caring and nursing practice from a caring science perspective.* Vaasa, Finland: Helsingin yliopistollinen keskussairaala: Institutionen för vårdvetenskap, Åbo Akademi & Vaasan sairaanhoitopiirin kuntayhtymä.]

Herberts, S., & Eriksson, K. (1995). Vårdarnas etiska profil. I K. Eriksson (red.), *Mot en caritativ vårdetik. Vårdforskning 5/1995* (s. 41-62). Vaasa, Finland: Institutionen för vårdvetenskap, Åbo Akademi. [The ethical profile of the carers. In K. Eriksson (Ed.), *Toward a caritative caring ethic. Caring research 5/1995* (pp. 41-

62). Vaasa, Finland: Department of Caring Science, Åbo Akademi.]

Secondary Sources
Doctoral Dissertations

Andersson, M. (1994). *Integritet som begrepp och princip. En studie av ett vårdetiskt ideal i utveckling.* Doktorsavhandling, Turku, Finland, Åbo Akademis Förlag. [*Integrity as a concept and as a principle in health care ethics.* Doctoral dissertation, Turku, Finland, Åbo Akademi University Press.]

Arman, M. (2003). *Lidande och existens i patientens värld. Kvinnors upplevelser av att leva med bröstcancer.* Doktorsavhandling, Turku, Finland, Åbo Akademis Förlag. [*Suffering and existence in the patient's world. Women's experiences of living with breast cancer.* Doctoral dissertation, Turku, Finland, Åbo Akademi University Press.]

Bondas, T. (2000). *Att vara med barn: en vårdvetenskaplig studie av kvinnors upplevelser under perinatal tid.* Doktorsavhandling, Turku, Finland, Åbo Akademis Förlag. [*To be with child: a study of women's lived experiences during the perinatal period from a caring science perspective.* Doctoral dissertation, Turku, Finland, Åbo Akademi University Press.]

Edlund, M. (2002). *Människans värdighet-ett grundbegrepp inom vårdvetenskapen.* Doktorsavhandling, Turku, Finland, Åbo Akademis Förlag. [*Human dignity—A basic caring science concept.* Doctoral dissertation, Turku, Finland, Åbo Akadem University Press.]

Ekebergh, M. (2001). *Tillägnandet av vårdvetenskaplig kunskap. Reflexionens betydelse för lärandet.* Doktorsavhandling, Turku, Finland, Åbo Akademis Förlag. [*Acquiring caring science knowledge—The importance of reflection for learning.* Doctoral dissertation, Turku, Finland, Åbo Akademi University Press.]

Fagerström, L. (1999). *The patient's caring needs. To understand and to measure the unmeasurable.* Doctoral dissertation, Turku, Finland, Åbo Akademi University Press.

Fredriksson, L. (2003). *Det vårdande samtalet.* Doktorsavhandling, Turku, Finland, Åbo Akademis Förlag. [*The caring conversation.* Doctoral dissertation, Turku, Finland, Åbo Akademi University Press.

Kasén, A. (2002). *Den vårdande relationen.* Doktorsavhandling, Turku, Finland, Åbo Akademis Förlag. [*The caring relationship.* Doctoral dissertation, Turku, Finland, Åbo Akademi University Press.

Lindholm, L. (1998). *Den unga människans hälsa och lidande.* Doktorsavhandling, Vaasa, Finland: Institutionen för vårdvetenskap, Åbo Akademi. [*The young person's health and suffering.* Doctoral dissertation, Vaasa, Finland: Department of Caring Science, Åbo Akademi University.]

Lindström, U. Å. (1992). *De psykiatriska specialsjukskötarnas yrkesparadigm.* Doktorsavhandling, Turku, Finland, Åbo Akademis Förlag. [*The professional paradigm of the qualified psychiatric nurses.* Doctoral dissertation, Turku, Finland, Åbo Akademi University Press.]

Lindwall, L. (2004). *Kroppen som bärare av hälsa och lidande.* Doktorsavhandling, Turku, Finland, Åbo Akademis Förlag. [*The body as a carrier of health and suffering.* Doctoral dissertation, Turku, Finland, Åbo Akademi University Press.]

Matilainen, D. (1997). *Idémönster i Karin Neuman-Rahns livsgärning och författarskap—En idéhistorisk-biografisk studie i psykiatrisk vård i Finland under 1900-talets första hälft.* Doktorsavhandling, Turku, Finland, Åbo Akademis Förlag. [*Patterns of ideas in Karin Neuman-Rahns' life-work and writings—A study of psychiatric care in Finland in the former part of the twentieth century, based on biography and the history of ideas.* Doctoral dissertation, Turku, Finland, Åbo Akademi University Press.]

Nilsson, B. (2004). *Savnets tone i ensomhetens melodi. Ensomhet hos aleneboende personer med alvorlig psykisk lidelse.* Doktorsavhandling, Turku, Finland, Åbo Akademis Förlag. [*The tune of want in the loneliness melody.* Doctoral dissertation, Turku, Finland, Åbo Akademi University Press.]

Nåden, D. (1998). *Når sykepleie er kunstutøvelse. En undersøkelse av noen nødvendige forutsetninger for sykepleie som kunst.* Doktorsavhandling, Vaasa, Finland: Institutionen för vårdvetenskap, Åbo Akademi. [*When caring is an exercise of art. An examination of some necessary preconditions of nursing as an art.* Doctoral dissertation, Vaasa, Finland: Department of Caring Science, Åbo Akademi University.]

Rehnsfeldt, A. (1999). *Mötet med patienten i ett livsavgörande skede.* Doktorsavhandling, Turku, Finland, Åbo Akademi. [*The encounter with the patient in a life-changing process.* Doctoral dissertation, Turku, Finland, Åbo Akademi University Press.]

Rundqvist, E. (2004). *Makt som fullmakt. Ett vårdvetenskapligt perspektiv.* Doktorsavhandling, Turku, Finland, Åbo Akademis Förlag. [*Power as authority. A caring science perspective.* Doctoral dissertation, Turku, Finland, Åbo Akademi University Press.]

Råholm, M-B. (2003). *I kampens och modets dialektik.* Doktorsavhandling, Turku, Finland, Åbo Akademis Förlag. [*In the dialectic of struggle and courage.* Doctoral dissertation, Turku, Finland, Åbo Akademi University Press.]

Sivonen, K. (2000). *Vården och det andliga. En bestämning av begreppet 'andlig' ur ett vårdvetenskapligt perspektiv.* Doktorsavhandling, Turku, Finland, Åbo Akademis Förlag. [*Features of spirituality in caring.* Doctoral dissertation, Turku, Finland, Åbo Akademi University Press.]

Söderlund, M. (2004). *Som drabbad av en orkan. Anhörigas tillvaro när en närstående drabbas av demens.* Doktorsavhandling, Turku, Finland, Åbo Akademis Förlag. [*As if struck by a hurricane: The situation of the relatives of someone suffering from dementia.* Doctoral dissertation, Turku, Finland, Åbo Akademi University Press.]

von Post, I. (1999). *Professionell naturlig vård ur anestes- och operationssjuksköterskors perspektiv.* Doktorsavhandling, Turku, Finland, Åbo Akademis Förlag. [*Professional natural care from the perspective of nurse anesthetists and operating room nurses.* Doctoral dissertation, Turku, Finland, Åbo Akademi University Press.]

Wiklund, L. (2000). *Lidandet som kamp och drama.* Doktorsavhandling, Turku, Finland, Åbo Akademis Förlag. [*Suffering as struggle and as drama.* Doctoral dissertation, Turku, Finland, Åbo Akademis Förlag.]

Wärnå, C. (2002). *Dygd och hälsa.* Doktorsavhandling, Turku, Finland, Åbo Akademis Förlag. [*Virtue and health.* Doctoral dissertation, Turku, Finland, Åbo Akademi University Press.]

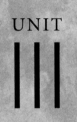

Nursing Models

- *Nursing conceptual models are concepts, definitions, and propositions that specify their interrelationships to form an organized perspective for viewing phenomena specific to the discipline.*

- *Conceptual models provide different ways of thinking about nursing and address the broad metaparadigm concepts that are central to its meaning.*

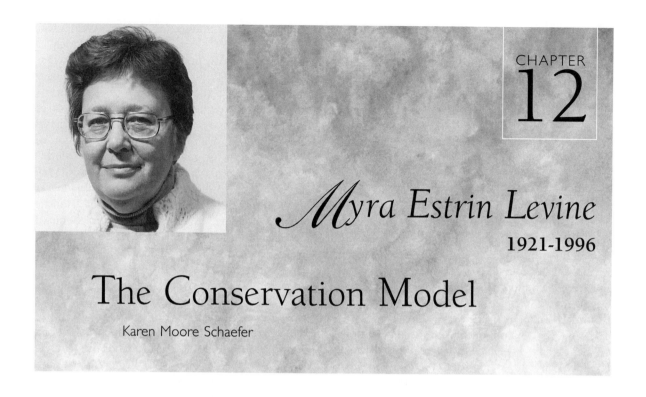

Myra Estrin Levine
1921-1996

The Conservation Model

Karen Moore Schaefer

CREDENTIALS AND BACKGROUND OF THE THEORIST*

Myra Estrin Levine obtained a diploma from Cook County School of Nursing in 1944, an S.B. from the University of Chicago in 1949, an M.S.N. from Wayne State University in 1962, and she took postgraduate courses at the University of Chicago. Hutchins' curriculum was being taught then to undergraduate students at the University of Chicago. All students took a year-long survey in the biological, physical, and social sciences and the humanities. The students read and analyzed primary work under the guidance of distinguished professors. Beland (1971) became Levine's mentor

Previous authors: Karen Moore Schaefer, Gloria S. Artigue, Karen J. Foil, Tamara Johnson, Ann Marriner Tomey, Mary Carolyn Poat, LaDema Poppa, Roberta Woeste, and Susan T. Zoretich.

*The information in this section is informed by Levine's autobiographical chapter (1988a), her curriculum vitae, and the program from the Mid-Year Convocation, Loyola University, Chicago (1992).

during her graduate studies at Wayne State and directed her attention to many of the authors who greatly influenced Levine's thinking (1988a).

Levine enjoyed a varied career. She was a private duty nurse (1944), a civilian nurse in the U.S. Army (1945), a preclinical instructor in the physical sciences at Cook County (1947 to 1950), the director of nursing at Drexel Home in Chicago (1950 to 1951), and a surgical supervisor at both the University of Chicago Clinics (1951 to 1952) and Henry Ford Hospital in Detroit (1956 to 1962). Levine worked her way up the academic ranks at Bryan Memorial Hospital in Lincoln, Nebraska (1951), Cook County School of Nursing (1963 to 1967), Loyola University (1967 to 1973), Rush University (1974 to 1977), and the University of Illinois (1962 to 1963, 1977 to 1987). She chaired the Department of Clinical Nursing at Cook County School of Nursing (1963 to 1967) and coordinated the graduate nursing program in oncology at Rush University (1974 to 1977). Levine was the director of the Department of Continuing Education at Evanston

Hospital (March to June 1974) and a consultant to the department (July 1974 to 1976). She was an adjunct associate professor of Humanistic Studies at the University of Illinois (1981 to 1987). In 1987, she became a Professor Emerita, Medical Surgical Nursing, at the University of Illinois at Chicago. In 1974, Levine went to Tel-Aviv University, Israel, as a visiting associate professor and returned as a visiting professor in 1982. She was also a visiting professor at Recanati School of Nursing, Ben Gurion University of the Negev, at Beer Sheva, Israel (March to April, 1982).

Levine received numerous honors, including charter fellow of the American Academy of Nursing (1973), honorary member of the American Mental Health Aid to Israel (1976), and honorary recognition from the Illinois Nurses Association (1977). She was the first recipient of the Elizabeth Russell Belford Award for excellence in teaching from Sigma Theta Tau (1977). Both the first and second editions of her book, *Introduction to Clinical Nursing* (Levine, 1969a; 1973), received *American Journal of Nursing* Book of the Year awards and her book, *Renewal for Nursing,* was translated into Hebrew (Levine, 1971a). Levine was listed in *Who's Who in American Women* (1977 to 1988) and in *Who's Who in American Nursing* (1987). She was elected fellow of the Institute of Medicine of Chicago (1987 to 1991). The Alpha Lambda Chapter of Sigma Theta Tau recognized Levine for her outstanding contributions to nursing in 1990. In January 1992, she was awarded an honorary doctorate of humane letters from Loyola University, Chicago (Mid-Year Convocation, Loyola University, 1992). Levine was an active leader in the American Nurses Association and the Illinois Nurses Association. After her retirement in 1987, she remained active in theory development and encouraged questions and research about her theory (Levine, 1996).

A dynamic speaker, Levine was a frequent presenter of programs, workshops, seminars, and panels and a prolific writer regarding nursing and education. She also served as a consultant to hospitals and schools of nursing. Although she never intended to develop theory, she provided an organizational structure for teaching medical-surgical

nursing and a stimulus for theory development (Stafford, 1996). "The Four Conservation Principles of Nursing" was the first statement of the conservation principles (Levine, 1967a). Other preliminary work included "Adaptation and Assessment: A Rationale for Nursing Intervention," "For Lack of Love Alone," and "The Pursuit of Wholeness" (Levine, 1966b, 1967b, 1969b). The first edition of her book using the conservation principles, *Introduction to Clinical Nursing,* was published in 1969 (Levine, 1969a). She addressed the consequences of the four conservation principles in "Holistic Nursing" (Levine, 1971b). The second edition of *Introduction to Clinical Nursing* was published in 1973 (Levine, 1973). After that, Levine (1984) presented the conservation principles at nurse theory conferences, some of which have been audiotaped, and at the Allentown College of St. Francis de Sales (now DeSales University) Conference.

Levine (1989) published a substantial change and clarification about her theory in "The Four Conservation Principles: Twenty Years Later." She elaborated on how redundancy characterizes availability of adaptive responses when stability is threatened. Adaptation processes establish a body economy to safeguard the individual's stability. The outcome of adaptation is conservation.

She explicitly linked health to the process of conservation to clarify that the Conservation Model views health as one of its essential components (Levine, 1991). Conservation, through treatment, focuses on integrity and the reclamation of oneness of the whole person.

Levine died on March 20, 1996, at the age of 75. She leaves a legacy as an administrator, educator, friend, mother, nurse, scholar, student of humanities, and wife (Pond, 1996). Dr. Baumhart (Mid-Year Convocation, Loyola University, 1992), President of Loyola University, said the following of Levine:

> Mrs. Levine is a renaissance woman . . . who uses knowledge from several disciplines to expand the vision of health needs of persons which can be met by modern nursing. In the Talmudic tradition of her ancestors, [she] has been a forthright spokesperson for social justice and the inherent dignity of human person as a child of God. (p. 6)

THEORETICAL SOURCES

From Beland's (1971) presentation of the theory of specific causation and multiple factors, Levine learned historical viewpoints of diseases and learned that the way people think about disease changes over time. Beland directed Levine's attention to numerous authors who became influential in her thinking, including Goldstein (1963), Hall (1966), Sherrington (1906), and Dubos (1961, 1965). Levine uses Gibson's (1966) definition of perceptual systems, Erikson's (1964) differentiation between total and whole, Selye's (1956) stress theory, and Bates' (1967) models of external environment. Levine was proud that Rogers (1970) was her first editor. She acknowledged Nightingale's contribution to her thinking about the "guardian activity" of observation used by nurses to "save lives and increase health and comfort" (Levine, 1992, p. 42).

MAJOR CONCEPTS & DEFINITIONS

The three major concepts of the Conservation Model are (1) wholeness, (2) adaptation, and (3) conservation.

WHOLENESS (HOLISM)

"Whole, health, hale are all derivations of the Anglo-Saxon word *hal*" (Levine, 1973, p. 11). Levine based her use of wholeness on Erikson's (1964, 1968) description of wholeness as an open system. Levine (as cited in 1969a) quotes Erikson, who states, "Wholeness emphasizes a sound, organic, progressive, mutuality between diversified functions and parts within an entirety, the boundaries of which are open and fluent" (p. 94). Levine (1996) believed that Erikson's definition set up the option of exploring the parts of the whole to understand the whole. Integrity means the oneness of the individuals, emphasizing that they respond in an integrated, singular fashion to environmental challenges.

ADAPTATION

"Adaptation is a process of change whereby the individual retains his integrity within the realities of his internal and external environment" (Levine, 1973, p. 11). Conservation is the outcome. Some adaptations are successful and some are not. Adaptation is a matter of degree, not an all-or-nothing process. There is no such thing as maladaptation.

Levine (1991) speaks of the following three characteristics of adaptation:
1. Historicity
2. Specificity
3. Redundancy

She states, "... every species has fixed patterns of responses uniquely designed to ensure success in essential life activities, demonstrating that adaptation is both historical and specific" (p. 5). In addition, adaptive patterns may be hidden in the individual's genetic code. Redundancy represents the fail-safe options available to individuals to ensure adaptation. Loss of redundant choices either through trauma, age, disease, or environmental conditions makes it difficult for the individual to maintain life. Levine (1991) suggests "the possibility exists that aging itself is a consequence of failed redundancy of physiological and psychological processes" (p. 6).

Environment

Levine (1973) also views each individual as having his or her own environment, both internally and externally. Nurses can relate the internal environment as the physiological and pathophysiological aspects of the patient. Levine uses Bates' (1967) definition of the external environment and suggests the following three levels:

Continued

MAJOR CONCEPTS & DEFINITIONS—cont'd

1. Perceptual
2. Operational
3. Conceptual

These levels give dimension to the interactions between individuals and their environments. The perceptual level includes the aspects of the world that individuals are able to intercept and interpret with their sense organs. The operational level contains things that affect individuals physically although they cannot directly perceive them, things such as microorganisms. At the conceptual level, the environment is constructed from cultural patterns, characterized by a spiritual existence, and mediated by the symbols of language, thought, and history (Levine, 1973).

Organismic Response

The capacity of the individual to adapt to his or her environmental condition is called the organismic response. It can be divided into the following four levels of integration:

1. Fight or flight
2. Inflammatory response
3. Response to stress
4. Perceptual awareness

Treatment focuses on the management of these responses to illness and disease (Levine, 1969a).

Fight or Flight. The most primitive response is the fight or flight syndrome. The individual perceives that he or she is threatened, whether or not a threat actually exists. Hospitalization, illness, and new experiences elicit a response. The individual responds by being on the alert to find more information and to ensure his or her safety and well-being (Levine, 1973).

Inflammatory Response. This defense mechanism protects the self from insult in a hostile environment. It is a way of healing. The response uses available energy to remove or keep out unwanted irritants or pathogens. It is limited in time because it drains the individual's energy reserves. Environmental control is important (Levine, 1973).

Response to Stress. Selye (1956) described the stress response syndrome to predictable, nonspecifically induced organismic changes. The wear and tear of life is recorded on the tissues and reflects long-term hormonal responses to life experiences that cause structural changes. It is characterized by irreversibility and influences the way patients respond to nursing care.

Perceptual Awareness. This response is based on the individual's perceptual awareness. It occurs only as the individual experiences the world around him or her. The individual uses this response to seek and maintain safety. It is information seeking (Levine, 1967a; 1969b).

Trophicognosis

Levine (1966a) recommended trophicognosis as an alternative to nursing diagnosis. It is a scientific method to reach a nursing care judgment.

CONSERVATION

Conservation is from the Latin word *conservatio*, meaning "to keep together" (Levine, 1973). "Conservation describes the way complex systems are able to continue to function even when severely challenged" (Levine, 1990, p. 192). Through conservation, individuals are able to confront obstacles, adapt accordingly, and maintain their uniqueness. "The goal of conservation is health and the strength to confront disability" as ". . . the rules of conservation and integrity hold" in all situations in which nursing is required (Levine, 1973, pp. 193-195). The primary focus of conservation is keeping together of the wholeness of the individual. Although nursing interventions may deal with one particular conservation principle, nurses must also recognize the influence of the other conservation principles (Levine, 1990).

Levine's (1973) model stresses nursing interactions and interventions that are intended to promote adaptation and maintain wholeness. These interactions are based on the scientific

MAJOR CONCEPTS *&* DEFINITIONS—cont'd

background of the conservation principles. Conservation focuses on achieving a balance of energy supply and demand within the biological realities unique to the individual. Nursing care is based on scientific knowledge and nursing skills. There are four conservation principles.

Conservation Principles

The goals of the Conservation Model are achieved through interventions that attend to the conservation principles.

Conservation of Energy. The individual requires a balance of energy and a constant renewal of energy to maintain life activities. Processes such as healing and aging challenge that energy. This second law of thermodynamics applies to everything in the universe, including people.

Conservation of energy has long been used in nursing practice even with the most basic procedures. Nursing interventions "scaled to the individual's ability are dependent upon providing care that makes the least additional demand possible" (Levine, 1990, pp. 197-198).

Conservation of Structural Integrity. Healing is a process of restoring structural and functional integrity through conservation in defense of wholeness (Levine, 1991). The disabled are guided to a new level of adaptation (Levine, 1996). Nurses can limit the amount of tissue involved in disease by early recognition of functional changes and by nursing interventions.

Conservation of Personal Integrity. Self-worth and a sense of identity are important. The most vulnerable become patients. This begins with the erosion of privacy and the creation of anxiety. Nurses can show patients respect by calling them by name, respecting their wishes, valuing personal possessions, providing privacy during procedures, supporting their defenses, and teaching them. "The nurse's goal is always to impart knowledge and strength so that the individual can resume a private life—no longer a patient, no longer dependent" (Levine, 1990, p. 199). The sanctity of life is manifested in all people. "The conservation of personal integrity includes recognition of the holiness of each person" (Levine, 1996, p. 40).

Conservation of Social Integrity. Life gains meaning through social communities and health is socially determined. Nurses fulfill professional roles, provide for family members, assist with religious needs, and use interpersonal relationships to conserve social integrity (Levine, 1967b; 1969a).

USE OF EMPIRICAL EVIDENCE

Levine (1973) believed that specific nursing activities could be deducted from scientific principles. The scientific theoretical sources have been well researched. She based much of her work on accepted science principles.

MAJOR ASSUMPTIONS

Introduction to Clinical Nursing is a text for beginning nursing students that uses the conservation principles as an organizing framework (Levine, 1969a, 1973). Although she didn't state them specifically as assumptions, Levine (1973) valued "a holistic approach to care of all people, well or sick" (p. 151). Her respect for the individuality of each person is noted in the following statements:

Ultimately, decisions for nursing interventions must be based on the unique behavior of the individual patient. . . . Patient centered nursing care means individualized nursing care . . . and as such he requires a unique constellation of skills, techniques, and ideas designed specifically for him. (1973, p. 6)

Schaefer (1996) identified the following statements as assumptions about the model:

- The person can be understood only in the context of his or her environment (Levine, 1973).
- "Every self-sustaining system monitors its own behavior by conserving the use of the resources required to define its unique identity" (Levine, 1991, p. 4).
- Human beings respond in a singular, yet integrated, fashion (Levine, 1971a).

Nursing

Levine (1973) stated the following about nursing:

Nursing is a human interaction. (p. 1)

Professional nursing should be reserved for those few who can complete a graduate program as demanding as that expected of professionals in any other discipline. . . . There will be very few professional nurses. (Levine, 1965, p. 214)

Nursing practice is based on nursing's unique knowledge and the scientific knowledge of other disciplines adjunctive to nursing knowledge (Levine, 1988b), as follows:

It is the nurse's task to bring a body of scientific principles, on which decisions depend, into the precise situation which she shares with the patient. Sensitive observation and the selection of relevant data form the basis for her assessment of his nursing requirements.

The nurse participates actively in every patient's environment and much of what she does supports his adjustments as he struggles in the predicament of illness. (Levine, 1966b, p. 2452)

The essence of Levine's theory is as follows:

. . . when nursing intervention influences adaptation favorably, or toward renewed social well-being, then the nurse is acting in a therapeutic sense; when

the response is unfavorable, the nurse provides supportive care. (1966b, p. 2450)

The goal of nursing is to promote adaptation and maintain wholeness. (1971b, p. 258)

Person

Person is described as a holistic being; wholeness is integrity (Levine, 1991). Integrity means that the person has freedom of choice and movement. The person has a sense of identity and self-worth. Levine also described person as a "system of systems, and in its wholeness expresses the organization of all the contributing parts" (pp. 8-9). Persons experience life as change through adaptation with the goal of conservation. According to Levine (1989), "The life process is the process of change" (p. 326).

Health

Health is socially determined by the ability to function in a reasonably normal manner (Levine, 1969b). Social groups predetermine health. Health is not just an absence of pathological conditions. Health is the return to self; individuals are free and able to pursue their own interests within the context of their own resources. Levine stressed the following:

It is important to keep in mind that health is also culturally determined—it is not an entity on its own, but rather a definition imparted by the ethos and beliefs of the groups to which individuals belong. (M. Levine, personal communication, February 21, 1995)

Even for a single individual, the definition of health will change over time.

Environment

Environment is conceptualized as the context in which individuals live their lives. It is not a passive backdrop. "The individual actively participates in his environment" (Levine, 1973, p. 443). Levine discussed the importance of the internal and external environment to the determinant of nursing interventions to promote adaptation. "All adaptations represent the accommodation that is possible between the internal and external environment" (p. 12).

THEORETICAL ASSERTIONS

Although many theoretical assertions can be generated from Levine's work, the four major assertions follow:

1. "Nursing intervention is based on the conservation of the individual patient's energy" (Levine, 1967a, p. 49).
2. "Nursing intervention is based on the conservation of the individual patient's structural integrity" (Levine, 1967a, p. 56).
3. "Nursing intervention is based on the conservation of the individual patient's personal integrity" (Levine, 1967a, p. 56).
4. "Nursing intervention is based on the conservation of the individual patient's social integrity" (Levine, 1967b, p. 57).

Levine (1991) provided some thoughts about two theories in their early stages of development. The theory of therapeutic intention is intended to provide the basis of nursing interventions that focus on the biological realities of the patient. Although not planned as such, the theory naturally flows from the conservation principles. The theory of redundancy expands the redundancy domain of adaptation and offers explanations for redundant options such as those found in aging and the physiological adaptation to a failing heart.

LOGICAL FORM

Levine primarily uses deductive logic. In developing her model, Levine integrates theories and concepts from the humanities and the sciences of nursing, physiology, psychology, and sociology. She uses the information to analyze nursing practice situations and describe nursing skills and activities. With the assistance of many of her students and colleagues and through her own personal health encounters, she has experienced the Conservation Model and its principles operating in practice.

ACCEPTANCE BY THE NURSING COMMUNITY
Practice

Levine helps define what nursing is by identifying the activities it encompasses and giving the scientific principles behind them. Conservation principles as a framework are not limited to nursing care in the hospital but can be generalized and used in every environment, hospital, or community (Levine, 1990, 1991). Conservation principles, levels of integration, and other concepts can be used in numerous contexts (Fawcett, 2000). Hirschfeld (1976) has used the principles of conservation in the care of the older adult. Savage and Culbert (1989) used the Conservation Model to establish a plan of care for infants. Dever (1991) based her care of children on the Conservation Model. Roberts, Fleming, and Yeates-Giese (1991) designed interventions for women in labor based on the Conservation Model. Mefford (2000) tested a theory of health promotion for preterm infants derived from Levine's Conservation Model of nursing and found a significant inverse relationship between the consistency of caregiver and the age at which the infant achieved health and an inverse relationship between the use of resources by preterm infants during the initial hospital stay and the consistency of caregivers. Cooper (1990) developed a framework for wound care focusing on structural integrity while integrating all the integrities. Webb (1993) used the Conservation Model to provide care for patients undergoing cancer treatment. Roberts, Brittin, and deClifford (1995) and Roberts, Brittin, Cook and deClifford (1994) used the Conservation Model to study the boomerang pillow technique effect on respiratory capacity. Taylor (1974) used it to measure the outcomes of nursing care and again in her textbook, *Neurological*

Dysfunction and Nursing Interventions (Taylor & Ballenger, 1980). Jost (2000) used the model to develop an assessment of the needs of staff during the experience of change.

Conservation principles have been used as frameworks for numerous practice settings in cardiology, obstetrics, gerontology, acute care (neurology), pediatrics, long-term care, emergency care, primary care, neonatology, critical care areas, and in the homeless community (Savage & Culbert, 1989; Schaefer & Pond, 1991).

Education

Levine (1973) wrote *Introduction to Clinical Nursing* as a textbook for beginning students. It introduced new material into the curricula. She presented an early discussion of death and dying and believed that women should be awakened after a breast biopsy and consulted about the next step.

Introduction to Clinical Nursing provides an organizational structure for teaching medical-surgical nursing to beginning students (Levine, 1969a, 1973). In both the 1969 and 1973 editions, Levine presents a model at the end of each of the first nine chapters. Each model contains objectives, essential science concepts, and nursing process to give nurses a foundation for nursing activities. These models are not part of the Conservation Model. The Conservation Model is addressed in the Introduction and in Chapter 10 of the introductory text. The teachers' manual that accompanies the text remains a timely source of educational principles that may be helpful to both beginning teachers and seasoned teachers who may benefit from a review of educational roots (Levine, 1971c).

Critics argue that although the text is labeled introductory, a beginning student would need a fairly extensive background in physical and social science to use it (*Canadian Nurse,* 1970). A critic of the second edition suggests that the emphasis of scientific principles is a definite strength, but the text's weakness is that it does not present adequate examples of pathological profiles when disturbances are discussed (*Canadian Nurse,* 1974). For this reason, this one reviewer recommends that the text be used

as a supplementary or complementary text, not a primary text.

Hall (1979) indicates that Levine's model is used as a curriculum model. The model has been integrated successfully into undergraduate and graduate curricula (Grindley & Paradowski, 1991; Schaefer, 1991a).

Research

Fitzpatrick and Whall (1983) state, "All in all, Levine's model served as an excellent beginning. Its contribution has added a great deal to the overall development of nursing knowledge" (p. 115). However, Fawcett (1995) states that to establish credibility, "more systematic evaluations of the use of the model in various clinical situations are needed, as are studies that test conceptual-theoretical-empirical structures directly derived from or linked with the conservation principles" (p. 208). Many research questions can be generated from Levine's model (Radwin & Fawcett, 2002; Schaefer, 1991b). Several graduate students have used the conservation principles as a framework for their research (Cox, 1988; Mefford, 2000; Nagley, 1984).

One of the most important questions to be asked about the model is, What are the human experiences not explained by the model? This question can provide guidance for continued testing of the model's application in nursing practice. For example, as health care providers use information from the human genome project, nurse researchers will want to test the ability of the model to explain comprehensive nursing care of the client undergoing genetic counseling. Based on the outcome of this testing, hypotheses can be developed and tested to support the prescription basis of the theories developed from the model.

FURTHER DEVELOPMENT

Levine and others have worked on using the conservation principles as the basis for a taxonomy of nursing diagnosis (Stafford, 1996; Taylor, 1989). Additional work has been done on use of Levine's model in administration and with the frail elderly. The model was used to develop a theory of health promotion in preterm infants (Mefford, 2000) and has great potential for studies of sleep disorders and in the development of collaborative and primary care practices as well (Fawcett, 2000). The philosophical, ethical, and spiritual implications of the model are research challenges yet to be realized (Stafford, 1996).

CRITIQUE
Clarity

Levine's model possesses clarity. Fitzpatrick and Whall (1983) believe that Levine's work is both internally and externally consistent. Fawcett (1995) states that "Levine's Conservation Model provides nursing with a logically congruent, holistic view of the person" (p. 208). The model has numerous terms; however, Levine adequately defines them for clarity.

Simplicity

Although the four conservation principles appear simple initially, they contain subconcepts and multiple variables. Nevertheless, this model is still one of the simpler ones developed.

Generality

The four conservation principles can be used in all nursing contexts.

Empirical Precision

Levine used deductive logic to develop her model, which can be used to generate research questions. As she lived her Conservation Model, she verified the use of inductive reasoning to further develop and inform her model (M. Levine, personal communication, May 17, 1989).

Derivable Consequences

Although some authors question the level of contribution Levine's model provides, the four conservation principles are recognized as one of the earliest nursing models. Furthermore, the model has continued to have utility for nursing practice and research and is receiving increased recognition in this twenty-first century.

SUMMARY

Levine developed her Conservation Model to provide a framework within which to teach beginning nursing students. In the first chapter of her book she introduced her assumptions about holism and that the conservation principles support a holistic approach to patient care (Levine, 1969a, 1973). The model is logically congruent, is externally and internally consistent, has breadth as well as depth and is understood, with few exceptions, by professionals and consumers of health care. Nurses using the Conservation Model can anticipate, explain, predict, and perform patient care. However, its ability to predict outcomes must be tested further. Levine (1990) said that everywhere that nursing is essential the rules of the conservation and the integrity hold" (p. 195).

*Case Study**

Yolanda is a 55-year-old married African-American mother of two adult children who has a history of breast cancer and was diagnosed with fibromyalgia 2 years ago, following years of unexplained muscle aches and what she thought was arthritis. The diagnosis was a relief for her because she was able to read about it and learn how to care for herself. Over the past 2 months Yolanda stopped taking all of her medicine because she was seeing a new physician and wanted to start her care at ground zero. In addition to her family responsibilities, she is completing her degree as an English major. At the

*This case study is based on raw data from a study in process titled "Fibromyalgia in African American Women: A Phenomenological Investigation," Philadelphia. Yolanda is a fictitious name used to protect the privacy and anonymity of the participant.

time of her appointment, she told the nurse practitioner that she was having the worst pain possible.

Using Levine's Conservation Model, the nurse practitioner completed a comprehensive assessment in preparation for developing a plan of care in consultation with the physician. Nursing care is organized according to the conservation principles with consideration of how the individual adapts to the internal and external environments. Yolanda's diagnosis of fibromyalgia was based on the exclusion of other illnesses with a cluster of symptoms including pain, fatigue, and sleeplessness (e.g., systemic lupus erythematosus, multiple sclerosis). Laboratory and other diagnostic results were all within normal limits.

The external environment includes the perceptual, operational, and conceptual factors. Perceptual factors are those that are perceived through the senses. Yolanda reported a history of unexplained fatigue and pain for years. She recently stopped her medications "to clean my body out." However she reported that the pain became almost unbearable and was making it difficult for her to sleep. She noted that when she sleeps at least 6 hours a night, her pain is less intense. With the current insomnia her pain is very intense.

Operational factors are threats to the environment that the client cannot perceive through the senses. Yolanda reported severe pain in response to both the cold weather and changes in the barometric pressure.

The conceptual environment includes the cultural and personal values about health care, the meaning of health and illness, knowledge about health care, education, language use, and spiritual beliefs. In response to breast cancer, Yolanda developed her spirituality through prayer and reading the bible. She believes that this is how she gets through the painful moments of her current illness.

The conservation of energy focuses on the balance of energy input and output to prevent excessive fatigue. Yolanda complains a fatigue that just "comes over me." She has difficulty doing housework. One day of work usually means one day in bed because of extreme fatigue. Her hemoglobin level and hematocrit are normal; her arterial blood gas results have always been within normal limits. Most diagnostic study values are within normal limits in patients with fibromyalgia, making treatment difficult.

The conservation of structural integrity involves maintaining the structure of the body to promote healing. Because there is no known cause of fibromyalgia, treatment focuses on reducing the symptoms. Yolanda's symptoms could not be traced to any physical or structural alteration, yet she reports severe pain and fatigue. The nurse practitioner knows that it is important to acknowledge the reality of the symptoms and work with the client to determine if activities of daily living result in changes in the pattern of illness. In addition, Yolanda thinks she is going through menopause and she is having trouble determining if her symptoms are caused by menopause or fibromyalgia.

With continued questioning, the nurse practitioner learns that Yolanda was diagnosed with irritable bowel syndrome several years earlier. She is not worried about constipation but is concerned about sudden diarrhea. She is afraid to go to school, because she does not know what might happen; she fears embarrassment because she might have an "accident." Yolanda was taking several medications for her discomfort. One of them made her feel so "hung over" that she stopped taking it after 2 weeks. She was given amitriptyline (Elavil) for sleep. It was the only medicine that helped her get 6 hours of continuous sleep.

Personal integrity involves the maintenance of one's sense of personal worth and self-esteem. Yolanda reported that she lost control when she was diagnosed with breast cancer. A dear friend convinced her to go to church and encouraged her to use prayer. When feeling sorry for herself, she would go into her bedroom and read her Bible, cry by herself, and pray. She believes that the prayer and her Bible reading helped her heal. She continues to pray and read her Bible to gain the strength she needs to live with her current illness. She also believes that she needs to be able to laugh at herself; humor helps her to feel better. She actively seeks health information, as indicated by her quest to learn about her new diagnosis of fibromyalgia.

She is most upset about not being able to walk like she used to walk. One of her favorite pastimes was shopping for shoes at the mall, which now is difficult for her.

Social integrity acknowledges that the patient is a social being. Yolanda is a married mother of three grown children. She keeps a lot of her feelings from her children but does share them with her husband. He is a major source of support for her. He takes her food shopping and makes sure that she gets to her appointments on time. She shared at the time of her visit that she wants to have a picnic for her birthday, but the only way she can do it is to ask her grandchildren to help her husband clean the yard.

Yolanda is a middle-aged woman with a history of severe pain, sleeplessness, and fatigue. Diagnostic studies have been unrevealing with the exception of multiple tender points. The history of pain and positive tender points supported the diagnosis of fibromyalgia. She has stopped taking all medications and reports that she may be going through menopause. She reports severe pain and fatigue that makes it difficult for her to sleep and to do normal housework. Her husband and grandchildren are available to help with chores at home and she seeks the support of prayer and reading her Bible to ease her discomfort. She also finds that humor helps her to feel better.

The initial plan of care includes (1) validate the illness experience, (2) encourage continued use of prayer, Bible reading, and humor to help her feel better, (3) discuss medication therapy and what might help her achieve restful sleep, (4) refer her for blood work to assess hormone levels, and (5) assist her with determining the meaning of the symptoms (e.g., menopause or fibromyalgia). Yolanda indicated that when she was able to get 6 hours of uninterrupted sleep, her pain was less intense and she felt better. Finding both medication-induced and nonpharmaceutical approaches to improve sleep is a high priority.

The nurse practitioner will assess the outcome of Yolanda's care based on the organismic responses. The following predicted responses suggest adaptation:

- Reports comfort as a result of prayer, Bible reading, and humor
- Distinguishes symptoms of menopause from symptoms of fibromyalgia
- Reports feeling rested after 6 hours of uninterrupted sleep
- Reports a perceived reduction in pain and fatigue
- Collaborates with health care providers to manage symptoms of menopause

CRITICAL THINKING *Activities*

1. Keep a reflective journal about a personal health or illness experience or that of someone very close. Reflect on the experience and its consistency with the Conservation Model. Consider how to modify, expand, or delimit the model to better provide a context in which to explain the experience.

2. Levine stated, "Health is culturally determined; it is not an entity on its own, but rather a definition imparted by the ethos and beliefs of groups to which the individual belongs" (M. Levine, personal communication, February, 21, 1995).

Visit a nearby museum and evaluate how artistic expression captures the beliefs of different ethnic groups. Explore how these beliefs may shape the definitions of health and compare it with Levine's approach to health and illness. On the basis of the ethnically derived definition of health, propose ethnically appropriate interventions using Levine's conservation principles.

3. Watch one of the following movies: *City of Joy, Soul Food,* or *The Secret Garden.* Use examples from the movie to support or refute the propositional statements that Levine made about the environment and the relationships with person, nursing, and health and illness.

4. Apply the Conservation Model to a pathography, such as *Love and Other Infectious Diseases* by Molly Haskell, to determine how well the model explains life with illness. Identify what is left unexplained and offer suggestions on how the model would need to be developed to encompass the entire experience of the subject in the book.

REFERENCES

Bates, M. (1967). A naturalist at large. *Natural History, 76*(6), 8-16.

Beland, I. (1971). *Clinical nursing: Pathophysiological and psychosocial implications* (2nd ed.). New York: Macmillan.

Cooper, D. H. (1990). Optimizing wound healing: A practice within nursing domains. *Nursing Clinics of North America, 25*(1), 165-180.

Cox, B. (1988). Pregnancy, anxiety, and time perception (Doctoral dissertation University of Illinois at Chicago, Health Science Center, 1988). *Dissertation Abstracts International, 48,* 2260B. (University Microfilms No. AA18724993)

Dever, M. (1991). Care of children. In K. M. Schaefer & J. B. Pond (Eds.), *The Conservation Model: A framework for nursing practice* (pp. 71-82). Philadelphia: F. A. Davis.

Dubos, R. (1961). *Mirage of health.* Garden City, NY: Doubleday.

Dubos, R. (1965). *Man adapting.* New Haven, CT: Yale University Press.

Erikson, E. H. (1964). *Insight and responsibility.* New York: W. W. Norton.

Erikson, E. H. (1968). *Identity: Youth and crisis.* New York: W. W. Norton.

Fawcett, J. (1995). Levine's Conservation Model. In J. Fawcett (Ed.), *Analysis and evaluation of conceptual models of nursing* (pp. 165-215). Philadelphia: F. A. Davis.

Fawcett, J. (2000). Levine's Conservation Model. In J. Fawcett (Ed.), *Analysis and evaluation of contemporary nursing knowledge: Nursing models and theories* (pp. 151-193). Philadelphia: F. A. Davis.

Fitzpatrick, J. J., & Whall, A. L. (1983). *Conceptual models of nursing: Analysis and application.* Bowie, MD: Robert J. Brady.

Gibson, J. E. (1966). *The senses considered as perceptual systems.* Boston: Houghton Mifflin.

Goldstein, K. (1963). *The organism.* Boston: Beacon Press.

Grindley, J., & Paradowski, M. B. (1991). Developing an undergraduate program using Levine's model. In K. M. Schaefer & J. B. Pond (Eds.), *Levine's Conservation Model: A framework for nursing practice* (pp. 199-208). Philadelphia: F. A. Davis.

Hall, E. T. (1966). *The hidden dimension.* Garden City, NY: Doubleday.

Hall, K. V. (1979). Current trends in the use of conceptual frameworks in nursing education. *Journal of Nursing Education, 18*(4), 26-29.

Hirschfeld, M. J. (1976). The cognitively impaired older adult. *American Journal of Nursing, 76,* 1981-1984.

Jost, S. G. (2000). An assessment and intervention strategy for managing. *Journal of Nursing Administration, 30*(1), 34-40.

Levine, M. E. (1965, June). The professional nurse and graduate education. *Nursing Science, 3,* 206.

Levine, M. E. (1966a). Trophicognosis: An alternative to nursing diagnosis. *American Nurses Association Regional Clinical Conferences, 2,* 55-70.

Levine, M. E. (1966b). Adaptation and assessment: A rationale for nursing intervention. *American Journal of Nursing, 66,* 2450-2454.

Levine, M. E. (1967a). The four conservation principles of nursing. *Nursing Forum, 6,* 45-59.

Levine, M. E. (1967b, Dec.). For lack of love alone. *Minnesota Nursing Accent, 39,* 179.

Levine, M. E. (1969a). *Introduction to clinical nursing.* Philadelphia: F. A. Davis.

Levine, M. E. (1969b). The pursuit of wholeness, *American Journal of Nursing, 69,* 93.

Levine, M. E. (1971a). *Renewal for nursing.* Philadelphia: F. A. Davis.

Levine, M. E. (1971b). Holistic nursing. *Nursing Clinics of North America, 6,* 253-263.

Levine, M. E. (1971c). Instructor's guide to introduction to clinical nursing. Philadelphia: F. A. Davis.

Levine, M. E. (1973). *Introduction to clinical nursing* (2nd ed.). Philadelphia: F. A. Davis.

Levine, M. E. (1984, April). *A conceptual model for nursing: The four conservation principles.* Proceedings from Allentown College of St. Francis Conference, Philadelphia.

Levine, M. E. (1988a). Myra Levine. In T. M. Schoor & A. Zimmerman (Eds.), *Making choices, taking chances: Nurse leaders tell their stories* (pp. 215-228). St. Louis: C. V. Mosby.

Levine, M. E. (1988b). Antecedents from adjunctive disciplines: Creation of nursing theory. *Nursing Science Quarterly, 1*(1), 16-21.

Levine, M. E. (1989). The four conservation principles: Twenty years later. In J. Riehl (Ed.), *Conceptual models for nursing practice* (3rd ed., pp. 325-337). New York: Appleton-Century-Crofts.

Levine, M. E. (1990). Conservation and integrity. In M. Parker (Ed.), *Nursing theories in practice* (pp. 189-201). New York: National League for Nursing.

Levine, M. E. (1991). The conservation principles: A model for health. In K. Schaefer & J. Pond (Eds.), *Levine's Conservation Model: A framework for nursing practice* (pp. 1-11). Philadelphia: F. A. Davis.

Levine, M. E. (1992). Nightingale redux. In B. S. Barnum (Ed.), *Nightingale's notes on nursing* (pp. 39-43). Philadelphia: J. B. Lippincott.

Levine, M. E. (1996). The conservation principles: A retrospective. *Nursing Science Quarterly, 9*(1), 38-41.

Mefford, L. C. (2000). *The relationships of nursing care to health outcomes of preterm infants: Testing a theory of health promotion for preterm infants based on Levine's Conservation Model.* Unpublished doctoral dissertation, University of Tennessee, Knoxville.

Mid-Year Convocation: Loyola University, Chicago. (1992). The Conferring of Honorary Degrees by R. C. Baumhart, Candidate for the degree of Doctor and Humane Letters, p. 6.

Nagley, S. J. (1984). Prevention of confusion in hospitalized elderly persons (Doctoral dissertation). *Dissertation Abstracts International, 48,* 1732B. (University Microfilms No. AA18420848) Case Western Reserve University.

Pond, J. B. (1996). Myra Levine, nurse educator and scholar dies. *Nursing Spectrum, 5*(8), 8.

Radwin, L., & Fawcett, J. (2002). A conceptual model based programme of nursing research: Retrospective and prospective applications. *Journal of Advanced Nursing, 40*(3), 355-360.

[Review of the book *Introduction to clinical nursing*]. (1970, Jan.). *Canadian Nurse, 66,* 42.

[Review of the book *Introduction to clinical nursing* (2nd ed.)]. (1974, May). *Canadian Nurse, 70,* 39.

Roberts, J. E., Fleming, N., & Yeates-Giese, D. (1991). Perineal integrity. In K. M. Schaefer & J. B. Pond (Eds.), *The Conservation Model: A framework for nursing practice* (pp. 61-70). Philadelphia: F. A. Davis.

Roberts, K. L., Brittin, M., Cook, M., & deClifford, J. (1994). Boomerang pillows and respiratory capacity. *Clinical Nursing Research, 3*(2), 157-165.

Roberts, K. L., Brittin, M., & deClifford, J. (1995). Boomerang pillows and respiratory capacity in frail elderly women. *Clinical Nursing Research, 4*(4), 465-471.

Rogers, M. E. (1970). *An introduction to the theoretical basis of nursing.* Philadelphia: F. A. Davis.

Savage, T. A., & Culbert, C. (1989). Early intervention: The unique role of nursing. *Journal of Pediatric Nursing, 4*(5), 339-345.

Schaefer, K. M. (1991a). Developing a graduate program in nursing: Integrating Levine's philosophy. In K. M. Schaefer & J. B. Pond (Eds.), *Levine's Conservation Model: A framework for nursing practice* (pp. 209-218). Philadelphia: F. A. Davis.

Schaefer, K. M. (1991b). Levine's conservation principles and research. In K. M. Schaefer & J. B. Pond (Eds.), *Levine's Conservation Model: A framework for nursing practice* (pp. 45-60). Philadelphia: F. A. Davis.

Schaefer, K. M. (1996). Levine's Conservation Model: Caring for women with chronic illness. In P. H. Walker & B. Neuman (Eds.), *Blueprint for use of nursing models: Education, research, practice and administration.* New York: National League for Nursing.

Schaefer, K. M., & Pond, J. B. (Eds.) (1991). *Levine's Conservation Model: A framework for nursing practice.* Philadelphia: F. A. Davis.

Selye, H. (1956). *The stress of life.* New York: McGraw-Hill.

Sherrington, A. (1906). *Integrative function of the nervous system.* New York: Charles Scribner's Sons.

Stafford, M. J. (1996). In tribute: Myra Estrin Levine, Professor Emerita, MSN, RN, FAAN. *Chart, 93*(3), 5-6.

Taylor, J. W. (1974). Measuring the outcomes of nursing care. *Nursing Clinics of North America, 9,* 337-348.

Taylor, J. W. (1989). Levine's conservation principles: Using the model for nursing diagnosis in a neurological setting. In J. P. Riehl-Sisca (Ed.), *Conceptual models for nursing practice* (3rd ed., pp. 349-358). Norwalk, CT: Appleton & Lange.

Taylor, J. W., & Ballenger, S. (1980). *Neurological dysfunction and nursing interventions.* New York: McGraw-Hill.

Webb, H. (1993). Holistic care following a palliative Hartmann's procedure. *British Journal of Nursing, 2*(2), 128-132.

BIBLIOGRAPHY
Primary Sources
Books

Levine, M. E. (1969). *Introduction to clinical nursing.* Philadelphia: F. A. Davis.

Levine, M. E. (1971). *Renewal for nursing.* Philadelphia: F. A. Davis. [Translated into Hebrew, Am Oved, Jerusalem, 1978.]

Levine, M. E. (1973). *Introduction to clinical nursing* (2nd ed.). Philadelphia: F. A. Davis.

Book Chapters

Levine, M. E. (1964). Nursing service. In M. Leeds & H. Shore (Eds.), *Geriatric institutional management.* New York: G. P. Putnam's Sons.

Levine, M. E. (1973). Adaptation and assessment: A rationale for nursing intervention. In M. E. Hardy (Ed.), *Theoretical foundations for nursing.* New York: Irvington.

Levine, M. E. (1988). Myra Levine. In T. M. Schorr & A. Zimmerman (Eds.), *Making choices, taking chances: Nursing leaders tell their stories.* St. Louis: Mosby.

Levine, M. E. (1989). The four conservation principles: Twenty years later. In J. Riehl (Ed.), *Conceptual models for nursing practice* (3rd ed.). New York: Appleton-Century-Crofts.

Levine, M. E. (1990). Conservation and integrity. In M. Parker (Ed.), *Nursing theories in practice* (pp. 189-201). New York: National League for Nursing.

Levine, M. E. (1991). The conservation principles: A model for health. In K. Schaefer & J. Pond (Eds.), *Levine's Conservation Model: A framework for nursing practice* (pp. 1-11). Philadelphia: F. A. Davis.

Levine, M. E. (1992). Nightingale redux. In B. S. Barnum (Ed.), *Nightingale's notes on nursing: Commemorative edition with commentaries by nursing theorists.* Philadelphia: J. B. Lippincott.

Levine, M. E. (1994). Some further thoughts on nursing rhetoric. In J. F. Kikuchi & H. Simmons (Eds.), *Developing a philosophy of nursing* (pp. 104-109). Thousand Oaks, CA: Sage.

Journal Articles

Levine, M. E. (1963). Florence Nightingale: The legend that lives. *Nursing Forum, 2*(4), 24-35.

Levine, M. E. (1964, Feb.). Not to startle, though the way were steep. *Nursing Science, 2,* 58-67.

Levine, M. E. (1964, Dec.). There need be no anonymity. *First, 18*(9), 4.

Levine, M. E. (1965). The professional nurse and graduate education. *Nursing Science, 3,* 206-214.

Levine, M. E. (1965). Trophicognosis: An alternative to nursing diagnosis. *ANA Regional Clinical Conferences, 2,* 55-70.

Levine, M. E. (1966.). Adaptation and assessment: A rationale for nursing intervention. *American Journal of Nursing, 66*(11), 2450-2453.

Levine, M. E. (1967, Dec.). For lack of love alone. Minnesota Nursing *Accent, 39*(7), 179-202.

Levine, M. E. (1967). Medicine-nursing dialogue belongs at patient's bedside. *Chart, 64*(5), 136-137.

Levine, M. E. (1967). The four conservation principles of nursing. *Nursing Forum, 6,* 45-59.

Levine, M. E. (1967). This I believe: About patient-centered care. *Nursing Outlook, 15,* 53-55.

Levine, M. E. (1968, Feb.). Knock before entering personal space bubbles (part 1). *Chart, 65*(2), 58-62.

Levine, M. E. (1968, March). Knock before entering personal space bubbles (part 2). *Chart, 65*(3), 82-84.

Levine, M. E. (1968). The pharmacist in the clinical setting: A nurse's viewpoint. *American Journal of Hospital Pharmacy, 25*(4), 168-171. [Also translated into Japanese and published in *Kyushu National Hospital Magazine* for Western Japan.]

Levine, M. E. (1969, Feb.). Constructive student power. *Chart, 66*(2), 42FF.

Levine, M. E. (1969, Oct.). Small hospital—Big nursing. *Chart, 66,* 265-269.

Levine, M. E. (1969, Nov.). Small hospital—Big nursing. *Chart, 66,* 310-315.

Levine, M. E. (1969). The pursuit of wholeness. *American Journal of Nursing, 69,* 93-98.

Levine, M. E. (1970). Dilemma. *ANA Clinical Conferences,* 338-342.

Levine, M. E. (1970). Breaking through the medications mystique. *American Journal of Hospital Pharmacy, 27*(4), 294-299; *American Journal of Nursing, 70*(4), 799-803.

Levine, M. E. (1970, July/Dec.). Symposium on a drug compendium: View of a nursing educator. *Drug Information Bulletin,* 133-135.

Levine, M. E. (1970). The intransigent patient. *American Journal of Nursing, 70,* 2106-2111.

Levine, M. E. (1971). Consider implications for nursing in the use of physician's assistant. *Hospital Topics, 49,* 60-63.

Levine, M. E. (1971). Holistic nursing. *Nursing Clinics of North America, 6,* 253-264.

Levine, M. E. (1971). The time has come to speak of health care. *AORN Journal, 13,* 37-43.

Levine, M. E. (1972). Benoni. *American Journal of Nursing, 72*(3), 466-468.

Levine, M. E. (1972). Nursing educators—An alienating elite? *Chart, 69*(2), 56-61.

Levine, M. E. (1973). On creativity in nursing. *Image: The Journal of Nursing Scholarship, 3*(3), 15-19.

Levine, M. E. (1974). The pharmacist's clinical role in interdisciplinary care: A nurse's viewpoint. *Hospital Formulary Management, 9,* 47.

Levine, M. E. (1975). On creativity in nursing. *Nursing Digest, 3,* 38-40.

Levine, M. E. (1977). Nursing ethics and the ethical nurse. *American Journal of Nursing, 77,* 845-849.

Levine, M. E. (1978). Cancer chemotherapy: A nursing model. *Nursing Clinics of North America, 13*(2), 271-280.

Levine, M. E. (1978). Does continuing education improve nursing practice? *Hospitals, 52*(21), 138-140.

Levine, M. E. (1978). Kapklavoo and nursing, too (Editorial). *Research in Nursing and Health, 1*(2), 51.

Levine, M. E. (1979). Knowledge base required by generalized and specialized nursing practice. *ANA Publications, (G-127),* 57-69.

Levine, M. E. (1980). The ethics of computer technology in health care. *Nursing Forum, 19*(2), 193-198.

Levine, M. E. (1982). Bioethics of cancer nursing. *Rehabilitation Nursing, 7,* 27-31, 41.

Levine, M. E. (1982). The bioethics of cancer nursing. *Journal of Enterostomal Therapy, 9,* 11-13.

Levine, M. E. (1988). Antecedents from adjunctive disciplines: Creation of nursing theory. *Nursing Science Quarterly, 1*(1), 16-21.

Levine, M. E. (1988, June). What does the future hold for nursing? 25th Anniversary Address, 18th District. *Illinois Nurses Association Newsletter, XXIV*(6), 1-4.

Levine, M. E. (1989). Beyond dilemma. *Seminars in Oncology Nursing, 5*, 124-128.

Levine, M. E. (1989). Ration or rescue: The elderly in critical care. *Critical Care Nursing, 12*(1), 82-89.

Levine, M. E. (1989). The ethics of nursing rhetoric. *Image: The Journal of Nursing Scholarship, 21*(1), 4-5.

Levine, M. E. (1995). The rhetoric of nursing theory. *Image: The Journal of Nursing Scholarship, 27*(1), 11-14.

Levine, M. E. (1996). On the humanities in nursing. *Canadian Journal of Nursing Research, 27*(2), 19-23.

Levine, M. E. (1996). The conservation principles: A retrospective. *Nursing Science Quarterly, 9*(1), 38-41.

Levine, M. E. (1997). On creativity in nursing. *Image: The Journal of Nursing Scholarship, 29*(3), 216-217.

Levine, M. E., Hallberg, C., Kathrein, M., & Cox, R. (1972). Nursing grand rounds: Congestive failure. *Nursing '72, 2*(10), 18-23.

Levine, M. E., Line, L., Boyle, A., & Kopacewski, E. (1972). Nursing grand rounds: Insulin reactions in a brittle diabetic. *Nursing '72, 2*(5), 6-11.

Levine, M. E., Moschel, P., Taylor, J., & Ferguson, G. (1972). Nursing grand rounds: Complicated case of CVA. *Nursing '72, 2*(3), 3-34.

Levine, M. E., Scanlon, M., Gregor, P., King, R., & Martin, N. (1972). Issues in rehabilitation: The quadriplegic adolescent. *Nursing '72, 2*, 6.

Levine, M. E., Zoellner, J., Ozmon, B., & Simunek, E. (1972). Nursing grand rounds: Severe trauma. *Nursing '72, 2*(9), 33-38.

Audiotapes

Levine, M. E. (1978, Dec.). *Nursing theory* (Audiotape). Paper presented at the Second Annual Nurse Educator Conference, New York. Available through Teach 'em Inc., 160 E. Illinois Street, Chicago, IL 60611.

Levine, M. E. (1984, May). *Application-practice/research/education* (Audiotape). Paper presented at Nursing Theory Conference, Boyle, Letoueneau Conference, Edmonton, Canada. Available through Ed Kennedy, Kennedy Recording, R. R. 5, Edmonton, Alberta, Canada T5P 4B7.

Videotape

Fawcett, J. (1988). *The nursing theorist: Portraits of excellence: Myra Levine* (Videotape). Oakland: Studio III. Available through Fuld Video Project, 370 Hawthorne Avenue, Oakland, CA 94609.

Proceedings

Levine, M. E. (1976). On the nursing ethnic and the negative command. *Proceedings of the Intensive Conference, Faculty of the University of Illinois Medical Center.* Philadelphia: Society for Health and Human Values.

Levine, M. E. (1977). History of nursing in Illinois. *Proceedings of the Bicentennial Workshop of the University of Illinois College of Nursing.* Chicago: University of Illinois Press.

Levine, M. E. (1977). Primary nursing: Generalist and specialist education. *Proceedings of the American Academy of Nursing.* Kansas City, MO: American Academy of Nursing.

Levine, M. E. (1984, April). A conceptual model for nursing: The four conservation principles. *Proceedings for a Conference on Nursing Education.* Allentown College of St. Francis de Sales, Philadelphia.

Levine, M. E. (1985). What's wrong about rights? In A. Carmi & S. Schneider (Eds.), *Proceedings of the 1st International Congress of Nursing Law and Ethics.* Berlin: Springer-Verlag.

SECONDARY SOURCES
Book Reviews

[Review of the book *Introduction to clinical nursing*]. (1969, Sept./Oct.). *Bedside Nurse, 2,* 4.

[Review of the book *Introduction to clinical nursing*]. (1970, Feb.). *Nursing Outlook, 18,* 20.

[Review of the book *Introduction to clinical nursing*]. (1970, Jan.). *American Journal of Nursing, 70,* 99.

[Review of the book *Introduction to clinical nursing*]. (1970, Jan.). *Canadian Nurse, 66,* 42.

[Review of the book *Introduction to clinical nursing*]. (1970, Oct.). *American Journal of Nursing, 70,* 2220.

[Review of the book *Introduction to clinical nursing*]. (1971, April). *Nursing Mirror, 132,* 43.

[Review of the book *Introduction to clinical nursing*]. (1971, Dec.). *Canadian Nurse, 76,* 47.

[Review of the book *Introduction to clinical nursing*]. (1971, Dec.). *Nursing Mirror, 133,* 16.

[Review of the book *Introduction to clinical nursing*]. (1974, Feb.). *American Journal of Nursing, 74,* 347.

[Review of the book *Introduction to clinical nursing*]. (1974, May). *Canadian Nurse, 70,* 39.

[Review of the book *Introduction to clinical nursing*]. (1974, May). *Nursing Outlook, 22,* 301.

[Review of the book *Introduction to clinical nursing*]. (1971, Nov.). *Bedside Nurse, 4,* 2.

[Review of the book *Renewal for nursing*]. (1971, Aug.). *Supervisor Nurse, 2,* 68.

[Review of the book *Renewal for nursing*]. (1971, Dec.). *AANA Journal, 49,* 495.

[Review of the book *Renewal for nursing*]. (1971, Dec.). *Canadian Nurse, 67,* 47.

[Review of the book *Renewal for nursing*]. (1971, Dec.). *Nursing Mirror, 133,* 16.

Book Chapters

Fawcett, J. (1995). Levine's Conservation Model. In J. Fawcett (Ed.), *Analysis and evaluating of conceptual models of nursing* (pp. 165-215). Philadelphia: F. A. Davis.

Leonard, M. K. (1990). Myra Estrin Levine. In J. B. George (Ed.), *Nursing theories: The base for professional nursing practice* (pp. 181-192). Englewood Cliffs, NJ: Prentice Hall.

MacLean, S. L. (1989). Activity intolerance: Cues for diagnosis. In R. M. Carroll-Johnson (Ed.), *Classification proceedings of the eighth annual conference of North American Nursing Diagnosis Association* (pp. 320-327). Philadelphia: J. B. Lippincott.

McLane, A. (1987). Taxonomy and nursing diagnosis, a critical view. In A. McLane (Ed.), *Classification proceedings of the seventh annual conference of Nursing of North America*. St. Louis: Mosby.

Meleis, A. I. (1985). Myra Levine. In A. I. Meleis (Ed.), *Theoretical nursing: Development and progress* (pp. 275-283). Philadelphia: J. B. Lippincott.

Peiper, B. A. (1983). Levine's nursing model. In J. J. Fitzpatrick & A. L. Whall (Eds.), *Conceptual models of nursing: Analysis and application* (pp. 101-115). Bowie, MD: Robert J. Brady.

Pond, J. B. (1990). Application of Levine's Conservation Model to nursing the homeless community. In M. E. Parker (Ed.), *Nursing theories in practice* (pp. 203-215). New York: National League for Nursing.

Schaefer, K. M. (1990). A description of fatigue associated with congestive heart failure: Use of Levine's Conservation Model. In M. E. Parker (Ed.), *Nursing theories in practice* (pp. 217-237). New York: National League for Nursing.

Schaefer, K. M. (1996). Levine's Conservation Model: Caring for women with chronic illness. In P. H. Walker & B. Neuman (Eds.), *Blueprint for use of nursing models: Education, research, practice and administration* (pp. 187-228). New York: National League for Nursing Press.

Schaefer, K. M. (2001). Levine's Conservation Model: A model for the future of nursing. In Parker, M. E. (Ed.), *Nursing theories and nursing practice* (pp. 103-124). Philadelphia: F. A. Davis.

Schaefer, K. M. (2001). Levine's Conservation Model: Use of the model in nursing practice. In M. R. Alligood & A. Marriner-Tomey (Eds.), *Nursing theory: Utilization & application* (pp. 89-108; Taiwanese ed.). St. Louis: Mosby.

Schaefer, K. M. (2002). Levine's Conservation Model in nursing practice. In M. R. Alligood & A.M. Tomey (Eds.), *Nursing theory: Utilization & application* (2nd ed., pp. 197-217). St. Louis: Mosby.

Taylor, J. W. (1989). Levine's conservation principles: Using the model for nursing diagnosis in a neurological setting. In J. P. Riehl-Sisca (Ed.), *Conceptual models for nursing practice* (3rd ed., pp. 349-358). Norwalk, CT: Appleton & Lange.

Books

Barnum, B. J. S. (1994). *Nursing theory: Analysis application evaluation* (4th ed.). Philadelphia: J. B. Lippincott.

Chinn, P. L., & Kramer, M. K. (1995). *Theory and nursing: A systematic approach* (4th ed.). St. Louis: Mosby.

Clark, M. J. (1992). *Nursing in the community.* Norwalk, CT: Appleton & Lange.

Dubos, R. (1961). *Miracle of health.* Garden City, NY: Doubleday.

Dubos, R. (1965). *Man adapting.* New Haven, CT: Yale University Press.

Erikson, E. H. (1964). *Insight and responsibility.* New York: W. W. Norton.

Erikson, E. H. (1968). *Identity: Youth and crisis.* New York: W. W. Norton.

Gibson, J. E. (1966). *The senses considered as perceptual systems.* Boston: Houghton Mifflin.

Goldstein, K. (1963). *The organism.* Boston: Beacon Press.

Griffith-Kenney, J. W., & Christensen, P. (1986). *Nursing process: Application of theories, frameworks, and models* (pp. 6, 24-25), St. Louis: Mosby.

Hall, E. (1966). *The hidden dimension.* Garden City, NY: Doubleday.

Rogers, M. E. (1970). An introduction to the theoretical basis of nursing. Philadelphia: F. A. Davis.

Selye, H. (1956). *The stress of life.* New York: McGraw-Hill.

Sherrington, A. (1906). *Integrative function of the nervous system.* New York: Charles Scribner's Sons.

Taylor, J. & Ballenger, S. (1980). *Neurological dysfunction and nursing interventions.* New York: McGraw-Hill.

Journal Articles

Bates, M. (1967). A naturalist at large. *Natural History, 76*(6), 8-16.

Brunner, M. (1985). A conceptual approach to critical care nursing using Levine's model. *Focus on Critical Care, 12*(2), 39-40.

Bunting, S. M. (1988, Nov.). The concept of perception in selected nursing theories. *Nursing Science Quarterly, 1*(4), 168-174.

Cooper, D. M. (1990, March). Optimizing wound healing: A practice within nursing's domain. *Nursing Clinics of North America, 25*(1), 165-180.

Crawford-Gamble, P. E. (1986). An application of Levine's conceptual model. *Perioperative Nursing Quarterly, 2*(1), 64-70.

Fawcett, J., Brophy, S. F., Rather, M. L., & Roos, J. (1997). Commentary about Levine's on creativity in nursing. *Image: The Journal of Nursing Scholarship, 29*(3), 218-219.

Fawcett, J., Tulman, L., & Samarel, N. (1995). Enhancing function in life transitions and serious illness. *Advance Practice Nursing Quarterly, 1,* 50-57.

Flaskerud, J. H., & Halloran, E. J. (1980). Areas of agreement in nursing theory development. *ANS Advances in Nursing Science, 3*(1), 1-7.

Foreman, M. D. (1989, Feb.). Confusion in the hospitalized elderly: Incidence, onset, and associated factors. *Research in Nursing and Health, 12*(1), 21-29.

Hall, K. V. (1979). Current trends in the use of conceptual frameworks in nursing education. *Journal of Nursing Education, 18*(4), 26-29.

Happ, M. B., Williams, C. C., Strumpf, N. E., & Burger, S. G. (1996). Individualized care for frail elderly: Theory and practice. *Journal of Gerontological Nursing, 22*(3), 6-14.

Hirschfeld, M. J. (1976). The cognitively impaired older adult. *American Journal of Nursing, 76,* 1981-1984.

Jost, S. G. (2000). An assessment and intervention strategy for managing staff needs during change. *Journal of Nursing Administration, 30*(1), 34-40.

Langer, V. S. (1990). Minimal handling protocol for the intensive care nursery. *Neonatal Network-Journal of Neonatal Nursing, 9*(3), 23-27.

Lynn-McHale, D. J., & Smith, A. (1991). Comprehensive assessment of families of the critically ill. *AACN Clinical Issues in Critical Care Nursing, 2*(2), 195-209.

Molchany, C. B. (1992). Ventricular septal and free wall rupture complicating acute MI. *Journal of Cardiovascular Nursing, 6*(4), 38-45.

Newport, M. A. (1984). Conserving thermal energy and social integrity in the newborn. *Western Journal of Nursing Research, 6*(2), 175-197.

O'Laughlin, K. M. (1986). Change in bladder function in the woman undergoing radical hysterectomy for cervical cancer. *Journal of Obstetrical, Gynecological and Neonatal Nursing, 15*(5), 380-385.

Piccoli, M., & Galvao, C. M. (2001). Perioperative nursing: Identification of the nursing diagnosis infection risk based on Levine's conceptual model (English abstract). *Revista Latino-Americana de Enfermagem, 9*(4), 37-43.

Roberts, K. L., Brittin, M., Cook, M., & deClifford, J. (1994). Boomerang pillows and respiratory capacity. *Clinical Nursing Research, 3*(2), 157-165.

Roberts, K. L., Brittin, M., & deClifford, J. (1995). Boomerang pillows and respiratory capacity in frail elderly women. *Clinical Nursing Research, 4*(4), 465-471.

Savage, T. V., & Culbert, C. (1989). Early intervention: The unique role of nursing. *Journal of Pediatric Nursing, 4*(5), 339-345.

Schaefer, K. M. (1997). Levine's Conservation Model in nursing practice. In M. R. Alligood & A. Marriner Tomey (Eds.), *Nursing theory: Utilization & application* (pp. 89-107). St. Louis: Mosby.

Schaefer, K. M., & Pond, J. (1994). Levine's Conservation Model as a guide to nursing practice. *Nursing Science Quarterly, 7*(2), 53-54.

Schaefer, K. M., & Shober-Potylycki, M. J. (1993). Fatigue in congestive heart failure: Use of Levine's Conservation Model. *Journal of Advanced Nursing, 18,* 260-268.

Schaefer, K. M., Swavely, D., Rothenberger, C., Hess, S., & Willistin, D. (1996). Sleep disturbances post coronary artery bypass surgery. *Progress in Cardiovascular Nursing, 11*(1), 5-14.

Stafford, M. J. (1996). In tribute: Myra Estrin Levine, Professor Emerita, MSN, RN, FAAN. *Chart, 93*(3), 5-6.

Taylor, J. W. (1974). Measuring the outcomes of nursing care. *Nursing Clinics of North America, 9,* 337-348.

Tillich, P. (1961). The meaning of health. *Perspectives in Biology and Medicine, 5,* 92-100.

Tompkins, E. S. (1980). Effect of restricted mobility and dominance on perceived duration. *Nursing Research, 29*(6), 333-338.

Tribotti, S. (1990). Admission to the neonatal intensive care unit: Reducing the risks. *Neonatal Network, 8*(4), 17-22.

Webb, H. (1993). Holistic care following a palliative Hartmann's procedure. *British Journal of Nursing, 2*(2), 128-132.

Web Sites

NurseScribe. Accessed December 20, 2004: http://*www. enursescribe.com/levine.htm*

Hahn School of Nursing and Health Science, University of San Diego. Accessed December 20, 2004: http://*www. sandiego.edu/nursing/theory/*

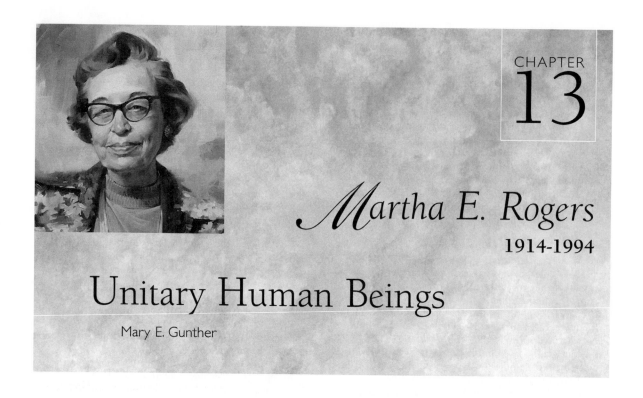

Martha E. Rogers
1914-1994

Unitary Human Beings

Mary E. Gunther

CREDENTIALS AND BACKGROUND OF THE THEORIST

Martha Elizabeth Rogers, eldest of four children of Bruce Taylor Rogers and Lucy Mulholland Keener Rogers, was born May 12, 1914, in Dallas, Texas. Soon after her birth, her family returned to Knoxville, Tennessee. She began her college education (1931 to 1933) studying science at the University of Tennessee. Receiving her nursing diploma from Knoxville General Hospital School of Nursing (1936), she quickly obtained a B.S. from George Peabody College in Nashville, Tennessee (1937). Her other degrees include an M.A. in public health nursing supervision from Teachers College,

Columbia University, New York (1945) and an M.P.H. (1952) and an Sc.D. (1954) from Johns Hopkins University in Baltimore.

Rogers' early nursing practice was in rural public health nursing in Michigan and in visiting nurse supervision, education, and practice in Connecticut. Rogers subsequently established the Visiting Nurse Service of Phoenix, Arizona. For 21 years (from 1954 to 1975), she was professor and head of the Division of Nursing at New York University. After 1975, she continued her duties as professor until she became Professor Emerita in 1979. She held this title until her death on March 13, 1994, at the age of 79.

Rogers' publications include three books and more than 200 articles. She lectured in 46 states, the District of Columbia, Puerto Rico, Mexico, the Netherlands, China, Newfoundland, Columbia, Brazil, and other countries (M. Rogers, personal communication, March 1988). Rogers received honorary doctorates from such renowned institutions as

Previous authors: Kaye Bultemeier, Mary Gunther, Joann Sebastian Daily, Judy Sporleder Maupin, Cathy A. Murray, Martha Carole Satterly, Denise L. Schnell, and Therese L. Wallace. Earlier editions of this chapter were critiqued by Dr. Lois Meier and Dr. Martha Rogers.

Duquesne University, University of San Diego, Iona College, Fairfield University, Emory University, Adelphi University, Mercy College, and Washburn University of Topeka. The numerous awards for her contributions and leadership in nursing include citations for Inspiring Leadership in the Field of Intergroup Relations by Chi Eta Phi Sorority, In Recognition of Your Outstanding Contribution to Nursing by New York University, and For Distinguished Service to Nursing by Teachers College. In addition, New York University houses the Martha E. Rogers Center for the Study of Nursing Science. In 1996, Rogers was posthumously inducted into the American Nurses Association Hall of Fame.

In 1988, colleagues and students joined her in forming the Society of Rogerian Scholars (SRS) and immediately began publishing *Rogerian Nursing Science News,* a members' newsletter, to disseminate theory developments and research studies (Malinski & Barrett, 1994). In 1993, SRS began publishing an annual refereed journal, *Visions: The Journal of Rogerian Nursing Science* (Malinski & Barrett, 1994). The society maintains and administers the Martha E. Rogers Fund. Keeping pace with the newest information technology, Rogers has a Web site and listserv based in Wales (*http://medweb.uwcm.uk. martha*). In 1995, New York University established the Martha E. Rogers Center (*http://education.nyu. edu/steinhardt/db/centers/9*) to provide a structure for continuation of Rogerian research and practice.

A verbal portrait of Rogers includes such descriptive terms as stimulating, challenging, controversial, idealistic, visionary, prophetic, philosophical, academic, outspoken, humorous, blunt, and ethical. Rogers remains a widely recognized scholar honored for her contributions and leadership in nursing.

Butcher (1999) noted, "Rogers, like Nightingale, was extremely independent, a determined, perfectionist individual who trusted her vision despite skepticism" (p. 114). Colleagues consider her one of the most original thinkers in nursing as she synthesized and resynthesized knowledge into "an entirely new system of thought" (Butcher, 1999, p. 111). Today she is thought of as "ahead of her time, in and out of this world" (Ireland, 2000, p. 59).

THEORETICAL SOURCES

Rogers' grounding in the liberal arts and sciences is apparent in both the origin and development of her conceptual model published in 1970 as *An Introduction to the Theoretical Basis of Nursing* (Rogers, 1970). Aware of the interrelatedness of knowledge, Rogers credited scientists from multiple disciplines with influencing the development of the Science of Unitary Human Beings. Rogerian science emerged from the knowledge bases of anthropology, psychology, sociology, astronomy, religion, philosophy, history, biology, physics, mathematics, and literature to create a model of unitary human beings and the environment as energy fields integral to the life process (Falco & Lobo, 1980). Within nursing, the origins of Rogerian science can be traced to Nightingale's proposals and statistical data, placing the human being within the framework of the natural world. This "foundation for the scope of modern nursing" began nursing's investigation of the relationship between human beings and the environment (Rogers, 1970, p. 30). Newman (1997) describes the Science of Unitary Human Beings as "the study of the moving, intuitive experience of nurses in mutual process with those they serve" (p. 9).

MAJOR CONCEPTS *&* DEFINITIONS

In 1970, Rogers' conceptual model of nursing rested on a set of basic assumptions that described the life process in human beings. Wholeness, openness, unidirectionality, pattern and organization, sentience, and thought characterized the life process (Rogers, 1970).

MAJOR CONCEPTS *&* DEFINITIONS—cont'd

Rogers postulates that human beings are dynamic energy fields integral with environmental fields. Both human and environmental fields are identified by pattern and characterized by a universe of open systems. In her 1983 paradigm, Rogers postulated four building blocks for her model: energy field, a universe of open systems, pattern, and four dimensionality (Rogers, 1983).

Rogers consistently updated the conceptual model through revision of the homeodynamic principles. Such changes corresponded with scientific and technological advances. In 1983, Rogers changed her wording from that of unitary man to unitary human being to remove the concept of gender. Additional clarification of unitary human beings as separate and different from the term *holistic* stressed the unique contribution of nursing to health care. In 1992, four dimensionality evolved into pandimensionality. Rogers' fundamental postulates have remained consistent since their introduction; her subsequent writings served to clarify her original ideas.

ENERGY FIELD

An energy field constitutes the fundamental unit of both the living and the nonliving. Field is a unifying concept and energy signifies the dynamic nature of the field. Energy fields are infinite and pandimensional. Two fields are identified: the human field and the environmental field (Rogers, 1983). "Specifically human beings and environment are energy fields" (Rogers, 1986b, p. 2). The unitary human being (human field) is defined as an irreducible, indivisible, pandimensional energy field identified by pattern and manifesting characteristics that are specific to the whole and that cannot be predicted from knowledge of the parts. The environmental field is defined as an irreducible, pandimensional energy field identified by pattern and integral with the human field. Each environmental field is specific to its given human field. Both change continuously, creatively, and integrally (Rogers, 1994a).

UNIVERSE OF OPEN SYSTEMS

The concept of the universe of open systems holds that energy fields are infinite, open, and integral with one another (Rogers, 1983). The human and the environmental field are in continuous process and are open systems.

PATTERN

Pattern identifies energy fields. It is the distinguishing characteristic of an energy field and is perceived as a single wave. The nature of the pattern changes continuously, innovatively, and these changes give identity to the energy field. Each human field pattern is unique and is integral with the environmental field (Rogers, 1983). Manifestations emerge as a human-environmental mutual process. Pattern is an abstraction; it reveals itself through manifestation. "Manifestations of pattern have been described as unique and refer to behaviors, qualities, and characteristics of the field" (Clarke, 1986, p. 30). A sense of self is a field manifestation, the nature of which is unique to each individual. Some variations in pattern manifestations have been described in phrases such as longer versus shorter rhythms, pragmatic versus imaginative, and time experienced as fast or slow. Pattern is continually changing and may manifest disease, illness, feelings, or pain (Wright, 1987). Pattern change is continuous, innovative, and relative.

PANDIMENSIONALITY

Rogers defines pandimensionality as a nonlinear domain without spatial or temporal attributes. The term *pandimensional* provides for an infinite domain without limit. It best expresses the idea of a unitary whole.

USE OF EMPIRICAL EVIDENCE

Being an abstract conceptual system, the Science of Unitary Human Beings does not directly identify testable empirical indicators. Rather it specifies a worldview and philosophy used to identify the phenomena of concern to the discipline of nursing. As mentioned previously, Rogers' model emerged from multiple knowledge sources; the most readily apparent of these are the nonlinear dynamics of quantum physics and general system theory.

Evident in her model are the influence of Einstein's (1961) theory of relativity in relation to space-time and Burr and Northrop's (1935) electro-dynamic theory relating to electrical fields. By the time von Bertalanffy (1960) introduced general system theory, theories regarding a universe of open systems were beginning to affect the development of knowledge within all disciplines. With general system theory, the term *negentropy* was brought into use to signify increasing order, complexity, and heterogeneity in direct contrast to the previously held belief that the universe was winding down. Rogers, however, refined and purified general system theory by denying hierarchical subsystems, the concept of single causation, and predictability of a system's behavior through investigations of its parts.

Introducing quantum theory and the theories of relativity and of probability fundamentally challenged the prevailing absolutism. As new knowledge escalated, the traditional meanings of homeostasis, steady state, adaptation, and equilibrium were questioned seriously. The closed-system, entropic model of the universe was no longer adequate to explain phenomena, and evidence accumulated in support of a universe of open systems (Rogers, 1994b). The continuing development within other disciplines of the acausal, nonlinear dynamics of life validated Rogers' model. Most notable of this development is that of chaos theory, quantum physics' contribution to the science of complexity (or wholeness), that blurs the boundaries between the disciplines, allowing an exploration and deepening of the understanding of the totality of human experience.

MAJOR ASSUMPTIONS
Nursing

Nursing is a learned profession, both a science and an art. It is an empirical science and, like that of other sciences, lies in the phenomenon central to its focus. Rogerian nursing focuses on concern with people and the world in which they live, a natural fit for nursing care, as it encompasses people and their environments. The integrality of people and their environments, operating from a pandimensional universe of open systems, points to a new paradigm and initiates the identity of nursing as a science. The purpose of nursing is to promote health and well-being for all persons. The art of nursing is the creative use of the science of nursing for human betterment (Rogers, 1994b). "Professional practice in nursing seeks to promote symphonic interaction between human and environmental fields, to strengthen the integrity of the human field, and to direct and redirect patterning of the human and environmental fields for realization of maximum health potential" (Rogers, 1970, p. 122). Nursing exists for the care of people and the life process of humans.

Person

Rogers defines *person* as an open system in continuous process with the open system that is the environment (integrality). She defines *unitary human being* as an "irreducible, indivisible, pandimensional energy field identified by pattern and manifesting characteristics that are specific to the whole" (Rogers, 1992, p. 29). Human beings "are not disembodied entities, nor are they mechanical aggregates. . . . Man is a unified whole possessing his own integrity and manifesting characteristics that are more than and different from the sum of his parts" (Rogers, 1970, pp. 46-47). Within a conceptual model specific to nursing's concern, people and their environment are perceived as irreducible energy fields integral with one another and continuously creative in their evolution.

Health

Rogers uses health in many of her earlier writings without clearly defining the term. She uses the term *passive health* to symbolize wellness and the absence of disease and major illness (Rogers, 1970). Her promotion of positive health connotes direction in helping people with opportunities for rhythmic consistency (Rogers, 1970). Later, she wrote that wellness "is a much better term . . . because the term health is very ambiguous" (Rogers, 1994b, p. 34).

Rogers uses health as a value term defined by the culture or individual. Health and illness are manifestations of pattern and are considered "to denote behaviors that are of high value and low value" (Rogers, 1980). Events manifested in the life process indicate the extent to which a human being achieves maximum health according to some value system. In Rogerian science, the phenomenon central to nursing's conceptual system is the human life process. The life process has its own dynamic and creative unity, inseparable from the environment, and is characterized by the whole (Rogers, 1970).

In "Dimensions of Health: A View from Space," Rogers (1986b) reaffirms the original theoretical assertions, adding philosophical challenges to the prevailing perception of health. Stressing a new world view that focuses on people and their environment, she lists iatrogenesis, nosocomial conditions, and hypochrondriasis as the major health problems in the United States. Rogers (1986b) writes, "A new world view compatible with the most progressive knowledge available is a necessary prelude to studying human health and to determining modalities for its promotion whether on this planet or in the outer reaches of space" (p. 2).

Environment

Rogers (1994a) defines environment as "an irreducible, pandimensional energy field identified by pattern and manifesting characteristics different from those of the parts. Each environmental field is specific to its given human field. Both change continuously and creatively" (p. 2). Environmental fields are infinite, and change is continuously innovative, unpredictable, and characterized by increasing diversity. Environmental and human fields are identified by wave patterns manifesting continuous change. Environmental and human fields are in continuous and mutual process (Barrett, 1990b).

THEORETICAL ASSERTIONS

The principles of homeodynamics postulate a way of perceiving unitary human beings. The evolution of these principles from 1970 to 1994 is depicted in Table 13-1. Rogers (1970) wrote, "The life process is homeodynamic. . . . These principles postulate the way the life process is and predict the nature of its evolving" (p. 96). Rogers identified the principles of change as helicy, resonancy, and integrality. The helicy principle describes spiral development in continuous, nonrepeating, and innovative patterning. Rogers' articulation of the principle of helicy describing the nature of change evolved from probabilistic to unpredictable, while remaining continuous and innovative. According to the principle of resonancy, patterning changes with development from lower to higher frequency, that is, with varying degrees of intensity. Resonancy embodies wave frequency and energy field pattern evolution. Integrality, the third principle of homeodynamics, stresses the continuous mutual process of person and environment. The principles of homeodynamics evolved into a concise and clear description of the nature, process, and context of change within human and environmental energy fields (Hills & Hanchett, 2001).

In 1970, Rogers identified the following five assumptions that are also theoretical assertions supporting her model derived from literature on human beings, physics, mathematics, and behavioral science:

1. "Man is a unified whole possessing his own integrity and manifesting characteristics more than and different from the sum of his parts" (energy field) (p. 47).
2. "Man and environment are continuously exchanging matter and energy with one another" (openness) (p. 54).

Table **13-1**

Evolution of Principles of Homeodynamics: 1970, 1983, 1986, and 1992

AN INTRODUCTION TO THE THEORETICAL BASIS OF NURSING, 1970	NURSING: A SCIENCE OF UNITARY MAN, 1980	SCIENCE OF UNITARY HUMAN BEINGS: A PARADIGM FOR NURSING, 1983	DIMENSIONS OF HEALTH: A VIEW FROM SPACE, 1986	NURSING SCIENCE AND THE SPACE AGE, 1992
RESONANCY				
Continuously propagating series of waves between man and environment	Continuous change from lower- to higher-frequency wave patterns in the human and environmental fields	Continuous change from lower- to higher-frequency wave patterns in the human and environmental fields	Continuous change from lower- to higher-frequency wave patterns in the human and environmental fields	Continuous change from lower- to higher-frequency wave patterns in the human and environmental fields
HELICY				
Continuous, innovative change growing out of mutual interaction of man and environment along a spiraling longitudinal axis bound in space-time	Nature of change between human and environmental fields is continuously innovative, probabilistic, and increasingly diverse, manifesting nonrepeating rhythmicities	Continuous innovative, probabilistic, increasing diversity of human and environmental field patterns, characterized by nonrepeating rhythmicities	Continuous, innovative, probabilistic, increasing human and environmental diversity characterized by nonrepeating rhythmicities	Continuous, innovative, unpredictable, increasing diversity of human and environmental field patterns
RECIPROCY				
Continuous mutual interaction between the human field and environmental field	—	—	—	—

Continued

Table **13-1**

Evolution of Principles of Homeodynamics: 1970, 1983, 1986, and 1992—cont'd				
AN INTRODUCTION TO THE THEORETICAL BASIS OF NURSING, 1970	NURSING: A SCIENCE OF UNITARY MAN, 1980	SCIENCE OF UNITARY HUMAN BEINGS: A PARADIGM FOR NURSING, 1983	DIMENSIONS OF HEALTH: A VIEW FROM SPACE, 1986	NURSING SCIENCE AND THE SPACE AGE, 1992
SYNCHRONY				
Change in the human field and simultaneous state of environmental field at any given point in space-time	Continuous, mutual, simultaneous interaction between human and environmental fields	Continuous, mutual human field and environmental field process	Continuous, mutual human field and environmental field process	Continuous, mutual human field and environmental field process

Conceptualized by Joann Daily from the following sources:

Riehl, J. P., & Roy, C. (Eds.). (1980). *Conceptual models for nursing practice* (2nd ed.). New York: Appleton-Century-Crofts.

Rogers, M. E. (1970). *An introduction to the theoretical basis of nursing*. Philadelphia: F. A. Davis.

Rogers, M. E. (1983). Science of unitary human beings: A paradigm for nursing. In I. W. Clements & F. B. Roberts (Eds.), *Family health: A theoretical approach to nursing care*. New York: John Wiley & Sons.

Table revised by Denise Schnell and Therese Wallace in 1988 to include the following source:

Rogers, M. E. (1986b). *Dimensions of health: A view from space* (obtained through personal correspondence with Martha Rogers, March 1988).

Table updated by Cathy Murray from the following source:

Rogers, M. E. (1992). Nursing science and the space age. *Nursing Science Quarterly, 5*(1), 27-34.

3. "The life process evolves irreversibly and unidirectionally along the space-time continuum" (helicy) (p. 59).
4. "Pattern and organization identify man and reflect his innovative wholeness" (pattern and organization) (p. 65).
5. "Man is characterized by the capacity for abstraction and imagery, language and thought, sensation, and emotion" (sentient, thinking being) (p. 73).

LOGICAL FORM

Rogers uses a dialectic method as opposed to a logistical, problematic, or operational method; that is,

Rogers explains nursing by referring to broader principles that explain human beings. She then explains human beings through principles that characterize the universe. The method is based on the perspective of a whole that organizes the parts (McHugh, 1986).

Rogers' model of unitary human beings is deductive and logical. The theory of relativity, general system theory, electrodynamic theory of life, and many other theories contributed ideas for Rogers' model. Unitary human beings and environment, the central components of the model, are integral with one another. The basic building blocks of her model are energy field, openness, pattern, and pandimensionality providing a new worldview. These concepts form the basis of an abstract conceptual system defining nursing and health. From the abstract conceptual system, Rogers derives the principles of homeodynamics, which postulate the nature and direction of human beings' evolution. Although Rogers invents the words *homeodynamics* (similar state of change and growth), *helicy* (evolution), *resonancy* (intensity of change), and *integrality* (wholeness), all definitions are etymologically consistent and logical.

ACCEPTANCE BY THE NURSING COMMUNITY

Practice

The Rogerian model is an abstract system of ideas from which to approach the practice of nursing. Rogers' model, stressing the totality of experience and existence, is relevant in today's health care system where continuum of care is more important than episodic illness and hospitalization. The model provides the abstract philosophical framework from which to view the unitary human-environmental field phenomenon. Within the Rogerian framework, nursing is based on theoretical knowledge that guides nursing practice. The professional practice of nursing is creative and imaginative and exists to serve people. It is rooted in intellectual judgment, abstract knowledge, and human compassion.

Historically, nursing has equated practice with the practical and theory with the impractical. More appropriately, theory and practice are two related components in a unified nursing practice. Alligood (1994) articulates how theory and practice direct and guide each other as they expand and increase nursing knowledge. Nursing knowledge provides the framework for the emergent artistic application of nursing care (Rogers, 1970).

Within Rogers' model, the critical thinking process directing practice can be divided into three components: pattern appraisal, mutual patterning, and evaluation. Cowling (1990) introduced a template for pattern-based nursing practice. The template emerged from Rogerian science and is widely

accepted by nurses functioning within the Rogerian model. Bultemeier (2002), who expanded on the ideas of Cowling and articulated Rogerian nursing from a theoretical and practice stance, outlined further clarification of practice from the unitary perspective.

Cowling (1993, 2000) states that pattern appraisal is meant to avoid, if not transcend, reductionistic categories of physical, mental, spiritual, emotional, cultural, and social assessment frameworks. Through observation and participation, the nurse focuses on human expressions of reflection, experience, and perception to form a profile of the patient. Mutual exploration of emergent patterns allows identification of unitary themes predominant in pandimensional human-environmental field process. Mutual understanding implies knowing participation but does not lead to the nurse prescribing change or predicting outcomes. As Cowling (2000) explains, "A critical feature of the unitary pattern appreciation process, and also of healing through appreciating wholeness, is a willingness on the part of the scientist or practitioner to let go of expectations about change" (p. 31). Evaluation centers on the perceptions emerging during mutual patterning.

Noninvasive patterning modalities used within Rogerian practice include, but are not limited to, therapeutic touch, massage, guided imagery, meditation, self-reflection, guided reminiscence, journal keeping, humor, hypnosis, sleep, hygiene, dietary manipulation, music, and physical exercise (Alligood, 1991a; Barrett, 2000; Bultemeier, 1993; Covington, 2001; Malinski, 1986; Smith, Kemp, Hemphill, & Vojir, 2002; Wright, 1987). Barrett (1998) notes that integral to these modalities are "meaningful dialogue, centering, and pandimensional authenticity (genuineness, trustworthiness, acceptance, and knowledgeable caring)" (p. 138). Nurses participate in the lived experience of health in a multitude of roles, including "facilitators and educators, advocates, assessors, planners, coordinators, and collaborators" by accepting diversity, recognizing patterns, viewing change as positive, and accepting the connectedness of life (Malinski, 1986, p. 27) These roles may require the nurse to "let go of traditional ideas of time, space, and outcome" (Malinski, 1997, p. 115).

The Rogerian model provides a challenging and innovative framework from which to plan and implement nursing practice, which Barrett (1998) defines as the "continuous process (of voluntary mutual patterning) whereby the nurse assists clients to freely choose with awareness ways to participate in their well-being" (p. 136).

Education

Rogers clearly articulated guidelines for the education of nurses within the Science of Unitary Human Beings. Rogers discusses structuring nursing education programs to teach nursing as a science and as a learned profession. Barrett (1990b) calls Rogers a "consistent voice crying out against antieducationalism and dependency" (p. 306). Rogers' model clearly articulates values and beliefs about human beings, health, nursing, and the educational process. As such, it has been used to guide curriculum development in all levels of nursing education (Barrett, 1990b; Hellwig & Ferrante, 1993; Mathwig, Young, & Pepper, 1990). Rogers (1990) stated that nurses must commit to lifelong learning and noted "The nature of the practice of nursing (the use of knowledge for human betterment)" (p. 111).

Rogers advocated separate licensure for nurses prepared with an associate degree and those with a baccalaureate degree, recognizing that there is a difference between the technically oriented and the professional nurse. In her view, the professional nurse needs to be well rounded and educated in the humanities, sciences, and nursing. Such a program would include a basic education in language, mathematics, logic, philosophy, psychology, sociology, music, art, biology, microbiology, physics, and chemistry; elective courses could include economics, ethics, political science, anthropology, and computer science (Barrett, 1990b). In regard to the research component of the curriculum, Rogers (1994b) stated the following:

> Undergraduate students need to be able to identify problems, to have tools of investigation and to do

studies that will allow them to use knowledge for the improvement of practice, and they should be able to read the literature intelligently. People with master's degrees ought to be able to do applied research. . . . The theoretical research, the fundamental basic research is going to come out of doctoral programs of stature that focus on nursing as a learned field of endeavor. (p. 34)

Barrett (1990b) notes that with increasing use of technology and severity of illness of hospitalized patients, students may be limited to observational experiences in these institutions. Therefore, the acquisition of manipulative technical skills must be accomplished in practice laboratories and alternative sites, such as clinics and home health agencies. Other sites for education include health-promotion programs, managed-care programs, homeless shelters, and senior centers.

Research

Rogers' conceptual model provides a stimulus and direction for research and theory development in nursing science. Fawcett (2000), who insists that the level of abstraction affects direct empirical observation and testing, endorses the designation of the Science of Unitary Human Beings as a conceptual model rather than a grand theory. She states clearly that the purpose of the work determines its category. If, as in the case of the Science of Unitary Human Beings, the purpose of the work is to "articulate a body of distinctive knowledge," the work is a conceptual model (Fawcett, 1995, p. 27).

Emerging from Rogers' model are theories that explain human phenomena and direct nursing practice. The Rogerian model, with its implicit assumptions, provides broad principles that conceptually direct theory development. The conceptual model provides a stimulus and direction for scientific activity. Relationships among identified phenomena generate both grand (further development of one aspect of the model) and middle range (description, explanation, or prediction of concrete aspects) theories (Fawcett, 1995).

Two prominent grand nursing theories grounded in Rogers' model are Newman's health as expanding consciousness and Parse's Human Becoming (Fawcett, 2000). Numerous middle range theories have emerged out of Rogers' three homeodynamic principles as follows: (1) helicy, (2) resonancy, and (3) integrality (Figure 13-1). Exemplars of middle range theories derived from the homeodynamic principles include power-as-knowing-participation-in-change (helicy) (Barrett, 1990a), the theory of perceived dissonance (resonancy) (Bultemeier, 1993), and the theory of interactive rhythms (integrality) (Floyd, 1983). Other middle range theories encompass the phenomena of human field motion (Ference, 1986b); creativity, actualization, and empathy (Alligood, 1991b); and self-transcendence (Reed, 1991).

Rogers (1986a) maintains that research in nursing must examine unitary human beings as integral with their environment. Therefore the intent of nursing research is to examine and understand a phenomenon and, from this understanding,

design patterning activities that promote healing. To obtain a clearer understanding of lived experiences, the person's perception and sentient awareness of what is occurring are imperative. The variety of events associated with human phenomena provides the experiential data for research that is directed toward capturing the dynamic, ever-changing life experiences of human beings. Selecting the correct methodology for examining the person and the environment as health-related phenomena is the challenge of the Rogerian researcher. Both quantitative and qualitative approaches have been used in the Science of Unitary Human Beings research, although not all researchers agree that both are appropriate. Researchers do agree that ontological and epistemological congruence between the model and the approach must be considered and reflected by the research question (Barrett, Cowling, Carboni, & Butcher, 1997). Quantitative experimental and

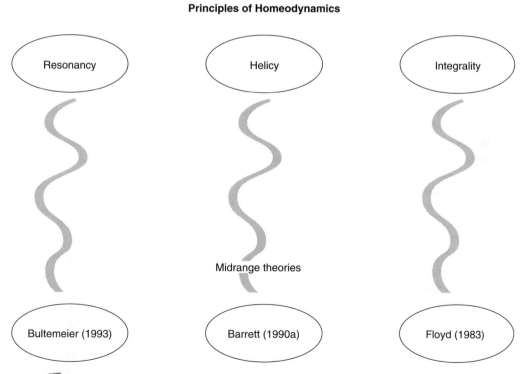

Principles of Homeodynamics

Resonancy   Helicy   Integrality

Midrange theories

Bultemeier (1993)   Barrett (1990a)   Floyd (1983)

Figure **13-1** Theory development within the Science of Unitary Human Beings.

quasi-experimental designs are not appropriate, because their purpose is to reveal causal relationships. Descriptive, explanatory, and correlational designs are more appropriate, because they recognize "the unitary nature of the phenomenon of interest" and may "propose evidence of patterned mutual change among variables" (Sherman, 1997, p. 132).

Specific research methodologies emerging from middle range theories based on the Rogerian model capture the human-environmental phenomena. As a means of capturing the unitary human being, Cowling (1998) describes the process of pattern appreciation using the combined research and practice case study method. Case study attends to the whole person (irreducibility), aims at comprehending the essence (pattern), and respects the inherent interconnectedness of phenomena. A pattern profile is composed through a synopsis and synthesis of the data (Barrett, et al., 1997). Other innovative methods of recording and entering the human-environmental field phenomenon include photodisclosure (Bultemeier, 1997), hermeneutic text interpretation (Alligood & Fawcett, 1999), and the measurement of the effect of dialogue combined with noninvasive modalities (Leddy & Fawcett, 1997).

Rogerian instrument development is extensive and ever-evolving. A wide range of instruments for measuring human-environmental field phenomena has emerged (Table 13-2). The continual emergence of middle range theories, methodologies, and instruments demonstrate recognition of the importance of Rogerian science to nursing.

FURTHER DEVELOPMENT

Rogers (1986a) believed that knowledge development within her model was a "never-ending process" using "a multiplicity of knowledge from many sources . . . to create a kaleidoscope of possibilities" (p. 4). Recent explorations by Rogerian scholars into Buddhist, Hindu, and aboriginal philosophies exemplify this belief in an essential unity (Madrid, 1997).

Fawcett (2000) identified the following three rudimentary theories developed by Rogers from the Science of Unitary Human Beings:
1. Theory of accelerating evolution
2. Theory of rhythmical correlates of change
3. Theory of paranormal phenomena

Further explication and testing of these theories and the homeodynamic principles will contribute to nursing science knowledge.

CRITIQUE
Simplicity

Ongoing studies and work within the model have served to simplify and clarify some of the concepts and relationships. However, when the model is examined in total perspective, some still classify it as complex. With its continued use in practice, research, and education, nurses will come to appreciate the model's elegant simplicity. As Whall (1987) notes, "With only three principles, a few major concepts, and five assumptions, Rogers has explained the nature of man and the life process" (p. 154).

Generality

Rogers' conceptual model is abstract and therefore generalizable and powerful. It is broad in scope, providing a framework for the development of nursing knowledge through the generation of grand and middle range theories.

Empirical Precision

Early criticisms of the model identified its major limitations as difficult-to-understand principles, lack of operational definitions, and inadequate tools for measurement (Butterfield, 1983). Drawing on knowledge from a multitude of scientific fields, Rogers' conceptual model is deductive in logic with the inherent lack of immediate empirical support (Barrett, 1990b). As Fawcett (1995) points out, failure to properly categorize the work as a conceptual model rather than a theory leads to "considerable misunderstandings and inappropriate

Table 13-2

Instruments Developed Within Rogers' Science of Unitary Human Beings

INSTRUMENT	CONSTRUCT	AUTHOR
Power-as-knowing-participation-in-change theory (PKPCT)	Power	Barrett (1990a)
Mutual exploration of the healing human-environmental field relationship	Healing human-environmental mutual process	Carboni (1992)
Human field motion test (HFMT)	Human field motion	Ference (1986a, 1986b)
Index of field energy (IFE)	Human field dynamics	Gueldner (1993)
Diversity of human field pattern scale (DHFPS)	Human field pattern diversity	Hastings-Tolsma (1992)
Human field image metaphor scale	Individual awareness of the infinite wholeness of the human field	Johnston (1994)
Person-environment participation scale (PEPS)	Experience of continuous human-environmental mutual process	Leddy (1995)
Leddy healthiness scale	Healthiness	Leddy (1996)
Temporal experience scale (TES)	Subjective experience of temporal awareness	Paletta (1990)
Assessment of dream experience	Dreaming as a beyond-waking experience	Watson (1993)
Perceived field motion (PFM) scale	Human field motion	Yarcheski & Mahon (1991)
Human field rhythms	Experience of rhythms in human-environmental field mutual process	Yarcheski & Mahon (1991)

Modified from Instruments developed within Rogers' science of unitary human beings. (1996). *Rogerian Nursing Science News*, *8*(4), 9-12.

expectations" (p. 29), which can result in the work being labeled inadequate.

As noted earlier, the development of the model by Rogerian scientists has resulted in the generation of testable theories accompanied by tools of measurement.

Derivable Consequences

Rogers' science has the fundamental intent of understanding human evolution and its potential.

It "coordinates a universe of open systems to identify the focus of a new paradigm and initiate nursing's identity as a science" (Rogers, 1989, p. 182).

Although all the metaparadigm concepts are explored, the emphasis is on the integrality of human-environmental field phenomena. Rogers (Ference, 1986b) suggested many ideas for future studies; on the basis of this and the research of others, it can be said that the conceptual model is useful. Such utility has been proven in the arenas of practice, education, and research.

SUMMARY

The Rogerian model emerged from a broad historical base and has moved to the forefront as scientific knowledge has evolved. Understanding the concepts and principles of the Science of Unitary Human Beings requires a foundation in general education, a willingness to let go of the traditional, and an ability to perceive the world in a new and creative way. Emerging from a strong educational base, the model provides a challenging framework from which to provide nursing care. The abstract ideas expounded in the Rogerian model and their congruence with modern scientific knowledge spur new and challenging theories that further the understanding of the unitary human being. Nursing scholars and practitioners are carrying Rogers' ideas into the next century.

Case Study

Charlie Dee is a 56-year-old male with a 30-year history of smoking two packs of cigarettes a day. He is seeing nurse practitioner, Sandra Gee, for the first time after being diagnosed with chronic obstructive pulmonary disease. Pattern appraisal begins with eliciting the client's description of his experience with this disease, his perceptions of his health, and how the disease is expressed (symptoms). Mr. Dee states that he has a productive cough that is worse in the morning, gets short of breath whenever he is physically active, and always feels tired. Through specific questions, the nurse practitioner discovers that Mr. Dee has experienced a change in his sleep patterns and nutritional intake. He is sleeping for shorter periods and eating less. She also learns that Mr. Dee's wife smokes and that they have indoor cats for pets. He does not think that his wife will be amenable to changing her habits or getting rid of the cats. During this appraisal, the nurse seeks to discover what is important to Mr. Dee and how he defines "healthy."

Mutual patterning involves sharing knowledge and offering choices. Upon completion of the appraisal, the nurse summarizes what she has been told and how she understands it. In this way, the nurse and client can reach consensus about what activities would be acceptable to Mr. Dee. Ms. Gee provides information about the disease and suggestions that will increase his comfort. Noninvasive interventions include breathing retraining, recommendations for a high protein–high calorie diet, eating smaller meals more frequently, sleeping with his head elevated, and using progressive relaxation exercises at bedtime. The nurse recommends that the Dees buy a HEPA filter and humidifier to assist in removing environmental pollutants and maintaining the proper humidity in the home.

Because Mr. Gee has expressed a desire to quit smoking, the nurse suggests that he use forms of centering, such as guided imagery and meditation, to supplement the nicotine patches prescribed by his physician. She also provides him with written material about the disease that he can share with his wife. At the end of the visit, Mr. Dee states that he feels better knowing that he has the power to change some things about his life.

CRITICAL THINKING *Activities*

1. Identify philosophical tenets from Nightingale that contributed to the basis for the development of the Rogerian model.

2. Discuss three main areas in which Rogerian science has had an impact on current nursing education.

3. Analyze your clinical practice and identify areas in which practice based on Rogerian science would improve nursing care. Enumerate what the changes would be and identify anticipated positive outcomes.

4. Review two research articles grounded in Rogerian science. If possible, identify the middle range theory that guided the research process. What principle of homeodynamics was the middle range theory derived from?

REFERENCES

Alligood, M. R. (1991a). Guided reminiscence: A Rogerian based intervention. *Rogerian Nursing Science News,* *3*(3), 1-3.

Alligood, M. R. (1991b). Testing Rogers' theory of accelerating change: The relationship among creativity, actualization, and empathy in persons 18 to 92 years of age. *Western Journal of Nursing Research, 13,* 84-96.

Alligood, M. R. (1994). Toward a unitary view of nursing practice. In M. Madrid & E. A. M. Barrett (Eds.), *Rogers' scientific art of nursing practice* (pp. 223-240). New York: National League for Nursing.

Alligood, M. R., & Fawcett, J. (1999). Acceptance of an invitation to dialogue: Examination of an interpretive approach for the science of unitary human beings. *Visions: Journal of Rogerian Nursing Science, 7*(1), 5-13.

Barrett, E. A. M. (1990a). An instrument to measure power-as-knowing-participation-in-change. In O. Strickland & C. Waltz (Eds.), *The measurement of nursing outcomes: Measuring clients self-care and coping skills* (Vol. 4, pp. 159-180). New York: Springer.

Barrett, E. A. M. (1990b). *Visions of Rogers' science-based nursing.* New York: National League for Nursing.

Barrett, E. A. M. (1998). A Rogerian practice methodology for health patterning. *Nursing Science Quarterly, 11*(4), 136-138.

Barrett, E. A. M. (2000). The theoretical matrix for a Rogerian nursing practice. *Theoria: Journal of Nursing Theory, 9*(4), 3-7.

Barrett, E. A. M., Cowling, W. R., Carboni, J. T., & Butcher, H. K. (1997). Unitary perspectives on methodological practices. In M. Madrid (Ed.), *Patterns of Rogerian knowing* (pp. 47-62). New York: National League for Nursing.

Bultemeier, K. (1993). Photographic inquiry of the phenomenon premenstrual syndrome within the Rogerian derived theory of perceived dissonance (Doctoral dissertation, University of Tennessee, Knoxville, 1993). *Dissertation Abstracts International, 54,* 2351A.

Bultemeier, K. (1997). Photo-disclosure: A research methodology for investigating the unitary human being. In M. Madrid (Ed.), *Patterns of Rogerian knowing.* New York: National League for Nursing Press.

Bultemeier, K. (2002). Rogers' science of unitary human beings in nursing practice. In M. R. Alligood & A. M. Tomey (Eds.), *Nursing theory: Utilization & application* (2nd ed., pp. 267-288). St. Louis: Mosby.

Burr, H. S., & Northrup, F. S. C. (1935). The electrodynamic theory of life. *Quarterly Review of Biology, 10,* 322-323.

Butcher, H. K. (1999). Rogerian ethics: An ethical inquiry into Rogers' life and science. *Nursing Science Quarterly, 5,* 111-118.

Butterfield, S. E. (1983). In search of commonalties: Analysis of two theoretical frameworks. *International Journal of Nursing Studies, 20*(1), 15-22.

Carboni, J. T. (1992). Instrument development and the measurement of unitary constructs. *Nursing Science Quarterly, 5,* 134-142.

Clarke, P. N. (1986). Theoretical and measurement issues in the study of field phenomena. *ANS Advances in Nursing Science, 9*(1), 29-39.

Covington, H. (2001). Therapeutic music for patients with psychiatric disorders. *Holistic Nursing Practice, 15*(2), 59-69.

Cowling, W. R. (1990). A template for nursing practice. In E. A. M. Barrett (Ed.), *Visions of Rogers' science-based nursing* (pp. 45-65). New York: National League for Nursing.

Cowling, W. R. (1993). Unitary knowing in nursing practice. *Nursing Science Quarterly, 6*(4), 201-207.

Cowling, W. R. (1998). Unitary case inquiry. *Nursing Science Quarterly, 11*(4), 139-141.

Cowling, W. R. (2000). Healing as appreciating wholeness. *ANS Advances in Nursing Science, 22*(3), 16-32.

Einstein, A. (1961). *Relativity.* New York: Crown.

Falco, S. M., & Lobo, M. L. (1980). Martha E. Rogers. In Nursing Theories Conference Group, *Nursing theories: The base for professional practice* (pp. 164-183). Englewood Cliffs, NJ: Prentice Hall.

Fawcett, J. (1995). *Analysis and evaluation of conceptual models of nursing* (3rd ed.). Philadelphia: F. A. Davis.

Fawcett, J. (2000). *Analysis and evaluation of contemporary nursing knowledge: Nursing models and theories.* Philadelphia: F. A. Davis.

Ference, H. M. (1986a). Foundations of a nursing science and its evolution: A perspective. In V. M. Malinski (Ed.), *Explorations in Martha Rogers' science of unitary human beings* (pp. 35-44). Norwalk, CT: Appleton-Century-Crofts.

Ference, H. M. (1986b). The relationship of time experience, creativity traits, differentiation, and human field motion. In V. M. Malinski (Ed.), *Explorations in Martha Rogers' science of unitary human beings* (pp. 95-106). Norwalk, CT: Appleton-Century-Crofts.

Floyd, J. A. (1983). Research using Rogers' conceptual system: Development of a testable theorem. *ANS Advances in Nursing Science, 5*(2), 37-48.

Gueldner, S. H. (1993). *Index of field energy: A psychometric analysis.* Unpublished manuscript.

Hastings-Tolsma, M. T. (1992). The relationship of diversity of human field pattern to risk-taking and time experience: An investigation of Rogers' principles of homeodynamics (Doctoral dissertation, New York University, 1992). *Dissertation Abstracts International, 53,* 4029B.

Hellwig, S. D., & Ferrante, S. (1993). Martha Rogers' model in associate degree education. *Nurse Educator, 18*(5), 25-27.

Hills, R. G. S., & Hanchett, E. (2001). Human change and individuation in pivotal life situations: Development and testing the theory of enlightenment. *Visions: The Journal of Rogerian Nursing Science, 9*(1), 6-19.

Ireland, M. (2000). Martha Rogers' odyssey. *American Journal of Nursing, 100*(10), 59.

Johnston, L. W. (1994). Psychometric analysis of Johnston's human field image metaphor scale. *Visions: The Journal of Rogerian Nursing Science, 2*(1), 7-11.

Leddy, S. K. (1995). Measuring mutual process: Development and psychometric testing of the person-environment participation scale. *Visions: The Journal of Rogerian Nursing Science, 3*(1), 20-31.

Leddy, S. K. (1996). Development and psychometric testing of the Leddy healthiness scale. *Research in Nursing and Health, 19*(5), 431-440.

Leddy, S. K., & Fawcett, J. (1997). Testing the theory of healthiness: Conceptual and methodological issues. In M. Madrid (Ed.), *Patterns of Rogerian knowing* (pp. 75-86). New York: National League for Nursing.

Madrid, M. (Ed.). (1997). *Patterns of Rogerian knowing.* New York: National League for Nursing.

Malinski, V. M. (Ed.). (1986). *Explorations on Martha Rogers' science of unitary human beings.* New York: Appleton-Century-Crofts.

Malinski, V. M. (1997). Rogerian health patterning: Evolving into the 21st century. *Nursing Science Quarterly, 10*(3), 115-116.

Malinski, V. M., & Barrett, E. A. M. (1994). *Martha E. Rogers: Her life and her work.* Philadelphia: F. A. Davis.

Mathwig, G. M., Young, A. A., & Pepper, J. M. (1990). Using Rogerian science in undergraduate and graduate nursing education. In E. A. M. Barrett (Ed.), *Visions of Rogers' science-based nursing* (pp. 319-334). New York: National League for Nursing.

McHugh, M. (1986). Nursing process: Musings on the method. *Holistic Nursing Practice, 1*(1), 21-28.

Newman, M. A. (1997). A dialogue with Martha Rogers and David Bohm about the science of unitary human beings. In M. Madrid (Ed.), *Patterns of Rogerian knowing* (pp. 3-10). New York: National League for Nursing.

Paletta, J. L. (1990). The relationship of temporal experience to human time. In E. A. M. Barrett (Ed.), *Visions of Rogers' science-based nursing* (pp. 239-254). New York: National League for Nursing.

Reed, P. G. (1991). Toward a nursing theory of self-transcendence: Deductive reformulation using developmental theories. *ANS Advances in Nursing Science, 13*(4), 64-77.

Rogers, M. E. (1970). *An introduction to the theoretical basis of nursing.* Philadelphia: F. A. Davis.

Rogers, M. E. (1980). *The science of unitary man. Tape V: Health and illness* (Audiotape). New York: Media for Nursing.

Rogers, M. E. (1983). Science of unitary human beings: A paradigm for nursing. In I. W. Clements & F. B. Roberts, *Family health: A theoretical approach to nursing care* (pp. 219-227). New York: John Wiley & Sons.

Rogers, M. E. (1986a). Science of unitary human beings. In V. M. Malinski (Ed.), *Explorations in Martha Rogers' science of unitary human beings* (pp. 3-8). Norwalk, CT: Appleton-Century-Crofts.

Rogers, M. E. (1986b). *Dimensions of health: A view from space.* Paper presented at the conference on "Law and Life in Space," September 12, 1986. Center for Aerospace Sciences, University of North Dakota.

Rogers, M. E. (1989). Nursing: A science of unitary human beings. In J. P. Riehl-Sisca (Ed.), *Conceptual models for nursing practice* (3rd ed., pp. 181-188). Norwalk, CT: Appleton-Century-Crofts.

Rogers, M. E. (1990). Space-age paradigm for new frontiers in nursing. In M. E. Parker (Ed.), *Nursing theories in practice* (pp. 105-114). New York: National League for Nursing.

Rogers, M. E. (1992). Nursing science and the space age. *Nursing Science Quarterly, 5*(1), 27-34.

Rogers, M. E. (1994a). Nursing science evolves. In M. Madrid & E. A. M. Barrett (Eds.), *Rogers' scientific art of nursing practice* (pp. 3-9). New York: National League for Nursing.

Rogers, M. E. (1994b). The science of unitary human beings: Current perspectives. *Nursing Science Quarterly, 7*(1), 33-35.

Sherman, D. W. (1997). Rogerian science: Opening new frontiers of nursing knowledge through its application in quantitative research. *Nursing Science Quarterly, 10*(3), 131-135.

Smith, M. C., Kemp, J., Hemphill, L., & Vojir, C. P. (2002). Outcomes of therapeutic massage for hospitalized cancer patients. *Journal of Nursing Scholarship, 34*(3), 257-262.

von Bertalanffy, L. (1960). *General system theory: Foundations, developments, application.* New York: George Braziller.

Watson, J. (1993). Relationship of sleep-wake rhythm, dream experience, human field motion, and time experience in older women. (Doctoral dissertation, New York University, 1993). *Dissertation Abstracts International, 54*(12), 6137B.

Whall, A. L. (1987). A critique of Rogers' framework. In R. R. Parse (Ed.), *Nursing science: Major paradigms, theories, and critiques* (pp. 147-158). Philadelphia: W. B. Saunders.

Wright, S. M. (1987). The use of therapeutic touch in the management of pain. *Nursing Clinics of North America, 22*(3), 705-713.

Yarcheski, A., & Mahon, N. E. (1991). An empirical test of Rogers' original and revised theory of correlates in adolescents. *Research in Nursing and Health, 14,* 447-455.

BIBLIOGRAPHY
Primary Sources
Books

Rogers, M. E. (1961). *Educational revolution in nursing.* New York: Macmillan.

Rogers, M. E. (1964). *Reveille in nursing.* Philadelphia: F. A. Davis.

Rogers, M. E. (1970). *An introduction to the theoretical basis of nursing.* Philadelphia: F. A. Davis.

Book Chapters

Rogers, M. E. (1977). Nursing: To be or not to be. In B. Bullough & V. Bullough (Eds.), *Expanding horizons for nursing.* New York: Springer.

Rogers, M. E. (1978). Emerging patterns in nursing education. In *Current perspectives in nursing education* (Vol. II, pp. 1-8). St. Louis: Mosby.

Rogers, M. E. (1980). Nursing: A science of unitary man. In J. P. Reihl & C. Roy, *Conceptual models for nursing practice* (2nd ed., pp. 329-337). New York: Appleton-Century-Crofts.

Rogers, M. E. (1981). Science of unitary man: A paradigm for nursing. In G. E. Laskar, *Applied systems and cybernetics* (Vol. IV, pp. 1719-1722). New York: Pergamon.

Rogers, M. E. (1983). Beyond the horizon. In N. L. Chaska, *The nursing profession: A time to speak.* New York: McGraw-Hill.

Rogers, M. E. (1983). The family coping with a surgical crisis: Analysis and application of Rogers' theory to nursing care. (Rogers' response). In I. W. Clements & F. B. Roberts, *Family health: A theoretical approach to nursing care.* New York: John Wiley & Sons.

Rogers, M. E. (1985). High touch in a high-tech future. In National League for Nursing, *Perspectives in nursing— 1985-1987* (pp. 25-31). New York: National League for Nursing.

Rogers, M. E. (1985). Nursing education: Preparing for the future. In National League for Nursing, *Patterns of education: The unfolding of nursing* (pp. 11-14). New York: National League for Nursing.

Rogers, M. E. (1985). Science of unitary human beings: A paradigm for nursing. In R. Wood & J. Kekhababh, *Examining the cultural implications of Martha E. Rogers' science of unitary human beings* (pp. 13-23). Lecompton, KS: Wood-Kekhababh Associates.

Rogers, M. E. (1986). Science of unitary human beings. In V. M. Malinski, *Explorations on Martha Rogers: Science of unitary human beings* (pp. 3-8). Norwalk, CT: Appleton-Century-Crofts.

Rogers, M. E. (1987). Nursing research in the future. In J. Roode (Ed.), *Changing patterns in nursing education* (pp. 121-123). New York: National League for Nursing.

Rogers, M. E. (1987). Rogers' science of unitary human beings. In R. R. Parse, *Nursing science: Major paradigms, theories, and critiques* (pp. 139-146). Philadelphia: W. B. Saunders.

Rogers, M. E. (1989). Nursing: A science of unitary human beings. In J. P. Riehl-Sisca (Ed.), *Conceptual models for nursing practice* (3rd. ed., pp. 181-188). Norwalk, CT: Appleton & Lange.

Rogers, M. E. (1990). Nursing: Science of unitary, irreducible, human beings: Update 1990. In E. A. M. Barrett, *Visions of Rogers' science-based nursing.* New York: National League for Nursing.

Rogers, M. E. (1992). Nightingale's notes on nursing: Prelude to the 21st century. In F. Nightingale, *Notes on nursing: What it is and what it is not* (Commemorative edition, pp. 58-62). Philadelphia: J. B. Lippincott.

Rogers, M. E., Doyle, M.B., Racolin, A., & Walsh, P. C. (1990). A conversation with Martha Rogers on nursing in space. In E. A. M. Barrett (Ed.), *Visions of Rogers' science-based nursing* (pp. 375-386). New York: National League for Nursing.

Journal Articles

Rogers, M. E. (1963). Building a strong educational foundation. *American Journal of Nursing, 63,* 94-95.

Rogers, M. E. (1963). Some comments on the theoretical basis of nursing practice. *Nursing Science, 1,* 11-13, 60-61.

Rogers, M. E. (1963). The clarion call. *Nursing Science, 1,* 134-135.

Rogers, M. E. (1964). Professional standards: Whose responsibility? *Nursing Science, 2,* 71-73.

Rogers, M. E. (1965). Collegiate education in nursing (Editorial). *Nursing Science, 3*(5), 362-365.

Rogers, M. E. (1965). Higher education in nursing (Editorial). *Nursing Science, 3*(6), 443-445.

Rogers, M. E. (1965). Legislative and licensing problems in health care. *Nursing Administration Quarterly, 2,* 71-78.

Rogers, M. E. (1965). What the public demands of nursing today. *RN, 28,* 80.

Rogers, M. E. (1966). Doctoral education in nursing. *Nursing Forum, 5*(2), 75-82.

Rogers, M. E. (1968). Nursing science: Research and researchers. *Teachers College Record, 69,* 469.

Rogers, M. E. (1969). Nursing education for professional practice. *Catholic Nurse, 18*(1), 28-37, 63-64.

Rogers, M. E. (1969). Preparation of the baccalaureate degree graduate. *New Jersey State Nurses Association Newsletter, 25*(5), 32-37.

Rogers, M. E. (1970). Yesterday a nurse, tomorrow a manager: What now? *Journal of New York State Nurses Association, 1*(1), 15-21.

Rogers, M. E. (1972). Nursing's expanded role . . . and other euphemisms. *Journal of New York State Nurses Association, 3*(4), 5-10.

Rogers, M. E. (1972). Nursing: To be or not to be? *Nursing Outlook, 20*(1), 42-46.

Rogers, M. E. (1975). Euphemisms and nursing's future. *Image: The Journal of Nursing Scholarship, 7*(2), 3-9.

Rogers, M. E. (1975). Forum: Professional commitment in nursing. *Image: The Journal of Nursing Scholarship, 2,* 12-13.

Rogers, M. E. (1975). Nursing is coming of age. *American Journal of Nursing, 75*(10), 1834-1843, 1859.

Rogers, M. E. (1975). Reactions to the two foregoing presentations. *Nursing Outlook, 20,* 436.

Rogers, M. E. (1975). Research is a growing word. *Nursing Science, 31,* 283-294.

Rogers, M. E. (1975). Yesterday a nurse, today a manager: What now? *Image: The Journal of Nursing Scholarship, 2,* 12-13.

Rogers, M. E. (1977). Legislative and licensing problems in health care. *Nursing Administration Quarterly, 2*(3), 71-78.

Rogers, M. E. (1978). A 1985 dissent (Peer review). *Health/PAC Bulletin, 80,* 32-35.

Rogers, M. E. (1979). Contemporary American leaders in nursing: An oral history. An interview with Martha E. Rogers. *Kango Tenbo, 4*(12), 1126-1138.

Rogers, M. E. (1985). The nature and characteristics of professional education for nursing. *Journal of Professional Nursing, 1*(6), 381-383.

Rogers, M. E. (1985). The need for legislation for licensure to practice professional nursing. *Journal of Professional Nursing, 1*(6), 384.

Rogers, M. E. (1988). Nursing science and art: A prospective. *Nursing Science Quarterly, 1*(3), 99-102.

Rogers, M. E. (1989). Creating a climate for the implementation of a nursing conceptual framework. *Journal of Continuing Education in Nursing, 20*(3), 112-116.

Rogers, M. E. (1990). AIDS: Reason for optimism. *Philippine Journal of Nursing, 60*(2), 2-3.

Rogers, M. E. (1994). The science of unitary human beings: Current perspectives. *Nursing Science Quarterly, 7*(1), 33-35.

Rogers, M. E., & Malinski, V. (1989). Vital signs in the science of unitary human beings. *Rogerian Nursing Science News, 1*(3), 6.

Audiotapes

Rogers, M. E. (1978). *Application of theory in education and service* (Audiotape). Available through Teach 'em Inc., 160 E. Illinois Street, Chicago, IL 60611.

Rogers, M. E. (1978). *Nursing science: A science of unitary mass* (Audiotape). Distinguished Lecture Series, Wright State University, Dayton, OH.

Rogers, M. E. (1980). *The science of unitary man. Tape I: Unitary man and his world: A paradigm for nursing* (Audiotape). New York: Media for Nursing.

Rogers, M. E. (1980). *The science of unitary man. Tape II: Developing an organized abstract system* (Audiotape). New York: Media for Nursing.

Rogers, M. E. (1980). *The science of unitary man. Tape III: Principles and theories* (Audiotape). New York: Media for Nursing.

Rogers, M. E. (1980). *The science of unitary man. Tape IV: Theories of accelerating change, paranormal phenomenon, and other events* (Audiotape). New York: Media for Nursing.

Rogers, M. E. (1980). *The science of unitary man. Tape V: Health and illness* (Audiotape). New York: Media for Nursing.

Rogers, M. E. (1980). *The science of unitary man. Tape VI: Interventive modalities: Translating theories into practice* (Audiotape). New York: Media for Nursing.

Rogers, M. E. (1984*). Paper presented at Nurses Theorist Conference, Edmonton, Alberta, Canada* (Audiotape). Available through Kennedy Recordings, R.R. 5, Edmonton, Alberta, Canada TSP 4B7 (Tel: 403-470-0013).

Rogers, M. E. (1987). *Rogers' framework* (Audiotape). Nurse Theorist Conference held in Pittsburgh, PA. Available through Meetings International, 1200 Delor Avenue, Louisville, KY 40217.

Videotapes

Distinguished leaders in nursing—Martha Rogers (Videotape). (1982). Capitol Heights, MD: The National Audiovisual Center. Available through National Institutes of Health, National Library of Medicine, Bethesda, MD 20894, and from Sigma Theta Tau International, 550 West North Street, Indianapolis, IN 46202.

The nurse theorist: Portraits of excellence—Martha Rogers (Videotape). (1988). Oakland, CA: Studio III. Available through Fuld Video Project, Studio III, 370 Hawthorne Avenue, Oakland, CA 94609.

National League for Nursing. (1987). *Nursing theory: A circle of knowledge* (Videotape). New York: National League for Nursing. Available through National League for Nursing, 10 Columbus Circle, New York, NY 10019.

Rogers, M. E. (1984). *The science of unitary man. An interview with Martha Rogers with E. Donnelly* (Videotape). Bloomington, IN: Indiana University School of Nursing.

Rogers, M. E. (1987). *Rogers' framework* (Videotape). Nurse Theorist Conference held in Pittsburgh, PA. Available through Meetings International, 1200 Delor Avenue, Louisville, KY 40217.

Lectures

Rogers M. E. (1962). *Viewpoints—Critical areas for nursing education in baccalaureate and higher degree programs.* An address given at the meeting of the Council of Member Agencies of the Department of Baccalaureate and Higher Degree Programs, Williamsburg, VA, March 26, 1962. New York: National League for Nursing, Department of Baccalaureate and Higher Degree Programs.

Rogers, M. E. (1969). Nursing research: Relevant to practice? *Proceedings of the Fifth Nursing Research Conference.* New York: American Nurses Association.

Rogers, M. E. (1984). *Current issues for nursing in the next decade.* Indiana Central University, Indianapolis.

Rogers, M. E. (1992). *Science and philosophy merge for a new reality.* Keynote speaker at the Fourth Annual Rosemary Ellis Scholars' Retreat, Case Western Reserve University, Cleveland, OH.

Dissertation

Rogers, M. E. (1954). *The association of maternal and fetal factors with the development of behavior problems among elementary school children.* (Doctoral dissertation, Baltimore: Johns Hopkins University, 1954).

Secondary Sources
Books

Alligood, M. R., & Tomey, A. M. (2002). *Nursing theory: Utilization and application* (2nd ed.). St. Louis: Mosby.

Barnum, B. J. (1998). *Nursing theory: Analysis, application, evaluation* (5th ed.). Philadelphia: J. B. Lippincott.

Barrett, E. A. M. (1990). *Visions of Rogers' science-based nursing.* New York: National League for Nursing.

Chinn, P. L., & Kramer, M. K. (2004). *Integrated knowledge development in nursing* (6th ed.). St. Louis: Mosby.

Fitzpatrick, J. J., & Whall, A. L. (1996). *Conceptual models of nursing: Analysis and application* (3rd ed.). Bowie, MD: Robert J. Brady.

George, J. B. (2002). *Nursing theories: The base for professional nursing practice* (5th ed.). Englewood Cliffs, NJ: Prentice-Hall.

Madrid, M., & Barrett, E. A. M. (1994). *Rogers' scientific art of nursing practice.* New York: National League for Nursing.

Malinski, V. M. (Ed.). (1986). *Explorations on Martha Rogers' science of unitary human beings.* Norwalk, CT: Appleton-Century-Crofts.

Sarter, B. (1988). *The stream of becoming: A study of Martha Rogers' theory.* New York: National League for Nursing.

Book Chapters

Andersen, M., & Hockman, E. M. (1997). Well-being and high-risk drug use among active drug users. In M. Madrid (Ed.), *Patterns of Rogerian knowing* (pp. 152-166). New York: National League for Nursing.

Barrett, E. A. M., Caroselli, C., Smith, A. S., & Smith, D. W. (1997). Power as knowing participation in change: Theoretical, practice, and methodological issues, insights, and ideas. In M. Madrid (Ed.), *Patterns of Rogerian knowing* (pp. 31-46). New York: National League for Nursing.

Bultemeier, K., Gunther, M., Daily, J. S., Maupin, J. S., Murray, C. A., Satterly, M. C., et al. (1998). Martha E. Rogers: Unitary human beings. In A. M. Tomey & M. R. Alligood (Eds.), *Nursing theorists and their work* (4th ed., pp. 207-226). St. Louis: Mosby.

Cowling, W. R. (1997). Pattern appreciation: The unitary science/practice for essence. In M. Madrid (Ed.), *Patterns of Rogerian knowing* (pp. 129-142). New York: National League for Nursing.

Field, S. (1997). The scientific art of medical practice. In M. Madrid (Ed.), *Patterns of Rogerian knowing* (pp. 267-284). New York: National League for Nursing.

Gold, J. (1997). Practicing medicine in the nineties with an emphasis on the unitary perspective of patient care. In M. Madrid (Ed.), *Patterns of Rogerian knowing* (pp. 257-266). New York: National League for Nursing.

Gold, J. (1997). The practice of nursing from a unitary perspective. In M. Madrid (Ed.), *Patterns of Rogerian knowing* (pp. 249-256). New York: National League for Nursing.

Gunther, M. E. (2002). Martha E. Rogers: Unitary human beings. In A. M. Tomey & M. R. Alligood (Eds.), *Nursing theorists and their work* (5th ed., pp. 226-249). St. Louis: Mosby.

Hanchett, E. S. (1997). Traditions of mysticism and Rogerian science. In M. Madrid (Ed.), *Patterns of Rogerian knowing* (pp. 103-111). New York: National League for Nursing.

Horvath, B. (1997). The pandimensional nurse manager. In M. Madrid (Ed.), *Patterns of Rogerian knowing* (pp. 211-217). New York: National League for Nursing.

Ireland, M. (1997). Pediatric acquired immunodeficiency syndrome (AIDS) studied from a Rogerian perspective: A sense of hope. In M. Madrid (Ed.), *Patterns of Rogerian knowing* (pp. 143-151). New York: National League for Nursing.

Malinski, V. M. (1986). Contemporary science and nursing: Parallels with Rogers. In V. M. Malinski (Ed.), *Explorations of Martha Rogers' science of unitary human beings* (pp. 15-24). Norwalk, CT: Appleton-Century-Crofts.

Malinski, V. M. (1986). Further ideas from Martha Rogers. In V. M. Malinski (Ed.), *Explorations of Martha Rogers' science of unitary human beings* (pp. 9-14). Norwalk, CT: Appleton-Century-Crofts.

Malinski, V. M. (1997). The relationship of temporal experience and power as knowing participation in change in depressed and nondepressed women. In M. Madrid (Ed.), *Patterns of Rogerian knowing* (pp. 197-208). New York: National League for Nursing.

Mandl, A. (1997). A plea to educate the public about Martha Rogers' science of unitary human beings. In

M. Madrid (Ed.), *Patterns of Rogerian knowing* (pp. 236-238). New York: National League for Nursing.

Matas, K. E. (1997). Therapeutic touch: A model for community-based health promotion. In M. Madrid (Ed.), *Patterns of Rogerian knowing* (pp. 218-229). New York: National League for Nursing.

McNiff, M. A. (1997). Power, perceived health, and life satisfaction in adults with long-term care needs. In M. Madrid (Ed.), *Patterns of Rogerian knowing* (pp. 177-186). New York: National League for Nursing.

Phillips, J. (1997). Evolution of the science of unitary human beings. In M. Madrid (Ed.), *Patterns of Rogerian knowing* (pp. 11-27). New York: National League for Nursing.

Reed, P. G. (1997). The place of transcendence in nursing's science of unitary human beings: Theory and practice. In M. Madrid (Ed.), *Patterns of Rogerian knowing* (pp. 187-196). New York: National League for Nursing.

Reeder, F. (1997). Mysticism/spirituality of Aborigine people and Rogerian science. In M. Madrid (Ed.), *Patterns of Rogerian knowing* (pp. 120-126). New York: National League for Nursing.

Sarter, B. (1997). Hindu mysticism: The realization of integrality. In M. Madrid (Ed.), *Patterns of Rogerian knowing* (pp. 112-119). New York: National League for Nursing.

Watson, J. (1997). Using Rogers' model to study sleep-wake pattern changes in older women. In M. Madrid (Ed.), *Patterns of Rogerian knowing* (pp. 167-176). New York: National League for Nursing.

Watson, J., Barrett, E. A. M., Hastings-Tolsma, M., Johnston, L., & Gueldner, S. (1997). Measurement in Rogerian science: A review of selected instruments. In M. Madrid (Ed.), *Patterns of Rogerian knowing* (pp. 87-99). New York: National League for Nursing.

Woodward, T. A., & Heggie, J. (1997). Rogers in reality: Staff nurse application of the science of unitary human beings in the clinical setting following changes in an orientation program. In M. Madrid (Ed.), *Patterns of Rogerian knowing* (pp. 239-248). New York: National League for Nursing.

Journal Articles

Alligood, M. R. (2002). A theory of the art of nursing discovered in Rogers' science of unitary human beings. *International Journal of Human Caring, 6*(2), 55-60.

Alligood, M. R., & McGuire, S. L. (2000). Perception of time, sleep patterns, and activity in senior citizens: A test of a Rogerian theory of aging. *Visions: The Journal of Rogerian Science, 8*(1), 6-14.

Armstrong, M. A., & Kelly, A. E. (1995). More than the sum of their parts: Martha Rogers and Hildegard Peplau. *Archives of Psychiatric Nursing, 9*(1), 40-44.

Atwood, J. R., & Gill-Rogers, B. P. (1984). Metatheory, methodology, and practicality: Issues in research uses of Rogers' science of unitary man. *Nursing Research, 33*(2), 88-91.

Barnes, S. J., & Adair, B. (2002). The cognitive-sensitive approach to dementia parallels with the science of unitary human beings. *Journal of Psychosocial Nursing and Mental Health Services, 40*(11), 30-37, 44-45.

Barrett, E. A. M. (1996). Canonical correlation analysis and its use in Rogerian science. *Nursing Science Quarterly, 9*(2), 50-52.

Barrett, E. A. M. (2000). Speculations on the unpredictable future of the science of unitary human beings. *Visions: The Journal of Rogerian Science, 8*(1), 15-25.

Batra, C. (1995). Theory based curricula and utilization of Martha Rogers' framework in undergraduate and graduate programs. *Rogerian Nursing Science News, 8*(2), 8-9.

Bernado, M. L. (1996). Parent-reported injury-associated behaviors and life events among injured, ill, and well preschool children. *Journal of Pediatric Nursing, 11*(2), 100-110.

Biley, F. C. (1996). Rogerian science, phantoms, and therapeutic touch: Exploring potentials. *Nursing Science Quarterly, 9*(4), 165-169.

Biley, F. C. (1998). The beat generation and beyond: Popular culture and the development of the science of unitary human beings. *Visions: The Journal of Rogerian Nursing Science, 6*(1), 5-12.

Biley, F. C. (2000). Nursing for the new millennium: Martha Rogers and the science of unitary human beings. *Theoria: Journal of Nursing Theory, 9*(3), 19-22.

Braunstein, M. S. (1998). Evaluation of nursing practice: Process and critique. *Nursing Science Quarterly, 11*(2), 64-68.

Bush, M. R. (1997). Influence of health locus of control and parental health perceptions as follow-through with school health nurse referral. *Issues in Comprehensive Pediatric Nursing, 20*(3), 175-182.

Butcher, H. K. (1996). A unitary field pattern portrait of dispiritedness in later life. *Visions: The Journal of Rogerian Nursing Science, 4*(1), 41-58.

Butcher, H. K. (1998). Crystallizing the processes of the unitary field pattern portrait research method. *Visions: The Journal of Rogerian Nursing Science, 6*(1), 13-26.

Butcher, H. K. (1999). The artistry of Rogerian practice. *Visions: The Journal of Rogerian Nursing Science, 7*(1), 49-54.

Butcher, H. K. (1999). Weaving a theoretical tapestry supporting pandimensionality: Deep connectedness in the multiverse. *Visions: The Journal of Rogerian Nursing Science, 6*(1), 51-55.

Butcher, H. K. (2000). Rogerian-praxis: A synthesis of Rogerian practice models and theories. *Rogerian Nursing Science News, 12*(1), 2.

Butcher, H. K. (2002). Living in the heart of helicy: An inquiry into the meaning of compassion and unpredictability within Rogers' nursing science. *Visions: The Journal of Rogerian Science, 10*(1), 6-22.

Butcher, H. K. (2003). Aging as emerging brilliance: Advancing Rogers' unitary theory of aging. *Visions: The Journal of Rogerian Science, 11*(1), 55-66.

Carboni, J. T. (1995). A Rogerian process of inquiry. *Nursing Science Quarterly, 5*(1), 22-34.

Carboni, J. T. (1995). Enfolding health-as-wholeness-and-harmony: A theory of Rogerian nursing practice. *Nursing Science Quarterly, 8*(2), 71-78.

Cowling, W. R. (2001). Unitary appreciative inquiry. *ANS Advances in Nursing Science, 23*(4), 32-48.

Cox, T. (2003). Theory and exemplars of advanced practice spiritual intervention. *Complementary Therapies in Nursing & Midwifery, 9*, 30-34.

Donahue, L., & Alligood, M. R. (1995). A description of the elderly from self-selected attributes. *Visions: The Journal of Rogerian Nursing Science, 3*(1), 12-19.

Fawcett, J. (1996). Issues of (in)compatibility between the worldview and research rules of the science of unitary human beings: An invitation to dialogue. *Visions: The Journal of Rogerian Nursing Science, 4*(1), 5-11.

Fawcett, J. (2003). The nurse theorists: 21st century updates—Martha E. Rogers. *Nursing Science Quarterly, 16*(1), 44-51.

Fawcett, J. (2003). The science of unitary human beings: Analysis of qualitative research approaches. *Visions: The Journal of Rogerian Science, 11*(1), 7-20.

Fawcett, J., & Alligood, M. R. (2001). SUHB instruments: An overview of research instruments and clinical tools derived from the science of unitary human beings. *Theoria: Journal of Nursing Theory, 10*(3), 5-12.

Frimel, T. J. (2001). Holistic modalities. Florence Nightingale, Martha Rogers and the art of feng shui. *Beginnings, 21*(1), 10.

Gibson, A. (1996). Personal experiences of individuals using meditations from a metaphysical source. *Visions: The Journal of Rogerian Nursing Science, 4*(1), 12-23.

Griffin, W. M., Moore, P., Ruge, C., & Weiler-Crespo, W. (1996). Martha E. Rogers' nursing science: Application to therapeutic touch. *Rogerian Nursing Science News, 8*(3), 9-12.

Halkitis, P. N., & Kirton, C. (1999). Self-strategies as means of enhancing adherence to HIV antiretroviral therapies: A Rogerian approach. *Journal of the New York State Nurses Association, 30*(2), 22-27.

Hanchett, E. S. (1999). Field phenomena and outcomes research on the brink of a quantum leap? *Visions: The Journal of Rogerian Nursing Science, 7*(1), 44-48.

Hardin, S. R. (1997). Culture: A manifestation of pattern. *Journal of Multicultural Nursing and Health, 3*(3), 21-23.

Hardin, S. R. (2003). Spirituality as integrality among chronic heart failure patients: A pilot study. *Visions: The Journal of Rogerian Science, 11*(1), 43-53.

Hikosaka, A., Hiramatsu, N., Oikawa, M., Shibata, M., & Hanchett, E. (2001). Martha Rogers and the polar bears: A cross-cultural study session on the principles of homeodynamics. *Visions: The Journal of Rogerian Nursing Science, 9*(1), 58-60.

Johnson, M. O. (1996). A mutual field manifestation: Substance abuse and nursing. *Visions: The Journal of Rogerian Nursing Science, 4*(1), 24-30.

Johnston, L. W. (2001). An exploration of individual preferences for audio enhancement of the dying environment. *Visions: The Journal of Rogerian Nursing Science, 9*(1), 20-26.

Kim, T.S. (2001). Relation of magnetic field therapy to pain and power over time in persons with chronic primary headache: A pilot study. *Visions: The Journal of Rogerian Nursing Science, 9*(1), 27-42.

Klemm, P. R., & Stashinko, E. E. (1997). Martha Rogers' science of unitary human beings: A participative teaching-learning approach. *Journal of Nursing Education, 36*(7), 341-343.

Leddy, S. K. (2003). A unitary-based nursing practice theory: Theory and application. *Visions: The Journal of Rogerian Science, 11*(1), 21-28.

Malinski, V. M. (1999). Participating, transforming, celebrating: The dance of unitary becoming. *Visions: The Journal of Rogerian Nursing Science, 7*(1), 14-23.

Malinski, V. M. (2002). Developing a nursing perspective on spirituality and healing. *Nursing Science Quarterly, 15*(4), 281-287.

Matas, K. E. (1997). Human patterning and chronic pain. *Nursing Science Quarterly, 10*(2), 88-96.

Novak, D. M. (1999). Perceptions of menopause and its application to Rogers' science of unitary human beings. *Visions: The Journal of Rogerian Nursing Science, 7*(4), 24-29.

O'Mathuna, D. P., Pryjmachuk, S., Spencer, W., & Matthiesen, S. (2002). A critical evaluation of the theory and practice of therapeutic touch. *Nursing Philosophy, 3*(2), 163-176.

Parse, R. R. (2000). Enjoy your flight: Health in the new millennium. *Visions: The Journal of Rogerian Science, 8*(1), 26-31.

Patty, C. M. (1999). Teaching affective competencies to surgical technologists. *AORN Journal, 70*(5), 778-781.

Perkins, J. B. (2003). Healing through spirit: The experience of the eternal in the everyday. *Visions: The Journal of Rogerian Science, 11*(1), 29-42.

Phillips, J. R. (2000). Rogerian nursing science and research: A healing process for nursing. *Nursing Science Quarterly, 13*(3), 196-201.

Porter, L. S. (1998). Reducing teenage and unintended pregnancies through client-centered and family-focused school-based family planning. *Journal of Pediatric Nursing, 13*(3), 158-163.

Reeder, F. (1999). Energy: Its distinctive meanings. *Nursing Science Quarterly, 12*(1), 6-8.

Rush, M. M. (1997). A study of the relations among perceived social support, spirituality, and power as knowing participation in change among sober female alcoholics within the science of unitary human beings. *Journal of Addiction Nursing, 9*(4), 146-155.

Salerno, E. M. (2002). Hope, power, and perception of self in individuals recovering from schizophrenia: A Rogerian perspective. *Visions: The Journal of Rogerian Science, 10*(1), 23-36.

Samarel, N. (1997). Therapeutic touch, dialogue, and women's experiences in breast cancer surgery. *Holistic Nursing Practice, 12*(1), 62-70.

Samarel, N., Fawcett, J., Davis, N. M., & Ryan, F. M. (1998). Effects of dialogue and therapeutic touch on preoperative and postoperative experiences of breast cancer surgery: An exploratory study. *Oncology Nursing Forum, 25*(8), 1369-1376.

Schaefer, P., Vaughn, G., Kenner, C., Donohue, F., & Longo, A. (2000). Revision of a parent satisfaction survey based on the parent perspective. *Journal of Pediatric Nursing: Nursing Care of Children and Families, 15*(6), 373-377.

Schneider, P. E. (1995). Focusing awareness: The process of extraordinary healing from a Rogerian perspective. *Visions: The Journal of Rogerian Nursing Science, 3*(1), 32-43.

Sherman, D. W. (1996). Nurses' willingness to care for AIDS patients and spirituality, social support, and death anxiety. *Image: The Journal of Nursing Scholarship, 28*(3), 205-213.

Smith, D. W. (1995). Power and spirituality in polio survivors: A study based on Rogers' science. *Nursing Science Quarterly, 8*(3), 133-139.

Smith, M. C. (1999). Caring and the science of unitary human beings. *ANS Advances in Nursing Science, 21*(4), 14-28.

Smith, M. C., & Reeder, F. (1998). Clinical outcomes research and Rogerian science: Strange or emergent bedfellows? *Visions: The Journal of Rogerian Nursing Science, 6*(1), 27-38.

Todaro-Franceschi, V. (1999). The idea of energy as phenomenon and Rogerian science: Are they congruent? *Visions: The Journal of Rogerian Nursing Science, 7*(1), 30-41.

Todaro-Franceschi, V. (2001). Energy: A bridging concept for nursing science. *Nursing Science Quarterly, 14*(2), 132-140.

Todaro-Franceschi, V. (2001). Pandimensional awareness, purposeful change and the kaleidoscopic cosmos. *Visions: The Journal of Rogerian Nursing Science, 9*(1), 52-57.

Ugarizza, D. N. (2002). Intentionality: Applications within selected theories of nursing. *Holistic Nursing Practice, 16*(4), 41-50.

Wall, L. M. (2000). Changes in hope and power in lung cancer patients who exercise. *Nursing Science Quarterly, 13*(3), 234-242.

Watson, J. (1996). Issues with measuring time experience in Rogers' conceptual model. *Visions: The Journal of Rogerian Nursing Science, 4*(1), 31-40.

Watson, J. (1999). Exploring the concept of beyond waking experience. *Visions: The Journal of Rogerian Nursing Science, 6*(1), 39-46.

Watson, J. (2002). Changing paradigms in epidemiology: Catching up with Martha Rogers. *Visions: The Journal of Rogerian Science, 10*(1), 37-50.

Watson, J., Sloyan, C. M., & Robalino, J. E. (2000). The time metaphor test re-visited: Implications for Rogerian research. *Visions: The Journal of Rogerian Science, 8*(1), 32-45.

Watson, J., & Smith, M. C. (2002). Caring science and the science of unitary human beings: A trans-theoretical discourse for nursing knowledge development. *Journal of Advanced Nursing, 37*(5), 452-461.

West, M. M. (2002). Early risk indicators of substance abuse among nurses. *Journal of Nursing Scholarship, 34*(2), 187-193.

Whall, L. M. (1999). Exercise: A unitary concept. *Nursing Science Quarterly, 12*(1), 68-72.

Winstead-Fry, P. (2000). Rogers' conceptual system and family nursing. *Nursing Science Quarterly, 13*(4), 278-280.

Yarcheski, A., & Mahon, N. E. (1995). Rogers's pattern manifestations and health in adolescents. *Western Journal of Nursing Research, 17*(4), 383-397.

Yarcheski, A., Mahon, N. E., & Yarcheski, T. J. (2002). Humor and health in early adolescents: Perceived field motion as a mediating variable. *Nursing Science Quarterly, 15*(2), 150-155.

Doctoral Dissertations

Bays, C. (1995). *Older adults' descriptions of hope after a stroke.* Unpublished doctoral dissertation, University of Cincinnati, Cincinnati, OH.

Bowles, D. J. N. (1999). *Exploring pattern manifestation through critical incident analysis of nurse educators and clinicians.* Unpublished doctoral dissertation, Spalding University, Louisville, KY.

Carboni, J. T. (1997). *Coming home: An investigation of the enfolding-unfolding movement of human environmental energy field patterns within the nursing home setting and the enfoldment of health-as-wholeness-and-harmony by the nurse and client.* Unpublished doctoral dissertation, University of Rhode Island, Kingston, RI.

Dominguez, L. M. (1996). *The lived experience of women with Mexican heritage with HIV/AIDS.* Unpublished doctoral dissertation, University of Arizona, Tucson, AZ.

Doyle, M. B. (1995). *Mental health nurses' imagination, power, and empathy: A descriptive study using Rogerian nursing science.* Unpublished doctoral dissertation, New York University, New York.

Dye, M. K. (2000). *"Getting back into the swing of things:" A Rogerian portrait of living with traumatic brain injury.* Unpublished doctoral dissertation, University of South Carolina, Columbia, SC.

Garrard, C. T. (1995). *The effect of therapeutic touch on stress reduction and immune function in persons with AIDS.* Unpublished doctoral dissertation, University of Alabama, Birmingham.

Girardin, B. W. (1990). *The relationship of lightwave frequency to sleepwakefulness frequency in well, full-term, Hispanic neonates.* Unpublished doctoral dissertation, Wayne State University, Detroit, MI.

Headley, J. A. (1997). *Chemotherapy-induced ovarian failure in women with breast cancer.* Unpublished doctoral dissertation, Texas Woman's University, Denton, TX.

Hills, R. G. S (1998). *Maternal field patterning of awareness, wakefulness, human field motion, and well-being in mothers with six-month-old infants: A Rogerian perspective.* Unpublished doctoral dissertation, Wayne State University, Detroit, MI.

Horvath, B. (1998). *The relation of the clinical application of music and mood in persons receiving treatment for alcoholism.* Unpublished doctoral dissertation, New York University, New York.

Hurley, M. (2002). *The relations of stress, power, and job satisfaction in female nurse managers within Rogers' Science of Unitary Human Beings (M. E. Rogers, E. A. M. Barrett).* Unpublished doctoral dissertation, New York University, New York.

Johnson, E. E. (1996). *Health choice-making: The experience, perception, expression of older women.* Unpublished doctoral dissertation, University of South Carolina, Columbia.

Jones, R. (2002). *The relations of dyadic trust, sensation-seeking, and sexual imposition with sexual risk behaviors in young, urban women with primary and non-primary male partners.* Unpublished doctoral dissertation, New York University, New York.

Kells, K. J. (1995). *Sensing presence as open or closed space: A phenomenological inquiry on blind individuals' experiences of obstacle detection.* Unpublished doctoral dissertation, University of Colorado Health Sciences Center, Denver.

Kim, T. S. (2000). *Magnetic field therapy: An exploration of its relation to pain and power in adults with chronic primary headache from a Rogerian perspective.* Unpublished doctoral dissertation, New York University, New York.

Larkin, D. M. (2001). *Ericksonian hypnotherapeutic approaches in chronic care support groups: A Rogerian exploration of power and self-defined health promoting goals.* Unpublished doctoral dissertation, New York University, New York.

Lewandowski, W. A. (2002). *Patterning of pain and power with guided imagery: An experimental study of persons experiencing chronic pain.* Unpublished doctoral dissertation, Case Western Reserve University, Cleveland, OH.

Mahoney, J. (1998). *The relationship of power and actualization to job satisfaction in female home health care nurses.* Unpublished doctoral dissertation, New York University, New York.

McNiff, M. A. (1995). *A study of the relationship of power, perceived health, and life satisfaction in adults with long-term care needs based on Martha E. Rogers' science of unitary human beings.* Unpublished doctoral dissertation, New York University, New York.

Nellett, G. H. (1998). *The caregiver's experience of deliberative mutual patterning with pain-ridden substance abusers.* Unpublished doctoral dissertation, Loyola University of Chicago, Chicago.

Noyes, L. E. (2001). *Stories of the oldest-old as they come to face death.* Unpublished doctoral dissertation, George Mason University, Fairfax, VA.

Pisarek, S. C. (2001). *Cross-cultural comparison of medical ethical decision making.* Unpublished doctoral dissertation, Walden University, Minneapolis.

Quinn-Griffin, M. T. (2001). *Quality of life of patients with mucosal ulcerative colitis following ileal pouch anal anastomosis surgery.* Unpublished doctoral dissertation, Case Western Reserve University, Cleveland, OH.

Rush, M. M. (1995). *A study of the relations among perceived social support, spirituality, and power as knowing participation in change among sober female alcoholics in Alcoholics Anonymous within the science of unitary human beings.* Unpublished doctoral dissertation, New York University, New York.

Salerno, E. M. (2000). *Hope, power, and perception of self in individuals recovering from schizophrenia: A Rogerian science perspective (Martha Rogers).* Unpublished doctoral dissertation, New York University, New York.

Shearer, N. B. C. (2000). *Facilitators of health empowerment in women.* Unpublished doctoral dissertation, University of Arizona, Tucson.

Smyth, P. E. (1999). *Reducing immunization pain perception in preschoolers with therapeutic touch.* Unpublished doctoral dissertation, University of Alabama, Birmingham.

Varela, T. (2001). *The mirror behind the mask: Experiences of five people living with HIV/AIDS (immune deficiency) who practice Santeria.* Unpublished doctoral dissertation, New York University, New York.

Wall, J. M. (1999). *An exploration of hope and power among lung cancer patients who have and have not participated in a preoperative exercise program.* Unpublished doctoral dissertation, New York University, New York.

West, M. M. (2000). *An investigation of pattern manifestations in substance abuse–impaired nurses.* Unpublished doctoral dissertation, Widener University School of Nursing, Chester, PA.

Wright, B. W. (1999). *An investigation of the relationship of trust and power in adults using Martha Rogers' science of unitary human beings.* Unpublished doctoral dissertation, New York University, New York.

Web Sites

Martha E. Rogers Home Page and Listserv: *http://medweb.uwcm.uk/martha*

New York University Martha E. Rogers Center: *http://education.nyu.edu/steinhardt/db/centers/9*

American Nurses Association Hall of Fame Inductee Page: Washburn University School of Nursing. Accessed December 20, 2004: *http://www.washburn.edu/sonu/rogers1.htm*

Martha E. Rogers Gravesite. Accessed December 20, 2004: *http://www.aahn.org/gravesites/rogers.html*

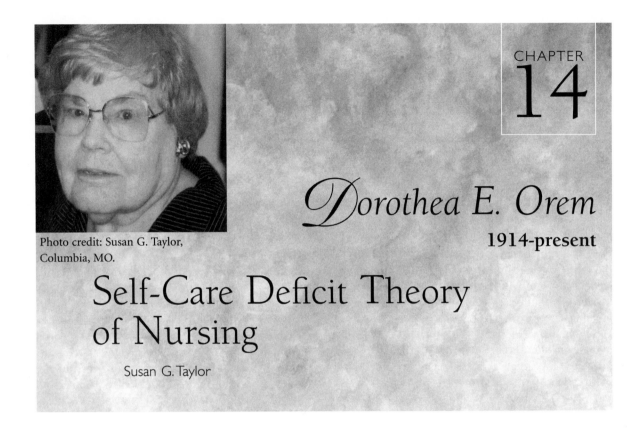

Dorothea E. Orem
1914-present

Photo credit: Susan G. Taylor,
Columbia, MO.

Self-Care Deficit Theory of Nursing

Susan G. Taylor

CREDENTIALS AND BACKGROUND OF THE THEORIST

Dorothea Elizabeth Orem, one of America's foremost nursing theorists, was born in Baltimore, Maryland, in 1914. Her father was a construction worker who liked fishing and her mother was a homemaker who liked reading. The younger of two daughters, Orem began her nursing career at Providence Hospital School of Nursing in Washington, D.C., where she received a diploma of nursing in the early 1930s. Orem later received a B.S. in Nursing

Previous authors: Susan G. Taylor, Angela Compton, Jeanne Donohue Eben, Sarah Emerson, Nergess N. Gashti, Ann Marriner Tomey, Margaret J. Nation, and Sherry B. Nordmeyer. The author acknowledges the research and editorial assistance of Sang-arun Isaramalai, M.S.N., R.N., doctoral student, School of Nursing, University of Missouri-Columbia.

Education from The Catholic University of America (CUA) in 1939, and in 1946, she received an M.S. in Nursing Education from the same university.

Her early nursing experiences included operating room nursing, private duty nursing (home and hospital), hospital staff nursing on pediatric and adult medical and surgical units, evening supervisor in the emergency room, and biological science teaching. Orem held the directorship of both the nursing school and the department of nursing at Providence Hospital, Detroit, from 1940 to 1949. After leaving Detroit, Orem spent 8 years (1949 to 1957) in Indiana working in the Division of Hospital and Institutional Services of the Indiana State Board of Health. Her goal was to upgrade the quality of nursing in general hospitals throughout the state. During this time, Orem developed her definition of nursing practice (Orem, 1956).

In 1957, Orem moved to Washington, D.C., to take a position at the Office of Education, U.S. Department of Health, Education, and Welfare as a curriculum consultant. From 1958 to 1960, she worked on a project to upgrade practical nurse training that stimulated a need to address the question: What is the subject matter of nursing? As a result, *Guides for Developing Curricula for the Education of Practical Nurses* was developed (Orem, 1959). Later that year, Orem became an assistant professor of nursing education at CUA. She subsequently served as acting dean of the School of Nursing and as associate professor of nursing education. She continued to develop her concepts of nursing and self-care at CUA. The formalization of the concepts was sometimes performed alone and sometimes with others. Members of the Nursing Models Committee at CUA and the Improvement in Nursing Group, which later became the Nursing Development Conference Group (NDCG), all contributed to the development of the theory. Orem provided the intellectual leadership throughout these collaborative endeavors.

In 1970, Orem left CUA and began her own consulting firm. Orem's first published book in 1971 was *Nursing: Concepts of Practice* (Orem, 1971). She was editor for the NDCG as they prepared and later revised *Concept Formalization in Nursing: Process and Product* (NDCG, 1972, 1979). Subsequent editions of *Nursing: Concepts of Practice* were published in 1980, 1985, 1991, 1995, and 2001. Orem retired in 1984 and resides in Savannah, Georgia. She continues working, alone and with colleagues, on the development of Self-Care Deficit Nursing Theory (SCDNT).

Georgetown University conferred on Orem the honorary degree of Doctor of Science in 1976. She received the CUA Alumni Association Award for Nursing Theory in 1980. Other honors received include Honorary Doctor of Science, Incarnate Word College, 1980; Doctor of Humane Letters, Illinois Wesleyan University, 1988; Linda Richards Award, National League for Nursing, 1991; and Honorary Fellow of the American Academy of Nursing, 1992. She was awarded the Doctor of Nursing Honoris Causae from the University of Missouri in 1998.

Orem's many papers and presentations provide insight into her views on nursing practice, nursing education, and nursing science. Some of these papers are now available to nursing scholars in a compilation edited by Renpenning and Taylor (2003). Other papers of Orem and scholars who worked with her in the development of the theory are archived in Johns Hopkins University.

THEORETICAL SOURCES

Well-versed in contemporary nursing literature and thought, Orem was not influenced directly by any particular nursing leader. Her association with nurses over the years provided many learning experiences, and she views her work with graduate students and her collaborative work with colleagues as valuable endeavors. Although she does not credit a major influence, she does cite many other nurses' works in terms of their contributions to nursing, including, but not limited to, Abdellah, Henderson, Johnson, King, Levine, Nightingale, Orlando, Peplau, Riehl, Rogers, Roy, Travelbee, and Wiedenbach. She also cites numerous authors in other disciplines including, but not limited to, Gordon Allport, Chester Barnard, René Dubos, Erich Fromm, Gartly Jaco, Robert Katz, Kurt Lewin, Ernest Nagel, Talcott Parsons, Hans Selye, Magda Arnold, William Wallace, Bernard Lonergan, and Ludwig von Bertalanffy. Familiarity with these sources is necessary to gain a full understanding of Orem's work.

Orem has identified her philosophical view as that of moderate realism, as described by Wallace (1979, 1996). Banfield (1997) presented an analysis of the metaphysical and epistemological foundations of Orem's work. Banfield concluded that "the view of human beings as dynamic, unitary beings who exist in their environments, who are in the process of becoming, and who possess free-will as well as other essential human qualities" (p. 204) are foundational to SCDNT. Taylor, Geden, Isaramalai, and Wongvatunyu (2000) also explored the philosophical foundations of the theory. Orem (1997) detailed her views of person in a recent work. The perspective of the person as a deliberate actor, or agent, forms the basis for the theory. This perspective applies to all persons in the nursing situation, including nurse, patient, and family. Concepts of speculative and practical science are also foundational (Orem, 1997). Gullifer (1997) suggests that Orem's "insights into the patient-nurse nexus . . . may be viewed as being partly built upon Kantian philosophy" (p. 155), including the categorical imperative and the fusion of mind and body.

Orem's views on nursing science as human practical science are basic to understanding how empirical evidence is gathered and interpreted.

Practical sciences include the speculatively practical, practically practical, and applied sciences. In the most recent edition, Orem (2001) identified two sets of speculative nursing sciences, nursing practice sciences and foundational sciences. Nursing practice sciences include sciences of wholly compensatory nursing, partly compensatory nursing, and supportive-educative or developmental nursing. Foundational nursing sciences include the sciences of self-care, self-care agency, and human assistance. She further suggests the development of applied nursing science and basic, non-nursing sciences as a part of the empirical evidence and knowledge base to be associated with nursing practice.

MAJOR CONCEPTS *&* DEFINITIONS

Orem labels her self-care deficit theory of nursing as a general theory composed of the following three related theories:

1. The theory of self-care, which describes why and how people care for themselves
2. The theory of self-care deficit, which describes and explains why people can be helped through nursing
3. The theory of nursing systems, which describes and explains relationships that must be brought about and maintained for nursing to be produced

The major concepts of these theories are identified here and discussed more fully in Orem's book, *Nursing: Concepts of Practice* (2001) (see Figure 14-1).

SELF-CARE

Self-care comprises the practice of activities that maturing and mature persons initiate and perform, within time frames, on their own behalf in the interest of maintaining life, healthful functioning, continuing personal development, and well-being through meeting known requisites for functional and developmental regulations (Orem, 2001, p. 522*).

SELF-CARE REQUISITES

A self-care requisite is a formulated and expressed insight about actions to be performed that are known or hypothesized to be necessary in the regulation of an aspect(s) of human functioning and development, continuously or under specified conditions and circumstances. A formulated self-care requisite names the following two elements:

1. The factor to be controlled or managed to keep an aspect(s) of human functioning and development within the norms compatible with life, health, and personal well-being
2. The nature of the required action

Formulated and expressed self-care requisite constitutes the formalized purposes of self-care. They are the reasons for which self-care is undertaken; they express the intended or desired

*Page numbers supplied throughout box refer the reader to the sections of the source publication in which the content may be located. They do not indicate direct excerpts from that publication.

Continued

MAJOR CONCEPTS & DEFINITIONS—cont'd

results—the goals of self-care (Orem, 2001, p. 522).

UNIVERSAL SELF-CARE REQUISITES

Universally required goals are to be met through self-care or dependent care and have their origins in what is known and what is validated or what is in the process of being validated about human structural and functional integrity at various stages of the life cycle. The following eight self-care requisites common to men, women, and children are suggested:

1. The maintenance of a sufficient intake of air
2. The maintenance of a sufficient intake of food
3. The maintenance of a sufficient intake of water
4. The provision of care associated with elimination processes and excrements
5. The maintenance of balance between activity and rest
6. The maintenance of balance between solitude and social interaction
7. The prevention of hazards to human life, human functioning, and human well-being
8. The promotion of human functioning and development within social groups in accordance with human potential, known human limitations, and the human desire to be normal. Normalcy is used in the sense of that which is essentially human and that which is in accordance with the genetic and constitutional characteristics and talents of individuals (Orem, 2001, p. 225).

DEVELOPMENTAL SELF-CARE REQUISITES

Developmental self-care requisites (DSCR) were separated from universal self-care requisites in the second edition of *Nursing: Concepts of Practice* (Orem, 1980). There are three sets of DSCR, as follows:

1. Provision of conditions that promote development

2. Engagement in self-development
3. Prevention of or overcoming effects of human conditions and life situations that can adversely affect human development (Orem, 1980, p. 231)

HEALTH DEVIATION SELF-CARE REQUISITES

These self-care requisites exist for persons who are ill or injured, who have specific forms of pathological conditions or disorders, including defects and disabilities, and who are under medical diagnosis and treatment. The characteristics of health deviation as conditions extending over time determine the kinds of care demands that individuals experience as they live with the effects of pathological conditions and live through their durations.

Disease or injury affects not only specific structures and physiological or psychological mechanisms, but also integrated human functioning. When integrated functioning is seriously affected (severe mental retardation, comatose states, or autism), the individual's developing or developed powers of agency are seriously impaired either permanently or temporarily. In abnormal states of health, self-care requisites arise from both the disease state and the measures used in its diagnosis or treatment.

Care measures to meet existent health-deviation self-care requisites must be made action components of individuals' systems of self-care or dependent care. The complexity of self-care or dependent-care systems is increased by the number of health-deviation requisites that must be met in specific time frames.

THERAPEUTIC SELF-CARE DEMAND

Therapeutic self-care demand consists of the summation of care measures necessary at specific times or over a duration of time for meeting all of an individual's known self-care requisites particularized for existent conditions and circumstances using methods appropriate for the following:

- Controlling or managing factors identified in the requisites, the values of which are regulatory of human functioning (sufficiency of air, water, and food)
- Fulfilling the activity element of the requisite (maintenance, promotion, prevention, and provision) (Orem, 2001, p. 523)

Therapeutic self-care demand at any time (1) describes factors in the patient or the environment that must be held steady within a range of values or brought within and held within such a range for the sake of the patient's life, health, or well-being, and (2) has a known degree of instrumental effectiveness derived from the choice of technologies and specific techniques for using, changing, or in some way controlling, patient or environmental factors.

SELF-CARE AGENCY

The self-care agency is a complex acquired ability of mature and maturing persons to know and meet their continuing requirements for deliberate, purposive action to regulate their own human functioning and development (Orem, 2001, p. 522).

AGENT

The agent engages in a course of action or has the power to do so (Orem, 2001, p. 514).

DEPENDENT-CARE AGENT

The dependent-care agent, a maturing adolescent or adult, accepts and fulfills the responsibility to know and meet the therapeutic self-care demand of relevant others who are socially dependent on them or to regulate the development or exercise of these persons' self-care agency (Orem, 2001, p. 515).

SELF-CARE DEFICIT

Self-care deficit is a relation between the persons' therapeutic self-care demands and their powers of self-care agency in which constituent developed self-care capabilities within self-care agency are not operable or not adequate for knowing and meeting some or all components of the existent or projected therapeutic self-care demand (Orem, 2001, p. 522).

NURSING AGENCY

Nursing agency comprises developed capabilities of persons educated as nurses that empower them to represent themselves as nurses and within the frame of a legitimate interpersonal relationship to act, to know, and to help persons in such relationships to meet their therapeutic self-care demands and to regulate the development or exercise of their self-care agency (Orem, 2001, p. 518).

NURSING DESIGN

Nursing design, a professional function performed both before and after nursing diagnosis and prescription, allows nurses, on the basis of reflective practical judgments about existent conditions, to synthesize concrete situational elements into orderly relations to structure operational units. The purpose of nursing design is to provide guides for achieving needed and foreseen results in the production of nursing toward the achievement of nursing goals; the units taken together constitute the pattern to guide the production of nursing (Orem, 2001, p. 519).

NURSING SYSTEMS

Nursing systems are series and sequences of deliberate practical actions of nurses performed at times in coordination with actions of their patients to know and meet components of their patients' therapeutic self-care demands and to protect and regulate the exercise or development of patients' self-care agency (Orem, 2001, p. 519).

Continued

HELPING METHODS

A helping method from a nursing perspective is a sequential series of actions which, if performed, will overcome or compensate for the health-associated limitations of persons to engage in actions to regulate their own functioning and development or that of their dependents. Nurses use all the methods, selecting and combining them in relation to the action demands on persons under nursing care and their health-associated action limitations, as follows:

- Acting for or doing for another
- Guiding and directing
- Providing physical or psychological support
- Providing and maintaining an environment that supports personal development
- Teaching (Orem, 2001, pp. 55-56)

USE OF EMPIRICAL EVIDENCE

Orem formulated her concept of nursing in relation to self-care as part of a study on the organization and administration of hospitals, which she conducted at the Indiana State Department of Health (Orem, 1956). This work enabled her to formulate and express her concept of nursing. Her knowledge of the features of nursing practice situations was acquired over many years. Orem used philosophical and scientific methods in developing her insights and validating her conclusions. Since the SCDNT was first published, extensive empirical evidence has contributed to the development of theoretical knowledge. Much of this is incorporated into the continuing development of the theory; however, the basics of the theory remain unchanged.

MAJOR ASSUMPTIONS

Assumptions basic to the general theory were formalized during the early 1970s and were first presented at Marquette University School of Nursing in 1973. Orem (2001) identifies the following five premises underlying the general theory of nursing:

1. Human beings require continuous, deliberate inputs to themselves and their environments to remain alive and function in accordance with natural human endowments.
2. Human agency, the power to act deliberately, is exercised in the form of care for self and others in identifying needs and making needed inputs.
3. Mature human beings experience privations in the form of limitations for action in care for self and others involving and making of life-sustaining and function-regulating inputs.
4. Human agency is exercised in discovering, developing, and transmitting ways and means to identify needs and make inputs to self and others.
5. Groups of human beings with structured relationships cluster tasks and allocate responsibilities for providing care to group members who experience privations for making required, deliberate input to self and others. (p. 140)

Orem lists presuppositions and propositions for the theory of self-care, the theory of self-care deficit, and the theory of nursing systems. These constitute the expression of the theories and are summarized below.

THEORETICAL ASSERTIONS

Presented as a general theory of nursing, one that represents a complete picture of nursing, the SCDNT is expressed in the following three theories:
1. Theory of nursing systems
2. Theory of self-care deficit
3. Theory of self-care

The three constituent theories, taken together in relationship, constitute the SCDNT. The theory of nursing systems is the unifying theory and includes all the essential elements. It subsumes the theory of self-care deficit and the theory of self-care. The theory of self-care deficit develops the reason why a person may benefit from nursing. The theory of self-care, foundational to the others, expresses the purpose, methods, and outcome of taking care of self.

Theory of Nursing Systems

The theory of nursing systems proposes that nursing is human action; nursing systems are action systems formed (designed and produced) by nurses through the exercise of their nursing agency for persons with health-derived or health-associated limitations in self-care or dependent care. Nursing agency includes concepts of deliberate action, including intentionality, and operations of diagnosis, prescription, and regulation. Figure 14-1 shows the basic nursing systems categorized according to the relationship between patient and nurse actions. Nursing systems may be produced for individuals, for persons who constitute a dependent-care unit, for groups whose members have therapeutic self-care demands with similar components or who have similar limitations for engagement in self-care or dependent care, or for families or other multiperson units.

Theory of Self-Care Deficit

The central idea of the theory of self-care deficit is that the requirements of persons for nursing are associated with the subjectivity of mature and maturing persons to health-related or health care–related action limitations. These limitations render them completely or partially unable to know existent and emerging requisites for regulatory care for themselves or their dependents. They also limit the ability to engage in the continuing performance of care measures to control or in some way manage factors that are regulatory of their own or their dependents' functioning and development.

Self-care deficit is a term that expresses the relationship between the action capabilities of individuals and their demands for care. Self-care deficit is an abstract concept that, when expressed in terms of

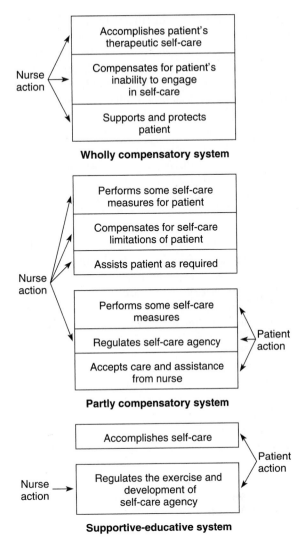

Wholly compensatory system

Partly compensatory system

Supportive-educative system

Figure **14-1** Basic nursing systems. (From Orem, D. E. [2001]. *Nursing: Concepts of practice* [6th ed., p. 351]. St. Louis: Mosby.)

action limitations, provides guides for the selection of methods for helping and understanding patient roles in self-care.

Theory of Self-Care

Self-care is a human regulatory function that individuals must, with deliberation, perform themselves or have performed for them to maintain life, health, development, and well-being. Self-care is an action system. The elaboration of the concepts of self-care, self-care demand, and self-care agency provide the foundation for understanding the action requirements and action limitations of persons who may benefit from nursing. Self-care, as a human regulatory function, is distinct from other types of regulation of human functioning and development, such as neuroendocrine regulation. Self-care must be learned and it must be performed deliberately and continuously in time and in conformity with the regulatory requirements of the individuals. These requirements are associated with their stages of growth and development, states of health, specific features of health or developmental states, levels of energy expenditure, and environmental factors. The theory of self-care is also extended to a theory of dependent care wherein the purpose, methods, and outcomes of care of others is expressed (Taylor, Renpenning, Geden, Neuman, & Hart, 2001).

LOGICAL FORM

Orem's insight led to her initial formalization and subsequent expression of a general concept of nursing. That generalization then made possible inductive and deductive thinking about nursing. The form of the theory is shown in the many models that Orem and others developed, such as those shown in Figures 14-1 and 14-2. Orem described the models and their importance to the development and understanding of the reality of the entities. The models are "directed toward knowing the structure of the processes that are operational or become operational in the production of nursing systems, systems of care for individuals or for dependent-care units or multiperson units served by nurses" (Orem, 1997, p. 31). The overall theory is logically congruent.

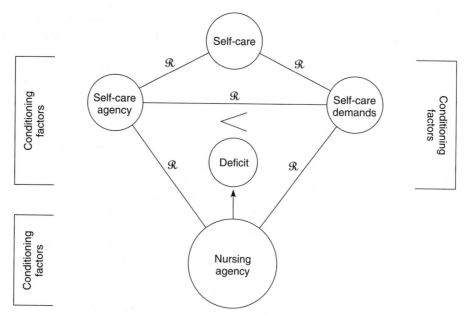

Figure **14-2 A conceptual framework for nursing. R,** Relationship; **<,** deficit relationship, current or projected. (From Orem, D. E. [2001]. *Nursing: Concepts of practice* [6th ed., p. 491]. St. Louis: Mosby.)

ACCEPTANCE BY THE NURSING COMMUNITY

Orem's SCDNT has achieved a significant level of acceptance by the nursing community as evidenced by the magnitude of published material. Over 800 references can be found through a computerized search dealing with a wide variety of subjects; therefore, the following is only a sample of this literature. In a review of research performed using SCDNT or components, the number of studies and the quality of work has improved over time (Taylor et al., 2000). In reviewing articles referenced as self-care, the searcher is cautioned that not all references to self-care are references to Orem's theory of nursing. However, much research on self-care, not directly citing Orem's theory, is pertinent and contributes to the body of knowledge. The reader is also cautioned that not all uses of Orem's theory accurately reflect the most current state of theory development as expressed in the sixth edition of *Nursing: Concepts of Practice* (2001).

The SCDNT has great appeal to practicing nurses, as evidenced by the literature and by phone calls and e-mail messages and questions received through the SCDNT Web page. Orem's theory has been translated into Italian, French, Spanish, Dutch, and Japanese; there are translations of some of her work in Germany, Thailand, and Norway, among others. Her work is used throughout the world. Practitioners of nursing in Great Britain, Taiwan, China, Hong Kong, Thailand, Japan, Korea, Canada, Australia, New Zealand, South Africa, Israel, Pakistan, Germany, Spain, Italy, France, Belgium, the Netherlands, Finland, Norway, Sweden, Switzerland, Slovenia, Brazil, Bolivia, Colombia, Uruguay, and Mexico report use of Orem's theory. The 8th International Congress on Self-Care Theory in 2004, Ulm, Germany, features presenters from Iran, the United States, South Africa, Germany, Norway, Thailand, Japan, Poland, Czech Republic, and others (G. Bekel, personal communication, January 15, 2004).

Practice

Nursing is a practice discipline; therefore, most research relates to questions of practice. There are an increasing number of case studies in the literature, but many more are needed (Cheung, 2002; Fialho, Pagliuca, & Soares, 2002; Garcia Velazquez, 2002; Silva, 2001). The first documented use of Orem's theory as the basis for structuring practice is found in descriptions of nurse-managed clinics at Johns Hopkins Hospital in 1973 (Allison, 1973; Backsheider, 1974). Since that time, there have been descriptions of the use of Orem's theory in a variety of clinical populations and age groups. The literature also includes the use of SCDNT in a number of ethnically and culturally diverse populations. For example, Villarruel & Denyes (1997) examined the experience of pain within Mexican-American culture, and Wang (1997) studied women in Taiwan. A reconstruction of one of the early studies focusing on self-care capabilities and nursing required to manage diabetes mellitus was published recently (Allison, 2003). Clinical situations or health problems that have been examined using SCDNT or components of SCDNT include all age groups, specific gender, families, homeless, oncology issues, psychiatric concepts, childbearing issues, health promotion, primary care, and specific disease-related concepts. Table 14-1 includes an array of current literature, illustrating the diversity and scope of work being done using SCDNT.

SCDNT has been used in a variety of settings (Allison, 1973; Taylor, 1989; Taylor & McLaughlin, 1991). Bekel (1998) described the use of the theory in practice in Germany. The Vancouver Health Department has done major work in designing community population-based care using Orem's conceptualizations (Duncan & Murphy, 1988). Newark Beth Israel was one of the first acute care hospitals where practitioners structured the nursing delivery and the documentation system from Orem's theory (NLN Editorial Review Board News, 1987). Some in occupational health nursing are basing their practice on SCDNT. There are many health hazards and job-related risk factors of which nurses must be aware. The ability to identify health problems, interpret findings, and draw correct conclusions is critical in occupational nursing (Komulainen, 1991). Binghamton General Hospital is using Orem's theory as part of the orientation

Text continued on p. 280.

Table 14-1

Survey of Current Literature		
CATEGORY	**TOPIC**	**AUTHOR, DATE**
AGE		
Infants/children	TSCD of normal newborns	Dennis & Jesek-Hale, 2003
	Autistic child case management	Oliver, 2003
	Health message design for children	Whitener, Cox, & Maglich, 1998
	Application of Orem's theory to the nursing management of pertussis	Logue, 1997
	Care of mentally and physically handicapped children	Hitejc, 2000
	Teaching health self-care skills to children	Betz, 2000
	Pediatric patient-controlled analgesia: enhancing the self-care construct	Vesely, 1995
	Child experiencing pain	Knigge-Demal, 1998
	Self-concept and self-care in children with cancer	Mosher & Moore, 1998
Adolescents	Homeless youth taking care of self	Rew, 2003
	Physical abuse, social support, self-care, and pregnancy outcomes of older adolescents	Renker, 1999
	Pregnant adolescent—case study	Torres, Davim, & da Nobrega, 1999
	Life change events, hope, and SCA in inner-city adolescents	Canty-Mitchell, 2001
	SCA and self-care practice of adolescents	Slusher, 1999
	Self-care in the adolescent	Rodriguez de la Parra & Baquero, 1999
	Adolescent self-esteem: a foundational disposition	Anderson & Olnhausen, 1999
	Self-care capabilities of abused/neglected and nonabused/nonneglected pregnant, low-socioeconomic adolescents	Warren, 1998
Elderly	Health beliefs, social support, and self-care behaviors, older Thai persons with diabetes	Surit, 2002
	Predictors of SCA, community-dwelling older adults	White, 2000
	A model of factors contributing to perceived abilities for health-promoting self-care of community-dwelling Thai older adults	Malathum, 2001
	Tai Chi, balance, functional mobility, health perception, older women	Taggert, 2000
	Nursing model for the aged in community	Deng & Xie, 2001

Table 14-1

Survey of Current Literature—cont'd

CATEGORY	TOPIC	AUTHOR, DATE
	Predictive model, well-being and self-care, rural elderly women, Taiwan	Wang & Laffrey, 2001
	Health-promoting lifestyle in rural elderly Taiwanese	Wang, 2001
	Structure of self-care in a group of elderly persons	Söderhamn & Cliffordson, 2001
	Nutrition and older adults, family caregivers	Biggs & Freed, 2000
	Self-care ability, home-dwelling elderly, Sweden	Söderhamn, Lindencrona, & Ek, 2000
GENDER		
Women	Self-care activities, quality of life, ovarian cancer survivors	Nicholson, 2002
	The art of watching out: vigilance in women who have migraine headaches	Meyer, 2000
	Women's self-care, a secondary concept	Weber, 2000
	Utilization of prenatal care, St. Thomas, U.S. Virgin Islands	Cooksey-James, 1999
	Self-care model of women's responses to battering	Campbell & Weber, 2000
	SCA, pregnant women	Hart & Foster, 1998
Men	Adherence to cardiac therapy for men with coronary artery disease	Baird & Pierce, 2001
HEALTH STATE		
Cancer	Self-care and health, cancer-related fatigue	Magnan, 2001
	Nurse's contribution, death at home for terminal cancer patients	Grov, 1999
	Family caregivers of cancer patients, predictors of emotion and perceived health	McKinney, 2000
	Intervention to increase self-care measures, breast cancer chemotherapy patients	Craddock, Adams, Usui, & Mitchell, 1999
	Case study, patient with hepatocellular carcinoma after extended right hepatectomy	Cheung, 2002
Mental health	Psychiatric patient and caregiver burden, a scale	Pipatananond & Hanucharurnkul, 2003
	Perceived social support, symptoms, and self-care actions, adults with schizophrenia, community living	Dato, 2002

Continued

Table 14-1

Survey of Current Literature—cont'd

CATEGORY	TOPIC	AUTHOR, DATE
	Assessing patients' perception of self-care agency in psychiatric care	Cutler, 2003
	SCA and symptom management in patients treated for mood disorder	Cutler, 2001
	Living with serious mental illness: the desire for normalcy	Pickens, 1999
	Self-neglect	Lauder, 2001
Diabetes	Self-care capabilities and nursing required to manage diabetes mellitus	Allison, 2003
	Self-care and dependent-care responsibility, adolescents with type I diabetes and their parents	Dashiff, 2003
	Health beliefs, social support, and self-care behaviors, older Thai persons, type 2 diabetes	Surit, 2002
Maternity	Nursing diagnosis in high-risk pregnant women	Farias & Nobrega, 2000
	Utilization of prenatal care by women	Cooksey-James, 1999
	Reducing incidence of teenage and unintended pregnancies, client-centered and family-focused school-based family planning programs	Porter, 1998
	The construct of thriving during pregnancy and postpartum	Walker & Grobe, 1999
Cardiology	Heart failure self-care inventory, instrument development	Ahrens, 2001
	Supportive-education nursing system for patients with advanced heart failure	Jaarsma, Halfens, Senten, Saad, & Dracup, 1998
	Adherence to cardiac therapy for men with coronary artery disease	Baird & Pierce, 2001
	Problems of cardiac patients in early recovery	Jaarsma, Kastermans, Dassen, & Philipsen, 1995
	Self-care and dependent-care experiences, Thai patients recovering from coronary artery bypass graft surgery	Asdornwised, 2000
	Self-care behaviors among patients with heart failure	Artinian, Magnan, Sloan, & Lange, 2002
	Quality of life in patients with pacemakers	Malm, Karlsson, & Fridlund, 1998

Table 14-1

Survey of Current Literature—cont'd

CATEGORY	TOPIC	AUTHOR, DATE
Renal/urology	Self-care of dialyzed patients, literature review	Ricka, Vanrenterghem, & Evers, 2002
	Self-care of well adult Canadians and adult Canadians with end-stage renal disease	Horsburgh, 1999
	Applying SCDNT to continence care	Bernier, 2002a
	Pelvic floor rehabilitation program for urinary incontinence	Bernier, 2002b
	Evaluation of a hemodialysis patient education and support program	Korniewicz & O'Brien, 1994
Asthma	Self-care and the adult with asthma	Monteiro, Nobrega, & Lima, 2002
	Partners views of asthma self-management and family environment, asthmatic adults' quality of life	Geden, Isaramalai, & Taylor, 2002
HIV	Effects of caffeine reduction on sleep and well-being in persons with HIV	Dreher, 2000
	Nursing management of anxiety in patients with HIV infection	Phillips & Morrow, 1998
NURSING FOCUS		
Patient education	Discharge planning and convalescence at home, same-day surgery patients	Young, O'Connell, & McGregor, 2000
	Evaluation of education materials	Wilson, Mood, Risk, & Kershaw, 2003
Supportive-educative nursing system	Developing a program for patients with advanced heart failure	Jaarsma, Halfens, Senten, Saad, & Dracup, 1998
Primary care	Nurse practitioners practice in primary care settings	Geden, Isaramalai, & Taylor, 2001
	The primary nurse practitioner: advocate for self-care	Thrasher, 2002
Health promotion	Health-promoting self-care behaviors, self-care self-efficacy, and self-care agency	Callaghan, 2003
	Adequacy of a health promotion self-care interview guide with healthy, middle-aged, Mexican-American women	Hartweg, 1996

HIV, Human immunodeficiency virus; *SCA,* self-care agency; *SCDNT,* Self-Care Deficit Nursing Theory; *TSCD,* therapeutic self-care demand.

process for new graduate nurses. For them, the first work experience is often the most difficult. There is some conflict with school teachings and work values. Educational programs based in SCDNT assist these nurses in combining their school teachings with the nursing work they perform after graduation (Feldsine, 1982).

Orem's theory has been used to define and describe various roles for nurses within multiple settings. The clinical nurse specialist role, the case management role, the advanced practice role, and the primary care role are documented as having gained meaning through the application of the theory (Geden, Isaramalai, & Taylor, 2001; Hurlock-Chorostecki, 1999; Issel, 1995; Mezinskis, 1998; Oliver, 2003). The administrative role and importance of SCDNT in designing systems of care are also described. Allison and Renpenning (1999) describe both the process of theory integration in practice and examples of products of that, including assessment and care planning. Evers (2000) explored quality assurance in clinical nursing. There are several reports of the use of Orem's SCDNT in the development of clinical measurement approaches. The first major work done in this area was a study by Horn and Swain (1978). They developed criteria measures of nursing care focused around the universal self-care requisites and health deviation self-care requisites. This work is still relevant and useful. Since then, a number of other clinical instruments have been developed. Moore and Gaffney (1989) developed the Dependent Care Agent questionnaire to measure mothers' performance of care activities for their children. Graff, Thomas, Hollingsworth, Cohen, and Rubin (1992) developed a postoperative self-assessment form with Orem's concept of the nurse assisting the patient in self-care. Riley (1996) developed a self-care action scale for chronic obstructive pulmonary disease. The Denyes Self-Care Agency Instrument (DSCAI) and the Denyes Self-Care Practice Instrument (DSCPI) are also useful in clinical practice (Denyes, 1980). Instruments have been developed to examine psychiatric patient and caregiver burden (Pipatananond & Hanucharurnkul, 2003), osteoporosis (Ailinger, Lasus, & Braun, 2003), heart failure self-care inventory (Ahrens, 2001), and women's self-care (Weber, 2000).

Much of the published literature is limited to Orem's theory of self-care and self-care deficit or other components of those theories as a way to explain practice. Orem cautions that the appropriate use of the SCDNT entails the use of all three theories as follows: (1) self-care, (2) self-care deficit, and (3) nursing systems. Supportive-educative nursing systems have been documented as effective with pregnant women, persons with advanced heart failure, and children with cancer (Betz, 2000; Hart & Foster, 1998; Jaarsma, Halfens, Senten, Saad, & Dracup, 1998; Rieg, 2000). Wholly compensatory nursing care was described by Evers related to enteral food intake (Evers, Viane, Sermeus, Simoens-De Smet, & Delesie, 2000). The theory of nursing systems can be inferred from the literature; however, it is not used explicitly, perhaps because of the complexity of practice. Orem (2001) notes that "nursing examined from the perspective of a human practical science is very complex" but should not be a reason to turn from a "vision of the wholeness of nursing science" (p. 179).

Education

This theory was first articulated in the 1950s; it was formalized and first published in 1972 for the purpose of "laying out the structure of nursing knowledge and explicating the domains of nursing knowledge" (Taylor, 1998). Orem began thinking about the need for a nursing-specific knowledge structure when she was director of the school at Providence Hospital in Detroit. She wrote the chapter on nursing for a report on nursing services for the Division of Hospital and Institutional Services of the Indiana State Board of Health (Orem, 1956). Orem returned to Washington, D.C., and took a position with the Office of Education, Vocational Section of the Technical Division, which had an ongoing project to upgrade practical nurse training. At this time, she began the more formal work of structuring her theory. She concluded that the following question needed to be answered: Why do people need nursing? Some of the elements of SCDNT emerged and were recorded in *Guides for*

Developing Curriculum for the Education of Practical Nurses (Orem, 1959).

After the publication of the *Guides for Developing Curriculum for the Education of Practical Nurses*, Orem began working on a book, *Foundations of Nursing and Its Practice* (Orem, 1967), which was published privately and used at Morris Harvey College (now the University of Charleston). Sections on education are found in each of Orem's subsequent book publications.

A number of reports in the literature describe the use of SCDNT as the basis for the curriculum (Berbiglia & Saenz, 2000; Hartweg, 1995, 2000; Raithel & Meyer, 2000). At least 45 schools of nursing have used SCDNT as the basis for their curricula (data from the International Orem Society). Taylor (1985a, 1985b) described the use of the theory in preservice nursing education and in teaching. The Sinclair School of Nursing, University of Missouri at Columbia, has used SCDNT as the framework for curriculum and teaching since 1978. The theory is used at all levels of the curriculum and in continuing education. Oakland University, College of St. Benedict, Oklahoma City University, and Anderson College are four schools with curricula designed within SCDNT. Samples of their courses may be accessed through the Internet by searching for SCDNT. Hartweg (2000) describes the 20-year experience with the theory at Illinois Wesleyan University, including the basic curriculum and the changes that have been made. Illinois Wesleyan University found the SCDNT a strong and effective framework for curricular design.

Research

The research related to or derived from Orem's theory can be classified as relating to the following three areas:

1. Development of research instruments for measuring the conceptual elements of the theory
2. Studies that test elements of the theory in specific populations
3. Development of new models or middle range theory

Research specific to the use of the theory in clinical situations is reviewed in the previous section on practice. This chapter is not to be considered a critical review of research literature. The complexity of such an analysis is beyond the scope of this chapter. Banfield (1997) and Taylor and colleagues (2000) examined the philosophical basis of Orem's work. They affirmed that moderate realism is foundational to Orem's work and hold the position that compatible research methods need to be used.

A number of instruments for research have been developed and critiqued (Carter, 1998; McBride, 1991; Moore & Pichler, 2000). Harris and Frey (2000) examined the measurement of concepts related to dependent-care and self-care practices. The SCDNT was the conceptual groundwork for the Exercise of Self-Care Agency (ESCA) (Kearney & Fleischer, 1972), the DSCAI (Denyes, 1980), and Hanson and Bickel's Perception of Self-Care Agency in 1981 (McBride, 1991). The SCDNT was a pivotal construct in the design of the Self-as-Carer Inventory (SCI) (Geden & Taylor, 1991). This inventory permits individuals to express their perceived capacity to care for self. McBride (1991) did a comparative analysis of the following three instruments designed to measure self-care agency: (1) DSCAI, (2) Kearney and Fleischer's ESCA, and (3) Hanson and Bickel's Perception of Self-Care Agency. To identify latent traits and their relationships, a common factor analysis and canonical correlation was performed. The results supported the multidimensionality of Orem's concept of self-care agency. McBride (1987) also points out that the use of only one instrument does not adequately reflect this multidimensionality. Geden and Taylor (1991, 1999) tested the construct and the empirical validity of the SCI and found that it seemed to possess strong theoretical validity, but they recommended further validity testing. The Appraisal of Self-Care Agency (ASA) scale was developed to measure the core concept of Orem's SCDNT (Evers, Isenberg, Philipsen, Senten, & Brouns, 1993). An extensive body of literature supports the use of ASA with well and ill populations in a number of cultures. The research instruments used most frequently include the ESCA, DSCAI, DSCPI, ASA, and SCI.

Some examples of the use of these tools follow. Moore (1995) used the Child and Adolescent Self-Care Practice Questionnaire, the DSCAI, and the ESCA when she measured the self-care practices of children and adolescents. McCaleb and Edgil (1994) used the DCSPI to measure self-concept and self-care practices of healthy adolescents. The ESCA and the ASA were used to assess basic conditioning factors and self-care abilities related to the health of pregnant women and their infants (Hart, 1995; Mapanga & Andrews, 1995). The SCI was used to describe collaborative care systems in adults (Geden & Taylor, 1999) and quality of life in ovarian cancer survivors (Nicholson, 2002) and community-dwelling older adults (White, 2000).

FURTHER DEVELOPMENT

Since the publication of the first edition of *Nursing: Concepts of Practice* in 1971, Orem has been engaged in the continual development of her conceptualizations. She has worked by herself and with colleagues. The sixth edition was completed and published in 2001. Orem presently works with a group of scholars, known as the Orem Study Group, to further develop the various conceptualizations and to structure nursing knowledge using the elements of the theory. This work led to the expression of a theory of dependent care (Taylor, et al., 2001) and the foundational science of self-care (Denyes, Orem, & Bekel, 2001). Other work that contributes to the development of SCDNT or to the understanding of theoretical components throughout the years is noteworthy. There is literature regarding nursing theory and nursing processes, including nursing diagnosis, from the perspective of SCDNT (Backsheider, 1974; Dennis & Jesek-Hale, 2003; Evers, 2001; Monteiro, Nobrega, & Lima, 2002; Taylor, 1988, 1991). The development of positive mental health from the perspective of the SCDNT was described by Orem and Vardiman (1995), contributing to both the knowledge base for psychiatric nursing and health promotion content.

Taylor (2001) examined theoretical concerns regarding Orem's general theory of nursing and families.

Other scholars have developed models that explain aspects of SCDNT. Some refer to these as middle range theory work. Examples include health promotion (Hartweg, 1990) and a model incorporating two new concepts—desired focal condition and regulatory outcome—to explain the relationship of self-care to health as an indirect one mediated by these concepts (Magnan, 2001). Models related to dependent care, family, and community (Taylor, 1989; Taylor et al., 2001; Taylor & McLaughlin, 1991; Taylor & Renpenning, 1995) have been developed. A model for collaborative care demonstrates the interaction of self-care systems in adults within enduring relationships (Geden, Isaramalai, & Taylor, 2002; Geden & Taylor, 1999). Weber (2000) developed a secondary concept of women's self-care. Weber also proposes an alternate method for concept analysis. Lauder (2001) explores the utility of self-care theory in understanding self-neglect. Burks (1999) proposes a model for chronic illness focused on enhanced self-management skills and the rehabilitation nurse's role in this process. A nursing practice theory of exercise as self-care is proposed by Ulbrich (1999). Philosophical and ethical considerations relative to SCDNT are also available (Banfield, 1997; Bekel, 1999; Taylor, 1998; Taylor et al., 2000; Taylor & Godfrey, 1999).

Nursing: Concepts of Practice (Orem, 2001) is organized with two focuses, nursing as a unique field of knowledge and nursing as practical science. It includes an expansion, from earlier editions, of content on nursing science and the theory of nursing systems. Important work has been done on the nature of person and interpersonal features of nursing. Orem identifies many areas for further development in her descriptions of the stages of theory development. She also describes the development of the science of self-care, which could include concepts such as elaboration of operational functions of self-care agency with the elements of sensation and perception, appraisal, and motivation and determining the relevance of the foundational capabilities and dispositions to discreet acts. There is a need to focus on person-in-the-situation and on capabilities for action and self-management. This content has been expanded in the description of the foundational nursing science of self-care (Denyes et al., 2001).

Allison and Renpenning (1999) further developed Orem's conceptualization of nursing administration. Based on their experiences, they presented a comprehensive approach to the use of the SCDNT within a health care organization, including all levels of the nursing service and care delivery. Ongoing research by many nursing scholars will clarify certain conceptualizations and will demonstrate the relationship of theory and practice.

The International Orem Society (IOS) for Nursing Science and Nursing Scholarship was established in 1993. Incorporated as a not-for-profit organization, the purpose of the IOS is to advance nursing science and scholarship through the use of Dorothea E. Orem's nursing conceptualizations in nursing education, practice, and research. The IOS publishes a semiannual newsletter. Some issues can be accessed through the Internet on the self-care deficit theory home page (*http://www.muhealth. org/nursing/scdnt/scdnt.html*), which is maintained by the University of Missouri at Columbia, Sinclair School of Nursing. In 2002, the IOS newsletter became the journal *Self Care, Dependent Care and Nursing.* The Sixth Inter-national Self-Care Deficit Theory Conference, which was held in Bangkok, Thailand, in February 2000, had more than 300 participants from many countries. There were over 70 research presentations that demonstrated the international use of Orem's theory. The Eighth International Self-Care Deficit Theory Conference was held in Ulm, Germany, October 2004.

CRITIQUE
Clarity

The terms Orem uses are defined precisely. The language of the theory is consistent with the language used in action theory and philosophy. The terminology of the theory is congruent throughout. The term *self-care* has multiple meanings across disciplines; Orem has defined the term and elaborated the substantive structure of the concept in a way that is unique, but also congruent with other interpretations. References have been made to the difficulty of Orem's language; however, the limitation generally resides in the reader's lack of familiarity with practical science and the field of action science.

Simplicity

Orem's theory is expressed in a limited number of terms. These terms are defined and used consistently in the expression of the theory. Orem's general theory, SCDNT, comprises the following three constituent theories: (1) self-care, (2) self-care deficit, and (3) nursing systems. The self-care deficit theory of nursing is a synthesis of knowledge about eight entities, which include self-care (and dependent-care), self-care agency (and dependent-care agency), therapeutic self-care demand, self-care deficit, nursing agency, and nursing system. The development of the theory using these entities is parsimonious. The relationship between and among these entities can be presented in a simple diagram. The substantive structure of the theory is found in the development of these entities. The depth of the concepts' development gives the theory the complexity necessary to describe and understand a human practice discipline.

Generality

Orem (1995) has commented on the generality or universality of the theory, as follows:

> The self-care deficit theory of nursing is not an explanation of the individuality of a particular concrete nursing practice situation, but rather the expression of a singular combination of conceptualized properties or features common to all instances of nursing. As a general theory, it serves nurses engaged in nursing practice, in development

and validation of nursing knowledge, and in teaching and learning nursing. (pp. 166-167)

A review of the research and other literature attests to the generality of the theory.

Empirical Precision

Orem's theory has been used for research using both qualitative and quantitative methodologies. The theoretical entities are well defined and lend themselves to measurement; however, instruments have not been developed for all entities. Empirical precision is dependent on the operational definitions constructed by the researcher for the population to be studied. Furthermore, the values of the theoretical entities are not constant across populations. Dennis and Jesek-Hale (2003) demonstrate this is in their work on the theory of self-care deficit. A self-care deficit is a function of the self-care requisites and basic conditioning factors. This necessitates the development of multiple instruments to measure the therapeutic self-care demand. Moore and Pichler (2000) examined research on basic conditioning factors and, noting the difficulty in gaining consensus on definition and measurement, suggest some strategies for measurement.

The most appropriate methods of inquiry for this theory and all nursing theories are evolving. There are reports of hermeneutic, ethnographic, phenomenological, and traditional quantitative methodologies used to test components of SCDNT or to test clinical phenomena by using components of SCDNT (Asdornwised, 2000; Wells-Biggs, 1985). The beauty of Orem's theory is in its scope, complexity, and clinical usefulness; it is useful for generating hypotheses and adding to the body of knowledge that is nursing.

Derivable Consequences

The SCDNT differentiates the focus of nursing from other disciplines. Although other disciplines find the theory of self-care helpful and contribute to its development, the theory of nursing systems provides the unique focus for nursing. The literature contains ample evidence that SCDNT is useful in developing and guiding practice and research. It gives direction to nursing-specific outcomes related to knowing and meeting the therapeutic self-care demands, regulating the development and exercise of self-care agency, and establishing self-care and self-management systems.

The theory is also useful in designing curricula for preservice, graduate, and continuing nursing education (Hartweg, 2000; Raithel & Meyer, 2000; Taylor, 1985a). The theory also gives direction to nursing administration. The significance of Orem's work extends far beyond the development of the SCDNT. In her works, she has provided the expression of the form of nursing science as practical science with a structure for ongoing development of nursing knowledge in the stages of theory development. She has presented a visionary view of contemporary nursing practice, education, and knowledge development expressed through the general theory.

SUMMARY

The critical question, what is the condition that indicates that a person needs nursing care, was the starting point for the development of the SCDNT. Orem noted that it was the inability of persons to maintain on a continuous basis their own care or the care of dependents. From this she began the process of formalizing knowledge about what persons need to do or have done for themselves to maintain health and well-being. When a person needs assistance, what are the appropriate nursing assistive actions? The theory of self-care describes what a person requires and what actions need to be taken to meet those requirements. The theory of self-care deficits describes the limitations in meeting the requirements for ongoing care and the effects these have on health and well-being of the person or dependent. The theory of nursing systems provides the structure for examining the actions and antecedent knowledge required to assist the person. These theories are also descriptive of situations involving families and communities.

Case Study

This case study documents an initial interaction between a nurse practitioner and clients, a married couple, in a primary care situation. The constituent units of design for the production of nursing (Orem, 2001, p. 296) provide the outline for the narrative.

Contract for Nursing

Betty is the wife and caregiver of George, who has had Parkinson's disease for 15 years. She is requesting information regarding the possibility of help with long-term care.

An initial assessment leads to the conclusion that there is no evidence of need for immediate regulatory action. This is always the first step and is based on information about universal self-care requisites focused particularly on maintaining adequate intake of oxygen, safety, or critical health states.

The husband indicates he is managing well but is frustrated by his inability to do things he used to be able to do (e.g., go out when or where he wished, to use hands for fine motor activities such as photography). George is a 71-year-old male of German origin, formerly an engineer. His wife expresses distress with high-risk behavior exhibited by her husband and frustration with her inability to help him recognize and accept the danger of his actions and the limitations present because of the disease and its treatment.

Legitimate Functional Unity of Care Providers

Until the last few years, George was a competent self-carer. He regularly sought medical help and followed physician instructions. Betty has been instrumental in helping him manage his illness. They have frequent contact with the neurologist and the nurse practitioner. George has been hospitalized several times for trauma related to falls. They are a well-groomed couple, well spoken, pleasant, cooperative, communicative, agreeable, responsive to questions, and able to answer questions.

George has stage 3 Parkinson's disease with postural instability (difficulty sitting, standing from sitting position, walking) and lymphedema, especially in his right leg. He has limited sensation and control of his fingers. He is a tall man, which makes it difficult for his wife to assist him.

Betty reports that her husband has stayed out late into early morning hours several times. She didn't know how to locate him. He didn't have needed medications along and required stranger assistance to return home; similar high-risk behavior is repeated regularly. Betty expresses difficulty dealing with these situations.

When out of the house, George behaves as if the environment is safe and his physical limitations don't put him at risk. His disease forced him into early retirement, with a drastic reduction in personal financial resources. He has cognitive limitations associated with disease and treatment, among them an inability to process new information, and he does not anticipate potential consequences of his behaviors. The couple lives in an apartment that is handicapped accessible.

Components of the Care System

The couple has an established collaborative care system (Geden & Taylor, 1999). George sees his self-care system as fine—what he can't do, his wife does, and if she is away, she arranges for somebody to help. If he needs help, he can and does get it. This perception is congruent with many collaborative care situations. However, Betty expresses the need for changes in their care system. Frustration with the current situation is evident. The apparent self-care system in place is generated primarily by dependent-care agent; George engages in some actions and makes some judgments within the system. No nursing system is in place. George says he manages well with assistance of his wife, physicians, and others who help out.

Therapeutic Self-Care Demand
Components Universal Self-Care Requisites
I. Maintain general good nutrition.
   A. Because of the medications, increased fluids and decreased protein are required.

B. Because of difficulty swallowing, attention to avoiding foods with high potential for choking is required.

C. Because of loss of fine motor control, adapted silverware is required.

II. Maintain intake of air using normal care measures.

III. Maintain elimination.

   A. Adaptive devices and personal assistance for getting to bathroom and managing clothing are required because of pathology and mobility limitations.

   B. Constipation is associated with the mobility limitations of parkinsonism and medication side effects, so measures such as increased fluid intake and laxatives may be required.

IV. Maintain a balance between solitude and social interaction.

   A. Neither solitude nor excessive social interaction is appropriate.

V. Maintain a balance between rest and activity.

   A. Neither excessive activity nor rest is appropriate.

   B. A lift chair may be required.

   C. There may need for a hospital bed in the home.

   D. Sleep is disturbed often.

VI. Maintain protection from hazards.

   A. There is a need for careful evaluation of potential hazards and means to address them.

VII. Promote normalcy.

   A. Create an environment that allows George to function as normally as possible (e.g., use of adaptive devices, lift chair).

Betty's requisites are those to be expected of a 65-year-old woman. In addition, she needs to make adjustments to her self-care in order to accommodate to her husband's demands.

Developmental Self-Care Requisites

Because of progressive chronic disease and unresolved issues, George is unable to progress developmentally; actions to date are unsuccessful in moving him forward with his developmental tasks. The progressive nature of the disease has led to changes in the collaborative care system such that the relationship is becoming more of a dependent-care system. This creates difficulties for both Betty and George. Although he accepts himself as having parkinsonism, he is not realistic about the effect it has on him.

Health Deviation Self-Care Requisites

They need to continue to seek medical attention regularly. Reliance on pharmacological management of pathology, to the exclusion of other management approaches, results in medication side effects that cause more problems to arise.

George accepts himself as a person with Parkinson's disease in need of health care but is frustrated with the progression and its effect on his ability to participate in activities. Both George and Betty are struggling to live with the effects of pathology that will not enable developmental progression. No additional needs were identified by George.

Self-Care and Dependent-Care Capabilities

George has severely limited abilities for decision making and self-care. George is unable to manage many activities of daily living, including both physical and decision-making activities; those he can manage require increasingly long periods. This will get progressively worse. Betty expresses a need for assistance in living with her husband in his current health state and with the associated care needs. Betty is well informed about the disease process, treatment modalities, and overall self-care requirements associated with the disease, and she is a skilled caregiver. She will continue to manage and control the care system but will find it more and more difficult to do the physical work of taking care of George.

Features of the Nursing System

The nursing system for George and Betty is periodic. It articulates with a dependent-care system as well as the self-care systems of both persons. As the disease progresses, there will be a need for assistance in accessing resources for care and, in some instances, providing care to George and support to Betty. As noted, Betty wishes to maintain management and control of the care system. She seeks a collaborative role with the nurse practitioner and others. As a first step, the nurse will assist the couple in getting appropriate adaptive equipment, such as a hospital bed and a powered wheelchair. Over time, when a need is identified, home care assistance will be initiated. The nurse and others will help Betty and George determine levels of assistance required. When it is not reasonable for Betty to continue to care for George at home, the physician, nurse, and others will aid them in relocating George to a residential facility.

The progressive nature of parkinsonism requires a long-term anticipatory approach to care. It will require many different persons as the problems change and new demands arise. Attention will need to be paid to Betty's self-care system while she increases her role as dependent caregiver.

CRITICAL THINKING *Activities*

1. Orem's writings are not all expositions of the SCDNT. Review some of her writings and identify works of theory and works of application or related ideas about nursing.

2. Review the definitions provided in the glossary of the sixth edition of *Nursing: Concepts of Practice* (Orem, 2001). Classify them as conceptual or operational, denotative or connotative. Explain.

3. Select a research article that purports to use SCDNT as the conceptual framework. Is the research question derived from the theory? What contribution does it make to further understanding of the theory?

4. Make a list of the definitions of nursing the theorists use. Which ones are specific to

nursing? Evaluate Orem's description of the proper object of nursing. How does that relate to others?

REFERENCES

Ahrens, S. L. G. (2001). The development and testing of the Heart Failure Self-Care Inventory: An instrument for measuring heart failure self-care. (Doctoral dissertation, Wayne State University). *Dissertation Abstracts International, 62,* 5636B.

Ailinger, R. L., Lasus, H., & Braun, M. A. (2003). Brief report. Revision of the Facts on Osteoporosis Quiz. *Nursing Research, 52*(3), 198-201.

Allison, S. E. (1973). A framework for nursing action in a nurse conducted diabetic managed clinic. *Journal of Nursing Administration, 3*(4), 53-60.

Allison, S. E. (2003). A posthumous reconstruction of an unpublished study by Joan E. Backscheider on self-care capabilities and nursing required to manage diabetes mellitus. *International Orem Society Newsletter, 11*(2), 5-14.

Allison, S. E., & Renpenning, K. (1999). *Nursing administration in the 21st century.* Thousand Oaks, CA: Sage.

Anderson, J. A., & Olnhausen, K. S. (1999). Adolescent self-esteem: A foundational disposition. *Nursing Science Quarterly, 12(1),* 62-67.

Artinian, N. T., Magnan, M., Sloan, M., & Lange, M. P. (2002). Self-care behaviors among patients with heart failure. *Heart & Lung: Journal of Acute & Critical Care, 31*(3),161-172.

Asdornwised, U. P. (2000). Self-care and dependent-care experiences of Thai patients recovering from coronary artery bypass graft surgery: An ethnographic study. *Dissertation Abstracts International, 61,* 1318B.

Backsheider, J. (1974). Self-care requirements, self-care capabilities and nursing systems in the diabetic nurse managed clinic. *American Journal of Public Health, 64*(12), 1138-1146.

Baird, K. K., & Pierce L. L. (2001). Adherence to cardiac therapy for men with coronary artery disease. *Rehabilitation Nursing, 26*(6), 233-237, 243, 251.

Banfield, B. E. (1997). A philosophical inquiry of Orem's self-care deficit nursing theory. *Dissertation Abstracts International, 58,* 5885B.

Bekel, G. (1998). Theory-based nursing practice in Germany. *International Orem Society Newsletter, 6*(2), 6-7.

Bekel, G. (1999). Statements on the object of science: A discussion paper. *International Orem Society Newsletter, 7*(1), 1-3.

Berbiglia, V. A., & Saenz, J. (2000). Design, implementation, and evaluation of a self-care undergraduate elective. *The International Orem Society Newsletter, 8*(1), 2-5.

Bernier, F. (2002a). Relationship of a pelvic floor rehabilitation program for urinary incontinence to Orem's self-care deficit theory of nursing: Part 1. *Urologic Nursing, 22*(6), 378-383, 390-391.

Bernier, F. (2002b). Applying Orem's self-care deficit theory of nursing to continence care: Part 2. *Urologic Nursing, 22*(6), 384-391.

Betz, C. L. (2000). California healthy and ready to work transition health care guide: Developmental guidelines for teaching health care self-care skills to children. *Issues in Comprehensive Pediatric Nursing, 23*(4), 203-244.

Biggs, A. J., & Freed, P. E. (2000). Nutrition and older adults: What do family caregivers know and do? *Journal of Gerontological Nursing, 26*(8), 6-14.

Burks, K. J. (1999). A nursing practice model for chronic illness. *Rehabilitation Nursing, 24*(5), 197-200.

Callaghan, D. M. (2003). Health-promoting self-care behaviors, self-care self-efficacy, and self-care agency. *Nursing Science Quarterly, 16*(3), 247-254.

Campbell, J. C., & Weber, N. (2000). An empirical test of a self-care model of women's responses to battering. *Nursing Science Quarterly, 13*(1), 45-53.

Canty-Mitchell, J. (2001). Life change events, hope, and self-care agency in inner-city adolescents [corrected]. *Journal of Child & Adolescent Psychiatric Nursing, 14*(1), 18-31. [Published erratum appears in *Journal of Child & Adolescent Psychiatric Nursing* (2001, Apr-Jun). *14*(2), 54.]

Carter, P. A. (1998). Self-care agency: The concept and how it is measured. *Journal of Nursing Measurement, 6*(2), 195-207.

Cheung, J. (2002). Applying Orem's self-care framework to the nursing care of a patient with hepatocellular carcinoma after extended right hepatectomy. *Hong Kong Nursing Journal, 38*(1), 20-26.

Cooksey-James, T. J. (1999). Utilization of prenatal care by women of St. Thomas, United States Virgin Islands: A descriptive study. *Dissertation Abstracts International, 61,* 2470B.

Craddock, R. B., Adams, P. F., Usui, W. M., & Mitchell, L. (1999). An intervention to increase use and effectiveness of self-care measures for breast cancer chemotherapy patients. *Cancer Nursing, 22*(4), 312-319.

Cutler, C. (2003). Assessing patients' perception of self-care agency in psychiatric care. *Issues in Mental Health Nursing, 24*(2), 199-211.

Cutler, C. G. (2001). Self-care agency and symptom management in patients treated for mood disorder. *Archives of Psychiatric Nursing, 15*(1), 24-31.

Dashiff, C. J. (2003). Self- and dependent-care responsibility of adolescents with IDDM and their parents. *Journal of Family Nursing, 9*(2), 166-183.

Dato, C. (2002). A. The relationship of perceived social support, positive symptoms, negative symptoms, and self-care actions in adults with schizophrenia living in the community. *Dissertation Abstracts International, 63,* 1266B.

Deng, X., & Xie, X. (2001). Apply Orem theory and theory of holistic nursing care to set up a nursing model for the aged in community [Chinese]. *Chinese Nursing Research, 15*(3), 173-174.

Dennis, C. M., & Jesek-Hale, S. (2003). Calculating therapeutic self-care demand for a nursing population of normal newborns. *Self Care, Dependent Care and Nursing, 11*(1), 3-10.

Denyes, M. J. (1980). Development of an instrument to measure self-care agency in adolescents. *Dissertation Abstracts International, 41,* 1716B.

Denyes, M. J., Orem, D. E., & Bekel, G. (2001). Self-care: A foundational science. *Nursing Science Quarterly, 14*(1), 48-54.

Dreher, H. M. (2000). The effect of caffeine reduction on sleep and well-being in persons with HIV (immune deficiency). *Dissertation Abstracts International, 61,* 4649B.

Duncan, S., & Murphy, F. (1988). Embracing a conceptual model. *Canadian Nurse, 84*(4), 24-26.

Evers, G. C. M. (2000). Clinical nursing research. Quality assurance revisited [German]. *Pflege, 13*(3), 133-138.

Evers, G. C. M. (2001). Viewpoint. Naming nursing: Evidence-based nursing. *Nursing Diagnosis, 2*(4), 137-142.

Evers, G. C. M., Isenberg, M. A., Philipsen, H., Senten, M., & Brouns, G. (1993). Validity testing of the Dutch translation of the appraisal of the self-care agency A.S.A. scale. *International Journal of Nursing Studies, 30*(4), 331-342.

Evers, G., Viane, A., Sermeus, W., Simoens-De Smet, A., & Delesie, L. (2000). Frequency of and indications for wholly compensatory nursing care related to enteral food intake: A secondary analysis of the Belgium National Nursing Minimum Data Set. *Journal of Advanced Nursing, 32*(1), 194-201.

Farias, M. C. A., & Nobrega, M. M. L. (2000). Nursing diagnoses in high-risk pregnant women based on Orem's self-care theory—A case study [Portuguese]. *Revista Latino-Americana de Enfermagem, 8*(6), 59-67.

Feldsine, F. T. (1982). Options for transition into practice: Nursing process orientation program . . . bicultural approach and Orem's conceptual framework of self-care. *Journal, New York State Nurses Association, 13*(1), 11-16.

Fialho, A. V. M., Pagliuca, L. M. F., & Soares, E. (2002). The Self-Care Deficit Theory adjustment in home-care in the light of Barnum's Model [Portuguese]. *Revista Latino-Americana de Enfermagem, 10*(5), 715-720.

Garcia Velazquez, M. C. (2002). A healthy old man: Plan of care based on D. Orem's theory [Spanish]. *Gerokomos, 13*(1), 17-26.

Geden, E., Isaramalai S., & Taylor, S. (2002). Influences of partners' views of asthma self-management and family environment on asthmatic adults' asthma quality of life. *Applied Nursing Research, 15*(4), 217-226.

Geden, E., Isaramalai, S., & Taylor, S. G. (2001). The value of self-care deficit nursing theory in informing the nurse practitioner's practice in primary care settings. *Nursing Science Quarterly, 14*(1), 29-33.

Geden, E., & Taylor, S. (1991). Construct and empirical validity of the self-as-carer inventory. *Nursing Research, 40*(1), 47-50.

Geden, E., & Taylor, S. G. (1999). Theoretical and empirical description of adult couples' collaborative care systems. *Nursing Science Quarterly, 12*(4), 329-334.

Graff, B. M., Thomas, J. S., Hollingsworth, A. O., Cohen, S. M., & Rubin, M. M. (1992). Development of a postoperative self-assessment form. *Clinical Nurse Specialist, 6*(1), 47-50.

Grov, E. K. (1999). Death at home—How can the nurse contribute in making death at home possible for people with terminal cancer? [Norwegian]. *Vard i Norden. Nursing Science & Research in the Nordic Countries, 19*(4), 4-9.

Gullifer, J. (1997). The acceptance of a philosophically based research culture? *International Journal of Nursing Practice, 3*, 153-158.

Harris, M. A., & Frey, M. A. (2000). Measurement corner. Measures of concepts from Orem's self-care deficit theory: Dependent-care actions and self-care practices. *Journal of Child & Family Nursing, 3*(5), 373-376.

Hart, M. A. (1995). Orem's self-care deficit theory: Research with pregnant women. *Nursing Science Quarterly, 8*(3), 120-126.

Hart, M. A., & Foster, S. N. (1998). Self-care agency in two groups of pregnant women. *Nursing Science Quarterly, 11*(4), 167-171.

Hartweg, D. L. (1990). Health promotion self-care within Orem's general theory of nursing. *Journal of Advance Nursing, 15*(1), 35-41.

Hartweg, D. L. (1995). Curricular decisions: Using Orem's conceptualizations to guide curriculum and student clinical practice. *International Orem Society Newsletter, 3*(1), 8-9.

Hartweg, D. L. (1996). Determining the adequacy of a health promotion self-care interview guide with healthy, middle-aged, Mexican-American women: A pilot study. *Health Care for Women International, 17*(1), 57-68.

Hartweg, D. L. (2000). Use of Orem's conceptualizations in a baccalaureate nursing program: 1980-2000. *International Orem Society Newsletter, 8*(1), 5-7.

Hitejc, Z. (2000). Application of the theory of Dorothy (sic) Orem in the process of nursing care of mentally and physically handicapped children [Slovenian]. *Obzornik Zdravstvene Nege, 34*(3/4), 121-125.

Horn, B. J., & Swain, M. A. (1978). *Development of criterion measures of nursing care* (Vols. 1 and 2; NTIS Publication No. 267-004 and 267-005). Washington, DC: National Center for Health Services Research, U.S. Department of Commerce.

Horsburgh, M. E. (1999). Self-care of well adult Canadians and adult Canadians with end stage renal disease. *International Journal of Nursing Studies, 36*(6), 443-453.

Hurlock-Chorostecki, C. (1999). Holistic care in the critical care setting: Application of a concept through Watson's and Orem's theories of nursing. *CACCN, 10*(4), 20-25.

Issel, M. (1995). Evaluating case management programs. *Maternal-Child Nursing, 20*, 67-74.

Jaarsma, T., Halfens, R., Senten, M., Saad, H. H. A., & Dracup, K. (1998). Developing a supportive-educative program for patients with advanced heart failure within Orem's general theory of nursing. *Nursing Science Quarterly, 11*(2), 79-85.

Jaarsma, T., Kastermans, M., Dassen, T., & Philipsen, H. (1995). Problems of cardiac patients in early recovery. *Journal of Advanced Nursing, 21*, 21-27.

Kearney, B., & Fleischer, B. J. (1972). Development of an instrument to measure exercise of self-care agency. *Research in Nursing and Health, 2*, 25-34.

Knigge-Demal, B. (1998).The child experiencing pain and coping with pain in situations of invasive diagnostics, therapy and nursing care [German]. *Pflege, 11*(6), 324-329.

Komulainen, P. (1991). Occupational health nursing based on self-care theory. *AAOHN Journal, 39*(7), 333-335.

Korniewicz, D. M., & O'Brien, M. E. (1994). Evaluation of a hemodialysis patient education and support program. *American Nephrology Nurses Association Journal, 21*(1), 33-38.

Lauder, W. (2001). The utility of self-care theory as a theoretical basis for self-neglect . . . including commentary by Orem D. E. *Journal of Advanced Nursing, 34*(4), 545-551.

Logue, G. A. (1997). An application of Orem's theory to the nursing management of pertussis. *Journal of School Nursing, 13*(4), 20-25.

Magnan, M. A. (2001). Self-care and health in persons with cancer-related fatigue: Refinement and evaluation of Orem's self-care framework. *Dissertation Abstracts International, 62*, 5644B.

Malathum, P. (2001). A model of factors contributing to perceived abilities for health-promoting self-care of community-dwelling Thai older adults. *Dissertation Abstracts International, 62*, 5034B.

Malm, D., Karlsson, J., & Fridlund, B. (1998). Quality of life in pacemaker patients from a nursing perspective. *Coronary Health Care, 2*(1), 17-27.

Mapanga, K. G., & Andrews, C. M. (1995). The influence of family and friends' basic conditioning factors and self-care agency on unmarried teenage primiparas' engagement in contraceptive practice. *Journal of Community Health, 12*(2), 89-100.

McBride, S. (1987). Validation of an instrument to measure exercise of self-care agency. *Research in Nursing and Health, 10,* 311-316.

McBride, S. (1991). Comparative analysis of three instruments designed to measure self-care agency. *Nursing Research, 40*(1), 12-16.

McCaleb, A. M., & Edgil, A. (1994). Self-concept and self-care practices of healthy adolescents. *Journal of Pediatric Nursing, 9*(4), 233-238.

McKinney, M. L. (2000). Hardiness, threat appraisal, self-care capability, and caregiving characteristics as predictors of emotions and perceived health in family caregivers of cancer patients. *Dissertation Abstracts International, 61,* 2992B.

Meyer, G. L. (2000). The art of watching out: Vigilance in women who have migraine headaches. *Dissertation Abstracts International, 61,* 0781B.

Mezinskis, P. M. (1998). Orem's self-care deficit theory. In A. S. Luggen (Ed.), *NGNA core curriculum for gerontological advanced practice nurses* (pp. 16-19). Thousand Oaks, CA: Sage.

Monteiro, E. M. L., Nobrega, M. M. L., & Lima, L. S. (2002). Self-care and the adult with asthma: The systematization (sic) of nursing assistance [Portuguese]. *Revista Brasileira de Enfermagem, 55*(2), 134-139.

Moore, J. B. (1995). Measuring the self-care practice of children and adolescents: Instrument development. *Maternal-Child Nursing Journal, 23*(3), 101-108.

Moore, J. B., & Gaffney, K. F. (1989). Development of an instrument to measure mothers' performance of self-care activities for children. *Advanced Nursing Science, 12*(1), 76-84.

Moore, J. B., & Pichler, V. H. (2000). Measurement of Orem's basic conditioning factors: A review of published research. *Nursing Science Quarterly, 13*(2), 137-142.

Mosher, R. B., & Moore, J. B. (1998). The relationship of self-concept and self-care in children with cancer. *Nursing Science Quarterly, 11*(3), 116-122.

National League for Nursing Editorial Review Board News. (1987, Dec.). Newark Beth Israel Medical Center adopts Orem's self-care model. *Nursing and Health Care, 8*(10), 593-594.

Nicholson, L. L. (2002). Self-care activities and quality of life in ovarian cancer survivors. *Dissertation Abstracts International, 63,* 1272B.

Nursing Development Conference Group (NDCG), Orem, D. E. (Ed.). (1972). *Concept formalization in nursing: Process and product.* Boston: Little, Brown & Co.

Nursing Development Conference Group (NDCG), Orem, D. E. (Ed.). (1979). *Concept formalization in nursing: Process and product* (2nd ed.). Boston: Little, Brown & Co.

Oliver, C. J. (2003). Triage of the autistic spectrum child utilizing the congruence of case management concepts and Orem's nursing theories. *Lippincott's Case Management, 8*(2), 66-82.

Orem, D. E. (1956). *Hospital nursing service: An analysis.* Report to the Division of Hospital and Institutional Services of the Indiana State Board of Health. Indianapolis: Division of Hospital and Institutional Services.

Orem, D. E. (1959). *Guides for developing curriculum for the education of practical nurses.* Washington, DC: U.S. Department of Health, Education, and Welfare.

Orem, D. E. (1967). *Foundations of nursing and its practice.* Unpublished manuscript distributed by author, Chevy Chase, Maryland, Catholic University of America.

Orem, D. E. (1971). *Nursing: Concepts of practice.* New York: McGraw-Hill.

Orem, D. E. (1980). *Nursing: Concepts of practice* (2nd ed.). New York: McGraw-Hill.

Orem, D. E. (1985). *Nursing: Concepts of practice* (3rd ed.). New York: McGraw-Hill.

Orem, D. E. (1988, May). The form of nursing science. *Nursing Science Quarterly, 1*(2), 75-79.

Orem, D. E. (1991). *Nursing: Concepts of practice* (4th ed.). St. Louis: Mosby.

Orem, D. E. (1995). *Nursing: Concepts of practice* (5th ed.). St. Louis: Mosby.

Orem, D. E. (1997). Views of human beings specific to nursing. *Nursing Science Quarterly, 10*(1), 26-31.

Orem, D. E. (2001). *Nursing: Concepts of practice* (6th ed.). St. Louis: Mosby.

Orem, D. E., & Vardiman, E. M. (1995). Orem's nursing theory and positive mental health: Practical considerations. *Nursing Science Quarterly, 8*(4), 165-173.

Phillips, K.D., & Morrow, J. H. (1998). Nursing management of anxiety in HIV infection. *Issues in Mental Health Nursing, 19*(4), 375-397.

Pickens, J. (1999). Living with serious mental illness: The desire for normalcy. *Nursing Science Quarterly, 12*(3), 233-239.

Pipatananond, P., & Hanucharurnkul, S. (2003). Development of the Psychiatric Patients' Caregiver Burden Scale (the PPCBS). *Thai Journal of Nursing Research, 7*(1), 37-48.

Porter, L. S. (1998). Reducing teenage and unintended pregnancies through client-centered and family-focused school-based family planning programs. *Journal of Pediatric Nursing, 13*(3), 158-163.

Raithel, A., & Meyer, G. (2000). Self care deficit nursing theory: Curriculum development project. *International Orem Society Newsletter, 8*(1), 7-12.

Renker, P. R. (1999). Physical abuse, social support, self-care, and pregnancy outcomes of older adolescents. *JOGNN Journal of Obstetric, Gynecologic, & Neonatal Nursing, 28*(4), 377-388.

Renpenning, K., & Taylor, S. G. (Eds.). (2003). *Self-care theory in nursing: Selected papers of Dorothea Orem.* New York: Springer.

Rew, L. (2003). A theory of taking care of oneself grounded in experiences of homeless youth. *Nursing Research, 52*(4), 234-241.

Ricka, R., Vanrenterghem, Y., & Evers, G. C. M. (2002). Adequate self-care of dialysed patients: A review of the literature. *International Journal of Nursing Studies, 39*(3), 329-339.

Rieg, L. C. (2000). Information retrieval of self-care and dependent-care agents using NetWellnessRTM, a consumer health information network. *Dissertation Abstracts International, 61,* 5801B.

Riley, P. (1996). Development of a COPD self-care action scale. *Rehabilitation Nursing Research, 5*(1), 3-8.

Rodriguez de la Parra, S., & Baquero, B. C. (1999). Autocuidado en el adolescente. *Revista Rol de Enfermia, 22*(4), 497-505. [Self-care in the adolescent. *Revista Rol de Enfermia, 22*(4), 497-505.]

Silva, L. M. G. (2001).A brief reflection on self-care in hospital discharge planning after a bone marrow transplantation (BMT): A case report [Portuguese]. *Revista Latino-Americana de Enfermagem, 9*(4), 75-82.

Slusher, I. L. (1999). Self-care agency and self-care practice of adolescents. *Issues in Comprehensive Pediatric Nursing, 22*(1), 49-58.

Söderhamn, O., & Cliffordson, C. (2001). The internal structure of the Appraisal of Self-care Agency (ASA) scale. *Theoria: Journal of Nursing Theory, 10*(4), 5-12.

Söderhamn, O., Lindencrona, C., & Ek, A. (2000). Ability for self-care among home dwelling elderly people in a health district in Sweden. *International Journal of Nursing Studies, 37*(4), 361-368.

Surit, P. (2002). Health beliefs, social support, and self-care behaviors of older Thai persons with non-insulin-dependent diabetes mellitus (NIDDM). *Dissertation Abstracts International, 63,* 1276B.

Taggert, H. M. (2000). Tai Chi, balance, functional mobility, fear of falling, and health perception among older women. *Dissertation Abstracts International, 61,* 2994B.

Taylor, S. G. (1985a). Curriculum development for pre-service programs using Orem's theory of nursing. In J. Riehl-Sisca (Ed.), *The science and art of self-care* (pp. 25-32). Norwalk, CT: Appleton-Century-Crofts.

Taylor, S. G. (1985b). Teaching self-care deficit theory to generic students. In J. Riehl-Sisca (Ed.), *The art and science of self-care.* Norwalk, CT: Appleton-Century-Crofts.

Taylor, S. G. (1988). Nursing theory and nursing process. *Nursing Science Quarterly, 1*(3), 111-119.

Taylor, S. G. (1989). The interpretation of family from the perspective of self-care deficit nursing theory. *Nursing Science Quarterly, 2*(3), 131-137.

Taylor, S. G. (1991). The structure of nursing diagnosis from Orem's theory. *Nursing Science Quarterly, 4*(1), 24-32.

Taylor, S. G. (1998). The development of self-care deficit nursing theory: An historical analysis. *International Orem Society Newsletter, 6*(2), 7-10.

Taylor, S. G. (2001). Theoretical concerns. Orem's general theory of nursing and families. *Nursing Science Quarterly, 14*(1), 7-9.

Taylor, S., Geden, E., Isaramalai, S., & Wongvatunyu, S. (2000). Orem's self-care deficit nursing theory: Its philosophical foundation and the state of the science. *Nursing Science Quarterly, 13*(2), 104-109.

Taylor, S. G., & Godfrey, N. S. (1999). Ethical issues. The ethics of Orem's theory—third in a series of articles. *Nursing Science Quarterly, 12*(3), 202-207.

Taylor, S. G., & McLaughlin, K. (1991, Winter). Orem's theory and community. *Nursing Science Quarterly, 4*(4), 153-160.

Taylor, S. G., & Renpenning, K. (1995). The practice of nursing in multiperson situations: Family and community. In D. E. Orem (Ed.), *Nursing: Concepts of practice* (5th ed., pp. 348-380). St. Louis: Mosby.

Taylor, S. G., Renpenning, K., Geden, E., Neuman, B., & Hart, M. (2001). A theory of dependent care. *Nursing Science Quarterly, 14*(1), 39-47.

Thrasher, C. (2002).The primary nurse practitioner: Advocate for self care. *Journal of the American Academy of Nurse Practitioners, 14*(3), 113-117.

Torres, G. O. V., Davim, R. M. B., & da Nobrega, M. M. L. (1999). Application of the nursing process based in Orem's theory: A case study with a pregnant adolescent [Spanish]. *Revista Latino-Americana de Enfermagem, 7*(2), 47-53.

Ulbrich, S. L. (1999). Theory. Nursing practice theory of exercise as self-care. *Image: The Journal of Nursing Scholarship, 31*(1), 65-70.

Vesely, C. (1995). Pediatric patient-controlled analgesia: Enhancing the self-care construct. *Pediatric Nursing, 21*(2), 124-128.

Villarruel, A. M., & Denyes, M. J. (1997). Testing Orem's theory with Mexican Americans. *Image: The Journal of Nursing Scholarship, 29*(3), 283-288.

Walker, L. O., & Grobe, S. J. (1999). The construct of thriving in pregnancy and postpartum. *Nursing Science Quarterly, 12*(2), 151-157.

Wallace, W. A. (1979). *From a realist point of view: Essays on the philosophy of science.* Washington, DC: Universal Press of America.

Wallace, W. A. (1996). *The modeling of nature: Philosophy of science and philosophy of nature in synthesis.* Washington, DC: The Catholic University of America Press.

Wang, C. (1997). The cross-cultural applicability of Orem's conceptual framework. *Journal of Cultural Diversity, 4*(2), 44-48.

Wang, H. (2001). A comparison of two models of health-promoting lifestyle in rural elderly Taiwanese women. *Public Health Nursing, 18*(3), 204-211.

Wang, H., & Laffrey, S. (2001). A predictive model of well-being and self-care for rural elderly women in Taiwan. *Research in Nursing & Health, 24*(2), 122-132.

Warren, J. K. (1998). Perceived self-care capabilities of abused/neglected and nonabused/non-neglected pregnant, low-socioeconomic adolescents. *Journal of Child & Adolescent Psychiatric Nursing, 11*(1), 30-37.

Weber, N. A. (2000). Explication of the structure of the secondary concept of women's self-care developed within Orem's self-care deficit theory: Instrumentation, psychometric evaluation and theory-testing. *Dissertation Abstracts International, 61,* 1331B.

Wells-Biggs, A. (1985). Hermeneutic interpretation of the work of Dorothea E. Orem: A nursing metaphor. *Dissertation Abstracts International, 47,* 0576B.

White, M. M. (2000). Predictors of self-care agency among community-dwelling older adults. *Dissertation Abstracts International, 61,* 1332B.

Whitener, L. M., Cox, K. R., & Maglich, S. A. (1998). Use of theory to guide nurses in the design of health messages for children. *ANS Advances in Nursing Science, 20*(3), 21-35.

Wilson, F. L., Mood, D. W., Risk, J., & Kershaw, T. (2003). Evaluation of education materials using Orem's self-care deficit theory. *Nursing Science Quarterly, 16*(1), 68-76.

Young, J., O'Connell, B., & McGregor, S. (2000). Day surgery patients' convalescence at home: Does enhanced discharge education make a difference? *Nursing & Health Sciences, 2*(1), 29-39.

BIBLIOGRAPHY
Primary Sources
Books

Nursing Development Conference Group (NDCG), Orem, D. E. (Ed.). (1972). *Concept formalization in nursing: Process and product.* Boston: Little, Brown & Co.

Nursing Development Conference Group (NDCG), Orem, D. E. (Ed.). (1979). *Concept formalization in nursing: Process and product* (2nd ed.). Boston: Little, Brown & Co.

Orem, D. E. (Ed.). (1959). *Guides for developing curriculum for the education of practical nurses.* Vocational Division #274. Trade and Industrial Education #68. Washington, DC: U.S. Department of Health, Education, and Welfare.

Orem, D. E. (1971). *Nursing: Concepts of practice.* New York: McGraw-Hill.

Orem, D. E. (1980). *Nursing: Concepts of practice* (2nd ed.). New York: McGraw-Hill.

Orem, D. E. (1985). *Nursing: Concepts of practice* (3rd ed.). New York: McGraw-Hill.

Orem, D. E. (1991). *Nursing: Concepts of practice* (4th ed.). St. Louis: Mosby.

Orem, D. E. (1995). *Nursing: Concepts of practice* (5th ed.). St. Louis: Mosby.

Orem, D. E. (2001). *Nursing: Concepts of practice* (6th ed.). St. Louis: Mosby.

Orem, D. E., & Parker, K. S. (Eds.). (1963). *Nurse practice education workshop proceedings.* Washington, DC: The Catholic University of America.

Orem, D. E., & Parker, K. S. (Eds.). (1964). *Nursing content in preservice nursing curriculum.* Washington, DC: The Catholic University of America Press.

Renpenning, K., & Taylor, S. G. (Eds.). (2003). *Self care theory in nursing: Selected papers of Dorothea Orem.* New York: Springer Publishing.

Book Chapters

Orem, D. E. (1966). Discussion of paper—Another view of nursing care and quality. In K. M. Straub & K. S. Parker (Eds.), *Continuity of patient care: The role of nursing.* Washington, DC: The Catholic University of America Press.

Orem, D. E. (1969). Inservice education and nursing practice forces effecting nursing practice. In D. K. Petrowski & K. M. Staub (Eds.), *School of nursing education.* Washington, DC: The Catholic University of America Press.

Orem, D. E. (1981). Nursing: A triad of action systems. In G. E. Lasker (Ed.), *Applied systems and cybernetics. Systems research in health care, biocybernetics, and ecology* (Vol. IV). New York: Pergamon Press.

Orem, D. E. (1982). Nursing: A dilemma for higher education. In Sr. A. Power (Ed.), *Words commemorated: Essays celebrating the centennial of Incarnate Word College.* San Antonio, TX: Incarnate Word College.

Orem, D. E. (1983). The self-care deficit theory of nursing: A general theory. In I. Clements & F. Roberts (Eds.), *Family health: A theoretical approach to nursing care.* New York: Wiley Medical Publications.

Orem, D. E. (1984). Orem's conceptual model and community health nursing. In M. K. Asay & C. C. Ossler (Eds.), *Proceedings of the Eighth Annual Community Health Nursing Conference: Conceptual models of nursing applications in community health nursing.* Chapel Hill, NC: University of North Carolina, Department of Public Health Nursing, School of Public Health.

Orem, D. E. (1988). Nursing administration: A theoretical approach. In B. Henry, C. Arndt, M. DiVincenti, & A. M. Tomey (Eds.), *Dimensions of nursing administration.* Boston: Blackwell Scientific.

Orem, D. E. (1990). A nursing practice theory in three parts, 1956-1989. In M. E. Parker (Ed.), *Nursing theories in practice.* New York: National League for Nursing.

Orem, D. E., & Taylor, S. (1986). Orem's general theory of nursing. In P. Winstead-Fry (Ed.), *Case studies in nursing theory* (pp. 37-71; Pub. No. 15-2152). New York: National League for Nursing.

Journal Articles

Denyes, M. J., Orem, D. E., & Bekel, G. (2001). Self-care: A foundational science. *Nursing Science Quarterly, 14*(1), 48-54.

Orem, D. E. (1962, Jan.). The hope of nursing. *Journal of Nursing Education, 1,* 5.

Orem, D. E. (1979, March). Levels of nursing education and practice. *Alumnae Magazine, 68,* 2-6.

Orem, D. E. (1985, May/June). Concepts of self-care for the rehabilitation client. *Rehabilitation Nursing, 10*(3), 33-36.

Orem, D. E. (1988, May). The form of nursing science. *Nursing Science Quarterly, 1*(2), 75-79.

Orem, D. E. (1997). Views of human beings specific to nursing. *Nursing Science Quarterly, 10*(1), 26-31.

Orem, D. E., & O'Malley, M. (1952, Aug.). Diagnosis of hospital nursing problems. *Hospitals, 26,* 63.

Orem, D. E., & Vardiman, E. (1995, Winter). Orem's nursing theory and positive mental health: Practical considerations. *Nursing Science Quarterly, 8*(4), 165-173.

Reports

Orem, D. E. (1955). *Indiana hospitals: A report. Author of three sections of 10-year report of status and problems of Indiana hospitals.* Indianapolis: Indiana State Board of Health.

Orem, D. E. (1956). *Hospital nursing service: An analysis and report of a study of administrative positions in one hospital nursing service.* Indianapolis: Indiana State Board of Health.

Orem, D. E., Dear, M., & Greenbaum, J. (1976). *Organization of nursing faculty responsibilities* (Project Report, Public Health Service Grant No. 03D-005-3666). Washington, DC: Georgetown University School of Nursing.

Audiotape

Orem, D. E. (1978, Dec.). *Paper presented at the Second Annual Nurse Educator Conference, New York* (Audiotape). Available through Teach 'em, Inc., 160 E. Illinois Street, Chicago, IL 60611.

Videotapes

Fawcett, J. (1988). *The nurse theorists. Portraits of excellence: Dorothea Orem* (Videotape). Available through Fuld Video Project, Studio III, 370 Hawthorne Avenue, Oakland, CA 94609.

Fawcett, J. (1992). *Excellence in action: Dorothea Orem* (Videotape). Oakland, CA: Studio III. Available through Fuld Video Project, Studio III, 370 Hawthorne Avenue, Oakland, CA 94609.

Fawcett, J. (1997). *Dorothea Orem: Self-care framework* (Videotape). Athens, OH: FITNE.

National League for Nursing. (1987). *Nursing theory: A circle of knowledge* (Videotape). Available through the author, 10 Columbus Circle, New York, NY 10019.

Secondary Sources
Dissertations

Ahrens, S. L. G. (2001). The development and testing of the Heart Failure Self-Care Inventory: An instrument for measuring heart failure self-care. *Dissertation Abstracts International, 62,* 5636B.

Anderson, J. A. M. (1996). Basic conditioning factors, self-care agency, self-care, and well-being in homeless adults. *Dissertation Abstracts International, 57,* 2473B.

Asdornwised, U. P. (2000). Self-care and dependent-care experiences of Thai patients recovering from coronary artery bypass graft surgery: An ethnographic study. *Dissertation Abstracts International, 61,* 1318B.

Baiardi, J. M. (1997).The influence of health status, burden, and degree of cognitive impairment on the self-care agency and dependent-care agency of caregivers of elders. *Dissertation Abstracts International, 58,* 5885B.

Banfield, B. E. (1997). A philosophical inquiry of Orem's self-care deficit nursing theory. *Dissertation Abstracts International, 58,* 5885B.

Bess, C. J. (1995). Abilities and limitation of adult type II diabetic patients with integrating of self-care practices into their daily lives. *Dissertation Abstracts International, 56,* 3688B.

Brown, K. L. G. (1996). Grief as a basic conditioning factor affecting the self-care agency and self-care of family caregivers of persons with neurotrauma. *Dissertation Abstracts International, 57,* 7447B.

Callaghan, D. M. (2000). The relationships among health-promoting self-care behaviors, self-care self-efficacy, and self-care agency. *Dissertation Abstracts International, 61,* 3504B.

Canty, J. L. (1993). An investigation of life change events, hope, and self-care agency in inner city adolescents. *Dissertation Abstracts International, 54,* 2992B.

Chen, Y. M. (1996). Relationships among health control orientation, self-efficacy, self-care, and subjective well-being in the elderly with hypertension. *Dissertation Abstracts International, 57,* 3652B.

Cooksey-James, T. J. (1999). Utilization of prenatal care by women of St. Thomas, United States Virgin Islands: A descriptive study. *Dissertation Abstracts International, 61,* 2470B.

Cull, V. V. (1995). Exposure to violence and self-care practices of adolescents. *Dissertation Abstracts International, 56,* 3690B.

Cutler, C. G. (1998). The relationship of self-care agency, self-efficacy, and social support to post-hospitalization adjustment of patients with a mood disorder. *Dissertation Abstracts International, 59,* 0600B.

Dato, C. (2002). A. The relationship of perceived social support, positive symptoms, negative symptoms, and self-care actions in adults with schizophrenia living in the community. *Dissertation Abstracts International, 63,* 1266B.

Demasters, J. J. (1999). Women and the hormone replacement therapy decision: A study of concerns, values, and behaviors using a multiattribute utility model. *Dissertation Abstracts International, 59,* 5784B.

Dennis, C. (1998). Self-care agency, learned helplessness, and health status in elderly adults. *Dissertation Abstracts International, 59,* 1582B.

Dreher, H. M. (2000). The effect of caffeine reduction on sleep and well-being in persons with HIV (immune deficiency). *Dissertation Abstracts International, 61,* 4649B.

Gallegos, E. C. (1997). The effect of social, family and individual conditioning factors on self-care agency and self-care of adult Mexican women. *Dissertation Abstracts International, 58,* 5889B.

Good, M. P. L. (1992). Comparison of the effects of relaxation and music on post-operative pain. *Dissertation Abstracts International, 53,* 1783B.

Haas, D. L. (1991). The relationship between coping dispositions and power components of dependent-care agency in parents of children with special health care needs. *Dissertation Abstracts International, 52,* 1351B.

Hoffart, M. B. (1995). Weaving the fabric of life: A phenomenological inquiry of solitude experienced by school age children (emotional control). *Dissertation Abstracts International, 56,* 5417B.

Isaramalai, S. (2002). Developing a cross-cultural measure of the Self-As-Carer Inventory questionnaire for the Thai population. *Dissertation Abstracts International, 63,* 2307B.

Keatley, V. M. (1998). Critical incident stress in generic baccalaureate students. *Dissertation Abstracts International, 59,* 2124B.

Kleinbeck, S. V. M. (1996). Postdischarge surgical recovery of adult laparoscope outpatients. *Dissertation Abstracts International, 57,* 989B.

Koster, M. K. (1995). A comparison of the relationship among self-care agency, self-determinism, and absenteeism in two groups of school-age children. *Dissertation Abstracts International, 56,* 541B.

Lee, M. B. (1996). Power, self-care, and health in women living in urban squatter settlements in Karachi, Pakistan: A test of Orem's theory. *Dissertation Abstracts International, 57,* 7451B.

Magnan, M. A. (2001). Self-care and health in persons with cancer-related fatigue: Refinement and evaluation of Orem's self-care framework. *Dissertation Abstracts International, 62,* 5644B.

Malathum, P. (2001). A model of factors contributing to perceived abilities for health-promoting self-care of community-dwelling Thai older adults. *Dissertation Abstracts International, 62,* 5034B.

McKinney, M. L. (2000). Hardiness, threat appraisal, self-care capability, and caregiving characteristics as predictors of emotions and perceived health in family caregivers of cancer patients. *Dissertation Abstracts International, 61,* 2992B.

Metcalfe, S. A. (1997). Self-care actions as a function of the therapeutic self-care demand and self-care agency in individuals with chronic obstructive pulmonary disease. *Dissertation Abstracts International, 57,* 7453B.

Meyer, G. L. (2000). The art of watching out: Vigilance in women who have migraine headaches. *Dissertation Abstracts International, 61,* 0781B.

Morgan, M. J. (1998). Self-care agency in people with end-stage renal disease. *Dissertation Abstracts International, 59,* 1048B.

Neuman, B. (1996). Relationship between children's descriptions of pain, self-care, and dependent-care and basic conditioning factors of development, gender, and ethnicity: "Bears in my throat." *Dissertation Abstracts International, 57,* 2482B.

Nicholson, L. L. (2002). Self-care activities and quality of life in ovarian cancer survivors. *Dissertation Abstracts International, 63,* 1272B.

O'Connor, N. A. (1995). Maieutic dimensions of self-care agency: Instrument development. *Dissertation Abstracts International, 56,* 2563B.

Pettine, A. (1995). Development of self-care: A problem for elementary-age children? *Dissertation Abstracts International, 56,* 3479B.

Raithel, J. A. (2000). Maintaining normalcy when managing the chronic physical illness of asthma. *Dissertation Abstracts International, 61,* 0782B.

Renker, P. R. (1998). Physical abuse, social support, self-care agency, self-care practices, and late adolescent pregnancy outcomes. *Dissertation Abstracts International, 58,* 5891B.

Rieg, L. C. (2000). Information retrieval of self-care and dependent-care agents using NetWellnessRTM, a consumer health information network. *Dissertation Abstracts International, 61,* 5801B.

Robinson, M. K. (1996). Determinants of functional status in chronically ill adults. *Dissertation Abstracts International, 56,* 5424B.

Schmidt, C. A. (1997). Mothers' views concerning the development of self-care agency in school-age children with diabetes. *Dissertation Abstracts International, 59,* 0162B.

Sonninen, A. L. (1997). Testing reliability and validity of the Finnish version of the Appraisal of Self-care Agency (ASA) scale with elderly Finns. *Dissertation Abstracts International, 60,* 0604C.

Surit, P. (2002). Health beliefs, social support, and self-care behaviors of older Thai persons with non-insulin-dependent diabetes mellitus (NIDDM). *Dissertation Abstracts International, 63,* 1276B.

Taggert, H. M. (2000). Tai Chi, balance, functional mobility, fear of falling, and health perception among older women. *Dissertation Abstracts International, 61,* 2994B.

Tiansawad, S. (1995). Self-care abilities and practices for prevention of HIV infection among rural Thai women who attended mobile family planning clinic. *Dissertation Abstracts International, 55,* 3241B.

Vogt, C. A. (1995). A comparison of educational models in determining patients' knowledge and behaviors concerning advance directives. *Dissertation Abstracts International, 55,* 3843B.

Wang, H. H. (1998). A model of self-care and well-being of rural elderly women in Taiwan. *Dissertation Abstracts International, 59,* 2689B.

Weber, N. A. (2000). Explication of the structure of the secondary concept of women's self-care developed within Orem's self-care deficit theory: Instrumentation, psychometric evaluation and theory-testing. *Dissertation Abstracts International, 61,* 1331B.

White, M. M. (2000). Predictors of self-care agency among community-dwelling older adults. *Dissertation Abstracts International, 61,*1332B.

Zehnder, N. R. (1996). The influence of basic conditioning factors on menopausal self-care agency and menopausal self-care in midlife women. *Dissertation Abstracts International, 57,* 7460B.

Books (since 1995)

Dennis, C. M. (1997). *Self-care deficit nursing theory: Concepts and applications.* St. Louis: Mosby.

Fawcett, J. (2000). *Analysis and evaluation of contemporary nursing knowledge: Nursing models and theories.* Philadelphia: F. A. Davis.

Meleis, A. J. (1997). *Theoretical nursing: Development and progress* (3rd ed.). Philadelphia: J. B. Lippincott.

Young, A., Taylor, S., & Renpenning, K. (2001). *Connections: Nursing research, theory and practice.* St. Louis: Mosby.

Book Chapters

Berbiglia, V. A. (1997). Orem's self-care deficit theory in nursing practice. In M. R. Alligood & A. M. Tomey (Eds.), *Nursing theory: Utilization & application* (pp. 129-152). St. Louis: Mosby.

Fawcett, J. (2000). Orem's self-care framework. In J. Fawcett (Ed.), *Analysis and evaluation of contemporary nursing knowledge* (pp. 259-360). Philadelphia: F. A. Davis.

Mezinskis, P. M. (1998). Orem's self-care deficit theory. In A. S. Luggen (Ed.), *NGNA core curriculum for gerontological advance practice nurses* (pp. 16-19). Thousands Oaks, CA: Sage.

Taylor, S. G., & Renpenning, K. (1995). Nursing in multi-person situations: Family and community. In D. E. Orem (Ed.), *Nursing: Concepts of practice* (5th ed., pp. 348-380). St. Louis: Mosby.

Other Resources

Copies of papers presented at the fifth, sixth, and seventh Annual Self-Care Deficit Nursing Theory Conferences and the first, second, third, and fourth International Self-Care Deficit Nursing Theory Conferences are available. These include papers by Orem and others. Also available are introductory videotapes. Order from the University of Missouri-Columbia, Sinclair School of Nursing, Nursing Outreach and Distance Education, S266 School of Nursing Building, Columbia, MO 65211, (573) 882-0216.

Web Sites

Département de Soins Infirmiers. French-language description of SCDNT and use. Accessed December 20, 2004: *http://www.colvir.net/departments/soins_infirmiers/pages/philosophie.html*

Eighth World Congress: Self-Care Deficit Nursing Theory. Official site for international conference. Accessed December 20, 2004: *http://www.worldcongress-scdnt.com*

GB Concept. German site focusing on SCDNT. Accessed December 20, 2004: *http://www.gbconcept.de*

Information & Resources for Nurses Worldwide: Dorothea Orem. Information sites and links. Accessed December 20, 2004: *http://www.nurses.info/nursing_theory_person_orem_dorothea.htm*

International Orem Society for Nursing Science and Scholarship Official Site. Information and newsletters. Accessed December 20, 2004: *http://www.muhealth.org/~nursing/scdnt/scdnt.html*

Labouré College, Caritas Christi Health Center. Associate-degree curriculum and course descriptions using SCDNT. Accessed December 20, 2004: *http://www.laboure.edu/*

Oklahoma City University, Kramer School of Nursing: Course Descriptions. Course descriptions for curriculum based in SCDNT. Accessed December 20, 2004: *http://www.okcu.edu/nursing/ksoncour.htm*

Imogene King

Interacting Systems Framework and Middle Range Theory of Goal Attainment

Christina L. Sieloff

CREDENTIALS AND BACKGROUND OF THE THEORIST

Imogene King earned a diploma in nursing from St. John's Hospital of Nursing in St. Louis, Missouri, in 1945. While working in a variety of staff nurse roles,

Previous authors: Christina L. Sieloff, Mary Lee Ackermann, Sallie Anne Brink, Jo Anne Clanton, Cathy Greenwell Jones, Ann Marriner Tomey, Sandra L. Moody, Gwynn Lee Perlich, Debra L. Price, and Beth Bruns Prusinski.
The author wishes to thank Dr. Imogene King for her past review of this chapter. The author and Dr. King strongly encourage all readers to read Dr. King's original materials in conjunction with this chapter.

she began course work toward a Bachelor of Science in Nursing Education, which she received from St. Louis University in 1948.

From 1947 to 1958, King worked as an instructor in medical-surgical nursing and as an assistant director at St. John's Hospital School of Nursing. She earned an M.S.N. (1957) from St. Louis University and a Doctor of Education (1961) from Teachers College, Columbia University, New York. King was awarded an honorary Ph.D. from Southern Illinois University in 1980.

From 1961 to 1966, King was an associate professor of nursing at Loyola University in Chicago, where she developed a master's degree program in nursing based on a nursing conceptual framework. Her first theory article appeared in 1964 in the journal *Nursing Science* edited by Dr. Martha Rogers. Between 1966 and 1968, King served as Assistant Chief of Research Grants Branch, Division of Nursing, in the United States Department of Health, Education, and Welfare. While she was in Washington, D.C., her article "A Conceptual Frame of Reference for Nursing" was published in *Nursing Research* (1968).

From 1968 to 1972, King was the director of the School of Nursing at Ohio State University in Columbus. While at Ohio State, her book, *Toward a Theory for Nursing: General Concepts of Human Behavior* (1971), was published. In this early work, King concluded, "a systematic representation of nursing is required ultimately for developing a science to accompany a century or more of art in the everyday world of nursing" (1971, p. 129). Her book subsequently was awarded the *American Journal of Nursing* Book of the Year Award in 1973 (King, 1995a).

King returned to Chicago in 1972 as a professor in the Loyola University graduate program. She also served as the Coordinator of Research in Clinical Nursing at the Loyola Medical Center, Department of Nursing, from 1978 to 1980.

From 1972 to 1975, she was a member of the Defense Advisory Committee on Women in the Services for the United States Department of Defense. She was elected alderman in Ward 2, Wood Dale, Illinois, in 1975 and served until 1979.

In 1980, King moved to Tampa, Florida, where she was appointed professor at the University of South Florida College of Nursing. The manuscript for her second book, *A Theory for Nursing: Systems, Concepts, Process,* was published in 1981. In addition to her first two books, she has authored multiple book chapters and articles in professional journals, and a third book, *Curriculum and Instruction in Nursing: Concepts and Process,* was published in 1986.

King retired in 1990 and is currently professor emeritus at the University of South Florida, where she continues to lecture. She also continues to provide community service and help plan care

through her framework and theory at various health care organizations. She was keynote speaker at two Sigma Theta Tau theory conferences in 1992 and continues to present at local, national, and international nursing education conferences. She consults with doctoral and master's students who are developing theories within the interacting systems framework. She has contributed to the development of instruments to measure the power of a nursing group within an organization (Sieloff, 1996) and patient satisfaction with professional nursing care (Killeen, 1996).

King has been an active member of the American Nurses Association, the Florida Nurses' Association, and Sigma Theta Tau International. She has held offices in various organizations and has served frequently as a delegate from the Florida Nurses' Association to the American Nurses Association House of Delegates. In 1994, she was inducted into the American Academy of Nursing. She was one of the founding members of a nursing organization, the King International Nursing Group (KING), established to facilitate the dissemination and utilization of her interacting systems framework, Theory of Goal Attainment, and related theories. Although the organization is currently inactive, King continues to consult with members of the organization. In 1996, she received the Jessie M. Scott Award at the American Nurses Association convention.

THEORETICAL SOURCES

King (1971) describes the purpose of her first book as follows:

> . . . propos[ing] a conceptual frame of reference for nursing. It is intended to be utilized specifically by students and teachers, and also by researchers and practitioners to identify and analyze events in specific nursing situations. The framework suggests that the essential characteristics of nursing are those properties that have persisted in spite of environmental changes. (p. ix)

King (1971) also identifies that the framework served is as follows:

MAJOR CONCEPTS & DEFINITIONS

"Concepts give meaning to our sense perceptions and permit generalizations about persons, objects, and things" (King, 1995a, p. 16). A limited number of definitions based on the systems framework are listed below. The remainder of King's definitions can be found in her 1981 book. To assist the reader, those concepts, the pages where the definitions can be found from the interacting systems framework, and the theory are listed alphabetically in Table 15-1.

HEALTH

"Health is defined as dynamic life experiences of a human being, which implies continuous adjustment to stressors in the internal and external environment through optimum use of one's resources to achieve maximum potential for daily living" (King, 1981, p. 5).

NURSING

"Nursing is defined as a process of action, reaction, and interaction whereby nurse and client share information about their perceptions in the nursing situation" (King, 1981, p. 2).

SELF

"The self is a composite of thoughts and feelings which constitute a person's awareness of his [/her] individual existence, his [/her] conception of who and what he [/she] is. A person's self is the sum total of all he [/she] can call his [/hers]. The self includes, among other things, a system of ideas, attitudes, values, and commitments. The self is a person's total subjective environment. It is a distinctive center of experience and significance. The self constitutes a person's inner world as distinguished from the outer world consisting of all other people and things. The self is the individual as known to the individual. It is that to which we refer when we say 'I'" (Jersild, 1952, p. 10).

. . . several purposes. . . . It is a way of thinking about the real world of nursing; . . . an approach for selecting concepts perceived to be fundamental for the practice of professional nursing; [and] shows a process for developing concepts that symbolize experiences within the physical, psychological, and social environment in nursing. (p. 125)

King clearly identified and referenced theoretical sources throughout her 1981 book.

USE OF EMPIRICAL EVIDENCE

King (1971) speaks of concepts as "abstract ideas that give meaning to our sense perceptions, permit generalizations, and tend to be stored in our memory for recall and use at a later time in new and different situations" (pp. 11-12). King (1984) defines theory as "a set of concepts, which, when defined, are interrelated and observable in the world of nursing practice" (p. 11). Theory serves to build "scientific knowledge for nursing" (King, 1995b, p. 24).

King (1975a) identifies at least two methods for developing theory as follows: (1) a theory can be developed and then tested in research, and (2) research can provide data from which a theory may be developed. King's opinion (1978) is that "in today's world of building knowledge for a complex profession such as nursing, one must consider these two strategies."

King cites many research studies in her 1981 book, especially regarding the development of her concepts. Within the personal system, King examines studies related to perception by Allport (1955), Kelley and Hammond (1964), Ittleson and Cantril (1954), and others. In developing her definition of space, she used studies from Sommer (1969) and Ardrey (1966) and noted Minckley's (1968) research. For the concept of time, she acknowledged Orme's (1969) work.

Within the interpersonal system, King presented communication theories and models, citing the studies of Watzlawick, Beavin, and Jackson (1967) and Krieger (1975). She examined studies by Whiting (1955), Orlando (1961), and Diers and Schmidt (1977) for information on interaction. She also noted Dewey and Bentley's (1949) theory of knowledge, which addressed self-action, interaction, and transaction in *Knowing and the Known,* and Kuhn's (1975) work on transactions.

Commenting on research existing at that time, particularly operations research regarding patient care, King (1975b) noted that ". . . most studies have centered on technical aspects of patient care and of the health care systems rather than on patient aspects directly. . . . Few problems have been stated that begin with what the patient's condition demands or what the patient wants" (p. 9).

In her 1981 book, King further discussed that "several theoretical formulations about interpersonal relations and nursing process have been described in nursing situations" (pp. 151-152), citing studies by Peplau (1952), Orlando (1961), Paterson and Zderad (1976), Yura and Walsh (1978), and herself.

Development of the Interacting Systems Framework

In preparation of her 1971 book, King posed the following questions:

- What is the goal of nursing?
- What are the functions of nurses?
- How can nurses continue to expand their knowledge to provide quality care? (pp. 30, 39)

As a result of a review of 20 years of nursing literature (before 1971), King identified multiple concepts used by nurses to describe nursing. Figure 15-1 demonstrates the interacting systems framework that provides "one approach to studying systems as a whole rather than as isolated parts of a system" (King, 1995a, p. 18) and is "designed to explain (the) organized wholes within which nurses are expected to function" (1995b, p. 23).

King (1981) used a systems approach in the development of her interacting systems framework and the subsequent middle range Theory of Goal Attainment, because systems have been used in the past to comprehend and respond to "changes and complexity in health care organizations" (p. 10). She added that "some scientists who have been studying systems have noted that the only way to study human beings interacting with the environment is

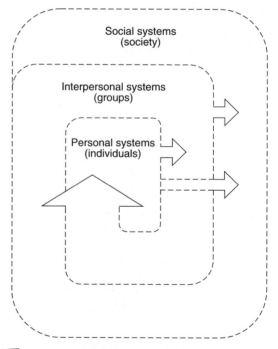

Figure **15-1 Dynamic interacting systems.** (From King, I. [1981]. *A theory for nursing: Systems, concepts, process* [p. 11]. New York: Delmar. Used with permission from I. King.)

to design a conceptual framework of interdependent variables and interrelated concepts" (King, 1981, p. 10). King (1995a) believes that her "framework differs from other conceptual schema in that it is concerned not with fragmenting human beings and the environment but with human transactions in different kinds of environments" (p. 21).

"An awareness of the complex dynamics of human behavior in nursing situations prompted [King's] formulation of a conceptual framework that represents personal, interpersonal and social systems as the domain of nursing" (King, 1981, p. 130). Each of the three systems identifies human beings as the basic element in the system. In addition, "the unit of analysis in [the] framework is human behavior in a variety of social environments" (King, 1995a, p. 18). Individuals exist within personal systems, and King provides an example of a total system as being a patient or a nurse. King believes that it is necessary to understand the concepts of body image, growth and development, perception, self, space, and time to comprehend human beings as persons.

Interpersonal systems are formed when two or more individuals interact, forming dyads (two people) or triads (three people). The dyad of a nurse and a patient is one type of interpersonal system. Families, when acting as small groups, can also be considered interpersonal systems. Comprehension of the interpersonal system requires an understanding of the concepts of communication, interaction, role, stress, and transaction.

A comprehensive interacting system consists of groups that make up society, and is referred to as a *social system*. Religious, educational, and health care systems are examples of social systems. The influential behavior of an extended family on an individual's growth and development in society is another example of the influence of a social system. Within a social system, the concepts of authority, decision making, organization, power, and status are essential for understanding of the type of system.

"The concepts in the framework are the organizing dimensions and represent knowledge essential for understanding the interactions between the three systems" (King, 1995a, p. 18). Concepts were placed in the personal system because they primarily related to individuals, whereas concepts were placed in the interpersonal system because they "emphasized interactions between two or more persons" (King, 1995a, p. 18). Concepts were placed in the social system because they "provided knowledge for nurses to function in larger systems" (King, 1995a, p. 18). However, King (1995a) clearly identifies that "the concepts in the framework are not limited to only one of the dynamic interacting systems but cut across all three systems" (p. 19). Table 15-1 lists the locations for the concepts from the systems framework and the Theory of Goal

Table **15-1**

Location of Concept Definitions in I.M. King's A Theory for Nursing: Systems, Concepts, Process

CONCEPTS	FROM SYSTEMS FRAMEWORK	FROM THEORY OF GOAL ATTAINMENT
Authority	p. 124	—
Body image	p. 33	—
Communication	—	p. 146
Decision making	p. 132	—
Growth and development	—	p. 148
Interaction	p. 32	p. 145
Nursing situation	p. 2	—
Organization (operational)	p. 119	—
Perception	p. 24	p. 146
Power	p. 127	—
Role	p. 93	—
Space	pp. 37-38	—
Status	p. 129	—
Stress	p. 32	—
Time	p. 44	—
Transaction	p. 82	p. 147

Data from King, I. M. (1981). *A theory for nursing: Systems, concepts, process.* New York: John Wiley & Sons.

Attainment in King's 1981 text, *A Theory for Nursing: Systems, Concepts, Process.*

Development of the Middle Range Theory of Goal Attainment From the Interacting Systems Framework

In 1981, King derived the middle range Theory of Goal Attainment from her interacting systems framework. The question that "motivated [King] to develop a theory was, what is the nature of nursing?" (King, 1995b, p. 25). The answer, "the way in which nurses, in their role, do with and for individuals that differentiates nursing from other health professionals (King, 1995b, p. 26)," guided the development of the Theory of Goal Attainment.

King (1995b) used the following criteria to develop the theory:

- What are the philosophical assumptions?
- Are the concepts clearly identified and defined?
- Are the concepts related in propositional statements or models?
- Does the theory generate questions to be answered, or hypotheses to be tested in research, to generate knowledge and affirm the theory?

"The human process of interactions formed the basis for designing a model of transactions that depicts theoretical knowledge used by nurses to help individuals and groups attain goals" (1995a, p. 27) (Figure 15-2).

King (1995b) stated the following:

> Mutual goal setting [between a nurse and a client] is based on (a) nurses' assessment of a client's concerns, problems, and disturbances in health; (b) nurse's and client's perceptions of the interference; and (c) their sharing of information whereby each functions to help the client attain the goals identified. In addition, nurses interact with family members when clients cannot verbally participate in the goal setting. (p. 28)

To test her theory, King (1981) conducted research, identifying that her study varied from previous studies in that it "described the nurse-patient interaction process that leads to goal attainment" (p. 153). King's research describes a process that leads to goal attainment and studied nurse-patient interactions to determine whether nurses made transactions. King used a method of nonparticipant observation to collect information of nurse-patient interactions in a patient care unit in a hospital setting. Patients and nurses volunteered to participate in the study. King then trained graduate students in the nonparticipant observation technique before collecting data. She examined multiple interactions and recorded verbal and nonverbal behaviors as raw data. King also developed a classification system that nurses can use to determine if they are making transactions that lead to goal attainment (I. King, personal communication, July 11, 1996).

MAJOR ASSUMPTIONS

King's personal philosophy about human beings and life influenced her assumptions, including those related to the environment, health, nursing, individuals, and nurse-patient interactions. Her interacting

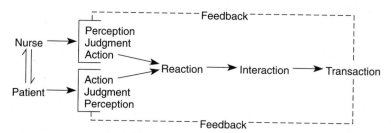

Figure 15-2 **A process of human interactions that lead to transactions: A model of transaction.** (From King, I. [1981]. *A theory for nursing: Systems, concepts, process* [p. 61]. New York: Delmar. Used with permission from I. King.)

systems framework and Theory of Goal Attainment are "based on an overall assumption that the focus of nursing is human beings interacting with their environment leading to a state of health for individuals, which is an ability to function in social roles" (King, 1981, p. 143).

Nursing

"Nursing is an observable behavior found in the health care systems in society" (King, 1971, p. 125). The goal of nursing "is to help individuals maintain their health so they can function in their roles" (King, 1981, pp. 3-4). Nursing is an interpersonal process of action, reaction, interaction, and transaction. Perceptions of a nurse and a patient also influence the interpersonal process.

Person

Specific assumptions relating to persons, or individuals, are detailed in *A Theory for Nursing: Systems, Concepts, Process* (King, 1981). In addition, the following assumptions are detailed in King's subsequent works:

- Individuals are spiritual beings (I. King, personal communication, July 11, 1996).
- Individuals have the capacity to think, know, make choices, and select alternative courses of action (King, 1981).
- Individuals have the ability through their language and other symbols to record their history and preserve their culture (King, 1986).
- Individuals are open systems in transaction with the environment. Transaction connotes that no separateness exists between human beings and the environment (King, 1981).
- Individuals are unique and holistic, are of intrinsic worth, and are capable of rational thinking and decision making in most situations (King, 1995b).
- Individuals differ in their needs, wants, and goals (King, 1995b).

Health

Health is a dynamic state in the life cycle; illness is an interference in the life cycle. Health "implies continuous adjustment to stress in the internal and external environment through optimum use of one's resources to achieve maximum potential for daily living" (King, 1981, p. 5).

Environment

King (1981) believes that "an understanding of the ways that human beings interact with their environment to maintain health is essential for nurses" (p. 2). Open systems imply that interactions occur between the system and the system's environment, inferring that the environment is constantly changing. "Adjustments to life and health are influenced by [an] individual's interactions with environment. . . . Each human being perceives the world as a total person in making transactions with individuals and things in the environment" (King, 1981, p. 141).

THEORETICAL ASSERTIONS

King's Theory of Goal Attainment (1981) focuses on the interpersonal system and the interactions that take place between individuals, specifically in the nurse-patient relationship. In the nursing process, each member of the dyad perceives the other, makes judgments, and takes actions. Together, these activities culminate in reaction. Interaction results and, if perceptual congruence exists and disturbances are conquered, transactions occur. The system is open to permit feedback because each phase of the activity potentially influences perception.

King (1981) developed eight propositions in her Theory of Goal Attainment. These propositions are detailed in Box 15-1 and describe the relationships between concepts. Diagrams follow each proposition. When the propositions were analyzed, 23 relationships were not specified; 22 relationships were positive and no relationship was negative (Austin & Champion, 1983) (Figure 15-3). In addition, King (1981) derived seven hypotheses from the Theory of Goal Attainment, which are found in *A Theory for Nursing: Systems, Concepts, Process.*

LOGICAL FORM

In the initial framework suggested in her 1968 article, King identified the following four com-

Box **15-1**

Propositions Within Kings Theory of Goat Attainment

1. If perceptual accuracy (PA) is present in nurse-client interactions (I), transactions (T) will occur.

$$PA(I) \xrightarrow{+} T$$

2. If nurse and client make transactions (T), goals will be attained (GA).

$$T \xrightarrow{+} GA$$

3. If goals are attained (GA), satisfactions (S) will occur.

$$GA \xrightarrow{+} S$$

4. If goals are attained (GA), effective nursing care (NC$_e$) will occur.

$$GA \xrightarrow{+} NC_e$$

5. If transactions (T) are made in nurse-client interactions (I), growth and development (GD) will be enhanced.

$$(I)T \xrightarrow{+} GD$$

6. If role expectations and role performance as perceived by nurse and client are congruent (RCN), transactions (T) will occur.

$$RCN \xrightarrow{+} T$$

7. If role conflict (RC) is experienced by nurse and client or both, stress (ST) in nurse-client interactions (I) will occur.

$$RC(I) \xrightarrow{+} ST$$

8. If nurses with special knowledge and skills communicate (CM) appropriate information to clients, mutual goal setting (T) and goal attainment (GA) will occur. [Mutual goal setting is a step in transaction and thus has been diagrammed as transaction.]

$$CM \xrightarrow{+} T \xrightarrow{+} GA$$

From Austin, J. K., & Champion, V.L. (1983). King's theory of nursing: Explication and evaluation. In P.L. Chinn (Ed.), *Advances in nursing theory development* (p. 55). Rockville, MD: Aspen.

	PA	T	GA	S	NC$_e$	GD	RCN	RC	ST	CM
PA		+	+	+	+	+	?	?	?	?
T			+	+	+	+	+	?	?	?
GA				+	+	+	+	?	?	+
S					?	?	+	?	?	+
NC$_e$						?	+	?	?	+
GD							+	?	?	+
RCN								?	?	?
RC									+	?
ST										?
CM										

Figure 15-3 Relationship table. *PA,* Perceptional accuracy; *T,* transactions; *GA,* goals attained; *S,* satisfactions; *NC$_e$,* effective nursing care; *GD,* growth and development; *RCN,* role congruency; *RC,* role conflict; *ST,* stress; *CM,* communicate. (From Austin, J. K., & Champion, V. L. [1983]. King's theory for nursing: Explication and evaluation. In P. L. Chinn [Ed.], *Advances in theory development* [p. 58]. Rockville, MD: Aspen.)

prehensive concepts that center around human beings:

1. Health
2. Interpersonal relationships
3. Perceptions
4. Social systems

She viewed individuals as open systems with energy exchange taking place within, and external to, human beings. Although King's original framework was abstract and dealt with "only a few elements of concrete situations" (King, 1981, p. 128), she believes that her four "universal ideas (social systems, health, perception, and interpersonal relations) are relevant in every nursing situation" (King, 1981, p. 128).

Later, King (1975a) identified that her "personal approach to synthesizing knowledge for nursing was to use data and information available from: a) research in nursing and related fields, and b) 25 years in active practice, teaching, and research. From all the knowledge available, a theoretical framework relevant for nursing was formulated" (p. 36). In 1978, King indicated that theory development is composed of inductive and deductive reasoning, with theory's primary purpose being the generation of knowledge through research.

King (1981) then began further development of her interacting systems framework and proposed the middle range Theory of Goal Attainment to describe "the nature of nurse-client interactions that lead to achievement of goals" (p. 142), as follows:

> Nurses purposely interact with clients to mutually establish goals, and to explore and agree on means to achieve goals. Mutual goal setting is based on nurses' assessment of clients' concerns, problems, and disturbances in health, their perceptions of problems, and their sharing information to move toward goal attainment. (pp. 142-143)

In her 1981 publication, King spoke of less dichotomy between health and illness, referring to illness as an interference in the life cycle. Through reformulation, King provided a more open system relationship between person and environment. King also revised her terminology, using adjustment instead of adaptation, and person, human being, and individual rather than man.

A logical progression of development existed in the framework from 1971 to 1981, with King deriving her middle range Theory of Goal Attainment from her interacting systems framework. The Theory of Goal Attainment "organize[d] elements in the process of nurse-client interactions that result in outcomes, that is, goals attained" (King, 1981, p. 143).

King (1971) had initially stated the following:

> . . . [i]f nurses are to assume the roles and responsibilities expected of them, . . . the discovery of knowledge must be disseminated in such a way that they are able to use it in their practice. . . . Descriptive data collected systematically provide cues for generating hypotheses for research in human behavior in nursing situations. (p. 128)

During a 1978 nursing theorist conference, King indicated that if nurses were taught this process, they could begin to predict outcomes in nursing. Later, in 1981, she added, "this [middle range] theory should serve as a standard of practice related to nurse-patient interactions and is, in this sense, a normative theory" (p. 145). Clements and Roberts expanded on these ideas in 1983 to show the process of the Theory of Goal Attainment in relation to various nursing situations, including the health of families.

ACCEPTANCE BY THE NURSING COMMUNITY

Practice

King's (1971) early publication led to nursing curriculum development and practice application at Ohio State and other universities. In her 1981 book, King identified that "theory, because it is abstract, cannot be immediately applied to nursing practice or to concrete nursing education programs. When empirical referents are identified, defined and described, . . . theory is useful and can be applied in concrete situations" (p. 157). However, "knowledge of the concepts can be applied in concrete situations" (p. 41).

Professionals in most specialty areas have used the concepts of King's (1981) Theory of Goal Attainment in nursing practice. Its relationship to practice is obvious because the nurse functions primarily through interactions with individuals and groups within the environment. Even before King's interacting systems framework was published, Brown and Lee (1980) stated that "this proposed intrasystems model provides an approach for stimulating continued learning, for establishing innovative foundations for nursing practice, and for generating inquiry through research" (p. 469). King (1984) believes that "nurses, who have knowledge of the concepts of this Theory of Goal Attainment, are able to accurately perceive what is happening to patients and family members and are able to suggest approaches for coping with the situations" (p. 12).

King also developed a documentation system, the Goal Oriented Nursing Record (GONR), to accompany the middle range Theory of Goal Attainment, and to record goals and outcomes. The GONR is a method of collecting data, identifying problems, and implementing and evaluating care. It has been used effectively in patient settings. The theory and the GONR are useful in practice, because nurses have the ability to provide individualized plans of care while encouraging active participation from patients in the decision-making phase (King, 1984).

Nurses can also use the GONR approach to document the effectiveness of nursing care. "The major elements in this record system are: (a) data base, (b) nursing diagnosis, (c) goal list, (d) nursing orders, (e) flow sheets, (f) progress notes, and (g) discharge summary" (King, 1995b, pp. 30-31).

Health care professionals have implemented King's (1981) interacting systems framework and middle range Theory of Goal Attainment in various national and international practice settings. The following briefly identifies some of the settings, and the bibliography details additional settings. Jolly and Winker (1995) described the application of the Theory of Goal Attainment within the context of nursing administration. Alligood (1995) applied the Theory of Goal Attainment to adult patients within orthopedic nursing settings. Laben, Sneed, and Seidel (1995) used goal attainment in short-term group psychotherapy. Coker and colleagues (1995) used the framework to implement nursing diagnoses in a Canadian community hospital, and Fawcett, Vaillancourt, and Watson (1995) used the

framework within a large Canadian tertiary care hospital. Viera and Rossi (2000) used King's interacting systems framework to study nursing diagnoses with puerperal women. Williams (2001) applied King's work in emergency and rural nursing. The Theory of Goal Attainment provided the framework for Daniel's (2002) descriptive study of the perceptions of young adults with chronic inflammatory bowel disease.

Education

Nursing faculty at several universities (Ohio State, Loyola in Chicago, and University of Texas in Houston) have used King's interacting systems framework to design curricula in nursing programs (I. King, personal communication, 1984). In 1980, Brown and Lee reported that King's concepts were useful in developing a framework for "use in nursing education, nursing practice, and for generating hypotheses for research. . . . [They] provide a systematic means of viewing the nursing profession, organizing a body of knowledge for nursing, and clarifying nursing as a discipline" (p. 468). King's framework and theory also have application for nursing education internationally as described by Rooke (1995b) for a Swedish educational setting and Bello (2000) for Portuguese undergraduate students. Additional publications detail the application of King's work in core curricula (Gold, Haas, & King, 2000).

Research

Many research studies have used King's work as a theoretical base. Several studies are mentioned here, and others are listed in the bibliography.

Many researchers have used concepts from King's interacting systems framework. Winker (1995) developed a system's view of health. Rooke (1995a) identified the implications of space for nursing. Sieloff (1995a) defined the health of a social system.

Other researchers have used King's (1981) framework as a theoretical base. This group includes the following:

■ Kemppainen (1990) analyzed a case study of a patient who had human immunodeficiency virus and was also experiencing psychotic symptoms.

- Alligood, Evans, and Wilt (1995) developed the concept of empathy within King's framework.
- Sharts-Hopko (1995) explored the perceived health status of women during the transition to menopause.
- McKinney & Dean (2000) applied the interacting systems framework to "study child abuse and the development of alcohol use/dependence in adult females" (p. 73).
- Gerstle (2001) explored relationships among nurses' moral judgments, their perceptions and judgments of pain, and selected nurse factors, using the interacting systems framework.

Researchers have also developed many middle range theories using King's interacting systems framework (King, 1978). Some of these theories include Frey's theory of families, children, and chronic illness (Frey, 1995), Killeen's theory of patient satisfaction with professional nursing care (1996), Sieloff's theory of departmental power (Sieloff, 1995b), Wicks' theory of family health (Wicks, 1995), Doornbos' (2000) theory related to family health, and Goodwin, Kiehl, and Peterson (2002) advance directive decision-making model.

Research has also been conducted using the concepts of the Theory of Goal Attainment (King, 1981). Hanucharurnkui and Vinya-nguag (1991) used goal attainment to study the outcomes of self-care on postoperative patients' recovery and satisfaction. Froman (1995) studied the perceptual congruency between nurses and patients experiencing medical-surgical conditions. Hanna's (1995) use of the Theory of Goal Attainment promoted the health behavior of adolescents, and Kameoka (1995) analyzed nurse-patient interactions. Anderson (2000) studied parental perceptions of family-centered care provided to children with cleft lip or palate, while Mahon (2001) studied the congruency of patient and nurse expectations and perceptions on postsurgical units.

FURTHER DEVELOPMENT

As early as 1971, King demonstrated consistently her belief in the need for further testing of the Theory of Goal Attainment. "Any profession that has as its primary mission the delivery of social services requires continuous research to discover new knowledge that can be applied to improve practice" (King, 1971, p. 112). "Because [the interacting] systems framework has been synthesized from basic elements in nursing, it will persist into the 21st century despite professional and social changes" (King, 1995a, p. 15).

In 1995, Fawcett and Whall identified the following five major areas in which further development of King's work would be helpful:

1. The concept of environment would benefit from additional definition and clarification. Although Zurakowski (2000) studied the social environment of nursing homes, additional work remains to be done in this area.
2. King's views of illness, health, and wellness will benefit from additional clarification and discussion. Although additional work needs to be done in this area, Gunther (2001) described the meaning of high-quality nursing care as derived from King's interacting systems, while Federowicz (2002) investigated clients' perceptions of quality nursing care.
3. Middle range theories that are implied rather than explicit, such as those of Alligood and colleagues (1995) and Rooke (1995b), will benefit from development into formal theories. Sieloff & Frey (2005) examine the status of middle range theory development from within King's interacting systems framework.
4. Future linkages between King's (1981) interacting systems framework and other existing middle range theories should continue to be done in a manner that ensures congruency between the framework and the specific middle range theory. Clarification of these linkages are described in the Sieloff and Frey (2005) text.
5. Empirical testing should continue for the Theory of Goal Attainment (King, 1981) and other middle range theories developed within King's interacting systems framework. Such testing will continue to "add to the evidence regarding the empirical adequacy of the theories and their generalizability across various situations and client

populations" (Fawcett & Whall 1995, p. 332). Empirical testing of relevant middle range theories has been demonstrated by researchers, such as Doornbos (2002) and Sieloff (2003), and are summarized in Sieloff & Frey's (2005) text. Additional empirical testing of the Theory of Goal Attainment has continued since 1995 but benefit would come from consolidation and reporting in a single text.

CRITIQUE

Simplicity

King maintains that her definitions are clear and conceptually derived from research literature that existed at the time the definitions were published. King's (1978) Theory of Goal Attainment presents 10 major concepts, making the theory complex. However, these concepts are easily understood and, with the exception of the concept of self, they have been derived from the research literature.

Generality

King's (1981) Theory of Goal Attainment has been criticized for having limited application in areas of nursing in which patients are unable to interact competently with the nurse. King has responded that 70% of communication is nonverbal and describes the following:

> Try observing a good nurse interact with a baby or a child who has not yet learned the language. If you systematically recorded your observations, you would be able to analyze the behaviors and find many transactions at a nonverbal level. I have a beautiful example of that when I was working side by side with a graduate student in a neuro unit with a comatose patient. I was talking to the patient, explaining everything that was happening and showing the graduate student what I believe to be important in nursing care. When the patient regained consciousness a few days later, she asked the nurse in the unit to find that wonderful nurse who was the only one who explained what was happening to her. She wanted to thank her. I made transactions. I could observe her muscle movement. She was trying to help us as a physician poked a tube down her throat.

A nurse midwife reports observing transactions between mothers and newborns. Psychiatric nurses have reported to me the value of my theory in their practice. So the need in nursing is to broaden nurses' knowledge of communication and that is what my theory is all about. (I. King, personal communication, 1985)

Health care professionals have documented additional examples of the application of the Theory of Goal Attainment with psychiatric patients (Kemppainen, 1990; Laben, et al, 1995; Ng & Tsang, 2002), patients with acute and chronic orthopedic problems (Alligood, 1995), and develop-mentally disabled patients (Messmer, 1995). King believes that critics assume that a theory will address every person, event, and situation, which is clearly impossible. She reminded critics that even Einstein's theory of relativity could not be tested completely until space travel made testing possible (I. King, personal communication, 1985).

Empirical Precision

King gathered empirical data on the nurse-patient interaction process that leads to goal attainment. A descriptive study was conducted to identify the characteristics of transaction and whether nurses made transactions with patients. From a sample of 17 patients, goals were attained in 12 cases (70% of the sample). King (1981) believes that if nursing students are taught the Theory of Goal Attainment and it is used in nursing practice, goal attainment can be measured and the effectiveness of nursing care can be demonstrated.

King continues to serve as a consultant to researchers who test hypotheses derived from her theory. Since the publication of her theory in 1981, multiple research studies provide additional and ongoing evidence of the empirical precision of the Theory of Goal Attainment.

Froman (1995) tested perceptual congruency between nurses and patients who were experiencing medical-surgical problems. Hanna (1995) tested the Theory of Goal Attainment in promoting health behaviors of adolescents. Using the Theory of Goal Attainment, Kameoka (1995) analyzed interactions between nurses and patients. Additional research projects are currently ongoing and others are listed in this chapter's bibliography.

Derivable Consequences

King's (1981) middle range Theory of Goal Attainment focuses on all aspects of the nursing process: assessment, planning, implementation, and evaluation. King believes that nurses must assess to set mutual goals, plan to provide alternative means to achieve goals, and evaluate to determine whether goals are attained. King has stated that she is "the only [nurse theorist] who has provided a theory that deals with choice, alternatives, participation of all individuals in decision making and specifically deals with outcomes of nursing care" (I. King, personal communication, 1985).

Health care professionals have used, and continue to use, King's interacting systems framework and middle range Theory of Goal Attainment to implement theory-based practice in various nursing practice settings in Canada, Japan, Portugal, Sweden, and the United States. In addition, King's work has been demonstrated over time to be a comprehensive frame for curriculum development at various educational levels. King and other nurse scientists and researchers have used her framework for theory testing and theory development at the grand and middle range levels.

SUMMARY

Imogene King contributed to the advancement of nursing knowledge through the development of her interacting systems framework and the middle range Theory of Goal Attainment. By focusing on the attainment of goals, or outcomes, by nurse-patient partnerships, King has provided a framework and middle range theory that has demonstrated its usefulness to nurses both in the present and in the future. Nurses from a variety of settings, working with different patient populations from around the world, continue to use Dr. King's work to improve the quality of patient care they provide.

Case Study

Upon receiving an assignment at the start of the shift, Colin Jennings, R.N., makes initial rounds of the patients. One patient, Amed Kyzeel, as reported by nurses on the previous shift, has been difficult to work with, demanding the attention of staff throughout the shift.

Mr. Jennings has decided to visit Mr. Kyzeel last during rounds so that additional time is available for an assessment. Upon entering Mr. Kyzeel's room, Mr. Jennings asks him how he is feeling. Mr. Kyzeel begins by complaining about a variety of concerns that could be considered minor by most nurses. Accepting that Mr. Kyzeel's perceptions are unique and valid to him, Mr. Jennings spends a few minutes just listening.

Because he knows that Mr. Kyzeel is to be discharged today, he asks the patient what he knows about his pending discharge and what his goals for the day might be. Mr. Kyzeel admits that he is concerned about leaving the hospital, because he does not know what he can expect during the first 24 hours at home. Mr. Jennings talks with the patient about the pending discharge, asking him what goals he might want to achieve both while in the hospital and upon return home. Mr. Kyzeel identifies two to three goals that he would like to achieve while in the hospital and says that he would like to make arrangements for someone to stay with him at his home, at least for the first night.

Of the goals identified, Mr. Jennings and Mr. Kyzeel identify which are the most important and the order in which Mr. Kyzeel would like to achieve them. Once this is done, Mr. Jennings and Mr. Kyzeel identify activities that can be done by the patient and the staff to achieve the goals. Before leaving the room, Mr. Jennings and Mr. Kyzeel agree on the goals, their priority, and the specific activities that are to be done.

Having established times when Mr. Jennings and Mr. Kyzeel would briefly talk to evaluate the achievement of the goals, Mr. Jennings leaves the room and Mr. Kyzeel begins working on the activities he needs to accomplish.

CRITICAL THINKING *Activities*

1. Think about and write your personal definitions of environment, health, nursing, and person. Compare your definitions with King's definitions. How are they similar? How are they different?

Are they more alike than different? If they are more alike, develop a plan to use King's framework and theory more extensively in your practice.

2. Analyze an interaction you have had with a patient. Were you able to achieve a transaction as King describes it? If so, think about what you did differently with this person? If not, think about the interaction and try to identify why the transaction was not achieved?

3. Does the philosophy of one of the agencies in which you have practiced encourage the involvement of the patients in their care? If so, does mutual goal setting occur? If not, what changes would you suggest to more actively involve patients in their own care?

4. Analyze the goal-setting process that occurs between the direct care staff and nursing management and administration in an agency where you have practiced. Does mutual goal setting occur? Discuss changes that could be made in the organizational culture to facilitate mutual goal setting and goal attainment among nurse managers, administrators, and registered nurses.

5. Develop a quality improvement plan to review patient outcomes based on whether mutual goal setting and attainment of patient goals occur. Document changes in the effectiveness and efficiency of the care provided, based on King's interacting systems framework and related theories.

REFERENCES

Alligood, M. R. (1995). Theory of goal attainment: Application to adult orthopedic nursing. In M. A. Frey & C. L. Sieloff (Eds.), *Advancing King's systems framework and theory of nursing* (pp. 209-222). Thousand Oaks, CA: Sage.

Alligood, M. R., Evans, G. W., & Wilt, D. L. (1995). King's interacting systems and empathy. In M. A. Frey & C. L. Sieloff (Eds.), *Advancing King's systems framework and theory of nursing* (pp. 66-78). Thousand Oaks, CA: Sage.

Allport, F. H. (1955). *Theories of perception and the concept of structure.* New York: John Wiley & Sons.

Anderson, K. G. (2000). Perceptions of family centered care of parents of children with cleft lip and/or palate. *Masters Abstracts International, 38-06,* 1580.

Ardrey, R. (1966). *The territorial imperative.* New York: Atheneum.

Austin, J. K., & Champion, V. L. (1983). King's theory for nursing: Explication and evaluation. In P. Chinn (Ed.), *Advances in nursing theory development* (pp. 49-61). Rockville, MD: Aspen.

Bello, I. T. R. (2000). Imogene King's theory as the foundation for the set of a teaching-learning process with undergraudation [sic] students [Portuguese]. *Texto & Contexto Enfermagem, 9*(2 Part 2), 646-657.

Brown, S. T., & Lee, B. T. (1980). Imogene King's conceptual framework: A proposed model for continuing nursing education. *Journal of Advanced Nursing, 5*(5), 467-473.

Clements, I. W., & Roberts, F. B. (1983). *Family health: A theoretical approach to nursing care.* New York: John Wiley & Sons.

Coker, E., Fridley, T., Harris, J., Tomarchio, D., Chan, V., & Caron, C. (1995). Implementing nursing diagnoses within the context of King's conceptual framework. In M. A. Frey & C. L. Sieloff (Eds.), *Advancing King's systems framework and theory of nursing* (pp. 161-175). Thousand Oaks, CA: Sage.

Daniel, J. M. (2002). Young adults' perceptions of living with chronic inflammatory bowel disease. *Gastroenterology Nursing, 25*(3), 83-94.

Dewey, J., & Bentley, A. (1949). *Knowing and the known.* Boston: Beacon Press.

Diers, D., & Schmidt, R. (1977). Interaction analysis in nursing research. In P. Verhonick (Ed.), *Nursing research II* (pp. 77-132). Boston: Little, Brown.

Doornbos, M. M. (2000). King's systems framework and family health: The derivation and testing of a theory. *Journal of Theory Construction & Testing, 4*(1), 20-26.

Doornbos, M. M. (2002). Predicting family health in families with young adults with severe mental illness. *Journal of Family Nursing, 8*(3), 241-263.

Fawcett, J. M., Vaillancourt, V. M., & Watson, C. A. (1995). Integration of King's framework into nursing practice.

In M. A. Frey & C. L. Sieloff (Eds.), *Advancing King's systems framework and theory of nursing* (pp. 176-191). Thousand Oaks, CA: Sage.

Fawcett, J. M., & Whall, A. L. (1995). State of the science and future directions. In M. A. Frey & C. L. Sieloff (Eds.), *Advancing King's systems framework and theory of nursing* (pp. 327-334). Thousand Oaks, CA: Sage.

Federowicz, M. L. (2002). An investigation of clients' perceptions of what constitutes quality nursing care: A phenomenological approach. *Masters Abstracts International, 40-06,* 1501.

Frey, M. A. (1995). Toward a theory of families, children, and chronic illness. In M. A. Frey & C. L. Sieloff (Eds.), *Advancing King's systems framework and theory of nursing* (pp. 109-125). Thousand Oaks, CA: Sage.

Froman, D. (1995). Perceptual congruency between clients and nurses: Testing King's theory of goal attainment. In M. A. Frey & C. L. Sieloff (Eds.), *Advancing King's systems framework and theory of nursing* (pp. 223-238). Thousand Oaks, CA: Sage.

Gerstle, D. S. (2001). Relationships among registered nurses' moral judgment and their perception and judgment of pain, and selected nurse factors (Imogene King). *Dissertation Abstracts International, 62-04B,* 1803.

Gold, C., Haas, S., & King, I. (2000). Conceptual frameworks: Putting the nursing focus into core curricula. *Nurse Educator, 25*(2), 95-98.

Goodwin, Z., Kiehl, E. M., & Peterson, J. Z. (2002). King's theory as foundation for an advance directive decision-making model. *Nursing Science Quarterly, 15*(3), 237-241.

Gunther, M. E. (2001). The meaning of high quality nursing care derived from King's interacting systems (Imogene King). *Dissertation Abstracts International, 62-04B,* 1804.

Hanna, K. M. (1995). Use of King's theory of goal attainment to promote adolescents' health behavior. In M. A. Frey & C. L. Sieloff (Eds.), *Advancing King's systems framework and theory of nursing* (pp. 239-250). Thousand Oaks, CA: Sage.

Hanucharurnkui, S., & Vinya-nguag, P. (1991). Effects of promoting patients' participation in self-care on postoperative recovery and satisfaction with care. *Nursing Science Quarterly, 4*(1), 14-20.

Ittleson, W., & Cantril, H. (1954). *Perception: A transactional approach.* Garden City, NY: Doubleday.

Jersild, A. T. (1952). *In search of self.* New York: Teachers College Press.

Jolly, M. L., & Winker, C. K. (1995). Theory of goal attainment in the context of organizational structure. In M. A. Frey & C. L. Sieloff (Eds.), *Advancing King's systems framework and theory of nursing* (pp. 305-316). Thousand Oaks, CA: Sage.

Kameoka, T. (1995). Analyzing nurse-patient interactions in Japan. In M. A. Frey & C. L. Sieloff (Eds.), *Advancing King's systems framework and theory of nursing* (pp. 251-260). Thousand Oaks, CA: Sage.

Kelley, K. J., & Hammond, K. R. (1964). An approach to the study of clinical inference. *Nursing Research, 13*(4), 314-322.

Kemppainen, J. K. (1990). Imogene King's theory: A nursing case study of a psychotic client with human immunodeficiency virus infection. *Archives of Psychiatric Nursing, 4*(6), 384-388.

Killeen, M. B. (1996). *Patient-consumer perceptions and responses to professional nursing care: Instrument development.* Unpublished doctoral dissertation, Wayne State University, Detroit.

King, I. M. (1964). Nursing theory: Problems and prospects. *Nursing Science, 1*(3), 394-403.

King, I. M. (1968). A conceptual frame of reference for nursing. *Nursing Research, 17*(1), 27-31.

King, I. M. (1971). *Toward a theory for nursing: General concepts of human behavior.* New York: John Wiley & Sons.

King, I. M. (1975a). A process for developing concepts for nursing through research. In P. Verhonick (Ed.), *Nursing research.* Boston: Little, Brown.

King, I. M. (1975b). Patient aspects. In L. J. Schumann, R. D. Spears, Jr., & J. P. Young (Eds.), *Operations research in health care: A critical analysis.* Baltimore: Johns Hopkins University Press.

King, I. M. (Speaker). (1978). *Speech presented at Second Annual Nurse Educators' Conference.* Chicago: Teach 'Em.

King, I. M. (1981). *A theory for nursing: Systems, concepts, process.* New York: John Wiley & Sons.

King, I. M. (1984). Effectiveness of nursing care: Use of a goal oriented nursing record in end stage renal disease. *American Association of Nephrology Nurses and Technicians Journal, 11*(2), 11-17, 60.

King, I. M. (1986). *Curriculum and instruction in nursing: Concepts and process.* Norwalk, CT: Appleton-Century-Crofts.

King, I. M. (1995a). A systems framework for nursing. In M. A. Frey & C. L. Sieloff (Eds.), *Advancing King's systems framework and theory of nursing* (pp. 14-22). Thousand Oaks, CA: Sage.

King, I. M. (1995b). The theory of goal attainment. In M. A. Frey & C. L. Sieloff (Eds.), *Advancing King's systems framework and theory of nursing* (pp. 23-32). Thousand Oaks, CA: Sage.

Krieger, D. (1975). Therapeutic touch: The imprimatur of nursing. *American Journal of Nursing, 75*(5), 784-787.

Kuhn, A. (1975). *Unified social science.* Homewood, IL: Dorsey.

Laben, J. K., Sneed, L. D., & Seidel, S. L. (1995). Goal attainment in short-term group psychotherapy settings: Clinical implications for practice. In M. A. Frey & C. L. Sieloff (Eds.), *Advancing King's systems framework and theory of nursing* (pp. 261-277). Thousand Oaks, CA: Sage.

Mahon, P. Y. (2001). Bridging the gap in patient satisfaction: Congruency of patient-nurse expectation and perception. *Dissertation Abstracts International, 61-10B,* 5237.

McKinney, N. L., & Dean, P. R. (2000). Application of King's theory of dynamic interacting systems to the study of child abuse and the development of alcohol use/dependence in adult females. *Journal of Addictions Nursing, 12*(2), 73-82.

Messmer, P. R. (1995). Implementation of theory-based nursing practice. In M. A. Frey & C. L. Sieloff (Eds.), *Advancing King's systems framework and theory of nursing* (pp. 294-304). Thousand Oaks, CA: Sage.

Minckley, B. B. (1968). Space and place in patient care. *American Journal of Nursing, 68*(3), 510-516.

Ng, B. F. L., & Tsang, H. W. H. (2002). A program to assist people with severe mental illness in formulating realistic life goals. *Journal of Rehabilitation, 68*(4), 59-66.

Orlando, I. J. (1961). *The dynamic nurse-patient relationship: Functions, process, principles.* New York: G. P. Putnam's Sons.

Orme, J. E. (1969). *Time, experience and behavior.* New York: American Elsevier.

Paterson, J., & Zderad, L. (1976). *Humanistic nursing.* New York: John Wiley & Sons.

Peplau, H. E. (1952). *Interpersonal relations in nursing.* New York: G. P. Putnam's Sons.

Rooke, L. (1995a). The concept of space in King's systems framework: Its implications for nursing. In M. A. Frey & C. L. Sieloff (Eds.), *Advancing King's systems framework and theory of nursing* (pp. 79-96). Thousand Oaks, CA: Sage.

Rooke, L. (1995b). Focusing on King's theory and systems framework in education by using an experiential learning model: A challenge to improve the quality of nursing care. In M. A. Frey & C. L. Sieloff (Eds.), *Advancing King's systems framework and theory of nursing* (pp. 278-293). Thousand Oaks, CA: Sage.

Sharts-Hopko, N. C. (1995). Using health, personal, and interpersonal system concepts within the King's systems framework to explore perceived health status during the menopause transition. In M. A. Frey & C. L. Sieloff (Eds.), *Advancing King's systems framework and theory of nursing* (pp. 147-160). Thousand Oaks, CA: Sage.

Sieloff, C. L. (1995a). Defining the health of a social system within Imogene King's framework. In M. A. Frey & C. L. Sieloff (Eds.), *Advancing King's systems framework and theory of nursing* (pp. 137-146). Thousand Oaks, CA: Sage.

Sieloff, C. L. (1995b). Development of a theory of departmental power. In M. A. Frey & C. L. Sieloff (Eds.), *Advancing King's systems framework and theory of nursing* (pp. 46-65). Thousand Oaks, CA: Sage.

Sieloff, C. L. (1996). *Development of an instrument to estimate the actualized power of a nursing department.* Unpublished doctoral dissertation, Wayne State University, Detroit.

Sieloff, C. L. (2003). Measuring nursing power within organizations. *Journal of Nursing Scholarship, 35*(2), 183-187.

Sieloff, C. L., & Frey, M. (2006). *Middle range theories for nursing practice: Using King's interacting systems framework.* New York: Springer.

Sommer, R. (1969). *Personal space.* Englewood Cliffs, NJ: Prentice-Hall.

Viera, C. S., & Rossi, L. (2000). Nursing diagnoses from NANDA's taxonomy in women with a hospitalized preterm child and King's Conceptual System [Portuguese]. *Revista Latin-Americana de Enfermagem, 8*(6), 110-116.

Watzlawick, P., Beavin, J. W., & Jackson, D. D. (1967). *Pragmatics of human communication.* New York: Norton.

Whiting, J. F. (1955). Q-sort technique for evaluating perceptions of interpersonal relationship. *Nursing Research, 4,* 71-73.

Wicks, M. N. (1995). Family health as derived from King's framework. In M. A. Frey & C. L. Sieloff (Eds.), *Advancing King's systems framework and theory of nursing* (pp. 97-108). Thousand Oaks, CA: Sage.

Williams, L. A. (2001). Imogene King's interacting systems theory—Application in emergency and rural nursing. *Online Journal of Rural Nursing and Health Care, 2*(1). Retrieved January 8, 2004, from CINAHL.

Winker, C. K. (1995). A systems view of health. In M. A. Frey & C. L. Sieloff (Eds.), *Advancing King's systems framework and theory of nursing* (pp. 35-45). Thousand Oaks, CA: Sage.

Yura, H., & Walsh, M. (1978). *The nursing process.* New York: Appleton-Century-Crofts.

Zurakowski, T. L. (2000). The social environment of nursing homes and the health of older residents. *Holistic Nursing Practice, 14*(4), 12-23.

BIBLIOGRAPHY
Primary Sources
Books

Fawcett, J., & King, I. (Eds.). (1997). *The language of nursing theory and metatheory.* Indianapolis: Sigma Theta Tau International Center Press.

King, I. M. (1971). *Toward a theory for nursing: General concepts of human behavior.* New York: John Wiley & Sons.

King, I. M. (1976). *Toward a theory of nursing: General concepts of human behavior* (Sugimori, M., Trans.). Tokyo: Igaku-Shoin.

King, I. M. (1981). *A theory for nursing: Systems, concepts, process.* New York: John Wiley & Sons.

King, I. M. (1985). *A theory for nursing: Systems, concepts, process* (Sugimori, M., Trans.). Tokyo: Igaku-Shoin.

King, I. M. (1986). *Curriculum and instruction in nursing: Concepts and process.* Norwalk, CT: Appleton-Century-Crofts.

King, I. M., & Fawcett, J. (1997). *The language of nursing theory and metatheory.* Indianapolis: Sigma Theta Tau International.

Book Chapter

King, I. M. (1995). The theory of goal attainment. In M. A. Frey & C. L. Sieloff (Eds.), *Advancing King's systems framework and theory of nursing* (pp. 23-32). Thousand Oaks, CA: Sage.

Journal Articles

Daubenmire, M. J., & King, I. M. (1973). Nursing process models: A systems approach. *Nursing Outlook, 21*(8), 512-517.

King, I. M. (1964). Nursing theory—Problems and prospect. *Nursing Science, 2*(5), 394-403.

King, I. M. (1968). Conceptual frame of reference for nursing. *Nursing Research, 17*(1), 27-31.

King, I. M. (1970). A conceptual frame of reference for nursing. *Japanese Journal of Nursing Research, 3,* 199-204.

King, I. M. (1987). Translating nursing research into practice. *Journal of Neuroscience Nursing, 19*(1), 44-48.

King, I. M. (1990, Fall). Health as the goal for nursing. *Nursing Science Quarterly, 3*(3), 123-128.

King, I. M. (1992). King's theory of goal attainment. *Nursing Science Quarterly, 5*(1), 19-26.

King, I. M. (1994). Quality of life and goal attainment. *Nursing Science Quarterly, 7*(1), 29-32.

King, I. M. (1996). The theory of goal attainment in research and practice. *Nursing Science Quarterly, 9*(2), 61-66.

King, I. M. (1997). King's theory of goal attainment in practice. *Nursing Science Quarterly, 10*(4), 180-185.

King, I. M. (1997). Reflections on the past and a vision for the future. *Nursing Science Quarterly, 10*(1), 15-17.

King, I. M. (1998). Nursing informatics: A universal nursing language. *Florida Nurse, 46*(1), 1-3, 5, 9.

King, I. M. (1998). The Bioethics Focus Group Report. *Florida Nurse, 46*(8), 24.

King, I. M. (1999). A theory of goal attainment: Philosophical and ethical implications. *Nursing Science Quarterly, 12*(4), 292-296.

King, I. M. (2000). Evidence-based nursing practice. *Theoria: Journal of Nursing Theory, 9*(2), 4-9.

Quigley, P., Janzen, S. K., King, I. M., & Goucher, E. (1999). Nurse staffing patient outcomes from one acute care setting within the Department of Veteran's Affairs. *Florida Nurse, 47*(2), 34.

Letter to the Editor

King, I. M., & Whelton, B. J. B. (2001). Reaction to "A nursing theory of person system empathy: Interpreting a conceptualization of empathy in King's Interacting Systems" by M. R. Alligood & B.A. May (Letter to the Editor). *Nursing Science Quarterly, 14*(1), 80-82.

Presented Papers

King, I. M. (1980, April). *Theory development in nursing.* Paper presented at Georgia State University, Atlanta.

King, I. M. (1989, May). *Health as a goal for nursing.* Paper presented at an International Theory Conference, Pittsburgh.

King, I. M. (1989, Nov.). *Theory: What it is and what it is not.* Paper presented at the Biennial Convention of Sigma Theta Tau International, Indianapolis.

King, I. M. (1990, Oct.). *Theory-based quality assurance in nursing.* Conference presented in Sedona, Arizona.

King, I. M. (1995, June). *Jessie M. Scott award presentation.* Paper presented at the 100th American Nurses Association Convention, Washington, DC.

King, I. M. (1997, Sept.). *Nursing's vision for the future.* Paper presented at the American Operating Room Nurses Convention, Sarasota, FL.

King, I. M. (1997, Sept./Oct.). *A theoretical basis for nursing informatics.* Paper presented at the International Nursing Informatics Conference, Stockholm.

King, I. M. (1999, Oct.). *Reflections of the past: Visions of the future.* Paper presented at the Inaugural Conference of the King International Nursing Group, Troy, MI.

King, I. M. (1999, Nov.). *Discovery, controversy, self-actualization.* Paper presented at the Ethics Conference, Loyola University, Chicago.

King, I. M. (1999, Nov.). *High tech, high touch: Nursing in the new millennium.* Paper presented at the Florida Nursing Student Association Annual Convention, St. Petersburg, FL.

King, I. M. (1999, Dec.). *Implementing a research program in a large medical center.* Paper presented at the Department of Nursing, Clearwater, FL.

King, I. M., & Fawcett, J. (1999, Oct.). *Charting the course for the new millennium.* Paper presented at the Inaugural Conference of the King International Nursing Group, Troy, MI.

King, I. M., & Killeen, M. (1999, Oct.). *Interaction, transaction, and new technology.* Paper presented at the Inaugural Conference of the King International Nursing Group, Troy, MI.

Secondary Sources
Books

Chinn, P. L., & Kramer, M. K. (1995). *Theory and nursing: A systematic approach* (3rd ed.). St. Louis: Mosby.

Fitzpatrick, J. J., & Whall, A. L. (1995). *Conceptual models of nursing: Analysis and application.* Bowie, MD: Robert J. Brady.

Frey, M. A., & Sieloff, C. L. (1995). *Advancing King's systems framework and theory of nursing.* Thousand Oaks, CA: Sage.

George, J. B. (1995). *Nursing theories: The base for professional nursing practice.* Englewood Cliffs, NJ: Prentice-Hall.

Polit, D., & Hungler, B. (1995). *Nursing research: Principles and methods* (5th ed.). Philadelphia: J. B. Lippincott.

Walker, L. O., & Avant, K. C. (1995). *Strategies for theory construction in nursing.* Norwalk, CT: Appleton-Century-Crofts.

Book Chapters

Alligood, M. R. (1995). Theory of goal attainment: Application to adult orthopedic nursing. In M. A. Frey & C. L. Sieloff (Eds.), *Advancing King's systems framework and theory of nursing* (pp. 209-222). Thousand Oaks, CA: Sage.

Alligood, M. R., Evans, G. W., & Wilt, D. L. (1995). King's interacting system and empathy. In M. A. Frey & C. L. Sieloff (Eds.), *Advancing King's systems framework and theory of nursing* (pp. 66-78). Thousand Oaks, CA: Sage.

Austin, J. K., & Champion, V. L. (1983). King theory for nursing: Explication and evaluation. In P. Chinn, *Advances in nursing theory development* (pp. 49-61). Rockville, MD: Aspen.

Benedict, M., & Frey, M. A. (1995). Theory-based practice in the emergency department. In M. A. Frey & C. L. Sieloff (Eds.), *Advancing King's systems framework and theory of nursing* (pp. 317-324). Thousand Oaks, CA: Sage.

Doornbos, M. M. (1995). Using King's systems framework to explore family health in the families of the young chronically mentally ill. In M. A. Frey & C. L. Sieloff (Eds.), *Advancing King's systems framework and theory of nursing* (pp. 192-205). Thousand Oaks, CA: Sage.

Fawcett, J. (1995). King's open systems model. In *Analysis and evaluation of conceptual models of nursing* (3rd ed., pp. 109-163). Philadelphia: F.A. Davis.

Fawcett, J. M., Vaillancourt, V. M., & Watson, C. A. (1995). Integration of King's framework into nursing practice. In M. A. Frey & C. L. Sieloff (Eds.), *Advancing King's systems framework and theory of nursing* (pp. 176-191). Thousand Oaks, CA: Sage.

Fawcett, J., & Whall, A. L. (1995). State of the science and future directions. In M. A. Frey & C. L. Sieloff (Eds.), *Advancing King's systems framework and theory of nursing* (pp. 327-334). Thousand Oaks, CA: Sage.

Frey, M. A. (1995). From conceptual framework to nursing knowledge. In M. A. Frey & C. L. Sieloff (Eds.), *Advancing King's framework and theory for nursing* (pp. 3-13). Thousand Oaks, CA: Sage.

Frey, M. A., & Norris, D. (1997). King's systems framework and theory in nursing practice. In M. R. Alligood & A. Marriner Tomey (Eds.), *Nursing theory: Utilization & application* (pp. 71-88). St. Louis: Mosby.

Froman, D. (1995). Perceptual congruency between clients and nurses: Testing King's theory of goal attainment. In M. A. Frey & C. L. Sieloff (Eds.), *Advancing King's systems framework and theory of nursing* (pp. 223-238). Thousand Oaks, CA: Sage.

Hanna, K. M. (1995). Use of King's theory of goal attainment to promote adolescents' health behavior. In M. A. Frey & C. L. Sieloff (Eds.), *Advancing King's systems framework and theory of nursing* (pp. 239-250). Thousand Oaks, CA: Sage.

Hobdell, E. F. (1995). Using King's interacting systems framework for research on parents of children with neural tube defects. In M. A. Frey & C. L. Sieloff (Eds.), *Advancing King's systems framework and theory of nursing* (pp. 126-136). Thousand Oaks, CA: Sage.

Jolly, M. L., & Winker, C. K. (1995). Theory of goal attainment in the context of organizational structure. In M. A. Frey & C. L. Sieloff (Eds.), *Advancing King's systems framework and theory of nursing* (pp. 305-316). Thousand Oaks, CA: Sage.

Kameoka, T. (1995). Analyzing nurse-patient interactions in Japan. In M. A. Frey & C. L. Sieloff (Eds.), *Advancing King's systems framework and theory of nursing* (pp. 251-260). Thousand Oaks, CA: Sage.

Laben, J. K., Sneed, L. D., & Seidel, S. L. (1995). Goal attainment in short-term group psychotherapy settings: Clinical implications for practice. In M. A. Frey & C. L. Sieloff (Eds.), *Advancing King's systems framework and theory of nursing* (pp. 261-277). Thousand Oaks, CA: Sage.

Messmer, P. R. (1995). Implementation of theory-based nursing practice. In M. A. Frey & C. L. Sieloff (Eds.), *Advancing King's systems framework and theory of nursing* (pp. 294-304). Thousand Oaks, CA: Sage.

Rooke, L. (1995a). Focusing on King's theory and systems framework in education by using an experiential learning model: A challenge to improve the quality of nursing care. In M. A. Frey & C. L. Sieloff (Eds.), *Advancing King's systems framework and theory of nursing* (pp. 278-293). Thousand Oaks, CA: Sage.

Rooke, L. (1995b). The concept of space in King's systems framework: Its implications for nursing. In M. A. Frey & C. L. Sieloff (Eds.), *Advancing King's systems framework and theory of nursing* (pp. 79-96). Thousand Oaks, CA: Sage.

Sharts-Hopko, N. C. (1995). Using health, personal and interpersonal system concepts within the King's systems framework to explore perceived health status during the menopause transition. In M. A. Frey & C. L. Sieloff (Eds.), *Advancing King's systems framework and theory of nursing* (pp. 147-160). Thousand Oaks, CA: Sage.

Wicks, M. N. (1995). Family health as derived from King's framework. In M. A. Frey & C. L. Sieloff (Eds.), *Advancing King's systems framework and theory of nursing* (pp. 97-108). Thousand Oaks, CA: Sage.

Winker, C. K. (1995). A systems view of health. In M. A. Frey & C. L. Sieloff (Eds.), *Advancing King's systems framework and theory of nursing* (pp. 35-45). Thousand Oaks, CA: Sage.

Journal Articles

Alligood, M. R., & May, B. A. (2000). A nursing theory of personal system empathy: Interpreting a conceptualization of empathy in King's interacting systems. *Nursing Science Quarterly, 13*(3), 243-247.

Baumann, S. L. (2000). Research issues: Family nursing: Theory-anemic, nursing theory–deprived. *Nursing Science Quarterly, 13*(4), 285-290.

Brooks, E. M., & Thomas, S. (1997). The perception and judgment of senior baccalaureate student nurses in clinical decision making. *ANS Advances in Nursing Science, 19*(3), 50-69.

Calladine, M. L. (1996). Nursing process for health promotion using King's theory. *Journal of Community Health Nursing, 13*(1), 51-57.

Campbell-Begg, T. (2000). A case study using animal-assisted therapy to promote abstinence in a group of individuals who are recovering from chemical addictions. *Journal of Addictions Nursing, 12*(1), 31-35.

Caris-Verhallen, W. M. C. M., Kerkstra, A., van der Heijden, P. G. M., & Bensing, J. M. (1998). Nurse–elderly patient communication in home care and institutional care: An explorative study. *International Journal of Nursing Studies, 35*(1/2), 95-108.

Carter, K. F., & Dufour, L. T. (1994). King's theory: A critique of the critiques. *Nursing Science Quarterly, 7*(3), 128-133.

Crossan, F., & Robb, A. (1998). Role of the nurse: Introducing theories and concepts. *British Journal of Nursing, 7*(10), 608-612.

David, G. L. B. (2000). Ethics in the relationship between nursing and AIDS-afflicted families [Portuguese]. *Texto & Contexto Enfermagem, 9*(2), 590-599.

Fawcett, J. (2001). Scholarly dialogue. The nurse theorists: 21st-century updates—Imogene M. King. *Nursing Science Quarterly, 14*(4), 311-315.

Frey, M. A. (1996). Behavioral correlates of health and illness in youths with chronic illness. *Advanced Nursing Research, 9*(4), 167-176.

Frey, M. A. (1997). Health promotion in youth with chronic illness: Are we on the right track? *Quality Nursing, 3*(5), 13-18.

Frey, M. A., Rooke, L., Sieloff, C. L., Messmer, P., & Kameoka, T. (1995). King's framework and theory in Japan, Sweden, and the United States. *Image: The Journal of Nursing Scholarship, 27*(2), 127-130.

Gill, J., Hopwood-Jones, L., Tyndall, J., Gregoroff, S., LeBlanc, P., Lovett, C., et al. (1995). Incorporating nursing diagnosis and King's theory in the O.R. documentation. *Canadian Operating Room Nursing Journal, 13*(1), 10-14.

Husting, P. M. (1997). A transcultural critique of Imogene King's theory of goal attainment. *The Journal of Multicultural Nursing & Health, 3*(3), 15-20.

Jones, S., Clark, V. B., Merker, A., & Palau, D. (1995). Changing behaviors: Nurse educators and clinical nurse specialists design a discharge planning program. *Journal of Nursing Staff Development, 11*(6), 291-295.

Kobayashi, F. T. (1970). A conceptual frame of reference for nursing. *Japanese Journal of Nursing Research, 3*(3), 199-204.

Kusaka, T. (1991). Application to the King's goal attainment theory in Japanese clinical setting. *Journal of the Japanese Academy of Nursing Education, 1*(1), 30-31.

Laramee, A. (1999). The building blocks of successful relationships. *Journal of Care Management, 5*(4), 40, 42, 44-45.

Lawler, J., Dowswell, G., Hearn, J., Forster, A., & Young, J. (1999). Recovering from stroke: A qualitative investigation of the role of goal setting in late stroke recovery. *Journal of Advanced Nursing, 30*(2), 401-409.

Lewinson, S. B. (2000). Professionally speaking: Interview with Imogene King. *Nursing Leadership Forum, 4*(3), 91-95.

Lockhart, J. S. (2000). Nurses' perceptions of head and neck oncology patients after surgery: Severity of facial disfigurement and patient gender. *Plastic Surgical Nursing, 20*(2), 68-80.

Long, J. M., Kee, C. C., Graham, M. V., Saethan, T. B., & Dames, F. D. (1998). Medication compliance and the older hemodialysis patient. *American Nephrology Nurses Association Journal, 25*(1), 43-49.

Mayer, B. W. (2000). Female domestic violence victims: Perspectives on emergency care. *Nursing Science Quarterly, 13*(4), 340-346.

McKinney, N., & Frank, D. I. (1998). Nursing assessment of adult females who are alcohol dependent and victims of sexual abuse. *Clinical Excellence for Nurse Practitioners, 2*(3), 152-158.

Milne, J. (2000). The impact of information on health behaviors of older adults with urinary incontinence. *Clinical Nursing Research, 9*(2), 161-176.

Moreira, T. M. M., & Arajo, T. L. (2002). The conceptual model of interactive open systems and the theory of goal attainment by Imogene King [Portuguese]. *Revista Latino-Americana deEnfermagem, 10*(1), 97-103.

Murray, R. L. E., & Baier, M. (1996). King's conceptual framework applied to a transitional living program. *Perspectives in Psychiatric Care, 32*(1), 15-19.

Nagano, M., & Funashima, N. (1995). Analysis of nursing situations in Japan: Using King's goal attainment theory. *Quality Nursing, 1*(1), 74-78.

Norgan, G. H., Ettipio, A. M., & Lasome, C. E. M. (1995). A program plan addressing carpal tunnel syndrome: The utility of King's goal attainment theory. *American Association of Occupational Health Nurses Journal, 43*(8), 407-411.

Olsson, H., & Forsdahl, T. (1996). Expectations and opportunities of newly employed nurses at the University Hospital, Tromso, Norway. *Social Sciences in Health: International Journal of Research and Practice, 2*(1), 14-22.

Petrich, B. (2000). Medical and nursing students' perceptions of obesity. *Journal of Addictions Nursing, 12*(10), 3-16.

Richard-Hughes, S. (1997). Attitudes and beliefs of Afro-Americans related to organ and tissue donation. *International Journal of Trauma Nursing, 3*(4), 119-123.

Riggs, C. J. (2001). A model of staff support to improve retention in long-term care. *Nursing Administration Quarterly, 25*(2), 43-54.

Scott, L. D. (1998). Perceived needs of parents of critically ill children. *Journal of the Society of Pediatric Nurses, 3*(1), 4-12.

Tripp-Reimer, T., Woodworth, G., McCloskey, J. C., & Bulechek, G. (1996). The dimensional structure of nursing interventions. *Nursing Research, 45*(1), 10-17.

Tritsch, J. M. (1996). Application of King's theory of goal attainment and the Carondelet St. Mary's case management model. *Nursing Science Quarterly, 11*(2), 69-73.

Ugarriza, D. N. (2002). Intentionality: Applications within selected theories of nursing. *Holistic Nursing Practice, 16*(4), 41-50.

Wadensten, B., & Carlsson, M. (2003). Nursing theory views on how to support the process of aging. *Journal of Advanced Nursing, 42*(2), 118-124.

Walker, K. M., & Alligood, M. R. (2001). Empathy from a nursing perspective: Moving beyond borrowed theory. *Archives of Psychiatric Nursing, 15*(3), 140-147.

Wilkinson, C. R., & Williams, M. (2002). Strengthening patient-provider relationships. *Lippincott's Case Management, 7*(3), 86-102.

Master's Theses

Allan, N. J. (1995). Goal attainment and life satisfaction among frail elderly. *Masters Abstracts International, 35-05,* 1486.

Aramburu-Drury, C. M. (1996). Exploring the association between body weight and health care avoidance. *Masters Abstracts International, 35-03,* 0725.

Arbeiter, N. A. (1998). The effect of a formal class on advance directives on nurses' perceptions. *Masters Abstracts International, 36-04,* 1059.

Brennan, K. M. (2000). Parents' perceptions of their roles during the treatment of their child's thermal injury. *Masters Abstracts International, 38-06,* 1581.

Dawson, B. W. (1996). The relationship between functional social support, social network and the adequacy of prenatal care. *Masters Abstracts International, 35-01,* 0361.

Genzel, M. C. (1998). Job satisfaction of the nursing staff development educator. *Masters Abstracts International, 36-04,* 1063.

Kahn, R. (1997). The number and types of interventions developed and employed for a population of ADHD students by an advanced nurse practitioner in a middle-sized urban school district in Michigan Title I Health Program during the 1995-1996 school year. *Masters Abstracts International, 36-01,* 0158.

Kaminski, L. A. (1999). Perceptions of home care nurses as facilitators of discussions and advance directives. *Masters Abstracts International, 37-04,* 1179.

Leonard, B. M. (1996). Team building using group and peer initiating processes within Imogene King's systems to facilitate CQI (Continuous Quality Improvement). *Masters Abstracts International, 34-06,* 2346.

McCartan, D. P. (2000). Measurement of the quality of life perceptions of in-home hospice patients: A descriptive/exploratory study. *Masters Abstracts International, 38-06,* 1586.

McGonigle, S. M. (1998). Evaluating outcomes: Client satisfaction with primary nursing in tertiary care. *Masters Abstracts International, 36-04,* 1066.

Mang, A. M. (2001). Parish nursing. *Masters Abstracts International, 40-03,* 674.

Phillips, E. L. (1995). Diploma nursing students' attitudes toward poverty. *Masters Abstracts International, 33-06,* 1846.

Pinnock-Philp, B. E. (1998). Attitudes toward restricting food in labor: Differences between caregivers in a tertiary care perinatal center and a birthing center. *Masters Abstracts International, 36-06,* 1600.

Ranta, M. (2000). The effect of mutual goal setting on the self-efficacy to manage heart failure in adults. *Masters Abstracts International, 39-01,* 196.

Rexford, D. S. (2001). Quality of life in a heart failure population. *Masters Abstracts International, 40-01,* 152.

Six, D. M. (1998). Patient satisfaction with prenatal care services in a rural setting: Time. *Masters Abstracts International, 36-06,* 1591.

Skariah, R. A. (1999). Analysis of first nation children's drawings of their perceptions of health. *Masters Abstracts International, 37-04,* 1184.

Sperry, E. J. (1999). Physician perceptions of behaviors associated with the nurse practitioner role. *Masters Abstracts International, 37-06,* 1821.

Stanley, J. M. (2000). Nurses' perceptions of hypnosis. *Masters Abstracts International, 38-03,* 685.

Stover, D. C. (1999). A change in patient satisfaction in the endoscopy laboratory. *Masters Abstracts International, 38-02,* 416.

Villanueva-Noble, N. S. (1998). Cross-cultural analysis of perceptions of health in children's drawings: A replicate study (Philippines, Canada). *Masters Abstracts International, 36-04,* 1070.

Doctoral Dissertations

Brooks, E. (1995). Exploring the perception and judgment of senior baccalaureate student nurses in clinical decision-making from a nursing theoretical perspective. *Dissertation Abstracts International, 56-12B,* 6667.

duMont, P. (1998). The effects of early menarche on health risk behaviors. *Dissertation Abstracts International, 60-07B,* 3200.

Ehrenberger, H. E. (1998). Testing a theory of decision making derived from King's systems framework in women eligible for a cancer clinical trial. *Dissertation Abstracts International, 60-07B,* 3201.

Killeen, M. (1996). Patient-consumer perceptions and responses to professional nursing care: Instrument development. *Dissertation Abstracts International, 57-04B,* 2479.

May, B. A. (2000). Relationships among basic empathy, self-awareness, and learning styles of baccalaureate pre-nursing students within King's personal system. *Dissertation Abstracts International, 61-06b,* 2991.

McKay, T. (1999). An examination of case management nurses' role strain, participative decision making, and their relationships to patient satisfaction: Utilization of King's theory of goal attainment in a managed care environment. *Dissertation Abstracts International, 60-09B,* 4522.

Sieloff, C. L. (1996). Development of an instrument to estimate the actualized power of a nursing department. *Dissertation Abstracts International, 57-04B,* 2484.

Sink, K. K. (2001). Perceptions, informational needs, and feelings of competency of new parents. *Dissertation Abstracts International, 62-01B,* 166.

Whelton, B. T. B. (1996). A philosophy of nursing practice: An application of the Thomistic-Aristotelian concept of nature to the science of nursing. *Dissertation Abstracts International, 57-03A,* 1176.

Winker, C. (1996). A descriptive study of the relationship of interaction disturbance to the organizational health of a metropolitan general hospital. *Dissertation Abstracts International, 57-07B,* 4306.

Web Sites

Clayton College and State University, Department of Nursing, Nursing Theory Link Page. Accessed December 20, 2004: *http://healthsci.clayton.edu/ eichelberger/nursing.htm*

Hahn School of Nursing and Health Science, University of San Diego. Accessed December 20, 2004: *http://www. sandiego.edu/nursing/theory/*

Mississippi University for Women. Accessed December 20, 2004: *http://www.muw.edu/nursing/tupelo/NU433KING'S. htm*

Nurses.info. Accessed December 20, 2004: *http://www. nurses.info/nursing_theory_person_king_imogene. htm*

NurseScribe. Accessed December 20, 2004: *http://www. enursescribe.com/imogene_king.htm*

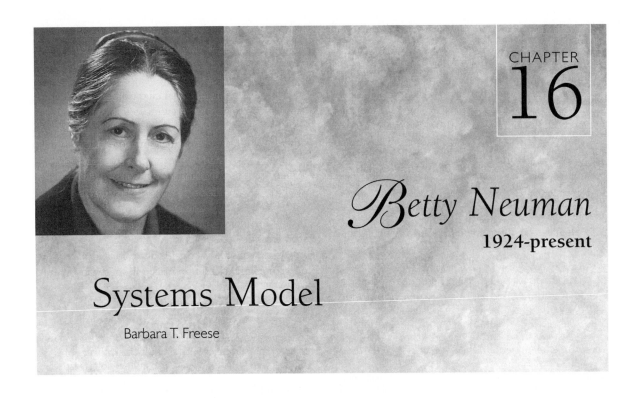

16

Betty Neuman

1924-present

Systems Model

Barbara T. Freese

CREDENTIALS AND BACKGROUND OF THE THEORIST

Betty Neuman was born in 1924 and grew up on a farm in Ohio. Her rural background helped her develop a compassion for people in need, which has been evident throughout her career. She completed her initial nursing education with double honors at Peoples Hospital School of Nursing (now General Hospital), Akron, Ohio, in 1947. As a young nurse, she moved to California and worked in a variety of roles that included hospital nurse, school nurse, industrial nurse, and clinical instructor at the University of Southern California Medical Center. She earned a baccalaureate degree in public health and psychology with honors (1957) and a master's degree in mental health, public health consultation

Previous authors: Barbara T. Freese, Sarah J. Beckman, Sanna Boxley-Harges, Cheryl Bruick-Sorge, Susan Matthews Harris, Mary E. Hermiz, Mary Meininger, and Sandra E. Steinkeler.

(1966), from the University of California, Los Angeles (UCLA). She completed a doctoral degree in clinical psychology from Pacific Western University in 1985 (B. Neuman, personal communication, June 3, 1984).

Neuman was a pioneer of nursing involvement in mental health. She and Donna Aquilina were the first two nurses to develop the nurse counselor role within community crisis centers in Los Angeles (B. Neuman, personal communication, June 21, 1992). She developed, taught, and refined a community mental health program for post–master's level nurses at UCLA. She developed her first explicit teaching and practice model for mental health consultation in the late 1960s, before the creation of her systems model. This teaching and practice model is cited in her first book publication, *Consultation and Community Organization in Community Mental Health Nursing* (Neuman, Deloughery, & Gebbie, 1971). Neuman designed a nursing conceptual model in 1970 for UCLA nursing students; the purpose was to expand understanding of client variables beyond the medical model (Neuman & Young, 1972). The Neuman model included behavioral science concepts such as problem identification and prevention. Neuman first published her model during the early 1970s (Neuman & Young, 1972; Neuman, 1974). She spent the following decade further defining and refining various aspects of the model in preparation for the first edition of *The Neuman Systems Model: Application to Nursing Education and Practice* (Neuman, 1982). Further development and revisions of the model are illustrated in the subsequent editions (Neuman, 1989, 1995b, 2002b).

Since developing the Neuman Systems Model, she has been involved in a wide variety of professional activities including numerous publications, paper presentations, consultations, lectures, and conferences on application and use of the model. Neuman has a wide range of teaching expertise and taught nurse continuing education at UCLA and in community agencies for 14 years. She is a Fellow of the American Association of Marriage and Family Therapy. She continues in active, private practice as a licensed clinical marriage and family therapist, with an emphasis on pastoral counseling. Neuman lives in Ohio and maintains a leadership role in the Neuman Systems Model Trustees Group. She serves as a consultant nationally and internationally regarding implementation of the model for nursing education programs and for clinical practice agencies (B. Neuman, personal communications, July 18, 2000; February 9, 2004).

THEORETICAL SOURCES

The Neuman Systems Model is based in general system theory and reflects the nature of living organisms as open systems (Bertalanffy, 1968) in interaction with each other and with the environment (Neuman, 1982). Within the model, Neuman synthesizes knowledge from several disciplines and incorporates her own philosophical beliefs and clinical nursing expertise, particularly in mental health nursing.

The model draws from gestalt theory (Perls, 1973), which describes homeostasis as the process by which an organism maintains its equilibrium, and consequently its health, under varying conditions. Neuman describes adjustment as the process by which the organism satisfies its needs. Many needs exist and each may disrupt client balance or stability; therefore, the adjustment process is dynamic and continuous. All life is characterized by this ongoing interplay of balance and imbalance within the organism. When the stabilizing process fails to some degree, or when the organism remains in a state of disharmony for too long and is consequently unable to satisfy its needs, illness may develop. When illness as a compensatory process fails completely, the organism may die (Neuman & Young, 1972). The gestalt approach considers the individual within the organism-environmental field and views behavior as a reflection of relatedness within that field (Perls, 1973).

The model is also derived from the philosophical views of de Chardin and Marx (Neuman, 1982). Marxist philosophy suggests that the properties of parts are determined partly by the larger wholes within dynamically organized systems. With this view, Neuman (1982) confirms that the patterns of the whole influence awareness of the part, which is drawn from de Chardin's philosophy of the wholeness of life.

Neuman used Selye's definition of stress, which is the nonspecific response of the body to any demand made on it. Stress increases the demand for readjustment. This demand is nonspecific; it requires adaptation to a problem, irrespective of the nature of the problem. Therefore, the essence of stress is the nonspecific demand for activity (Selye, 1974). Stressors are the tension-producing stimuli that result in stress; they may be positive or negative.

Neuman adapts the concept of levels of prevention from Caplan's conceptual model (1964) and relates these prevention levels to nursing. Primary prevention is used to protect the organism before it encounters a harmful stressor. Primary prevention involves reducing the possibility of encountering the stressor or strengthening the client's normal line of defense to decrease the reaction to the stressor. Secondary and tertiary prevention are used following the client's encounter with a harmful stressor.

Secondary prevention attempts to reduce the effect or possible effect of stressors through early diagnosis and effective treatment of illness symptoms; Neuman describes this as strengthening the internal lines of resistance. Tertiary prevention attempts to reduce the residual stressor effects and return the client to wellness after treatment (Capers, 1996; Neuman, 2002b).

MAJOR CONCEPTS *&* DEFINITIONS

Betty Neuman (2001) describes the Neuman systems model by stating the following:

> The Neuman systems model reflects nursing's interest in well and ill people as holistic systems and in environmental influences on health. Clients' and nurses' perceptions of stressors and resources are emphasized, and clients act in partnership with nurses to set goals and identify relevant prevention interventions. The individual, family or other group, community, or a social issue all are client systems, which are viewed as composites of interacting physiological, psychological, sociocultural, developmental, and spiritual variables. (p. 322)

The major concepts identified in the model [see Figure 16-1] are wholistic approach, open system (including function, input and output, feedback, negentropy, entropy, and stability), environment, created environment, wellness and illness, client system (including five client variables, basic structure, lines of resistance, normal line of defense, and flexible line of defense), stressors, degree of reaction, prevention as intervention, and recon-stitution (Neuman, 2002b, pp. 12-30; see also Neuman, 1982, 1989, 1995b).

WHOLISTIC APPROACH

The Neuman Systems Model is a dynamic, open, systems approach to client care originally developed to provide a unifying focus for nursing problem definition and for best understanding the client in interaction with the environment. The client as a system may be defined as a person, family, group, community, or social issue (Neumann, 2002b, p. 15).

Clients are viewed as wholes whose parts are in dynamic interaction. The model considers all variables simultaneously affecting the client system: physiological, psychological, sociocultural, developmental, and spiritual. Neuman included the spiritual variable in the second edition (1989). She changed the spelling of the term *holistic* to *wholistic* in the second edition to enhance understanding of the term as referring to the whole person (B. Neuman, personal communication, June 20, 1988).

OPEN SYSTEM

A system is open when its elements are continuously exchanging information and energy within its complex organization. Stress and reaction to stress are basic components of an open system (Neuman, 2002c, p. 323; see also Neuman, 1982, 1989, 1995b).

Function or Process

The client as a system exchanges energy, information, and matter with the environment as it uses available energy resources to move toward stability and wholeness (Neuman, 2002c, p. 323; see also Neuman, 1982, 1989, 1995b).

Input and Output

For the client as a system, input and output are the matter, energy, and information that are exchanged between the client and the environment (B. Neuman, personal communication, January 20, 1988).

Feedback

System output in the form of matter, energy, and information serves as feedback for future input for corrective action to change, enhance, or stabilize the system (B. Neuman, personal communication, January 20, 1988).

MAJOR CONCEPTS & DEFINITIONS—cont'd

Negentropy

Neuman defines *negentropy* as ". . . a process of energy conservation utilization that assists system progression toward stability or wellness" (Neuman, 2002c, p. 323; see also Neuman, 1982, 1989, 1995b).

Entropy

She likewise defines *entropy* as ". . . a process of energy depletion and disorganization that moves the system toward illness or possible death" (Neuman, 1982, p. 8; Perls, 1973).

Stability

According to Neuman, *stability* is ". . . a desired state of balance in which the system copes with stressors to maintain an optimal level of health and integrity" (Neuman, 2002c, p. 324; see also Neuman, 1982, 1989, 1995b).

ENVIRONMENT

As defined by Neuman, ". . . internal and external forces surrounding and affecting the client at any time comprise the environment" (Neuman, 2002c, p. 322; see also Neuman, 1982, 1989, 1995b).

CREATED ENVIRONMENT

The created environment is developed unconsciously by the client to express system wholeness symbolically. Its purpose is to provide a safe arena for client system functioning, and to insulate the client from stressors (Neuman, 2002b, pp. 19-20; see also Neuman, 1982, 1989, 1995b).

CLIENT SYSTEM

The five variables (physiological, psychological, sociocultural, developmental, and spiritual) of the client in interaction with the environment comprise the client as a system. The physiological variable refers to body structure and function. The psychological variable refers to mental processes in interaction with the environment.

The sociocultural variable refers to the effects and influences of social and cultural conditions. The developmental variable refers to age-related processes and activities. The spiritual variable refers to spiritual beliefs and influences (Neuman, 2002b, pp. 16-17; see also Neuman, 1982, 1989, 1995b).

Basic Client Structure

The client as a system is composed of a central core surrounded by concentric rings. The inner circle of the diagram (see Figure 16-1) represents the basic survival factors or energy resources of the client. This core structure ". . . consists of basic survival factors common to all members of the species", such as innate or genetic features (Neuman, 1982, p. 15; 2002c, p. 322; see also Neuman, 1982, 1989, 1995b).

Lines of Resistance

The series of broken rings surrounding the basic core structure are called *the lines of resistance*. These rings represent resource factors that help the client defend against a stressor. An example is the body's immune response system (Neuman, 2002c, p. 323; see also Neuman, 1982, 1989, 1995b).

When the lines of resistance are effective, the client system can reconstitute; if they are ineffective, death may ensue. The amount of resistance to a stressor is determined by the interrelationship of the five variables of the client system (Neuman, 2001, p. 322).

Normal Line of Defense

The normal line of defense is the model's outer solid circle. It represents a stability state for the individual or system. It is maintained over time and serves as a standard to assess deviations from the client's usual wellness. It includes system variables and behaviors such as the individual's usual coping patterns, lifestyle, and developmental stage (Neuman, 2002c, p. 323; see also Neuman, 1982, 1989, 1995b). Expansion of the normal line

Continued

MAJOR CONCEPTS *&* DEFINITIONS—cont'd

of defense reflects an enhanced wellness state; contraction, a diminished state of wellness (Neuman, 2001, p. 322).

Flexible Line of Defense

The model's outer broken ring is called the flexible line of defense. It is dynamic and can be altered rapidly over a short time. It is perceived as a protective buffer for preventing stressors from breaking through the usual wellness state as represented by the normal line of defense. The relationship of the variables (physiological, psychological, sociocultural, developmental, and spiritual) can affect the degree to which individuals are able to use their flexible line of defense against possible reaction to a stressor or stressors, such as loss of sleep (Neuman, 2002c, p. 323; see also Neuman, 1982, 1989, 1995b).

Neuman describes the flexible line of defense as the client system's first protective mechanism. "When the flexible line of defense expands, it provides greater short-term protection against stressor invasion; when it contracts, it provides less protection" (Neuman, 2001, p. 322).

WELLNESS

Wellness exists as a stable condition when the parts of the client system interact in harmony with the whole system. System needs are met (Neuman, 2002c, p. 324; see also Neuman, 1982, 1989, 1995b).

ILLNESS

Illness occurs when needs are not satisfied, resulting in a state of instability and energy depletion (Neuman, 2002c, p. 324; see also Neuman, 1982, 1989, 1995b).

STRESSORS

Stressors are tension-producing stimuli that have the potential to disrupt system stability. They may be:

- Intrapersonal forces occurring within the individual, such as conditioned responses
- Interpersonal forces occurring between one or more individuals, such as role expectations
- Extrapersonal forces occurring outside the individual, such as financial circumstances (Neuman, 2002c, p. 324; see also Neuman, 1982, 1989, 1995b)

DEGREE OF REACTION

The degree of reaction is the amount of energy required for the client to adjust to the stressor(s) (Neuman, 2002c, p. 322; see also Neuman, 1982, 1989, 1995b).

PREVENTION AS INTERVENTION

Interventions are purposeful actions to help the client retain, attain, or maintain system stability. They can occur before or after protective lines of defense and resistance are penetrated in both reaction and reconstitution phases. Neuman supports beginning intervention when a stressor is either suspected or identified. Interventions are based on possible or actual degree of reaction, resources, goals, and the anticipated outcome. Neuman identifies the following three levels of intervention: (1) primary, (2) secondary, and (3) tertiary (Neuman, 2002c, p. 323; see also Neuman, 1982, 1989, 1995b).

Primary Prevention

Primary prevention is carried out when a stressor is suspected or identified. A reaction has not yet occurred, but the degree of risk is known. Neuman (1982) states the following:

The actor or intervener would perhaps attempt to reduce the possibility of the individual's encounter with the stressor or in some way attempt to strengthen the individual's encounter with the stressor or attempt to strengthen the individual's flexible line of defense to decrease the possibility of a reaction. (p. 15; see also Neuman, 2002, p. 14)

MAJOR CONCEPTS & DEFINITIONS—cont'd

Secondary Prevention

Secondary prevention involves interventions or treatment initiated after symptoms from stress have occurred. Both the client's internal and external resources are used toward system stabilization to strengthen internal lines of resistance, reduce the reaction, and increase resistance factors (Neuman, 1982, p. 15; see also Neuman, 2002, p. 14).

Tertiary Prevention

Tertiary prevention occurs after the active treatment or secondary prevention stage. It focuses on readjustment toward optimal client system stability. A primary goal is to strengthen resistance to stressors to help prevent recurrence of reaction or regression. This process leads back in a circular fashion toward primary prevention. An example would be avoidance of stressors known to be hazardous to the client (Neuman, 1982, p. 16; see also Neuman, 2002b, p. 14).

RECONSTITUTION

Reconstitution occurs following treatment of stressor reactions. It represents return of the system to stability, which may be at a higher or lower level of wellness than prior to stressor invasion (Neuman, 2002c, p. 324).

It includes interpersonal, intrapersonal, extrapersonal, and environmental factors interrelated with client system variables (physiological, psychological, sociocultural, developmental, and spiritual) (see also Neuman, 1982, 1989, 1995b).

USE OF EMPIRICAL EVIDENCE

Neuman conceptualized the model from sound theories rather than from nursing research. She initially evaluated the utility of the model by submitting a tool to her nursing students at UCLA who were beginning their master's programs. The outcome data were published in *Nursing Research* (Neuman & Young, 1972). The tool was developed for use by students rather than through the use of statistical evidence; therefore, the model originally lacked empirical support. However, subsequent nursing research has produced sound empirical evidence in support of the Neuman Systems Model (Figure 16-1).

MAJOR ASSUMPTIONS
Nursing

Neuman (1982) believes nursing is concerned with the whole person. She views nursing as a "unique profession in that it is concerned with all of the variables affecting an individual's response to stress" (p. 14). The nurse's perception influences the care given; therefore, Neuman (1995b) states that the perceptual field of the caregiver and the client must be assessed. She has developed an assessment and intervention tool to help with this task.

Person as Client or Client System

The Neuman Systems Model presents the concept of client as a system that may be an individual, family, group, community, or social issue. The client system is a dynamic composite of interrelationships among physiological, psychological, sociocultural, developmental, and spiritual factors. The client system is viewed as being in constant change or motion and is seen as an open system in reciprocal interaction with the environment (Neuman, 2002b).

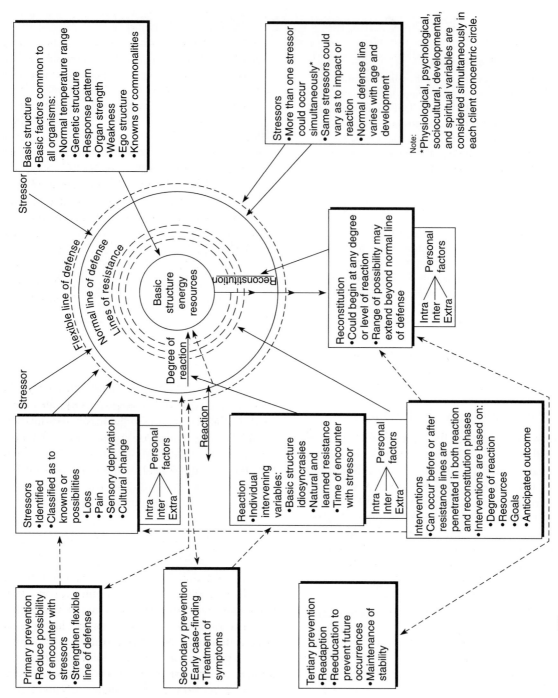

Figure 16-1 The Neuman Systems Model. (Original copyright 1970 by Betty Neuman. Used with permission.)

Health

Neuman considers her work a wellness model. She views health as a continuum of wellness to illness that is dynamic in nature and is constantly subject to change, as follows: "Optimal wellness or stability indicates that total system needs are being met. A reduced state of wellness is the result of unmet system needs. The client is in a dynamic state of either wellness or illness, in varying degrees, at any given point in time" (1995b, p. 46).

Environment

Environment and person are identified as the basic phenomena of the Neuman Systems Model, with the relationship between environment and person being reciprocal. Environment is defined as being all the internal and external factors that surround or interact with person and client. Stressors (intrapersonal, interpersonal, and extrapersonal) are significant to the concept of environment and are described as environmental forces that interact with and potentially alter system stability.

Neuman (1995b) identifies the following three relevant environments: (1) internal, (2) external, and (3) created. The internal environment is intrapersonal, with all interaction contained within the client. The external environment is interpersonal or extrapersonal, with all interactions occurring outside the client. The created environment is unconsciously developed and is used by the client to support protective coping. It is primarily intrapersonal. The created environment is dynamic in nature and mobilizes all system variables to create an insulating effect that helps the client cope with the threat of environmental stressors by changing the self or the situation. Examples are the use of denial (psychological variable) and life cycle continuation of survival patterns (developmental variable). The created environment perpetually influences and is influenced by changes in the client's perceived state of wellness (Neuman, 1995b).

THEORETICAL ASSERTIONS

Theoretical assertions are the relationships among the essential concepts of a model (Torres, 1986). The Neuman model depicts the nurse as an active participant with the client and as "concerned with all the variables affecting an individual's response to stressors" (Neuman, 1982, p. 14). The client is in a reciprocal relationship with the environment in that "he interacts with this environment by adjusting himself to it or adjusting it to himself" (Neuman, 1982, p. 14). Neuman links the four essential concepts of person, environment, health, and nursing in her statements regarding primary, secondary, and tertiary prevention. Earlier publications by Neuman stated basic assumptions that linked essential concepts of the model. These statements, listed in Box 16-1, have also been identified as propositions and serve to define, describe, and link the concepts of the model.

LOGICAL FORM

Neuman used both deductive and inductive logic in developing her model. As previously discussed, Neuman derived her model from other theories and disciplines. The model is also a product of her philosophy and of observations made in teaching mental health nursing and clinical counseling (Fawcett, Carpenito, et al., 1982).

ACCEPTANCE BY THE NURSING COMMUNITY

Alligood and Tomey (2002) state that a conceptual model provides a frame of reference for practice, while a grand theory proposes a set of truths that can be tested. Neuman's model can be described as both a model and as a grand nursing theory. As a model, it provides a conceptual framework for nursing practice, research, and education (Freese, Neuman, & Fawcett, 2002; Louis, Neuman, & Fawcett, 2002; Newman, Neuman, & Fawcett, 2002). As a grand theory, it proposes diverse ways of viewing nursing phenomena in the form of basic

Box 16-1

Basic Assumptions of the Neuman Systems Model

1. Although each individual client or group as a client system is unique, each system is a composite of common known factors or innate characteristics within a normal, given range of response contained within a basic structure.

2. Many known, unknown, and universal environmental stressors exist. Each differs in its potential for disturbing a client's usual stability level, or normal line of defense. The particular interrelationships of client variables—physiological, psychological, sociocultural, developmental, and spiritual—at any time can affect the degree to which a client is protected by the flexible line of defense against possible reaction to a single stressor or a combination of stressors.

3. Each individual client or client system has evolved a normal range of response to the environment that is referred to as a *normal line of defense,* or *usual wellness-stability state.* The normal line of defense can be used as a standard from which to measure health deviation.

4. When the cushioning, accordion-like effect of the flexible line of defense is no longer capable of protecting the client or client system against an environmental stressor, the stressor breaks through the normal line of defense. The interrelationships of variables—physiological, psychological, sociocultural, developmental, and spiritual— determine the nature and degree of system reaction or possible reaction to the stressor.

5. The client, whether in a state of wellness or illness, is a dynamic composite of the inter-relationships of variables (physiological, psychological, sociocultural, developmental, and spiritual). Wellness is on a continuum of available energy to support the system in an optimal state of system stability.

6. Implicit within each client system are internal resistance factors known as *lines of resistance,* which function to stabilize and return the client to the usual wellness state (normal line of defense) or possibly to a higher level of stability following an environmental stressor reaction.

7. Primary prevention relates to general knowledge that is applied in client assessment and intervention in identification and reduction or mitigation of possible or actual risk factors associated with environmental stressors to prevent possible reaction. The goal of health promotion is included in primary prevention.

8. Secondary prevention relates to symptomatology following a reaction to stressors, appropriate ranking of intervention priorities, and treatment to reduce their noxious effects.

9. Tertiary prevention relates to the adjustive processes taking place as reconstitution begins and maintenance factors move the client back in a circular manner toward primary prevention.

10. The client as a system is in dynamic, constant energy exchange with the environment.

From Neuman, B. (1995). *The Neuman systems model* (3rd ed., pp. 20-21). Norwalk, CT: Appleton & Lange, with permission from Pearson Education.

assumptions (Neuman, 2002b). The model is used extensively in the United States and Canada, and in other countries throughout the world (Australia, Brazil, Costa Rica, Denmark, Egypt, England, Finland, Ghana, Holland, Hong Kong, Iceland, Japan, Korea, New Zealand, Portugal, Puerto Rico, the Republic of China, Spain, Sweden, Taiwan, Wales, and Yugoslavia). As an example, the model was used to structure the World Health Organization's Collaborative Center for Primary Health Care Nursing in Maribor, Yugoslavia (Slovenia) (Neuman, 1995a).

The model has been adapted equally well to all levels of nursing education and to a wide variety of practice areas. It adapts well transculturally and is used extensively for public health nursing in other countries. It is the most widely accepted model for community health nursing in the United States and Canada (L. Lowry, personal communication, June 4, 1992).

The ongoing development and universal appeal of the model are reflected in the international Biennial Neuman Systems Model Symposium, which provides a forum across cultures for practitioners, educators, researchers, and students to share information about their use of the model. The first symposium was held in 1986 at Neumann College in Aston, Pennsylvania. Subsequent symposia have been held in Kansas City, Missouri (1988), Dayton, Ohio (1990), Rochester, New York (1993), Orlando (1995), Boston (1997), Vancouver, British Columbia (1999), Salt Lake City, Utah (2001), Willow Grove, Pennsylvania (2003), and Akron, Ohio (2005). Each symposium attracts participation from countries throughout the world and from disciplines beyond nursing.

Practice

The Neuman Systems Model has broad relevance for nursing practice. Use of the model by nurses facilitates goal-directed, unified, wholistic approaches to client care, yet it is also appropriate for multidisciplinary use to prevent fragmentation of client care. The model delineates a client system and

classification of stressors that can be understood and used by all members of the health care team (Mirenda, 1986). Guidelines have been published for use of the model in clinical nursing practice (Freese, et al., 2002) and for the administration of health care services (Shambaugh, Neuman, & Fawcett, 2002).

Neuman has developed several instruments to facilitate use of the model. These instruments include an assessment and intervention tool to assist nurses in collecting and synthesizing client data, a format for prevention as intervention, and a format for application of the nursing process within the framework of the Neuman Systems Model (Neuman, 2002a; Russell, 2002). The Neuman Nursing Process Format consists of the following three steps: (1) nursing diagnosis, (2) nursing goals, and (3) nursing outcomes. Nursing diagnosis involves obtaining a broad, comprehensive database from which variances from wellness can be determined. Goals are then established by negotiation with the client for desired prescriptive changes to correct variances from wellness. Nursing outcomes are determined by nursing intervention through the use of one or more of the three prevention as intervention modes. Evaluation then takes place either to confirm the desired outcome goals or to reformulate nursing goals.

Fawcett (1995a) has incorporated Neuman's nursing process format and prevention as intervention format into an outline (Box 16-2) to illustrate steps of the nursing process based on the Neuman Systems Model. Russell (2002) provides a review of clinical tools using the model to guide nursing practice with individuals, families, communities, and organizations.

The breadth of the Neuman model has resulted in its application and adaptation in a variety of nursing practice settings with individuals, families, groups, and communities. Numerous examples are cited in Neuman's books (1982, 1989, 1995b, 2002b). The model has been used successfully with clients in many settings, including hospitals, nursing homes, rehabilitation centers, hospices, and childbirth centers. The model's wholistic approach makes

Box 16-2

The Neuman Systems Model: Nursing Process Format

I. Nursing diagnosis

A. Establish database that includes the simultaneous consideration of the dynamic interactions of physiological, psychological, sociocultural, developmental, and spiritual variables

1. Identify client's or client system's perceptions

a. Assess condition and strength of basic structure factors and energy resources

b. Assess characteristics of the flexible and normal lines of defense, lines of resistance, degree of potential or actual reaction, and potential for reconstitution following a reaction

c. Assess internal and external environments

(1) Identify and evaluate potential or actual stressors that pose a threat to the stability of the client or client system

(2) Classify stressors that threaten stability of client or client system

(a) Deprivation

(b) Excess

(c) Change

(d) Intolerance

d. Identify, classify, and evaluate potential or actual intrapersonal, interpersonal, and extrapersonal interactions between the client or client system and the environment, considering all five variables

e. Assess the created environment

(1) Discover the nature of client's or client system's created environment

(a) Assess client's or client system's perception of stressors

(b) Identify client's or client system's major problem, stress areas, or areas of concern

(c) Identify client's or client system's perception of how present circumstances differ from usual pattern of living

(d) Identify ways in which client or client system handled similar problems in the past

(e) Identify what client or client system anticipates for self in the future as a consequence of the present situation

(f) Determine what client or client system is doing and what he or she can do to help self

(g) Determine what client or client system expects caregivers, family, friends, or others to do for him or her

(2) Determine degree of protection provided

(3) Uncover cause of client's or client system's created environment

f. Evaluate influence of past, present, and possible future life process and coping patterns on client or client system stability

g. Identify and evaluate actual and potential internal and external resources for optimal state of wellness

2. Identify caregiver's perceptions (repeat steps I. A. 1. a. to g. from caregiver's perspective)

3. Compare client's or client system's and caregiver's perceptions

a. Identify similarities and differences in perceptions

Box 16-2

The Neuman Systems Model: Nursing Process Format—cont'd

b. Facilitate client awareness of major perceptual distortions
c. Resolve perceptual differences

B. Variances from wellness
  1. Synthesize client database with relevant theories from nursing and adjunctive disciplines
  2. State a comprehensive nursing diagnosis
  3. Prioritize goals
    a. Consider client or client system wellness level
    b. Consider system stability needs
    c. Consider total available resources
  4. Postulate outcome goals and interventions that will facilitate the highest possible level of client or client system stability or wellness (maintain the normal line of defense and retain the flexible line of defense)

II. Nursing goals
  A. Negotiate desired prescriptive changes or outcome goals to correct variances from wellness with the client or client system
    1. Consider needs identified in I. B. 3. b.
    2. Consider resources identified in I. B. 3. c.
  B. Negotiate prevention as intervention modalities and actions with client or client system

III. Nursing outcomes
  A. Implement nursing interventions through use of one or more of three prevention modalities
    1. Primary prevention nursing actions to retain system stability
      a. Prevent stressor invasion
      b. Provide information to retain or strengthen existing client or client system strengths
      c. Support positive coping and functioning
      d. Desensitize existing or possible noxious stressors
      e. Motivate toward wellness

    f. Coordinate and integrate interdisciplinary theories and epidemiological input
    g. Educate or reeducate
    h. Use stress as a positive intervention strategy
    2. Secondary prevention nursing actions to attain system stability
      a. Protect basic structure
      b. Mobilize and optimize internal or external resources to attain stability and energy conservation
      c. Facilitate purposeful manipulation of stressors and reactions to stressors
      d. Motivate, educate, and involve client or client system in health care goals
      e. Facilitate appropriate treatment and intervention measures
      f. Support positive factors toward wellness
      g. Promote advocacy by coordination and integration
      h. Provide primary prevention intervention as required
    3. Perform tertiary prevention nursing actions to maintain system stability
      a. Attain and maintain highest possible level of wellness and stability during reconstitution
      b. Educate, reeducate, or reorient as needed
      c. Support client or client system toward appropriate goals
      d. Coordinate and integrate health service resources
      e. Provide primary or secondary preventive intervention as required
  B. Evaluate outcome goals
    1. Confirm attainment of outcome goals
    2. Reformulate goals
  C. Set intermediate and long-range goals for subsequent nursing action that are structured in relation to short-term goal outcomes

it particularly applicable for clients who are experiencing complex stressors that affect multiple client variables. For example, Black, Deeny, and McKenna (1997) used the model as a framework to guide nurses in preventing and alleviating sensoristrain in intensive care patients.

The model is used to guide nursing practice in countries throughout the world. As an example, it is being used in Holland to guide Emergis, a comprehensive program of mental health that provides psychiatric care for children, adolescents, adults and elderly, addiction care, and social services (Munck & Merks, 2002). The Neuman model was selected because it is holistic, is focused on the uniqueness of the client within his or her environment, is aimed toward prevention, and provides for collaboration with other disciplines. A research-based approach to implementation of the model for Emergis has been used, which will enable evaluation of how using the model affects quality of care, employee job satisfaction, and client satisfaction. The final goal for the project is to integrate a taxonomy of nursing diagnoses as described by Zeigler (1982) into nursing practice at Emergis.

Neuman's model provides a systems perspective that enables nurses to assess and care for the family unit as a client. Issel (1995) used it as the theoretical framework for a comprehensive case management program for obstetrical client families. Within the broader context of the caregiver unit as a system, Jones (1996) identified the intrapersonal, interpersonal, and extrapersonal stressors of primary caregivers of persons with traumatic head injuries. Lin, Ku, Leu, Chen, and Lin (1996) described the interrelationships among stress, coping behavior, and health status in family caregivers of patients with hepatoma. Picton (1995) used the model with emergency care patients to assist nurses to view them wholistically as part of a family system.

The Neuman Systems Model is used in community-based practice with groups and in public health nursing. Anderson, McFarland, and Helton (1986) were the first to adapt the model to develop a community health needs assessment in which they identified violence toward women as a major community health concern. Dwyer, Walker, Suchman, and Coggiola (1995) used it as the basis for a collaborative practice by nurse practitioners and physicians at the University of Rochester Community Nursing Center. It is used for describing services and cost-effectiveness in a senior citizens health center in Pennsylvania (Wollman, 2004).

The Neuman Systems Model is used effectively to enhance advanced practice nursing. Barker, Robinson, and Brautigan (1999) used the model to evaluate if psychiatric nurse home visits could decrease hospital readmission rates of patients with depression, and they found a substantial reduction in readmissions in the group which received psychiatric nurse home follow-up. Hassell (1996) integrated the Neuman Systems Model and medical perspectives to improve the management of depression by nurse practitioners. Martin (1996) applied the model to the practice of nurse anesthesia using specific examples of the nurse anesthetist's role.

The model has been studied and applied in other disciplines such as physical therapy (Beckman et al., 1994; Toot & Schmull, 1995). Further research continues to validate its applicability beyond nursing.

Education

The model has been accepted in academic circles and is used widely as a curriculum guide. It has been used at all levels of nursing education throughout the United States and in other countries, including Australia, Canada, Denmark, England, Korea, Kuwait, Portugal, Taiwan, Holland, and Japan (Beckman et al., 1994; Lowry, 2002). In an integrative review of use of the model in educational programs at all levels, Lowry (2002) reports that "although the trend is toward eclecticism in nursing education today, the Neuman Systems Model has served many programs well . . ." and is frequently selected in other countries to facilitate student learning (p. 231). Guidelines have been published for use of the model in education for the health professions (Newman, et al., 2002).

The model's wholistic perspective provides an effective framework for nursing education at all levels. It is used for a practical nursing program at the Community College of Baltimore County (CCBC, n.d.) and for associate degree nursing education at Central Florida Community College (CFCC, n.d.). Lowry and Newsome (1995) reported on a study of 12 associate degree programs that use the model as a conceptual framework for curriculum development. The results indicated that graduates use the model most often in the roles of teacher and care provider and that they tend to continue practice from a Neuman Systems Model–based perspective following graduation. Recent interest has been expressed regarding translation of the model into Arabic for use in nursing education (B. Neuman, personal communication, February 23, 2005).

Neuman's model has been selected for baccalaureate programs on the basis of its theoretical and comprehensive perspectives for a wholistic curriculum, and because of its potential for use with individuals, families, small groups, and the community. Neumann College Division of Nursing was the first school to select the Neuman Systems Model as its conceptual base for its curriculum and approach to client care in 1976. The faculty has developed an assessment and intervention tool based on Neuman's framework and has developed clinical evaluation tools based on Neuman's model and Bondy's evaluation format (Lowry & Newsome, 1995). The University of Pittsburgh in Pennsylvania was one of the first baccalaureate nursing programs to implement the model in an integrated curriculum (Knox, Kilchenstein, & Yakulis, 1982). The model has been used at Lander University in Greenwood, South Carolina, as the framework for baccalaureate nursing education since 1987 (Freese & Lander University Nursing Faculty, 1995).

The model is used as a comprehensive framework to organize data collected from maternity patients by undergraduate nursing students at the University of South Florida (Lowry, 2002). At the University of Texas at Tyler, Neuman's levels of prevention as intervention are used to level content in courses across the curriculum (Klotz, 1995). The Minnesota Intercollegiate Nursing Consortium, composed of three private church-related colleges, has developed a cooperative baccalaureate nursing program that uses the Neuman Systems Model as its organizing curriculum framework (Glazebrook, 1995). The model provided the framework for developing a baccalaureate nursing program at Palm Beach Atlantic University, with graduation of the first class in 2007 (Alligood, 2004). It is used at Malone College in Ohio (Malone College, n.d.), at Missouri Southern State University (MSSU, n.d.), and at Saint Anselm College in New Hampshire (Saint Anselm College, n.d.).

The model's effectiveness has been demonstrated in supporting the conceptual transition among levels of nursing education. Hilton and Grafton (1995) discussed its application as the framework for the transition from diploma to associate degree education at the Los Angeles County Medical Center School of Nursing. Sipple and Freese (1989) described the transition from associate degree to Neuman Systems Model–based baccalaureate education at Lander College in Greenwood, South Carolina. At the University of Tennessee at Martin, the model provided the curriculum framework for a Bachelor of Science in Nursing degree program initiated in 1988; Strickland-Seng (1995) described its use as the basis for clinical evaluation of students in their Bachelor of Science in Nursing degree program.

The Neuman Systems Model has been used effectively in postbasic nursing education and beyond. Bunn (1995) described the development and implementation of a community mental health nursing course based on Canadian health care principles for registered nurses enrolled in a Bachelor of Science in Nursing program at the University of Ottawa. The model enabled students to study selected client populations, such as elderly Chinese, as a high-risk aggregate and to plan culturally relevant health prevention activities at primary, secondary, and tertiary levels. Martin (1996) stated that the transition of nurse anesthesia education into graduate nursing programs will require incorporation of advanced nursing theory and applied the Neuman Systems Model to the practice of nurse anesthesia.

The model's inclusion of both client perception and nurse perception makes it particularly relevant for teaching culture concepts, and for teaching across cultures. The model is used at California State University, Fresno, to study the significance of culture and how culture influences each of the five client system variables (Stittich, Flores, & Nuttall, 1995). Bloch and Bloch (1995) described a format that uses the model to assist students to assess clients across cultural barriers and then to provide appropriate care. Capers (1996) stated that the model can foster the delivery of culturally relevant care, because its wholistic perspective includes the cultural aspects of client systems. Neuman (2001) notes that several faculty experts are facilitating use of the model in diverse cultures in countries that include Guatemala, Kuwait, Thailand, and Taiwan, and that it is used to guide nursing curricula in Jordan, Taiwan, Guam, and Iceland.

Multidisciplinary use of the model continues to grow. For example, the model has been implemented beyond nursing in Kuwait and Jordan (B. Neuman, personal communication, July 18, 1996). The model's emphasis on wholism, systems, prevention, and wellness prompted the Commission on Accreditation in Physical Therapy Education (CAPTE) to adapt it to conceptualize sections of the CAPTE evaluative criteria that address the organization and resources required for a physical therapy program (Toot & Schmull, 1995). Lowry, Burns, Smith, and Jacobson (2000) described an interdisciplinary approach to training health professionals based on experiences with a multidisciplinary team of faculty from four disciplines.

The Neuman Systems Model is used to provide the conceptual framework for multiple levels of nursing and health-related curricula around the world. Acceptance by the nursing education community is clearly evident.

Research

Testing the efficacy and usefulness of nursing models through controlled research is imperative for nursing to advance as a scientific discipline. Research on the components of the model for additional explication and generation of testable nursing

theories through research are examples of the Neuman model's potential contribution to research activity and nursing knowledge (Fawcett, 1990, 1995a; Mirenda, 1986; Ross & Bourbannais, 1985; J. Russell, personal communication, Jan. 10, 1988). Rules for Neuman Systems Model–based nursing research have been specified by Fawcett, a Neuman model trustee, based on the content of the model and related literature (Fawcett & Gigliotti, 2001). Guidelines have been published to guide use of the model for nursing research (Louis et al., 2002).

Neuman reports that hers is one of the three models most frequently used for nursing research (B. Neuman, personal communication, July 18, 1996). Research reported by the nursing community supports increasing empirical use of the model. In the third edition of *The Neuman Systems Model,* Louis (1995) discussed its use in nursing research and identified nearly 100 studies conducted between 1989 and 1993, for which the model provided the organizing framework. The third edition also contains an annotated bibliography of selected studies conducted from 1989 to 1993, with an appendix listing research studies published in journals, dissertations, and master's theses. In the fourth edition of *The Neuman Systems Model,* Fawcett and Giangrande (2002) present an integrated review of 200 research reports of model use that were published through 1997. An updated list compiled by Fawcett of published research using the model is located on the Neuman Systems Model Web site at *http://www.neumansystemsmodel.com.*

Review of current research using the Neuman Systems Model indicates that it continues to be selected frequently as the conceptual framework for research by practitioners and graduate students. Recent examples include studies of the effects of spirituality, resourcefulness, and arthritis on the health perceptions of elderly adults with rheumatoid arthritis (Potter & Zauszniewski, 2000), of caregiving and help-seeking in mothers of low-birthweight and of normal infants (May, 2000), of cardiovascular disease as a health concern (Wilson, 2000), of the quality of life in persons with chronic nonmalignant pain (Gerstle, 2001), of the nursing care of patients undergoing alcohol detoxification (Norrish, 2001), of the created environment for case managers (Skillen, 2001), and of the effect of preoperative teaching on anxiety levels for patients having cataract surgery (Morrell, 2001).

The model is used frequently by graduate students as a conceptual framework for dissertations and theses. Recent examples include studies of the use of condoms among black women (Simpson, 2000), of coping behaviors and drug use among middle school children (Wallom, 2000), of the effects of guided imagery on blood pressure (Young, 2000), of the relationship of family environment characteristics and cardiovascular risk (Riley-Lawless, 2000), and of military health care providers' adherence to national patient guidelines for managing hypertension (Collins, 2000).

The model can be adapted well for studying areas of interest across cultural barriers. Examples include studies of breastfeeding in India (Vijaylak-shmi, 2002), of adapting the model to nursing in Malaysia (Shamsudin, 2002), of selected aspects of the spiritual variable of Israeli oncology nurses (Musgrave, 2001), of risk assessment for low birthweight in Thai mothers (Lapvongwatana, 2000), and of beliefs about smoking among teens (Hanson, 1999).

Earlier research studies using the Neuman Systems Model are reported in earlier editions of this chapter. Additional studies using the model are listed in the bibliography following this chapter.

The Biennial Neuman Systems Model Symposium provides a rich forum for presentation of research (completed and in progress). At the eighth (2001) and ninth (2003) symposia, nurses from the United States, Canada, Holland, and Sweden reported the outcomes of numerous studies using the model. Four studies were reported on women's and children's health issues (Gehrling, 2003; Gigliotti, 2003a; Hemphill, 2001; Zavala-Onyett & Komnenich, 2001). Seven studies were reported on adult health issues (Breckenridge, 2001, 2003; Cammuso & Shambaugh, 2001; Casalenuovo,

2003; Elmore, 2003; Geib, 2003; Traver, 2003). Two studies related to nursing management issues were reported (Breckenridge & Van Parys, 2003; Hanson, 2001). Four studies were reported on aspects of nursing education (Aylward, 2001; Cammuso, 2003; Kennett, 2001; Newman, 2001). Three studies that reflect continued development of the spiritual variable were reported (Lowry, 2001, 2003; Vito & Farahmand, 2003). In addition, seven studies were reported using the model for research across cultures (Abegglen & Bond, 2001; Agren, 2001, 2003; Callister & Coverston, 2001; Crawford & Tarko, 2001; Kartchner & Callister, 2001; Merks, 2003). Research projects that were reported at the fourth, fifth, sixth, and seventh symposia (1993 through 1999) are cited in previous editions of this chapter.

The Neuman Systems Model is used extensively to provide the conceptual framework for research projects in the United States and in other countries. Acceptance by the nursing research community is clearly evident.

FURTHER DEVELOPMENT

A conceptual model identifies relevant phenomena and describes the interrelationships in general and abstract terms, representing the initial step in the development of theoretical statements (Fawcett, et al., 1982). In 1983, the Neuman Systems Model was described as being at a very early stage of theory development (Walker & Avant, 1983). However, subsequent publications (Breckenridge, 1995; Fawcett, 1995b; Louis & Koertvelyessy, 1989) support increasing utility of the model for theory development in nursing.

The model diagram has remained unchanged because Neuman has received continuous positive feedback on its completeness. The breadth of the model appeals to those in nursing because it allows for much creativity within its structure (Neuman, 1982).

For most nursing models, the process of establishing full validity through research is still in progress. Although the Neuman Systems Model has proved itself empirically, additional research is indicated to clarify and validate several components of the model.

Earlier evaluation of the model stated that two components needed further development as follows: (1) the spiritual variable and (2) the created environment (Beckman, et al., 1994). Description of the spiritual variable was expanded significantly in *The Neuman Systems Model,* third edition (Curran, 1995; Fulton, 1995). More recent research studies on the spiritual variable have been reported at Neuman Systems Model symposia held between 1997 and 2003, and at the Spiritual Care Research Conference held by the Nurses Christian Fellowship in 2001 (Artinian, 2001).

Neuman's concept of health and her view of the relationship between client and environment are two of the areas identified for further development and clarification. Fawcett (1995b) suggests clarification of the concept of health by identification of wellness and illness as polar ends of a continuum rather than as dichotomous conditions. She also states that viewing client-environment interactions as a dynamic equilibrium, as a steady state, and as homeostasis is logically incompatible and that Neuman should specify which view best represents her conceptualization of client-environmental interaction.

Further research is indicated in several other areas, including the lines of resistance and of defense, vulnerable aggregate client populations, and development and evaluation of primary prevention programs (B. Neuman, personal communication, July 18, 1996). Although significant application of the model to provide culturally sensitive nursing care has occurred over the past few years, this remains an area for continued enhancement of the model's utility.

Establishing full credibility of the model depends on extending the development and testing of middle range theory from it. Neuman and Koertvelyessy have identified the following two theories that are being generated from the model: (1) the theory of optimal client system stability and (2) the theory of prevention as intervention (Fawcett, 1995b). Breckenridge (1995) has described the use of the model to develop middle range theory through research based on practice with nephrology patients. However, Gigliotti (2003b) has stated that ". . . to date, no explicit NSM-derived middle range theories have been developed" (p. 202).

The Neuman Systems Model Trustee Group was established in 1988 to preserve, protect, and perpetuate the integrity of the model for the future of nursing (Neuman, 2002d). Its international members, personally selected by Neuman, are dedicated professionals. The Neuman Archives are housed at Neuman College Library at Aston, Pennsylvania. A description of the Neuman Systems Model as it is used in the Neuman College nursing program can be found at *http://www.neuman. edu/academics/undergraduate/nursing/model.asp.*

Smith and Edgil (1995) proposed the creation of an Institute for the Study of the Neuman Systems Model to formulate and test theories derived from the model. In response, a program for the systematic study of the model has been organized, and preliminary work has been completed consisting of assembling resources, of identifying concepts and the relationships among them, and of synthesizing existing research based on Neuman Systems Model concepts (Gigliotti, 2003b).

CRITIQUE

Neuman developed a comprehensive nursing conceptual model that operationalizes systems concepts that are relevant to the breadth of nursing phenomena. It should remain relevant for use by nursing in the future, and by other health care professions. The model's wholistic perspective allows for a wide range of creativity in its use. Neuman's own critique notes that prior criticisms, such as those claiming its concepts are too broad, have been discounted (B. Neuman, personal communication, June 21, 1992). The model provides an appropriate conceptual framework for nursing, while its comprehensive and flexible nature will allow it to remain adaptable for use in the future to deal with health care delivery issues in the twenty-first century (Mirenda, 1986).

Clarity

Neuman presents abstract concepts that are familiar to nurses. The model's essential concepts of client, environment, health, and nursing are congruent with traditional understanding of these concepts within nursing. Concepts defined by Neuman and those borrowed from other disciplines are used consistently throughout the model.

Simplicity

The model consists of concepts that are organized in a complex, yet logical manner. Multiple interrelationships exist among concepts, and variables tend to overlap to some degree. Distinctions between concepts tend to blur at several points, but a loss of theoretical meaning would occur if they were separated completely. Neuman states that the concepts can be separated for analysis, specific goal setting, and interventions (B. Neuman, personal communication, June 21, 1992). The model can be used to enhance use of systems theory for nursing, as well as for other health care professions. It can be used to explain the client's dynamic state of equilibrium and the reaction or possible reaction to stressors. The concept of prevention as intervention can be used to describe or predict nursing phenomena. The model is complex in nature; therefore, it cannot be described as a simple framework, yet nurses using the model describe it as easy to understand and use across cultures and in a wide variety of practice settings.

Generality

The Neuman Systems Model has been used in a wide variety of nursing situations; it is both comprehensive and adaptable. Some concepts are broad and represent the phenomenon of "client," which may be one person or a larger system. Other concepts are more definitive and identify specific modes of action, such as primary prevention. The model's broad scope allows it to be useful to nurses and to other health care professionals in working with individuals, families, groups, or communities in all health care settings.

Health professionals beyond nursing can use the model as a framework for care because its wholistic perspective can accommodate varied approaches to client assessment and care. Its systems approach and its emphasis on involving the client as an active participant fit well with contemporary health care values (for example, client-centered care, prevention, and integrated care management).

Empirical Precision

Although the model has not been tested completely to date, nursing scientists are demonstrating significant interest in the model and are using it to guide nursing research. Early work by Hoffman (1982) described a list of variables and selected operational definitions that were derived from the model. Louis and Koertvelyessy's survey (1989) on the use of the model in nursing research and subsequent research reports provides further documentation of increasing empiricism of the model. Continued testing and refinement will increase the model's empirical precision as research continues and the findings from multiple studies are synthesized (Gigliotti, 1999, 2003b).

Derivable Consequences

The derivable consequences of Neuman's conceptual model include guidelines for the professional nurse for assessment of the client system, utilization of the nursing process, and implementation of preventive interventions. The focus on primary prevention and interdisciplinary care is futuristic and serves to improve quality of care. The Neuman nursing process fulfills current health mandates by involving the client actively in negotiating the goals of nursing care (Neuman, 2002a).

Another derivable consequence of the model is its potential to generate nursing theory, for example, the theories of optimal client stability and prevention as intervention (Fawcett, 1995a). The model concepts are relevant to twenty-first century health professional trends. Through continued theory development and research with the model, the nursing profession can expand its scientific knowledge base. According to Fawcett (1989, 1995b), the model meets social considerations of congruence, significance, and utility. The model is broad and systemically based. It lends itself well to a comprehensive view within which nursing can be responsive to the world's rapidly changing health care needs.

SUMMARY

The Neuman Systems Model is derived from general systems theory. Its focus is on the client as a system (which may be an individual, family, group, or community) and on the client's responses to stressors. The client system includes five variables (physiological, psychological, sociocultural, developmental, spiritual), and is conceptualized as an inner core (basic energy resources) surrounded by concentric circles that include lines of resistance, a normal line of defense, and a flexible line of defense. Each of the five variables is considered part of each of the concentric circles. Stressors are tension-producing stimuli which may be intrapersonal, interpersonal, or extrapersonal in nature.

The model suggests three levels for nursing interventions (primary prevention, secondary prevention, tertiary prevention), which are based on Caplan's concept of levels of prevention (1964). The purpose of prevention as intervention is to achieve the maximum possible level of client system stability. Neuman suggests a format for the nursing process in which the client as recipient of care participates actively with the nurse as caregiver to set goals and select interventions.

The model has been well accepted by the nursing community and is used in administration, practice, education, and research. A Neuman Systems Model Trustees Group is actively involved in protecting the integrity of the model and advancing its development. An Institute for the Study of the Neuman Systems Model has begun work to derive and test middle range theories based on the model.

Case Study

Family as Client

Nadia Williams is a 35-year-old African-American woman who is approximately 40 pounds overweight and has hypertension. She divorced her husband, Robert, last year after being married for 15 years. Robert abused Nadia verbally and emotionally for most of their married life. Nadia and Robert have two children—Emily, age 13, and Justin, age 10. After Nadia left Robert, she and her children lived for 6 weeks in a shelter for abused women. While they were in the shelter, Emily told one of the counselors that Robert had abused her sexually on numerous occasions during the past year, but that Nadia would not listen when Emily tried to tell her about it. Following this revelation, Emily was admitted to an adolescent psychiatric hospital, where she was diagnosed with posttraumatic stress disorder. Nadia now lives in a small apartment with the children and works part time in a local restaurant. She is being treated medically for hypertension and type II diabetes. She and Emily are in counseling.

Use the Neuman Systems Model as a conceptual framework to respond to the following:

- Describe the Williams family as a client system.
- Describe the environment of the Williams family during the year before Nadia left Robert; differentiate Nadia's created environment from Emily's perception of the family's environment.
- What stressors, actual and potential, now threaten the family?
- What additional assessment data are needed related to Nadia's medical diagnoses?
- What level(s) of prevention as intervention are appropriate to assist the Williams family? What specific strategies can you suggest to retain, attain, and maintain stability for the family system?

CRITICAL THINKING *Activities*

Community as Client

1. Select one organization with which you are familiar and which would be considered a community, based on having face-to-face interaction and a shared set of interests or values. This could be a church, an employing organization, or a civic group. Use the Neuman Systems Model as a conceptual framework to analyze the organization as a community-client and to support organizational planning, as follows:

- What is the basic structure (core)? What factors in the lines of resistance support the status quo? What factors in the lines of defense support healthy organizational functioning?

- What stressors, actual or potential, that are impacting the organization may disrupt it as a system and result in change?

- What perception of goals by members of the organization would be appropriate for this change?

- What perception of goals by leaders of the organization would be appropriate for this change?

- If these perceptions differ, how can the differences be resolved for mutual goal setting that will be beneficial for the organization?

- What prevention as intervention strategies will support the organization in making the changes successfully?

REFERENCES

Abegglen, J. A., & Bond, E. (2001, March). *Wellness and stressors that interfere with the Bedouin woman's pursuit of wellness for self and family*. Paper presented at the Eighth Biennial Neuman Systems Model Symposium, Salt Lake City, UT.

Agren, C. (2001, March). *Identification and description for stress factors with heads of the departments in somatic and psychiatric care. A preliminary study*. Paper presented at the Eighth Biennial Neuman Systems Model Symposium, Salt Lake City, UT.

Agren, C. (2003, April). *How head nurses handle problems and difficulties related to their work*. Paper presented at the Ninth Biennial Neuman Systems Model Symposium, Willow Grove, PA.

Alligood, M. R. (2004). *Welcome: Palm Beach Atlantic University School of Nursing*. West Palm Beach, FL: Palm Beach Atlantic University. Retrieved January 30, 2004, from *http://www.pba.edu/Academic/Nursing*.

Alligood, M. R., & Tomey, A. M. (2002). Introduction to nursing theory: History, terminology and analysis. In A. M. Tomey & M. R. Alligood (Eds.), *Nursing theorists and their works* (5th ed., pp. 3-13). St. Louis: Mosby.

Anderson, E., McFarland, J., & Helton, A. (1986). Community-as-client: A model for practice. *Nursing Outlook, 34*(5), 220-224.

Artinian, B. (2001, June). *Testing of a nursing model: using the intersystem model for providing spiritual care*. Paper presented at Spiritual Care Research Conference, Azusa Pacific University, Azusa, CA.

Aylward, P. (2001, March). *Survey of nursing faculty educational needs related to a curriculum adaptation of the Neuman systems model*. Paper presented at the Eighth Biennial Neuman Systems Model Symposium, Salt Lake City, UT.

Barker, E., Robinson, D., & Brautigan, R. (1999). The effect of psychiatric home nurse follow-up on readmission rates of patients with depression. *Journal of American Psychiatric Nurses Association, 5*(4), 111-116.

Beckman, S. J., Boxley-Harges, S., Bruick-Sorge, C., Harris, S. M., Hermiz, M. E., Meininger, M., et al. (1994). Betty Neuman systems model. In A. Marriner Tomey (Ed.), *Nursing theorists and their work* (3rd ed., pp. 269-304). St. Louis: Mosby.

Bertalanffy, L. (1968). *General system theory*. New York: George Braziller.

Black, P., Deeny, P., & McKenna, H. (1997). Sensoristrain: An exploration of nursing interventions in the context of the Neuman systems theory. *Intensive and Critical Care Nursing, 13*(5), 249-258.

Bloch, C., & Bloch, C. (1995). Teaching content and process of the Neuman systems model. In B. Neuman (Ed.), *The Neuman systems model* (3rd ed., pp. 175-182). Norwalk, CT: Appleton & Lange.

Breckenridge, D. M. (1995). Nephrology practice and directions for nursing research. In B. Neuman (Ed.), *The Neuman systems model* (3rd ed., pp. 499-507). Norwalk, CT: Appleton & Lange.

Breckenridge, D. M. (2001, March). *Nephrology and oncology nursing*. Paper presented at the Eighth Biennial

Neuman Systems Model Symposium, Salt Lake City, UT.

Breckenridge, D. M. (2003, April). *Decisions regarding prostate cancer treatment modality: A holistic perspective.* Paper presented at the Ninth Biennial Neuman Systems Model Symposium, Willow Grove, PA.

Breckenridge, D. M., & Van Parys, E. (2003, April). *A secondary analysis of survey results of the AMH nursing initiative to attract, recruit, retain, and support nurses to determine Neuman system variables reflected.* Paper presented at the Ninth Biennial Neuman Systems Model Symposium, Willow Grove, PA.

Bunn, H. (1995). Preparing nurses for the challenge of the new focus on community mental health nursing. *The Journal of Continuing Education in Nursing, 26*(2), 55-59.

Callister, L. C., & Coverston, C. (2001, March). *Cultural research: Application of the Neuman systems model.* Paper presented at the Eighth Biennial Neuman Systems Model Symposium, Salt Lake City, UT.

Cammuso, B. S. (2003, April). *The implementation of strategies to develop critical thinking skills in freshmen nursing students.* Paper presented at the Ninth Biennial Neuman Systems Model Symposium, Willow Grove, PA.

Cammuso, B. S., & Shambaugh, B. F. (2001, March). *The Neuman systems model applied to family caregivers of clients with Alzheimer's Disease.* Paper presented at the Eighth Biennial Neuman Systems Model Symposium, Salt Lake City, UT.

Capers, C. F. (1996). The Neuman systems model: A culturally relevant perspective. *ABNF Journal, 7*(5), 113-117.

Caplan, G. (1964). *Principles of preventive psychiatry.* New York: Basic Books.

Casalenuovo, G. (2003, April). *Testing a middle range theory of well-being derived from Neuman's theory of optimal client system stability and the Neuman systems model in adults living with diabetes mellitus.* Paper presented at the Ninth Biennial Neuman Systems Model Symposium, Willow Grove, PA.

Central Florida Community College (CFCC). (n.d.). *Programs of study: Associate in arts degree.* Lecanto, FL: CFCC. Retrieved on January 30, 2004, from *http://www.cf.edu/catalog/programs.htm#asreq.*

Collins, T. J. (2000). *Adherence to hypertension management recommendations for patient follow-up care and lifestyle modifications made by military healthcare providers. Masters Abstracts International, 06,* 1603. (University Microfilms No. AAI1399503). Retrieved February 23, 2005 from *www.cebcmd.edu/allied-health/pn/vision.html.*

Community College of Baltimore County (CCBC). (n.d.). *School of health professions—Practical nursing: Vision.* Baltimore, MD: CCBC. Retrieved January 30, 2004, from *http://www.ccbcmd.edu/allied_health/pn/vision.html.*

Crawford, J. A., & Tarko, M. A. (2001). *Psychiatric nurses' narratives: Application of the Neuman systems model from a Canadian perspective.* Paper presented at the Eighth Biennial Neuman Systems Model Symposium, Salt Lake City, UT.

Curran, G. (1995). The Neuman systems model revisited. In B. Neuman (Ed.), *The Neuman systems model* (3rd ed., pp. 93-99). Norwalk, CT: Appleton & Lange.

Dwyer, C. M., Walker, P. H., Suchman, A., & Coggiola, P. (1995). Opportunities and obstacles: Development of a true collaborative practice with physicians. In B. Murphy (Ed.), *Nursing centers: The time is now* (pp. 134-155, NLN Pub. No. 41-2629). New York: National League for Nursing.

Elmore, D. (2003, April). *Delirium in the hospitalized elderly: Clinical indicators found in the medical record.* Paper presented at the Ninth Biennial Neuman Systems Model Symposium, Willow Grove, PA.

Fawcett, J. (1989). *Analysis and evaluation of conceptual models of nursing* (2nd ed., pp. 172-177). Philadelphia: F. A. Davis.

Fawcett, J. (1990, Nov.). *Neuman systems model: Directions for research.* Keynote address presented at the Third International Neuman Systems Model Symposium, Dayton, OH.

Fawcett, J. (1995a). Constructing conceptual-theoretical-empirical structures for research. In B. Neuman (Ed.), *The Neuman systems model* (3rd ed., pp. 459-471). Norwalk, CT: Appleton & Lange.

Fawcett, J. (1995b). *Neuman's systems model: Analysis and evaluation of conceptual models of nursing* (3rd ed., pp. 217-275). Philadelphia: F. A. Davis.

Fawcett, J., Carpenito, L. J., Efinger, J., Goldblum-Graff, D., Groesbeck, M., Lowry, L. W., et al. (1982). A framework for analysis and evaluation of conceptual models of nursing with an analysis of the Neuman systems model. In B. Neuman (Ed.), *The Neuman systems model: Application to nursing education and practice* (pp. 30-43). Norwalk, CT: Appleton-Century-Crofts.

Fawcett, J., & Giangrande, S. (2002). The Neuman systems model and research: An integrative review. In B. Neuman & J. Fawcett, (Eds.), *The Neuman systems model* (4th ed., pp. 120-149). Upper Saddle River, NJ: Pearson Education.

Fawcett, J., & Gigliotti, E. (2001). Using conceptual models to guide nursing research: The case of the Neuman systems model. *Nursing Science Quarterly, 14,* 339-345.

Freese, B. T., & Lander University Faculty (1995, Feb.). *Application of the Neuman systems model to education: Baccalaureate workshop.* Paper presented at the Fifth International Neuman Systems Model Symposium, Orlando, FL.

Freese, B. T., Neuman, B., & Fawcett, J. (2002). Guidelines for Neuman systems model–based clinical practice. In B. Neuman & J. Fawcett (Eds.), *The Neuman systems model* (4th ed., pp. 37-42). Upper Saddle River, NJ: Pearson Education.

Fulton, R. A. B. (1995). The spiritual variable: Essential to the client system. In B. Neuman (Ed.), *The Neuman systems model* (3rd ed., pp. 77-92). Norwalk, CT: Appleton & Lange.

Gehrling, K. Reed. (2003, April). *Development of the Neuman family assessment measure: Preliminary data.* Paper presented at the Ninth Biennial Neuman Systems Model Symposium, Willow Grove, PA.

Geib, K. (2003, April). *The Neuman systems model and nursing vigilance: The relationships among nursing vigilance by nurses, patient satisfaction with nursing vigilance, and patient length of stay in a surgical cardiac care unit.* Paper presented at the Ninth Biennial Neuman Systems Model Symposium, Willow Grove, PA.

Gerstle, D. S. (2001). Quality of life and chronic non-malignant pain. *Pain Management Nursing, 2*(3), 98-109.

Gigliotti, E. (1999). Women's multiple role stress: Testing Neuman's flexible line of defense. *Nursing Science Quarterly, 12*(1), 36-44.

Gigliotti, E. (2003a, April). *Maternal-student role stress during concurrent transitions.* Paper presented at the Ninth Biennial Neuman Systems Model Symposium, Willow Grove, PA.

Gigliotti, E. (2003b). The Neuman systems model institute: Testing middle-range theories. *Nursing Science Quarterly, 16*(3), 201-206.

Glazebrook, D. S. (1995). The Neuman systems model in cooperative baccalaureate nursing education: The Minnesota Intercollegiate Nursing Consortium experience. In B. Neuman (Ed.), *The Neuman systems model* (3rd ed., pp. 227-230). Norwalk, CT: Appleton & Lange.

Hanson, M. J. S. (1999). Cross-cultural study of beliefs about smoking among teenaged females . . . including commentary by Laffrey S. C. with author response. *Western Journal of Nursing Research, 21*(5), 635-651.

Hanson, P. A. (2001, March). *An application of Bowen family systems theory and the Neuman systems model: Triangulation, differentiation of self and nurse manager job stress responses.* Paper presented at the Eighth Biennial Neuman Systems Model Symposium, Salt Lake City, UT.

Hassell, J. S. (1996). Improved management of depression through nursing model application and critical thinking. *Journal of the American Academy of Nurse Practitioners, 8*(4), 161-166.

Hemphill, J. C. (2001, March). *A nursing intervention designed to increase resilience in homeless abused women.* Paper presented at the Eighth Biennial Neuman Systems Model Symposium, Salt Lake City, UT.

Hilton, S. A., & Grafton, M. D. (1995). Curriculum transition based on the Neuman systems model: Los Angeles County Medical Center School of Nursing. In B. Neuman (Ed.), *The Neuman systems model* (3rd ed., pp. 163-174). Norwalk, CT: Appleton & Lange.

Hoffman, M. K. (1982). From model to theory construction: An analysis of the Neuman health-care system model. In B. Neuman (Ed.), *The Neuman systems model: Application to nursing education and practice* (pp. 44-54). Norwalk, CT: Appleton-Century-Crofts.

Issel, L. M. (1995). Evaluating case management programs. *Maternal/Child Nursing Journal, 29,* 67-74.

Jones, W. R. (1996). Stressors in the primary caregivers of traumatic head injured persons. *AXON, 18*(1), 9-11.

Kartchner, R., & Callister, L. C. (2001, March). *Giving birth: Voices of Chinese women.* Paper presented at the Eighth Biennial Neuman Systems Model Symposium, Salt Lake City, UT.

Kennett, J. (2001, March). *Nursing utilizing the internet in the advancement toward professionalization: An application of the Neuman systems theory.* Paper presented at the Eighth Biennial Neuman Systems Model Symposium, Salt Lake City, UT.

Klotz, L. D. (1995). Integration of the Neuman systems model into the BNS curriculum at the University of Texas at Tyler. In B. Neuman (Ed.), *The Neuman systems model* (3rd ed., pp. 183-190). Norwalk, CT: Appleton & Lange.

Knox, J. E., Kilchenstein, L., & Yakulis, I. M. (1982). Utilization of the Neuman model in an integrated baccalaureate program: University of Pittsburgh. In B. Neuman (Ed.), *The Neuman systems model: Application to nursing education and practice* (pp. 117-124). Norwalk, CT: Appleton-Century-Crofts.

Lapvongwatana, P. (2000). Perinatal risk assessment for low birthweight in Thai mothers: using the Neuman systems model. *Dissertation Abstracts International, 61,* 1328B. (University Microfilms No. AA19965512)

Lin, M., Ku, N., Leu, J., Chen, J., & Lin, L. (1996). An exploration of the stress aspects, coping behaviors, health status, and related aspects in family caregivers of hepatoma patients. *Nursing Research (China), 4*(2), 171-185.

Louis, M. (1995). The Neuman model in nursing research: An update. In B. Neuman (Ed.), *The Neuman systems model* (3rd ed., pp. 473-495). Norwalk, CT: Appleton & Lange.

Louis, M., & Koertvelyessy, A. (1989). Neuman model: Use in research. In B. Neuman (Ed.), *The Neuman systems model* (2nd ed., pp. 93-114). Norwalk, CT: Appleton & Lange.

Louis, M., Neuman, B., & Fawcett, J. (2002). Guidelines for Neuman systems model–based nursing research. In B. Neuman & J. Fawcett (Eds.), *The Neuman systems model*

(4th ed., pp. 113-119). Upper Saddle River, NJ: Pearson Education.

Lowry, L. W. (2001, March). *Exploring the meaning of spirituality with ageing adults.* Paper presented at the Eighth Biennial Neuman Systems Model Symposium, Salt Lake City, UT.

Lowry, L. W. (2002). The Neuman systems model and education: An integrative review. In B. Neuman & J. Fawcett (Eds.), *The Neuman systems model* (4th ed., pp. 216-237). Upper Saddle River, NJ: Pearson Education.

Lowry, L. W. (2003, April). *Exploring the meaning of spirituality with aging adults in Appalachia.* Paper presented at the Ninth Biennial Neuman Systems Model Symposium, Willow Grove, PA.

Lowry, L. W., Burns, C. M., Smith, A. A., & Jacobson, H. (2000). Compete or complement? An interdisciplinary approach to training health professionals. *Nursing and Health Care Perspectives, 21*(2), 76-80.

Lowry, L. W., & Newsome, G. G. (1995). Neuman-based associate degree programs: Past, present, and future. In B. Neuman (Ed.), *The Neuman systems model* (3rd ed., pp. 197-214). Norwalk, CT: Appleton & Lange.

Malone College. (n.d.). *School of nursing.* Canton, OH: Malone College. Retrieved January 30, 2004, from *http://www.malone.edu/2242.*

Martin, S. A. (1996). Applying nursing theory to the practice of nurse anesthesia. *American Association of Nurse Anesthetists Journal, 64*(4), 369-372.

May, K. M. (2000). Caregiving and help seeking by mothers of low birthweight infants and mothers of normal birthweight infants. *Public Health Nursing 17*(4), 273-279.

Merks, A. A. (2003, April). *A diagnosis of the organizational culture as important condition for successful implementation of the Neuman systems model.* Paper presented at the Ninth Biennial Neuman Systems Model Symposium, Willow Grove, PA.

Mirenda, R. M. (1986). The Neuman systems model: Description and application. In P. Winstead-Fry (Ed.), *Case studies in nursing theory* (pp. 127-167). New York: National League for Nursing.

Missouri Southern State University (MSSU). (n.d.). *Department of nursing.* Joplin, MO: MSSU. Retrieved January 23, 2005, from *http://www.mssu.edu/technology/Nursl.*

Morrell, G. (2001). Effect of structured preoperative teaching on anxiety levels of patients scheduled for cataract surgery. *Insight, 26*(1), 4-9.

Munck, C. K., & Merks, A. (2002). Using the Neuman systems model to guide administration of nursing services in Holland: The case of Emergis, institute for mental health care. In B. Neuman & J. Fawcett (Eds.), *The Neuman systems model* (4th ed., pp. 300-316). Upper Saddle River, NJ: Prentice-Hall.

Musgrave, C. F. (2001). Religiosity, spiritual well-being, and attitudes toward spiritual care of Israeli oncology nurses. *Dissertation Abstracts International, 61*(11B), 5799. (University Microfilms No. AA199995617)

Neuman, B. (1974). The Betty Neuman health care systems model: A total person approach to patient problems. In J. P. Riehl & C. Roy (Eds.), *Conceptual models for nursing practice* (2nd ed., pp. 119-134). NY: Appleton-Century-Crofts.

Neuman, B. (1982). *The Neuman systems model: Application to nursing education and practice.* Norwalk, CT: Appleton-Century-Crofts.

Neuman, B. (1989). *The Neuman systems model* (2nd ed.). Norwalk, CT: Appleton & Lange.

Neuman, B. (1995a). In conclusion—Toward new beginnings. In B. Neuman (Ed.), *The Neuman systems model* (3rd ed., pp. 671-703). Norwalk, CT: Appleton & Lange.

Neuman, B. (1995b). *The Neuman systems model* (3rd ed.). Norwalk, CT: Appleton & Lange.

Neuman, B. (2001). The Neuman systems model: A futuristic care perspective. In N. L. Chaska (Ed.), *The nursing profession: Tomorrow and beyond* (pp. 321-329). Thousand Oaks, CA: Sage Publications.

Neuman, B. (2002a). Assessment and intervention based on the Neuman systems model. In B. Neuman & J. Fawcett (Eds.), *The Neuman systems model* (4th ed., pp. 347-359). Upper Saddle River, NJ: Prentice-Hall.

Neuman, B. (2002b). The Neuman systems model. In B. Neuman & J. Fawcett (Eds.), *The Neuman systems model* (4th ed., pp. 3-34). Upper Saddle River, NJ: Prentice-Hall.

Neuman, B. (2002c). The Neuman systems model definitions. In B. Neuman & J. Fawcett (Eds.), *The Neuman systems model* (4th ed., pp. 322-324). Upper Saddle River, NJ: Prentice-Hall.

Neuman, B. (2002d). The Neuman Systems Model Trustees Group. In B. Neuman & J. Fawcett (Eds.), *The Neuman systems model* (4th ed., pp. 360-363). Upper Saddle River, NJ: Prentice-Hall.

Neuman, B., Deloughery, G. W., & Gebbie, M. (1971). *Consultation and community organization in community mental health nursing.* Baltimore: Williams & Wilkins.

Neuman, B., & Young, R. J. (1972, May/June). A model for teaching total person approach to patient problems. *Nursing Research, 21,* 264-269.

Newman, D. M. L. (2001, March). *A descriptive study of the Neuman systems model as applied to undergraduate nursing student practice.* Paper presented at the Eighth Biennial Neuman Systems Model Symposium, Salt Lake City, UT.

Newman, D. M. L., Neuman, B., & Fawcett, J. (2002). Guidelines for Neuman systems model–based education for the health professions. In B. Neuman & J.

Fawcett (Eds.), *The Neuman systems model* (4th ed., pp. 193-215). Upper Saddle River, NJ: Pearson Education.

Norrish, M. E. (2001). Nursing care of the patient undergoing alcohol detoxification. *Curationis, 24*(3), 36-48.

Perls, F. (1973). *The gestalt approach: Eye witness to therapy.* Palo Alto, CA: Science and Behavior Books.

Picton, C. E. (1995). An explanation of family-centered care in Neuman's model with regard to the care of the critically ill adult in an accident and emergency setting. *Accident and Emergency Nursing, 3,* 33-37.

Potter, M. L., & Zauszniewski, J. A. (2000). Spirituality, resourcefulness, and arthritis impact on health perception of elders with rheumatoid arthritis. *Journal of Holistic Nursing, 18*(4), 311-331.

Riley-Lawless, K. (2000). The relationship among characteristics of the family environment and behavioral and physiologic cardiovascular risk factors in parents and their adolescent twins. *Dissertation Abstracts International, 61,* 1328B. (University Microfilms No. AA19965555)

Ross, M. M., & Bourbannais, F. F. (1985). The Neuman systems model in nursing practice: A case study approach. *Journal of Advanced Nursing, 10,* 199-207.

Russell, J. (2002). The Neuman systems model and clinical tools. In B. Neuman & J. Fawcett (Eds.), *The Neuman systems model* (4th ed., pp. 61-73). Upper Saddle River, NJ: Prentice-Hall.

Saint Anselm College. (n.d.). *Department of nursing: Philosophy.* Manchester, NH: Saint Anselm College.

Selye, H. (1974). *Stress without distress.* Philadelphia: J. B. Lippincott.

Shambaugh, B. F., Neuman, B., & Fawcett, J. (2002). Guidelines for Neuman systems model–based administration of health care services. In B. Neuman & J. Fawcett (Eds.), *The Neuman systems model* (4th ed., pp. 265-270). Upper Saddle River, NJ: Pearson Education.

Shamsudin, N. (2002). Can the Neuman systems model by adapted to the Malaysian nursing context? *International Journal of Nursing Practice, 8*(2), 99-105.

Simpson, E. M. (2000). Condom use among black women: A theoretical basis for HIV prevention guided by Neuman systems model and theory of planned behavior (immune deficiency). *Dissertation Abstracts International, 61,* 5240B. (University Microfilms No. AA19989654)

Sipple, J. A., & Freese, B. T. (1989). Transition from technical to professional level education. In B. Neuman (Ed.), *The Neuman systems model* (2nd ed., pp. 193-200). Norwalk, CT: Appleton & Lange.

Skillen, D. L. (2001). The created environment for physical assessment by case managers. *Western Journal of Nursing Research, 23*(1), 72-89.

Smith, M. C., & Edgil, A. E. (1995). Future directions for research with the Neuman systems model. In B.

Neuman (Ed.), *The Neuman systems model* (3rd ed., pp. 509-517). Norwalk, CT: Appleton & Lange.

Stittich, E. M., Flores, F. C., & Nuttall, P. (1995). Cultural considerations in a Neuman-based curriculum. In B. Neuman (Ed.), *The Neuman systems model* (3rd ed., pp. 147-162). Norwalk, CT: Appleton & Lange.

Strickland-Seng, V. (1995). The Neuman systems model in clinical evaluation of students. In B. Neuman (Ed.), *The Neuman systems model* (3rd ed., pp. 215-223). Norwalk, CT: Appleton & Lange.

Toot, J. L., & Schmull, B. J. (1995). The Neuman systems model and physical therapy educational curricula. In B. Neuman (Ed.), *The Neuman systems model* (3rd ed., pp. 231-246). Norwalk, CT: Appleton & Lange.

Torres, G. (1986). *Theoretical foundations of nursing.* Norwalk, CT: Appleton-Century-Crofts.

Traver, B. A. (2003, April). *Nurses' levels of knowledge to promote the health of clients experiencing stressors related to pathological gambling.* Paper presented at the Ninth Biennial Neuman Systems Model Symposium, Willow Grove, PA.

Vijaylakshmi, S. (2002). Breastfeeding technique in prevention of nipple sore—A study. *Nursing Journal of India, 93*(8), 173-174.

Vito, K. O., & Farahmand, J. M. (2003, April). *The relationship of spiritual well-being to physiological well-being in adults with diabetes.* Paper presented at the Ninth Biennial Neuman Systems Model Symposium, Willow Grove, PA.

Walker, L. O., & Avant, K. (1983). *Strategies for theory construction in nursing.* Norwalk, CT: Appleton-Century-Crofts.

Wallom, B. L. L. (2000). Coping behaviors and drug use among fifth- and sixth-grade students. *Dissertation Abstracts International, 61,* 08A, p. 3076. (University Microfilms No. AA19982666)

Wilson, L. C. (2000). Implementation and evaluation of church-based health fairs. *Journal of Community Nursing, 17*(1), 39-48.

Wollman, K. (2004). *The community nursing center of Chester and vicinity.* Philadelphia: National Nursing Centers Consortium. Retrieved January 23, 2005, from *http://www.rncc.us/NNCC_Member_Centers/member_community_Health_Center_of_Chester_and_Vicinity.htm.*

Young, L. M. (2000). The effects of guided mental imagery on the blood pressure of clients experiencing mild to moderate essential hypertension. *Dissertation Abstracts International, 61,* 02B, p. 787. (University Microfilms No. AA19961229)

Zavala-Onyett, N., & Komnenich, P. (2001, March). *The impact of a school-based health clinic on school absence.* Paper presented at the Eighth Biennial Neuman Systems Model Symposium, Salt Lake City, UT.

Zeigler, S. M. (1982). Taxonomy for nursing diagnosis derived from the Neuman systems model. In B. Neuman (Ed.), *The Neuman Systems Model: Application to nursing education and practice* (pp. 55-68). Norwalk, CT: Appleton-Century-Crofts.

BIBLIOGRAPHY
Primary Sources
Books

Hinton Walker, P., & Neuman, B. (Eds.). (1996). *Blueprint for use of nursing models.* New York: National League for Nursing Press.

Neuman, B. (1982). *The Neuman systems model: Application to nursing education and practice.* Norwalk, CT: Appleton-Century-Crofts.

Neuman, B. (1989). *The Neuman systems model* (2nd ed.). Norwalk, CT: Appleton & Lange.

Neuman, B. (1995). *The Neuman systems model* (3rd ed.). Norwalk, CT: Appleton & Lange.

Neuman, B., Deloughery, G. W., & Gebbie, M. (1971). *Consultation and community organization in community mental health nursing.* Baltimore: Williams & Wilkins.

Neuman, B., & Fawcett, J. (2002). *The Neuman systems model* (4th ed.). Upper Saddle River, NJ: Pearson Education.

Neuman, B. M., & Walker, P. H. (1996). *Blueprint for use of nursing models: Education, research, practice, and administration.* New York: National League for Nursing Press.

Book Chapters

Freese, B. T., Neuman, B., & Fawcett, J. (2002). Guidelines for Neuman systems model–based clinical practice. In B. Neuman & J. Fawcett (Eds.), *The Neuman systems model* (4th ed., pp. 37-42). Upper Saddle River, NJ: Pearson Education.

Louis, M., Neuman, B., & Fawcett, J. (2002). Guidelines for Neuman systems model–based nursing research. In B. Neuman & J. Fawcett (Eds.), *The Neuman systems model* (4th ed., pp. 113-119). Upper Saddle River, NJ: Pearson Education.

Neuman, B. (1974). The Betty Neuman health care systems model: A total person approach to patient problems. In J. P. Riehl & C. Roy (Eds.), *Conceptual models for nursing practice* (pp. 94-104). New York: Appleton-Century-Crofts.

Neuman, B. (1980). The Betty Neuman health care systems model: A total person approach to patient problems. In J. P. Riehl & C. Roy (Eds.), *Conceptual models for nursing practice* (2nd ed., pp. 119-134). New York: Appleton-Century-Crofts.

Neuman, B. (1983). Analysis and application of Neuman's health care model. In I. W. Clements & F. B. Roberts (Eds.), *Family health: A theoretical approach to nursing care* (pp. 239-254, 353-367). New York: John Wiley & Sons.

Neuman, B. (1986). The Neuman systems model explanation: Its relevance to emerging trends toward wholism in nursing. In I. B. Engberg & K. Kuld (Eds.), *Omvårdnad 1986* [Nursing care book]. Mullsjö: Sweden: Omvårdnad's Forum HB.

Neuman, B. (1989). The Neuman nursing process format: Adapted to a family case study. In J. P. Riehl & C. Roy (Eds.), *Conceptual models for nursing practice* (pp. 49-62). Norwalk, CT: Appleton & Lange.

Neuman, B. (1990). The Neuman systems model: A theory for practice. In M. E. Parker (Ed.), *Nursing theories in practice* (pp. 24-26). New York: National League for Nursing.

Neuman, B. (1995). In conclusion—Toward new beginnings. In B. Neuman (Ed.), *The Neuman systems model* (3rd ed., pp. 671-703). Norwalk, CT: Appleton & Lange.

Neuman, B. (1995). The Neuman systems model. In B. Neuman (Ed.), *The Neuman systems model* (3rd ed., pp. 3-62). Norwalk, CT: Appleton & Lange.

Neuman, B. (2001). The Neuman systems model: A futuristic care perspective. In N. L. Chaska, (Ed.), *The nursing profession: Tomorrow and beyond* (pp. 321-329). Thousand Oaks, CA: Sage Publications.

Neuman, B. (2002). Assessment and intervention based on the Neuman systems model. In B. Neuman & J. Fawcett (Eds.), *The Neuman systems model* (4th ed., pp. 347-359). Upper Saddle River, NJ: Pearson Education.

Neuman, B. (2002). Betty Neuman's autobiography and chronology of the development and utilization of the Neuman systems model. In B. Neuman & J. Fawcett (Eds.), *The Neuman systems model* (4th ed., pp. 325-346). Upper Saddle River, NJ: Pearson Education.

Neuman, B. (2002). The future and the Neuman systems model. In B. Neuman & J. Fawcett (Eds.), *The Neuman systems model* (4th ed., pp. 319-321). Upper Saddle River, NJ: Pearson Education.

Neuman, B. (2002). The Neuman systems model definitions. In B. Neuman & J. Fawcett (Eds.), *The Neuman systems model* (4th ed., pp. 322-324). Upper Saddle River, NJ: Pearson Education.

Neuman, B. (2002). The Neuman systems model. In B. Neuman & J. Fawcett (Eds.), *The Neuman systems model* (4th ed., pp. 3-33). Upper Saddle River, NJ: Pearson Education.

Neuman, B. (2002). The Neuman Systems Model Trustees Group. In B. Neuman & J. Fawcett (Eds.), *The Neuman systems model* (4th ed., pp. 360-363). Upper Saddle River, NJ: Pearson Education.

Neuman, B., & Wyatt, M. (1980). The Neuman stress/adaptation systems approach to education for nurse administrators. In J. P. Riehl & C. Roy (Eds.), *Conceptual models for nursing practice* (2nd ed., pp. 142-150). New York: Appleton-Century-Crofts.

Newman, D. M. L., Neuman, B., & Fawcett, J. (2002). Guidelines for Neuman systems model–based education for the health professions. In B. Neuman & J. Fawcett (Eds.), *The Neuman systems model* (4th ed., pp. 193-215). Upper Saddle River, NJ: Pearson Education.

Shambaugh, B. F., Neuman, B., & Fawcett, J. (2002). Guidelines for Neuman systems model–based administration of health care services. In B. Neuman & J. Fawcett (Eds.), *The Neuman systems model* (4th ed., pp. 265-270). Upper Saddle River, NJ: Pearson Education.

Journal Articles

Deloughery, G. W., Neuman, B. M., & Gebbie, K. M. (1971, Oct.). Nurses in community mental health: An informative interpretation for employees of professional nurses. *Public Personnel Review, 32*(4), 215-218.

Neuman, B. (1985, Sept.). The Neuman systems model: Its importance for nursing. *Senior Nurse, 3,* 3.

Neuman, B. (1990). Health: A continuum based on the Neuman systems model. *Nursing Science Quarterly, 3,* 129-135.

Neuman, B. (1996). The Neuman systems model in research and practice. *Nursing Science Quarterly, 9*(2), 67-70.

Neuman, B. (1998). NDs should be future coordinators of health care (Letter to the Editor). *Image: The Journal of Nursing Scholarship, 30,* 106.

Neuman, B. (2000). Leadership-scholarship integration: Using the Neuman systems model for 21st century professional nursing practice. *Nursing Science Quarterly, 13*(1), 60-63.

Neuman, B., Chadwick, P. L., Beynon, C. E., Craig, D. M., Fawcett, J., Chang, N. J., et al. (1997). The Neuman systems model: Reflections and projections. *Nursing Science Quarterly, 10*(1), 18-21.

Neuman, B., Deloughery, G. W., & Gebbie, K. M. (1974, Jan.). Teaching organizational concepts to nurses in community mental health. *Journal of Nursing Education, 13,* 1.

Neuman, B. M., Deloughery, G. W., & Gebbie, K. M. (1970). Changes in problem solving ability among nurses receiving mental health consultation: A pilot study. *Communicating Nursing Research, 3,* 41-52.

Neuman, B. M., Deloughery, G. W., & Gebbie, K. M. (1970, Jan./Feb.). Levels of utilization: Nursing specialists in community mental health. *Journal of Psychiatric Nursing and Mental Health Services, 8*(1), 37-39.

Neuman, B. M., Deloughery, G. W., & Gebbie, K. M. (1972, Feb.). Mental health consultation as a means of improving problem solving ability in work groups: A pilot study. *Comparative Group Studies, 3*(1), 81-97.

Neuman, B. M., & Martin, K. S. (1998). Neuman systems model and the Omaha system. *Image: The Journal of Nursing Scholarship, 30*(1), 8.

Neuman, B. M., & Young, R. J. (1972, May/June). A model for teaching total person approach to patient problems. *Nursing Research, 21,* 264-269.

Neuman, B., Newman, D. M. L., & Holder, P. (2000). Leadership-scholarship integration: Using the Neuman systems model for 21st-century professional nursing practice. *Nursing Science Quarterly, 13*(1), 60-63.

Neuman, B., & Wyatt, M. A. (1981). Prospects for change: Some evaluative reflections by faculty members from one articulated baccalaureate program. *Journal of Nursing Education, 20,* 40-46.

Secondary sources
Books

Bertalanffy, L. (1968). *General system theory.* New York: George Braziller.

Caplan, G. (1964). *Principles of preventive psychiatry.* New York: Basic Books.

Fawcett, J. (1989). *Analysis and evaluation of conceptual models of nursing.* Philadelphia: F. A. Davis.

Fawcett, J. (1999). *The relationship of theory and research* (3rd ed.). Philadelphia: Davis.

Fawcett, J. (2000). *Analysis and evaluation of contemporary nursing knowledge: Nursing models and theories.* Philadelphia: Davis.

Lowry, Lois W. (1998). *The Neuman systems model and nursing education: Teaching strategies and outcomes.* Indianapolis: Sigma Theta Tau International: Center Nursing Press.

Meleis, A. I. (1997). *Theoretical nursing: Development and progress* (3rd ed.). Philadelphia: Lippincott.

Perls, F. (1973). *The gestalt approach: Eye witness to therapy.* Palo Alto, CA: Science and Behavior Books.

Reed, K. S. (1993). *Betty Neuman: The Neuman systems model.* Newbury Park, CA: Sage.

Selye, H. (1974). *Stress without distress.* Philadelphia: J. B. Lippincott.

Torres, G. (1986). *Theoretical foundations of nursing.* Norwalk, CT: Appleton-Century-Crofts.

Walker, L. O., & Avant, K. (1983). *Strategies for theory construction in nursing.* Norwalk, CT: Appleton-Century-Crofts.

Book Chapters

Alligood, M. R., & Tomey, A. M. (2002). Introduction to nursing theory: History, terminology and analysis. In A. M. Tomey & M. R. Alligood (Eds.), *Nursing theorists and their works* (5th ed., pp. 3-13). St. Louis: Mosby.

Amaya, M. A. (2002). The Neuman systems model and clinical practice: An integrative review 1974-2000. In B. Neuman & J. Fawcett (Eds.), *The Neuman systems model* (4th ed., pp. 43-60). Upper Saddle River, NJ: Pearson Education.

Beckman, S. J., Boxley-Harges, S., Bruick-Sorge, C., & Eichenaur, J. (1998). Critical thinking, the Neuman systems model, and associate degree education. In L. Lowry (Ed.), *The Neuman systems model and nursing education: Teaching strategies and outcomes* (pp. 53-58). Indianapolis: Center Nursing Press.

Beckman, S. J., Boxley-Harges, S., Bruick-Sorge, C., & Eichenaur, J. (1998). Evaluation modalities for assessing student and program outcomes. In L. Lowry (Ed.), *The Neuman systems model and nursing education: Teaching strategies and outcomes* (pp. 149-160). Indianapolis: Center Nursing Press.

Beddome, G. (1989). Application of the Neuman systems model to the assessment of community-as-client. In B. Neuman (Ed.), *The Neuman systems model* (2nd ed., pp. 363-374). Norwalk, CT: Appleton & Lange.

Beddome, G. (1995). Community-as-client assessment: A Neuman-based guide for education and practice. In B. Neuman (Ed.), *The Neuman systems model* (3rd ed., pp. 567-580). Norwalk, CT: Appleton & Lange.

Beynon, C. E. (1995). Neuman-based experiences of the Middlesex-London health unit. In B. Neuman (Ed.), *The Neuman systems model* (3rd ed., pp. 537-549). Norwalk, CT: Appleton & Lange.

Bloch, C., & Bloch, C. (1995). Teaching content and process of the Neuman systems model. In B. Neuman (Ed.), *The Neuman systems model* (3rd ed., pp. 175-182). Norwalk, CT: Appleton & Lange.

Breckenridge, D. M. (1995). Nephrology practice and directions for nursing research. In B. Neuman (Ed.), *The Neuman systems model* (3rd ed., pp. 499-507). Norwalk, CT: Appleton & Lange.

Breckenridge, D. M. (2002). Using the Neuman systems model to guide nursing research in the United States. In B. Neuman & J. Fawcett (Eds.), *The Neuman systems model* (4th ed., pp. 176-182). Upper Saddle River, NJ: Pearson Education.

Bueno, M. M., & Sengin, K. K. (1995). The Neuman systems model for critical care nursing: A framework for practice. In B. Neuman (Ed.), *The Neuman systems model* (3rd ed., pp. 275-292). Norwalk, CT: Appleton & Lange.

Busch, P., & Lynch, M. (1998). Creative teaching strategies in a Neuman-based baccalaureate curriculum. In L. Lowry (Ed.), *The Neuman systems model and nursing education: Teaching strategies and outcomes* (pp. 59-70). Indianapolis: Center Nursing Press.

Cammuso, B. S., & Wallen, A. J. (2002). Using the Neuman systems model to guide nursing education in the United States. In B. Neuman & J. Fawcett (Eds.), *The Neuman systems model* (4th ed., pp. 244-253). Upper Saddle River, NJ: Pearson Education.

Capers, C. F. (1995). Editorial comments. In B. Neuman (Ed.), *The Neuman systems model* (3rd ed., pp. 496-497). Norwalk, CT: Appleton & Lange.

Chang, N. J., & Freese, B. T. (1998). Teaching culturally competent care: A Korean-American experience. In L. Lowry (Ed.), *The Neuman systems model and nursing education: Teaching strategies and outcomes* (pp. 85-90). Indianapolis: Center Nursing Press.

Chiverton, P., & Flannery, J. C. (1995). Cognitive impairment: Use of the Neuman systems model. In B. Neuman (Ed.), *The Neuman systems model* (3rd ed., pp. 249-262). Norwalk, CT: Appleton & Lange.

Cookfair, J. M. (1996). Community as client. In J. M. Cookfair (Ed.), *Nursing care in the community* (2nd ed., pp. 19-37). St. Louis: Mosby.

Craig, D., & Beynon, C. (1996). Nursing administration and the Neuman systems model. In P. H. Walker (Ed.), *Blueprint for use of nursing models: Education, research, practice, and administration* (pp. 251-274). New York: National League for Nursing Publications.

Craig, D. M. (1995). The Neuman model: Examples of its use in Canadian educational programs. In B. Neuman (Ed.), *The Neuman systems model* (3rd ed., pp. 521-527). Norwalk, CT: Appleton & Lange.

Craig, D. M., & Morris-Coulter, C. (1995). Neuman implementation in a Canadian psychiatric facility. In B. Neuman (Ed.), *The Neuman systems model* (3rd ed., pp. 397-406). Norwalk, CT: Appleton & Lange.

Crawford, J. A., & Tarko, M. (2002). Using the Neuman systems model to guide nursing practice in Canada. In B. Neuman & J. Fawcett (Eds.), *The Neuman systems model* (4th ed., pp. 90-110). Upper Saddle River, NJ: Pearson Education.

Cross, J. R. (1995). Nursing process of the family client: Application of Neuman's systems model. In P. J. Christensen & J. W. Kenney (Eds.), *Nursing process: Application of conceptual models* (4th ed., pp. 246-269). St. Louis: Mosby–Year Book.

Curran, G. (1995). The Neuman systems model revisited. In B. Neuman (Ed.), *The Neuman systems model* (3rd ed., pp. 93-99). Norwalk, CT: Appleton & Lange.

Curran, G. (1995). The spiritual variable: A world view. In B. Neuman (Ed.), *The Neuman systems model* (3rd ed., pp. 581-590). Norwalk, CT: Appleton & Lange.

Damant, M. (1995). Community nursing in the United Kingdom: A case for reconciliation using the Neuman systems model. In B. Neuman (Ed.), *The Neuman systems model* (3rd ed., pp. 607-620). Norwalk, CT: Appleton & Lange.

Davies, P., & Proctor, H. (1995). In Wales: Using the model in community mental health nursing. In B. Neuman (Ed.), *The Neuman systems model* (3rd ed., pp. 621-628). Norwalk, CT: Appleton & Lange.

de Kuiper, M. (2002). Using the Neuman systems model to guide nursing education in Holland. In B. Neuman & J. Fawcett (Eds.), *The Neuman systems model* (4th ed., pp. 254-262). Upper Saddle River, NJ: Pearson Education.

Dwyer, C. M., Walker, P. H., Suchman, A., & Coggiola, P. (1995). Opportunities and obstacles: Development of a true collaborative practice with physicians. In B. Murphy (Ed.), *Nursing centers: The time is now* (pp. 135-155, NLN Pub. No. 41-2629). New York: National League for Nursing Press.

Engberg, I. B. (1995). Brief abstracts: Use of the Neuman systems model in Sweden. In B. Neuman (Ed.), *The Neuman systems model* (3rd ed., pp. 653-656.) Norwalk, CT: Appleton & Lange.

Engberg, I. B., Bjalming, E., & Bertilson, B. (1995). A structure for documenting primary health care in Sweden using the Neuman systems model. In B. Neuman (Ed.), *The Neuman systems model* (3rd ed., pp. 637-654). Norwalk, CT: Appleton & Lange.

Evans, B. (1998). Fourth-generation evaluation and the Neuman systems model. In L. Lowry (Ed.), *The Neuman systems model and nursing education: Teaching strategies and outcomes* (pp. 117-128). Indianapolis: Center Nursing Press.

Fashinpaur, D. (2002). Using the Neuman systems model to guide nursing practice in the United States: Nursing prevention interventions for postpartum mood disorders. In B. Neuman & J. Fawcett (Eds.), *The Neuman systems model* (4th ed., pp. 74-89). Upper Saddle River, NJ: Pearson Education.

Fawcett, J. (1989). Neuman systems model. In J. Fawcett, *Analysis and evaluation of conceptual models of nursing* (2nd ed., pp. 169-204). Philadelphia: F. A. Davis.

Fawcett, J. (1995). Constructing conceptual-theoretical-empirical structures for research: Future implications for use of the Neuman systems model. In B. Neuman (Ed.), *The Neuman systems model* (3rd ed., pp. 459-472). Norwalk, CT: Appleton & Lange.

Fawcett, J. (1995). Neuman's systems model. In J. Fawcett (Ed.), *Analysis and evaluation of conceptual models of nursing* (3rd ed., pp. 217-275). Philadelphia: F. A. Davis.

Fawcett, J. (1997). Conceptual models as guides for psychiatric nursing practice. In A. W. Burgess (Ed.), *Psychiatric nursing: Promoting mental health* (pp. 627-642). Stamford, CT: Appleton & Lange.

Fawcett, J. (1998). Conceptual models and therapeutic modalities in advanced psychiatric nursing practice. In A. W. Burgess (Ed.), *Advanced practice psychiatric nursing* (pp. 41-48). Stamford, CT: Appleton & Lange.

Fawcett, J. (2002). Neuman systems model bibliography. In B. Neuman & J. Fawcett (Eds.), *The Neuman systems model* (4th ed., pp. 364-400). Upper Saddle River, NJ: Pearson Education.

Fawcett, J., & Giangrande, S. K. (2002). The Neuman systems model and research: An integrative review. In B. Neuman & J. Fawcett (Eds.), *The Neuman systems model* (4th ed., pp. 120-149). Upper Saddle River, NJ: Pearson Education.

Felix, M., Hinds, C., Wolfe, Sr. C., & Martin, A. (1995). The Neuman systems model in a chronic care facility: A Canadian experience. In B. Neuman (Ed.), *The Neuman systems model* (3rd ed., pp. 549-566). Norwalk, CT: Appleton & Lange.

Freese, B., Beckman, S. J., Boxley-Harges, S., Bruick-Sorge, C., Harris, S. M., Hermiz, et al. (1998). Betty Neuman: Systems model. In A. M. Tomey & M. R. Alligood (Eds.), *Nursing theorists and their work* (4th ed., pp. 267-299). St. Louis: Mosby.

Freese, B. T. (2002). Betty Neuman: Systems model. In A. M. Tomey & M. R. Alligood (Eds.), *Nursing theorists and their work* (5th ed., pp. 299-335). St. Louis: Mosby.

Freese, B. T., & Scales, C. J. (1998). NSM-based care as an NLN program evaluation outcome. In L. Lowry (Ed.), *The Neuman systems model and nursing education: Teaching strategies and outcomes* (pp. 135-139). Indianapolis: Center Nursing Press.

Frieburger, O. A. (1998). Overview of strategies that integrate the Neuman systems model, critical thinking, and cooperative learning. In L. Lowry (Ed.), *The Neuman systems model and nursing education: teaching strategies and outcomes* (pp. 31-26). Indianapolis: Center Nursing Press.

Frieburger, O. A. (1998). The Neuman systems model, critical thinking, and cooperative learning in a nursing issues course. In L. Lowry (Ed.), *The Neuman systems model and nursing education: Teaching strategies and outcomes* (pp. 79-84). Indianapolis: Center Nursing Press.

Frioux, T. D., Roberts, A. G., & Butler, S. J. (1995). Oklahoma state public health nursing: Neuman-based. In B. Neuman (Ed.), *The Neuman systems model* (3rd ed., pp. 407-414). Norwalk, CT: Appleton & Lange.

Fulton, R. A. B. (1995). The spiritual variable: Essential to the client system. In B. Neuman (Ed.), *The Neuman systems model* (3rd ed., pp. 77-92). Norwalk, CT: Appleton & Lange.

George, J. B. (1995). Betty Neuman. In J. B. George (Ed.), *Nursing theories: The base for professional nursing practice* (4th ed., pp. 251-279). Norwalk, CT: Appleton & Lange.

Gigliotti, E., & Fawcett, J. (2002). The Neuman systems model and research instruments. In B. Neuman & J. Fawcett (Eds.), *The Neuman systems model* (4th ed., pp. 150-175). Upper Saddle River, NJ: Pearson Education.

Glazebrook, D. S. (1995). The Neuman systems model in cooperative baccalaureate nursing education: The Minnesota intercollegiate nursing consortium experience. In B. Neuman (Ed.), *The Neuman systems model* (3rd ed., pp. 227-230). Norwalk, CT: Appleton & Lange.

Hassell, J. S. (1998). Critical thinking strategies for family and community client systems. In L. Lowry (Ed.), *The Neuman systems model and nursing education: Teaching strategies and outcomes* (pp. 71-78). Indianapolis: Center Nursing Press.

Hilton, S. A., & Grafton, M. D. (1995). Curriculum transition based on the Neuman systems model: Los Angeles County Medical Center School of Nursing. In B. Neuman (Ed.), *The Neuman systems model* (3rd ed., pp. 163-174). Norwalk, CT: Appleton & Lange.

Hinton Walker, P. (1995). Neuman-based education, practice, and research in a community nursing center. In B. Neuman (Ed.), *The Neuman systems model* (3rd ed., pp. 415-430). Norwalk, CT: Appleton & Lange.

Hinton Walker, P. (1995). TQM and the Neuman systems model: Education for health care administration. In B. Neuman (Ed.), *The Neuman systems model* (3rd ed., pp. 365-376). Norwalk, CT: Appleton & Lange.

Hinton Walker, P. (1996). Blueprint example: An integrated model for evaluation, research, and policy analysis in the context of managed care. In P. Hinton Walker & B. Neuman (Eds.), *Blueprint for use of nursing models* (pp. 11-30). New York: National League for Nursing Press.

Kelley, J. A., & Sanders, N. F. (1995). A systems approach to the health of nursing and health care organizations. In B. Neuman (Ed.), *The Neuman systems model* (3rd ed., pp. 347-364). Norwalk, CT: Appleton & Lange.

Klotz, L. C. (1995). Integration of the Neuman systems model into the BSN curriculum at the University of Texas at Tyler. In B. Neuman (Ed.), *The Neuman systems model* (3rd ed., pp. 183-190). Norwalk, CT: Appleton & Lange.

Lancaster, D. R. (1996). Neuman's systems model. In J. J. Fitzpatrick & A. L. Whall (Eds.), *Conceptual models of nursing: Analysis and application* (3rd ed., pp. 199-223). Stamford, CT: Appleton & Lange.

Leddy, S., & Pepper, J. M. (1985). Models of nursing. In S. Leddy & J. M. Pepper (Eds.), *Conceptual bases of professional nursing* (pp. 135-149). Philadelphia: J. B. Lippincott.

Louis, M. (1995). The Neuman model in nursing research: An update. In B. Neuman (Ed.), *The Neuman systems model* (3rd ed., pp. 473-495). Norwalk, CT: Appleton & Lange.

Lowry, L. W. (1998). Creative teaching and effective evaluation. In L. Lowry (Ed.), *The Neuman systems model and nursing education: Teaching strategies and outcomes* (pp. 17-30). Indianapolis: Center Nursing Press.

Lowry, L. W. (1998). Efficacy of the Neuman systems model as a curriculum framework: A longitudinal study. In L. Lowry (Ed.), *The Neuman systems model and nursing education: Teaching strategies and outcomes* (pp. 139-148). Indianapolis: Center Nursing Press.

Lowry, L. W. (1998). Vision, values, and verities. In L. Lowry (Ed.), *The Neuman systems model and nursing education: Teaching strategies and outcomes* (pp. 167-174). Indianapolis: Center Nursing Press.

Lowry, L. W. (2002). The Neuman systems model and education: An integrative review. In B. Neuman & J. Fawcett (Eds.), *The Neuman systems model* (4th ed., pp. 216-237). Upper Saddle River, NJ: Pearson Education.

Lowry, L. W., Bruick-Sorge, C., Freese, B. T., & Sutherland, R. (1998). Development and renewal of faculty for Neuman-based teaching. In L. Lowry (Ed.), *The Neuman systems model and nursing education: Teaching strategies and outcomes* (pp. 161-166). Indianapolis: Center Nursing Press.

Lowry, L. W., & Newsome, G. G. (1995). Neuman-based associate degree programs: Past, present, and future. In B. Neuman (Ed.), *The Neuman systems model* (3rd ed., pp. 197-214). Norwalk, CT: Appleton & Lange.

Lowry, L. W., Walker, P. H., & Mirenda, R. (1995). Through the looking glass back to the future. In B. Neuman (Ed.), *The Neuman systems model* (3rd ed., pp. 63-76). Norwalk, CT: Appleton & Lange.

McCulloch, S. J. (1995). Utilization of the Neuman systems model: University of South Australia. In B. Neuman (Ed.), *The Neuman systems model* (3rd ed., pp. 591-598). Norwalk, CT: Appleton & Lange.

McGee, M. (1995). Implications for use of the Neuman systems model in occupational health nursing. In B. Neuman (Ed.), *The Neuman systems model* (3rd ed., pp. 657-668). Norwalk, CT: Appleton & Lange.

Meleis, A. I. (1995). Theory testing and theory support: Principles, challenges, and a sojourn into the future. In B. Neuman (Ed.), *The Neuman systems model* (3rd ed., pp. 447-458). Norwalk, CT: Appleton & Lange.

Mirenda, R. M. (1986). The Neuman systems model: Description and application. In P. Winsted Fry (Ed.), *Case studies in nursing theory* (pp. 127-166). New York: National League for Nursing Press.

Munck, C. K., & Merks, A. (2002). Using the Neuman systems model to guide administration of nursing services in Holland: The case of Emergis, institute for mental health care. In B. Neuman & J. Fawcett (Eds.), *The Neuman systems model* (4th ed., pp. 300-316). Upper Saddle River, NJ: Pearson Education.

Newsome, G. G., & Lowry, L. W. (1998). Evaluation in nursing: History, models, and Neuman's framework. In L. Lowry (Ed.), *The Neuman systems model and nursing education: Teaching strategies and outcomes* (pp. 37-52). Indianapolis: Center Nursing Press.

Nuttall, P. R., Stittich, E. M., & Flores, F. C. (1998). The Neuman systems model in advanced practice nursing. In L. Lowry (Ed.), *The Neuman systems model and nursing education: Teaching strategies and outcomes* (pp. 109-116). Indianapolis: Center Nursing Press.

Peirce, A. G., & Fulmer, T. T. (1995). Application of the Neuman systems model to gerontological nursing. In B. Neuman (Ed.), *The Neuman systems model* (3rd ed., pp. 293-308). Norwalk, CT: Appleton & Lange.

Poole, V. L., & Flowers, J. S. (1995). Care management of pregnant substance abusers using the Neuman systems model. In B. Neuman (Ed.), *The Neuman systems model* (3rd ed., pp. 377-386). Norwalk, CT: Appleton & Lange.

Pothiban, L. (2002). Using the Neuman systems model to guide nursing research in Thailand. In B. Neuman & J. Fawcett (Eds.), *The Neuman systems model* (4th ed., pp. 183-190). Upper Saddle River, NJ: Pearson Education.

Proctor, N. G., & Cheek, J. (1995). Nurses' role in world catastrophic events: War dislocation effects on Serbian Australians. In B. Neuman (Ed.), *The Neuman systems model* (3rd ed., pp. 119-132). Norwalk, CT: Appleton & Lange.

Reed, K. S. (2002). The Neuman systems model and educational tools. In B. Neuman & J. Fawcett (Eds.), *The Neuman systems model* (4th ed., pp. 238-243). Upper Saddle River, NJ: Pearson Education.

Rodriguez, M. L. (1995). The Neuman systems model adapted to a continuing care retirement community. In B. Neuman (Ed.), *The Neuman systems model* (3rd ed., pp. 431-442). Norwalk, CT: Appleton & Lange.

Russell, J. (2002). The Neuman systems model and clinical tools. In B. Neuman & J. Fawcett (Eds.), *The Neuman systems model* (4th ed., pp. 61-73). Upper Saddle River, NJ: Pearson Education.

Russell, J., Hileman, J. W., & Grant, J. S. (1995). Assessing and meeting the needs of home caregivers using the Neuman systems model. In B. Neuman (Ed.), *The Neuman systems model* (3rd ed., pp. 331-342). Norwalk, CT: Appleton & Lange.

Sanders, N. F., & Kelley, J. A. (2002). The Neuman systems model and administration of nursing services: An integrative review. In B. Neuman & J. Fawcett (Eds.), *The Neuman systems model* (4th ed., pp. 271-287). Upper Saddle River, NJ: Pearson Education.

Scicchitani, B., Cox, J., Heyduk, L. J., Maglicco, P. A., & Sargent, N. A. (1995). Implementing the Neuman model in a psychiatric hospital. In B. Neuman (Ed.), *The Neuman systems model* (3rd ed., pp. 387-396). Norwalk, CT: Appleton & Lange.

Seng, V. S. (1998). Clinical evaluation: The heart of clinical performance. In L. Lowry (Ed.), *The Neuman systems model and nursing education: Teaching strategies and outcomes* (pp. 129-134). Indianapolis: Center Nursing Press.

Seng, V. S., Mirenda, R., & Lowry, L. W. (1996). The Neuman systems model in nursing education. In P. H. Walker, (Ed.), *Blueprint for use of nursing models: Education, research, practice, and administration* (pp. 91-140). New York: National League for Nursing Publications.

Smith, M. C., & Edgil, A. E. (1995). Future directions for research with the Neuman systems model. In B. Neuman (Ed.), *The Neuman systems model* (3rd ed., pp. 509-517). Norwalk, CT: Appleton & Lange.

Sohier, R. (1995). Nursing care for the people of a small planet: Culture and the Neuman systems model. In B. Neuman (Ed.), *The Neuman systems model* (3rd ed., pp. 101-118). Norwalk, CT: Appleton & Lange.

Sohier, R. (1997). Neuman's systems model in nursing practice. In M. R. Alligood & A. Marriner Tomey (Eds.), *Nursing theory: Utilization & application* (pp. 109-127). St. Louis: Mosby.

Stittich, E. M., Flores, F. C., & Nuttall, P. (1995). Cultural considerations in a Neuman-based curriculum. In B. Neuman (Ed.), *The Neuman systems model* (3rd ed., pp. 147-162). Norwalk, CT: Appleton & Lange.

Strickland-Seng, V. (1995). The Neuman systems model in clinical evaluation of students. In B. Neuman (Ed.), *The Neuman systems model* (3rd ed., pp. 215-223). Norwalk, CT: Appleton & Lange.

Strickland-Seng, V. (1998). Clinical evaluation: The heart of clinical performance. In L. Lowry (Ed.), *The Neuman systems model and nursing education: Teaching strategies and outcomes* (pp. 129-134). Indianapolis: Sigma Theta Tau International Center Nursing Press.

Strickland-Seng, V., Mirenda, R., & Lowry, L. W. (1996). The Neuman systems model in nursing education. In P. Hinton Walker & B. Neuman (Eds.), *Blueprint for use of nursing models* (pp. 91-140). New York: National League for Nursing Press.

Stuart, G. W., & Wright, L. K. (1995). Applying the Neuman systems model to psychiatric nursing practice. In B. Neuman (Ed.), *The Neuman systems model* (3rd ed., pp. 263-274). Norwalk, CT: Appleton & Lange.

Sutherland, R., & Forrest, D. L. (1998). Primary prevention in an associate of science curriculum. In L. Lowry (Ed.), *The Neuman systems model and nursing education: Teaching strategies and outcomes* (pp. 99-108). Indianapolis: Center Nursing Press.

Tomlinson, P. S., & Anderson, K. S. (1995). Family health and the Neuman systems model. In B. Neuman (Ed.), *The Neuman systems model* (3rd ed., pp. 133-144). Norwalk, CT: Appleton & Lange.

Toot, J. L. & Schmull, B. J. (1995). The Neuman systems model and physical therapy educational curricula. In B. Neuman (Ed.), *The Neuman systems model* (3rd ed., pp. 231-246). Norwalk, CT: Appleton & Lange.

Torakis, M. L. (2002). Using the Neuman systems model to guide administration of nursing services in the United States: Redirecting nursing practice in a freestanding pediatric hospital. In B. Neuman & J. Fawcett (Eds.), *The Neuman systems model* (4th ed., pp. 288-299). Upper Saddle River, NJ: Pearson Education.

Trepanier, M. J., Dunn, S. J., & Sprague, A. E. (1995). Application of the Neuman systems model to perinatal nursing. In B. Neuman (Ed.), *The Neuman systems model* (3rd ed., pp. 309-329). Norwalk, CT: Appleton & Lange.

Vaughn, B., & Gough, P. (1995). Use of the Neuman systems model in England: Abstracts. In B. Neuman (Ed.), *The Neuman systems model* (3rd ed., pp. 599-606). Norwalk, CT: Appleton & Lange.

Verbeck, F. (1995). In Holland: Application of the Neuman model in psychiatric nursing. In B. Neuman (Ed.), *The Neuman systems model* (3rd ed., pp. 629-636). Norwalk, CT: Appleton & Lange.

Ware, L. A., & Shannahan, M. K. (1995). Using Neuman for a stable support group in neonatal intensive care. In B. Neuman (Ed.), *The Neuman systems model* (3rd ed., pp. 321-330). Norwalk, CT: Appleton & Lange.

Weitzel, A. R., & Wood, K. C. (1998). Community health nursing: Keystone of baccalaureate education. In L. Lowry (Ed.), *The Neuman systems model and nursing education: Teaching strategies and outcomes* (pp. 91-98). Indianapolis: Center Nursing Press.

Journal Articles

August-Brady, M. (2000). Prevention as intervention. *Journal of Advanced Nursing, 31*(6), 1304-1308.

Barker, E., Robinson, D., & Brautigan, R. (1999). The effect of psychiatric home nurse follow-up on readmission rates of patients with depression. *Journal of American Psychiatric Nurses Association, 5*(4), 111-1116.

Beebe, L. H. (2003). Theory-based research in schizophrenia. *Perspectives in Psychiatric Care, 39*(2), 67-75.

Bennett, S., Hulkes, C., Jones, J., Marden, B., Richards, A., Stone, A., et al. (1998). Models of care: Developing a trust-wide philosophy. *Community Practitioner, 71*(10), 334, 336.

Black, P., Deeny, P., & McKenna, H. (1997). Sensoristrain: An exploration of nursing interventions in the context of the Neuman systems theory. *Intensive and Critical Care Nursing, 13*(5), 249-258.

Bowles, L., Oliver, N., & Stanley, S. (1995, Jan.). A fresh approach. *Nursing Times, 91*(1), 40-41.

Bowman, A. M. (1997). Sleep satisfaction, perceived pain, and acute confusion in elderly clients undergoing orthopaedic procedures. *Journal of Advanced Nursing, 26*(3), 550-564.

Breckenridge, D. M. (1997). Decisions regarding dialysis treatment modality: A holistic perspective. *Holistic Nursing Practice, 12*(1), 54-61.

Breckenridge, D. M. (1997). Patients' perceptions of why, how, and by whom dialysis treatment modality was chosen . . . including commentary by Whittaker, A. A. and Locking-Cusolito, H. with author response. *American Nephrology Nurses Association Journal, 24*(3), 313-321.

Bunn, H. (1995). Preparing nurses for the challenge of the new focus on community mental health nursing. *The Journal of Continuing Education in Nursing, 26*(2), 55-59.

Butts, J. B. (2001). Outcomes of comfort touch in institutionalized elderly female residents. *Geriatric Nursing, 22*(4), 180-184.

Capers, C. F. (1996). The Neuman systems model: A culturally relevant perspective. *ABNF Journal, 7*(5), 113-117.

Carrigg, K. C., & Weber, R. (1997). Development of the spiritual care scale. *Image: The Journal of Nursing Scholarship, 29*(3), 293.

Cheung, Y. L. (1997). Student forum. The application of the Neuman system model to nursing in Hong Kong? *Hong Kong Nursing Journal, 33*(4), 17-21.

Chiverton, P., Tortoretti, D., LaForest, M., & Walker, P. H. (1999). Bridging the gap between psychiatric hospitalization and community care: Cost and quality outcomes. *Journal of the American Psychiatric Nurses Association, 5*(2), 46-53.

Collins, M. A. (1996). The relation of work stress, hardiness, and burnout among full-time hospital staff nurses. *Journal of Nursing Staff Development, 12*(2), 81-85.

Cowperthwaite, B., LaPlante, K., Mahon, B., & Markowski, T. (1997). Latex allergy in the nursing population. *Canadian Operating Room Nursing Journal, 15*(2), 23-24, 26-28, 30-32.

Dale, J. L., & Savala, S. M. (1990). A new approach to the senior practicum. *Nursing Connections, 3*(1), 45-51.

Denson, V. L. (2002). Maternal serum screening: women's experiences. 35th annual communicating nursing research conference/16th. Annual WIN assembly. *Community Nursing Research, 35*(10), 394.

Edelman, M. A. (2000). You make the diagnosis. A diabetic educator's use of the Neuman systems model. *Nursing Diagnosis, 11*(4), 179-182.

Fawcett, J. (2001). Neuman systems model–based research: An integrative review project. *Nursing Science Quarterly, 14*(3), 231-238.

Fawcett, J. (2001). Scholarly dialogue. The nurse theorists: 21st century updates—Betty Neuman. *Nursing Science Quarterly, 14*(3), 211-214.

Fawcett, J. (2001). Using conceptual models of nursing to guide nursing research: The case of the Neuman systems model. *Nursing Science Quarterly, 14*(4), 339-345.

Fawcett, J., & Giangrande, S. K. (2001). Neuman systems model–based research: An integrative review project. *Nursing Science Quarterly, 14*(3), 231-238.

Fawcett, J., & Gigliotti, E. (2001). Using conceptual models to guide nursing research: The case of the Neuman systems model. *Nursing Science Quarterly, 14*(4), 339-345.

Fawcett, J., Tulman, L., & Samarel, N., (1995). Enhancing function in life transitions and serious illness. *Advanced Practice Quarterly, 1*(3), 50-57.

Flanders-Stepans, M. B., & Fuller, S. G. (1999). Physiological effects of infant exposure to environmental tobacco smoke: A passive observation study. *Journal of Perinatal Education, 8*(1), 10-21.

Flannery, J. (1995). Cognitive assessment in the acute care setting: Reliability and validity of the levels of cognitive function assessment scale (LOCFAS). *Journal of Nursing Measurement, 3*(1), 43-58.

Fuller, C. C., & Hartley, B. (2000). Linear scleroderma: A Neuman nursing perspective. *Journal of Pediatric Nursing, 15*(3), 168-174.

George, J. (1997). Nurses' perceived autonomy in a shared governance setting. *Journal of Shared Governance, 3*(2), 17-21.

Gerstle, D. S. (2001). Quality of life and chronic nonmalignant pain. *Pain Management Nursing, 2*(3), 98-109.

Gibson, M. (1996). Health promotion for a group of elderly clients. *Perspectives, 20*(3), 2-5.

Gifford, D. K. (1997). Monthly incidence of stroke in rural Kansas. *Kansas Nurse, 71*(5), 3-4.

Gigliotti, E. (1997). Use of Neuman's lines of defense and resistance in nursing research: Conceptual and empirical considerations. *Nursing Science Quarterly, 10*(3), 136-143.

Gigliotti, E. (1998). You make the diagnosis. Case study: Integration of the Neuman systems model with the theory of nursing diagnosis in postpartum nursing . . . including commentary by Lunney, M. *Nursing Diagnosis: The Journal of Nursing Language and Classification, 9*(1), 14.

Gigliotti, E. (1999). Women's multiple role stress: Testing Neuman's flexible line of defense. *Nursing Science Quarterly, 12*(1), 36-44.

Gigliotti, E. (2001). Empirical tests of the Neuman systems model: Relational statement analysis. *Nursing Science Quarterly, 14*(2), 149-157.

Gigliotti, E. (2002). A theory-based clinical nurse specialist practice exemplar using Neuman's systems model and nursing's taxonomies. *Clinical Nurse Specialist, 16*(1), 10-16.

Gigliotti, E. (2003). The Neuman systems model institute: Testing middle-range theories. *Nursing Science Quarterly, 16*(3), 201-206.

Goodman, H. (1995). Patients' views count as well. *Nursing Standard, 9*(40), 55.

Hainsworth, D. S. (1996). Research briefs. The effect of death education on attitudes of hospital nurses toward care of the dying. *Oncology Nursing Forum, 23*(6), 963-967.

Hanson, M. J. S. (1999). Cross-cultural study of beliefs about smoking among teenaged females . . . including commentary by Laffery S. C. with author response. *Western Journal of Nursing Research, 21*(5), 635-651.

Hassell, J. S. (1996). Improved management of depression through nursing model application and critical thinking. *Journal of the American Academy of Nurse Practitioners, 8*(4), 161-166.

Imamura, E. (2002). Amy's chat room: Health promotion programmes for community dwelling elderly adults. *International Journal Nursing Practice, 8*(1), 61-64.

Issel, L. M. (1995). Evaluating case management programs. *Maternal/Child Nursing Journal, 29*, 67-74.

Jones, W. R. (1996). Stressors in the primary caregivers of traumatic head injured persons. *AXON, 18*(1), 9-11.

Kain, H. B. (2000). Care of the older adult following hip fracture. *Holistic Nursing Practice, 14*(4), 24-39.

Kinservik, M. A., & Friedhoff, M. M. (2000). Control issues in toilet training. *Pediatric Nursing, 26*(3), 267-274.

Kottwitz, D. (2003). A pilot study of the Elder Abuse Questionnaire. *Kansas Nurse, 78*(7), 4-6.

Lin, M., Ku, N., Leu, J., Chen, J., & Lin, L. (1996). An exploration of the stress aspects, coping behaviors, health status, and related aspects in family caregivers of hepatoma patients. *Nursing Research (China), 4*(2), 171-185.

Lowry, L. W. (2000). Compete or complement? An interdisciplinary approach to training health professionals. *Nursing and Health Care Perspectives, 21*(2), 76-80.

Lowry, L. W. (2001). Using computer simulations and focus groups for planned change in prenatal clinics. *Outcomes Management Nursing Practice, 5*(3), 134-139.

Lowry, L. W. (2004). Conceptual models of nursing: international in scope and substance? The case of the Neuman systems model. Interview by Jacqueline Fawcett. *Nursing Science Quarterly, 17*(1), 50-54.

Lowry, L. W., Burns, C. M., Smith, A. A., & Jacobson, H. (2000). Compete or complement? An interdisciplinary approach to training health professionals. *Nursing and Health Care Perspectives, 21*(2), 76-80.

Lowry, L. W., Saeger, J., & Barnett, S. (1997). Client satisfaction with prenatal care and pregnancy outcomes. *Outcomes Management for Nursing Practice, 1*(1), 29-35.

Mackenzie, S., & Spence-Laschinger, H. K. (1995). Correlates of nursing diagnosis quality in public health nursing. *Journal of Advanced Nursing, 21*, 800-808.

Madrid, M. (2001). Research issues. Nursing research on the health patterning modalities of therapeutic touch and imagery . . . including commentary by Malinski, V. M. *Nursing Science Quarterly, 14*(3), 187-194.

Malinski, V. M. (2002). Research issues. Developing a nursing perspective on spirituality and healing. *Nursing Science Quarterly, 15*(4), 281-287.

Malinski, V. M. (2003). Nursing research and nursing conceptual models: Betty Neuman's systems model. *Nursing Science Quarterly, 16*(3), 201.

Mannina, J. (1997). Finding an effective hearing testing protocol to identify hearing loss and middle ear disease in school-aged children. *Journal of School Nursing, 13*(5), 23-28.

Marsh, V., Beard, M. T., & Adams, B. N. (1999). Job stress and burnout: The mediational effect of spiritual well-being and hardiness among nurses. *Journal of Theory Construction and Testing, 3*(1), 13-19.

Martin, S. A. (1996). Applying nursing theory to the practice of nurse anesthesia. *American Association of Nurse Anesthetists Journal, 64*(4), 369-372.

Martsolf, D. S., & Mickley, J. R. (1998). The concept of spirituality in nursing theories: Differing world-views and extent of focus. *Journal of Advanced Nursing, 27*(2), 294-303.

May, K. M. (2000). Caregiving and help seeking by mothers of low birthweight infants and mothers of normal birthweight infants. *Public Health Nursing 17*(4), 273-279.

McHolm, F. A., & Geib, K. M. (1998). Application of the Neuman systems model to teaching health assessment and nursing process. *Nursing Diagnosis: The Journal of Nursing Language and Classification, 9*(1), 23-33.

Melton, L. (2001). Resources for practice. A community needs assessment for a SANE program using Neuman's model. *Journal American Academy Nurse Practitioners, 13*(4), 178-186.

Memmott, R. J. (2000). Use of the Neuman systems model for interdisciplinary teams. *Online Journal of Rural Nursing and Health Care, 1*(2), 9p.

Mill, J. E. (1997). The Neuman systems model: Application in a Canadian HIV setting. *British Journal of Nursing, 6*(3), 163-166.

Miner, J. (1995). Incorporating the Betty Neuman systems model into HIV clinical practice. *AIDS Patient Care, 9*(1), 37-39.

Molassiotis, A. (1997). A conceptual model of adaptation to illness and quality of life for cancer patients treated with bone marrow transplants. *Journal of Advanced Nursing, 26*(3), 572-579.

Moody, N. B. (1996). Nurse faculty job satisfaction: A national survey. *Journal of Professional Nursing, 12*(5), 277-288.

Morrell, G. (2001). Effect of structured preoperative teaching on anxiety levels of patients scheduled for cataract surgery. *Insight, 26*(1), 4-9.

Narsavage, G. (2003). Education and support needs of young and older cancer survivors. *Applied Nursing Research, 16*(2), 103-109.

Narsavage, G. L. (1997). Promoting function in clients with chronic lung disease by increasing their perception of control. *Holistic Nursing Practice, 12*(1), 17-26.

Norrish, M. E. (2001). Nursing care of the patient undergoing alcohol detoxification. *Curationis, 24*(3), 36-48.

Nuttall, P., & Flores, F. C. (1997). Hmong healing practices used for common childhood illnesses. *Pediatric Nursing, 23,* 247-251.

Olson, R. S. (2001). Community re-entry after critical illness. *Critical Care Clinics of North America, 13*(3), 449-461.

Owens, M. (1995). Care of a woman with Down's syndrome using the Neuman systems model. *British Journal of Nursing, 4*(13), 752-758.

Peternelj-Taylor, C. A., & Johnson, R. (1996). Custody and caring: Clinical placement of student nurses in a forensic setting. *Perspectives in Psychiatric Care: The Journal for Nurse Psychotherapists, 32*(4), 23-29.

Picot, S. J. F., Zauszniewski, J. A., Debanne, S. M., & Holston, E. C. (1999). Mood and blood pressure in black female caregivers and noncaregivers. *Nursing Research, 48*(3), 150-161.

Picton, C. E. (1995). An explanation of family-centered care in Neuman's model with regard to the care of the critically ill adult in an accident and emergency setting. *Accident and Emergency Nursing, 3,* 33-37.

Potter, M. L., & Zauszniewski, J. A. (2000). Spirituality, resourcefulness, and arthritis impact on health perception of elders with rheumatoid arthritis. *Journal of Holistic Nursing, 18*(4), 311-336.

Reed, K. S. (1993). Adapting the Neuman systems model for family nursing. *Nursing Science Quarterly, 6*(2), 93-97.

Reed, K. S. (2003). Grief is more than tears. *Nursing Science Quarterly, 16*(1), 77-81.

Reitano, J. K. (1997, Fall). Learning through experience—Chester Community Nursing Center: A healthy partnership. *Accent,* 11. Available from Neumann College, Aston, PA.

Sabo, C. E., & Michael, S. R. (1996). The influence of personal message with music on anxiety and side effects associated with chemotherapy. *Cancer Nursing, 19*(4), 283-289.

Semple, O. D. (1995). The experiences of family members of persons with Huntington's disease. *Perspectives, 19*(4), 4-10.

Shamsudin, N. (2002). Can the Neuman systems model be adapted to the Malaysian nursing context? *International Journal of Nursing Practice, 8*(2), 99-105.

Skillen, D. L. (2001). The created environment for physical assessment by case managers. *Western Journal of Nursing Research, 23*(1), 72-89.

Smith, N. C. (2001). Review of the book Analysis and evaluation of contemporary nursing knowledge: Nursing models and theories. Nursing and Health Care Perspectives, 22(2), 92-93.

Smith, N. H. (2003). The impact of education on the use of physical restraints in the acute care setting. *Journal of Continuing Education in Nursing, 34*(1), 26-33, 46-47.

Stephans, M. B. F. (2002). Application of Neuman's framework: Infant exposure to environmental tobacco smoke. *Nursing Science Quarterly, 15*(4), 327-334.

Taggart, L., & Mattson, S. (1996). Delay in prenatal care as a result of battering in pregnancy: Cross-cultural implications. *Health Care for Women International, 17*(1), 25-34.

Torakis, M. L., & Smigielski, C. M. (2000). Documentation of model-based practice: One hospital's experience. *Pediatric Nursing, 26*(4), 394-399.

Tourville, C., & Ingalls, K. (2003). The living tree of nursing theories. *Nursing Forum, 38*(3), 21-36.

Vijaylakshmi, S. (2002). Breastfeeding technique in prevention of nipple sore—A study. *Nursing Journal of India, 93*(8), 173-174.

Villarruel, A. M. (2001). Borrowed theories, shared theories, and the advancement of nursing knowledge. *Nursing Science Quarterly, 14*(2), 158-163.

Wilson, L. C. (2000). Implementation and evaluation of church-based health fairs. *Journal of Community Nursing, 17*(1), 39-48.

Wormald, L. (1995). Samuel—The boy with tonsillitis: A care study. *Intensive and Critical Care Nursing, 11*(3), 157-160.

Wright, K. B. (1998). Professional, ethical, and legal implications for spiritual care in nursing. *Image: The Journal of Nursing Scholarship, 30,* 81-83.

Newsletter

Neuman News. (1992-present). The Neuman Systems Model Trustee Group. Available through Neumann College, c/o Director of Library Media and Archives, One Neumann Drive, Aston, PA 19014.

Electronic Media

Burns-Vandenberg, J., & Jones, E. (1999). *Evaluating postpartum home visits by student nurses.* Tucson, AZ: University of Arizona College of Nursing. Retrieved January 30, 2004, from *http://juns.nursing.arizona.edu/Burns-Van.htm.*

Central Florida Community College (CFCC). (n.d.). *Programs of study: Associate in arts degree.* Lecanto, FL: CFCC. Retrieved on January 30, 2004, from *http://www.cf.edu/catalog/programs.htm#asreq.*

Community College of Baltimore County (CCBC). (n.d.). *School of health professions—Practical nursing: Vision.* Baltimore, MD: CCBC. Retrieved January 30, 2004, from *http://www.ccbcmd.edu/allied_health/pn/vision.html.*

Malone College. (n.d.). *School of nursing.* Canton, OH: Malone College. Retrieved January 30, 2004, from *http://www.malone.edu/2242.*

Missouri Southern State University (MSSU). (n.d.). *Department of nursing.* Joplin, MO: MSSU. Retrieved February 23, 2005, from *http://www.mssu.edu*

Palm Beach Atlantic University (PBA). (n.d.). Palm Beach Atlantic University School of Nursing. West Palm Beach, FL: PBA. Retrieved January 30, 2004, from *http://www.pba.edu/Academic/Nursing.*

Saint Anselm College. (n.d.). *Department of nursing: Philosophy.* Manchester, NH: Saint Anselm College.

Wollman, K. (2004). *The community nursing center of Chester and vicinity.* Philadelphia: National Nursing Centers Consortium. Retrieved February 23, 2005, from *http://www.rncc.us/NNCC_Member_Centers/member_Community_Health_of_Chester_and_Vicinity.htm.*

Dissertations and Theses

Allen, K. S. (1997). The effect of cancer diagnosis information on the anxiety of patients with an initial diagnosis of first cancer. *Masters Abstracts International, 35*(04), 0996. (University Microfilms No. AAG1384216)

Ark, P. D. (1997). Health risk behaviors and coping strategies of African-American sixth graders. *Dissertation Abstracts International, 58*(03B), 1205. (University Microfilms No. AAG9726999)

Barnes-McDowell, B. M. (1997). Home apnea monitoring: Family functioning, concerns, and coping. *Dissertation Abstracts International, 58-03B,* 1205. (University Microfilms No. AAG9726731)

Bemker, M. A. (1996). Adolescent female substance abuse: Risk and resiliency factors. *Dissertation Abstracts International, 57,* 7544B. (University Microfilms No. AAG9714858)

Bittinger, J. P. (1995). Case management and satisfaction with nursing care of patients hospitalized with congestive heart failure. *Dissertation Abstracts International, 56-07B,* 3688. (University Microfilms No. AA19537111)

Butts, M. J. (1998). Outcomes of comfort touch in institutionalized elderly female residents. *Dissertation Abstracts International, 59-07B,* 3344. (University Microfilms No. AAG9839828)

Cagle, R. (1996). The relationship between health care provider advice and the initiation of breast-feeding. *Dissertation Abstracts International, 57-08B,* 4974. (University Microfilms No. AAG9700009)

Chilton, L. L. A. (1997). The influence of behavioral cues on immunization practices of elders. *Dissertation Abstracts International, 57,* 5572(B). (University Microfilms No. AAG9704005)

Collins, C. R. (1999). The older widow-adult child relationship as an influence upon health promoting behaviors. *Dissertation Abstracts International, 60*(04), 1527B. (University Microfilms No. AAG9926389)

Collins, T. J. (2000). Adherence to hypertension management recommendations for patient follow-up care and lifestyle modifications made by military healthcare providers. *Masters Abstracts International, 06*(2000), 1603. (University Microfilms No. AAI1399503) Available at http://lrcgwf.usuf2.usuhs.mil.

Doherty, D. C. (1997). Spousal abuse: An African-American female perspective. *Dissertation Abstracts International, 58-04B,* 1798. (University Microfilms No. AAG9729466)

Downing, B. H. (1995). Evaluation of a computer assisted intervention for musculoskeletal discomfort, strength, and flexibility and job satisfaction of video display operators. *Dissertation Abstracts International, 55,* 3237B. (University Microfilms No. AAG9434186)

Ferguson, M. J. (1995). Relationship between quiz game participation and final exam performance for nursing models. *Masters Abstracts International, 33,* 173. (University Microfilms No. AAG1358291)

Fukuzawa, M. (1996). Nursing care behaviors which predict patient satisfaction. *Masters Abstracts International, 28,* 408. (University Microfilms No. AA1378670)

Gibson, M. H. (1996). The quality of life of adult hemodialysis patients. *Dissertation Abstracts International, 56,* 5416B. (University Microfilms No. AA19603848)

Gigliotti, E. (1997). The relations among maternal and student role involvement, perceived social support and perceived multiple role stress in mothers attending college: A study based on Betty Neuman's systems model. *Dissertation Abstracts International 58,* 135B. (University Microfilms No. AAG9718709)

Gray, R. (1998). The lived experience of children, ages 8-12 years, who witness family violence in the home. *Masters Abstracts International, 36-05,* 1327. (University Microfilms No. AAG1389149)

Gullivar, K. M. (1997). Hopelessness and spiritual well-being in persons with HIV infection. *Masters Abstracts International, 35-05,* 1374. (University Microfilms No. AAG-1385172)

Hanson, M. J. S. (1995). Beliefs, attitudes, subjective norms, perceived behavioral control, and cigarette smoking in white, African-American, and Puerto Rican-American teenage women. *Dissertation Abstracts International, 56-08B,* 4240. (University Microfilms No. AA19543082)

Hanson, P. A. (1997). An application of Bowen family systems theory: Triangulation, differentiation of self and nurse manager job stress. *Dissertation Abstracts International, 58-11B,* 5889. (University Microfilms No. AAG9815103)

Higgs, K. T. (1995). Preterm labor risk factors identified in an ambulatory perinatal setting with home uterine activity monitoring support. *Masters Abstracts International, 33,* 1490. (University Microfilms No. AAI1360323)

Holloway, C. (1995). Stress perceived among nurse managers in community health settings. *Masters Abstracts International, 33-05,* 1490. (University Microfilms No. AAI1361519)

Hood, L. J. (1997). The effects of nurse faculty hardiness and sense of coherence on perceived stress, scholarly productivity, and job satisfaction. *Dissertation Abstracts International, 58-09B,* 4720. (University Microfilms No. AAG9809243)

Jennings, K. M. (1997). Predicting intention to obtain a pap smear among African-American and Latina women. *Dissertation Abstracts International, 58-07B,* 3557. (University Microfilms No. AAG9800878)

Johnson, K. M. (1996). Stressors of local Ontario Nurses' Association presidents. *Masters Abstracts International, 29,* 645. (University Microfilms No. AAI1376934)

Klimek, S. C. (1995). Identification and comparison of factors affecting breast self-examination between professional nurses and non-nursing professional women. *Masters Abstracts International, 33,* 516. (University Microfilms No. AAG1358568)

Lamb, K. A. (1998). Baccalaureate nursing students' perception of empathy and stress in their interactions with clinical instructors: Testing a theory of optimal student system stability according to the Neuman systems model. *Dissertation Abstracts International, 60-03B,* 1028. (University Microfilms No. AAG9923301)

Lapvongwatana, P. (2000). Perinatal risk assessment for low birthweight in Thai mothers: Using the Neuman systems model. *Dissertation Abstracts International, 61*(03), 1325B. (University Microfilms No. AAI9965512)

Larino, E. A. (1997). Determining the level of care provided by a family nurse practitioner during deployment. *Masters Abstracts International, 35-05,* 1376. (University Microfilms No. AAG1385132)

Lee, P. L. (1995). Caregiver stress as experienced by wives of institutionalized and in-home dementia husbands. *Dissertation Abstracts International, 56-08B,* 4241. (University Microfilms No. AAI9541861)

Lijauco, C. C. (1997). Factors related to length of stay in coronary artery bypass graft patients. *Masters Abstracts International, 36-02,* 0512. (University Microfilms No. AAG1387418)

Mann, N. J. (1996). Risk behavior of adolescents who have liver disease. *Masters Abstracts International, 29,* 648. (University Microfilms No. AAI1376930)

Marlett, L. A. (1998). The breast feeding practices of women with a history of breast cancer. *Masters Abstracts International, 37-04,* 1180.

Marsh, V. (1997). Job stress and burnout among nurses: The mediational effect of spiritual well-being and hardiness. *Dissertation Abstracts International, 58-08B,* 4142. (University Microfilms No. AAG9804907)

McMillan, D. E. (1995). Impact of therapeutic support of inherent coping strategies on chronic low back pain: A nursing intervention study. *Masters Abstracts International, 35-02,* 0520. (University Microfilms No. AAGMM13363)

Micevski, V. (1997). Gender differences in the presentation of physiological symptoms of myocardial infarction. *Masters Abstracts International, 35-02,* 0520. (University Microfilms No. AAG1382268)

Mirenda, R. M. (1995). A conceptual-theoretical strategy for curriculum development in baccalaureate nursing programs. *Dissertation Abstracts International, 56-10B,* 5421. (University Microfilms No. AAI9601825)

Monahan, G. L. (1996). A profile of pregnant drug-using female arrestees in California: The relationships among sociodemographic characteristics, reproductive and drug addiction histories, HIV/STD risk behaviors, and utilization of prenatal care services and substance abuse programs. *Dissertation Abstracts International, 57-09B,* 5576. (University Microfilms No. AAG9704608)

Moynihan, B. A. (1995). A descriptive study of three male adolescent sex offenders. *Masters Abstracts International, 28,* 275. (University Microfilms No. AAI1359536)

Musgrave, C. F. (2001). Religiosity, spiritual well-being, and attitudes toward spiritual care of Israeli oncology nurses. *Dissertation Abstracts International, 61*(11B), 5799. (University Microfilms No. AA199995617)

Neabel, B. (1998). A comparison of family needs perceived by nurses and family members of acutely brain-injured patients. *Masters Abstracts International, 37-02,* 0592. (University Microfilms No. AAGMQ32546)

Newman, S. K. (1995). Perceived stressors between partnered and unpartnered women. *Masters Abstracts International, 33,* 873. (University Microfilms No. AAG1357431)

Nicholson, C. H. (1995). Clients' perceptions of preparedness for discharge home following total hip or knee replacement surgery. *Masters Abstracts International, 33-03,* 0873. (University Microfilms No. AAI1359739)

Parker, V. J. (1995). Stress of discharge in men and women following cardiac surgery. *Masters Abstracts International, 33,* 518. (University Microfilms No. AAG1358788)

Parodi, V. A. (1998). Neuman based analysis of women's health needs aboard a deployed Navy ship: Can nursing make a difference? *Dissertation Abstracts International, 58,* 6491B. (University Microfilms No. AAG9818848)

Peters, M. R. (1998). An exploratory study of job stress and stressors in hospice administration. *Masters Abstracts International, 36-02,* 0502. (University Microfilms No. AAG1387515)

Peterson, G. A. (1997). Nursing perceptions of the spiritual dimensions of patient care: The Neuman systems model in curricular formations. *Dissertation Abstracts International, 59-02B,* 0605. (University Microfilms No. AAG9823988)

Ramsey, B. A. (1999). Can a multidisciplinary team decrease hospital length of stay for elderly trauma patients? *Masters Abstracts International, 37-04,* 1182. (University Microfilms No. AAG1393701)

Riley-Lawless, K. (2000). The relationship among characteristics of the family environment and behavioral and physiologic cardiovascular risk factors in parents and their adolescent twins. *Dissertation Abstracts International, 61*(03B), 1328. (University Microfilms No. AA19965555)

Robinson, C. A. (1998). The difference in perception of quality of life in patients one year after an infrainguinal bypass for critical limb ischemia. *Masters Abstracts International, 37-03,* 0914. (University Microfilms No. AAG1392664)

Sabati, N. (1994). Relationships between Neuman's systems model's buffering property of the flexible line of defense and active participation in support groups for women. *Masters Abstracts International, 33,* 179. (University Microfilms No. MA133 no 01 (1994) 0179)

Semple, O. D. (1995). The experiences of family members of patients with Huntington's disease. *Masters Abstracts International, 33,* 1847. (University Microfilms No. AAI1374651)

Simpson, E. M. (2000). Condom use among black women: A theoretical basis for HIV prevention guided by Neuman systems model and theory of planned behavior (immune deficiency). *Dissertation Abstracts International, 6-10,* 5240B. (University Microfilms No. AA19989654)

Smith, J. A. (1995). Caregiver wellness following interventions based on interdisciplinary geriatric assessment. *Masters Abstracts International, 33,* 1707. (University Microfilms No. AAI1361952)

South, L. D. (1995). The relationship of self-concept and social support in school age children with leukemia. *Dissertation Abstracts International, 56,* 1939B. (University Microfilms No. AAI9527022)

Thomas, Y. M. (1996). *Measuring the diabetes knowledge of senior nursing students attending a bachelor of science in nursing program.* Unpublished master's thesis, Pittsburgh State University, Pittsburgh.

Vitthuhn, K. M. (1999). Delivery of analgesics for the postoperative thoracotomy patient. *Masters Abstracts International, 37-04,* 1185. (University Microfilms No. AAG1393446)

Wallom, B. L. L. (2000). Coping behaviors and drug use among fifth- and sixth-grade students. *Dissertation Abstracts International, 61-08A,* 3076. (University Microfilms No. AA19982666)

Wright, J. G. (1996). The impact of preoperative education on health locus of control, self-efficacy, and anxiety for patients undergoing total joint replacement surgery.

Masters Abstracts International, 35-01, 0216. (University Microfilms No. AAG1382185)

Yoder, R. E. (1995). Primary prevention emphasis and self-reported health behaviors of nursing students. *Dissertation Abstracts International, 56,* 747B. (University Microfilms No. AAI9520576)

Young, L. M. (2000). The effects of guided mental imagery on the blood pressure of clients experiencing mild to moderate essential hypertension. *Dissertation Abstracts International, 61-02B,* 787. (University Microfilms No. AA19961229)

Computer Software

Fuld Institute for Technology in Nursing Education. (1997). Betty Neuman: Neuman systems model (Computer software). In Fuld Institute for Technology in Nursing Education, *The nurse theorists, portraits of excellence.* Athens, OH: The Institute.

Web Sites

Neuman Systems Model. Accessed December 20, 2004: *http://www.neumansystemsmodel.com*

Neumann College. Accessed December 20, 2004: *http://www.neumann.edu*

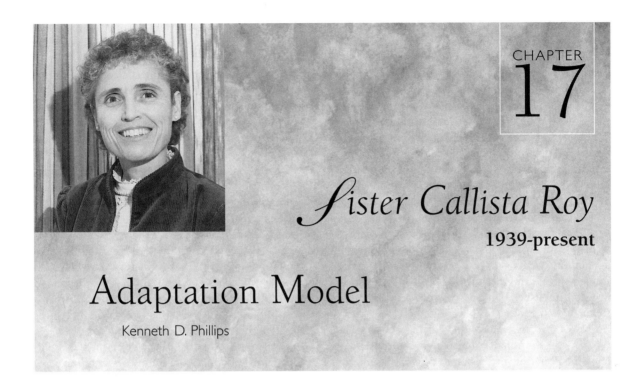

Sister Callista Roy
1939-present

Adaptation Model

Kenneth D. Phillips

CREDENTIALS AND BACKGROUND OF THE THEORIST

Sister Callista Roy, a member of the Sisters of Saint Joseph of Carondelet, was born on October 14, 1939, in Los Angeles, California. She received a bachelor's degree in nursing in 1963 from Mount Saint Mary's College in Los Angeles and an master's degree in nursing from the University of California, Los Angeles, in 1966. After earning her nursing degrees, Roy began her education in sociology, receiving both a master's degree in sociology in 1973 and a doctorate in sociology in 1977 from the University of California.

While working toward her master's degree, Roy was challenged in a seminar with Dorothy E.

Previous authors: Kenneth D. Phillips, Carolyn L. Blue, Karen M. Brubaker, Julia M.B. Fine, Martha J. Kirsch, Katherine R. Papazian, Cynthia M. Riester, and Mary Ann Sobiech.
The author wishes to express appreciation to Sister Callista Roy for critiquing the chapter.

Johnson to develop a conceptual model for nursing. While working as a pediatric staff nurse, Roy had noticed the great resiliency of children and their ability to adapt in response to major physical and psychological changes. Roy was impressed by adaptation as an appropriate conceptual framework for nursing. Roy developed the basic concepts of the model while she was a graduate student at the University of California, Los Angeles, from 1964 to 1966. Roy began operationalizing her model in 1968 when Mount Saint Mary's College adopted the adaptation framework as the philosophical foundation of the nursing curriculum. The Roy Adaptation Model was first presented in the literature in an article published in *Nursing Outlook* in 1970 entitled "Adaptation: A Conceptual Framework for Nursing" (Roy, 1970).

Roy was an associate professor and chairperson of the Department of Nursing at Mount Saint Mary's College until 1982. She was promoted to the rank of professor in 1983 at both Mount Saint

Mary's College and the University of Portland. She helped initiate and taught in a summer master's program at the University of Portland. From 1983 to 1985, she was a Robert Wood Johnson postdoctoral fellow at the University of California, San Francisco, as a clinical nurse scholar in neuroscience. During this time, she conducted research on nursing interventions for cognitive recovery in head injuries and on the influence of nursing models on clinical decision making. In 1987, Roy began the newly created position of nurse theorist at Boston College School of Nursing.

Roy has published many books, chapters, and periodical articles and has presented numerous lectures and workshops focusing on her nursing adaptation theory (Roy & Andrews, 1991). The refinement and restatement of the Roy Adaptation Model is published in her 1999 book, *The Roy Adaptation Model* (Roy & Andrews, 1999).

Roy is a member of Sigma Theta Tau, and she received the National Founder's Award for Excellence in Fostering Professional Nursing Standards in 1981. Her achievements include an Honorary Doctorate of Humane Letters by Alverno College (1984), honorary doctorates from Eastern Michigan University (1985) and St. Joseph's College in Maine (1999), and an *American Journal of Nursing* Book of the Year Award for *Essentials of the Roy Adaptation Model* (Andrews & Roy, 1986). Roy has been recognized in the World Who's Who of Women (1979), Personalities of America (1978), as a fellow of the American Academy of Nursing (1978), recipient of a Fulbright Senior Scholar Award from the Australian-American Educational Foundation (1989), and the Martha Rogers Award for Advancing Nursing Science from the National League for Nurses (1991). Roy received the Outstanding Alumna award and the prestigious Carondelet Medal from her alma mater, Mount Saint Mary's.

THEORETICAL SOURCES

Derivation of the Roy Adaptation Model for nursing included a citation of Harry Helson's work in psychophysics that extended to social and behavioral sciences (Roy, 1984). In Helson's adaptation theory, adaptive responses are a function of the incoming stimulus and the adaptive level (Roy, 1984). A stimulus is any factor that provokes a response. Stimuli may arise from either the internal or the external environment (Roy, 1984). The adaptation level is made up of the pooled effect of the following three classes of stimuli:

1. Focal stimuli, which immediately confront the individual
2. Contextual stimuli, which are all other stimuli present that contribute to the effect of the focal stimulus
3. Residual stimuli, environmental factors of which the effects are unclear in a given situation

Helson's work developed the concept of the adaptation level zone, which determines whether a stimulus will elicit a positive or a negative response. According to Helson's theory, adaptation is a process of responding positively to environmental changes (Roy & Roberts, 1981).

Roy (Roy & Roberts, 1981) combined Helson's work with Rapoport's definition of system to view the person as an adaptive system. With Helson's adaptation theory as a foundation, Roy (1970) developed and further refined the model with concepts and theory from Dohrenwend, Lazarus, Mechanic, and Selye. Roy gave special credit to co-authors Driever, for outlining subdivisions of self-integrity, and Martinez and Sato, for identifying common and primary stimuli affecting the modes. Other co-workers also elaborated the concepts. Poush-Tedrow and Van Landingham made contributions to the interdependence mode, and Randell made contributions to the role function mode.

After the development of her model, Roy presented it as a framework for nursing practice, research, and education (Walker & Avant, 1983). According to Roy (1971), more than 1500 faculty and students have contributed to the theoretical development of the adaptation model. By 1987, it was estimated that over 100,000 nurses in the United States and Canada had been prepared to practice using the Roy model.

In *Introduction to Nursing: An Adaptation Model*, Roy (1976a) discussed self-concept and group identity mode. She and her collaborators cited the work of Coombs and Snygg regarding self-consistency and major influencing factors of self-concept (Roy, 1984). Social interaction theories are cited to provide a theoretical basis. For example, Roy (1984) notes that Cooley indicates in Epstein's publication that self-perception is influenced by perceptions of other's responses. She points out that Mead expands the idea by hypothesizing that self-appraisal uses the generalized other. Roy builds on Sullivan's suggestion that self arises from social interaction (Roy, 1984). Gardner and Erickson support Roy's developmental approaches (Roy, 1984). The other modes—physiological-physical, role function, and interdependence—were drawn similarly from biological and behavioral sciences for an understanding of the person.

Additional development of the model occurred during the later 1900s and into the twenty-first century. These developments included updated scientific and philosophical assumptions; a redefinition of adaptation and adaptation levels; extension of the adaptive modes to group-level knowledge development; and analysis, critique, and synthesis of the first 25 years of research based on the Roy Adaptation Model. Roy agrees with other theorists who believe that changes in the person-environment systems of the earth are so extensive that a major epoch is ending (Davies, 1988; De Chardin, 1966). During the 67 million years of the Cenozoic era, the Age of Mammals and an era of great creativity, human life appeared on Earth. During this era, humankind has had little or no influence on the universe (Roy, 1997). "As the era closes, humankind has taken extensive control of the life systems of the earth. Roy claims that we are now in the position of deciding what kind of universe we will inhabit" (Roy, 1997, p. 42). Roy "has made the foci of assumptions of the twenty-first century mutual complex person and environment self-organization and a meaningful destiny of convergence of the universe, persons, and environment in what can be considered a supreme being or God" (Roy & Andrews, 1999, p. 395). According to Roy (1997), "persons are coextensive with their physical and social environments" (p. 34), and they "share a destiny with the universe and are responsible for mutual transformations" (Roy & Andrews, 1999, p. 395). Developments of the model related to the integral relationship between person and the environment have been influenced by Pierre Teilhard de Chardin's law of progressive complexity and increasing consciousness (De Chardin, 1959, 1965, 1966, 1969) and the work of Swimme and Berry (1992).

MAJOR CONCEPTS & DEFINITIONS

SYSTEM

A system is "a set of parts connected to function as a whole for some purpose and that does so by virtue of the interdependence of its parts" (Roy & Andrews, 1999, p. 32). In addition to having wholeness and related parts, "systems also have inputs, outputs, and control and feedback processes" (Andrews & Roy, 1991, p. 7).

ADAPTATION LEVEL

"Adaptation level represents the condition of the life processes described on three levels as integrated, compensatory, and compromised" (Roy & Andrews, 1999, p. 30). A person's adaptation level is "a constantly changing point, made up of focal, contextual, and residual stimuli, which represent the person's own standard of the range of stimuli to which one can respond with ordinary adaptive responses" (Roy, 1984, pp. 27-28).

ADAPTATION PROBLEMS

Adaptation problems are "broad areas of concern related to adaptation. These describe the difficulties related to the indicators of positive

Continued

MAJOR CONCEPTS & DEFINITIONS—cont'd

adaptation" (Roy & Andrews, 1999, p. 65). Roy (1984) states the following:

> It can be noted at this point that the distinction being made between adaptation problems and nursing diagnoses is based on the developing work in both of these fields. At this point, adaptation problems are seen not as nursing diagnoses, but as areas of concern for the nurse related to adapting person or group (within each adaptive mode). (pp. 89-90)

FOCAL STIMULUS

The focal stimulus is "the internal or external stimulus most immediately confronting the human system" (Roy & Andrews, 1999, p. 31).

CONTEXTUAL STIMULI

Contextual stimuli "are all other stimuli present in the situation that contribute to the effect of the focal stimulus" (Roy & Andrews, 1999, p. 31). That is, "contextual stimuli are all the environmental factors that present to the person from within or without but which are not the center of the person's attention and/or energy" (Andrews & Roy, 1991, p. 9).

RESIDUAL STIMULI

Residual stimuli "are environmental factors within or without the human system with effects in the current situation that are unclear" (Roy & Andrews, 1999, p. 32).

COPING PROCESSES

Coping processes "are innate or acquired ways of interacting with the changing environment" (Roy & Andrews, 1999, p. 31).

INNATE COPING MECHANISMS

Innate coping mechanisms "are genetically determined or common to the species and are generally viewed as automatic processes; humans do not have to think about them" (Roy & Andrews, 1999, p. 46).

ACQUIRED COPING MECHANISMS

Acquired coping mechanisms "are developed through strategies such as learning. The experiences encountered throughout life contribute to customary responses to particular stimuli" (Roy & Andrews, 1999, p. 46).

REGULATOR SUBSYSTEM

Regulator is "a major coping process involving the neural, chemical, and endocrine systems" (Roy & Andrews, 1999, p. 32).

COGNATOR SUBSYSTEM

Cognator is "a major coping process involving four cognitive-emotive channels: perceptual and information processing, learning, judgment, and emotion" (Roy & Andrews, 1999, p. 31).

ADAPTIVE RESPONSES

Adaptive responses are those "that promote integrity in terms of the goals of human systems" (Roy & Andrews, 1999, p. 31).

INEFFECTIVE RESPONSES

Ineffective responses are those "that do not contribute to integrity in terms of the goals of the human system" (Roy & Andrews, 1999, p. 31).

INTEGRATED LIFE PROCESS

Integrated life process refers to the "adaptation level at which the structures and functions of a life process are working as a whole to meet human needs" (Roy & Andrews, 1999, p. 31).

PHYSIOLOGICAL-PHYSICAL MODE

The physiological mode "is associated with the physical and chemical processes involved in the function and activities of living organisms" (Roy & Andrews, 1999, p. 102). Five needs are identified in the physiological-physical mode relative to the basic need of physiological integrity as follows: (1) oxygenation, (2) nutrition, (3) elimination, (4) activity and rest, and (5) protection. Complex

MAJOR CONCEPTS *&* DEFINITIONS—cont'd

processes that include the senses; fluid, electrolyte, and acid-base balance; neurological function; and endocrine function contribute to physiological adaptation. The basic need of the physiological mode is physiological integrity (Roy & Andrews, 1999). The physical mode is "the manner in which the collective human adaptive system manifests adaptation relative to basic operating resources, participants, physical facilities, and fiscal resources" (Roy & Andrews, 1999, p. 104). The basic need of the physical mode is operating integrity.

SELF-CONCEPT–GROUP IDENTITY MODE

The self-concept–group identity mode is one of the three psychosocial modes and "it focuses specifically on the psychological and spiritual aspects of the human system. The basic need underlying the individual self-concept mode has been identified as psychic and spiritual integrity, or the need to know who one is so that one can be or exist with a sense of unity, meaning, and purposefulness in the universe" (Roy & Andrews, 1999, p. 107). "Self-concept is defined as the composite of beliefs and feelings about oneself at a given time and is formed from internal perceptions and perceptions of others' reactions" (Roy & Andrews, 1999, p. 107). Its components include the following: (1) the physical self, which involves sensation and body image and (2) the personal self, which is made up of self-consistency, self-ideal or expectancy, and the moral-ethical-spiritual self. The group identity mode "reflects how people in groups perceive themselves based on environmental feedback. The group identity mode is comprised of interpersonal relationships, group self-image, social milieu, and culture" (Roy & Andrews, 1999, p. 108). The basic need of the group identity mode is identity integrity (Roy & Andrews, 1999).

ROLE FUNCTION MODE

The role function mode "is one of two social modes and focuses on the roles the person occupies in society. A role, as the functioning unit of society, is defined as a set of expectations about how a person occupying one position behaves toward a person occupying another position. The basic need underlying the role function mode has been identified as social integrity—the need to know who one is in relation to others so that one can act" (Hill & Roberts, 1981, pp. 109-110). Persons perform primary, secondary, and tertiary roles. These roles are carried out with both instrumental and expressive behaviors. Instrumental behavior is "the actual physical performance of a behavior" (Andrews, 1991, p. 348). Expressive behaviors are "the feelings, attitudes, likes or dislikes that a person has about a role or about the performance of a role" (Andrews, 1991, p. 348).

> The primary role determines the majority of behavior engaged in by the person during a particular period of life. It is determined by age, sex, and developmental stage. (Andrews, 1991, p. 349)

> Secondary roles are those that a person assumes to complete the task associated with a developmental stage and primary role. (Andrews, 1991, p. 349)

> Tertiary roles are related primarily to secondary roles and represent ways in which individuals meet their role associated obligations . . . . Tertiary roles are normally temporary in nature, freely chosen by the individual, and may include activities such as clubs or hobbies. (Andrews, 1991, p. 349)

The major roles that one plays can be analyzed by imagining a tree formation. The trunk of the tree is one's primary role, or developmental level such as generative adult female. Secondary roles branch off from this—for example, wife,

Continued

mother, teacher. Finally, tertiary roles branch off from secondary roles—for example, the mother role might involve the role of parent-teacher association president for a given period. Each of these roles is seen as occurring in a dyadic relationship, that is with a reciprocal role (Roy & Andrews, 1981).

INTERDEPENDENCE MODE

"The interdependence mode focuses on close relationships of people (individually and collectively) and their purpose, structure, and development. . . . Interdependent relationships involve the willingness and ability to give to others and accept from them aspects of all that one has to offer such as love, respect, value, nurturing, knowledge, skills, commitments, material possessions, time, and talents." (Roy & Andrews, 1999, p. 111)

The basic need of this mode is termed *relational integrity* (Roy & Andrews, 1999).

Two specific relationships are the focus of the interdependence mode as it applies to individuals. The first is with significant others, persons who are the most important to the individual. The second is with support systems, that is, others contributing to meeting interdependence needs. (Roy & Andrews, 1999, p. 112)

Two major areas of interdependence behaviors have been identified, receptive behavior and contributive behavior. These behaviors apply respectively to the "receiving and giving of love, respect and value in interdependent relationships" (Roy & Andrews, 1999, p. 112).

PERCEPTION

"Perception is the interpretation of a stimulus and the conscious appreciation of it" (Pollock, 1993, p.169). Perception links the regulator with the cognator and connects the adaptive modes (Rambo, 1983).

USE OF EMPIRICAL EVIDENCE

The use of the Roy Adaptation Model in nursing practice led to further clarification and refinement. A 1971 pilot research study and a survey research study from 1976 to 1977 led to some tentative confirmations of the model (Roy, 1980).

From this beginning, the Roy Adaptation Model has been supported through research in practice and in education (Brower & Baker, 1976; Farkas, 1981; Mastal & Hammond, 1980; Meleis, 1986; Roy & Obloy, 1978; Wagner, 1976). In 1999 (Roy & Andrews, 1999), a group of seven scholars working with Roy conducted an analysis, critique, and synthesis of 163 studies based on the Roy Adaptation Model that had been published in 44 English-language journals on five continents and dissertations and theses from the United States. Of the 163

studies, 116 met the criteria established for testing propositions from the model. Twelve generic propositions based on Roy's earlier work were derived. To synthesize the research, the findings of each study were used to state ancillary and practice propositions, and support for the propositions was examined. Of the 265 propositions tested, 216 (82%) were supported.

MAJOR ASSUMPTIONS

Assumptions from systems theory and assumptions from adaptation-level theory have been combined into a single set of scientific assumptions. From systems theory, human adaptive systems are viewed as interactive parts that act in unity for some purpose. Human adaptive systems are complex, multifaceted, and respond to myriad environmental stimuli to achieve adaptation. With their ability to adapt to environmental stimuli, humans have the capacity to create changes in the environment (Roy & Andrews, 1999). Drawing on characteristics of creation spirituality by Swimme and Berry (1992), Roy combined the assumptions of humanism and veritivity into a single set of philosophical assumptions. Humanism asserts that the person and human experiences are essential to knowing and valuing and that they share in creative power. Veritivity affirms the belief in the purpose, value, and meaning of all human life. These scientific and philosophical assumptions have been refined for use of the model in the twenty-first century (Box 17-1).

Adaptation

Roy has further defined adaptation for use in the twenty-first century (Roy & Andrews, 1999). According to Roy, adaptation refers to "the process and outcome whereby thinking and feeling persons as individuals or in groups, use conscious awareness and choice to create human and environmental integration" (Roy & Andrews, 1999, p. 30). Rather than a system simply striving to respond to environmental stimuli to maintain integrity, every human life is purposeful in a universe that is creative and persons are inseparable from their environment.

Nursing

Roy defines nursing broadly as a "health care profession that focuses on human life processes and patterns and emphasizes promotion of health for individuals, families, groups, and society as a whole" (Roy & Andrews, 1999, p. 4). Specifically, Roy defines nursing according to her model as the science and practice that expands adaptive abilities and enhances person and environmental transformation. She identifies nursing activities as the assessment of behavior and the stimuli that influence adaptation. Nursing judgments are based on the assessment, and interventions are planned to manage the stimuli (Roy & Andrews, 1999). Roy differentiates nursing as a science from nursing as a

Box **17-1**

Vision Basic to Concepts for the Twenty-First Century

SCIENTIFIC ASSUMPTIONS

- Systems of matter and energy progress to higher levels of complex self-organization.
- Consciousness and meaning are constitutive of person and environment integration.
- Awareness of self and environment is rooted in thinking and feeling.
- Humans, by their decisions, are accountable for the integration of creative processes.
- Thinking and feeling mediate human action.
- System relationships include acceptance, protection, and fostering of interdependence.
- Persons and the earth have common patterns and integral relationships.
- Persons and environment transformations are created in human consciousness.
- Integration of human and environment meanings results in adaptation.

PHILOSOPHICAL ASSUMPTIONS

- Persons have mutual relationships with the world and God.
- Human meaning is rooted in an omega point convergence of the universe.
- God is ultimately revealed in the diversity of creation and is the common destiny of creation.
- Persons use human creative abilities of awareness, enlightenment, and faith.
- Persons are accountable for the processes of deriving, sustaining, and transforming the universe.

From Roy, C., and Andrews, H. (1999). *The Roy Adaptation Model* (2nd ed., p. 35). Upper Saddle River, NJ: Pearson Education, Inc.

practice discipline. Nursing science is "a developing system of knowledge about persons that observes, classifies, and relates the processes by which persons positively affect their health status" (Roy, 1984, pp. 3-4). Nursing as a practice discipline is "nursing's scientific body of knowledge used for the purpose of providing an essential service to people, that is, promoting ability to affect health positively" (Roy, 1984, pp. 3-4). "Nursing acts to enhance the interaction of the person with the environment—to promote adaptation" (Andrews & Roy, 1991, p. 20).

Roy's goal of nursing is "the promotion of adaptation for individuals and groups in each of the four adaptive modes thus contributing to health, quality of life, and dying with dignity" (Roy & Andrews, 1999, p. 19). Nursing fills a unique role as a facilitator of adaptation by assessing behavior in each of these four adaptive modes and factors influencing adaptation and by intervening to promote adaptive abilities and to enhance environment interactions (Roy & Andrews, 1999).

Person

According to Roy, humans are holistic, adaptive systems. "As an adaptive system, the human system is described as a whole with parts that function as unity for some purpose. Human systems include people as individuals or in groups including families, organizations, communities, and society as a whole" (Roy & Andrews, 1999, p. 31). Despite their great diversity, all persons are united in a common destiny (Roy & Andrews, 1999). "Human systems have thinking and feeling capacities, rooted in consciousness and meaning, by which they adjust effectively to changes in the environment and, in turn, affect the environment" (Roy & Andrews, 1999, p. 36). Persons and the earth have common patterns and mutuality of relations and meaning (Roy & Andrews, 1999). Roy (Roy & Andrews, 1999) defined the person as the main focus of nursing, the recipient of nursing care, a living, complex, adaptive system with internal processes (cognator and regulator) acting to maintain adaptation in the four adaptive modes (physiological, self-concept, role function, and interdependence).

Health

"Health is a state and a process of being and becoming integrated and a whole person. It is a reflection of adaptation, that is, the interaction of the person and the environment" (Andrews & Roy, 1991, p. 21). Roy (1984) derived this definition from the thought that adaptation is a process of promoting physiological, psychological, and social integrity and that integrity implies an unimpaired condition leading to completeness or unity. In her earlier work, Roy viewed health along a continuum flowing from death and extreme poor health to high-level and peak wellness (Brower & Baker, 1976). During the late 1990s, Roy's writings focused more on health as a process in which health and illness can coexist (Roy & Andrews, 1999). Drawing on the writings of Illich (1974, 1976), Roy wrote "health is not freedom from the inevitability of death, disease, unhappiness, and stress, but the ability to cope with them in a competent way" (Roy & Andrews, 1999, p. 52).

Health and illness are one inevitable, coexistent dimension of the person's total life experience (Riehl & Roy, 1980). Nursing is concerned with this dimension. When mechanisms for coping are ineffective, illness results. Health ensues when humans continually adapt. As people adapt to stimuli, they are free to respond to other stimuli. The freeing of energy from ineffective coping attempts can promote healing and enhance health (Roy, 1984).

Environment

According to Roy, environment is "all the conditions, circumstances, and influences surrounding and affecting the development and behavior of persons or groups, with particular consideration of the mutuality of person and earth resources that includes focal, contextual, and residual stimuli" (Roy & Andrews, 1999, p. 81). "It is the changing environment [that] stimulates the person to make adaptive responses" (Andrews & Roy, 1991, p. 18). Environment is the input into the person as an adaptive system involving both internal and external factors. These factors may be slight or large, negative or positive. However, any environmental change demands increasing energy to adapt to the situation. Factors in the environment that affect the person are categorized as focal, contextual, and residual stimuli.

THEORETICAL ASSERTIONS

Roy's model focuses on the concept of adaptation of the person. Her concepts of nursing, person, health, and environment are all interrelated to this central concept. The person continually experiences environmental stimuli. Ultimately, a response is made and adaptation occurs. That adaptive response may be either an adaptive or an ineffective response. Adaptive responses promote integrity and help the person to achieve the goals of adaptation; that is, they achieve survival, growth, reproduction, mastery, and person and environmental transformations. Ineffective responses fail to achieve or threaten the goals of adaptation. Nursing has a unique goal to assist the person's adaptation effort by managing the environment. The result is attainment of an optimal level of wellness by the person (Andrews & Roy, 1986; Randell, Tedrow, & Van Landingham, 1982; Roy, 1970, 1971, 1980, 1984; Roy & Roberts, 1981).

As an open living system, the person receives inputs or stimuli from both the environment and the self. The adaptation level is determined by the combined effect of the focal, contextual, and residual stimuli. Adaptation occurs when the person responds positively to environmental changes. This adaptive response promotes the integrity of the person, which leads to health. Ineffective responses to stimuli lead to the disruption of the integrity of the person (Andrews & Roy, 1986; Randell et al., 1982; Roy, 1970, 1971, 1980; Roy & McLeod, 1981).

There are two interrelated subsystems in Roy's model (Figure 17-1). The primary, functional, or control processes subsystem consists of the regulator and the cognator. The secondary, effector subsystem consists of the following four adaptive modes: (1) physiological needs, (2) self-concept, (3) role function, and (4) interdependence (Andrews & Roy, 1986; Limandri, 1986; Mastal, Hammond, & Roberts, 1982; Meleis, 1986; Riehl & Roy, 1980; Roy, 1971, 1975).

Roy views the regulator and cognator as methods of coping. The regulator coping subsystem, by way of the physiological adaptive mode, "responds automatically through neural, chemical, and endocrine coping processes" (Andrews & Roy, 1991, p. 14). The cognator coping subsystem, by way of the self-concept, interdependence, and role function adaptive modes "responds through four cognitive-emotive channels: perceptual information processing, learning, judgment, and emotion" (Andrews & Roy, 1991, p. 14). Perception is the interpretation of a stimulus, and perception links the regulator with the cognator in that "input into the regulator is transformed into perceptions. Perception is a process of the cognator. The

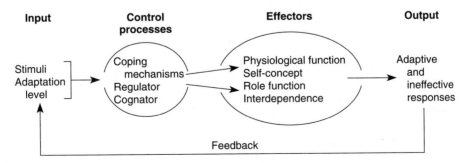

Figure **17-1 Person as an adaptive system.** (From Roy, C. [1984]. *Introduction to nursing: An adaptation model* [2nd ed., p. 30]. Englewood Cliffs, NJ: Prentice Hall.)

responses following perception are feedback into both the cognator and the regulator" (Galligan, 1979, p. 67).

The four adaptive modes of the two subsystems in Roy's model provide form or manifestations of cognator and regulator activity. Responses to stimuli are carried out through four adaptive modes. The physiological-physical adaptive mode is concerned with the way humans interact with the environment through physiological processes to meet the basic needs of oxygenation, nutrition, elimination, activity and rest, and protection. The self-concept–group identity adaptive mode is concerned with the need to know who one is and how to act in society. An individual's self-concept is defined by Roy as "the composite of beliefs or feelings that an individual holds about him or her self at any given time" (Roy & Andrews, 1999, p. 49). An individual's self-concept is comprised of the physical self (body sensation and body image) and personal self (self-consistency, self-ideal, and moral-ethical-spiritual self). The role function adaptive mode describes the primary, secondary, and tertiary roles that an individual performs in society. A role describes the expectations about how one person behaves toward another person. The interdependence adaptive mode describes the interactions of people in society. The major task of the interdependence adaptive mode is for persons to give and receive love, respect, and value. The most important components of the interdependence adaptive mode are a person's significant other (spouse, child, friend, or God) and his or her social support system. The purpose of the four adaptive modes is to achieve physiological, psychological, and social integrity. The four adaptive modes are interrelated through perception (Roy & Andrews, 1999) (Figure 17-2).

The person as a whole is made up of six subsystems. These subsystems (the regulator, cognator, and the four adaptive modes) are interrelated to form a complex system for the purpose of adaptation. Relationships among the four adaptive modes occur when internal and external stimuli affect more than one mode, when disruptive behavior occurs in more than one mode, or when one mode becomes the focal, contextual, or residual stimulus for another

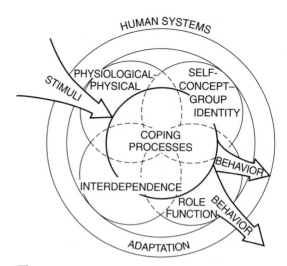

Figure 17-2 Diagrammatic representation of human adaptive systems. (From Roy, C., & Andrews, H. [1999]. *The Roy adaptation model* [2nd ed.]. Upper River Saddle, NJ: Pearson Education, Inc.)

mode (Brower & Baker, 1976; Chinn & Jacobs, 1987; Mastal & Hammond, 1980).

In regard to human social systems, Roy broadly categorizes the control processes into the stabilizer and innovator subsystems. The stabilizer system is analogous to the regulator subsystem of the individual and is concerned with stability. To maintain the system, the stabilizer subsystem involves organizational structure, cultural values, and regulation of daily activities of the system. The innovator subsystem is associated with the cognator subsystem of the individual and is concerned with creativity, change, and growth (Roy & Andrews, 1999).

LOGICAL FORM

The Roy Adaptation Model of nursing is both deductive and inductive. It is deductive in that much of Roy's theory is derived from Helson's psychophysics theory. Helson developed the concepts of focal, contextual, and residual stimuli, which Roy (1971) redefined within nursing to form a typology of factors related to adaptation levels of persons. Roy also uses other concepts and theory outside the discipline of nursing and synthesizes these within her adaptation theory.

Roy's adaptation theory is inductive in that she developed the four adaptive modes from research and nursing practice experiences of herself, her colleagues, and her students. Roy built on the conceptual framework of adaptation and developed a step-by-step model by which nurses use the nursing process to administer nursing care to promote adaptation in situations of health and illness (Roy, 1976a, 1980, 1984).

ACCEPTANCE BY THE NURSING COMMUNITY

Practice

The Roy Adaptation Model is deeply rooted in nursing practice and this, in part, contributes to its continued success (Fawcett, 2002). It remains one of the most frequently used conceptual frameworks to guide nursing practice, and it is used nationally and internationally (Roy & Andrews, 1999; Fawcett, 2005).

Roy's model is useful for nursing practice, because it outlines the features of the discipline and provides direction for practice, education, and research. The model considers goals, values, the patient, and practitioner interventions. Roy's nursing process is well developed. The two-level assessment assists in identification of nursing goals and diagnoses (Brower & Baker, 1976).

It is a valuable theory for nursing practice, because it includes a goal that is specified as the aim for activity and prescription for activities to realize the goal (Dickoff, James, & Wiedenbach, 1968a, 1968b). The goal of nursing and of the model is the person's adaptation in four adaptive modes in situations of health and illness. The prescriptions or interventions are the management of stimuli by removing, increasing, decreasing, or altering them. These prescriptions can be obtained by listing practice-related hypotheses generated by the model (Roy, 1984).

With use of Roy's six-step nursing process, the nurse performs the following six functions:

1. Assesses the behaviors manifested from the four adaptive modes
2. Assesses the stimuli for those behaviors and categorizes them as focal, contextual, or residual stimuli
3. Makes a statement or nursing diagnosis of the person's adaptive state
4. Sets goals to promote adaptation
5. Implements interventions aimed at managing the stimuli to promote adaptation
6. Evaluates whether the adaptive goals have been met

By manipulating the stimuli and not the patient, the nurse enhances "the interaction of the person with their environment, thereby promoting health" (Andrews & Roy, 1986, p. 51). The nursing process is well suited for use in a practice setting. The two-level assessment is unique to this model and leads to the identification of adaptation problems or nursing diagnoses.

Roy and colleagues have developed a typology of nursing diagnoses from the perspective of the Roy Adaptation Model (Roy, 1984; Roy & Roberts, 1981). In this typology, commonly recurring problems have been related to the basic needs of the four adaptive modes (Andrews & Roy, 1991).

Intervention is based specifically on the model, but there is a need to develop an organization of categories of nursing interventions (Roy & Roberts, 1981). Nurses provide interventions that alter, increase, decrease, remove, or maintain stimuli (Roy & Andrews, 1999). The nursing judgment model outlined by McDonald and Harms (1966) is recommended by Roy to guide selection of the best intervention for modifying a particular stimulus. According to this model, a number of alternative interventions are generated that may be appropriate for modifying the stimulus. Each possible intervention is judged for the expected consequences of modifying a stimulus, the probability that a consequence will occur (high, moderate, or low), and the value of the change (desirable or undesirable).

Senesac (2003) reviewed the literature for evidence that the Roy Adaptation Model is being implemented in nursing practice. She reported that the Roy Adaptation Model has been used to the greatest extent by individual nurses to understand, plan, and direct nursing practice in the care of individual patients. Although there are fewer examples of implementation of the adaptation model in institutional practice settings, such examples do exist. She concluded that if the model is to be implemented successfully as a practice philosophy that it should be reflected in the mission and vision statements of the institution, recruitment tools, assessment tools, nursing care plans, and other documents related to patient care.

The Roy Adaptation Model is useful in guiding nursing practice in institutional settings. It has been implemented in a neonatal intensive care unit, an acute surgical ward, a rehabilitation unit, two general hospital units, an orthopedic hospital, a neurosurgical unit, and a 145-bed hospital, among others (Roy & Andrews, 1999).

De Villers (1998) demonstrated the way in which clinical nurse specialists could use the Roy Adaptation Model to help delineate their roles as expert practitioners in the obstetrical and gynecological setting. She applied Roy's steps of the nursing process and gave specific examples or expert care from each of the adaptive modes.

The Roy Adaptation Model has been applied to the nursing care of individual groups of patients. Examples of the wide range of applications of the Roy Adaptation Model are found in the literature. Villareal (2003) applied the Roy Adaptation Model to the care of young women who were contemplating smoking cessation. The author provides a comprehensive discussion of the use of Roy's six-step nursing process to guide the nursing care for young women in their mid-20s who smoked and were members of a closed support group. The researcher performed a two-level assessment. In the first level, stimuli were identified for each of the four adaptive modes. In the second level, the nurse made a judgment about the focal (nicotine addiction), contextual (belief that smoking is enjoyable, makes them feel good, relaxes them, brings them a sense of comfort, and is part of their routine), and residual stimuli (beliefs and attitudes about their body image and that smoking cessation causes weight gain). The

nurse made the nursing diagnosis that for this group there was a lack of motivation to quit smoking related to dependency. The women in the support group and the nurse mutually established short-term goals to change behaviors, rather than the long-term goal of smoking cessation. The intervention focused on discussion of the effects of smoking on the body, reasons and beliefs about smoking and smoking cessation, stress management, nutrition, physical activity, and self-esteem. During the evaluation phase it was determined that the women had moved from precontemplation to the contemplation phase of smoking cessation. The author concluded that the Roy Adaptation Model provided a useful framework for providing care to women who smoke.

Samarel, Tulman, and Fawcett (2002) examined the effects of two types of social support (telephone and group social support) and education on adaptation to early-stage breast cancer in a sample of 125 women. Women in the experimental group received both types of social support and education ($n = 34$), while women in the first control group received only telephone support and education, and women in the second control group received only education. Mood disturbance and loneliness were reduced significantly for the experimental group and the first control group, but were not reduced for the second control group. No differences were observed among the groups for cancer-related worry or well-being. This study provides an excellent example of how to use the Roy Adaptation Model to guide the conceptualization, literature review, theory construction, and development of an intervention.

Samarel and colleagues (1999) developed a resource kit for women with breast cancer. The contents of the kit were derived from the Roy Adaptation Model. The kit contains *The Resource Manual for Women With Breast Cancer,* which collects pertinent information into one source. The manual is divided into eight chapters that are theoretically based on the four adaptive modes. It contains a variety of practice activities to reinforce the information contained in the chapters. The kit contains pamphlets, audiotapes, and videotapes that supplement the narrative in the manual.

Newman (1997a) applied the Roy Adaptation Model to caregivers of chronically ill family members. With a thorough review of the literature, Newman demonstrated how the Roy Adaptation Model can be used to provide care for this population. Newman views the chronically ill family member as the focal stimulus. Contextual stimuli include the caregiver's age, gender, and relationship to the chronically ill family member. The caregiver's physical health status is a manifestation of the physiological adaptive mode. The caregiver's emotional responses to caregiving (shock, fear, anger, guilt, increased anxiety) are effective or ineffective responses of the self-concept mode. Relationships with significant others and support indicate adaptive responses in the interdependence mode. Caregivers' primary, secondary, and tertiary roles are strained by the addition of the caregiving role. Practice and research implications illuminate the applicability of the Roy Adaptation Model for providing care to caregivers of chronically ill family members.

The Roy Adaptation Model has been applied to the care of persons with chronic renal failure who require hemodialysis (Keen et al. 1998), women in menopause (Cunningham, 2002), and to the assessment of an elderly man undergoing a right, below-the-knee amputation. The Roy Adaptation Model has been applied to the care of adolescents with asthma (Hennessy-Harstad, 1999) and inflammatory bowel disease (Decker, 2000) and a 10-month-old child with tracheomalacia (Lankester & Sheldon, 1999). Cook (1999) delineates nursing assessment related to the self-concept of cancer patients and provides specific interventions to promote adaptation in this group of patients.

Araich (2001) uses a case study to illustrate how theory can be integrated into a cardiac care unit. In this effort, Araich conducts a two-level assessment and describes possible nursing interventions to promote adaptation of persons in cardiac care. Dixon (1999) demonstrates how community health nursing can be guided by the Roy Adaptation Model.

Education

The Roy Adaptation Model defines the distinct purpose of nursing for students, which is to promote adaptation of persons in each of the adaptive modes in situations of health and illness. The model also distinguishes nursing science from medical science by having the content of these areas taught in separate courses. She stresses collaboration but delineates separate goals for nurses and physicians. According to Roy (1971), it is the nurse's goal to help the patient put his or her energy into getting well, whereas the medical student focuses on the patient's position on the health-illness continuum with the goal of causing movement along the continuum. She views the model as a valuable tool to analyze the distinctions between the two professions of nursing and medicine. Roy (1979) believes that curricula based on this model help in theory development by the students, who also learn how to test theories and recognize new theoretical insights. Roy (1971) suggests that the model clarifies objectives, identifies content, and specifies patterns for teaching and learning.

The adaptation model has been useful in the educational setting and had guided nursing education at Mount Saint Mary's College Department of Nursing in Los Angeles since 1970. As early as 1987, more than 100,000 student nurses had been educated in nursing programs based on the Roy Adaptation Model in the United States and abroad. The Roy Adaptation Model provides educators with a systematic way of teaching students to assess and care for patients within the context of their lives rather than just as victims of illness.

Dobratz (2003) evaluated the learning outcomes of a nursing research course designed from the perspective of the Roy Adaptation Model. The author describes in some detail the theoretical content of the course that was taught to students in a senior nursing research course. The evaluation tool was a Likert-type scale that contained seven statements. Students were asked to disagree, agree, or strongly agree with seven statements. Four open-ended questions were included to elicit information from the students about the most helpful learning activity, the least helpful learning activity, methods used by the instructor that enhanced learning and grasp of research, and what the instructor could have done to increase learning. The researcher concluded that a research course based on the Roy Adaptation Model helped students to put the pieces of the research puzzle together. A future study would be strengthened by the inclusion of a control or comparison group.

Research

If research is to affect practitioners' behavior, it must be directed toward testing and retesting theories derived from conceptual models for nursing practice. Roy (1984) has stated that theory development and the testing of developed theories are the highest priorities for nursing. The model generates many testable hypotheses that need to be researched.

Roy's theory has generated a number of general propositions. From these general propositions, specific hypotheses can be developed and tested. Hill and Roberts (1981) have demonstrated the development of testable hypotheses from the model, as has Roy. Data to validate or support the model are created by the testing of such hypotheses; the model continues to generate more of this type of research. The Roy Adaptation Model has been used extensively to guide knowledge development through nursing research (Frederickson, 2000).

Roy (1970) has identified a set of concepts forming a model from which the process of observation and classification of facts would lead to postulates. The postulates concern the occurrence of adaptation problems, coping mechanisms, and interventions based on laws derived from factors making up the response potential of the focal, contextual, and residual stimuli. Roy and colleagues have outlined a typology of adaptation problems or nursing diagnoses (Roy, 1973, 1975, 1976b). Research and testing are needed in the area of typology and categories of interventions that have been derived from the model. General propositions that need to be tested have also been developed (Roy & McLeod, 1981).

Practice-based research. DiMattio and Tulman (2003) described changes in functional status and correlates of functional status of 61 women during the 6-week postoperative period following a coronary artery bypass graft. Functional status was measured at 2, 4, and 6 weeks after surgery, using the Inventory of Functional Status in the Elderly and the Sickness Impact Profile. Significant increases were found in all dimensions of functional status except personal at the three measurement points. The greatest increases in functional status occurred between 2 and 4 weeks after surgery. However, none of the dimensions of functional status had returned to the baseline values at the 6-week point. This information will help women who have undergone coronary artery bypass graft surgery to better understand the recovery period and to set more realistic goals.

Young-McCaughan and colleagues (2003) studied the effects of a structured aerobic exercise program on exercise tolerance, sleep patterns, and quality of life in patients with cancer from the perspective of the Roy Adaptation Model. The subjects exercised for 20 minutes, twice a week, for 12 weeks. Significant improvements in exercise tolerance, subjective sleep quality, and psychological and physiological quality of life were demonstrated.

Yeh (2002) tested the Roy Adaptation Model in a sample of 116 Taiwanese boys and girls with cancer (7 to 18 years of age at the time of diagnosis). Two of Roy's propositions were tested. The first proposition is that environmental stimuli (severity of illness, age, gender, understanding of illness, and communication with others) influence biopsychosocial responses (health-related quality of life [HRQOL]). The second proposition is that the four adaptive modes are interrelated. Using structural equation modeling, the researcher found that severity of illness provided an excellent fit with stage of illness, laboratory values (white blood cell count, hemoglobin, platelets, absolute neutrophil count), and the total number of hospitalizations. Although it is not altogether clear how the focal and contextual stimuli were defined, this study showed that environmental stimuli (severity of illness, age, gender, understanding of illness, and communication with others) influence the biopsychosocial adaptive responses of children to cancer. Finally, this study demonstrated the interrelatedness of the physiological (physical HRQOL), self-concept (disease and symptoms HRQOL), interdependence (social HRQOL), and role function (cognitive HRQOL) adaptive modes.

Woods and Isenberg (2001) provide an example of theory synthesis. In their study of intimate abuse and traumatic stress in battered women, they developed a middle range theory by synthesizing the Roy Adaptation Model with current literature related to intimate abuse and posttraumatic stress disorder. A predictive correlational model was used to examine adaptation as a mediator of intimate abuse and posttraumatic stress disorder. The focal stimulus of this study was the severity of intimate abuse, emotional abuse, and risk of homicide by an intimate partner. Adaptation was operationalized within the four adaptive modes and tested as a mediator between intimate abuse and posttraumatic stress disorder. Direct relationships were detected between the focal stimulus and intimate abuse, and adaptation in each of the four modes mediated the relationships between the focal stimulus and traumatic stress.

Chiou (2000) conducted a meta-analysis of the interrelationships among Roy's four adaptive modes. Using well-defined inclusion and exclusion criteria, a literature search of the *Cumulative Index to Nursing and Allied Health Literature* yielded eight research reports with diverse samples. One in-press report was included. The convenience samples for the nine studies included only adults, some of whom were elderly. The meta-analysis revealed small to medium correlations between each two-mode set, except for a nonsignificant association between the interdependence and physiological modes. The small to moderate relationships provide support that the four adaptive modes are related but independent.

Zhan (2000) found support for Roy's proposition that cognitive adaptive processes help maintain self-consistency. Using Roy's Cognitive Adaptation Processing Scale (Roy & Zhan, 2001) to measure cognitive adaptation and the Self-Consistency Scale (Zhan & Shen, 1994), Zhan found that cognitive adaptation plays an important role in helping older adults maintain self-consistency in the face of hearing loss. Self-consistency was higher for hearing impaired men than for hearing impaired women, but it did not vary for age, educational level, race, marital status, or income.

Nuamah, Cooley, Fawcett, and McCorkle (1999) studied quality of life in 515 cancer patients. The researchers clearly established theoretical linkages among the concepts of the Roy Adaptation Model, the middle range theory concepts, and the empirical indicators. Focal and contextual stimuli were identified. Variables in each of the adaptive modes were operationalized. Using structural equation modeling, the researchers found that two of the environmental stimuli (adjuvant cancer treatment and severity of the disease) explained 59% of the variance in the biopsychosocial indicators of the latent variable health-related quality of life. Their findings supported the proposition of the Roy Adaptation Model that environmental stimuli influence biopsychosocial responses.

Samarel and colleagues (1999) used the Roy Adaptation Model to study women's perceptions of adaptation to breast cancer in a sample of 70 women who were participating in an experimental support and education group. The experimental group received coaching; the control group received no coaching. Using quantitative content analysis of structured telephone interviews, the researchers found that 51 of 70 women (72.9%) experienced a positive change toward their breast cancer over the study period, which was indicative of adaptation to the breast cancer. The researchers report qualitative indicators of adaptation for each of Roy's four adaptive modes.

Modrcin-Talbott and colleagues have studied self-esteem from the perspective of the Roy Adaptation Model in 140 well adolescents (Modrcin-Talbott, Pullen, Ehrenberger, Zandstra, & Muenchen, 1998) and 77 adolescents in an outpatient mental health setting (Modrcin-Talbott, Pullen, Zandstra, Ehrenberger, & Muenchen, 1998). Well adolescents were grouped in early (12 to 14 years), middle (15 to 16 years), or late adolescence (17 to 19 years). Well adolescents were conveniently recruited from a large, southeastern church. Self-esteem in well adolescents did not differ by age group, gender, or whether or not they smoked tobacco. Well adolescents who exercised regularly did score higher on self-esteem. Significant negative relationships were found between self-esteem and depression, state anger, trait anger, anger-in, anger-out, anger control, and anger expression. In the second study, the adolescents were sampled from participants of regularly scheduled group sessions as part of an outpatient psychiatric treatment program. Self-esteem significantly differed by age group, with older adolescents scoring lowest on self-esteem. Self-esteem did not differ by gender or whether or not they smoked tobacco. A significant negative relationship was observed between self-esteem and depression. Unlike their study in well adolescents, no statistically significant relationship was found between self-esteem and the dimensions of anger. Self-esteem was not significantly related to parental alcohol use in either group.

Modrcin-Talbott, Harrison, Groer, and Younger (2003) tested the effects of gentle human touch on the biobehavioral adaptation of preterm infants based on the Roy Adaptation Model. According to Roy, infants are born with two adaptive modes, the physiological and interdependence modes. Premature infants often are deprived of human touch, and an environment filled with machines, noxious stimuli, and invasive procedures surrounds them. These researchers found that gentle human touch (focal stimulus) promotes physiological adaptation for premature infants. Heart rate, oxygen saturation stability, increased quiet sleep, less active sleep and drowsiness, decreased motor activity, increased time not moving, and decreased behavioral distress cues were identified as effective responses in the physiological adaptive mode. This study supports Roy's conceptualization of adaptation in infants.

Gallagher (1998) conducted a pilot study to discern if a relationship exists between urogenital distress and the psychosocial impact of urinary incontinence in 17 elderly women. The researcher found significant relationships between urogenital distress and physical activity, social relationships, and travel, which are dimensions of the psychosocial impact of urinary incontinence. Although the findings are inconclusive because there was a small sample size, the study was framed well in the Roy Adaptation Model and provided important information for future studies.

The University of Montreal Research Team in Nursing Science (Ducharme, Ricard, Duquette, Levesque, & Lachance, 1998; Levesque, Ricard, Ducharme, Duquette, & Bonin, 1998) is studying adaptation to a variety of environmental stimuli. Four groups of individuals were included in their studies as follows: (1) informal family caregivers of a demented relative at home, (2) informal family caregivers of a psychiatrically ill relative at home, (3) nurses as professional caregivers in geriatric institutions, and (4) aged spouses in the community. Using linear structural relations (LISREL), perceived stress (focal stimulus), social support (contextual stimulus), and passive and avoidance coping (coping mechanism) were directly or indirectly linked to psychological distress. This finding supports Roy's proposition that coping promotes adaptation.

Bournaki (1997) studied pain-related responses to venipuncture in school-age children from the perspective of the Roy Adaptation Model. Based on Roy's assumption that "adaptive behavior is a function of the stimulus and adaptation level, that is, the pooled effects of the focal, contextual, and residual stimuli" (Roy & Corliss, 1993, p. 217), Bournaki tested the hypothesis that age, gender, past painful experiences, temperament, medical fears, general fears, and childrearing practices are related to pain location, pain intensity, pain quality, observed behaviors, and heart rate. The findings of this study provided partial support for Roy's proposition that focal and contextual stimuli influence adaptive responses. In this study, pain related to venipuncture was the focal stimulus, and age, gender, past painful experiences, temperament, medical fears, general fears, and childrearing practices were contextual stimuli. Canonical correlation revealed that age (developmental stage), medical fears (self-concept), and two dimensions of temperament, (1) distractibility and (2) threshold (parent-child interdependence), were related to pain quality, behavioral responses, and heart rate responses. Gender was related to behavioral responses, in that girls cried more often than boys.

Development of adaptation research instruments. The Roy Adaptation Model has provided the theoretical basis for the development of a number of research instruments. Newman (1997b) developed the Inventory of Functional Status—Caregiver of a Child in a Body Cast to measure the extent to which parental caregivers continue their usual activities while a child is in a body cast. Reliability testing indicates that the subscales for household, social, and community childcare of the child in a body cast, childcare of other children, and personal care (rather than the total score) are reliable measures of these constructs. Modrcin-McCarthy, McCue, and Walker (1997) used the Roy Adaptation Model to develop a clinical tool that may be used to identify actual and potential stressors of fragile premature infants and to implement care for them. This tool measures the signs of stress, touch interventions, reduction of pain, environmental considerations, state, and stability (STRESS).

Development of middle range theories of adaptation. Silva (1986) has pointed out that using a conceptual framework for a research study is not theory testing. Many researchers who used Roy's model did not actually test propositions or hypotheses of her model but have provided face validity for its usefulness as a framework to guide their studies. Theory derived from a conceptual framework must be made explicit; therefore, the need is for the development and testing of middle range theories derived from the Roy Adaptation Model. Some research of this nature has been conducted on the model, but more is needed for further validation and development of new areas. The model does generate many testable hypotheses related to both practice and nursing theory. The success of a conceptual framework is evaluated, in part, by the number and quality of middle range theories it generates. The Roy Adaptation Model has been the theoretical source for a number of middle range theories.

Dunn (2004) used theoretical substruction to derive a middle range theory of adaptation to chronic pain from the Roy Adaptation Model. In Dunn's model of adaptation to chronic pain, pain intensity is specified as the focal stimulus. Contextual stimuli include age, race, and gender. Religious and nonreligious coping are functions of the cognator subsystem. Manifestations of adaptation to chronic pain are its effects on functional ability and psychological and spiritual well-being.

Frame, Kelly, and Bayley (2003) developed the Frame theory of adolescent empowerment by synthesizing the Roy Adaptation Model, Murrell-Armstrong's empowerment matrix, and Harter's developmental perspective. The theory of adolescent empowerment was tested using a quasi-experimental design in which children diagnosed with attention deficit–hyperactivity disorder (ADHD) were randomly assigned to a treatment or a control group. Ninety-two fifth and sixth grade students were assigned to either the treatment or control group. Children in the treatment group attended an eight-session, school nurse–led, support group intervention (twice weekly for 4 weeks). The treatment was designed to teach the children about ADHD, the gifts of having ADHD, powerlessness versus empowerment, empowerment with one's feelings, teachers, family, and classmates, and how to learn to relax. Children in the control group received no intervention. Using analysis of covariance, the children in the treatment group reported significantly higher perceived social acceptance, perceived athletic competence, perceived physical appearance, and perceived global self-worth.

Jirovec, Jenkins, Isenberg, and Baiardi (1999) have proposed a middle range urine control theory derived from the Roy Adaptation Model, intended to explicate the phenomenon of urine control and to decrease urinary incontinence. According to the theory of urine control, the focal stimulus for urine control is bladder distention. Contextual stimuli include accessible facilities and mobility skills. A residual stimulus is the intense socialization about bladder and sanitary habits that begin in childhood. This theory takes into account the physiological coping mechanisms, regulator (spinal reflex mediated by S2 to S4, and coordinated detrusor muscle contraction and sphincter relaxation) and cognator (perception, learning judgment, and awareness of urgency or dribbling). Adaptive responses to prevent urinary incontinence are described for the four adaptive modes. Effective adaptation is defined as continence and ineffective adaptation is defined as incontinence. The authors provide limited support for the theory of urine control through case studies. The theory of urine control illuminates the complexity, multidimensionality, and holistic nature of adaptation.

Researchers at the University of Montreal have proposed a middle range theory of adaptation to caregiving that is based on the Roy Adaptation Model. This middle range theory has been tested in a number of published studies of informal caregivers of demented relatives at home, informal caregivers of psychiatrically ill relatives at home, professional caregivers of elderly institutionalized patients, and aged spouses in the community. Perceived stress is conceptualized as the focal stimulus. Contextual stimuli include gender, conflicts, and social support. Coping mechanisms include active, passive, and avoidant coping strategies. In this middle range theory, the adaptive (nonadaptive) response (psychological distress) is manifested in the self-concept mode. LISREL analyses have provided support for many of the propositions of this middle range theory of adaptation to caregiving and for the Roy Adaptation Model (Ducharme et al., 1998; Levesque et al., 1998).

Tsai, Tak, Moore, and Palencia (2003) derived a middle range theory of pain from the Roy Adaptation Model. In the theory of chronic pain, chronic pain is the focal stimulus, disability and social support are contextual stimuli, and age and gender are residual stimuli. Perceived daily stress is a coping process. Depression is an outcome variable manifested in all four adaptive modes. Path analysis provided partial support for the theory of chronic pain. Greater chronic pain and disability were associated with greater daily stress, and greater social support was associated with less daily stress. These three variables accounted for 35% of the variance in daily stress. Greater daily stress explained 35% of the variance in depression.

Other middle range theories derived from the Roy Adaptation Model have been proposed, but research reports testing the theories were not found at the time of this literature review. Tsai (2003) has proposed a middle range theory of caregiver stress. Whittemore and Roy (2002) developed a middle range theory of adapting to diabetes mellitus using theory synthesis. Based on an analysis of Pollock's (1993) middle range theory of chronic illness and a thorough review of the literature, reconceptualization of the chronic illness model and the addition of concepts such as self-management, integration, and health-within-illness more specifically extend the Roy Adaptation Model to adapting to diabetes mellitus.

FURTHER DEVELOPMENT

The Roy Adaptation Model is an approach to nursing that has made and continues to make a significant contribution to the body of nursing knowledge, but a few areas remain for development of the model. A more thoroughly defined typology of nursing diagnoses and an organization of categories of interventions would facilitate its use in nursing practice. Overlap in the psychosocial categories of self-concept, role function, and interdependence continues to be noted by scientists who do research from the perspective of the Roy Adaptation Model. Roy recently has redefined health, deemphasizing the concept of a health-illness continuum and conceptualizing health as integration and wholeness of the person. This approach incorporates the adaptive mechanisms of the comatose patient in response to tactile and verbal stimuli more clearly. However, because health was not conceptualized in this manner in the earlier work, this opens up a new area for research. Following an integrative review of the literature, Frederickson (2000) concluded that there is good empirical support for Roy's conceptualization of person and health. She made the following recommendations for future research. First, there is a need to design studies to test propositions related to environment and nursing. Second, interventions based on the concepts and propositions that have been supported previously should be tested.

CRITIQUE
Clarity

According to Chinn and Jacobs, "clarity requires the semantic and structural organization of goals, assumptions, concepts, definitions, relationships, and structure into a logically coherent whole" (Chinn & Jacobs, 1987, p. 140). In an early critique of the Roy Adaptation Model, Duldt and Giffin (1985) stated that Roy's arrangement of concepts is logical, but that the development of definitions is inadequate related to her original format. Terms and concepts borrowed from other disciplines are not redefined for nursing. Roy's theory examples tend to use a biopsychosocial set as the principle for organizing rather than the adaptive modes and the internal processors. One limitation Duldt and Giffin cited is that Roy claimed to follow a holistic view, but omitted spiritual, humanistic, and existential aspects of being a person. Instead, "man is defined as a survival-oriented, behaviorist (condition-response), amoral, living system" (Duldt & Giffin, 1985, p. 246).

In recent writings, Roy has acknowledged the holistic nature of persons who exist in a universe that is "progressing in structure, organization, and complexity. Rather than a system acting to maintain itself, the emphasis shifts to the purposefulness of human existence in a universe that is creative" (Roy & Andrews, 1999, p. 35). Roy contends that persons have mutual, integral, and simultaneous relationships with the universe and God and that as humans they "use their creative abilities of awareness, enlightenment, and faith in the processes of deriving, sustaining, and transforming the universe" (Roy & Andrews, 1999, p. 35). Using these creative abilities, persons (sick or well) are active participants in their care and are able to achieve a higher level of adaptation (health).

Mastal and Hammond (1980) discussed difficulties with Roy's model in classifying certain behaviors because concept definitions overlapped. The problem dealt with theory conceptualization and the need for mutually exclusive categories to classify human behavior. Conceptualizing a person's position on the health-illness continuum is no longer a problem because Roy redefined health as personal integration. Other researchers have referred to difficulty in classifying behavior exclusively in one adaptive mode (Bradley & Williams, 1990; Limandri, 1986; Nyqvist & Sjoden, 1993; Silva, 1987). However, this observation supports Roy's proposition that behavior in one adaptive mode affects and is affected by the other modes.

Simplicity

The Roy model includes the concepts of nursing, person, health-illness, environment, adaptation, and nursing activities. It also includes two subconcepts (regulator and cognator) and four effector modes (physiological, self-concept, role function, and interdependence). This model has several major concepts and subconcepts; therefore, it has numerous relational statements and is complex.

Generality

Roy (1984) defines her model as drawn from multiple middle range theories and advocates multiple middle range theories for use in nursing. Middle range theories are testable and have sufficient generality to be scientifically interesting (Walker & Avant, 1983). The Roy Adaptation Model's broad scope is an advantage, because it may be used for other theory building and testing in studying smaller ranges of phenomena (Reynolds, 1971). Roy's model (Roy & Corliss, 1993) is generalizable to all settings in nursing practice, but it is limited in scope because it primarily addresses the concept of person-environment adaptation and focuses primarily on the patient. Information on the nurse is implied.

Empirical Precision

Increasing complexity within theories often helps increase empirical precision. When subcomponents are designated within the theory, the empirical precision increases, assuming the broad concepts are based in reality (Chinn & Jacobs, 1987).

Roy's broad concepts stem from theory in physiological psychology, psychology, sociology, and nursing; empirical data indicate that this general theory base has substance. Roy's model offers direction for researchers who want to incorporate physiological phenomena in their studies. Roy (1980) studied and analyzed 500 samples of patient behaviors collected by nursing students. From this analysis, Roy proposed her four adaptive modes in humans.

Roy (Roy & McLeod, 1981; Roy & Roberts, 1981) identifies many propositions in relation to the regulator and cognator mechanisms and the self-concept, role function, and interdependence modes. These propositions have varying degrees of support from general theory and empirical data. Most of the propositions are relational statements and can be tested (Tiedeman, 1983). Over the years, many testable hypotheses have been derived from the model (Hill & Roberts, 1981).

The greatest needs to increase empirical precision of the Roy Adaptation Model are for researchers to continue to build middle range theory based on the Roy Adaptation Model and to develop empirical referents specifically designed to measure concepts proposed in the derived theory. Roy has explicated a great number of propositions, theorems, and axioms that serve well in the development of middle range theory. The holistic nature of the model serves well for nurse researchers who are interested in the complex reaction between physiological and psychosocial adaptive processes.

Derivable Consequences

Derivable consequences refer to how practically useful, important, and generally sufficient the theory is in relation to achieving valued nursing outcomes. The theory needs to guide research and practice, generate ideas, and differentiate the focus of nursing from other service professions (Chinn & Jacobs, 1987).

The Roy Adaptation Model has a clearly defined nursing process and can be useful in guiding clinical practice. The model provides direction in providing nursing care that addresses the holistic needs of the patient. The model is also capable of generating new information through the testing of the hypotheses that have been derived from it (Roy & Corliss, 1993; Smith, Garvis, & Martinson, 1983).

SUMMARY

The Roy Adaptation Model has greatly influenced the profession of nursing. It is one of the most frequently used models to guide nursing research, education, and practice. The model is taught as part of the curriculum of most baccalaureate, master's, and doctoral programs of nursing. The influence of the Roy Adaptation Model on nursing research is evidenced by the number of qualitative and quantitative research studies it has guided. The Roy Adaptation Model has inspired the development of many middle range nursing theories and the development of adaptation instruments. Sister Callista Roy continues to refine the adaptation model for nursing research, education, and practice.

According to Roy, persons are holistic adaptive systems and the focus of nursing. The internal and external environment consists of all phenomena that surround the human adaptive system and affect their development and behavior. Persons are in constant interaction with the environment and exchange information, matter, and energy; that is, persons affect and are affected by the environment. The environment is the source of stimuli that either threaten or promote a person's existence. For survival, the human adaptive system must respond positively to environmental stimuli. Humans make effective or ineffective adaptive responses to environmental stimuli. Adaptation promotes survival, growth, reproduction, mastery, and transformations of persons and the environment. Roy defines health as a state of becoming an integrated and whole human being.

Three types of environmental stimuli are described in the Roy Adaptation Model. The focal stimulus is that which most immediately confronts the individual and demands the most attention and adaptive energy. Contextual are all other stimuli present in the situation that contribute positively or negatively to the strength of the focal stimulus. Residual stimuli affect the focal stimulus, but their effects are not readily known. These three types of stimuli together form the adaptation level. A person's adaptation level may be integrated, compensatory, or compromised.

Coping mechanisms refer to innate or acquired processes that a person uses to deal with environmental stimuli. Coping mechanisms may be categorized broadly as the regulator or cognator subsystem. The regulator subsystem responds automatically through innate neural, chemical, and endocrine coping processes. The cognator subsystem responds through innate and acquired cognitive-emotive processes that include perceptual and information processing, learning, judgment, and emotion.

Behaviors that manifest adaptation can be observed in four adaptive modes. The physiological mode refers to the person's physical responses to the environment, and the underlying need is physiological integrity. The self-concept mode refers to a person's thoughts, beliefs, or feelings about himself or herself at any given time. The basic need of the self-concept mode is psychic or spiritual integrity. The self-concept is a composite belief about self that is formed from internal perceptions and the perceptions of others. The self-concept is comprised of the physical self (body sensation and body image) and the personal self (self-consistency, self-ideal, and the moral-ethical-spiritual self). The role function mode refers to the primary, secondary, and tertiary roles a person performs in society.

The basic need of the role function adaptive mode is social integrity or for one to know how to behave and what is expected of him or her in society. The interdependence adaptive mode refers to relationships among people. The basic need of the interdependence adaptive mode is social integrity or to give and receive love, respect, and value from significant others and social support systems (Table 17-1).

The goal of nursing is to promote adaptive responses. This is accomplished through a six-step nursing process: assessment of behavior, assessment of stimuli, nursing diagnosis, goal setting, intervention, and evaluation. Nursing interventions focus on managing environmental stimuli by "altering, increasing, decreasing, removing, or maintaining them" (Roy & Andrews, 1999, p. 86).

Table 17-1

Overview of the Adaptive Modes		
SUBSYSTEM	**ADAPTIVE MODE**	**COPING NEED**
REGULATOR Neural Chemical Endocrine	PHYSIOLOGICAL The physiological adaptive mode refers to the way a person, as a physical being, responds to and interacts with the internal and external environment **Basic need:** Physiological integrity	**Oxygenation:** To maintain appropriate oxygenation through ventilation, gas exchange, and gas transport **Nutrition:** To maintain function, promote growth, and to replace tissue through ingestion and assimilation of food **Elimination:** To excrete metabolic wastes primarily through the intestines and kidney **Activity and rest:** To maintain a balance between physical activity and rest **Protection:** To defend the body against infection, trauma, and temperature changes primarily by way of integumentary structures and innate and acquired immunity

Continued

Table 17-1

	Overview of the Adaptive Modes—cont'd	
SUBSYSTEM	**ADAPTIVE MODE**	**COPING NEED**
		Senses: To enable persons to interact with their environment by sight, hearing, touch, taste, and smell
		Fluid and electrolyte and acid-base balance: To maintain homeostatic fluid, electrolyte, and acid-base balance to promote cellular, extracellular, and systemic function
		Neurological function: To coordinate and control body movements, consciousness, and cognitive-emotional processes
		Endocrine function: To integrate and coordinate body functions
COGNATOR	SELF-CONCEPT	PHYSICAL SELF
	The self-concept adaptive mode refers to the psychological and spiritual characteristics of a person	**Body sensation:** To maintain a positive feeling about one's physical being (i.e., physical functioning, sexuality, or health)
	The self-concept consists of the composite of a person's feelings about himself or herself at any given time	**Body image:** To maintain a positive view of one's physical body and physical appearance
	The self-concept is formed from internal perceptions and the perceptions of others' reactions	PERSONAL SELF
		Self-consistency: To maintain consistent self-organization and to avoid dysequilibrium
	The self-concept has two major dimensions: the physical self and the personal self	**Self-ideal or self-expectancy:** To maintain a positive or hopeful view of what one is, what one expects to be, and what one hopes to do
	Basic need: Psychic and spiritual integrity	**Moral-spiritual-ethical self:** To maintain a positive evaluation of who one is
	INTERDEPENDENCE	To maintain close, nurturing relationships with people who are willing to give and receive love, respect, and value
	Basic need: Relational integrity or security in nurturing relationships	To know who one is and what society's expectations are so that one can act appropriately within society
	ROLE FUNCTION	
	Basic need: Social integrity	

Meleis (1986) asserts that there are three types of nursing theorists, as follows:

1. Those who focus on needs
2. Those who focus on interaction
3. Those who focus on outcome

The Roy Adaptation Model is classified as an outcome theory, defined by Meleis (1986) as "a well-articulated conception of man as a nursing client and of nursing as an external regulatory mechanism" (p. 180). Roy, in applying the concepts of system and adaptation to person as the patient of nursing, has presented her articulation of the person for nurses to use as a tool in practice, education, and research. Her conceptions of person and of the nursing process contribute to the science and the art of nursing. The Roy Adaptation Model deserves further study and development by nursing educators, researchers, and practitioners.

Case Study

A 23-year-old male patient is admitted with a fracture of C6 and C7 that has resulted in quadriplegia. He was injured during a football game at the university where he is currently a senior. His career as quarterback had been very promising. At the time of the injury, contract negotiations were in progress with a leading professional football team.

1. Use Roy's criteria to identify focal and contextual stimuli for each of the four adaptive modes.
2. Consider what adaptations would be necessary in each of the following four adaptive modes: (1) physiological, (2) self-concept, (3) interdependence, and (4) role function.
3. Create an intervention for each of the adaptive modes that will promote adaptation.

CRITICAL THINKING *Activities*

1. Karen, a recent graduate from a nursing program based on the Roy Adaptation Model, is performing her morning assessments. She enters Mr. Shadeed's room. Mr. Shadeed is awaiting preoperative preparation for a laparotomy to explore an unknown mass. Mr. Shadeed is very irritable this morning. He says that he is thirsty. Karen continues her assessment of Mr. Shadeed. What further data will she need from each of the four adaptive modes before implementing nursing interventions? What are the focal stimuli, contextual stimuli, and residual stimuli? What is the nursing diagnosis? What are possible interventions? What process can Karen use to select the best nursing intervention?

2. Although it would be easy to assume that Mr. Shadeed's nursing care needs stem from anxiety during the preoperative period, this assumption may or may not be true. Assessment of stimuli in each of the four adaptive modes will enable Karen to assess the focal, contextual, and residual stimuli and come to the correct diagnosis. Identify the additional assessment data Karen will need to collect for each of the following adaptive modes.
   - Physiological adaptive mode
   - Self-concept adaptive mode
   - Role function adaptive mode
   - Interdependence adaptive mode

REFERENCES

Sr. Callista Roy to assume nurse theorist post at Boston College (1987). *Nursing and Health Care, 8,* 536.

Andrews, H. (1991). Overview of the role function mode. In C. Roy & H. Andrews (Eds.), *The Roy adaptation model: The definitive statement* (pp. 347-361). Norwalk, CT: Appleton & Lange.

Andrews, H., & Roy, C. (1986). *Essentials of the Roy adaptation model.* Norwalk, CT: Appleton-Century-Crofts.

Andrews, H., & Roy, C. (1991). Essentials of the Roy adaptation model. In C. Roy & H. Andrews (Eds.), *The Roy adaptation model: The definitive statement* (pp. 3-25). Norwalk, CT: Appleton & Lange.

Araich, M. (2001). Roy's adaptation model: Demonstration of theory integration into process of care in coronary care unit. *ICUs and Nursing Web Journal, 7,* 1-12.

Bournaki, M. C. (1997). Correlates of pain-related responses to venipunctures in school-age children. *Nursing Research, 46,* 147-154.

Bradley, K. M., & Williams, D. M. (1990). A comparison of the preoperative concerns of open heart surgery patients and their significant others. *Journal of Cardiovascular Nursing, 5,* 43-53.

Brower, H. T., & Baker, B. J. (1976). The Roy adaptation model. Using the adaptation model in a practitioner curriculum. *Nursing Outlook, 24,* 686-689.

Chinn, P., & Jacobs, M. K. (1987). *Theory and nursing: A systematic approach.* St. Louis: Mosby.

Chiou, C. P. (2000). A meta-analysis of the interrelationships between the modes in Roy's adaptation model. *Nursing Science Quarterly, 13,* 252-258.

Cook, N. F. (1999). Self-concept and cancer: Understanding the nursing role. *British Journal of Nursing, 8,* 318-324.

Cunningham, D. A. (2002). Application of Roy's adaptation model when caring for a group of women coping with menopause. *Journal of Community Health Nursing, 19,* 49-60.

Davies, P. (1988). *The cosmic blueprint.* New York: Simon & Schuster.

De Chardin, P. T. (1959). *The phenomenon of man.* New York: Harper & Row.

De Chardin, P. T. (1965). *Hymn of the universe.* New York: Harper & Row.

De Chardin, P. T. (1966). *Man's place in nature.* New York: Harper & Row.

De Chardin, P. T. (1969). *Human energy.* New York: Harper & Row.

Decker, J. W. (2000). The effects of inflammatory bowel disease on adolescents. *Gastroenterology Nursing, 23,* 63-66.

De Villers, M. J. (1998). The clinical nurse specialist as expert practitioner in the obstetrical/gynecological setting. *Clinical Nurse Specialist, 12,* 193-199.

Dickoff, J., James, P., & Wiedenbach, E. (1968a). Theory in a practice discipline. I. Practice oriented discipline. *Nursing Research, 17,* 415-435.

Dickoff, J., James, P., & Wiedenbach, E. (1968b). Theory in a practice discipline. II. Practice oriented research. *Nursing Research, 17,* 545-554.

DiMattio, M. J., & Tulman, L. (2003). A longitudinal study of functional status and correlates following coronary artery bypass graft surgery in women. *Nursing Research, 52,* 98-107.

Dixon, E. L. (1999). Community health nursing practice and the Roy adaptation model. *Public Health Nursing, 16,* 290-300.

Dobratz, M. C. (2003). Putting the pieces together: Teaching undergraduate research from a theoretical perspective. *Journal of Advanced Nursing, 41,* 383-392.

Ducharme, F., Ricard, N., Duquette, A., Levesque, L., & Lachance, L. (1998). Empirical testing of a longitudinal model derived from the Roy adaptation model. *Nursing Science Quarterly, 11,* 149-159.

Duldt, B., & Giffin, K. (1985). *Theoretical perspectives for nursing.* Boston: Little, Brown.

Dunn, K. S. (2004). Toward a middle-range theory of adaptation to chronic pain. *Nursing Science Quarterly, 17,* 78-84.

Farkas, L. (1981). Adaptation problems with nursing home application for elderly persons: An application of the Roy adaptation nursing model. *Journal of Advanced Nursing, 6,* 363-368.

Fawcett, J. (2002). The nurse theorists: 21st-century updates—Callista Roy. *Nursing Science Quarterly, 15,* 308-310.

Fawcett, J. (2005). Roy's adaptation model. In J. Fawcett (Ed.), *Analysis and evaluation of contemporary nursing knowledge: Nursing models and theories* (2nd ed.) (pp. 364–437). Philadelphia: F. A. Davis.

Frame, K., Kelly, L., & Bayley, E. (2003). Increasing perceptions of self-worth in preadolescents diagnosed with ADHD. *Journal of Nursing Scholarship, 35,* 225-229.

Frederickson, K. (2000). Nursing knowledge development through research: Using the Roy adaptation model. *Nursing Science Quarterly, 13,* 12-16.

Gallagher, M. S. (1998). Urogenital distress and the psychosocial impact of urinary incontinence on elderly women. *Rehabilitation Nursing, 23,* 192-197.

Galligan, A. C. (1979). Addressing small children. Using Roy's concept of adaptation to care for young children. *MCN: American Journal of Maternal Child Nursing, 4,* 24-28.

Hennessy-Harstad, E. B. (1999). Empowering adolescents with asthma to take control through adaptation. *Journal of Pediatric Health Care, 13,* 273-277.

Hill, B. J., & Roberts, C. S. (1981). Formal theory construction: An example of the process. In C. Roy & S. L. Roberts (Eds.), *Theory construction in nursing: An adaptation model.* Englewood Cliffs, NJ: Prentice-Hall.

Illich, I. (1974). Medical nemesis. *Lancet, 1,* 918-921.

Illich, I. (1976). *Limits to medicine: Medical nemesis, the expropriation of health.* London: Boyars.

Jirovec, M. M., Jenkins, J., Isenberg, M., & Baiardi, J. (1999). Urine control theory derived from Roy's conceptual framework. *Nursing Science Quarterly, 12,* 251-255.

Keen, M., Breckenridge, D., Frauman, A. C., Hartigan, M. F., Smith, L., & Butera, E. (1998). Nursing assessment and intervention for adult hemodialysis patients: Application of Roy's adaptation model. *American Nephrology Nurses' Association Journal, 25,* 311-319.

Lankester, K., & Sheldon, L. M. (1999). Health visiting with Roy's model: A case study. *Journal of Child Health Care, 3,* 28-34.

Levesque, L., Ricard, N., Ducharme, F., Duquette, A., & Bonin, J. P. (1998). Empirical verification of a theoretical model derived from the Roy adaptation model: Findings from five studies. *Nursing Science Quarterly, 11,* 31-39.

Limandri, B. J. (1986). Research and practice with abused women—Use of the Roy adaptation model as an explanatory framework. *ANS Advances in Nursing Science, 8,* 52-61.

Mastal, M. F., & Hammond, H. (1980). Analysis and expansion of the Roy adaptation model: A contribution to holistic nursing. *ANS Advances in Nursing Science, 2,* 71-81.

Mastal, M. F., Hammond, H., & Roberts, M. P. (1982). Theory into hospital practice: A pilot implementation. *Journal of Nursing Administration, 12,* 9-15.

McDonald, F. J., & Harms, M. (1966). Theoretical model for and experimental curriculum. *Nursing Outlook, 14,* 48-51.

Meleis, A. I. (1986). *Theoretical nursing development and process.* Philadelphia: J. B. Lippincott.

Modrcin-McCarthy, M. A., McCue, S., & Walker, J. (1997). Preterm infants and STRESS: A tool for the neonatal nurse. *Journal of Perinatal & Neonatal Nursing, 10,* 62-71.

Modrcin-Talbott, M. A., Harrison, L. L., Groer, M. W., & Younger, M. S. (2003). The biobehavioral effects of gentle human touch on preterm infants. *Nursing Science Quarterly, 16,* 60-67.

Modrcin-Talbott, M. A., Pullen, L., Ehrenberger, H., Zandstra, K., & Muenchen, B. (1998). Self-esteem in adolescents treated in an outpatient mental health setting. *Issues in Comprehensive Pediatric Nursing, 21,* 159-171.

Modrcin-Talbott, M. A., Pullen, L., Zandstra, K., Ehrenberger, H., & Muenchen, B. (1998). A study of self-esteem among well adolescents: Seeking a new direction. *Issues in Comprehensive Pediatric Nursing, 21,* 229-241.

Newman, D. M. (1997a). Responses to caregiving: A reconceptualization using the Roy adaptation model. *Holistic Nursing Practice, 12,* 80-88.

Newman, D. M. (1997b). The Inventory of Functional Status—Caregiver of a Child in a Body Cast. *Journal of Pediatric Nursing, 12,* 142-147.

Nuamah, I. F., Cooley, M. E., Fawcett, J., & McCorkle, R. (1999). Testing a theory for health-related quality of life in cancer patients: A structural equation approach. *Research in Nursing & Health, 22,* 231-242.

Nyqvist, K. H., & Sjoden, P. O. (1993). Advice concerning breast-feeding from mothers of infants admitted to a neonatal intensive-care unit—The Roy adaptation model as a conceptual structure. *Journal of Advanced Nursing, 18,* 54-63.

Pollock, S. E. (1993). Adaptation to chronic illness: A program of research for testing nursing theory. *Nursing Science Quarterly, 6,* 86-92.

Rambo, B. (1983). *Adaptation nursing: Assessment and intervention.* Philadelphia: W. B. Saunders.

Randell, B., Tedrow, M. P., & Van Landingham, J. (1982). *Adaptation nursing: The Roy conceptual model applied.* St. Louis: Mosby.

Reynolds, P. D. (1971). *A primer in theory construction.* Indianapolis: Bobbs-Merrill.

Riehl, J. P., & Roy, C. (1980). *Conceptual models for nursing practice* (2nd ed.) New York: Appleton-Century-Crofts.

Roy, C. (1970). Adaptation: A conceptual framework for nursing. *Nursing Outlook, 18,* 42-45.

Roy, C. (1971). Adaptation: A basis for nursing practice. *Nursing Outlook, 19,* 254-257.

Roy, C. (1975). A diagnostic classification system for nursing. *Nursing Outlook, 23,* 90-94.

Roy, C. (1976a). *Introduction to nursing: An adaptation model.* Englewood Cliffs, NJ: Prentice-Hall.

Roy, C. (1976b). The impact of nursing diagnosis. *Nursing Digest, 4,* 67-69.

Roy, C. (1979). Relating nursing theory to nursing education: A new era. *Nurse Educator, 4,* 16-21.

Roy, C. (1980). The Roy adaptation model. In J. P. Riehl & C. Roy (Eds.), *Conceptual models for nursing practice* (2nd ed., pp. 179-188). New York: Appleton-Century-Crofts.

Roy, C. (1984). *Introduction to nursing: An adaptation model* (2nd ed.). Englewood Cliffs, NJ: Prentice-Hall.

Roy, C. (1997). Future of the Roy model: Challenge to redefine adaptation. *Nursing Science Quarterly, 10,* 42-48.

Roy, S. C. (1973). Adaptation: Implications for curriculum change. *Nursing Outlook, 21,* 163-168.

Roy, C., & Andrews, H. (1991). *The Roy adaptation model: The definitive statement.* Norwalk, CT: Appleton & Lange.

Roy, C., & Andrews, H. (1999). *The Roy adaptation model* (2nd ed.). Upper Saddle River, NJ: Pearson Education, Inc.

Roy, C., & McLeod, D. (1981). Theory of the person as an adaptive system. In C. Roy & S. Roberts (Eds.), *Theory construction in nursing: An adaptation model* (pp. 49-69). Englewood Cliffs, NJ: Prentice-Hall.

Roy, C., & Obloy, M. (1978). The practitioner movement. *American Journal of Nursing, 78,* 1698-1702.

Roy, C., & Roberts, S. (1981). *Theory construction in nursing: An adaptation model.* Englewood Cliffs, NJ: Prentice-Hall.

Roy, C., & Zhan, L. (2001). The Roy adaptation model: Theoretical update and knowledge for practice. In M. E. Parker (Ed.), *Nursing theories and nursing practice* (pp. 315-342). Philadelphia: F. A. Davis.

Roy, S. C., & Corliss, C. P. (1993). The Roy adaptation model: Theoretical update and knowledge for practice. In M. E. Parker (Ed.), Patterns of nursing theories in practice. (Press Pub. 15-2548). New York: National League for Nursing Press.

Samarel, N., Fawcett, J., Tulman, L., Rothman, H., Spector, L., Spillane, P. A., et al. (1999). A resource kit for women with breast cancer: Development and evaluation. *Oncology Nursing Forum, 26,* 611-618.

Samarel, N., Tulman, L., & Fawcett, J. (2002). Effects of two types of social support and education on adaptation to early-stage breast cancer. *Research in Nursing & Health, 25,* 459-470.

Senesac, P. (2003, Spring). Implementing the Roy adaptation model: From theory to practice. *Roy Adaptation Review,* v4, No 2, Chestnut Hill, MA.

Silva, M. C. (1986). Research testing nursing theory: State of the art. *ANS Advances in Nursing Science, 9,* 1-11.

Silva, M. C. (1987). Needs of spouses of surgical patients: A conceptualization within the Roy adaptation model. *Scholarly Inquiry for Nursing Practice, 1,* 29-44.

Smith, C. E., Garvis, M. S., & Martinson, I. M. (1983). Content analysis of interviews using a nursing model: A look at parents adapting to the impact of childhood cancer. *Cancer Nursing, 6,* 269-275.

Swimme, B., & Berry, T. (1992). *The universe story.* San Francisco: Harper.

Tiedeman, M. E. (1983). The Roy adaptation model. In J. Fitzpatrick & A. Whall (Eds.), *The Roy adaptation model* (pp. 157-180). Bowie, MD: Brady.

Tsai, P. F. (2003). Middle-range theory of caregiver stress. *Nursing Science Quarterly, 16,* 137-145.

Tsai, P. F., Tak, S., Moore, C., & Palencia, I. (2003). Testing a theory of chronic pain. *Journal of Advanced Nursing, 43,* 158-169.

Villareal, E. (2003). Using Roy's adaptation model when caring for a group of young women contemplating quitting smoking. *Public Health Nursing, 20,* 377-384.

Wagner, P. (1976). The Roy adaptation model. Testing the adaptation model in practice. *Nursing Outlook, 24,* 682-685.

Walker, L. O., & Avant, K. C. (1983). *Strategies for theory construction in nursing.* Norwalk, CT: Appleton-Century-Crofts.

Whittemore, R., & Roy, C. (2002). Adapting to diabetes mellitus: A theory synthesis. *Nursing Science Quarterly, 15,* 311-317.

Woods, S. J., & Isenberg, M. A. (2001). Adaptation as a mediator of intimate abuse and traumatic stress in battered women. *Nursing Science Quarterly, 14,* 215-221.

Yeh, C. H. (2002). Health-related quality of life in pediatric patients with cancer—A structural equation approach with the Roy adaptation model. *Cancer Nursing, 25,* 74-80.

Young-McCaughan, S., Mays, M. Z., Arzola, S. M., Yoder, L. H., Dramiga, S. A., Leclerc, K. M., et al. (2003). Research and commentary: Change in exercise tolerance, activity and sleep patterns, and quality of life in patients with cancer participating in a structured exercise program. *Oncology Nursing Forum, 30,* 441-454.

Zhan, L. (2000). Cognitive adaptation and self-consistency in hearing-impaired older persons: testing Roy's adaptation model. *Nursing Science Quarterly, 13,* 158-165.

Zhan, L., & Shen, C. (1994). The development of an instrument to measure self-consistency. *Journal of Advanced Nursing, 20,* 509-516.

BIBLIOGRAPHY
Primary Sources
Books

Andrews, H., & Roy, C. (1986). *Essentials of the Roy adaptation model.* Norwalk, CT: Appleton-Century-Crofts.

Boston-Based Adaptation Research in Nursing Society. (1999). *Roy adaptation model-based research: 25 years of contributions to nursing science.* Indianapolis: Sigma Theta Tau International Center Nursing Press.

Riehl, J. P., & Roy, C. (Eds.). (1974). *Conceptual models for nursing practice.* Englewood Cliffs, NJ: Prentice-Hall.

Riehl, J. P., & Roy, C. (Eds.). (1980). *Conceptual models for nursing practice* (2nd ed.). New York: Appleton-Century-Crofts.

Roy, C. (1976). *Introduction to nursing: An adaptation model.* Englewood Cliffs, NJ: Prentice-Hall.

Roy, C. (1982). *Introduction to nursing: An adaptation model* (Japanese translation by Yuriko Kanematsu). Tokyo, Japan: UNI Agency.

Roy, C. (1984). *Introduction to nursing: An adaptation model* (2nd ed.). Englewood Cliffs, NJ: Prentice-Hall.

Roy, C., & Andrews, H. A. (1991). *The Roy adaptation model: The definitive statement.* Norwalk, CT: Appleton & Lange.

Roy, C., & Andrews, H. A. (1999). *The Roy adaptation model* (2nd ed.). Upper Saddle River, NJ: Pearson Education, Inc.

Roy, C., & Roberts, S. (1981). *Theory construction in nursing: An adaptation model.* Englewood Cliffs, NJ: Prentice-Hall.

Book Chapters

Barone, S. H., & Roy, C. (1996). The Roy adaptation model in research: Rehabilitation nursing. In P. H. Walker & B. Neuman (Eds.), *Blueprint for use of nursing models: Education, research, practice, and administration* (pp. 64-87). New York: National League for Nursing.

Roy, C. (1974). The Roy adaptation model. In J. P. Riehl & C. Roy (Eds.), *Conceptual models for nursing practice* (pp. 135-144). New York: Appleton-Century-Crofts.

Roy, C. (1980). The Roy adaptation model. In J. P. Riehl & C. Roy (Eds.), *Conceptual models for nursing practice* (2nd ed., pp. 179-188). New York: Appleton-Century-Crofts.

Roy, C. (1981). A systems model of nursing care and its effect on the quality of human life. In G. E. Lasker (Ed.),

Applied systems and cybernetics. Vol. 4. Systems research in health care, biocybernetics, and ecology (pp. 1705-1714). New York: Pergamon.

Roy, C. (1983). A conceptual framework for clinical specialist practice. In A. B. Hamrick & J. Spross (Eds.), *The clinical nurse specialist in theory and practice* (pp. 3-20). New York: Grune & Stratton.

Roy, C. (1983). Roy adaptation model. In I. Clements & F. Roberts (Eds.), *Family health: A theoretical approach to family health* (pp. 255-278). New York: Wiley.

Roy, C. (1983). Theory development in nursing: A proposal for direction. In N. Chaska (Ed.), *The nursing profession: A time to speak* (pp. 453-467). New York: McGraw-Hill.

Roy, C. (1983). The expectant family: Analysis and application of the Roy adaptation model, and the family in primary care—Analysis and application of the Roy adaptation model. In I. W. Clements & F. B. Roberts (Eds.), *Family health: A theoretical approach to nursing care* (pp. 298-303). New York: John Wiley & Sons.

Roy, C. (1987). Roy's adaptation model. In R. R. Parse (Ed.), *Nursing science: Major paradigms, theories, and critiques* (pp. 35-45). Philadelphia: Saunders.

Roy, C. (1987). The influence of nursing models on clinical decision making II. In K. J. Hannah, M. Reimer, W. C. Mills, & S. Letourneau (Eds.), *Clinical judgment and decision making. The future of nursing diagnosis* (pp. 42-47). New York: Wiley.

Roy, C. (1988). Sister Callista Roy. In T. M. Schorr & A. Zimmerman (Eds.). *Making choices: Taking chances* (pp. 291-298). St. Louis: Mosby.

Roy, C. (1989). The Roy adaptation model. In J. P. Riehl (Ed.), *Conceptual models for nursing practice* (3rd ed., pp. 105-114). Norwalk, CT: Appleton & Lange.

Roy, C. (1991). Altered cognition: An information processing approach. In P. H. Mitchell, L. C. Hodges, M. Muwaswes, & C. A. Walleck (Eds.), *AANN's neuroscience nursing: Phenomenon and practice—Human responses to neurological health problems* (pp. 185-211). Norwalk, CT: Appleton & Lange.

Roy, C. (1991). Structure of knowledge: Paradigm, model, and research specifications for differentiated practice. In I. E. Goertzen (Ed.), *Differentiating nursing practice: Into the twenty-first century* (pp. 31-39). Kansas City, MO: American Academy of Nursing.

Roy, C. (1992). Vigor, variables, and vision: Commentary of Florence Nightingale. In F. Nightingale (Ed.), *Notes on nursing: What it is, and what it is not* (Commemorative edition, pp. 63-71). Philadelphia: Lippincott.

Roy, C. (2000). Alteration in cognitive processing. In C. Stewart-Amidei, J. Kunkel, & K. Bronstein (Eds.), *AANN's neuroscience nursing: Human responses to neurologic dysfunction* (2nd ed., pp. 275-323). Philadelphia: Saunders.

Roy, C. (2000). NANDA and the nurse theorists: The truth of nursing theory. In North American Nursing Diagnosis Association, *Classification of nursing diagnoses* (pp. 59-57). St. Louis: Mosby.

Roy, C., & Anway, J. (1989). Roy's adaptation model: Theories and hypotheses for nursing administration. In B. Henry, M. DiVincenti, C. Arndt, & A. Marriner Tomey (Eds.), *Dimensions of nursing administration: Theory, research, education, and practice* (pp. 75-88). Boston: Blackwell Scientific.

Roy, C., & Corliss, C. P. (1993). The Roy adaptation model. Theoretical update and knowledge for practice. In M. E. Parker (Ed.), *Patterns of nursing theories in practice* (pp. 215-229). New York: National League for Nursing Press.

Roy, C., & McLeod, D. (1981). Theory of the person as an adaptive system. In C. Roy & S. L. Roberts (Eds.), *Theory construction in nursing: An adaptation model* (pp. 49-69). Englewood Cliffs, NJ: Prentice-Hall.

Roy, C., & Zhan, L. (2001). The Roy adaptation model: A basis for developing knowledge for practice with the elderly. In M. Parker, (Ed.), *Nursing theories and nursing practice* (pp. 315-342). Philadelphia: F. A. Davis.

Journal Articles

Artinian, N. T., & Roy, C. (1990). Strengthening the Roy adaptation model through conceptual clarification. Commentary (Artinian) and response (Roy). *Nursing Science Quarterly, 3,* 60-66.

Hanna, D. R., & Roy C. (2001). Roy adaptation model perspectives on family. *Nursing Science Quarterly, 14*(1), 9-13.

Pollock, S. E., Frederickson, K., Carson, M. A., Massey, V. H., & Roy, C. (1994). Contributions to nursing science: Synthesis of findings from adaptation model research. *Scholarly Inquiry for Nursing Practice, 8*(4), 361-374.

Roy, C. (1970). Adaptation: A conceptual framework in nursing. *Nursing Outlook, 18,* 42-45.

Roy, C. (1971). Adaptation: A basis for nursing practice. *Nursing Outlook, 19,* 254-257.

Roy, C. (1973). Adaptation: Implications for curriculum change. *Nursing Outlook, 21,* 163-168.

Roy, C. (1975). A diagnostic classification system for nursing. *Nursing Outlook, 23,* 90-94.

Roy, C. (1975). The impact of nursing diagnosis. *AORN Journal, 21,* 1023-1030.

Roy, C. (1976). The Roy adaptation model: Comment. *Nursing Outlook, 24,* 690-691.

Roy, C. (1979). Nursing diagnosis from the perspective of a nursing model. *Nursing Diagnosis Newsletter, 6*(3), 1-3.

Roy, C. (1979). Relating nursing theory to nursing education: A new era. *Nurse Educator, 4*(2), 16-21.

Roy, C. (1980). Exposé de Callista Roy sur theories. Exposé de Callista Roy sur l'utilisation de sa theories au nouveau de la recherche. *Acta Nursologica, 3.* [Essay by

Castilla Roy on theories. Essay by Castilla Roy on utilization of her theories in new research. *Acta Nursologica, 3.*]

Roy, C. (1987). Response to "Needs of spouses of surgical patients, a conceptualization within the Roy adaptation model." *Scholarly Journal for Nursing Practice, 1*(1), 45-50.

Roy, C. (1988). An explication of the philosophical assumptions of the Roy adaptation model. *Nursing Science Quarterly, 1*, 26-34.

Roy, C. (1988). Human information processing and nursing research. *Annual Review of Nursing Research, 6*, 237-262.

Roy, C. (1990). Case reports can provide a standard for care in nursing practice. *Journal of Professional Nursing, 6*(3), 179-180.

Roy, C. (1990). Strengthening the Roy adaptation model through conceptual clarification. *Nursing Science Quarterly, 3*(2), 64-66.

Roy, C. (1991). Theory and research for clinical knowledge development. *Journal of Japanese Nursing Research, 14*(1), 21-29.

Roy, C. (1995). Developing nursing knowledge: Practice issues raised from four philosophical perspectives. *Nursing Science Quarterly, 8*(2), 79-85.

Roy, C. (1997). Future of the Roy model: Challenge to redefine adaptation. *Nursing Science Quarterly, 10*(1), 42-48.

Roy, C. (2000). A theorist envisions the future and speaks to nursing administrators. *Nursing Administration Quarterly, 24*(2), 1-12.

Roy, C. (2000). Critique: Research on cognitive consequences of treatment for childhood acute lymphoblastic leukemia. *Seminars in Oncology Nursing, 16*(4), 291.

Roy, C. (2000). The visible and invisible fields that shape the future of the nursing care system. *Nursing Administration Quarterly, 25*(1), 119-131.

Roy, C. (2003). Reflections on nursing research and the Roy adaptation model. *Japanese Journal of Nursing Research, 36*(1), 7-11.

Dissertation

Roy, C. (1977). *Decision-making by the physically ill and adaptation during illness.* Unpublished doctoral dissertation, University of California, Los Angeles.

Booklet

Roy, S. C. (1978). The future of nursing. In Forum of Nursing Service, *Administrators in the West* (Pub. No. 52-1805). San Diego: National League for Nursing.

Audiotapes

Roy, C. (1978). *Paper presented at the second annual nurse educator conference* (Audiotape). Available through Teach 'em Inc., 160 E. Illinois Street, Chicago, IL 60611.

Roy, C. (1984). *Nurses' theorist conference at Edmonton, Alberta* (Audiotape). Available through Kennedy Recordings, R. R. 5, Edmonton, Alberta, Canada TSP 4B7.

Interviews

Professional profile: Sister Callista Roy: Influencing the direction of nursing. (1985). *Focus on Critical Care Nursing, 12*(3), 45-46.

Keighly, T. (1997). The interview: Callista Roy. Nursing Management: Nursing Standard Journal for Nurse Leaders, 4(5), 16-19.

Secondary Sources
Book Chapters

Fawcett, J. (2005). Roy's adaptation model. In J. Fawcett (Ed.), *Analysis and evaluation of contemporary nursing knowledge: Nursing models and theories* (pp. 364-437). Philadelphia: F. A. Davis.

Galbreath, J. (2002). Roy adaptation model: Sister Callista Roy. In J. B. George (Ed.), *Nursing theories: The base for professional nursing practice* (pp. 295-338). Upper Saddle River, NJ: Prentice Hall.

Lutjens, L. R. J. (1995). Callista Roy: An adaptation model. In C. M. McQuiston & A. A. Webb (Eds.), *Foundations of nursing theory: Contributions of twelve key theorists* (pp. 91-138). Thousand Oaks, CA: Sage Publications.

Pearson, A., Vaughan, B., & Fitzgerald, M. (1996). An adaptation model for nursing. In *Nursing models for practice* (pp. 110-129). Oxford: Reed Educational and Professional Publishing.

Phillips, K. D. (2002). Roy's adaptation model in nursing practice. In M. R. Alligood & A. M. Tomey (Eds.), *Nursing theory: Utilization & application* (pp. 289-314). St. Louis: Mosby.

Tiedeman, M. E. (2005). Roy's adaptation model. In J. J. Fitzpatrick & A. L. Whall (Eds.), *Conceptual models of nursing: Analysis and application* (4th ed., pp. 146-176). Englewood Cliffs, NJ: Prentice Hall.

Dissertations

Beck-Little, R. (2000). Sleep enhancement interventions and the sleep of institutionalized older adults (Doctoral dissertation, University of South Carolina, 2000). *Dissertation Abstracts International, 61*, 3503.

Burns, D. P. (1997). Coping with hemodialysis: A midrange theory deduced from the Roy adaptation model (Doctoral dissertation, Wayne State University, 1997). *Dissertation Abstracts International, 58*, 1206.

Cacchione, P. Z. (1998). Assessment of acute confusion in elderly persons who reside in long-term care facilities (Doctoral dissertation, St. Louis University, 1998). *Dissertation Abstracts International, 59*, 156.

Cheng, S. (2002). A multi-method study of Taiwanese children's pain experience (Doctoral dissertation, University of Colorado Health Sciences Center, 2002). *Dissertation Abstracts International, 63,* 1265.

Chiou, C. P. (1997). Correlates of functional status of hemodialysis patients in Taiwan (Doctoral dissertation, University of Pennsylvania, 1997). *Dissertation Abstracts International, 58,* 5887.

Chung, C. (1999). Sense of coherence, self-care, and self-actualizing behaviors of Korean menopausal women (Doctoral dissertation, Case Western Reserve University Health Sciences, 1999). *Dissertation Abstracts International, 61,* 776.

Domico, V. D. (1998). The impact of social support and meaning and purpose in life on quality of life of spousal caregivers of persons with dementia (Doctoral dissertation, University of Alabama, 1998). *Dissertation Abstracts International, 58,* 776.

Dunn, K. S. (2001). Adaptation to chronic pain: Religious and non-religious coping in Judeo-Christian elders (Doctoral dissertation, Wayne State University, 2001). *Dissertation Abstracts International, 62,* 5640.

Frame, K. R. (2002). The effect of a support group on perceptions of scholastic competence, social acceptance and behavioral conduct in preadolescents with attention deficit hyperactivity disorder (Doctoral dissertation, Widener University School of Nursing, 2002). *Dissertation Abstracts International, 63,* 737.

Giedt, J. F. (1999). The psychoneuroimmunological effects of guided imagery in patients on hemodialysis for end-stage renal disease (Doctoral dissertation, Wayne State University, 1999). *Dissertation Abstracts International, 61,* 192.

Harner, H. M. (2001). Obstetrical outcomes of teenagers with adult and peer age partners (Doctoral dissertation, University of Pennsylvania, 2001). *Dissertation Abstracts International, 62,* 2256.

Henderson, P. D. (2002). African-American women coping with breast cancer (Doctoral dissertation, Hampton University, 2002). *Dissertation Abstracts International, 63,* 5764.

Hinkle, J. L. (1999). A descriptive study of variables explaining functional recovery following stroke (Doctoral dissertation, University of Pennsylvania, 1999). *Dissertation Abstracts International, 60,* 6021.

Huang, C. M. (2002). Sleep and daytime sleepiness in first-time mothers during early postpartum in Taiwan (Doctoral dissertation, University of Texas, 2002). *Dissertation Abstracts International,* DAJ-B 64-07, p. 3189, January 2004.

Kittiwatanapaisan, W. (2002). Measurement of fatigue in myasthenia gravis patients (Doctoral dissertation, University of Alabama, 2002). *Dissertation Abstracts International, 63,* 4595.

Klein, G. J. M. (2000). The relationships among anxiety, self-concept, the impostor phenomenon, and generic senior baccalaureate nursing students' perceptions of clinical competency (Doctoral dissertation, Widener University School of Nursing, 2000). *Dissertation Abstracts International, 61,* 5236.

Kline, N. E. (1999). Sleep disturbances in children receiving short-term, high dose glucocorticoid therapy for acute lymphoblastic leukemia (Doctoral dissertation, Texas Women's University, 1999). *Dissertation Abstracts International, 61,* 194.

Kruszewski, A. Z. (1999). Psychosocial adaptation to termination of pregnancy for fetal anomaly (Doctoral dissertation, Wayne State University, 1999). *Dissertation Abstracts International, 61,* 194.

Lu, Y. (2001). Caregiving stress effects on functional capability and self-care behavior for elderly caregivers of persons with Alzheimer's disease (Doctoral dissertation, Case Western Reserve University, Health Sciences, 2001). *Dissertation Abstracts International, 62,* 1807.

Mahoney, E. T. (2000). The relationships among social support, coping, self-concept, and stage of recovery in alcoholic women (Doctoral dissertation, Catholic University of America, 2000). *Dissertation Abstracts International, 61,* 1872.

Salazar-Gonzalez, B. C. (1999). Responses to exercise in elderly Mexican women (Doctoral dissertation, Wayne State University, 1999). *Dissertation Abstracts International, 61,* 197.

Taival, A. S. (1998). The older person's adaptation and the promotion of adaptation in home nursing care: Action research of intervention through training based on the Roy adaptation model (Doctoral dissertation, Tampereen Teknillinen Korkeakoulu, 1998). *Dissertation Abstracts International, 60,* 113.

Thomas-Hawkins, C. (1998). Correlates of changes in functional status in chronic in-center hemodialysis patients (age, gender) (Doctoral dissertation, University of Pennsylvania, 1998). *Dissertation Abstracts International, 59,* 5792.

Toughill, E. H. (2001). Quality of life: The impact of age, severity of urinary incontinence and adaptation (Doctoral dissertation, New York University, 2001). *Dissertation Abstracts International, 61,* 5240.

Tsai, P. F. (1998). Development of a middle-range theory of caregiver stress from the Roy adaptation model (Doctoral dissertation, Wayne State University, 1998). *Dissertation Abstracts International, 60,* 133.

Velos Weiss, J. C. (1998). Lifestyle and angina in the elderly following elective coronary artery bypass graft surgery (Doctoral dissertation, University of Pennsylvania, 1998). *Dissertation Abstracts International, 59,* 1589.

Wood, A. F. (1998). An investigation of stimuli related to baccalaureate nursing students' transition toward role mastery (Roy adaptation model) (Doctoral dissertation, University of Tennessee, 1998). *Dissertation Abstracts International, 59,* 4023.

Woods, S. J. (1997). Predictors of traumatic stress in battered women: A test and explication of the Roy adaptation model (Doctoral dissertation, Wayne State University, 1997). *Dissertation Abstracts International, 58,* 1220.

Journal Articles

Chiou, C. (2000). A meta-analysis of the interrelationships between the modes in Roy's adaptation model. *Nursing Science Quarterly, 13*(3), 252-258.

Dawson, S. (1998). Adult/elderly care nursing: Pre-amputation assessment using Roy's adaptation model. *British Journal of Nursing, 7*(9), 536, 538-542.

Decker, J. W. (2000). The effects of inflammatory bowel disease on adolescents. *Gastroenterology Nursing, 23*(2), 63-66.

Dixon, E. L. (1999). Community health nursing practice and the Roy adaptation model. *Public Health Nursing, 16,* 290-300.

Dunn, H. C., & Dunn D. G. (1997). The Roy adaptation model and its application to clinical nursing practice. *Journal of Ophthalmic Nursing and Technology, 6*(2), 74-78.

Harding-Okimoto, M. B. (1997). Pressure ulcers, self-concept, and body image in spinal cord injury patients. *SCI Nursing, 14*(4), 111-117.

Hennessy-Harstad, E. B. (1999). Empowering adolescents with asthma to take control through adaptation. *Journal of Pediatric Health Care, 13*(6 Part 1), 273-277.

Ingram, L. (1995). Roy's adaptation model and accident and emergency nursing. *Accident and Emergency Nursing, 3,* 150-153.

LeMone, P. (1995). Assessing psychosexual concerns in adults with diabetes: Pilot project using Roy's modes of adaptation. *Issues in Mental Health Nursing, 16*(1), 67-78.

Modrcin-McCarthy, M. A., McCue, S., & Walker, J. (1997). Preterm infants and STRESS: A tool for the neonatal nurse. *Journal of Perinatal & Neonatal Nursing, 10,* 62-71.

Modrcin-Talbott, M. A., Pullen, L., Ehrenberger, H., Zandstra, K., & Muenchen, B. (1998). Self-esteem in adolescents treated in an outpatient mental health setting. *Issues in Comprehensive Pediatric Nursing, 21,* 159-171.

Modrcin-Talbott, M. A., Pullen, L., Zandstra, K., Ehrenberger, H., & Muenchen, B. (1998). A study of self-esteem among well adolescents: Seeking a new direction. *Issues in Comprehensive Pediatric Nursing, 21,* 229-241.

Newman, D. M. L., & Fawcett, J. (1995). Caring for a young child in a body cast: Impact on the care giver. *Orthopedic Nursing, 14*(1), 41-46.

Niska, K. J. (1999). Family nursing interventions: Mexican American early family formation: Third part of a three-part study. *Nursing Science Quarterly, 12*(4), 335-340.

Niska, K. J. (2001). Mexican American family survival, continuity, and growth: The parental perspective. *Nursing Science Quarterly, 14*(4), 322-329.

Orsi, A. J., Grandy, C., Tax, A., & McCorkle, R. (1997). Nutritional adaptation of women living with HIV: A pilot study. *Holistic Nursing Practice, 12*(1), 71-79.

Robinson, J. H. (1995). Grief responses, coping processes, and social support of widows: Research with Roy's model. *Nursing Science Quarterly, 8*(4), 158-164.

Samarel, N., Fawcett, J., Krippendorf, K., Piacentino, J. C., Eliasof, B., Hughes, P., et al. (1998). Women's perception of group support and adaptation to breast cancer. *Journal of Advanced Nursing, 28*(6), 1259-1268.

Samarel, N., Fawcett, J., Tulman, L., Rothman, H., Spector, L., Spillane, P. A., et al. (1999). A resource kit for women with breast cancer: Development and evaluation. *Oncology Nursing Forum, 26,* 611-618.

Sheppard, V. A., & Cunnie, K. L. (1996). Incidence of diuresis following hysterectomy. *Journal of Post Anesthesia Nursing, 11,* 20-28.

Woods, S. J., & Isenberg, M. A. (2001). Adaptation as a mediator of intimate abuse and traumatic stress in battered women. *Nursing Science Quarterly, 14*(3), 215-221.

Yeh, C. H. (2001). Adaptation in children with cancer: Research with Roy's model. *Nursing Science Quarterly, 14,* 141-148.

Zhan, L. (2000). Cognitive adaptation and self-consistency in hearing-impaired older persons: Testing Roy's adaptation model. *Nursing Science Quarterly, 13*(2), 158-165.

Other Sources

Cooley, C. H. (1902). *Human nature and social order.* New York: Scribner's.

Coombs, A., & Snygg, D. (1959). *Individual behavior: A perceptual approach to behavior.* New York: Harper Brothers.

Davies, P. (1988). *The cosmic blueprint.* New York: Simon & Schuster.

De Chardin, P. T. (1959). *The phenomenon of man.* New York: Harper & Row.

De Chardin, P. T. (1965). *Hymn of the universe.* New York: Harper & Row.

De Chardin, P. T. (1966). *Man's place in nature.* New York: Harper & Row.

De Chardin, P. T. (1969). *Human energy.* New York: Harcourt Brace Jovanovich.

Dohrendwend, B. P. (1961). The social psychological nature of stress: A framework for causal inquiry. *Journal of Abnormal and Social Psychology, 62*(2), 294-302.

Driever, M. J. (1976). Theory of self-concept. In C. Roy (Ed.), *Introduction to nursing: An adaptation model.* Englewood Cliffs, NJ: Prentice-Hall.

Ellis, R. (1968, May/June). Characteristics of significant theories. *Nursing Research, 17,* 217-223.

Epstein, S. (1973, May). The self-concept revisited or a theory of a theory. *American Psychologist, 28*(5), 404-416.

Erikson, E. H. (1963). *Childhood and society* (2nd ed.). New York: W. W. Norton.

Gardner, B. D. (1964). *Development in early childhood.* New York: Harper & Row.

Helson, H. (1964). *Adaptational-level theory: An experimental and systematic approach to behavior.* New York: Harper & Row.

Illich, I. (1976). *Limits to medicine: Medical nemesis, the expropriation of health.* London: Boyars.

Lazarus, R. S. (1966). *Psychological stress and the coping process.* New York: McGraw-Hill.

Lazarus, R. S., Averill, J. R., & Opton, E. M., Jr. (1974). The psychology of coping: Issues of research and assessment. In G. V. Coelho, D. A. Hamburg, & J. E. Adams (Eds.), *Coping and adaptation.* New York: Basic Books.

Malaznik, N. (1976). Theory of role function. In C. Roy (Ed.), *Introduction to nursing: An adaptation model.* Englewood Cliffs, NJ: Prentice-Hall.

Maslow, A. H. (1968). *Toward a psychology of being* (2nd ed.). New York: Van Nostrand Reinhold.

Mead, G. H. (1934). *Mind, self, and society.* Chicago: University of Chicago.

Mechanic, D. (1970). Some problems in developing a social psychology of adaptation to stress. In J. McGrath (Ed.), *Social and psychological factors in stress.* New York: Holt, Rinehart, & Winston.

Mechanic, D. (1974). Social structure and personal adaptation: Some neglected dimensions. In G. V. Coelho, D. A. Hamburg, & J. E. Adams (Eds.), *Coping and adaptation.* New York: Basic Books.

Miller, J. G. (1965, July). Living systems: Basic concepts. *Behavioral Science, 10,* 193-237.

Selye, H. (1978). *The stress of life.* New York: McGraw-Hill.

Sullivan, H. S. (1953). *The interpersonal theory of psychiatry.* New York: W. W. Norton.

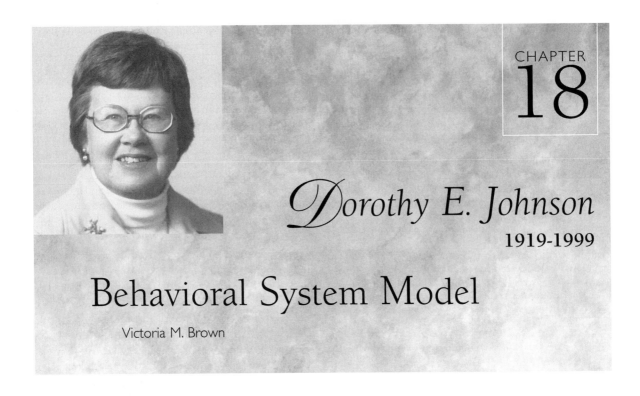

Dorothy E. Johnson
1919-1999

Behavioral System Model

Victoria M. Brown

CREDENTIALS AND BACKGROUND OF THE THEORIST

Dorothy E. Johnson was born on August 21, 1919, in Savannah, Georgia. She received her A.A. from Armstrong Junior College in Savannah, Georgia (1938), her B.S.N. from Vanderbilt University in Nashville, Tennessee (1942), and her M.P.H. from Harvard University in Boston (1948).

Johnson's professional experiences involved mostly teaching, although she was a staff nurse at the Chatham-Savannah Health Council from 1943 to 1944. She was an instructor and an assistant professor in pediatric nursing at Vanderbilt University School of Nursing. From 1949 until her retirement in 1978 and her subsequent move to Key Largo, Florida, Johnson was an assistant professor of pediatric nursing, an associate professor of nursing,

Previous authors: Victoria M. Brown, Sharon S. Conner, Linda S. Harbour, Jude A. Magers, and Judith K. Watt.

and a professor of nursing at the University of California in Los Angeles (D. Johnson, curriculum vitae, 1984).

In 1955 and 1956, Johnson was a pediatric nursing advisor assigned to the Christian Medical College School of Nursing in Vellore, South India. From 1965 to 1967, she served as chairperson on the committee of the California Nurses Association that developed a position statement on specifications for the clinical specialist. Johnson's publications include four books, more than 30 articles in periodicals, and many papers, reports, proceedings, and monographs (Johnson, 1980).

Of the many honors she received, Johnson (personal correspondence, 1984) was proudest of the 1975 Faculty Award from graduate students, the 1977 Lulu Hassenplug Distinguished Achievement Award from the California Nurses Association, and the 1981 Vanderbilt University School of Nursing Award for Excellence in Nursing. She died in February 1999 at the age of 80 (B. Holaday, personal correspondence, 2000). She was pleased that her Behavioral System Model had been found useful in furthering the development of a theoretical basis for nursing and was being used as a model for nursing practice on an institution-wide basis, but she reported that her greatest source of satisfaction came from following the productive careers of her students (D. Johnson, personal communication, 1996).

THEORETICAL SOURCES

Johnson's Behavioral System Model springs from Nightingale's belief that nursing's goal is to help individuals prevent or recover from disease or injury (Loveland-Cherry & Wilkerson, 1983). The science and art of nursing should focus on the patient as an individual and not on the specific disease entity (Johnson, 1992). Johnson reported that the Behavioral System Model was based on a preexistent body of knowledge developed over years by researchers from a number of disciplines.

She used the work of behavioral scientists in psychology, sociology, and ethnology to develop her theory. Talcott Parsons is acknowledged specifically in early developmental writings presenting concepts of the Behavioral System Model (Johnson, 1961b). Johnson relied heavily on the systems theory and used concepts and definitions from Rapoport, Chinn, and Buckley (Johnson, 1980). The structure of the Behavioral System Theory is patterned after a systems model; a system is defined as consisting of interrelated parts functioning together to form a whole. In her writings, Johnson conceptualized a person as a behavioral system in which the functioning outcome is the observed behavior. An analogy to the Behavioral System Model is the biological system theory, in which a person is viewed as a biological system consisting of biological parts and disease is an outcome of biological system disorder.

Johnson noted that, although the literature indicates others support the idea that a person is a behavioral system and that a person's specific response patterns form an organized and integrated whole, as far as she knew, the idea was original with her. Just as the development of knowledge of the whole biological system was preceded by knowledge of the parts, the development of knowledge of behavioral systems was focused on specific behavioral responses. Empirical literature supporting the notion of the behavioral system as a whole and its usefulness as a framework for nursing decisions in research, education, and nursing practice has accumulated since it was introduced (Benson, 1997; Derdiarian, 1991; Grice, 1997; Holaday, 1980; Lachicotte & Alexander, 1990; Poster, Dee, & Randell, 1997; Turner-Henson, 1992; Wilkie, 1990).

Developing the Behavioral System Model from a philosophical perspective, Johnson (1980) wrote that nursing contributes by facilitating effective behavioral functioning in the patient before, during, and after illness. She used concepts from other disciplines, such as social learning, motivation, sensory stimulation, adaptation, behavioral modification, change process, tension, and stress to expand her theory for the practice of nursing.

MAJOR CONCEPTS *&* DEFINITIONS

BEHAVIOR

Johnson accepted the definition of behavior as expressed by the behavioral and biological scientists; that is, the output of intraorganismic structures and processes as they are coordinated and articulated by and responsive to changes in sensory stimulation. Johnson (1980) focused on behavior affected by the actual or implied presence of other social beings that has been shown to have major adaptive significance.

SYSTEM

Using Rapoport's 1968 definition of system, Johnson (1980) stated, "A system is a whole that

Continued

functions as a whole by virtue of the interdependence of its parts" (p. 208). She accepted Chinn's statement that there is "organization, interaction, interdependency, and integration of the parts and elements" (Johnson, 1980, p. 208). In addition, a person strives to maintain a balance in these parts through adjustments and adaptations to the impinging forces.

BEHAVIORAL SYSTEM

A behavioral system encompasses the patterned, repetitive, and purposeful ways of behaving. These ways of behaving form an organized and integrated functional unit that determines and limits the interaction between the person and his or her environment and establishes the relationship of the person to the objects, events, and situations within his or her environment. Usually the behavior can be described and explained. A person as a behavioral system tries to achieve stability and balance by adjustments and adaptations that are successful to some degree for efficient and effective functioning. The system is usually flexible enough to accommodate the influences affecting it (Johnson, 1980).

SUBSYSTEMS

The behavioral system has many tasks to perform; therefore, parts of the system evolve into subsystems with specialized tasks. A subsystem is "a minisystem with its own particular goal and function that can be maintained as long as its relationship to the other subsystems or the environment is not disturbed" (Johnson, 1980, p. 221). The seven subsystems identified by Johnson are open, linked, and interrelated. Input and output are components of all seven subsystems (Grubbs, 1980).

Motivational drives direct the activities of these subsystems, which are continually changing through maturation, experience, and learning. The systems described appear to exist cross culturally and are controlled by biological,

psychological, and sociological factors. The seven identified subsystems are attachment-affiliative, dependency, ingestive, eliminative, sexual, achievement, and aggressive-protective (Johnson, 1980).

Attachment-Affiliative Subsystem

The attachment-affiliative subsystem is probably the most critical, because it forms the basis for all social organization. On a general level, it provides survival and security. Its consequences are social inclusion, intimacy, and formation and maintenance of a strong social bond (Johnson, 1980).

Dependency Subsystem

In the broadest sense, the dependency subsystem promotes helping behavior that calls for a nurturing response. Its consequences are approval, attention or recognition, and physical assistance. Developmentally, dependency behavior evolves from almost total dependence on others to a greater degree of dependence on self. A certain amount of interdependence is essential for the survival of social groups (Johnson, 1980).

Ingestive Subsystem

The ingestive and eliminative subsystems should not be seen as the input and output mechanisms of the system. All subsystems are distinct subsystems with their own input and output mechanisms. The ingestive subsystem "has to do with when, how, what, how much, and under what conditions we eat" (Johnson, 1980, p. 213). "It serves the broad function of appetitive satisfaction" (Johnson, 1980, p. 213). This behavior is associated with social, psychological, and biological considerations (Johnson, 1980).

Eliminative Subsystem

The eliminative subsystem addresses "when, how, and under what conditions we eliminate" (Johnson, 1980, p. 213). As with the ingestive subsystem, the social and psychological factors

MAJOR CONCEPTS *&* DEFINITIONS—cont'd

are viewed as influencing the biological aspects of this subsystem and may be, at times, in conflict with the eliminative subsystem (Loveland-Cherry & Wilkerson, 1983).

Sexual Subsystem

The sexual subsystem has the dual functions of procreation and gratification. Including, but not limited to, courting and mating, this response system begins with the development of gender role identity and includes the broad range of sex-role behaviors (Johnson, 1980).

Achievement Subsystem

The achievement subsystem attempts to manipulate the environment. Its function is control or mastery of an aspect of self or environment to some standard of excellence. Areas of achievement behavior include intellectual, physical, creative, mechanical, and social skills (Johnson, 1980).

Aggressive-Protective Subsystem

The aggressive-protective subsystem's function is protection and preservation. This follows the line of thinking of ethologists such as Lorenz (1966) and Feshbach (1970) rather than the behavioral reinforcement school of thought, which contends that aggressive behavior is not only learned, but has a primary intent to harm others. Society demands that limits be placed on modes of self-protection and that people and their property be respected and protected (Johnson, 1980).

EQUILIBRIUM

Johnson (1961c) stated that equilibrium is a key concept in nursing's specific goal. It is defined as "a stabilized but more or less transitory, resting state in which the individual is in harmony with himself and with his environment" (p. 65). "It implies that biological and psychological forces are in balance with each other and with impinging social forces" (Johnson, 1961b, p. 11). It is "not synonymous with a state of health, since it may be found either in health or illness" (Johnson, 1961b, p. 11).

TENSION

"The concept of tension is defined as a state of being stretched or strained and can be viewed as an end-product of a disturbance in equilibrium" (Johnson, 1961a, p. 10). Tension can be constructive in adaptive change or destructive in inefficient use of energy, hindering adaptation and causing potential structural damage (Johnson, 1961a). Tension is the cue to disturbance in equilibrium (Johnson, 1961b).

STRESSOR

Internal or external stimuli that produce tension and result in a degree of instability are called *stressors*. "Stimuli may be positive in that they are present; or negative in that something desired or required is absent. [Stimuli] . . . may be either endogenous or exogenous in origin [and] may play upon one or more of our linked open systems" (Johnson, 1961b, p. 13). The open-linked systems are in constant interchange. The open-linked systems include the physiological, personality, and meaningful small group (the family) systems and the larger social system (Johnson, 1961b).

USE OF EMPIRICAL EVIDENCE

Some of the concepts Johnson identified and defined in her theory are supported in the literature. Leitch and Escolona point out that tension produces behavioral changes and that the manifestation of tension by an individual depends on both internal and external factors (Johnson, 1980). Johnson (1959b) used the work of Selye, Grinker, Simmons, and Wolff to support the idea that specific patterns of behavior are reactions to stressors from biological, psychological, and sociological sources, respectively. Johnson (1961a) suggested a difference in her model from Selye's conception of stress. Johnson's concept of stress "follows rather closely Caudill's conceptualization; that is, that stress is a process in which there is interplay between various stimuli and the defenses erected against them. Stimuli may be positive in that they are present, or negative in that something desired or required is absent" (Johnson, 1961a, pp. 7-8). Selye "conceives stress as 'a state manifested by the specific syndrome which consists of all the nonspecifically induced changes within a biologic system'" (Johnson, 1961a, p. 8).

In *Conceptual Models for Nursing Practice*, Johnson (1980) described seven subsystems that make up her behavioral system. To support the attachment-affiliative subsystem, she cited the work of Ainsworth and Robson. Heathers, Gerwitz, and Rosenthal have described and explained dependency behavior, another subsystem defined by Johnson. The response systems of ingestion and elimination, as described by Walike, Mead, and Sears, are also parts of Johnson's behavioral system. The work of Kagan and Resnik were used to support the sexual subsystem. The aggressive-protective subsystem, which functions to protect and preserve, is supported by Lorenz and Feshbach (Feshbach, 1970; Johnson, 1980; Lorenz, 1966). According to Atkinson, Feather, and Crandell, physical, creative, mechanical, and social skills are manifested by achievement behavior, another subsystem identified by Johnson (1980).

Another subsystem, restorative, has been suggested by faculty and clinicians to include behaviors such as sleep, play, and relaxation (Grubbs, 1980). Although Johnson (personal communication, 1996) agreed that "there may be more or fewer subsystems" than originally identified, she did not accept restorative as a subsystem of the Behavioral System Model. She believed that sleep is primarily a biological force, not a motivational behavior. She suggested that many of the behaviors identified in infants during their first years of life, such as play, are actually achievement behaviors. Johnson (personal communication, 1996) stated that there may be a need to examine the possibility of an eighth subsystem that addresses explorative behaviors; further investigation may delineate it as a subsystem separate from the achievement subsystem.

MAJOR ASSUMPTIONS
Nursing

Nursing, as perceived by Johnson, is an external force acting to preserve the organization of the patient's behavior by means of imposing regulatory mechanisms or by providing resources while the patient is under stress (Loveland-Cherry & Wilkerson, 1983). An art and a science, it supplies external assistance both before and during system balance disturbance and therefore requires knowledge of order, disorder, and control (Herbert, 1989; Johnson, 1980). Nursing activities do not depend on medical authority, but they are complementary to medicine.

Person

Johnson (1980) viewed the person as a behavioral system with patterned, repetitive, and purposeful ways of behaving that link the person to the environment. An individual's specific response patterns form an organized and integrated whole (Johnson, 1968b). A person is a system of interdependent parts that requires some regularity and adjustment to maintain a balance (Johnson, 1980).

Johnson (1980) further assumed that a behavioral system is essential to the individual. When strong forces or lower resistance disturb behavioral system balance, the individual's integrity is threatened. A person's attempt to reestablish balance may require an extraordinary expenditure of energy, which leaves a shortage of energy to assist biological processes and recovery (Loveland-Cherry & Wilkerson, 1983).

Health

Johnson perceived health as an elusive, dynamic state influenced by biological, psychological, and social factors. Health is a desired value by health professionals and focuses on the person rather than the illness (Loveland-Cherry & Wilkerson, 1983). Health is reflected by the organization, interaction, interdependence, and integration of the subsystems of the behavioral system (Johnson, 1980). An individual attempts to achieve a balance in this system, which will lead to functional behavior. A lack of balance in the structural or functional requirements of the subsystems leads to poor health. When the system requires a minimal amount of energy for maintenance, a larger supply of energy is available to affect biological processes and recovery (Loveland-Cherry & Wilkerson, 1983).

Environment

In Johnson's theory, the environment consists of all the factors that are not part of the individual's behavioral system, but influence the system, some of which can be manipulated by the nurse to achieve the health goal for the patient (Loveland-Cherry & Wilkerson, 1983). The individual links to and interacts with the environment (Johnson, 1959a). The behavioral system attempts to maintain equilibrium in response to environmental factors by adjusting and adapting to the forces that impinge on it. Excessively strong environmental forces disturb the behavioral system balance and threaten the person's stability. An unusual amount of energy is required for the system to reestablish equilibrium in the face of continuing forces (Loveland-Cherry & Wilkerson, 1983). When the environment is stable, the individual is able to continue with successful behaviors.

THEORETICAL ASSERTIONS

Johnson's Behavioral System Theory addresses two major components as follows: (1) the patient and (2) nursing. The patient is a behavioral system with seven interrelated subsystems (Figure 18-1).

Each subsystem can be described and analyzed in terms of structure and functional requirements. The four structural elements that have been identified include the following: (1) drive, or goal, (2) set, predisposition to act, (3) choice, alternatives for action, and (4) behavior (Johnson, 1980).

Each of the subsystems has the same three functional requirements as follows: (1) protection, (2) nurturance, and (3) stimulation (Loveland-Cherry & Wilkerson, 1983). The system and subsystems tend to be self-maintaining and self-perpetuating as long as internal and external conditions remain orderly and predictable. If the conditions and resources necessary to their functional requirements are not met, or the interrelationships among the subsystems are not harmonious, dysfunctional behavioral results (Johnson, 1980).

The responses by the subsystems are developed through motivation, experience, and learning and are influenced by biological, psychological, and social factors (Johnson, 1980). The behavioral system attempts to achieve balance by adapting to internal and environmental stimuli. The behavioral system is made up of "all the patterned, repetitive, and purposeful ways of behaving that characterize each man's life" (Johnson, 1980, p. 209). This functional unit of behavior "determines and limits the interaction of the person and his environment and establishes the relationship of the person with the objects, events, and situations in his environment" (Johnson, 1980, p. 209). "The behavioral system manages its relationship with its environment" (Johnson, 1980, p. 209). The behavioral system appears to be active and not passive. The nurse is external to and interactive with the behavioral system.

A state of instability in the behavioral system results in a need for nursing intervention. Identification of the source of the problem in the system

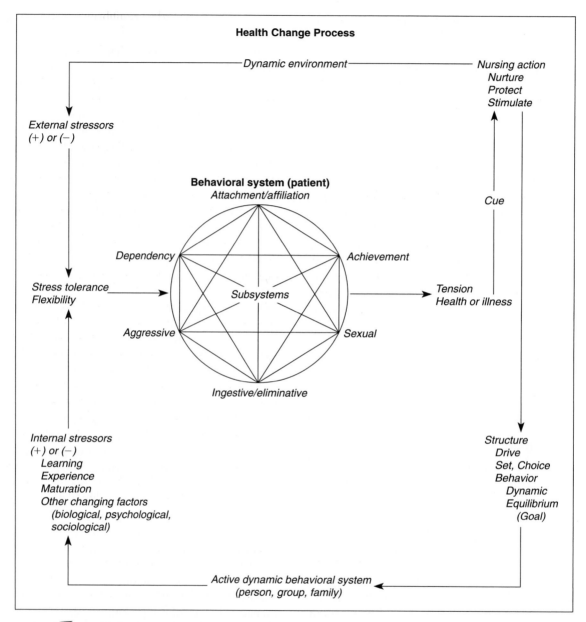

Figure **18-1** Johnson's Behavioral System Model. (Conceptualized by Jude A. Magers, Indianapolis.)

leads to appropriate nursing action that results in the maintenance or restoration of behavioral system balance (Loveland-Cherry & Wilkerson, 1983). Nursing is seen as an external regulatory force that acts to restore the balance in the behavioral system (Johnson, 1980).

LOGICAL FORM

By studying the literature of other disciplines and observing specifics in her practice, nursing literature, and research, Johnson used the logical forms of deductive and inductive reasoning to develop her theory. She stated that a common core exists in nursing, a core that practitioners use in many settings and with varying populations (Johnson, 1959a). Johnson (1974) used her observations of behavior over many years to formulate a general theory of the person as a behavioral system.

ACCEPTANCE BY THE NURSING COMMUNITY
Practice

According to Johnson (1980), the Behavioral System Model provides direction for practice, education, and research. The goal of the theory is to use protection, nurturing, and stimulation to maintain and restore balance in the patient and achieve an optimal level of functioning. This is congruent with the goals of nursing.

Johnson does not use the term *nursing process*. Assessment, disorders, treatment, and evaluation are concepts referred to in a variety of Johnson's works. "For the practitioner, conceptual models provide a diagnostic and treatment orientation, and thus are of considerable practical import" (Johnson, 1968a, p. 2). The nursing process becomes applicable in the Behavioral System Model when behavioral malfunction occurs "that is in part disorganized, erratic, and dysfunctional. Illness or other sudden internal or external environmental change is most frequently responsible for such malfunctions" (Johnson, 1980, p. 212). "Assistance is appropriate at those times the individual is experiencing stress of a health-illness

nature which disturbs equilibrium, producing tension" (Johnson, 1961a, p. 6).

Johnson (1959a) implied that the initial nursing assessment begins when the cue tension is observed and signals disequilibrium. Sources for assessment data can be through history taking, testing, and structural observations (Johnson, 1980). "The behavioral system is thought to determine and limit the interaction between the person and his environment" (Johnson, 1968a, p. 3). This suggests that the accuracy and quantity of the data obtained during nursing assessment are not controlled by the nurse, but by the patient (system). The only observed part of the subsystems structure is behavior. Six internal and external regulators have been identified that "simultaneously influence and are influenced by behavior" including biophysical, psychological, developmental, sociocultural, family, and physical environmental regulators (Randell, 1991, p. 157).

The nurse must be able to access information related to goals, sets, and choices that make up the structural subsystems. "One or more of [these] subsystems is likely to be involved in any episode of illness, whether in an antecedent or a consequential way or simply in association, directly or indirectly with the disorder or its treatment" (Johnson, 1968a, p. 3). Accessing the data is critical to accurate statement of the disorder.

Johnson did not define specific disorders, but she did state two general categories of disorders on the basis of the relationship to the biological system (Johnson, 1968a).

> Disorders are those which are related tangentially or peripherally to disorder in the biological system; that is, they are precipitated simply by the fact of illness or the situational context of treatment; and ... those [disorders] which are an integral part of a biological system disorder in that they are either directly associated with or a direct consequence of a particular kind of biological system disorder or its treatment. (Johnson, 1968a, p. 7)

The "means of management" or interventions do consist in part of the provision of nurturance, protection, and stimulation (Johnson, 1968a, 1980).

The nurse may provide "temporary imposition of external regulatory and control mechanisms, such as inhibiting ineffective behavioral responses, and assisting the patient to acquire new responses" (Johnson, 1968a, p. 6). Johnson (1980) suggested that techniques may include "teaching, role modeling, and counseling" (p. 211). If a problem or disorder is anticipated, preventive nursing action is appropriate with adequate methodologies (Johnson, 1980). Nurturance, protection, and stimulation are as important for preventive nursing care or health promotion as they are for managing illness.

The outcome of nursing intervention is behavioral system equilibrium. "More specifically, equilibrium can be said to have been achieved at that point at which the individual demonstrates a degree of constancy in his pattern of functioning, both internally and interpersonally" (Johnson, 1961a, p. 9). The evaluation of the nursing intervention is based on whether it made "a significant difference in the lives of the persons involved" (Johnson, 1980, p. 215).

The Behavioral System Model has been operationalized through the development of several assessment instruments. In 1974, Grubbs (1980) used the theory to develop an assessment tool and a nursing process sheet based on Johnson's seven subsystems. Questions and observations related to each subsystem provided tools with which to collect important data that assist in discovering other choices of behavior that will enable the patient to accomplish his or her goal of health.

That same year, Holaday (1980) used the theory as a model to develop an assessment tool when caring for children. This tool allowed the nurse to describe objectively the child's behavior and to guide nursing action.

Derdiarian (1990) investigated the effects of using two systematic assessment instruments on patient and nurse satisfaction. The Johnson Behavioral System Model was used to develop a self-report and observational instrument to be implemented with the nursing process. The Derdiarian Behavioral System Model instrument included assessment of the restorative subsystem and the seven subsystems advocated by Johnson. The results indicated that implementation of the instruments provided a more comprehensive and systematic approach to assessment and intervention, thereby increasing patient and nurse satisfaction with care.

Lanouette and St-Jacques (1994) used Johnson's model to compare the coping abilities and perceptions of families with premature infants with those of families with full-term infants. The results indicated that positive coping skills were relative to bonding with the infant, using resources, solving problems, and making decisions. Lanouette and St-Jacques suggested that improvement in nursing care practices in nursery, hospital, and community settings might have contributed to this outcome. This supported Johnson's (personal correspondence, 1996) statement that "the effective use of nurturance, protection, and stimulation during maternal contact at birth could significantly reduce the behavioral system problems we see today."

Case studies have documented the use and evaluation of the Johnson Behavioral System Model in clinical practice. In 1980, Rawls used the theory to assess systematically a patient who was facing the loss of function in one arm and hand. Herbert (1989) reported the outcomes of a nursing care plan developed for an elderly stroke patient. Rawls and Herbert concluded that Johnson's theory provided a theoretical base that predicted the results of nursing interventions, formulated standards for care, and administered holistic care. Fruehwirth (1989) found it equally effective in assessing and intervening with a support group for the caregivers of patients with Alzheimer's disease.

Recent studies of nursing practice using Johnson's model have focused on decision making and evaluation of outcomes. Grice (1997) found that the nurse, patient, and situational characteristics influenced assessment and decision making for the administration of antianxiety and antipsychotic medication for psychiatric inpatients at certain hours. Benson (1997) conducted a review of research literature on the fear of crime among older adults. The Behavioral System Model was used to describe the "hazards of fear of crime" that could cause disturbances in the ingestive, dependency, achievement, affiliative, and aggressive-protective subsystems (Benson, 1997, p. 26). Patient- and community-focused interventions were presented to improve quality of care and quality of life of older adults.

Lachicotte and Alexander (1990) examined the use of Johnson's Behavioral System Model as a framework for nursing administrators to use when making decisions concerning the management of impaired nurses. They suggested that, by viewing all levels of the environment, the framework encouraged the nurse administrators to assess the imbalance in the nursing system when nurse impairment exists and evaluate the "system's state of balance in relationship to the method chosen to deal with nurse impairment" (Lachicotte & Alexander, 1990, p. 103). The results of the study indicated that nurse administrators preferred an assistive approach when dealing with nurse impairment. It was believed that "when the impaired nurse is confronted and assisted, equilibrium begins to be restored and balance brought back to the system" (Lachicotte & Alexander, 1990, p. 103).

At the University of California, Los Angeles, the Neuropsychiatric Institute and Hospital has used Johnson's Behavioral System Model as the basis of their psychiatric nursing practice for many years (Poster, et al., 1997). "Patients are assessed and behavioral data are classified by subsystem. Nursing diagnoses are formulated that reflect the nature of the ineffective behavior and its relationship to the regulators in the environment" (Randell, 1991, p. 154). A study comparing the diagnostic labels generated from the Johnson Behavioral System Model with those on the North American Nursing Diagnosis Association list indicated that the Johnson Behavioral System Model was better at distinguishing the problems and the etiology (Randell, 1991).

It has become increasingly important to document nursing care and demonstrate the effectiveness of the care on patient outcomes. Using Johnson's model, Poster and colleagues (1997) found a positive relationship between nursing interventions and the achievement of patient outcomes at discharge. They concluded "a nursing theoretical framework made it possible to prescribe nursing care as a distinction from medical care" (Poster, et al., 1997, p. 73).

Dee, van Servellen, and Brecht (1998) examined the effects of managed health care on patient outcomes using Johnson's Behavioral System Model. Upon admission, nurses develop a behavioral profile by assessing the eight subsystems, determine the balance or imbalance of the subsystems, and rate the impact of the six regulators. This is used to determine the nursing diagnoses, plan of action, and evaluation of care for each patient. The results of this study indicated significant improvement in the level of functioning upon discharge for patients with shorter hospital stays.

Education

Loveland-Cherry and Wilkerson (1983) analyzed Johnson's theory and concluded that it has utility in nursing education. A curriculum based on a person as a behavioral system would have definite goals and straightforward course planning. Study would center on the patient as a behavioral system and its dysfunction, which would require use of the nursing process. In addition to an understanding of systems theory, the student would need knowledge from the social and behavioral disciplines and the physical and biological sciences. The model has been used in practice and educational institutions in the United States, Canada, and Australia (Grice, 1997; Orb & Reilly, 1991).

Research

Johnson (1968a) stated that nursing research would need to "identify and explain the behavioral system disorders which arise in connection with illness, and develop the rationale for the means of management" (p. 7). Theory derived from the Behavioral System Model leads the researcher in one of two directions. One researcher might investigate the functioning of the system and subsystems by focusing on the basic sciences (Loveland-Cherry & Wilkerson, 1983). In addition to the growing body of knowledge concerning the patterning of behavior from infancy to adolescence and during aging, there is a need for more knowledge about the response systems within the behavioral systems of individuals between adolescence and aging. Another researcher might concentrate on investigating methods of gathering diagnostic data or problem-solving activities as they influence the behavioral system (Randell, 1992).

Small (1980) used Johnson's theory as a conceptual framework when caring for visually impaired children. By evaluating and comparing the perceived body image and spatial awareness of normally sighted children with those of visually impaired children, Small found that the sensory deprivation of visual impairment affected the normal development of the child's body image and the awareness of his body in space. She concluded that when the human system is subjected to excessive stress, the goals of the system can not be maintained.

Wilkie, Lovejoy, Dodd, and Tesler (1988) examined cancer pain control behaviors using Johnson's Behavioral System Model. The results of the study demonstrated that persons used known behaviors to protect themselves from high-intensity pain. This supported the assumption that "aggressive/protective subsystem behaviors are developed and modified over time to protect the individual from pain and these behaviors represent some of the patient's pain control choices" (Wilkie et al., 1988, p. 729).

These findings were supported in a recent study that examined the "meanings associated with self-report and self-management decision-making" of cancer patients with metastatic bone pain (Coward & Wilkie, 2000, p. 101). Pain provided an incentive to seek treatment from health care providers; therefore, it was a protective mechanism. Yet the results indicated that most of the cancer patients did not take pain medication as often as prescribed and preferred nonpharmacological methods, such as positioning or distraction, as their pain control choices.

Believing the model had potential in preventive care, Majesky, Brester, and Nishio (1978) used it to construct a tool to measure patient indicators of nursing care. Holaday (1980), Rawls (1980), and Stamler (1971) have conducted research using one subsystem. Derdiarian (1991) examined the relationships between the aggressive and protective

subsystem and the other subsystems. Her findings supported the proposition that the subsystems are interactive, interdependent, and integrated; therefore, Derdiarian supported Johnson's contention that "changes in a subsystem resulting from illness cannot be well understood without understanding their relationship to changes in the other subsystems" (Johnson, 1980, p. 219).

Damus (1980) tested the validity of Johnson's theory by comparing serum alanine aminotransferase (ALT) values in patients who had various nursing diagnoses and had been exposed to hepatitis B. Damus correlated the physiological disorder of elevated ALT values with behavioral disequilibrium and found that disorder in one area reflected disorder in another area.

Nurse researchers have demonstrated the usefulness of Johnson's theory in clinical practice. Most of these studies have been conducted with individuals with long-term illnesses or chronic illnesses, such as those with urinary incontinence, chronic pain, cancer, acquired immunodeficiency syndrome, and psychiatric illnesses (Colling, Owen, McCreedy, & Newman, 2003; Coward & Wilkie, 2000; Derdiarian, 1988; Derdiarian & Schobel, 1990; Grice, 1997). Studies have documented the effectiveness of using the model with children, adolescents, and the elderly population. Based on extensive practice, instrument development, and research, Holaday (1980) concluded that the user of Johnson's theory was provided with a guide for planning and giving care based on scientific knowledge.

FURTHER DEVELOPMENT

Johnson (1961a) believed that people are active beings constantly seeking to adjust to their environments and that they adjust their environments to achieve better functioning for themselves. Therefore, she viewed the behavioral system as active rather than merely reactive. As the model allows for this belief, it can also be studied.

Primarily, the theory has been associated with individuals. Johnson believed that groups of individuals can be considered groups of interactive behavioral systems. Use of her theory with families and other groups needs more visibility (Johnson, 1965).

As a result of the current emphasis on health promotion and maintenance and illness and injury prevention, theory could be derived from the model recognizing behavioral disorders in these areas. This could be an important area for further development.

It should be noted that preventive nursing (to prevent behavioral system disorder) is not the same as preventive medicine (to prevent biological system disorders), and disorders in both cases must be identified and explicated before approaches to prevention can be developed. At this point, not even medicine has developed very many specific preventive measures (immunizations for some infectious diseases and protection against some vitamin deficiency diseases are notable exceptions). A number of general approaches to better health, including adequate nutrition, safe water, and exercise, are applicable, contributing to prevention of some disorders. It is small wonder that preventive nursing remains to be developed; this is true no matter what model or theory for nursing is used (D. Johnson, personal correspondence, 1984).

Riegel (1989) reviewed the literature to identify major factors that predict "cardiac crippled behaviors or dependency following a myocardial infarction" (p. 74). Social support, self-esteem, anxiety, depression, and perceptions of functional capacity were considered the primary factors affecting psychological adjustment to chronic coronary heart disease. This emphasized the effect of social support or nurturing on the structure and function of the dependency subsystem. Johnson stated, "If care takers were aware of how their behaviors and family behaviors interact with patients to encourage dependency behaviors at the beginning of illness, they could easily prevent many dysfunctional problems" (D. Johnson, personal communication, 1996).

Further development could identify nursing actions that would facilitate appropriate functioning of the system toward disease prevention and health maintenance. Rather than expending energy developing nursing interventions in response to the consequences of disequilibrium, nurses need to learn how to identify precursors of disequilibrium and respond with preventive interventions.

Assuming that a community is a geographical area, a subpopulation, or any aggregate of people and assuming that a community can benefit from nursing interventions, the behavioral system framework can be applied to community health. A community can be described as a behavioral system with interacting subsystems that have structural elements and functional requirements. For example, mothers of chronically ill children have functional requirements needed to maintain stability within the achievement subsystem. The interaction of environmental factors such as "economic, educational, and employment influence mothers' caretaking skills" (Turner-Henson, 1992, p. 97).

Communities have goals, norms, choices, and actions in addition to needing protection, nurturance, and stimulation. The community reacts to internal and external stimuli, which results in functional or dysfunctional behavior. An example of an external stimulus is health policy and an example of dysfunctional behavior is a high infant mortality rate. The behavioral system consists of yet undefined subsystems that are organized, interacting, interdependent, and integrated. Physical, biological, and psychosocial factors also affect community behavior.

CRITIQUE
Simplicity

Johnson's theory is relatively simple in relation to the number of concepts. A person is described as a behavioral system composed of seven subsystems. Nursing is an external regulatory force. However, the theory is potentially complex because there are a number of possible interrelationships between and among the behavioral system, its subsystems, and the forces impinging on them. At this point, however, only a few of the potential relationships have been explored.

Generality

Johnson's theory is relatively unlimited when applied to sick individuals, but it has not been used as much with well individuals or groups. Johnson perceived a person as a behavioral system comprised of seven subsystems, aggregates of interactive behavioral systems. Initially, Johnson did not clearly address nonillness situations or preventive nursing (D. Johnson, curriculum vitae, 1984). In later publications, Johnson (1992) emphasized the role of nurses in preventive health care of individuals and for society. She stated, "Nursing's special responsibility for health is derived from its unique social mission. Nursing needs to concentrate on developing preventive nursing to fulfill its social obligations" (Johnson, 1992, p. 26).

Empirical Precision

Empirical precision is achieved by identifying empirical indicators for the theory because models contain abstract concepts. Empirical precision improves when the subconcepts and the relationships between and among them become better defined and empirical indicators are introduced to the science. The units and the relationships between the units in Johnson's theory are consistently defined and used. So far, a moderate degree of empirical precision has been demonstrated in research using Johnson's model. However, throughout Johnson's writings, terms such as balance, stability, and equilibrium, adjustments and adaptations, disturbances, disequilibrium, and behavioral disorders are used interchangeably, which confounds their meanings. The clarity of definitions in the subsystems improves the model's empirical precision.

Derivable Consequences

Johnson's model guides nursing practice, education, and research; generates new ideas about nursing; and differentiates nursing from other health professions. By focusing on behavior rather than biology, the theory clearly differentiates nursing from medicine, although the concepts overlap with those of the psychosocial professions.

Johnson's Behavioral System Model provides a conceptual framework for nursing education, practice, and research. The theory has directed questions for nursing research. It has been analyzed and judged to be appropriate as a basis for the development of a nursing curriculum. Practitioners and patients have judged the resulting nursing actions to be satisfactory (Johnson, 1980). The theory has potential for continued utility in nursing to achieve valued nursing goals.

SUMMARY

Johnson's Behavioral System Model describes the person as a behavioral system with seven subsystems: the achievement, attachment-affiliative, aggressive-protective, dependency, ingestive, eliminative, and sexual subsystems. Each of the seven subsystems is interrelated with the others and the environment and specific structural elements and functions that help maintain the integrity of the behavioral system. The structural components of the behavioral system describe how individuals are motivated (drive) to obtain specified goals using the individual's predisposition to act in certain ways (set) using available choices to produce an action or patterned behavior. The functional requirements protect, nurture, and stimulate the behavioral system. When the behavioral system has balance and stability, the individual's behaviors will be purposeful, organized, and predictable. Imbalance and instability in the behavioral system occur when there are tension and stressors that affect the relationship of the subsystems or the internal and external environments.

Nursing is an external regulatory force that acts to restore balance and stability by inhibiting, stimulating, or reinforcing certain behaviors (control mechanisms), changing the structural components (patient goals, choices, actions), or fulfilling function requirements. Health is the result of the behavioral system having stability, balance, and equilibrium (Johnson, 1980).

Case Study

A 67-year-old man is admitted to the hospital for diagnostic tests after experiencing severe abdominal pain and streaks of blood in his stool. He is alert and oriented. He has a history of type II diabetes and hypertension. His blood glucose level is 187 mg/dl and blood pressure is 188/100 mm Hg. He is 5′10″ and weighs 145 pounds. He is currently taking antihypertensive, anticoagulant, antiinflammatory, and antidiabetic medications.

His recent history reveals that he had an acute cerebral vascular accident (CVA) 6 weeks ago that resulted in partial paralysis and numbness of the right arm and leg, expressive aphasia, and slurred speech. He completed 4 weeks of inpatient rehabilitation and is able to walk short distances with a cane and moderate assistance. He is weak and becomes fatigued quickly. Although he can move his right arm, he guards it due to pain with movement. He receives acetaminophen (Extra Strength Tylenol) for his right arm prior to therapy and before sleep. He also continues to exhibit slight expressive aphasia. He is anxious about continuing his therapy and indicates concern about missing his appointment with the orthopedic physician who was to evaluate his right arm. He reports that food doesn't taste right anymore and he has no appetite. With encouragement from his family, he eats small portions of each meal and drinks fluids without difficulty.

The patient is a college graduate who recently retired. He has been married for 45 years and has two adult children who live in the same city. He is a leader in the church and social community. His family and friends visit him frequently in the hospital. He is cheerful and attempts to talk with them when they visit. When he doesn't have visitors, he sits quietly in a dark room or sleeps. He is tearful each time his family hugs him prior to leaving. He expresses appreciation for each visit and apologizes each time he "gets emotional."

Behavioral Assessment

Using Johnson's Behavioral System Model, the following behavioral assessment is identified:

- *Achievement:* The patient has achieved many developmental goals of adulthood. He is relearning how to do activities of daily living (ADLs), walk, talk, as well as other cognitive-motor skills such as reading, writing, and speaking.
- *Attachment-affiliative:* The patient is married with two adult children who are supportive and live in the same city. He has many friends and social contacts who visit frequently.
- *Aggressive-protective:* The patient worries about his wife traveling to the hospital at night and he worries that she doesn't eat well while staying with him in the hospital.
- *Dependency:* His recent stroke, resulting in decreased use of his right arm and leg, has affected his mobility and independent completion of ADLs. His potential for falling, inability to feel his arm or leg if injured, and weakness are safety concerns. His wife has taken on the financial and home maintenance responsibilities.
- *Ingestive:* Since the stroke, the patient has had a decreased appetite. He has lost 20 pounds in 6 weeks. Studies reveal no swallowing difficulties. He is able to feed himself with his left hand but needs assistance with cutting foods.
- *Eliminative:* The patient is able to urinate without difficulty in a urinal but prefers walking to the bathroom. He becomes constipated easily due to decreased fluid and food intake.
- *Sexual:* There are changes in the patient's sexual relationship with his wife due to pain, limited use of his right side, and fatigue.

Environmental Assessment

The assessment of internal and external environmental factors indicates that several are creating tension and threatening the balance and stability of the behavioral system. This hospitalization and diagnostic testing adds additional stress to the already weakened biological and psychological stability of the behavioral system. The stroke produced several physical and cognitive impairments that affect independence, self-care, learning, maturation, and socialization. Hospitalization at this time can delay or decrease the prognosis of the patient's physical and speech rehabilitation. He will need assistance to move safely in the hospital environment.

The patient and his wife are active in their church and participate in many social activities. The patient taught classes in Sunday school. The recent illnesses, hospitalizations, and fatigue have decreased his ability to participate in previous activities. Although he has adapted to his right-sided weakness and decreased motor function by performing his ADLs with his left hand and walking with a cane, he still needs assistance. The patient and his wife live in a suburban neighborhood. Family members installed a ramp to facilitate access to the home. His wife states that neighbors watch the house when she is away and watch for her return to be sure she is safe.

Structural Components

- *Drive or goal:* The patient seems motivated to complete the diagnostic tests and return home. He is eager to get back into his outpatient rehabilitation program. It seems equally important for him to decrease stress on his wife. His wife provides positive encouragement and support for him. He looks to her for assistance with decisions.
- *Set:* It is evident that the patient is accustomed to making his own decisions and being a leader. It is also evident that he is accustomed to conferring with his wife to ensure that she is comfortable with decisions being made.
- *Choice:* Although the patient agrees to the diagnostic tests, he is no longer in pain and has had no bleeding since his hospitalization. Therefore, he is more focused on achieving his rehabilitation goals. He initiates activities and seeks assistance from his family in walking to the bathroom, walking in the hall, and completing his ADLs.
- *Actions:* The patient socializes with visitors and family by actively participating in conversations. He requests assistance as needed for physical and cognitive needs. He asks for prayers from his family and friends for spiritual guidance in managing his illness.

Functional Requirements

The patient needs outside assistance for all three functional requirements including protection, nurturance, and stimulation. His inability to feel his right side and his impaired mobility increase his potential for injury. Protective devices such as hand bars and a shower chair can be used. The patient needs assistance with preparing meals but has adapted to using his left hand for eating and drinking. Socialization and performance expectations at the outpatient rehabilitation facility are important methods of providing stimulation for the patient. Stimulation is also provided by friends and family who visit the patient. Continued social stimulation is vital for this patient, because he has difficulty understanding other forms of stimulation such as radio, television, and reading.

Nursing

Nursing actions are external regulatory forces that should protect, stimulate, and nurture to preserve the organization and integration of the patient's behavioral system. Nursing actions for this patient should focus on providing explanation of diagnostic tests to be performed and the results of the tests. Identification of favorite foods and encouragement of small frequent meals with sufficient fluids to prevent constipation will be needed. The nurse should advocate for inpatient physical and speech therapy to stimulate functional abilities and reinforce the patient's achievement behaviors and to decrease dependency requirements. It will be equally important to encourage ongoing socialization with friends and family. The patient and his wife will need support and teaching to identify methods of adapting to and managing system imbalance and instability and to identify actions that will enhance behaviors to create system balance and stability.

CRITICAL THINKING *Activities*

1. In a practice setting, use Johnson's Behavioral System Model to guide your practice for one day. Describe how the use of this model affected your approach to assessing needs, making and prioritizing nursing decisions, and evaluating outcomes.

2. Identify the strengths and limitations of the model for preventive care in a community setting.

3. Develop a teaching plan for a patient with a recent CVA and his or her family using Johnson's Behavioral System Model.

4. Design a research study to examine the evaluation outcomes of managed care in your practice setting using this model.

REFERENCES

Benson, S. (1997). The older adult and fear of crime. *Journal of Gerontological Nursing, 23*(10), 24-31.

Colling, J., Owen, T., McCreedy, M., & Newman, D. (2003). The effects of a continence program on frail community-dwelling elderly persons. *Urologic Nursing, 23*(2), 117-131.

Coward, D. D., & Wilkie, D. J. (2000). Metastatic bone pain: Meanings associated with self-report and self-management decision making. *Cancer Nursing, 23*(2), 101-108.

Damus, K. (1980). An application of the Johnson behavioral system model for nursing practice. In J. P. Riehl & C. Roy (Eds.), *Conceptual models for nursing practice* (2nd ed.). New York: Appleton-Century-Crofts.

Dee, V., van Servellen, G., & Brecht, M. (1998). Managed behavioral health care patients and their nursing care problems, level of functioning, and impairment on discharge. *Journal of American Psychiatric Nurses Association, 4*(2), 57-66.

Derdiarian, A. K. (1988). Sensitivity of the Derdiarian behavioral system model instrument to age, site, and stage of cancer: A preliminary validation study. *Scholarly Inquiry for Nursing Practice, 2*(2), 103-124.

Derdiarian, A. K. (1990). Effects of using systematic assessment instruments on patient and nurse satisfaction with nursing care. *Oncology Nursing Forum, 17*(1), 95-100.

Derdiarian, A. K. (1991). Effects of using a nursing model-based assessment instrument on quality of nursing care. *Nursing Administration Quarterly, 15*(3), 1-16.

Derdiarian, A. K., & Schobel, D. (1990). Comprehensive assessment of AIDS patients using the behavioral systems model for nursing practice instrument. *Journal of Advanced Nursing, 15*(4), 436-446.

Feshbach, S. (1970). Aggression. In P. Mussen (Ed.), *Carmichael's manual of child psychology* (3rd ed.). New York: John Wiley & Sons.

Fruehwirth, S. E. S. (1989). An application of Johnson's behavioral model: A case study. *Journal of Community Health Nurse, 6*(2), 61-71.

Grice, S. L. (1997). *Nurses' use of medication for agitation for the psychiatric inpatient.* Unpublished doctoral dissertation, Catholic University of America, Washington, DC.

Grubbs, J. (1980). *An interpretation of the Johnson behavioral system model for nursing practice* (2nd ed.). New York: Appleton-Century-Crofts.

Herbert, J. (1989). A model for Anna . . . using the Johnson model of nursing in the care of one 75-year-old stroke patient. *The Journal of Clinical Practice, Education and Management, 3*(42), 30-34.

Holaday, B. (1980). Implementing the Johnson model for nursing practice. In J. P. Riehl & C. Roy (Eds.), *Conceptual models for nursing practice* (2nd ed.). New York: Appleton-Century-Crofts.

Johnson, D. E. (1959a). A philosophy of nursing. *Nursing Outlook, 7,* 198-200.

Johnson, D. E. (1959b). The nature of a science of nursing. *Nursing Outlook, 7,* 291-294.

Johnson, D. E. (1961a). *Nursing's specific goal in patient care.* Unpublished lecture, Faculty Colloquium, School of Nursing, University of California, Los Angeles.

Johnson, D. E. (1961b). *A conceptual basis for nursing care.* Unpublished lecture, Third Conference, C. E. Program, University of California, Los Angeles.

Johnson, D. E. (1961c). The significance of nursing care. *American Journal of Nursing Studies, 61,* 63-66.

Johnson, D. E. (1965). *Is nursing meeting the challenge of family needs?* Unpublished lecture, Wisconsin League for Nursing, Madison, WI.

Johnson, D. E. (1968a). *One conceptual model of nursing.* Unpublished lecture, Vanderbilt University, Nashville, TN.

Johnson, D. E. (1968b). Theory in nursing: Borrowed and unique. *Nursing Research, 17,* 206-209.

Johnson, D. E. (1974). Development of theory: A requisite for nursing as a primary health profession. *Nursing Research, 23,* 372-377.

Johnson, D. E. (1980). The behavioral system model for nursing. In J. P. Riehl & C. Roy (Eds.), *Conceptual models for nursing practice* (2nd ed.). New York: Appleton-Century-Crofts.

Johnson, D. E. (1992). Origins of behavioral system model. In F. Nightingale (Ed.), *Notes on nursing* (Commemorative edition, pp. 23-28). Philadelphia: J. B. Lippincott.

Lachicotte, J. L., & Alexander, J. W. (1990). Management attitudes and nurse impairment. *Nursing Management, 21*(9), 102-110.

Lanouette, M., & St-Jacques, A. (1994). Premature infants and their families. *Canadian Nurse, 90*(9), 36-39.

Lorenz, K. (1966). *On aggression.* New York: Harcourt.

Loveland-Cherry, C., & Wilkerson, S. (1983). Dorothy Johnson's behavioral systems model. In J. Fitzpatrick & A. Whall (Eds.), *Conceptual models of nursing: Analysis and application.* Bowie, MD: Robert J. Brady.

Majesky, S. J., Brester, M. H., & Nishio, K. T. (1978). Development of a research tool: Patient indicators of nursing care. *Nursing Research, 27*(6), 365-371.

Orb, A., & Reilly, D. E. (1991). Changing to a conceptual base curriculum. *International Nursing Review, 38*(2), 56-60.

Poster, E. C., Dee, V., & Randell, B. P. (1997). The Johnson behavioral systems model as a framework for patient outcome evaluation. *Journal of American Psychiatric Nurses Association, 3*(3), 73-80.

Randell, B. P. (1991). NANDA versus the Johnson behavioral systems model: Is there a diagnostic difference? In R. M. Carroll-Johnson (Ed.), *Classification of nursing diagnosis: Proceedings of the ninth conference.* Philadelphia: J. P. Lippincott.

Randell, B. P. (1992). Nursing theory: The 21st century. *Nursing Science Quarterly, 5*(4), 176-184.

Rawls, A. (1980). Evaluation of the Johnson behavioral model in clinical practice: Report of a test and evaluation of the Johnson theory. *Image: The Journal of Nursing Scholarship, 12,* 13-16.

Riegel, B. (1989). Social support and psychological adjustment to chronic coronary heart disease: Operationalization of Johnson's behavioral system model. *ANS Advances in Nursing Science, 11*(2), 74-84.

Small, B. (1980). Nursing visually impaired children with Johnson's model as a conceptual framework. In J. P. Riehl & C. Roy (Eds.), *Conceptual models for nursing practice* (2nd ed.). New York: Appleton-Century-Crofts.

Stamler, C. (1971). Dependency and repetitive visits to nurses' office in elementary school children. *Nursing Research, 20*(3), 254-255.

Turner-Henson, A. (1992). *Chronically ill children's mothers' perceptions of environmental variables.* Unpublished doctoral dissertation, University of Alabama at Birmingham.

Wilkie, D. J. (1990). Cancer pain management: State-of-the-art nursing care. *Nursing Clinics of North America, 25*(2), 331-343.

Wilkie, D., Lovejoy, N., Dodd, M., & Tesler, M. (1988). Cancer pain control behaviors: Description and correlation with pain intensity. *Oncology Nursing Forum, 15*(6), 723-731.

BIBLIOGRAPHY
Primary Sources
Book Chapters

Johnson, D. E. (1964, June). Is there an identifiable body of knowledge essential to the development of a generic professional nursing program? In M. Maker (Ed.), *Proceedings of the first interuniversity faculty work conference.* Stowe, VT: New England Board of Higher Education.

Johnson, D. E. (1973). Medical-surgical nursing: Cardiovascular care in the first person. In American Nurses Association, *ANA Clinical Sessions* (pp. 127-134). New York: Appleton-Century-Crofts.

Johnson, D. E. (1976). Foreword. In J. R. Auger (Ed.), *Behavioral systems and nursing.* Englewood Cliffs, NJ: Prentice-Hall.

Johnson, D. E. (1978). State of the art of theory development in nursing. In National League for Nursing, *Theory development: What, why, how?* (NLN Pub. No. 15-1708). New York: National League for Nursing.

Johnson, D. E. (1980). The behavioral system model for nursing. In J. P. Riehl & C. Roy (Eds.), *Conceptual models for nursing practice* (2nd ed.). New York: Appleton-Century-Crofts.

Johnson, D. E. (1990). The behavioral system model for nursing. In M. E. Parker (Ed.), *Nursing theories in practice.* New York: National League for Nursing.

Johnson, D. E. (1992). Origins of behavioral system model. In F. Nightingale (Ed.), *Notes on nursing* (Commemorative ed., pp. 23-28). Philadelphia: J. B. Lippincott.

Journal Articles

Johnson, D. E. (1943, March). Learning to know people. *American Journal of Nursing, 43,* 248-252.

Johnson, D. E. (1954). Collegiate nursing education. *College Public Relations Quarterly, 5,* 32-35.

Johnson, D. E. (1959, April). A philosophy of nursing. *Nursing Outlook, 7,* 198-200.

Johnson, D. E. (1959, May). The nature of a science of nursing. *Nursing Outlook, 7,* 291-294.

Johnson, D. E. (1961, Oct.). Patterns in professional nursing education. *Nursing Outlook, 9,* 608-611.

Johnson, D. E. (1961, Nov.). The significance of nursing care. *American Journal of Nursing, 61,* 63-66.

Johnson, D. E. (1962, July/Aug.). Professional education for pediatric nursing. *Children, 9,* 153-156.

Johnson, D. E. (1964, Dec.). Nursing and higher education. *International Journal of Nursing Studies, 1,* 219-225.

Johnson, D. E. (1965, Sept.). Today's action will determine tomorrow's nursing. *Nursing Outlook, 13,* 38-41.

Johnson, D. E. (1965, Oct.). Crying in the newborn infant. *Nursing Science, 3,* 339-355.

Johnson, D. E. (1966, Jan.). Year round programs set the pace in health careers promotion. *Hospitals, 40,* 57-60.

Johnson, D. E. (1966, Oct.). Competence in practice: Technical and professional. *Nursing Outlook, 14,* 30-33.

Johnson, D. E. (1967). Professional practice in nursing. *NLN Convention Papers, 23,* 26-33.

Johnson, D. E. (1967, April). Powerless: A significant determinant in patient behavior? *Journal of Nursing Educators, 6,* 39-44.

Johnson, D. E. (1968). Critique: Social influences on student nurses in their choice of ideal and practiced solutions to nursing problems. *Communicating Nursing Research, 1,* 150-155.

Johnson, D. E. (1968, April). Toward a science in nursing. *Southern Medical Bulletin, 56,* 13-23.

Johnson, D. E. (1968, May/June). Theory in nursing: Borrowed and unique. *Nursing Research, 17,* 206-209.

Johnson, D. E. (1974, Sept./Oct.). Development of theory: A requisite for nursing as a primary health profession. *Nursing Research, 23,* 372-377.

Johnson, D. E. (1982, Spring). Some thoughts on nursing. *Clinical Nurse Specialist, 3,* 1-4.

Johnson, D. E. (1987, July/Aug.). Evaluating conceptual models for use in critical care nursing practice. *Dimensions of Critical Care Nursing, 6,* 195-197.

Johnson, D. E., Wilcox, J. A., & Moidel, H. C. (1967). The clinical specialist as a practitioner. *American Journal of Nursing, 67,* 2298-2303.

McCaffery, M., & Johnson, D. E. (1967). Effect of parent group discussion upon epistemic responses. *Nursing Research, 16,* 352-358.

Audiotape

Johnson, D. E. (1978, Dec.). *Paper presented at the Second Annual Nurse Educator Conference, New York* (Audiotape). Available through Teach 'em Inc., 160 E. Illinois Street, Chicago, IL 60611.

Videotape

The nurse theorists: Portraits of excellence: Dorothy Johnson (Videotape). (1988). Oakland, CA: Studio III. Available through Fuld Video Project, 370 Hawthorne Avenue, Oakland, CA 94609.

Unpublished Lectures

Johnson, D. E. (1961). *A conceptual basis for nursing care.* Presentation given at the Third Conference, C. E. Program, University of California, Los Angeles.

Johnson, D. E. (1961). *Nursing's specific goal in patient care.* Presentation given at Faculty Colloquium, University of California, Los Angeles.

Johnson, D. E. (1965). *Is nursing meeting the challenge of family needs?* Presentation given to the Wisconsin League for Nursing, Madison, WI.

Johnson, D. E. (1968). *One conceptual model of nursing.* Lecture given at Vanderbilt University, Nashville, TN.

Johnson, D. E. (1976). *The search for truth.* Presentation to Sigma Theta Tau, University of California, Los Angeles.

Johnson, D. E. (1977). *The behavioral system model for nursing.* Sigma Theta Tau Conference, University of California, Los Angeles.

Johnson, D. E. (1978). *The behavioral system model: Then and now.* Presentation given to Vanderbilt University, Nashville, TN.

Johnson, D. E. (1982). *Conceptual frameworks or models.* Presentation at Wheeling College, Wheeling, WV.

Johnson, D. E. (1986). *The search for truth.* Presentation to Sigma Theta Tau, University of Miami, Miami, FL.

Secondary Sources
Books

Fawcett, J. (1995). *Analysis and evaluation of conceptual models of nursing* (3rd ed.). Philadelphia: F. A. Davis.

Fitzpatrick, J. J., & Whall, A. L. (1996). *Conceptual models of nursing: Analysis and application* (3rd ed.). Norwalk, CT: Appleton & Lange.

Hoeman, S. P. (1996). Conceptual bases for rehabilitation nursing. In S. P. Hoeman (Ed.), *Rehabilitation nursing: Process and application* (2nd ed., p. 7). St. Louis: Mosby.

Dissertations

Aita, V. A. (1995). Toward improved practice: Formal prescriptions and informal expressions of compassion in American nursing during the 1950s. Unpublished doctoral dissertation, University of Nebraska Medical Center, Omaha, NE.

Dee, V. (1986). Validation of a patient classification instrument for psychiatric patients based on the Johnson model for nursing. *Dissertation Abstracts International, 47,* 4822B.

Grice, S. L. (1997). *Nurses' use of medication for agitation for the psychiatric inpatient.* Unpublished doctoral dissertation, The Catholic University of America, Washington, DC.

Lovejoy, N. C. (1981). *An empirical verification of the Johnson behavioral system model for nursing.* Unpublished doctoral dissertation, University of Alabama, Birmingham.

Riegal, B. J. (1991). *Social support and cardiac invalidism following myocardial infarction.* Unpublished doctoral dissertation, University of California, Los Angeles.

Turner-Henson, A. (1992). *Chronically ill children's mothers' perceptions of environmental variables.* Unpublished doctoral dissertation, University of Alabama, Birmingham.

Book Chapters

Fawcett, J. (1995). Johnson's behavioral systems model. In J. Fawcett (Ed.), *Analysis and evaluation of conceptual models of nursing* (3rd ed., pp. 67-107). Philadelphia: F. A. Davis.

Fawcett, J. (2000). Johnson's behavioral system model. In J. Fawcett (Ed.), *Analysis and evaluation of contemporary knowledge: Nursing models and theories* (pp. 73-104). Philadelphia: F. A. Davis.

Holaday, B. (1997). Johnson's behavioral system model in nursing practice. In M. R. Alligood & A. Marriner Tomey (Eds.), *Nursing theory: Utilization & application* (pp. 49-70). St. Louis: Mosby.

Holaday, B., Turner-Henson, A., & Swan, J. (1996). The Johnson behavioral system model: Explaining activities of chronically ill children. In P. H. Walker & B. Neuman (Eds.), *Blueprint for use of nursing models: Education, research, practice and administration* (pp. 33-63, Pub. No. 14-2696). New York: National League for Nursing.

Directional and Biographical Source

Henderson, J. (1957-1959). *Nursing studies index* (Vol. IV). Philadelphia: J. B. Lippincott.

Journal Articles

Benson, S. (1997). The older adult and fear of crime. *Journal of Gerontological Nursing, 23*(10), 24-31.

Colling, J., Owen, T., McCreedy, M., & Newman, D. (2003). The effects of a continence program on frail community-dwelling elderly persons. *Urologic Nursing, 23*(2), 117-131.

Coward, D. D., & Wilkie, D. J. (2000). Metastatic bone pain: Meanings associated with self-report and self-management decision making. *Cancer Nursing, 23*(2), 101-108.

Dee, V., van Servellen, G., & Brecht, M. (1998). Managed behavioral health care patients and their nursing care problems, level of functioning, and impairment on discharge. *Journal of American Psychiatric Nurses Association, 4*(2), 57-66.

Derdiarian, A. K. (1991). Effects of using a nursing model-based assessment instrument on quality of nursing care. *Nursing Administration Quarterly, 15*(3), 1-16.

Derdiarian, A. K., & Forsythe, A. B. (1983, Sept. /Oct.). An instrument for theory and research development using the behavioral systems model for nursing: The cancer patient. Part II. *Nursing Research, 32,* 260-266.

Derdiarian, A. K., & Schobel, D. (1990). Comprehensive assessment of AIDS patients using the behavioral systems model for nursing practice instrument. *Journal of Advanced Nursing, 15*(4), 436-446.

Dhasaradhan, I. (2001). Application of nursing theory into practice. *Nursing Journal of India, 92*(10), 224, 236.

D'Huyvetter, D. (2000). The trauma disease. *Journal of Trauma Nursing, 7*(1), 5-12.

Lanouette, M., & St-Jacques, A. (1994). Premature infants and their families. *Canadian Nurse, 90*(9), 36-39.

Ma T., & Gandet, D. (1997). Assessing the quality of our end-stage renal disease client population. *Journal of the Canadian Association of Nephrology Nurses and Technicians, 7*(2), 13-16.

Newman, M. A. (1994). Theory for nursing practice. *Nursing Science Quarterly, 7*(4), 153-157.

Poster, E. C., Dee, V., & Randell, B. P. (1997). The Johnson behavioral systems model as a framework for patient outcome evaluation. *Journal of American Psychiatric Nurses Association, 3*(3), 73-80.

Rawls, A. C. (1980, Feb.). Evaluation of the Johnson behavioral model in clinical practice. *Image: The Journal of Nursing Scholarship, 12,* 13-16.

Urh, I. (1998). Dorothy Johnson's theory and nursing care of a pregnant woman. *OBZORNIK ZDRAVSTVENE NEGE, 32*(516), 199-203.

Wilkie, D., Lovejoy, N., Dodd, M., & Tesler, M. (1988). Cancer pain control behaviors: Description and correlation with pain intensity. *Oncology Nursing Forum, 15*(6), 723-731.

Web Site

Johnson Behavioral System Model. Accessed December 20, 2004: *http://healthsci.clayton.edu/eichelberger/theory/johnson_behavioral_system.htm*

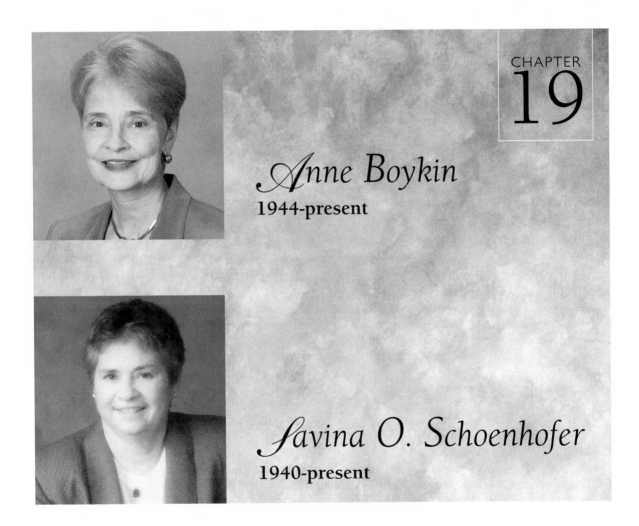

Anne Boykin
1944-present

Savina O. Schoenhofer
1940-present

Nursing as Caring: A Model for Transforming Practice

Marguerite J. Purnell

CREDENTIALS AND BACKGROUND OF THE THEORISTS

Anne Boykin

Anne Boykin grew up in Kaukauna, Wisconsin, the eldest of six children. She began her career in nursing in 1966, graduating from Alverno College in Milwaukee, Wisconsin. She received her master's degree from Emory University in Atlanta, Georgia, and her doctorate from Vanderbilt University in Nashville, Tennessee. South Florida became her home in 1981 and, today, continues to enchant and nourish her love for the natural life. Dr. Boykin is married to Steve Staudenmeyer, and they have four children.

Anne Boykin is dean and professor of the Christine E. Lynn College of Nursing at Florida Atlantic University. She is director of the Christine E. Lynn Center for Caring, which is housed in the College of Nursing. This center was created for the purpose of humanizing care through the integration of teaching, research, and service. Boykin has demonstrated a longstanding commitment to the advancement of knowledge in the discipline, especially regarding the phenomenon of caring.

Positions she has held within the International Association for Human Caring include president elect (1990 to 1993), president (1993 to 1996), and member of the nominating committee (1997 to 1999). As immediate past president, she served as coeditor of the journal, *International Association for Human Caring,* from 1996 to 1999.

Boykin's scholarly work is centered on caring as the grounding for nursing. This is evidenced in her book (coauthored with Schoenhofer), *Nursing as Caring: A Model for Transforming Practice* (1993, 2001a), and the book, *Living a Caring-Based Program* (1994b). The latter book illustrates how caring grounds the development of a nursing program from creating the environment for study through evaluation. In addition to these books, Dr. Boykin is editor of *Power, Politics and Public Policy: A Matter of Caring* (1995) and coeditor (along with Gaut) of *Caring as Healing: Renewal Through Hope* (1994). She has also written numerous book chapters and articles and serves as a consultant locally, regionally, nationally, and internationally on the topic of caring.

Savina O. Schoenhofer

Savina Schoenhofer was born the second child and eldest daughter in a family of nine children and spent her formative years on the family cattle ranch in Kansas. She is named for her maternal grandfather, who was a classical musician in Kansas City, Missouri. She has a daughter, Carrie, and a granddaughter, Emma.

During the 1960s, Schoenhofer spent 3 years in the Amazon region of Brazil, working as a volunteer in community development. Her initial nursing study was at Wichita University, where she earned undergraduate and graduate degrees in nursing, psychology, and counseling. She completed a Ph.D. in educational foundations and administration at Kansas State University in 1983. In 1990, Schoenhofer co-founded *Nightingale Songs,* an early venue for communicating the beauty of nursing in poetry and prose. An early study made it apparent to Schoenhofer that caring was the service that patients overwhelmingly recognized. In addition to her work on caring, including coauthorship with Boykin of *Nursing as Caring: A Model for Transforming Practice* (1993, 2001a), Schoenhofer has written numerous articles on nursing values, primary care, nursing education, support, touch, personnel management in nursing homes, and mentoring.

Her career in nursing has been influenced significantly by three colleagues: Lt. Col. Ann Ashjian (Ret.), whose community nursing practice in Brazil presented an inspiring model of nursing; Marilyn E. Parker, Ph.D., a faculty colleague who mentored her in the idea of nursing as a discipline, the academic role in higher education, and the world of nursing theories and theorists; and Anne Boykin, Ph.D., who introduced her to caring as a substantive field of nursing study. Schoenhofer created and manages the Web site and discussion forum on the theory of Nursing as Caring (*http://www.nursingascaring.com*). She is currently a professor of graduate nursing at the Cora S. Balmat School of Nursing, Alcorn State University, Natchez, Mississippi, and lives her commitment and passion for illuminating the study of nursing as caring.

THEORETICAL SOURCES

The theory of Nursing as Caring was borne out of the early curriculum development work in the College of Nursing at Florida Atlantic University. Authors Anne Boykin and Savina Schoenhofer were among the faculty group revising the caring-based curriculum. When the revised curriculum was instituted, each recognized the importance and human necessity of continuing to develop ideas toward a comprehensive conceptual framework that expressed the meaning and purpose of nursing as a discipline and a profession. The point of departure from traditional thought was the acceptance that caring is the end, rather than the means, of nursing, and the intention of nursing rather than merely its instrument. This work led Boykin and Schoenhofer to conceptualizing the focus of nursing as "nurturing persons living caring and growing in caring" (Boykin & Schoenhofer, 1993, p. 22).

Further work to identify foundational assumptions about nursing clarified the idea of the nursing situation as a shared lived experience in which the "caring between" (Boykin & Schoenhofer, 1993, p. 26) enhances personhood. Personhood is illuminated as living grounded in caring. The clarified notions of nursing situation and focus of nursing bring to life the meaning of the assumptions underlying the theory and permit the practical understanding of nursing as both a discipline and a profession. As critique and refinement of the theory and study of nursing situations progressed, the notion of nursing as being primarily concerned with health was seen as limiting. Boykin and Schoenhofer now understand nursing to be concerned with the broad spectrum of human living.

Three bodies of work significantly influenced the initial development of the theory. Paterson and Zderad's (1988) existential phenomenological theory of humanistic nursing, viewed by Boykin and Schoenhofer as the historical antecedent of Nursing as Caring, was the source for such germinal ideas as "the between," "call for nursing," "nursing response," and "personhood," and served as substantive and structural bases for their conceptualization of Nursing as Caring. Roach's (1987, 2002) thesis that caring is the human mode of being finds its natural expression and domain in the assumptions of the theory. Her "6 C's"—commitment, confidence, conscience, competence, compassion, and comportment—contribute to providing a language of caring (Roach, 2002). Mayeroff's (1971) work, *On Caring,* provided a rich, elemental language that facilitated the recognition and description of the practical meaning of living caring in the ordinariness of life. Mayeroff's (1971) major ingredients of caring—knowing, alternating rhythms, patience, honesty, trust, humility, hope, and courage—describe the wellspring of human living. In the theory of Nursing as Caring, these concepts are essential for understanding living as caring, and for coming to appreciate their unique expression in the reciprocal relationship of the nurse and nursed.

Boykin and Schoenhofer's conception of nursing as a discipline was influenced directly by Phenix (1964), King and Brownell (1976), and the Nursing Development Conference Group (Orem, 1979), and as a profession by Flexner's (1910) ideas. In addition to the work of these thinkers, Anne Boykin and Savina Schoenhofer are longstanding members of the community of nursing scholars whose study focuses on caring. Their collegial association and

mutual support also undoubtedly brought subtle influence to bear on their work.

Nascent forms of the theory of Nursing as Caring were first published in 1990 and 1991, with the first complete exposition of the theory presented at a theory conference in 1992 (Boykin & Schoenhofer, 1990, 1991; Schoenhofer & Boykin, 1993). These expositions were followed by the work, *Nursing as Caring: A Model for Transforming Practice*, published in 1993 (Boykin & Schoenhofer, 1993) and re-released with an epilogue in 2001 (Boykin & Schoenhofer, 2001a).

Gaut notes that the contemporary theory is an excellent example of growth by intension, or gradual illumination, characterized by "the development of an extant bibliography, categorization of caring conceptualizations, and the further development of human care/caring theories" (Boykin & Schoenhofer, 2001a, p. xii).

Text continues on p. 412

MAJOR CONCEPTS *&* DEFINITIONS

FOCUS AND INTENTION OF NURSING

Disciplines of knowledge are described as *communities of scholars* who develop a particular perspective on the world and what it means to be in the world (King & Brownell, 1976). Each disciplinary community holds in common a value system that is expressed in its unique focus on knowledge and practice. From the perspective of Nursing as Caring, the focus of nursing is nurturing person living and growing in caring. The general intention of nursing is to know persons as caring and to support and sustain them as they live caring (Boykin & Schoenhofer, 2000). This intention is expressed when the nurse enters the relationship with the nursed with the intention of knowing the other as a caring person, and affirming and celebrating the person as caring (Boykin & Schoenhofer, 2001a). Caring is an expression of nursing and is "the intentional and authentic presence of the nurse with another who is recognized as living in caring and growing in caring" (Boykin &

Schoenhofer, 1993, p. 24). Sensitivity and skill in creating unique and effective ways of communicating caring are developed through intention to care.

PERSON

Person is recognized as an individual living caring and growing in caring. Through the lens of Nursing as Caring, persons are complete and whole in the moment: There is no deficit, deficiency, insufficiency, or brokenness. To encounter person as less than whole is not to encounter person.

NURSING SITUATION

Nursing takes place in the nursing situation. The idea of the nursing situation is conceptualized as "the shared, lived experience in which *caring between* nurse and nursed enhances personhood" (Boykin & Schoenhofer, 1993, p. 33) and is the locus of all that is known and done in nursing

MAJOR CONCEPTS *&* DEFINITIONS—cont'd

(Boykin & Schoenhofer, 2001a). Nursing situation is a construct in the mind of the nurse and is present whenever the intent of the nurse is "to nurse" (Boykin & Schoenhofer, 2001a). The practice of nursing, and thus the practical knowledge of nursing, is situated in the relational locus of person-with-person caring in the nursing situation. The nursing situation involves the expression of values, intentions, and actions of two or more persons choosing to live a nursing relationship. In this lived relationship, all knowledge of nursing is created and understood (Boykin & Schoenhofer, 2000).

STORY AS METHOD FOR KNOWING NURSING

As the repository of all nursing knowledge, any single nursing situation has the potential to illuminate the depth and complexity of the experience as lived, that is, the caring that takes place between the nurse and the one nursed. Nursing situations are best communicated through aesthetic media such as storytelling, poetry, graphic arts, and dance to preserve the lived meaning of the situation and the openness of the situation through text. These media provide time and space for reflecting and for creativity in advancing understanding (Boykin & Schoenhofer, 1991, 2001a; Boykin, Parker, & Schoenhofer, 1994).

The nursing situation as a unit of knowledge and practice is recreated in narrative or story (Boykin & Schoenhofer, 1991). Story is a method for knowing nursing through which "the content of nursing knowledge . . . is generated, conserved and known through the lived experience of the nursing situation" (p. 246) and is the medium for all forms of nursing inquiry.

Nursing stories embody the lived experience of a nursing situation involving the nurse and nursed. Story as method "re-creates and re-presents" the essence of the experience, making the knowledge of nursing available for further

study (Boykin & Schoenhofer, 2001a). The following poem exquisitely portrays the tender nurturing within the nursing situation.

Seasons

Tell me a story
Not just any story, one from your soul
That animates my spirit and dances in your eyes
Tell me a story from days of old,
Before time began and patience lost
You don't speak that much, if at all.
Your attention is on the changing seasons,
Today, during your bath,
I was allowed into your world.
As I washed your back,
Your uninterrupted gaze at a soldier's picture and
your daughter's meek, soft voice broke the silence.
She met him when she was a nurse in the war.
I turned to find your daughter standing in the
doorway.
How spiffy my dad looked in his hat
And uniform, adorned with shiny buttons.
He was off-duty and candidly said,
"I'm going to need a nurse one day, and you're the
prettiest little lady I've seen in all my 22 years,
What's your name baby doll?"
We always spent time together and watched the
seasons change.
She prayed every day that he'd be safe
And return to her.
Season after season he did
First as nurse and soldier
then as boyfriend and girlfriend,
finally as husband and wife
Again they watched the seasons change but one
year in particular, he didn't return to her.
His life was lost in battle.
His season had come.
As I dress you after your bath, I feel your fragile
body and hear your shallow breathing
You stare at me with teary eyes as I slip your cap onto
your head gently feeling where your hair was lost

Continued

MAJOR CONCEPTS *&* DEFINITIONS—cont'd

from Chemotherapy
You grasp my hand and your gaze returns to the
photo
And I hear your last breath
Your season had come
You allowed me into an intimate part of your life
my first caring situation that transcended the
natural.
I experienced your season change.

Jennifer M. Thorpe
Coconut Creek, FL

The story is told through the eyes of a beginning nurse. With loving intention, the nurse transforms the giving of a bath into a final ritual of caring. The poem begins with the nurse inviting the one nursed to share her story, reaching deep into memories of the past that matter so much in the moment: "Tell me a story . . . one from your soul." The nurse knows that the one nursed speaks little, and so connects with her eyes, bathing, connecting with the photograph, and bathing again in a circle of shared understanding.

The daughter, who had been watching unseen, comes to join in the nurturance of the caring between by breaking the water-splashed silence with, "She met him when she was a nurse in the war," and by recounting what only her mother can reveal with her steadfast connection to the photograph: love, living caring together in life, profound loss, "His season had come," and soon, living caring together again after her own death. The nurse shares in the reliving of the story, becoming one with past and present as she tenderly cares until the end: "You grasp my hand and your gaze returns to the photo. And I hear your last breath. Your season had come."

In this story within a story, all are nursed. The mother was affirmed with the retelling of a life of devotion and with the tender ministrations of the nurse. The nurse was cared for in the deeper knowing of the nursed and in the gift of sharing the life of the one she was nursing. The daughter was nursed in the final walking through her life with her mother and the living caring together, within the intimacy of the ritual of the bath. All grew within the caring that connects past and present, nurse and nursed, season with season, living in the present, with living long gone.

PERSONHOOD

Personhood is understood to mean living grounded in caring. From the perspective of Nursing as Caring, personhood is the universal human call. This implies that the fullness of being human is expressed in living caring uniquely day to day and enhanced through participation in caring relationships (Boykin & Schoenhofer, 2001a). Personhood is a process of living caring and growing in caring and implies being authentic, demonstrating congruence between beliefs and behaviors, and living out the meaning of one's life (Boykin & Schoenhofer, 2001a). The shared, lived experience of caring within the nursing situation enhances personhood, and both the nurse and nursed grow in caring. In the intimacy of caring, respect for self as person and respect for other are values that affirm personhood. "A profound understanding of personhood communicates the paradox of person-as-person and person-in-communion all at once" (Boykin & Schoenhofer, 2000, p. 393).

In the poem "Seasons" the personhood of the one nursed was nurtured, living out of her life in loving, caring connections until the very end. The personhood of the daughter was enhanced by her appreciation of her mother and father, expressing and recounting their story as a gift of her own. For the nurse, personhood was enhanced by growth in caring and in greater understanding of the meaning of life as lived by one who was dying and one who was living.

DIRECT INVITATION

The direct invitation opens the relationship to truly caring between. The nurse risks entering the

MAJOR CONCEPTS & DEFINITIONS—cont'd

other's world and directly invites the one nursed to share what matters most in the moment. "What matters most to you in this moment, at this time?" and "How might I nurse you in ways that are meaningful to you?" are communicated in the personal language of the nurse and call forth responses for mutual valuing in the beauty of the caring between. The power of the direct invitation reaches deep into the humility of the nursing situation, uniting and guiding the intention of both the nurse and the one nursed.

In the poem "Seasons" the direct invitation of the nurse calls forth meaning and value in the unspeaking of the nursed and, with sensitive understanding, sees the response in her eyes. The daughter is conjoined with her mother as they respond, one for the other, one silent, one anticipating, together.

CALL FOR NURSING

"A call for nursing is a call for acknowledgement and affirmation of the person living caring in specific ways in the immediate situation" (Boykin & Schoenhofer, 1993, p. 24). Intentionality (Schoenhofer, 2002a) and authentic presence open the nurse to hearing calls for nursing. Calls for nursing are calls for nurturance (Boykin & Schoenhofer, 2001a, 2001b) to which the nurse responds uniquely with a deliberately developed knowledge of what it means to be human. Because calls for nursing are unique, situated personal expressions, they cannot be predicted, but originate within persons who are living caring in their lives and who hold hopes and aspirations for growing in caring. "Calls for nursing are individually relevant ways of saying 'Know me as caring person in the moment and be with me as I try to live fully who I truly am'" (Boykin & Schoenhofer, 2000, p. 393).

In the nursing situation in "Seasons," the call for nursing was for affirmation of a caring life and of a love that transcended time. The nurse responded with authenticity and creativity,

redrawing the close connections with the call for nursing of the daughter, who needed both to tell the story and to hear.

CARING BETWEEN

When the nurse enters the world of the other person with the intention of knowing the other as a caring person, the encountering of the nurse and the one nursed gives rise to the phenomenon of caring between, within which personhood is nurtured (Boykin & Schoenhofer, 2001a). Through presence and intentionality, the nurse comes to know the other, living and growing in caring. Constant and mutual unfolding enhances this loving relation. Without the caring between the nurse and nursed, unidirectional activity or reciprocal exchange can occur, but nursing in its fullest sense does not occur. It is in the context of the caring between that personhood is nurtured, each expressing self and recognizing the other as caring person (Boykin & Schoenhofer, 2001a).

In the nursing situation in "Seasons," the caring between was the loving intention for expressing caring in the nursing situation. Although the nursed was unable to talk, the nurse enhanced the caring between by living understanding through her eyes and through the recitation of her history, shared by her daughter.

NURSING RESPONSE

As an expression of nursing, "Caring is the intentional and authentic presence of the nurse with another who is recognized as living caring and growing in caring" (Boykin & Schoenhofer, 1993, p. 25). In responding to the nursing call, the nurse enters the nursing situation with the intention of knowing the other person as caring. This knowing of person clarifies the call for nursing and shapes the nursing response, transforming the knowledge brought by the nurse to the situation from general, to the particular and unique (Boykin & Schoenhofer, 2001a). The nursing response is co-created

Continued

in the immediacy of what truly matters and is a specific expression of caring nurturance to sustain and enhance the other living and growing in caring. Nursing responses to calls for caring evolve as nurses clarify their understandings of calls through presence and dialogue. Such responses are uniquely created for the moment and cannot be predicted or applied as preplanned protocols (Boykin & Schoenhofer, 1997).

Nursing responses in "Seasons" are shaped by the growing understanding between the nurse and nursed, and revolve around what matters to the nursed. As the caring relationship develops during the bath, the nurse's response to the call to be recognized as living and growing in caring, even though dying, embraces both mother and daughter, holding, listening, waiting together, and transcending.

USE OF EMPIRICAL EVIDENCE

The assumptions of theory of Nursing as Caring ground the practice of nursing in knowing, enhancing, and illuminating the caring between and, as such, do not directly provide empirical variables from which hypotheses and testable predictions are made; rather, the theory of Nursing as Caring qualitatively transforms practice. In the theory, persons are unique and unpredictable in the moment, and therefore cannot, and should not, be manipulated or objectified as testable, researchable, variables. Ellis believed that theories should reveal the knowledge that nurses must, and should, spend time pursuing (Algase & Whall, 1993). Nursing as Caring reveals the essentiality of recognizing the caring between the nurse and the one nursed as the substantive knowledge that nurses must pursue. From this perspective, outcomes of nursing care reflect the valuing of person in ways that communicate the "value added" richness of the nursing experience (Boykin, Schoenhofer, Smith, St. Jean, & Aleman, 2003, p. 225). Characteristics of personhood essential to the theory, such as unity, whole, awareness, and intention, are inconsonant with the objective terms of normative science that permeate language outcomes currently in use. In Nursing as Caring, outcomes are articulated instead in terms that are subjective and descriptive, rather than objective and predictive (Boykin & Schoenhofer, 1997).

MAJOR ASSUMPTIONS

Fundamental beliefs about what it means to be human undergird the theory of Nursing as Caring. Boykin and Schoenhofer (2001a) address six major assumptions that reflect a set of values to provide a basis for understanding and explicating the meaning of nursing.

Persons Are Caring by Virtue of Their Humanness

The belief that persons are caring by virtue of their humanness sets forth the ontological and ethical bases in which the theory is grounded. Being a person means living caring, through which being and possibilities are able to be known to their fullest. Each person, throughout his or her life, grows in the capacity to express caring. The assumption that all persons are caring does not require that each act of a person be caring, but it does require the acceptance that "fundamentally, potentially, and actually, each person is caring" (Boykin & Schoenhofer, 2001a, p. 2). The belief that all persons are caring involves a commitment to know self and other as caring persons. Through entering, experiencing, and appreciating the life-world of other, the nature of being human is understood more fully. From the perspective of the theory of Nursing as Caring, the understanding of person as caring "centers on valuing and celebrating human wholeness, the human person as living and growing in caring, and active personal engagement with others" (Boykin & Schoenhofer, 2001a, p. 5).

Persons Are Whole and Complete in the Moment

Respect for the total person is communicated in the notion of person as whole or complete in the moment. Being complete in the moment signifies that there is no insufficiency, no brokenness or absence of something. Wholeness, or the fullness of being, is forever present. The view of person as caring and complete is intentional, offering a unifying lens for being with other that prevents segmenting into parts such as mind, body, and spirit. Through this lens, the person is at all times whole, with no insufficiency, brokenness, or absence of something. The idea of wholeness does not preclude the idea of complexity of being. Instead, from the perspective of Nursing as Caring, to encounter a person as less than whole fails to truly encounter the person.

Persons Live Caring, Moment to Moment

Caring is a lifetime process that is lived moment to moment and is constantly unfolding. In the rhythm of life experiences, we continually develop expressions of ourselves as caring persons. Actualization of the potential to express caring varies in the moment. As competency in caring is developed through life, we come to understand what it means to be a caring person, to live caring, and to nurture each other as caring. This awareness of self as caring person draws forth to consciousness the valuing of caring and becomes the moral imperative, directing the "oughts" of actions with the persistent question, "How ought I act as caring person?" (Boykin & Schoenhofer, 2001a, p. 4).

Personhood Is Living Life Grounded in Caring

Personhood is living out who we are, demonstrating congruence between beliefs and behaviors, and living out the meaning of our lives. Personhood acknowledges the potential for unfolding caring possibilities moment to moment.

Personhood Is Enhanced Through Participating in Nurturing Relationships With Caring Others

Personhood is being authentic, being who I am as caring person in the moment, and is enhanced through participation in nurturing relationships with caring others. The nature of relationships is transformed through caring. Caring is living in the context of relational responsibilities and possibilities, and acknowledges the importance of knowing person as person. Through knowing self as caring person, I am able to be authentic to self, freeing me to truly be with others (Boykin & Schoenhofer, 2001a, p. 4).

Nursing Is Both a Discipline and a Profession

Nursing is an "exquisitely interwoven" (Boykin & Schoenhofer, 2001a, p. 6) unity of aspects of the discipline and profession of nursing. As a discipline, nursing is a way of knowing, being, valuing, and living in the world, and is envisaged as a unity of knowledge within a larger unity. The discipline of nursing attends to the discovery, creation, development, and refinement of knowledge needed for the practice of nursing. The profession of nursing attends to the application of that knowledge in response to human needs.

Nursing as caring focuses on the knowledge needed for plenary understanding of what it means to be human and on the distinctive methods needed to verify this knowledge. As a human science, knowing nursing means knowing in the realms of personal, empirical, ethical, and aesthetic all at once (Carper, 1978; Phenix, 1964). These patterns of knowing provide an organizing framework for asking epistemological questions of caring in nursing.

THEORETICAL ASSERTIONS

The broad philosophical framework of the theory assures its congruence in a variety of nursing situations. As a general theory, Nursing as Caring is an appropriate model for various nursing roles, such as individual practice, group or institutional practice, or a variety of practice venues such as acute care, long-term care, nursing administration, and nursing education.

The fundamental assumptions of the theory of Nursing as Caring underpin all assertions and concepts of the theory. They are as follows: (1) to be human is to be caring and (2) the purpose of the discipline and profession is to come to know persons and nurture them as persons living caring and growing in caring. These assumptions give rise to the concept of respect for persons as caring individuals and respect for that which matters to them. The notion of respect grounds and characterizes relationships and is the starting place for all activities.

Dance of Caring Persons

The Dance of Caring Persons is a visual representation of the lived caring between the nurse and the nursed and expresses underlying relationships (Figure 19-1). The concept of a hierarchical ladder is inconsistent with Nursing as Caring. Instead, the egalitarian spirit of caring respect characterizes each participant in the dance of caring persons, in which the contributions of each dancer, including the nursed, are honored.

Dancers enter the nursing situation, visualized as a circle of caring that provides organizing purpose and integrated functioning (Boykin, et al., 2003). Dancers move freely; some dancers touch, some dance alone, but all dance in relation to each other and to the circle. Each dancer brings special gifts as the nursing situation evolves. Some dancers may hear different notes and a different rhythm, but all harmonize in the unity of the dance and the oneness of the circle. Personal knowing of self and other is integral to the connectedness of persons in the dance, in which the nature of relating in the circle is grounded in valuing and respecting person (Boykin

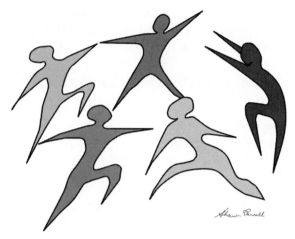

Figure **19-1 The Dance of Caring Persons.** (From Boykin, A., & Schoenhofer, S. O. [2001]. *Nursing as caring: A model for transforming practice* [p. 37] [Re-release of original volume, with epilogue added]. Sudbury, MA: Jones & Bartlett; graphic created by Shawn Pennell, Florida Atlantic University, Boca Raton, FL.)

& Schoenhofer, 2001a). All in the nursing situation, including the nurse and the nursed, sustain the dance, being energized and resonating with the music of caring.

Outcomes of Nursing Care

In considering outcomes of care, the notion of predictable evidence-based outcomes is incompatible with the significance of values experienced in caring nursing. Outcomes of nursing care are conceptualized from values experienced in the nursing relationship and are unacknowledged in normative documentation. Boykin and Schoenhofer (1997) note that it is the responsibility of the courageous advanced practice nurse to "go beyond what is currently accepted in delimiting and languaging the value expressed by persons who participate in nursing situations" (p. 63). Work is underway in identifying and clarifying the "value added" unique outcomes of nursing care (Thomas, Finch, Green, & Schoenhofer, 2004).

LOGICAL FORM

The framework of the theory is presented in logical form, grounded in general assumptions related to persons as caring and in nursing as a discipline of knowledge and a profession. The theory is a broad-based, general theory of nursing rendered in everyday language. Mayeroff's (1971) work, *On Caring,* and Roach's (1987) "5 C's" provided a language that illuminated the practical meaning of caring in nursing situations.

Key concepts of caring, nursing, intention, nursing situation, direct invitation, call for nursing as caring, caring between, and nursing response are described in context of the general assumptions, and interrelated meanings are illustrated in the model of the dance of caring persons. The direct invitation, introduced in the 2001 edition of *Nursing as Caring: A Model for Transforming Practice,* is an elaboration of the nursing situation and further clarifies the role of the nurse in initiating and sustaining caring responses. Story as a method for knowing nursing continues to focus on the nursing situation as the locus for all nursing knowledge and is a fluid and logical extension of the framework.

ACCEPTANCE BY THE NURSING COMMUNITY

Practice

Nursing is a way of living caring in the world and is revealed in personal patterns of caring. Foundations for practice of the theory of Nursing as Caring become illumined when the nurse comes to know self as caring person "in ever deepening and broadening dimensions" (Boykin & Schoenhofer, 2001a, p. 23). Practicing nursing within this framework requires the acknowledgment that knowing self as caring matters, especially in the light of practice environments which depersonalize and support the notion of the nurse as instrument and as a means to an end. In reflecting upon their caring, nurses describe "Aha!" moments, signal realizations of self as always having been caring, and rediscover freedom in caring possibilities within the nursing situation:

"freedom to be, freedom to choose, and freedom to unfold" (Boykin & Schoenhofer, 2001a, p. 23).

Often, plenary realization of the self as caring person does not occur until the story of the caring transpiring in the nursing situation is articulated and shared. Reentering moments of caring through articulation of the nursing story allows the nurse to frame outcomes of caring in the language and substance of caring that is meaningful for nursing. Through the sharing of story, new possibilities arise for living nursing as caring. Honoring caring values in explicit ways reaffirms the substance of nursing and refreshes the caring intention of the nurse.

Nursing service administration. In living Nursing as Caring, the nursing administrator makes decisions through a lens in which activities are infused with a concern for shaping a transformative culture that embodies the fundamental values expressed within nursing as caring. All activities of the nursing administrator must be connected to the direct work of nursing and be "ultimately directed to the person(s) being nursed" (Boykin & Schoenhofer, 2001a, p. 33). These activities include creating, maintaining, and supporting an environment open to hearing calls for nursing and to providing nurturing responses.

Boykin and Schoenhofer (2001a) state that contrary to the perception of being removed from the direct care of the nursed, the nursing administrator instead is able to directly or indirectly enter the world of the nursed, respond uniquely, and assist the nurse in securing resources to nurture persons as they live and grow in caring. The nursing administrator is also able to enter the world of the nursed indirectly, through the stories of colleagues in other roles. Other activities of the nursing administrator within the interdisciplinary environment of the organization include facilitating understanding and clarity of the focus of nursing and also informing other members of the interdisciplinary health care team of the unique contributions of nursing. Sharing the depth of nursing with others through nursing situations illuminates meanings and allows for a fluid reciprocity among colleagues.

The work of the nursing administrator must also reflect the uniqueness of the discipline so that it is nursing which is being reflected, portraying respect for persons as caring and extending through mission statements, goals, objectives, standards of practice, policies, and procedures (Boykin & Schoenhofer, 2001a). The following story, related by a nursing administrator practicing from the perspective of Nursing as Caring, reflects the complexity and intentional caring expressed in living caring amid the multitude of daily activities:

> As a nursing administrator, the concept of caring for others is complex. Although I do not take direct care of patients in my role as director of nursing, I do take responsibility for the direct care of many, that is, patients, families, staff, colleagues, students, and my ownership for each practicing RN/LPN that I supervise with other nurse leaders. I make it a priority to see each nurse manager daily, speak to them throughout the day, visit their patients and staff, and be constantly visible throughout any given day.
>
> How do I live and practice? Commitment—always to the well-being of others. Wearing my business hat as nurse leader in a profit driven world with dwindling reimbursement practices, this is difficult to meet facility goals for the fiscal performance, however, I must never lose sight of the patient and the family and the dedicated nurses caring for them. I must make certain that each project I work on, each deadline to meet, takes into account the impact this will have on the nurse delivering care, the patient receiving the care and the outcome.
>
> Currently, I am working on a project relating to job analysis and the activity of nurse managers and the impact that has on their role and trying to put in place a support system for them to better manage their activities. This I believe will give them more time to directly engage each nurse in living in caring more freely and more consistently. I talk to them daily about work balance and how I can assist them: They grow with me in the moment of learning something new, or how to incorporate into their practice a new way to deliver care. (Courtesy Joseph St. Jean, RN, Boca Raton, FL)

Education

Nursing as Caring is a transformation model for all arenas, including nursing practice, nursing service organization, nursing inquiry, and nursing educa-

tion. Assumptions grounding Nursing as Caring also ground the practice of nursing education and nursing education administration (Boykin & Schoenhofer, 2001a). As expressions of the discipline, the structure and practices of the education program, including the curriculum, should reflect the values and assumptions inherent in the statement of focus and domain of the discipline, that is, nurturing persons living caring and growing in caring. Through the lens of Nursing as Caring, fundamental assumptions should be reflected. They are that persons are caring by virtue of their humanness, knowing the person as whole or complete in the moment and living caring uniquely, understanding that personhood is a process of living grounded in caring and is enhanced through participation in nurturing relationships with caring other, and affirming nursing as a discipline and profession. Schoenhofer (2001) asserts that caring, as one of the significant components of nursing knowledge, should not be limited to a single course but should be taught, studied, and infused throughout the curriculum. All activities of the program of study should therefore be directed toward developing, organizing, and communicating nursing knowledge, the knowledge of nurturing persons living caring and growing in caring.

Caring is posited as the link between spirituality and higher education and as an ethic for being in relationship (Boykin & Parker, 1997). Caring is the framework for knowing and the moral basis for relating. Self-discovery through an ongoing search for truth prepares learners "to receive a greater understanding of his/her reality as well as the reality of others; to develop a sense of identification, connectedness and compassion with others, and a deeper understanding of truth" (Boykin & Parker, 1997, p. 32). The challenge is to create an environment that can sustain and nurture the living of caring and spirituality in higher education (Boykin & Parker, 1997).

From the perspective of Nursing as Caring, the model for organizational design of nursing education is analogous to the dance of caring persons. Faculty, students, and administrators dance together in the study of nursing. Each dancer is recognized, prized, and celebrated for the gifts he or she brings. The role of each influences how the commitment to nursing education is lived out. The role of the dean of a caring-based nursing program is "intrinsically linked" (Boykin, 1994a, p. 17) to an understanding of nursing as both a discipline and profession and focuses actions on developing and maintaining a caring environment in which the knowledge of the discipline can be discovered. As administrator, the dean "nurtures ideas, secures resources, communicates the nature of the discipline, models living and growing in caring, co-creates a culture in which the study of nursing can be achieved freely and fully, grounds all actions in a commitment to caring as a way of being, and treats others with the same care, concern, and understanding as those entrusted to our nursing care" (Boykin, 1994a, pp. 17-18). Such a broad scope of responsibility rests on the moral obligation inherent in the role of the dean to ensure that all actions originate in caring and that an environment is created that fosters development of the capacity to care (Boykin, 1990).

Research

Methodology. Boykin and Schoenhofer (2001a) assert that because the nature of nursing exemplified in the Nursing as Caring theory is one of reciprocal relation, where persons are united in oneness in caring, then sciencing in nursing must also be commensurate with this perspective. As a human science, nursing must call for methods of inquiry that assure the dialogic circle in the nursing situation and fully encompass that which can be known of nursing. The ontology of nursing, with its locus in person as caring in community with others and with the universe, therefore requires an epistemology consonant with human science values and methods, with "methods and techniques that honor freedom, creativity, and interconnectedness" (Boykin & Schoenhofer, 2001a, p. 53). Traditional or normative methods of research that are derived from mathematics are not amenable to study of the fullness of the nursing situation. Using phenomenology, likewise, one is unable to achieve a full understanding of nursing, because phenomena for

study are removed from the context of the nursing situation and must be reintegrated into the nursing situation in order to understand nursing.

Boykin and Schoenhofer (2001a) state that the systematic study of nursing should include a new, creative methodology that recognizes the locus of study in the nursing situation. They postulate that a methodology fully adequate to tap into the vein of nursing knowledge within the nursing situation would include a "phenomenological-hermeneutical process within an action research orientation" (Boykin & Schoenhofer, 2001a, p. 62). Such a method would allow the study of nursing meaning as it is being co-created within the lived experience of the nursing situation. An effort was made to develop a philosophical underpinning for these two research approaches (Schoenhofer, 2002b). The idea of praxis and the theory of communicative action were explored initially as possible underpinnings for an emergent research methodology; however, aspects of both views were found to require further consideration.

Research studies. Research guided by the theory of Nursing as Caring is ongoing. The practicality of Nursing as Caring is being tested and implemented in several nursing practice settings. Executive personnel, directors of nursing, and nurse administrators are calling for practice models that speak to the essentiality of caring in nursing. Nursing practice models have been developed and are continuing to be refined in acute and long-term care settings.

In separate research inquiries within units of two major regional hospitals, JFK Medical Center and Boca Raton Community Hospital, each described below, values and outcomes of caring were reframed and rearticulated to reflect integration of the theory of Nursing as Caring. The significant courage of administrators collaborating in this caring research reflected growing realization that caring for person as person is the value to which persons respond. Outcomes of care that nurses documented were within reframed institutional values of caring that nurses contributed from their practice.

In 2002, a 2-year study entitled Demonstration of a Caring-Based Model for Health Care Delivery Based on the Theory of Nursing as Caring was completed at JFK Medical Center, Atlantis, Florida, funded by the Quantum Foundation. The practice model based on the theory of Nursing as Caring was implemented in a telemetry unit. Many persons from all stakeholder groups were invited to tell a story illustrating caring as it was lived in a nursing situation on the pilot unit. The model evolved from shared values of Nursing as Caring and included those expressed by patients, patients' families, nurses, other members and staff of the pilot unit, and members of the administrative team. Themes were uncovered in a narrative analysis and synthesis and served as explicit components of the model. Major themes of the nursing practice model were based on the theory of Nursing as Caring, and strategies and operational structures were created to reflect these themes (Boykin, Bulfin, Southern, & Baldwin, 2004). The core of the caring-based model arises from the direct invitation (Boykin & Schoenhofer, 2001a, 2001b) and is a new and renewed focus on "responding to that which matters" (Boykin et al., 2003, p. 229), which is now being incorporated more actively into the nursing situation.

This project demonstrated that when nursing practice is focused intentionally on coming to know person as caring, and on nurturing and supporting those nursed as they live their caring, transformation of care occurs. Within this new model, those nursed were able to articulate the experience of being cared for, patient and nurse satisfaction increased dramatically, retention increased, and the environment for care became grounded in the values of and respect for person (Boykin et al., 2003). Continuing outcomes of the model reveal that the unit is sought after as a satisfying place to work among caring others. When nurses transfer from the demonstration unit to other floors, the values of the model are transferred with them and are beginning to be self-generated in other areas of practice.

A similar project was begun in 2003 in the emergency department of Boca Raton Community Hospital, Boca Raton, Florida. The first phase of a model based on the theory of Nursing as Caring is entitled Emergency Department: Transformation from Object Centered Care to Person Centered Care Through Caring. In creating the model, staff realized that changes in conceptualizations of nursing practice were needed. Initially, all emergency services staff, including physicians, nurses, and support services staff, were included, emulating organization of the dance of caring persons. Evaluation of the model is beginning early, because of the success of the model in the busy venue of the emergency department. Plans are already being made to extend the model to other areas of the hospital. Early results of the study have been presented formally in an international venue (Boykin et al., 2004).

Caring from the heart (Touhy, Strews, & Brown, 2002) is a model for practice based on the theory of Nursing as Caring in a long-term care facility. The model was designed through collaboration between project personnel and all stakeholders. All persons on the model unit participated in the process to create an innovative approach that blends into the existing facility design. Major themes revolve around responding to that which matters, caring as a way of expressing spiritual commitment, devotion inspired by love for others, commitment to creating a home environment, and coming to know and respect person as person. The major building blocks of the nursing models for acute care hospitals and the long-term care facility each reflect central themes of Nursing as Caring, but those themes are drawn out in ways unique to the setting and to the persons involved in each setting. The differences and similarities in these practice models demonstrate the power of Nursing as Caring to transform practice in a way that reflects unity without conformity and uniqueness within oneness (Touhy et al., 2002).

More Alike Than Different: Caring Across Cultures in Nursing Homes (Touhy 2003) is the first phase of a study of cultural harmony based on Boykin and Schoenhofer's (2001a) theory of Nursing as Caring. Major themes emerging from the study are respect, coming to know person, and caring and love unite us (Touhy, 2003). The study was funded by the Quantum Foundation in Palm Beach County, Florida.

In a study entitled The Phenomenology of Everyday Caring, also based on the theory of Nursing as Caring, Schoenhofer, Bingham, and Hutchins

(1998) examined the lived experience of caring at the essential level of everyday life. They created an innovative research methodology that elicited a rich description of caring through a group process. Hermeneutic phenomenology, employed to illuminate the meaning of lived experience embedded in text, was coupled with guided reflection in a collaborative, developmental process. Data were generated by 13 small groups of 3 to 5 persons who shared common characteristics such as age, role, setting, or circumstance. Participants included co-researchers who were involved not only in data generation but in the data synthesis process as well. Participants were asked to reflect on a situation in which they expressed themselves uniquely as caring persons in their everyday lives. The following essential themes emerged from the action narratives shared by the participants:

(a) Caring is evidenced by empathetic understanding, actions, and patience on another's behalf.

(b) Caring for one another by actions, words, and being there leads to happiness and touches the heart.

(c) Caring is giving of self while preserving the importance of self (Schoenhofer et al., 1998, p. 27).

The metatheme that emerged from the stories of everyday caring is "Caring is a fulfilling giving of oneself on another's behalf" (Schoenhofer, et al., 1998, p. 27). The understandings arising from this study of everyday caring have the potential to inform the nurse's understanding of the one nursed and to enhance effective nurse-patient caring.

The theory of Nursing as Caring also underpinned Schoenhofer and Boykin's (1998b) study entitled The Value of Caring Experienced in Nursing, which took place in the context of home health nursing. A client family, a nurse associated with a rural, community-based home health agency, a nursing supervisor, and an executive director of the agency participated in dialogic interviews. Caring expressed and values experienced were illuminated by the nursed, the nurse, the nursing supervisor, and the agency executive. Major themes that emerged include trust, honesty, authentic presence,

commitment, intention, reciprocity-mutuality, and quality indicators of outcomes of caring (Schoenhofer & Boykin, 1998b). Schoenhofer and Boykin (1998b) note that under many systems of quality indicators and outcomes, most of the value experienced within the nursing relationship could be relegated to categories of patient satisfaction and nurse satisfaction, for which no adequate nomenclature is available to reflect outcomes.

In a 2004 study entitled The Value Experienced in Relationships Involving Nurse Practitioner–Nursed Dyads, Thomas, Finch, Green, and Schoenhofer sought to describe the shared experience of caring between nurse practitioners and those they nurse and to uncover the caring experienced in the relationship. The research approach used was praxis, in which dialogue ensued between the nurse practitioner, nursed, and nurse researcher. A portrait of the caring between the nurse practitioner and nursed manifests the caring experienced as the following:

> . . . mutuality of love, trust and respect. The caring between them is built on a foundation of respect—an acceptance of and authentic appreciation for the other as caring person. The commitment of respect engenders an empowering trust—trust in self, trust in other, commitment to trustworthiness. The depth and meaning of the caring between the nurse practitioner and the one nursed is communicated in expressions of spiritual connectedness. These profound expressions of caring—respect, trust, mutuality, spirituality, reflect enhanced personhood as each grows in strengthening and expanding loving ways of living grounded in caring. (S. Schoenhofer, personal communication, May 8, 2004)

Acceptance of the theory of Nursing as Caring by the community of scholars in nursing is evidenced by increasing discussion and critique in the literature. Nursing as Caring has been included in several collected and edited works on nursing theories (George, 2002; Parker, 1993, 2000). George's (2002) collection of general nursing theories employs Fawcett's (1993) metaparadigm concepts for analysis and evaluation. Parker's (1993) *Patterns of*

Nursing Theories in Practice and (2000) *Nursing Theories and Nursing Practice* are collections of vibrant chapter dyads, each with an original chapter authored by the nurse theorist and accompanied by a chapter written by a nurse living out the theory in practice. Nursing as Caring is represented in both of these books by authors Schoenhofer and Boykin (1993), Boykin and Schoenhofer (2001a), and by practitioners Kearney and Yeager (1993) and Linden (2000).

McCance, McKenna, and Boore (1999) included Nursing as Caring in their comparative analysis of four caring theories. The analysis was based on factors that included origin, scope, and key concepts of the theory, definition of caring, description of nursing, goal or outcome of nursing from the perspective of the theory, and simplicity of the internal structure. Results of the analysis were reported in terms of the utility of the theory in practice.

Smith (1999) analyzed concepts of caring in nursing from the literature, seeking to find areas of congruence from the literature with the perspective of the Science of Unitary Human Beings. The theory of Nursing as Caring contributed to four of the five identified constitutive meanings of caring: manifesting intentions, appreciating pattern, attuning to dynamic flow, and inviting creative emergence (Smith, 1999).

Kiser-Larson (2000) analyzed concepts of caring and story through the lens of Newman, Sime, and Corcoran-Perry's three nursing paradigms: particulate-deterministic, interactive-integrative, and unitary-transformative. Nursing as Caring contributed to the author's understanding of the complexity of caring in the literature and the basis for the author's thesis that "caring and story become reciprocal as caring invites story and story enhances caring" (Kiser-Larson, 2000, p. 28).

FURTHER DEVELOPMENT
Theory

As a general theory of nursing, Nursing as Caring serves as a broad, conceptual framework underpinning middle range theory development. Drawing on Nursing as Caring as an underlying theoretical framework, Locsin (1995) created a model of machine technologies and caring in nursing. In the model, competence in machine technology and caring is presented as nursing practice if grounded in a caring perspective, without which nursing simply becomes the practice of machine proficiency. Locsin (1998) further developed this critical understanding in the theory of technological competence as caring in critical care nursing. In this theory, the intention to care and to nurture the other as caring is actualized through direct knowing, as well as through the medium of technologically produced data and technological competence.

Dunphy (1998) developed a model, the circle of caring, for advanced practice nursing. The core component of the model, caring processes, focuses on ways of knowing the person as caring and of truly being with the person in advanced practice nursing situations. This core provides the crucial link of caring as the central focus of both traditional nursing and advanced practice nursing.

Research

Research and development efforts are focused on expanding the language of caring by uncovering personal ways of living caring in everyday life (Schoenhofer et al., 1998) and on reconceptualizing nursing outcomes as "value experienced in nursing situations" (Boykin & Schoenhofer, 1997; Schoenhofer & Boykin, 1998a, 1998b). In consultation with graduate students, nursing faculties and health care agencies are using aspects of the theory to ground research, teaching, and practice. Developmental efforts include the following areas: (1) clarification of the concept of personhood, (2) expansion of the understanding of enhancing personhood as the general outcome of nursing, (3) innovations in nursing research, (4) use of the theory in middle range theory work, and (5) use of the theory in the critical analysis of caring.

In a development that signifies grass roots acceptance of the theory, Nursing as Caring has been translated into Japanese. The process is also underway with translation of the theory into Spanish and Portuguese.

CRITIQUE

Clarity

Boykin and Schoenhofer achieve semantic clarity by developing the theory of Nursing as Caring with everyday language. The major assumptions that undergird the theory are clearly stated and interrelated. Meanings are understood intuitively and reflectively. The assumption that all persons are caring is necessary for understanding the theory, because Boykin and Schoenhofer assert that the caring between the nurse and nursed is the source and ground of nursing. The assumption that nursing is both a discipline and profession provides a conceptual locus for the creation of research methodologies that fluidly unite both the discipline and profession within the notion of research within praxis, or praxis as research. Boykin and Schoenhofer assert that a methodology fully adequate to tap into the vein of nursing knowledge within the nursing situation would include a phenomenological-hermeneutical process within an action research orientation. Such a methodology permits the study of nursing meaning as it is being co-created within the lived experience of the nursing situation.

Simplicity

The simplicity of the theory rests in the everyday language and in the reciprocal nature of nursing characterized by the fundamental grounding in person as caring. The assumptions of the theory encompass a broad sweep of human understanding and lay plainly the conceptual groundwork for living caring. In this regard, however, the theory becomes more complex, in that assumptions and concepts become richer in meaning and densely interconnected as the nurse comes to know self as caring person in ever greater dimensions (Boykin & Schoenhofer, 2001a). The lived meaning of Nursing as Caring is illuminated best in a nursing situation in which the notion of living caring enhances knowing of self and other.

Generality

Boykin and colleagues (2003) describe the theory of Nursing as Caring as a general or grand nursing theory that offers a broad philosophical framework with practical implications for transforming practice. From the perspective of Nursing as Caring, the focus of nursing knowledge and nursing action is nurturing persons living caring and growing in caring. The theory may be used to guide individual practice or to guide the larger perspective of the organizational practice of institutions. The theory of Nursing as Caring underpins middle range frameworks such as Locsin's (1998) theory of technological competence as caring and Dunphy's (1998) model for advanced practice nursing.

Empirical Precision

The theory of Nursing as Caring does not lend itself to research methodologies of traditional science. The testability and ultimate use of the theory rest in the methods used for testing. Because the locus of nursing inquiry is the nursing situation, the systematic study of nursing calls for a method of inquiry that can encompass the dialogic circle of understanding of persons connected in caring. Boykin and Schoenhofer distinguish clearly between inquiry about nursing and inquiry of nursing. The fullness of the nursing situation is not amenable to study by measurement techniques, even though the information derived can be useful to the nurse and to the client of nursing. Aspects or variables of only the nursing situation become known.

Derivable Consequences

When integrated into nursing practice, the theory of Nursing as Caring illuminates and brings into consciousness and articulation the values of nursing care. These include the direct, unmediated worth of nursing care in economic terms, the value of nursing as a social and human service, the value of nursing caring as a rich, satisfying practice for nurses, and the value of regenerative nursing for the discipline. The significance of Nursing as Caring is evidenced by the adoption of the theory at multiple levels ranging from individual practice to hospital department, to nursing administration and, in the future, to the entire institution. Nursing values are being translated into values for general well-being, and caring is being infused into the domains of non-nursing personnel.

SUMMARY

The theory of Nursing as Caring is a general or grand nursing theory that offers a broad philosophical framework with practical implications for transforming practice (Boykin, et al., 2003). From the perspective of Nursing as Caring, the focus and aim of nursing as a discipline of knowledge and a professional service is "nurturing persons living caring and growing in caring" (Boykin & Schoenhofer, 2001a, p. 12). The theory is grounded in fundamental assumptions that (1) to be human is to be caring, and (2) the activities of the discipline and profession of nursing coalesce in coming to know persons as caring, and nurturing them as persons living and growing in caring.

Formed intention and authentic presence guide the nurse in selecting and organizing empirically based knowledge for practical use in each unique and unfolding nursing situation. Because caring is uniquely created in the moment in response to a uniquely experienced call for nursing caring, there can be no prescribed, expected outcome of nursing as caring. However, the caring that is experienced by the nursed and others in the nursing situation can be described and valued (Boykin & Schoenhofer, 1997; Schoenhofer & Boykin, 1998a, 1998b).

Caring in nursing is "an altruistic, active expression of love, and is the intentional and embodied recognition of value and connectedness" (Boykin & Schoenhofer, 2000, p. 393). Although caring is not unique to nursing, it is uniquely lived in nursing. The understanding of nursing as a discipline and a profession uniquely focuses on caring as its central value, its primary interest, and the direct intention of its practice.

Models for practice are being developed in several institutional practice areas, and Nursing as Caring is being used as a conceptual basis for developing middle range theories. As the theory of Nursing as Caring has become more widely known, consideration and referential inclusion in disciplinary journals has steadily increased. The theory is also beginning to be used as theoretical basis for master's and doctoral research (Herrington, 2002; Linden, 1996).

Case Study

Study of the Nursing Situation

From the perspective of Nursing as Caring, the concept of case study is not consonant with the notion of personhood as a process of living grounded in caring (Boykin & Schoenhofer, 1991). The mutual relationship shared by the nurse and nursed is one of reciprocity and subjectivity. Studying a case with a problem, need, or deficit does not reflect the respect for person as person grounded in the assumptions of Nursing as Caring. Because all nursing knowledge is found in the nursing situation, the shared, lived experience in which the caring between nurse and nursed enhances personhood, and the nursing situation becomes the unit of knowledge studied.

Carper's (1978) fundamental patterns of knowing, personal, empirical, ethical, and aesthetic, open useful pathways for organizing and understanding the rich content of the nursing situation. Each of these patterns may be seen below in the nursing situation in the poem, "Unseen."

Personal knowing centers on encountering, experiencing, and knowing of self and other. Empathy, the shared knowing of other, is an expression of personal knowing. Empirical knowing is impersonal and factual and addresses the science of caring in nursing. Ethical knowing is concerned with moral obligations inherent in the nursing situation and what ought to be.

Each pathway transforms knowledge in the creation of aesthetic knowing. Aesthetic knowing is the subjective appreciation of phenomena and is the synthesis of all knowing as lived in the nursing situation. Nursing stories, therefore, represent both the process of aesthetic knowing (creative appreciation) and the product of aesthetic knowing (illumination and integration) (Boykin &

Schoenhofer, 1991). The outcomes of nursing then become the values experienced within the nursing situation.

You are invited to participate in the following, which is a nursing situation for study. Enter into a quiet inner space of contemplation. Put all thoughts and distractions aside, and allow yourself to be one with the nurse and the one nursed.

Unseen

You slump in the wheelchair listing to the right
Drool slides down from the corner of your mouth
Your shirt is askew with buttons and holes mismatched
Your trousers are baggy and it is increasingly
Difficult to get into them without help
You wear new slippers your daughter sent you as a
reminder of her love.
Your days are now filled with waiting, hoping, and
reminiscing.
Waiting for someone, anyone to come into your room
To leisurely sit and chat,
And not just rush
Away after completing their required task.
Hoping for a phone call to come for you
So you can hear the sweet voices of your grandchildren
To share in the lives of your loved ones
In the outside world.
Reminiscing of the days, not so long ago,
When you were directing the board meeting,
Lunching with clients,
And landing the contracts.
As you sit in the chair, and watch the day's activities
You wonder
Does anyone really see me?
Do they know I have wishes and hopes?
Do they care?
And then the gentle touch of a hand,
The soft spoken hello
The conversation where one takes the time
To truly listen.
In this you see someone does care
And in these moments, however brief, you are not unseen.

Cheri L. Larese
Stuart, FL

CRITICAL THINKING *Activities*

Reflecting Upon the Nursing Situation

Pause for a moment. Close your eyes and reflect upon the meaning and the caring of the nursing situation in "Unseen."

1. What were calls for nursing perceived by the nurse?

2. What were some of the ways in which the nurse's personal knowing sustained and nurtured the one nursed? What was the personal knowing of the nursed?

3. Can you describe the empirical knowing of the nurse as captured in her poignant description of the nursed? How did this influence her nurturing responses? Look out at the world through the eyes of the nursed. What was his empirical knowing of the situation? How did this influence his hope in the moment?

4. Seat yourself in the wheelchair, with the one nursed. What was his ethical knowing? How did he feel he ought to be? What was the ethical knowing of the nurse?

5. Place yourself in the nurse's shoes and see the one nursed through her eyes. What were the nurse's responses to the calls for nursing? How did her aesthetic knowing shape her response to the calls?

6. What were the values experienced in the nursing situation by the one nursed? By his family? What were values experienced by the nurse?

As you come to a quiet rest in your reflections, honor your understandings and your own expressions of personal caring. Remember a special story of your own caring and record it in a journal. Appreciate your life's journey and the unique expression of your caring in nursing.

REFERENCES

Algase, D. L., & Whall, A. F. (1993). Rosemary Ellis' views on the substantive structure of nursing. *Image: The Journal of Nursing Scholarship, 25*(1), 69-72.

Boykin, A. (1990). Creating a caring environment: Moral obligations in the role of dean. In M. Leininger & J. Watson (Eds.), *The caring imperative in education* (pp. 247-254). New York: National League for Nursing.

Boykin, A. (1994a). Creating a caring environment for nursing education. In A. Boykin (Ed.), *Living a caring-based program* (pp. 11-25). New York: National League for Nursing Press.

Boykin, A. (Ed.). (1994b). *Living a caring-based program.* New York: National League for Nursing.

Boykin, A. (Ed.). (1995). *Power, politics and public policy: A matter of caring.* New York: National League for Nursing.

Boykin, A., Bulfin, S., Southern, B., & Baldwin, J. (2004, June). *Emergency department: Transformation from object centered care to person centered care through caring. Phase 1 of study funded by the Center for Excellence in Nursing, Boca Raton Community Hospital.* Paper presented at 26th Annual Conference of the International Association for Human Caring, Montreal, Quebec.

Boykin, A., & Parker, M. E. (1997). Illuminating spirituality in the classroom. In M. S. Roach (Ed.), *Caring from the heart: The convergence of caring and spirituality* (pp. 21-33). Mahwah, NJ: Paulist Press.

Boykin, A., Parker, M., & Schoenhofer, S. (1994). Aesthetic knowing grounded in an explicit conception of nursing. *Nursing Science Quarterly, 7*(4), 158-161.

Boykin, A., & Schoenhofer, S. (1993). *Nursing as caring: A model for transforming practice.* New York: National League for Nursing Press.

Boykin, A. & Schoenhofer, S. O. (1990). Caring in nursing: Analysis of extant theory. *Nursing Science Quarterly, 3*(4), 149-155.

Boykin, A., & Schoenhofer, S. O. (1991). Story as link between nursing practice, ontology, and epistemology. *Image: The Journal of Nursing Scholarship, 23*(4), 245-248.

Boykin, A., & Schoenhofer, S. O. (1997). Reframing nursing outcomes. *Advanced Practice Nursing Quarterly, 1*(3), 60-65.

Boykin, A., & Schoenhofer, S. O. (2000). Nursing as caring: An overview of a general theory of nursing. In M. E. Parker (Ed.), *Nursing theories and nursing practice* (pp. 391-402). Philadelphia: F. A. Davis.

Boykin, A., & Schoenhofer, S. O. (2001a). *Nursing as caring: A model for transforming practice* [Rerelease of original volume, with epilogue added]. Sudbury, MA: Jones & Bartlett Publishers.

Boykin, A., & Schoenhofer, S. O. (2001b). The role of nursing leadership in creating caring environments in health care delivery systems. *Nursing Administration Quarterly, 25*(3), 1-7.

Boykin, A., Schoenhofer, S. O., Smith, N., St. Jean, J., & Aleman, D. (2003). Transforming practice using a caring-based nursing model. *Nursing Administration Quarterly, 27,* 223-230.

Carper, B. A. (1978). Fundamental patterns of knowing in nursing. *ANS Advances in Nursing Science, 1*(1), 113-124.

Dunphy, L. H. (1998). *The circle of caring: A transformative model of advanced practice nursing.* 20th Research Conference of the International Association for Human Caring, Philadelphia.

Fawcett, J. (1993). *Analysis and evaluation of nursing theories.* Philadelphia: F. A. Davis.

Flexner, A. (1910). *Medical education in the United States and Canada.* New York: The Carnegie Foundation for the Advancement of Teaching.

Gaut, D. A., & Boykin, A. (Eds.). (1994). *Caring as healing: Renewal through hope.* New York: National League for Nursing.

George, J. B. (2002). Nursing as caring: Anne Boykin and Savina Schoenhofer. In J. B. George (Ed.), *Nursing theories: The basis for professional nursing practice* (pp. 539-554). Upper Saddle River, NJ: Prentice Hall.

Herrington, C. L. (2002). *The meaning of caring: From the perspective of homeless women* (Master's thesis, University of Nevada, Reno, 2002). *Masters Abstracts International, 41*(01), 191.

Kearney, C., & Yeager, V. (1993). Practical applications of nursing as caring theory. In M. E. Parker (Ed.), *Patterns of nursing theories in practice* (pp. 93-102). New York: National League for Nursing.

King, A., & Brownell, J. (1976). *The curriculum and the disciplines of knowledge.* Huntington, NY: Robert E. Krieger Publishing.

Kiser-Larson, N. (2000). The concepts of caring and story viewed from three nursing paradigms. *International Journal for Human Caring, 4*(2), 26-32.

Linden, D. (1996). *Philosophical exploration in search of the ontology of authentic presence* (Master's thesis, Florida Atlantic University, West Palm Beach, FL, 1996). *Masters Abstracts International, 35*(2), 519.

Linden, D. (2000). The lived experience of nursing as caring. In M. E. Parker (Ed.), *Nursing theories and nursing practice* (pp. 403-407). Philadelphia, PA: F. A. Davis.

Locsin, R. C. (1995). Machine technologies and caring in nursing. *Image: The Journal of Nursing Scholarship, 27*(3), 201-203.

Locsin, R. C. (1998). Technologic competence as caring in critical care nursing. *Holistic Nursing Practice, 12*(4), 50-56.

Mayeroff, M. (1971). *On caring.* New York: Harper Collins.

McCance, T. V., McKenna, H. P., & Boore, J. R. (1999). Caring: Theoretical perspectives of relevance to nursing. *Journal of Advanced Nursing, 30,* 1388-1395.

Nightingale Songs. Retrieved March 10, 2005, from *http://www.fau.edu/nursing/ngsongs/nighting.htm*

Orem, D. E. (Ed.). (1979). *Concept formalization in nursing. Process and product* (2nd ed.). Boston: Little, Brown and Company.

Parker, M. E. (Ed.). (1993). *Patterns of nursing theories in practice.* New York: National League for Nursing.

Parker, M. E. (Ed.). (2000). *Nursing theories and nursing practice.* Philadelphia: F. A. Davis.

Paterson, J. G., & Zderad, L. T. (1988). *Humanistic nursing.* New York: National League for Nursing Press.

Phenix, P. (1964). *Realms of meaning.* New York: McGraw Hill.

Roach, M. S. (1987). *Caring, the human mode of being.* Ottawa, Ontario, Canada: CHA Press.

Roach, M. S. (2002). *Caring, the human mode of being* (2nd revised ed.). Ottawa, Ontario, Canada: CHA Press.

Schoenhofer, S. O. (2001). Infusing the nursing curriculum with literature on caring: An idea whose time has come. *International Journal for Human Caring, 5*(2), 7-14.

Schoenhofer, S. O. (2002a). Choosing personhood: Intentionality and the theory of nursing as caring. *Holistic Nursing Practice, 16*(4), 36-40.

Schoenhofer, S. O. (2002b). Philosophical underpinnings of an emergent methodology for nursing as caring inquiry. *Nursing Science Quarterly, 15*(4), 275-280.

Schoenhofer, S. O., Bingham, V., & Hutchins, G. (1998). Giving of oneself on another's behalf: The phenomenology of everyday caring. *International Journal for Human Caring, 2*(2), 23-29.

Schoenhofer, S. O., & Boykin, A. (1993). *Nursing as caring: An emerging general theory of nursing.* In M. E. Parker (Ed.), *Patterns of nursing theories in practice* (pp. 83-92). New York: National League for Nursing Press.

Schoenhofer, S. O., & Boykin, A. (1998a). Discovering the value of nursing in high-technology environments: Outcomes revisited. *Holistic Nursing Practice, 12*(4), 31-39.

Schoenhofer, S. O., & Boykin, A. (1998b). The value of caring experienced in nursing. *International Journal for Human Caring, 2*(4), 9-15.

Smith, M. C. (1999). Caring and the science of unitary human beings. *ANS Advances in Nursing Science, 21*(4), 14-28.

Thomas, J., Finch, L. P., Green, A., & Schoenhofer, S. O. (2004). The caring relationships created by nurse practitioners and the ones nursed: Implications for practice. *Topics in Advanced Nursing Practice, eJournal 4*(4), Retrieved March 9, 2005, from *http://www.medscape.com.*

Touhy, T. A. (2003). *More alike than different: Caring across cultures in nursing homes.* Unpublished study of cultural harmony based on Boykin and Schoenhofer's theory of nursing as caring. Funding by Quantum Foundation, West Palm Beach, FL.

Touhy, T. A., Strews, W., & Brown, C. (2002). *Caring from the heart.* Unpublished study. Christine E. Lynn College of Nursing, Boca Raton, FL.

BIBLIOGRAPHY
Primary Sources
Books

Boykin, A. (Ed.). (1994). *Living a caring-based program.* New York: National League for Nursing.

Boykin, A. (Ed.). (1995). *Power, politics and public policy: A matter of caring.* New York: National League for Nursing.

Boykin, A., & Schoenhofer, S. O. (1993). *Nursing as caring: A model for transforming practice.* New York: NLN Publications.

Boykin, A., & Schoenhofer, S. O. (2001). *Nursing as caring: A model for transforming practice* [Rerelease of original volume, with epilogue added]. Sudbury, MA: Jones & Bartlett Publishers.

Gaut, D. A., & Boykin, A. (Eds.). (1994). *Caring as healing: Renewal through hope.* New York: National League for Nursing.

Book Chapters

Beckerman, A., Boykin A., Folden S., & Winland-Brown, J. (1994). The experience of being a student in a caring-based program. In A. Boykin (Ed.), *Living a caring-based program* (pp. 79-92). New York: National League for Nursing.

Boykin A. (1990). Creating a caring environment: Moral obligations in the role of dean. In M. Leininger & J. Watson (Eds.), *The caring imperative in education* (pp. 247-254). New York: National League for Nursing.

Boykin, A. (1994). Creating a caring environment for nursing education. In A. Boykin (Ed.), *Living a caring-based program* (pp. 11-25). New York, National League for Nursing.

Boykin, A., & Parker, M. (1997). Illuminating spirituality in the classroom. In S. Roach (Ed.), *Caring from the heart.* Mahwah, NJ: Paulist Press.

Boykin, A., & Schoenhofer, S. O. (2000). Nursing as caring: An overview of a general theory of nursing. In M. E. Parker (Ed.), *Nursing theories and nursing practice.* Philadelphia: F. A. Davis.

Schoenhofer, S. O. (2001). A framework for caring in a technologically dependent nursing practice environment. In R. C. Locsin (Ed.), *Advancing technology, caring and nursing* (pp. 3-11). Westport, CT: Auburn House.

Schoenhofer, S. O. (2001). Outcomes of nurse caring in high technology practice environments. In R. C. Locsin (Ed.), *Advancing technology, caring, and nursing* (pp. 79-87). Westport, CT: Auburn House.

Schoenhofer, S. O., & Boykin, A. (1993). Nursing as caring: An emerging general theory of nursing. In M. E. Parker (Ed.), *Patterns of nursing theories in practice* (pp. 83-92). New York: National League for Nursing Press.

Schoenhofer, S. O., & Boykin, A. (2001). Caring and the advanced practice nurse. In L. Dunphy & J. Winland-Brown (Eds.), *Primary care: The art and science of advanced practice nursing.* Philadelphia: F. A. Davis.

Schoenhofer, S. O., & Coffman, S. (1993). Valuing, prizing and growing in a caring based program. In A. Boykin (Ed.), *Living a caring based program* (pp. 127-165). New York: National League for Nursing.

Journal Articles

Boykin, A., & Dunphy, L. (2002). Reflective essay: Justice-making: Nursing's call . . . Florence Nightingale. *Policy, Politics and Nursing Practice, 3*(1), 14-19.

Boykin, A., Parker, M., & Schoenhofer, S. (1994). Aesthetic knowing grounded in an explicit conception of nursing. *Nursing Science Quarterly, 7*(4), 158-161.

Boykin, A., & Schoenhofer, S. O. (l990). Caring in nursing: Analysis of extant theory. *Nursing Science Quarterly, 3*(4), l49-l55.

Boykin, A., & Schoenhofer, S. O. (1991). Story as link between nursing practice, ontology, and epistemology. *Image: The Journal of Nursing Scholarship, 23*(4), 245-248.

Boykin, A., & Schoenhofer, S. O. (1997). Reframing nursing outcomes. *Advanced Practice Nursing Quarterly, 1*(3), 60-65.

Boykin, A., & Schoenhofer, S. O. (2000). Is there really time to care? *Nursing Forum, 35*(4), 36-38.

Boykin, A., & Schoenhofer, S. O. (2001). The role of nursing leadership in creating caring environments in health care delivery systems. *Nursing Administration Quarterly, 25*(3), 1-7.

Boykin, A., Schoenhofer, S. O., Smith, N., St. Jean, J., & Aleman, D. (2003). Transforming practice using a caring-based nursing model. *Nursing Administration Quarterly, 27,* 223-230.

Boykin, A., & Winland-Brown, J. (1995). The dark side of caring: Challenges of caregiving. *Journal of Gerontological Nursing, 21*(5), 13-18.

Schoenhofer, S. O. (1989). Love, beauty, and truth: Fundamental nursing values. *Journal of Nursing Education, 28*(8), 382-384.

Schoenhofer, S. O. (1994). Transforming visions for nursing in the timeworld of Einstein's dreams. *ANS Advances in Nursing Science, 16*(4), 1-8.

Schoenhofer, S. O. (1995). Rethinking primary care: Connections to nursing. *ANS Advances in Nursing Science, 17*(4), 12-21.

Schoenhofer, S. O. (2001). Infusing the nursing curriculum with literature on caring: An idea whose time has come. *International Journal for Human Caring, 5*(2), 7-14.

Schoenhofer, S. O. (2002). Philosophical underpinnings of an emergent methodology for nursing as caring inquiry. *Nursing Science Quarterly, 15*(4), 275-280.

Schoenhofer, S. O. (2002). Choosing personhood: Intentionality and the theory of nursing as caring. *Holistic Nursing Practice, 16*(4), 36-40.

Schoenhofer, S., Bingham, V., & Hutchins, G. (1998). Giving of oneself on another's behalf: The phenomenology of everyday caring. *International Journal for Human Caring, 2*(2), 23-29.

Schoenhofer, S. O., & Boykin, A. (1998). The value of caring experienced in nursing. *International Journal for Human Caring, 2*(4), 9-15.

Schoenhofer, S. O., & Boykin, A. (1998). Discovering the value of nursing in high-technology environments: Outcomes revisited. *Holistic Nursing Practice, 12*(4), 31-39.

Secondary Sources
Books

Locsin, R. C. (Ed.). (2001). *Advancing technology, caring, and nursing.* Westport, CT: Greenwood Publishing.

Locsin, R. C. (2005). *Technological competency as caring in nursing: A model for practice.* Indianapolis: Sigma Theta Tau International Honor Society of Nursing.

Book Chapters

George, J. (2002). Nursing as caring. Anne Boykin and Savina Schoenhofer. In J. George (Ed.), *Nursing theories.* Upper Saddle River, NJ: Prentice-Hall.

Linden, D. (2000). The lived experience of nursing as caring. In M. E. Parker (Ed.), *Nursing theories and nursing practice* (pp. 403-407). Philadelphia: F. A. Davis.

Locsin, R. C. (1995). Technology and caring in nursing. In A. Boykin (Ed.), *Power, politics, and public policy: A matter of caring* (pp. 24-36). New York: National League for Nursing.

Locsin, R., & Campling, A. (2005). Techno sapiens and post humans: Nursing, caring, and technology. In R. Locsin (Ed.), *Technological competency as caring in nursing: A model for practice* (pp. 142-155). Indianapolis: Center Nursing Press, Sigma Theta Tau International Honor Society of Nursing.

Journal Articles

Barry, C. D. (2001). Creating a quilt: An aesthetic expression of caring for nursing students. *International Journal for Human Caring, 6*(1), 25-29.

Carter, M. A. (1994). [Book reviews: *Nursing as caring: A model for transforming practice*]. *Nursing Science Quarterly, 7,* 183-184.

Kiser-Larson, N. (2000). The concepts of caring and story viewed from three nursing paradigms. *International Journal for Human Caring, 4*(2), 26-32.

Locsin, R. C. (1995). Machine technologies and caring in nursing. *Image: The Journal of Nursing Scholarship, 27*(3), 201-203.

Locsin, R. C. (1997). Expressing nursing as caring through music. *The Silliman Journal, 8*(1 & 2), 1-10.

Locsin, R. C. (1998). Music as expression of nursing: A co-created moment. *International Journal for Human Caring, 2*(3), 40-42.

Locsin, R. C. (1998). Technological competence as caring in critical care nursing. *Holistic Nursing Practice, 12*(4), 50-56.

Locsin, R. C. (2000). Technological competency as caring: Perceptions of professional nurses. *The Silliman Journal, 40 & 41,* 100-104.

Locsin, R. C. (2002). Aesthetic expressions of the lived world of people waiting to know: Ebola at Mbarara, Uganda. *Nursing Science Quarterly, 15*(2), 123-130.

McCance, T. V., McKenna, H. P., & Boore, J. R. P. (1999). Caring: Theoretical perspectives of relevance to nursing. *Journal of Advanced Nursing, 30,* 1388-1395.

Smith, M. C. (1994). [Book review: *Nursing as caring: A model for transforming practice*]. *Nursing Science Quarterly, 7,* 184-185.

Smith, M. C. (1999). Caring and the science of unitary human beings. *ANS Advances in Nursing Science, 21*(4), 14-28.

Touhy, T. A. (2001). Touching the spirit of elders in nursing homes: Ordinary yet extraordinary care. *International Journal for Human Caring, 6*(1), 12-17.

Touhy, T. A. (2004). Dementia, personhood, and nursing: Learning from a nursing situation. *Nursing Science Quarterly, 17*(1), 43-49.

Winland-Brown, J. E. (1996). Can caring for critically ill patients be taught by reading a novel? *Nurse Educator, 21*(5), 23-27.

Other Sources

Herrington, C. L. (2002). The meaning of caring: From the perspective of homeless women (Masters thesis, University of Nevada, Reno, 2002). *Masters Abstracts International, 41*(01), 191.

Linden, D. (1996). Philosophical exploration in search of the ontology of authentic presence (Masters thesis, Florida Atlantic University, West Palm Beach, FL, 1996). *Masters Abstracts International, 35*(2), 519.

Touhy, T. A. (2003). *More alike than different: Caring across cultures in nursing homes.* Unpublished study of cultural harmony based on Boykin and Schoenhofer's theory of nursing as caring. Funding by Quantum Foundation, West Palm Beach, FL.

Web Site

Nursing as Caring. Accessed December 20, 2004: *http://www.nursingascaring.com*

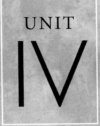

UNIT

IV

Nursing Theories

- Grand nursing theories are conceptual structures that are nearly as abstract as the nursing models from which they are derived, but they propose outcomes based on use and application of the model in nursing practice.

- Theories are ways of looking at a phenomenon to describe, explain, predict, or control it.

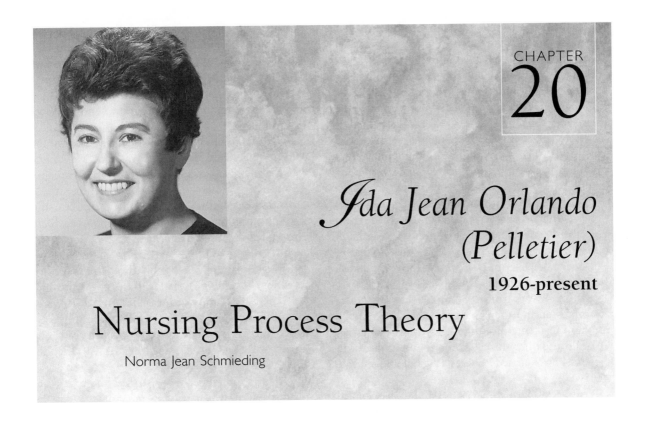

CHAPTER
20

*Ida Jean Orlando
(Pelletier)*
1926-present

Nursing Process Theory

Norma Jean Schmieding

CREDENTIALS AND BACKGROUND OF THE THEORIST

Ida Jean Orlando was born August 12, 1926. She received a diploma in nursing from New York Medical College, Flower Fifth Avenue Hospital School of Nursing, in New York in 1947. In 1951, she received a B.S. in public health nursing from St. John's University in Brooklyn, New York, and an M.A. in mental health consultation from Columbia University Teachers College in 1954. While pursuing

Previous authors: Larry P. Schumacher, Susan Fisher, Ann Marriner Tomey, Deborah I. Mills, and Marcia K. Sauter. The author expresses appreciation to Ida Jean Orlando (Pelletier) for her continuing insightful contributions to this chapter. Orlando continually supports endeavors to extend the use of her theory and encouraged the author's interpretation of the theory. Patients, nurses, and the profession continue to benefit from her theoretical contributions.

her education, Orlando worked intermittently, and sometimes concurrently, as a staff nurse in obstetrical, medical, surgical, and emergency nursing services. She also worked as a supervisor in a general hospital. In addition, as an assistant director of nursing, she was responsible for a general hospital's nursing service and for teaching several courses in the hospital's nursing school.

After receiving her master's degree in 1954, Orlando was employed by Yale School of Nursing in New Haven, Connecticut, for 8 years. Until 1958, she was a research associate and principal investigator of a federal project grant entitled Integration of Mental Health Concepts in a Basic Curriculum. The project focused on identifying factors influencing the integration of mental health principles in a basic nursing curriculum. Orlando conducted this project by observing and participating in student experiences with patients and medical, nursing, and instructional personnel throughout the students' basic curriculum. For 3 years, she recorded her observations and spent a fourth year analyzing the accumulated data. Orlando reported her findings in 1958 in her first book, *The Dynamic Nurse-Patient Relationship: Function, Process and Principles of Professional Nursing Practice* (1961). Although completed in 1958, this book remained unpublished until 1961. The formulation in this publication provides the foundation for Orlando's nursing theory.

There are five consecutive foreign-language editions of Orlando's theory: Japanese, Hebrew, French, Portuguese, and Dutch. Two sections of the book were written in German (Mischo-Kelling & Wittneben, 1995, pp. 50-59, 184-186). Orlando's 1972 book was published in Japanese.

During 4 years from 1958 to 1961, as an associate professor and then as director of the graduate program in mental health and psychiatric nursing, Orlando used her theory as the foundation of the program. She married Robert J. Pelletier and left Yale in 1961.

From 1962 through 1972, Orlando was Clinical Nursing Consultant at McLean Hospital in Belmont, Massachusetts. While in this position, she studied interactions of nurses with patients, peers, and other staff members. She also examined how these interactions affected the processes that nurses use to help patients. Orlando convinced the hospital director that a training program for nurses was needed. As a result, the McLean Hospital nursing service was reorganized and a training program based on her theory was implemented. Orlando subsequently applied for and received federal funding to evaluate training in the nursing process discipline.

While at McLean Hospital, Orlando published The Patient's Predicament and Nursing Function in *Psychiatric Opinion* in 1967 (Pelletier, 1967). Orlando reported 10 years of work at the hospital in her second book, *The Discipline and Teaching of Nursing Process: An Evaluative Study* (Orlando, 1972).

From 1972 to 1981, Orlando lectured, served as a consultant, and conducted about 60 workshops about her theory throughout the United States and Canada. She served on the board of the Harvard Community Health Plan in Boston, Massachusetts, from 1972 to 1984 and served on the hospital committee of the board from 1979 to 1985. Since then, she has served in various capacities, such as on the membership, program, and services committees.

In 1981, Orlando was hired as Nurse Educator for Metropolitan State Hospital in Waltham, Massachusetts, and held various administrative nursing positions from 1984 to 1987. In September 1987, Orlando became the Assistant Director of Nursing for Education and Research at Metropolitan State Hospital. She retired from nursing in 1992.

In 1990, the National League for Nursing (NLN) reprinted Orlando's 1961 publication. In the preface to the NLN edition, Orlando states the following: "If I had been more courageous in 1961, when this book was first written, I would have proposed it as 'nursing process theory' instead of as a 'theory of effective nursing practice'" (Orlando, 1990, p. vii).

Orlando's nursing theory stresses the reciprocal relationship between patient and nurse. What the nurse and patient say and do affects both. She is one of the first nursing leaders to identify and emphasize the elements of nursing process and the critical importance of the patient's participation in the nursing process. Orlando views nursing as a distinct profession and separate from medicine (Hilton, 1997). Orlando believes physicians' orders are for patients, not for nurses. However, the nurse helps the patient carry out the order or, if the patient is unable, the nurse does it for patient. Likewise, the nurse may help patients avoid adhering to physicians' orders if data support it. The nurse would, however, communicate the rationale for this to the physician (Pelletier, 1967). Orlando may have facilitated the development of nurses as logical thinkers (Nursing Theories Conference Group & George, 1980). Orlando views nurses as determining nursing action rather than being prompted by physician's orders, organizational needs, and past personal experiences. Therefore, nursing action is derived from the patient's immediate experience and immediate need for help.

Orlando states that her search for facts in observing nursing situations influenced her most before the development of her theory and that she derived her theory from the conceptualization of those facts (I. Pelletier, personal communication, 1984). Her overall goal was to develop "a theory of effective nursing practice" (Orlando, 1961, p. viii) that would identify a distinctive role for professional nurses that would provide a systematic foundation for the study of nursing.

Orlando made major contributions to nursing theory and practice. Her conceptualizations of the deliberative nursing process fulfill the criteria of a theory. In her theory, she does the following:

- Presents interrelated concepts that represent a systematic view of nursing phenomena
- Specifies relationships among the concepts
- Explains what happens during the nursing process and why
- Prescribes how nursing phenomena can be controlled
- Explains how the control leads to the prediction of outcome

Although nurses such as Fitzpatrick and Whall (1989) note the debate about whether models are theory and conclude they are not, numerous other theorists such as Fawcett (1993), George (1995), and Walker and Avant (1995) classify Orlando's theory at various levels of accepted theory. Despite these diverging views, Orlando's theory has substantial merit for its application to practice, research, education, and administration. Orlando's views about nursing, nurses, and patients remain the same as when she developed her theory (I. Orlando, personal interview, May 27, 2000).

THEORETICAL SOURCES

Orlando does not acknowledge any theoretical sources for the development of her theory. None of her publications includes a bibliography. However, Schmieding (1986) traced similarities of her formulations to those of John Dewey and to some of the nurse colleagues and educators with whom Orlando was associated at Columbia (Schmieding, 1993).

MAJOR CONCEPTS & DEFINITIONS

Orlando describes her model as revolving around the following five major interrelated concepts (Schmieding, 1986):

1. The function of professional nursing
2. The presenting behavior of the patient
3. The immediate or internal response of the nurse
4. The nursing process discipline
5. Improvement

NURSE'S RESPONSIBILITY

The nurse's responsibility consists of "whatever help the patient may require for his needs to be met (i.e., for his physical and mental comfort to be assured as far as possible while he is undergoing some form of medical treatment or supervision" (Orlando, 1990, p. 5). It is the nurse's responsibility to see that "the patient's needs for help are met, either directly by her own activity or indirectly by calling in the help of others" (Orlando, 1961, p. 29).

NEED

Need is "situationally defined as a requirement of the patient which, if supplied, relieves or diminishes his immediate distressor and improves his immediate sense of adequacy or well-being" (Orlando, 1990, p. 6).

PRESENTING BEHAVIOR OF PATIENT

The presenting behavior is any observable verbal or nonverbal behavior (Forchuk, 1991).

IMMEDIATE REACTIONS

Immediate reactions include both the nurse's and patient's individual perceptions, thoughts, and feelings (Forchuk, 1991).

Continued

MAJOR CONCEPTS *&* DEFINITIONS—cont'd

NURSING PROCESS DISCIPLINE

Nursing process discipline includes the nurse communicating to the patient his or her own immediate reaction, clearly identifying that the item expressed belongs to the nurse, and then asking for validation or correction (Forchuk, 1991). Nursing process discipline was called *deliberative nursing process* in Orlando's first book, *The Dynamic Nurse-Patient Relationship: Function, Process and Principles of Professional Nursing Practice* (Orlando, 1961), and also is called *nursing process* and *process discipline*.

IMPROVEMENT

According to Orlando (1961), improvement "means to grow better, to turn to profit, to use to advantage" (p. 6).

PURPOSE OF NURSING

"The purpose of nursing is to supply the help a patient requires in order for his needs to be met" (Orlando, 1990, p. 9).

AUTOMATIC NURSING ACTION

Automatic actions are "those (nursing actions) decided upon for reasons other than the patient's immediate need" (Crane, 1985, p. 167).

DELIBERATIVE NURSING ACTION

Deliberative actions are those decided upon after ascertaining a need and then meeting this need (Crane, 1985).

USE OF EMPIRICAL EVIDENCE

Orlando was the first nurse to develop her theory from actual nurse-patient situations. Orlando recorded the content of 2000 nurse-patient contacts and created her theory based on the analysis of these data (Schmieding, 1993). Orlando asserts that her theory was valid, and she applied it in her work with patients and nurses and in teaching students. She used a qualitative method to obtain data from which she developed her theory. According to Meleis (1997), "Orlando used field methodology before it became a world view in research" (p. 348).

At McLean Hospital, Orlando implemented the nursing process theory that she had developed at Yale. During her last 3 years there, she received a research grant to perform evaluative research of the training program to test her formulations. Orlando published these results in her second book, *The Discipline and Teaching of Nursing Process: An Evaluative Study,* in 1972. In it, Orlando clearly and succinctly presents the components of her theory, describes a person's process of action, and specifies which types of action facilitate or hinder the nurse from finding out the patient's immediate need for help. Several Yale faculty members used Orlando's theory as a basis for discussing and developing a nursing practice theory (Henderson, 1987).

MAJOR ASSUMPTIONS

Nearly all the assumptions in Orlando's theory are implicit. Meleis (1991) thinks that one of the major problems with Orlando's assumptions is that it is not totally clear how they were derived, because no documentation exists. However, Orlando, similar to other early theorists, did not specify assumptions. Various authors have extrapolated them. Schmieding (1993) derived assumptions from Orlando's writings in the following four areas and elaborated on Orlando's view about each:

1. **Assumptions about nursing**
   "Nursing is a distinct profession separate from other disciplines" (p. 10).
   "Professional nursing has a distinct function and product (outcome)" (p. 10).

"There is a difference between lay and professional nursing" (p. 11).

"Nursing is aligned with medicine" (p. 12).

2. **Assumptions about patients**

"Patients' needs for help are unique" (p. 12).

"Patients have an initial ability to communicate their needs for help" (p. 12).

"When patients cannot meet their own needs they become distressed" (p. 13).

"The patient's behavior is meaningful" (p. 13).

"Patients are able and willing to communicate verbally (and nonverbally when unable to communicate verbally)" (p. 13).

3. **Assumptions about nurses**

"The nurse's reaction to each patient is unique" (p. 14).

"Nurses should not add to the patient's distress" (p. 14).

"The nurse's mind is the major tool for helping patients" (p. 14).

"The nurse's use of automatic responses prevents the responsibility of nursing from being fulfilled" (p. 15).

"Nurse's practice is improved through self-reflection" (p. 15).

4. **Assumptions about the nurse-patient situation**

"The nurse-patient situation is a dynamic whole" (p. 15).

"The phenomenon of the nurse-patient encounter represents a major source of nursing knowledge" (p. 16).

The metaparadigm assumptions of Orlando's theory follow in the next section.

Nursing

Orlando's major assumption about nursing is that it should be a distinct profession that functions autonomously. Although nursing has been historically aligned with medicine and continues to have a close relationship with medicine, nursing and the practice of medicine are clearly separate professions (Orlando, 1961). These assumptions are reflected in Orlando's definition of the function of professional nursing.

Orlando (1972) denotes "the function of professional nursing is conceptualized as finding out and meeting the patient's immediate need for help" (p. 20). It is the nurse's responsibility to see that "the patient's needs for help are met, either directly by her own activity or indirectly by calling in the help of others" (Orlando, 1961, p. 22). This is more fully amplified by Orlando's approach to nursing process discipline, which she proposes is composed of the following basic elements: "(1) the behavior of the patient, (2) the reaction of the nurse, and (3) the nursing actions, which are designed for the patient's benefit. The interaction of these elements with each other is nursing process" (Orlando, 1961, p. 36).

Another assumption Orlando (1972) makes is that nurses should help relieve physical or mental discomfort and should not add to the patient's distress. This assumption is evident in Orlando's concept of improvement in the patient's behavior as the intended outcome of nursing actions. Orlando is concerned with providing direct assistance to individuals in whatever setting for the purpose of avoiding, relieving, diminishing, or curing the person's sense of helplessness (Forchuk, 1991).

Person

Orlando assumes that persons behave verbally and nonverbally. Evidence of this assumption is found in Orlando's emphasis on behavior, in observing changes in the patient's behavior. Orlando assumes that people are sometimes able to meet their own need for help in some situations; however, they become distressed when they are unable to do so. This is the basis for Orlando's assertion (1961) that professional nurses should be concerned only with those persons who are unable to meet their need for help independently. However, nurses observe and communicate with patients periodically to determine if there are new needs for help. She also states that each patient is unique and individual in his or her response; a professional nurse can recognize that the same behavior in different patients can signal quite different needs.

Health

Orlando (1961) did not define health, but she assumes that freedom from mental or physical discomfort and feelings of adequacy and well-being contribute to health. "Orlando implicitly assumed feelings of adequacy and well-being from fulfilled needs contribute to health" (Jones & Meleis, 1993, p. 4). Orlando (1961) notes which "repeated experiences of having been helped undoubtedly culminate over periods of time in greater degrees of improvement" (p. 90). Therefore these cumulative changes are fertile areas for further research.

Environment

Orlando (1961) does not define environment. She assumes that a nursing situation occurs when there is a nurse-patient contact and that both nurse and patient perceive, think, feel, and act in the immediate situation. However, she does specify that a patient may react with distress to any aspect of an environment that was designed for therapeutic and helpful purposes. When the nurse observes any patient behavior, it needs to be viewed as a signal of distress. Any aspect of the environment, even though it is designed for therapeutic and helpful purposes, can cause the patient to become distressed.

THEORETICAL ASSERTIONS

Orlando (1961) views the professional function of nursing as finding out and meeting the patient's immediate need for help. This function is fulfilled when the nurse finds out and meets a patient's immediate need for help. Orlando's theory focuses on how to produce improvement in the patient's behavior. Evidence of relieving the patient's distress is determined by positive changes in the patient's observable behavior.

According to Orlando (1961), a person becomes a patient requiring nursing care when he or she has needs for help that cannot be met independently because he or she has physical limitations, has a negative reaction to an environment, or has an experience that prevents the patient from communicating his or her needs. Orlando asserts that these limitations on the patient's ability to meet his or her needs are most likely to occur while the patient is

receiving medical care or supervision. The restrictions Orlando frequently has placed on the concept of patient can be viewed as a function of the impediments that people have in meeting their own needs.

Patients experience distress or feelings of helplessness because of unmet needs for help (Orlando, 1961). Orlando believes there is a positive correlation between the length of time the patient experiences the unmet needs and the degree of distress. Therefore, immediacy is emphasized throughout her theory. In Orlando's view, when people are able to meet their own needs, they do not feel distress and do not require care from a professional nurse at that time. For a person who does have a need for help, it is crucial that the nurse obtain the patient's correction or verification of the nurse's perceptions, thoughts, or feelings to determine whether the patient is in need of help.

Individuals in contact with each other go through an action process that involves the observation of the other's behavior, the resulting thought about this observation, a feeling originating from the person's thought, and an action chosen by each individual in response to the reaction (Orlando, 1972). When the nurse acts, an action process transpires. This action process by the nurse in a nurse-patient contact is called *nursing process*. The nurse's action may be automatic or deliberative. Any patient behavior observed by the nurse must be viewed as a signal of distress, because the patient may become distressed by any aspect of an environment that was designed for therapeutic and helpful purposes. The nurse's perception of a patient's behavior produces thoughts that cause the nurse to experience a feeling. Orlando (1961) identifies and defines the elements of this immediate reaction as follows:

- Perception, a physical stimulation of any one of a person's five senses
- The automatic thought about the perception that occurs in an individual's mind
- A feeling stimulated by the thought that inclines a person toward or against a perception, thought, or feeling

The nurse's reaction then precipitates a nursing action.

The nurse's asking the patient about his or her perception of the patient's behavior rather than first exploring his or her own thoughts and feelings is more effective and less time consuming, because the physical stimulus for perception has objective validity. Nursing actions that are not deliberative are automatic (Orlando, 1961). Automatic nursing actions are those having nothing to do with finding out and meeting the patient's need for help. Deliberative nursing actions are those designed to identify and meet the patient's immediate needs for help and to fulfill the professional nursing function. Deliberative nursing actions require that the nurse seek verification or correction of his or her thoughts and the origin of the feelings with the patient before the nurse and the patient can know what nursing action will meet the patient's need for help.

In Orlando's (1972) second book, *The Discipline and Teaching of Nursing Process: An Evaluative Study*, she renamed deliberative nursing action a process discipline with three specific requirements. Application of the nursing process discipline qualifies as a disciplined professional response. Despite this change in terminology, Orlando provides clear guidelines for nurses to find out and meet a patient's immediate needs for help. First, the nurse expresses to the patient any or all of the items contained in his or her reaction to the patient's behavior. Second, the nurse states to the patient that the expressed item belongs to the nurse by use of the personal pronoun (an "I" message which indicates it is the nurse's perception). Finally, the nurse asks about the item expressed, attempting to verify or correct his or her perceptions, thoughts, or feelings (Schmieding, 1987).

The value of the nursing process discipline is its accuracy in determining whether the patient experiences distress and, if so, finding out what help is required to relieve the distress (McCann-Flynn & Heffron, 1984). Without the investigation required by use of the nursing process discipline, the nurse does not have a reliable database for action (Orlando, 1972). When the nurse responds automatically, the perceptions, thoughts, and feelings of each person are not available to the other. When the nurse uses the nursing process discipline, the perceptions, thoughts, and feelings of the nurse are available to the patient and vice versa. Orlando (1961) views this latter type of response as a form of "continuous reflection as the nurse tries to understand the meaning to the patient of the behavior she observed and what he needs from her in order to be helped" (p. 67). The nurse evaluates his or her actions at the end of the contact by comparing the patient's verbal and nonverbal behavior with that which was present when the process started.

LOGICAL FORM

Orlando's theory was developed inductively. She collected records of her observations of nurse-patient situations during a 3-year period. After various attempts to categorize these data, Orlando recognized that they were either good or bad patient outcomes. Good outcomes were defined as those that improved the patient's behavior. Bad outcomes were defined as those associated with absence of improvement. Orlando concluded that the nurse's use of the nursing process discipline was an effective means of achieving a good outcome. On this basis, Orlando formulated her nursing process theory from these qualitative data (Schmieding, 1986).

If Walker and Avant's (1995) criteria are used for theory analysis, Orlando's theory is logically adequate. Although inductive argument can produce false conclusions even when the premises are true, Orlando's conclusions are logically sound. The structure of relationships is clear and sufficiently precise; it is possible to represent the relationships schematically. The relationships progress from existence and conditional statement to prediction and control. The predictions Orlando makes are acceptable to the nursing profession, because improvement in patient care is always considered valuable. There are no logical fallacies within Orlando's theory, because relationships are developed sufficiently.

ACCEPTANCE BY THE NURSING COMMUNITY

Henderson (1964) accepted Orlando's theory early in its development. Orlando's conclusions convinced her that "the most effective nursing involves a continuous analysis and validation of the nurse's interpretation of patient's needs" (p. 65). Orlando's theory is readily applicable to nursing practice. Orlando's theory and the research by her students provided the foundation for behavioral and social practice in the late 1960s (Wooldridge, Skipper, & Leonard, 1968). Orlando's ideas were also evident in the writings of Dickoff and James (1986).

Practice

There is early and increasing evidence of its application in practice as indicated by the literature. Schmidt (1972) reports using Orlando's theory as a basis for practice in 1972. Peitchinis (1972) suggests that Orlando's nursing process discipline reflects the elements of the therapeutic relationship, which includes expression of empathy, warmth, and genuineness. She proposes that nursing practice based on Orlando's theory would increase the therapeutic effectiveness of nursing. Its use continues in a variety of clinical practices. Rosenthal (1996) recommends Orlando's theory as the basis for perioperative nursing. She believes that because patients are in the operating room for a short duration, rapid and accurate assessment is paramount.

A case study illustrates application of the theory. A patient's procedure was rescheduled twice and surgery was postponed. The caretakers did not capture the incongruities between verbal and nonverbal communication. The type of anesthesia was changed from general anesthesia to epidural and heavy sedation. The patient tolerated the 6-hour surgery without anxiety. According to Rosenthal (1996), this supports Orlando's theory of the dynamic patient-nurse relation.

Orlando's theory was used successfully in psychiatric and general hospitals. Early examples of acceptance by the psychiatric nursing community include the Mid-Missouri Mental Health Center and a new psychiatric unit located within a general hospital in Antigonish, Nova Scotia.

The former Boston's Beth Israel Hospital Division of Nursing Statement of Philosophy and Purpose had been based on their nursing service on the formulations of Henderson, Wiedenbach, and Orlando. There is evidence that Orlando's theory is used at the patient care, managerial, and nursing division levels within this organization.

Since 1994, the New Hampshire Hospital Nursing Department selected Orlando's theory for use in both nursing practice and nursing administration. Houle (1997) describes the process of learning to apply the theory in practice. Barbara Bockenhauer, Assistant Director of Nursing Education and Research, is a leader in the hospital and a resource to the staff. Notable is that patients clearly receive benefits from staff reinforcement of the use of Orlando's theory. Additionally, introducing students to Orlando's theory makes their connections to patients much more meaningful. Mimi Dye, M.N., M.S.N., A.R.N.P. (written communication, April 28, 2004), who was a student of Orlando at Yale, is a consultant to the New Hampshire Hospital Orlando Project, which involves educating people throughout the hospital. Working with a committee she implements training, consults monthly with supervisors, and is a member of the Nursing Educational Resource Service Department.

Although Orlando's theory has been used as an overall framework for practice, its predominant use is focused on immediate nurse-patient contacts. If the process discipline is used, observation of the patient's verbal and nonverbal behavior provides the nurse with immediate data for determining the patient's level of distress. With the patient, the nurse explores what action is to be taken to meet the patient's immediate needs for help. Finally, the nurse investigates the patient's new behavior to determine whether the action actually relieved the patient's distress (evaluation). If the distress is not relieved, the process begins again until the patient's needs for help are determined.

Administration-leadership. Increasingly more nurse administrators and nurse leaders are writing about Orlando's theory, and their work is being published in journals and on the Schmieding Web site. Schmieding used Orlando's theory simultaneously in both practice and administration in several hospitals during the early 1970s. Schmieding (1984) reported the advantages of adopting Orlando's theory throughout a nursing department. Implementation of Orlando's theory produced substantial benefits. Its use increased effectiveness in meeting patient needs; improved decision-making skills among staff nurses, particularly in determining what constituted nursing versus nonnursing functions; facilitated more effective conflict resolution among staff nurses and between staff and physicians; and influenced a more positive nursing identity and unity among staff. Schmieding (1987) discussed "how specific types of actions facilitate or thwart problem identification" (pp. 435-436) and, by using Orlando's theory, analyzed managerial responses in face-to-face contacts.

With few exceptions, nursing theorists focus on management of patients. Recently nurses recognize that a manager and a leader are not the same. Several nurses have written intriguing articles to help managers become leaders. Although nursing practice foundation is based on numerous nursing theories, its focus has been on effective management of patient care, not on leadership. Laurent (2000) proposed a leadership theory using Orlando's nursing model that provides a foundation of both management of patient care and leadership. Nurses manage things rather than lead people. According to Laurent, Orlando advocates exploration to identify the patient's immediate needs for help. From Orlando's perspective, she concurs with the nursing leadership process components. Orlando's "dynamic leadership-follower relationship model" (Laurent, 2000, p. 85) is based on the dynamic nurse-patient relationship theory. Laurent provides numerous ways for using Orlando's theory as the basis of practice.

Based on Orlando's leadership, Faust (2002) demonstrated the use of her theory in an extended care facility. There were two older adult women: one constantly called for staff or used the call bell whereas the other woman removed her oxygen, crawled into the other client's bed, and called out at night. When staff met, they identified the women's unmet needs. Using Orlando's theory, Faust's staff was able to find out what the women were thinking and why they had been behaving as they had. Consequently, the staff was able to meet their needs after

determining the special requirements for help. Faust recommends research-based evidence to conduct interventions of stressful behaviors to bring about positive outcomes through leadership practices.

Valentine's (2002) nursing leadership theory is modeled after Orlando's nursing theory. She identifies patients' distress and their immediate needs for help. Valentine draws on interpersonal process to draw cues to reach the objectives. Interaction between managers and new nurses can develop basic leadership principles by interactions with established nurse leaders.

Reflexive principle. The process between the patient and the nurse is referred to as a *reflexive principle* (Barnum, 1994). The patient's input is required before the nurse's final judgment is made. Its reciprocal principle causes Orlando's theory to require four steps, "patient action, nurse reaction, nurse-patient validation, and nurse action" (Barnum, 1994, p. 206). Therefore, it is more complicated than theories without specific guidelines. However, as an interaction theory, behaviors not previously recognized are brought to the forefront. Orlando's theory continues to be used, because it effectively facilitates inquiry and discovery in nurse-patient contacts. Therefore, in both nursing practice and research, Oiler Boyd (1993) recommends the "reconsideration of the centrality of the nurse-patient relationship" (p. 18).

Individual nurse's practice. Individual nurses use Orlando's theory to guide their practice. Martha Brown, staff nurse, uses it with both English-speaking and non–English-speaking patients in the public health department in Lincoln, Nebraska. Orlando (I. Pelletier, telephone interview, April 21, 2000) clarified how the nurse meets the requirements of the discipline process with non–English-speaking persons. Examples of Brown's work appear in Alligood and Marriner Tomey's (2002) second edition of *Nursing Theory: Utilization & Application.* In the Boston area, Julie Felty, a psychiatric nurse, uses Orlando's theory in private practice with patients who range in age from 17 to 96 and have various diagnoses. In 1993, Julie Felty and Susan Donaldson, M.D., used Orlando's theory in establishing a 12-bed mental health unit in Waltham, Massachusetts. The use of physical restraints has been essentially eliminated (J. Felty, e-mail communication, June 27, 2000). Janice Logan has been a nurse in community health for many years. She uses Orlando's theory because it is logical and makes common sense. Logan notes that her use of Orlando's theory has shaped her career as a nurse (J. Logan, e-mail correspondence, 2004; e-mail address: logja@gis.net). Mimi Dye, an advanced registered nurse practitioner, uses Orlando's theory with patients in her private practice. She also does clinical teaching at Yale University School of Nursing and Rivier College (M. Dye, personal communication, April 26, 2004).

Education

Orlando's nursing process theory is a conceptual framework which, if taught and practiced, would enhance professional nursing. Orlando's process recording form has made a significant contribution to nursing education. Orlando (1972) found that training in the nursing process discipline was necessary for the nurse to be able to control the nursing process and achieve improvement in the patient's behavior. Therefore, she developed the process recording, a tool to facilitate self-evaluation to determine whether or not the nursing process discipline was used. This "systematic repetitious examination and study of the nursing process" (Orlando, 1972) was designed for students to facilitate their learning about how to express their immediate reactions to patients and to ask for correction or verification. The process recording is an educational tool still used in nursing education. Larson's (1977) research confirms the need for teaching student nurses to perceive patients as individuals rather than to stereotype them by categories.

The use of Orlando's theory permeates nursing education and practice (Meleis, 1997). However, acknowledgement that the theory comes from Orlando is not often known or cited. To many users of Orlando's theory, its creator remains unknown. Pamela Greene noted that, although she used this theory in teaching beginning students at Midwestern State University in Texas, it was only when

examining nursing theories in her doctoral program that she recognized that its origin was from Orlando (P. Greene, e-mail correspondence, June 9, 2000).

Orlando's is one of the theories Greene uses while working in the Menninger Clinic in Wichita Falls, Texas (P. Greene, e-mail correspondence, March 21, 2004; e-mail: pgreene3@houston.rr.com). According to her, Orlando's theory involves understanding the meaning of the experience and the importance of perceptions; it seems to fit quite well in her practice. Greene asks questions to gain information about nurses' perceptions, their thoughts, and their feelings. She returns to the participants at least twice, once to transcribe the interview. Each patient has the opportunity to add or clarify information. During the second interview, Greene analyzes and compiles the analysis or interpretation. It allows participants to give input as to whether or not the comprehensive summation with the analysis and interpretation "ring true."

Schmieding discovered serendipitously in 2000 that for more than 10 years South Dakota State University has used Haggerty's (1985) communication model, which is based on Orlando's theory, to teach beginning students. Joyce Fjelland, a professor at South Dakota State University, uses Orlando's theory in the junior mental health experience to reinforce communication skills. She requires students to apply Orlando's theory in their interpersonal recording analysis. Senior students study it again during their last semester. Fjelland believes that students understand the theory as they intervene with clients needing interventions. It also helps them recognize their own automatic behaviors and their need to use deliberate behaviors that result in behavioral change in both clients and students (Fjelland, e-mail correspondence, March 2, 2004).

Orlando (1961) wrote her first book "to offer the professional nursing student a theory of effective practice" (p. viii). Since 1961, many psychiatric nursing texts have included Orlando's theory. Orlando has written chapters in numerous textbooks on nursing theories. Orlando deserves credit for providing clear guidelines for the nurse to use in contacts with patients. Orlando's theory was instrumental in the development of the interaction theory currently used in psychiatric nursing (Artinian, 1983), and nursing master's programs are increasing use of Orlando's theory in their courses.

Winder (1984) identifies the need to provide a facilitating environment for implementing the caring process in the nursing curriculum. He suggests that Orlando's theory provides a model for such a training process, which is presented clearly in her book, *The Discipline and Teaching of Nursing Process: An Evaluative Study* (1972).

Studying student nurses, Haggerty (1987) analyzed their responses to distressed patients based on Orlando's nursing process concept. She found that "emphasis on communication and psychosocial foundations in baccalaureate curricula may not translate into more effective exploratory skills in these students" (p. 451). She recommends Orlando's model for teaching these students to conceptualize the interaction process and its goals.

In 1982, Henderson wrote that Orlando's insistence on validation was an important contribution to nursing practice. Recently, Mohr (1999) reiterated this insistence by Orlando, for "without this validation the nurse is working with an inadequate data base" (p. 1058).

International nursing. In Sweden, Orlando's theory was considered useful for students in helping elderly patients cope with needs and maintaining patients' identity and autonomy (Fagerberg & Ekman, 1997).

A project was developed in Kristianstad, Sweden, for a nursing ward, to bridge the theory-practice gap for students throughout their education and practice (Johansson, Blomquist, Nilsson, & Olsson, 1996-1998).

The project's purpose was to support reflective thinking. Orlando's nursing theory was selected, because it was developed inductively. Students were asked the following four questions: (1) What do I see? (2) What do I think? (3) What do I feel? and (4) How do I act? The first three were inside the person's inner content. The forth question was visible. Consequently assumptions could be verified or revised from this question. Assumptions have quite different ideas and needs by different nurses.

Reflective tools were developed so that they were done in two separate steps. Additionally, teachers

were trained in reflective thinking (Selanders, Schmieding, & Hartweg, 1995). In a national conference where they presented the results, they shared how to integrate theory and practice. Supervisors, students, and teachers found Orlando's reflective process of nursing very useful. Orlando's method was easy to introduce, and they expressed that it was exactly how they thought and could now put it into words.

In England, Price (2003) examined the understanding and origin of practice problems. Also of concern was reflective practice. It is not sufficient to recognize a problem without inquiry. Along with other colleagues, he addressed various types of problems. Price used Schmieding's (1999) inquiry process for decision making. It focused on observations and thought, using patients' past experiences, a back-and-forth gathering of information, and collaboration with others.

In Australia, at the University of Southern Queensland, Perrin and Reilly (2002) developed a management course. Previously, little management preparation had been provided. The instructors used, among other references, Schmieding's (1999) reflective framework for administration (Perrin & Reilly, 2002).

Schmieding and Kokuyama (1995) addressed cross-cultural and comparative research. The purpose was to identify universal theories and practice in two different cultures. Primomo (2000) in Japan published information about how the Japanese are preparing for the nursing care needs of elderly people during the coming century.

Kawamura, Shijiki, & Mastsuo (2004) note that Orlando's theory focuses on patients' immediate needs; other theories did not. According to Toshiko Yokuyama, before becoming the Chief of School of Nursing, Dean at the Ehime University Faculty of Health Science in Japan, she used Orlando's theory for teaching both undergraduate and master's-level students (T. Yokuyama, e-mail correspondence, 2004; e-mail address: t.kokuya@nurse.medic.mie-u.ac.jp). Tomoyo Matsui (2004) based her master's thesis on Orlando's theory at the university where Yokuyama is employed. Orlando's theory was also used by Kobayshi (1998) and Kumata and Goto (1984).

In Germany, Mischo-Kelling and Wittneben (1995) included a section on Orlando's theory that highlighted Orlando's focus on problematic situations, the investigation of these situations, and the investigation of the patient's immediate need for help (pp. 184-187).

Ana Mendes, Ana Pinheiro, Isabel Viola, Jose Elias, Paula Malveiro, and Virginio Pateiro (Mendes and colleagues, e-mail communication, 2003) are nurses from Portugal who contacted Schmieding about Orlando's work. These six nurses developed an extensive paper using Orlando's theory.

Rocio Ganan, Rocio Berraco, Isabel Redondo, Maite Algovia, and Maria Lozano, nursing students at the University of Alcala de Henares in Madrid, Spain, sought information from Schmieding about Orlando's theory for their project. Their comment was "we would love to obtain more information about this nurse and her work." There have been several communications with them (M. Lozano Munoz, e-mail communication, March 8, 2004; e-mail address: mariainalaska@yahoo.es).

Brazilian nurses Ana Claudia de Souza Toniolli and Lorita Marlena Freitag Pagli (2002) wrote about Orlando's theory in the journal *Revista Brasileira de Enfermagem*. The English title is "Analysis of Orlando Theory Applied in the Brazilians' Nursing Magazines" [sic] [Portuguese]. This publication uses Orlando's theory in descriptive and exploratory research study (Patricia Gomes, e-mail communication, 2002; e-mail: reben@abennacional.org.br).

Research

Orlando's theory continues to have considerable acceptance in the area of nursing research and has been applied to a variety of research settings. Many of the studies provided empirical evidence that Orlando's theoretical assertions are valid. These are discussed later in this chapter, in the section "Empirical Precision."

Dracup and Breu (1978) used Orlando's definition of the need for help in their study of the needs of grieving spouses. Hampe (1975) used the definition in a similar study. In studying patients with cancer, Pienschke (1973) found adequacy of care

enhanced by openness of approach, perception of patient needs, and congruity between patient and nurse on patient's need and adequacy of care.

Orlando's nursing process discipline has been designated the experimental approach in several studies to examine its effects on a patient's distress during admission and before surgery. Anderson, Mertz, and Leonard (1965) found that deliberative nursing actions promoted stress reduction during admission. Wolfer and Visintainer (1975) demonstrated this same result with both children and their parents. Dumas and Johnson (1972) concluded that preoperative exploration with patients to determine the real source of distress permitted the nurse to take appropriate action to relieve the distress and that less distress before surgery correlated with fewer postoperative complications. In their study of postoperative vomiting, Dumas and Leonard (1963) used nursing process discipline as the experimental nursing action. Thibaudeau and Reidy (1977) found that when nurses used deliberative nursing, mothers had more knowledge of illness and complications and complied more fully with treatments prescribed than did mothers who did not receive deliberative nursing.

Although Olson and Hanchett (1997) considered five other nursing theories, they selected Orlando's theory because it was best suited to studying the relationship between nurse empathy and patient outcome. Results indicated support for the relationships proposed by the theory. As was noted earlier, Haggerty (1987) used Orlando's nursing process concept to conduct research on nursing students' responses to distressed patients. Princeton (1986) tested the effects of the nursing process discipline with breast-feeding mothers and their infants. These research studies can be considered both theory testing and theory generating. They provide empirical support for Orlando's theory (theory testing) and have produced new principles for practice and education, especially in the area of preoperative teaching and student nurse communication (theory generating).

Schmieding (1988) used Orlando's theory to investigate the action process of nurse administrators in realistic hypothetical situations presented to them by their staff. The findings indicated the administrators' first thought was seldom about their staff member's reaction to the situation, and most administrators would tell the nurse what to do rather than inquire about what the nurse thought about the situation. Schmieding concludes that the quality of nursing is reflected in the quality of help nurses receive from their administrators in the problem-solving process. The results of this study indicate that the quality of this help may be less than optimal. In a review of this study, Sheafor (1991) concludes that Orlando's theory should be included in a graduate program for nursing administrators. These studies also suggest that the use of Orlando's theory in the graduate education of advanced practice nurses is important.

In a study of adult patients with cancer, Ponte-Reid (1992) examined the relationship between empathy and Orlando's nursing process discipline. A positive relationship was found between primary nurses' empathy skills and the use of nursing process discipline. Ponte-Reid encourages further research in the area of nurses' interpersonal skills and patient outcomes.

In a Veterans Administration (V.A.) ambulatory psychiatric practice, Shea, McBride, Gavin, and Bauer (1997) used Orlando's theoretical model with patients ($N = 76$) who had bipolar disorder. Their research results indicate that there was higher patient retention, reduced emergency service, decreased hospital stay, and increased satisfaction when the model was used. They recommended its use throughout the V.A. system. Orlando's model is being used in a multimillion-dollar research study of patients with bipolar disorder at 12 sites in the V.A. system (L. McBride, telephone interview, July 21, 2000).

Bauer and McBride (2002) continue their work on bipolar disease, incorporating Orlando's theory in the treatment protocol. They encourage illness self-management skills and social and occupational experiences. Theirs is an empowering program that seeks wellness-based issues.

Potter has written extensively on research about Orlando's theory, including a chapter focusing on middle range theories (Potter, 2004). Many publications have evolved from her experience at the New Hampshire Hospital. Potter's quest for research validation for clinical practice is most worthy. She makes it easier for nurses to explore the assumptions and proposition of Orlando's deliberative nursing practice. Potter's research is used in practice in various types of patient situations.

As Potter (2004) realizes Orlando's theory, although the words are easy to read, "the theory's complexity involves learning how to use it. Being proficient in the use of Deliberative Nursing Process necessitates time, practice, and self-reflection, often in the form of a supervisor experience" (p. 310). Potter's chapter contains much information that is useful when putting Orlando's theory into practice, including instrumentation, application, and empirical testing.

In a pilot study, Potter and Bockenhauer (2000) found positive results after implementing Orlando's theory. These included positive, patient-centered outcomes, a model for staff to use in their approach to patients, and a decrease in the patients' immediate distress. The study provides variable measurements that might be used in other research studies.

Potter and Dawson (2001) noted concern about the definition of safety contracts. Orlando's theory was used to develop a safety agreement that is more concise and more patient-nurse friendly in promoting safety and decreasing patients' immediate stress than the contract they had been using. Through the nurse-patient relationship, the value of the safety agreement involves communication and collaboration.

The diversity of the research using Orlando's theory attests to its breadth of application in various types of patients. It also indicates its utility for application in any clinical setting.

FURTHER DEVELOPMENT

The nursing process discipline needs to be an integral part of student nurses' education so that it can be implemented in any practice setting. Orlando's theory has provided the basis of both clinical and administrative practice in general and psychiatric settings. Its disciplined nursing process is also relevant to community and long-term nursing and in other areas where nursing is practiced. Orlando's study could be replicated to validate that the process discipline is directly related to the effectiveness of a nursing system. As nurses obtain advanced degrees, more are expanding Orlando's theory and publishing their findings.

Schmieding (1999) expanded the theory by incorporating criteria of a reflective inquiry framework for nursing administration. These theoretical formulations could be tested in both clinical and administrative practice and used in undergraduate and advanced practice in nursing education.

Whereas nursing theories reflect distinct patterns of conceptual frameworks and theoretical perspectives, Cody (1996) criticizes the mania of using borrowed theory only remotely connected to health care. He recommends that nursing theories, Orlando's included, be developed further. Unquestionably, Orlando's theory, which is accepted by the nursing community, warrants continuing development. Fawcett (2000) agrees and notes that despite impressive evidence, continued study is needed to test Orlando's predictions of her theory. As the numbers of nurses using Orlando's theory increases, more research is being generated. An example of this is Bauer and McBride's (2002) treatment process that uses Orlando's theory in aspects of bipolar disease.

CRITIQUE
Clarity

In her first book, *The Dynamic Nurse-Patient Relationship: Function, Process and Principles of Professional Nursing Practice* (1961), Orlando presented concepts clearly. She consistently used the same terms in her theory. In her second book, *The Discipline and Teaching of Nursing Process: An Evaluative Study* (1972), she redefined and renamed deliberative nursing process as nursing process discipline. Other than this change, Orlando consistently used the same word for her major components and processes. However, many continue to use the deliberative nursing process for its clarity of meaning.

Orlando defined concepts minimally at first and then developed them throughout the book. The evolution of the theory requires the reader to be familiar with both books if one is to evaluate it thoroughly. Although her writing is clear and concise, some repetition might facilitate easier comprehension.

Simplicity

Because Orlando deals with relatively few concepts and their relationships with each other, her theory would be considered simple. However, it is elegant in its simplicity. Her theory may also be viewed as simplistic, because she is able to make some predictive statements as opposed to only description and explanation. The simplicity of Orlando's theory has benefited research application.

Walker and Avant (1995) use Orlando's theory as an example of grand nursing theory; however, not all grand theories are at the same level of abstraction. They state that grand nursing theories provide a global perspective, but by virtue of their generality and abstractness, most grand theories are untestable in their current form. Although Orlando's theory has undergone testing, its global perspective could support labeling this work as a grand theory. However, there is controversy among theorists in terms of its level. Orlando's theory has also been described as a practice theory. Practice theories provide a framework to specify when the guidelines should be applied, describe the means to be used, and specify the goals to be used for outcome evaluation (George, 1995).

Generality

Orlando discusses and illustrates nurse-patient contacts in which the patient is conscious, able to communicate, and in need of help. Although she did not focus on unconscious patients and groups, application of her theory to them is feasible. Nonverbal behavior is an element of her formulations; therefore, nurses would focus on this for determining the patient's needs for help and observing for nonverbal behavioral changes after the nursing action.

It is possible that anyone could make use of the nursing process discipline with any group, if educated properly. Although Orlando's theory, at the time of development, focused on a moderate number of situations, their types are increasing. Schmieding (2004) has written extensively on nursing administration. Conceivably, the theory can be adapted to other nursing situations and other professional fields in which the focus is on identifying patients' immediate needs for help. For example, Orlando's theory has been used in public health nursing and by other nurses practicing independently, both within the United States and internationally.

Empirical Precision

Two thirds of Orlando's second book, *The Discipline and Teaching of Nursing Process: An Evaluative Study* (1972), is a report of a research project designed to test the validity of her nursing formulations. A training program based on her formulations had been in progress for 3 years before the project began. Nurses were trained to use the nursing process discipline in nurse-patient contacts. Those nurses who became clinical nursing supervisors were trained to use the nursing process discipline in their supervisory and other contacts. The following is a brief description of the research methodology.

The purpose of the project was to evaluate the effectiveness of the nursing process discipline in the nurses' contacts at work and the effectiveness of the training program. However, these evaluations could not take place before hypothetical measures were identified for the nursing process discipline and the effectiveness of the nursing process discipline. A discipline variable was defined (Orlando, 1972). Effectiveness was determined by the presence or absence of a helpful outcome, as judged by two reliable outcome coders. The outcome coders compared the beginning behavior of the subject with the behavior at the end of the record. Testing of the relationship of the nursing process discipline (in use) with the presence or absence of a helpful outcome in patient, staff, and supervisee contacts was also completed. The training program participants were

evaluated by testing whether nurses increased their use of the nursing process discipline after being trained. Two groups of nurses were included in the study. The control group consisted of veterans (previously trained supervisors and staff nurses). The experimental group consisted of novices (untrained supervisors and staff nurses). Transcripts were made of the novices' and veterans' contacts at work from tape-recorded, 20-minute periods (six for each subject).

This report is extensive and detailed and may be difficult to read and interpret for those without a good understanding of statistics and research methodology. The study concludes that training in the nursing process discipline and its use achieves helpful outcomes in patients, supervisees, and staff contacts.

Although precise understanding of Orlando's theory is required to develop research based on it, numerous studies by Orlando's first graduate students at Yale during the 1960s supported the validity of her theory (Anderson et al., 1965; Bochnak, 1963; Cameron, 1963; Dumas, 1963; Dumas & Johnson, 1972; Dumas & Leonard, 1963; Dye, 1963a, 1963b). Several studies that incorporated Orlando's nursing process discipline approach have previously been mentioned in this section on research application. Others who specifically tested the usefulness of the nursing process discipline approach include the following: Pienschke (1973), who also found that nursing intervention was more effective under conditions of open disclosure because patients' needs were perceived more accurately; Bochnak (1963), who found that the nursing process discipline was more effective in relieving patients' pain; Dye (1963a), who controlled for staff-patient ratios and amount of nursing time and still demonstrated that deliberative nursing actions met patient needs effectively; and Cameron (1963), who revealed that the nursing process discipline led to the most consistent, effective results in verifying patient needs.

Orlando asserts that patient distress stems from a reaction to the environment that the patient cannot control alone. Dye (1963b) provides empirical evidence for this assertion in her study on clarifying patient needs. She found that patients experienced distress more as a reaction to the hospital setting than to their illnesses.

Orlando also asserts that patient distress stems from the nurse's misinterpretation of the patient's experience or from the patient's initial inability to communicate clearly the needs for help. Both necessitate the use of the nursing process discipline to find out the specific needs for help. Two studies, one by Elder (1963) and the other by Gowan and Morris (1964), provide support for this assertion. Both studies demonstrated that, although patients often did not express their needs clearly, deliberative nursing actions alleviated their problems.

Other research studies cited earlier in this chapter add to the empirical precision of Orlando's theory.

Derivable Consequences

Orlando's theory remains effective and efficient in achieving valued outcomes. Identifying the patient's immediate needs for help and the nurse's ability to meet these needs are critically important to patient outcomes and the advancement of nursing practice.

Incorporating validation into the nursing process discipline, as Orlando suggests, allows for maximal participation by the patient in his or her care. Numerous researchers have also demonstrated that the use of a disciplined professional response enables the nurse to find out and meet the patient's immediate needs for help. The study of what nurses say and do in their practice, and the resulting effect manifested by the patient, is valuable content for use in nursing education and developing further research studies. The nursing process discipline allows nurses to view the patient from a nursing perspective rather than from a medical disease orientation. Use of Orlando's theory benefits the patient, enhances the nurse's professional identity, and helps to advance the nursing profession.

SUMMARY

Ida Orlando's 1961 book, *The Dynamic Nurse-Patient Relationship*, presents a classic nursing theory. Her theory is simple to understand but requires that the nurse focus on the patient to find out the immediate needs for help. Nurses need to explore patients' perceptions, thoughts, and feelings to find out what help patients need, which is not as easy as it appears. Because each patient is unique, the nurse must find out what help the individual requires. Orlando describes this as the deliberative nursing process.

Orlando's theory is used in various practices, from psychiatric to public health nursing, and her book describes individual nurses who use her theory. Orlando's theory is used in various hospitals, notably the New Hampshire Hospital. There a psychiatric nurse-physician pair works with people who have bipolar disease, using Orlando's theory.

As Orlando's theory expands, it is used in education, administration, and nursing leadership. Regardless of where the nurse practices, the focus is on the patient. For example, nurse administrators base their thinking on the patient to determine practice changes, to hire nurses, and to make decisions while using her theory.

Research using Orlando's theory is steadily increasing. Schmieding and Potter have written extensive research publications. The breadth of the research attests to its diversity in other practice areas.

The number of nurses using Orlando's theory internationally is increasing. Some are in England, Germany, Japan, and Sweden. They add new ideas, thus enhancing the theory. Other nursing students from Portugal and Spain have used Orlando's theory, and there is a publication about Orlando's theory in a Brazilian journal (*Revista Brasileira de Enfermagen*, 2002).

Conceivably, it can be adapted to other nursing situations in which the focus is on identifying and finding out patients' immediate needs for help. For example, Orlando's theory has been used in public health nursing and by nurses practicing independently in the United States and internationally.

Orlando's disciplined nursing process is relevant to community and long-term nursing and in other areas where nursing is practiced. Orlando's 1972 evaluative study could be replicated to validate that the process discipline is directly related to the effectiveness of a nursing system. As nurses obtain advanced degrees, the number of publications about

Orlando's theory will be growing. Orlando's theory remains vital in 2004 and beyond.

Case Study

George is a 70-year-old patient who has been assigned to you, his community-based nurse case manager. George has severe congestive heart failure, peripheral vascular disease, and no family or social support. George has had 15 hospital admissions and 35 visits to the emergency department this year because of noncompliance with his medication and diet regimen. He receives a monthly Social Security check, which he spends on food, gambling (primarily bingo), and medications (in that order).

1. Describe your immediate reactions to George, who is uncertain of the need for a nurse.
2. Place yourself in George's situation and describe the immediate reactions he would have as a patient.
3. What would your first interaction with George be like? Describe the dialogue.
4. State your automatic nursing actions in relation to George.
5. State your deliberative nursing actions in relation to George.

CRITICAL THINKING *Activities*

1. Select two situations in which a patient would not require medical intervention but would require professional nursing action.
   a. List two deliberative nursing actions for each situation.
   b. List two automatic nursing actions for each situation.

2. Describe how Orlando's theory can be used in practice when the nurse-patient relationship is extremely short term, as in the extremely short lengths of stay experienced by hospitalized patients.

REFERENCES

Alligood, M. R., & Marriner Tomey, A. (2002). *Nursing theory: Utilization & application* (2nd ed.). St. Louis: Mosby.

Anderson, B., Mertz, H., & Leonard, R. (1965). Two experimental tests of a patient-centered admission process. *Nursing Research, 14,* 151-157.

Artinian, B. (1983). Implementation of the intersystem patient-care model in clinical practice. *Journal of Advanced Nursing, 8,* 117-124.

Barnum, B. J. S. (1994). *Nursing theory—Analysis, application, evaluation* (4th ed.). Philadelphia: J. B. Lippincott.

Bauer, S., & McBride, L. (2002). *Structured group psychotherapy for bipolar disorder. The life goal program* (2nd ed.). New York: Springer Publishing.

Bochnak, M. (1963). The effect of an automatic and deliberative process of nursing activity on the relief of patients' pain: A clinical experiment. *Abstract in Nursing Research, 12,* 191-192.

Cameron, J. (1963). An exploratory study of the verbal responses of the nurses in twenty nurse-patient interactions. *Abstract in Nursing Research, 12,* 192.

Cody, W. K. (1996). Drowning in eclecticism. *Nursing Science Quarterly, 9*(3), 86-88.

Crane, M. (1985). Ida Jean Orlando. In J. B. George (Ed.), *Nursing theories: The base for professional nursing practice* (pp. 158-179). Englewood Cliffs, NJ: Prentice-Hall.

de Souza Toniolli, A. C., & Freitag Pagli, L. M. (2002). Analysis of Orlando theory applied in the Brazilians' nursing magazines. *Revista Brasileira de Enfermagem, 55*(5), 489-494.

Dickoff, J., & James, P. (1986). A theory of theories: A position paper. In L. H. Nicoll (Ed.), *Perspectives on nursing theory* (pp. 101-112). Boston: Little, Brown.

Dracup, K., & Breu, C. (1978). Using nursing research findings to meet the needs of grieving spouses. *Nursing Research, 27,* 212-216.

Dumas, R. (1963). Psychological preparation for surgery. *American Journal of Nursing, 63,* 52-55.

Dumas, R., & Johnson, B. (1972). Research in nursing practice: A review of five clinical experiments. *International Journal of Nursing Studies, 9,* 137-149.

Dumas, R., & Leonard, R. (1963). The effect of nursing on the incidence of postoperative vomiting. *Nursing Research, 12,* 12-15.

Dye, M. (1963a). A descriptive study of conditions conducive to an effective process of nursing activity. *Abstract in Nursing Research, 12,* 194.

Dye, M. (1963b). Clarifying patients' communications. *American Journal of Nursing, 63,* 56-59.

Elder, R. (1963). What is the patient saying? *Nursing Forum, 11,* 25-37.

Fagerberg, I., & Ekman, S. (1997). First-year Swedish nursing students' experiences with elderly patients. *Western Journal of Nursing Research, 19*(2), 177-189.

Faust, C. (2002). Orlando's deliberative nursing process theory. A practice application in an extended care facility. *Journal of Gerontological Nursing, 28*(7), 14-18.

Fawcett, J. (1993). *Orlando's theory of the deliberative nursing process. Analysis and evaluation of nursing theories.* Philadelphia: F. A. Davis.

Fawcett, J. (2000). *Analysis and evaluation of contemporary nursing knowledge: Nursing models and theories* (pp. 603-626). Philadelphia: F. A. Davis.

Fitzpatrick, J., & Whall, A. L. (1989). *Conceptual models of nursing: Analysis and application* (2nd ed.). Norwalk, CT: Appleton & Lange.

Forchuk, C. (1991). A comparison of the works of Peplau and Orlando. *Archives of Psychiatric Nursing, 5*(1), 38-45.

George, J. B. (Ed.). (1995). *Nursing theories: The base for professional nursing practice* (4th ed.). Norwalk, CT: Appleton & Lange.

Gowan, N., & Morris, M. (1964). Nurses' responses to expressed patient needs. *Nursing Research, 13,* 68-71.

Haggerty, L. A. (1985). A theoretical model for developing students' communication skills. *Journal of Nursing Education, 24*(7), 296-298.

Haggerty, L. A. (1987). An analysis of senior nursing students' immediate responses to distressed patients. *Journal of Advanced Nursing, 12,* 451-461.

Hampe, S. (1975). Needs of the grieving spouse in a hospital setting. *Nursing Research, 24,* 113-120.

Henderson, V. (1964, Aug.). The nature of nursing. *American Journal of Nursing, 64*(8), 62-68.

Henderson, V. (1982). The nursing process—Is the title right? *Journal of Advanced Nursing, 7,* 103-109.

Henderson, V. (1987). Nursing process—A critique. *Holistic Nursing Practice, 1*(3), 7-18.

Hilton, P. A. (1997). Theoretical perspectives of nursing: A review of the literature. *Journal of Advanced Nursing, 26,* 1211-1220.

Houle, P. (1997). Ida in action. *BayState Nurse News, 5*(10), 12.

Johansson, B., Blomquist, K., Nilsson, S., & Olsson, A. (1996-1998). *The reference ward—An important source of knowledge in nursing education. Bridging the gap between theory and practice in nursing education* (pp. 1-9). Skane, Sweden: Kristianstad University Department of Health Sciences.

Jones, P. S., & Meleis, A. I. (1993). Health is empowerment. *Advance Nursing Science, 15*(3), 1-14.

Kawamura, S., Shijiki, Y., & Mastsuo, M. (2004). *Kangogakugairon [An introduction of nursing]* (p. 138). Osaka, Japan: Medicus Shuppan.

Kobayshi, M. (1998). Skills of how to find out patients who have need for nurses' help in OPD nursing. *Kanko Gijutsu, 44*(13), 20-27.

Kumata, M., & Goto, H. (1984). What I learned from Orlando—Individuality and determination in actual interaction with a patient. *Gekkan Nursing, 4*(4), 129-133.

Larson, P., Sr. (1977). Nurse perceptions of patient characteristics. *Nursing Research, 26,* 416-421.

Laurent, C. L. (2000). A nursing theory for nursing leadership. *Journal of Nursing Management, 8,* 83-87.

Matsui, K. (2004). *Descriptive study about negotiation competence of care-giving practitioner.* Unpublished Master's thesis, Dean of School of Nursing, Faculty of Health Sciences, Ehime University, Mie-ken, Japan.

McCann-Flynn, J., & Heffron, B. (1984). *Nursing: From concept to practice.* Bowie, MD: Robert J. Brady.

Meleis, A. I. (1991). *Theoretical nursing: Development and progress* (2nd ed., pp. 343-379). New York: J. B. Lippincott.

Meleis, A. I. (1997). Ida Orlando theory description. In A. I. Meleis (Ed.), *Theoretical nursing: Development and progress* (3rd ed.). New York: J. B. Lippincott.

Mischo-Kelling, M., & Wittneben, K. (Eds.). (1995). *Ida Jean Orlando Pelletier: Zur bedeutungproblematischer situationen. Pfledgebidung und pflegetheorien* (pp. 50-67, 184-186). Baltimore: Urban & Schwarzenberg.

Mohr, W. K. (1999). Deconstructing the language of psychiatric hospitalization. *Journal of Advanced Nursing, 29*(5), 1052-1059.

Nursing Theories Conference Group, & George, J. B. (Chairperson). (1980). *Nursing theories: The base for professional practice.* Englewood Cliffs, NJ: Prentice-Hall.

Oiler Boyd, C. (1993). Toward a nursing practice research method. *Advanced Nursing Science, 16*(2), 9-25.

Olson, J., & Hanchett, E. (1997). Nurse-expressed empathy, patient outcomes, and development of a middle-range theory. *Image: The Journal of Nursing Scholarship, 29*(1), 71-76.

Orlando, I. J. (1961). *The dynamic nurse-patient relationship: Function, process and principles of professional nursing practice.* New York: G. P. Putnam's Sons.

Orlando, I. J. (1972). *The discipline and teaching of nursing process: An evaluative study.* New York: G. P. Putnam's Sons.

Orlando, I. J. (1990). *The dynamic nurse-patient relationship: Function, process, and principles* (Pub. No. 15-2341). New York: National League for Nursing.

Peitchinis, L. (1972). Therapeutic effectiveness of counseling by nursing personnel. *Nursing Research, 21,* 138-148.

Pelletier, I. O. (1967). The patient's predicament and nursing function. *Psychiatric Opinion, 4*(1), 25-30.

Perrin, C., & Reilly, R. (2002). *Management in specialist nursing practice* (pp. 1-5). Toowoomba, Australia: The University of Southern Queensland.

Pienschke, D., Sr. (1973). Guardedness or openness on the cancer unit. *Nursing Research, 22,* 484-490.

Ponte-Reid, P. A. (1992). Distress in cancer patients and primary nurses' empathy skills. *Cancer Nursing, 15*(4), 283-292.

Potter, M. L. (2004). Deliberative nursing process. In S. J. Peterson & T. S. Bredow, *Middle range theories: Application to nursing research.* Philadelphia: Lippincott Williams & Wilkins.

Potter, M. L., & Bockenhauer, B. J. (2000). Implementing Orlando's nursing theory: A pilot study. *Journal of Psychosocial Nursing and Mental Health Services, 38*(3), 14-21.

Potter, M. L., & Dawson, A. (2001). From safety contract to safety agreement. *Journal of Psychosocial Nursing and Mental Health Services, 39*(8), 38-45.

Price, B. (2003). Understanding the origins of practice problems. *Nursing Standards, 17*(50), 47-53.

Primomo, J. (2000, May 31). Nursing around the world: Japan—Preparing for the century of the elderly. *Online Journal of Issues in Nursing, 5*(2), 1-16. Retrieved September 3, 2004, from *http://www.nursingworld.org/ojin/topic12/tpc12_1.htm.*

Princeton, J. (1986). Incorporating a deliberative nursing care approach with breast-feeding mothers. *Health Care for Women International, 7,* 277-293.

Revista Brasileira de Enfermagen. (2002). *Brasila, 5,* n. 5, pp. 489-494.

Rosenthal, B. C. (1996). An interactionist's approach to perioperative nursing. *AORN Journal, 62*(2), 254-260.

Schmidt, J. (1972). Availability: A concept of nursing practice. *American Journal of Nursing, 72,* 1086-1089.

Schmieding, N. (1984). Putting Orlando's theory into practice. *American Journal of Nursing, 84*(6), 759-761.

Schmieding, N. J. (1986). Orlando's theory. In P. Winstead-Fry (Ed.), *Case studies in nursing theory* (pp. 1-36). New York: National League for Nursing.

Schmieding, N. J. (1987). Problematic situations in nursing: Analysis of Orlando's theory based on Dewey's theory of inquiry. *Journal of Advanced Nursing, 12*(4), 431-440.

Schmieding, N. J. (1988). Action process of nurse administrators to problematic situations based on Orlando's theory. *Journal of Advanced Nursing, 13*(1), 99-107.

Schmieding, N. J. (1993). *Ida Jean Orlando: A nursing process theory.* Newbury Park, CA: Sage Publications.

Schmieding, N. J. (1999). Reflective inquiry framework for nurse administrators. *Journal of Advanced Nursing, 30*(3), 631-639.

Schmieding, N. J. (2004). *Ida J. Orlando.* Kingston, RI: Norma Jean Schmieding, University of Rhode Island College of Nursing. Retrieved September 3, 2004, from *http://www.uri.edu/nursing/schmieding/orlando/.*

Schmieding, N. J., & Kokuyama, T. (1995). The need for and process of collaborative international research; a replication of Japanese staff nurse perceptions of head nurses' actions. *Journal of Advanced Nursing, 2,* 820-826.

Selanders, L. C., Schmieding, N. J, & Hartweg, D. L. (1995). *Antechningar om Omvardnadsteorier IV.* Lund, Germany: Studentlitteratur.

Shea, N. M., McBride, L., Gavin, C., & Bauer, M. (1997). The effects of an ambulatory collaborative practice model on process and outcome of care for bipolar disorder. *Journal of the American Psychiatric Nurses Association, 3*(2), 49-57.

Sheafor, M. (1991). Productive work groups in complex hospital units. *Journal of Nursing Administration, 21*(5), 25-30.

Thibaudeau, M., & Reidy, M. (1977). Nursing makes a difference: A comparative study of the health behavior of mothers in three primary care agencies. *International Journal of Nursing Studies, 14,* 97-107.

Valentine, S. O. (2002). Nursing leadership and the new nurse. *Journal of Undergraduate Nursing Scholarship* (online journal published by the University of Arizona College of Nursing), *4*(1). Retrieved September 3, 2004, from juns.nursing.arizona.edu/articlesn/Fall% 202002/Valentine.htm.

Walker, L. O., & Avant, K. C. (1995). *Strategies for theory construction in nursing* (3rd ed.). Norwalk, CT: Appleton & Lange.

Winder, A. (1984). A mental health professional looks at nursing care. *Nursing Forum, 21,* 184-188.

Wolfer, J., & Visintainer, M. (1975). Pediatric surgical patients' and parents' stress responses and adjustment. *Nursing Research, 24,* 244-255.

Wooldridge, P. J., Skipper, J. K., Jr., & Leonard, R. C. (1968). *Behavioral science, social practice, and the nursing profession.* Cleveland, OH: The Case Western Reserve University.

BIBLIOGRAPHY
Primary Sources
Books

Orlando, I. (1961). *The dynamic nurse-patient relationship.* New York: G. P. Putnam's Sons.

Orlando, I. (1972). *The discipline and teaching of nursing process.* New York: G. P. Putnam's Sons.

Orlando, I. J. (1990). *The dynamic nurse-patient relationship* (Pub. No. 15-2341). New York: National League for Nursing.

Book Chapter

Orlando, I. (1962). Function, process and principle of professional nursing practice. In *Integration of mental health concepts in the human relations professions* (pp. 87-106). New York: Bank Street College of Education.

Journal Articles

Orlando, I. (1987). Nursing in the 21st century: Alternate path. *Journal of Advanced Nursing, 12,* 405-412.

Orlando, I. J., & Dugan, A. (1989, Feb.). Independent and dependent paths: The fundamental issue for the nursing profession. *Nursing and Health Care, 2,* 77-80.

Pelletier, I. O. (1967). The patient's predicament and nursing function. *Psychiatric Opinion, 4,* 25-30.

Videotape and CD-ROM

Ida Orlando the deliberative nursing process. (1997). In *The nurse theorists portraits of excellence* (CD-ROM). Athens, OH: Fuld Institute for Technology in Nursing Education.

Pelletier, I. O. (1988). *The nurse theorist: Portraits of excellence. Ida Orlando Pelletier* (Videotape). Athens, OH: Fuld Institute for Technology in Nursing Education.

Secondary Sources
Books

Chinn, P. L., & Kramer, M. K. (1991). *Theory and nursing: A systematic approach* (3rd ed., pp. 177-178). St. Louis: Mosby.

Chinn, P. L., & Kramer, M. K. (1999). *Theory and nursing—Integrated knowledge development* (5th ed.). St. Louis: Mosby.

Chinn, P. L., & Kramer, M. K. (2004). *Integrated knowledge development in nursing* (6th ed.). St. Louis: Mosby.

Fawcett, J. (2000). *Analysis and evaluation of contemporary nursing knowledge: Nursing models and theories.* Philadelphia: F. A. Davis.

Kim, H. S., & Kollack, I. (1999). *Nursing theories—Conceptual and philosophical foundations.* New York: Springer Publishing.

Meleis, A. (1985). *Theoretical nursing: Development and progress.* Philadelphia: J. B. Lippincott.

Meleis, A. (1998). *Theoretical nursing: Development and progress* (3rd ed.). New York: J. B. Lippincott.

Nursing Theories Conference Group, & J. B. George (Chairperson). (1980). *Nursing theories: The base for professional nursing* practice. Englewood Cliffs, NJ: Prentice-Hall.

Schmieding, N. J. (1993). *Ida Jean Orlando: A nursing process theory.* Newbury Park, CA: Sage.

Book Chapters

Andrews, C. M. (1989). Ida Orlando's model of nursing practice. In J. J. Fitzpatrick & A. L. Whall (Eds.), *Conceptual models of nursing—Analysis and application* (2nd ed.). Norwalk, CT: Appleton & Lange.

Boyd, M. A. (1998). Theoretical basis of psychiatric nursing. In M. A. Boyd & M. A. Nihart (Eds.), *Psychiatric nursing—Contemporary practice.* Philadelphia: Lippincott.

Burgess, A. W. (1997). Psychiatric nursing. In A. W. Burgess (Ed.), *Psychiatric nursing: Promoting mental health.* Stamford, CT: Appleton & Lange.

Crane, M. D. (1985). Ida Jean Orlando. In J. B. George (Ed.), *Nursing theories: The base for professional nursing practice* (3rd ed.). Englewood Cliffs, NJ: Prentice-Hall.

Diers, D. (1997). What is nursing? In J. C. McCloskey & H. K. Grace (Eds.), *Current issues in nursing* (5th ed., pp. 5-12). St. Louis: Mosby.

Leonard, M. K., & George, J. B. (1995). Ida Jean Orlando. In J. B. George (Ed.), *Nursing theories: The base for professional nursing practice* (4th ed.). Norwalk, CT: Appleton & Lange.

Meleis, A. I. (1991). Ida Orlando theory description. In A. I. Meleis (Ed.), *Theoretical nursing: Development and progress* (2nd ed.). Philadelphia: J. B. Lippincott.

Meleis, A. I. (1997). Ida Orlando theory description. In A. I. Meleis (Ed.), *Theoretical nursing: Development and progress* (3rd ed.). New York: J. B. Lippincott.

Mertz, H. (1962). *Nurse actions that reduce stress in patients.* In *Emergency intervention by the nurse* (Monograph 1). New York: American Nurses Association.

Mischo-Kelling, M., & Wittneben, K. (1995). In M. Mischo-Kelling (Ed.), *Ida Jean Orlando Pelletier: Zur bedeutungproblematischer situationen. Pfledgebidung und pflegetheorien* (pp. 184-187). Baltimore: Urban & Schwarzenberg.

Schmieding, N. J. (1983). An analysis of Orlando's theory based on Kuhn's theory of science. In P. L. Chinn (Ed.), *Advances in nursing theory development.* Rockville, MD: Aspen.

Schmieding, N. J. (1986). Orlando's theory. In P. Winstead-Fry (Ed.), *Case studies in nursing theory.* New York: National League for Nursing.

Schmieding, N. J. (2000). Orlando's nursing process theory. In M. R. Alligood & A. M. Tomey (Eds.), *Nursing theory: Utilization & application* (2nd ed.). St. Louis: Mosby.

Schumacher, L. P., Fisher, S., Marriner Tomey, A., Mills, D. I., & Sauter, M. K. (1998). Ida Jean Orlando (Pelletier)—Nursing process theory. In A. M. Tomey & M. R. Alligood (Eds.), *Nursing theorists and their work* (4th ed.). St. Louis: Mosby.

Wesley, R. L. (1995). Orlando's theory of the deliberative nursing process. In R. L. Wesley (Ed.), *Nursing theories and models* (2nd ed.). Springhouse, PA: Springhouse.

Dissertations

Olson, J. K. (1993). *Relationships between nurse expressed empathy, patient perceived empathy and patient distress.* Unpublished doctoral dissertation, Wayne State University, Detroit.

Ponte-Reid, P. A. (1988). *The relationships among empathy and the use of Orlando's deliberative process by the primary nurse and the distress of the adult cancer patient.* Unpublished doctoral dissertation. Boston University, Boston.

Schmieding, N. (1983). *A description and analysis of the directive process used by directors of nursing, supervisors, and head nurses in problematic situations based on Orlando's theory of nursing experience.* Unpublished doctoral dissertation, Boston University, Boston.

Sellers, S. C. (1991). *A philosophical analysis of conceptual models of nursing.* Unpublished doctoral dissertation, Iowa State University, Ames, IA.

Journal Articles

Dumas, R. (1963). Psychological preparation for surgery. *American Journal of Nursing, 63,* 52-55.

Dye, M. (1963). Clarifying patients' communications. *American Journal of Nursing, 63,* 56-59.

Eisler, J., Wolfer, J., & Diers, D. (1972). Relationship between need for social approval and postoperative recovery and welfare. *Nursing Research, 21,* 520-525.

Elder, R. (1963). What is the patient saying? *Nursing Forum, 11,* 25-37.

Elms, R., & Leonard, R. (1966). Effects of nursing approaches during admission. *Nursing Research, 15,* 39-48.

Haggerty, L. (1987). An analysis of senior nursing students' immediate response to distressed patients. *Journal of Advanced Nursing, 12,* 451-461.

Harrison, C. (1966). Deliberative nursing process versus automatic nurse action—The care of a chronically ill man. *Nursing Clinics of North America, 1*(3), 387-397.

Henderson, V. (1978). The concept of nursing. *Journal of Advanced Nursing, 3,* 113-130.

Larson, P., Sr. (1977). Nursing perceptions of patient characteristics. *Nursing Research, 26,* 416-421.

Lipson, J. G., & Meleis, A. I. (1983). Issues in health care of Middle Eastern patients. *The Western Journal of Medicine, 139,* 854-861.

Meleis, A. I. (1998). Revisions in knowledge development: A passion for substance. *Scholarly Inquiry for Nursing Practice: An International Journal, 12*(1), 65-77.

Nagle, L. M. (1999). A matter of extinction or distinction. *Western Journal of Nursing Research, 32,* 71-82.

Ponte-Reid, P. A. (1992). Distress in cancer patients and primary nurses' empathy skills. *Cancer Nursing, 15*(4), 283-292.

Princeton, J. (1986). Incorporating a deliberative nursing approach with breast-feeding mothers. *Health Care for Women International, 7,* 277-293.

Schmieding, N. (1987). Analyzing managerial responses in face-to-face contacts. *Journal of Advanced Nursing, 12,* 357-365.

Schmieding, N. (1987). Problematic situations in nursing: Analysis of Orlando's theory based on Dewey's theory of inquiry. *Journal of Advanced Nursing, 12,* 431-440.

Schmieding, N. (1988). Action process of nurse administrators to problematic situations based on Orlando's theory. *Journal of Advanced Nursing, 13,* 99-107.

Schmieding, N. (1990). A model for assessing nurse administrator's actions. *Western Journal of Nursing, 12*(3), 293-306.

Schmieding, N. (1990). An integrative nursing theoretical framework. *Journal of Advanced Nursing, 15,* 463-467.

Schmieding, N. (1990). Do head nurses include staff in problem solving? *Nursing Management, 21*(3), 58-60.

Schmieding, N. (1991). Relationship between head nurse responses to staff nurses and staff nurse responses to patients. *Western Journal of Nursing Research, 13*(6), 746-760.

Schmieding, N. J. (1970). Relationship of nursing to the process of chronicity. *Nursing Outlook, 18*(2), 58-62.

Schmieding, N. J. (1984). Putting Orlando's theory into practice. *American Journal of Nursing, 83,* 759-761.

Schmieding, N. J. (1993). Nurse empowerment through context, structure and process. *Journal of Professional Nursing, 9*(4), 239-245.

Schmieding, N. J. (1993). Successful superior-subordinate relationships require mutual management. *Health Care Supervisor, 11*(4), 52-63.

Schmieding, N. J. (1999). Reflective inquiry framework for nurse administrators. *Journal of Advanced Nursing, 30*(3), 631-639.

Sheafor, M. (1991). Productive work groups in complex hospital units. *Journal of Nursing Administration, 21*(5), 25-30.

Tryon, P. A., & Leonard, R. C. (1964). The effect of patients' participation on the outcome of a nursing procedure. *Nursing Forum, 3*(2), 79-89.

Web Site

Ida J. Orlando's Nursing Process Theory. Accessed December 20, 2004: *http://www.uri.edu/nursing/schmieding/orlando/*

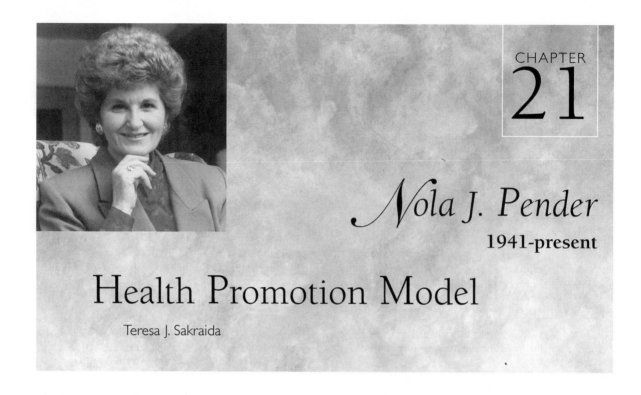

$\mathcal{N}$ola J. Pender

1941-present

Health Promotion Model

Teresa J. Sakraida

CREDENTIALS AND BACKGROUND OF THE THEORIST

Nola J. Pender's first encounter with professional nursing occurred at the age of 7, when she observed the nursing care given to her hospitalized aunt. "The experience of watching the nurses caring for my aunt in her illness created in me a fascination with the work of nursing," noted Pender (personal interview, May 6, 2004). This experience and her subsequent education instilled in her a desire to care for others and influenced her belief that the goal of nursing was to help people care for themselves. Pender contributes to nursing knowledge of health promotion through her research, teaching, presentations, and writings.

Previous author: Lucy Anne Tillett.

The author wishes to express appreciation to Nola J. Pender for reviewing the chapter.

Pender was born August 16, 1941, in Lansing, Michigan (N. Pender, personal interview, May 6, 2004). She was the only child of parents who were advocates of education for women. Family encouragement for her goal of becoming a registered nurse led her to attend the School of Nursing at West Suburban Hospital in Oak Park, Illinois. This school was chosen for its ties with Wheaton College and its strong Christian foundation. She received her nursing diploma in 1962 and began working on a medical-surgical unit and subsequently in a pediatric unit in a Michigan hospital.

In 1964, Pender completed her baccalaureate in nursing at Michigan State University in East Lansing. She credits Helen Penhale, the assistant to the dean, for helping to streamline her program and foster her options for further education. As was common in the 1960s, Pender changed her major from nursing as she pursued her graduate degrees.

She earned her master's degree in human growth and development at Michigan State University in 1965. "The M.A. in growth and development influenced my interest in health over the human lifespan. This background contributed to the formation of a research program for children and adolescents," stated Pender (personal interview, May 6, 2004). She completed her Ph.D. in psychology and education in 1969 at Northwestern University in Evanston, Illinois. Pender's (1970) dissertation investigated developmental changes in encoding processes of short-term memory in children. Dr. Pender credits Dr. James Hall, a doctoral program advisor, with "introducing me to considerations of how people think and how a person's thoughts motivate behavior" (N. Pender, personal interview, May 6, 2004). Several years later, she completed master's-level work in community health nursing at Rush University in Chicago.

After earning her Ph.D., Pender notes a shift in her thinking toward defining the goal of nursing care as the optimal health of the individual. A series of conversations with Dr. Beverly McElmurry at Northern Illinois University and reading *High-Level Wellness* by Halpert Dunn (1961) inspired expanded notions of health and nursing. Her marriage to Albert Pender, an associate professor of business and economics who has collaborated with his wife in writing about the economics of health care, and the birth of a son and daughter, provided increased personal motivation to learn more about optimizing human health.

In 1975, Pender published "A Conceptual Model for Preventive Health Behavior," which was a basis for studying how individuals made decisions about their own health care in a nursing context. This article identified factors that were found in earlier research to influence decision making and actions of individuals in preventing disease. The original Health Promotion Model (HPM) was presented in the first edition of the text, *Health Promotion in Nursing Practice*, published in 1982 (Pender). Based on subsequent research, the HPM was revised and is presented in the second edition, published in 1987, and in the third edition, published in 1996. A fourth edition of *Health Promotion in Nursing Practice*,

jointly authored by Pender with Carolyn L. Murdaugh (Ph.D.) and Mary Ann Parsons (Ph.D.), was published in 2002.

A 6-year study funded by the National Institutes of Health was conducted at Northern Illinois University in DeKalb by Pender and her colleagues Susan Walker (Ed.D.), Karen Sechrist (Ph.D.), and Marilyn Frank-Stromborg (Ed.D.) (1988). The study tested the validity of the HPM (Pender, Walker, Sechrist, & Stromborg, 1988). An instrument, the Health Promoting Lifestyle Profile, was developed by the research team to study the health-promoting behavior of working adults, older adults, patients undergoing cardiac rehabilitation, and ambulatory patients with cancer (Pender et al., 2002). Results from these studies support the HPM (N. Pender, personal interview, July 19, 2000). Subsequently, more than 40 studies have tested the predictive capability of the model for health-promoting lifestyle, exercise, nutrition practices, use of hearing protection, and avoidance of exposure to environmental tobacco smoke (Pender, 1996; Pender et al., 2002).

Pender has provided important leadership in the development of nursing research in the United States. Her work in support of the National Center for Nursing Research in the National Institutes of Health was instrumental to its formation in 1981. She has promoted scholarly activity in nursing through her involvement with Sigma Theta Tau International, as a past president of the Midwest Nursing Research Society (1985 to 1987), and as chairperson of the Cabinet on Nursing Research of the American Nurses Association. Inducted as a fellow of the American Academy of Nursing in 1981, she served as president of the academy from 1991 until 1993 (N. Pender, curriculum vitae, 2000). In 1998, she was appointed to a 4-year term on the U.S. Preventive Services Task Force, an independent panel charged to evaluate scientific evidence and make age-specific and risk-specific recommendations for clinical preventive services (Pender, 2000).

A recipient of many awards and honors, Dr. Pender has served as a distinguished scholar at a number of universities. She received an honorary doctoral degree from Widener University in 1992. In 1988, she received the Distinguished Research Award from the Midwest Nursing Research Society for her contributions to research and research leadership, and in 1997 she received the American Psychological Association Award for outstanding contributions to nursing and health psychology. In 1998, the University of Michigan School of Nursing honored Pender with the Mae Edna Doyle Award for excellence in teaching (N. Pender, personal interview, May 24, 2004). Her widely used text, *Health Promotion in Nursing Practice* (Pender et al., 2002), was honored as the ANA Book of the Year for contributions to community health nursing (Pender, 2000).

Pender was the Associate Dean for Research at the University of Michigan School of Nursing from 1990 to 2001. In this position, Dr. Pender facilitated external funding of faculty research, supported emerging centers of research excellence in the School of Nursing, promoted interdisciplinary research, supported translating research into science-based practice, and linked nursing research to the formulation of health policy (Pender, 2000). A child and adolescent health behavior research center initiated at the University of Michigan in 1991 represents Pender's efforts to build a large interdisciplinary research team to study and influence the health-promoting behaviors of individuals by understanding how these behaviors are established in youth (N. Pender, personal interview, May 24, 2000). Her current and future program of research has two major foci, as follows:

1. Understanding how self-efficacy effects the exertion and affective (activity-related affect) responses of adolescent girls to the physical activity challenge
2. Developing an interactive computer program as an intervention to increase physical activity among adolescent girls (Pender, 2000)

The Design of a Computer Based Physical Activity Counseling Intervention for Adolescent Girls is an ongoing research program led by Dr. Lorraine Robbins (N. Pender, personal interview, May 6, 2004).

Pender has published numerous articles on exercise, behavior change, and relaxation training as aspects of health promotion and has served as an editor for journals and books. Pender is recognized as a scholar, presenter, and consultant on health-promotion topics. She has consulted with nurse scientists in Japan, Korea, Mexico, Thailand, the Dominican Republic, Jamaica, England, New Zealand, and Chile (N. Pender, curriculum vitae 2000; Pender, 2000). Her book is now available in the Japanese and Korean languages (Pender, 1997a, 1997b).

As Professor Emeritus at the University of Michigan School of Nursing, Pender is currently involved in influencing the nursing profession by providing leadership as a consultant to research centers and providing early scholars consultation (Pender, 2000). As a nationally and internationally known leader, Pender speaks at conferences and seminars. She collaborates with Dr. Michael O'Donnell, editor of the *American Journal of Health Promotion*, to advocate for legislation to fund health promotion research (N. Pender, personal interview, May 6, 2004).

Pender's future plans include continuing with travel to offer consultation and to engage in speaking opportunities. She expects to do some graduate teaching on occasion. Pender plans to continue active mentoring through e-mail exchanges with scholars beginning research programs (N. Pender, personal interview, May 6, 2004).

THEORETICAL SOURCES

Pender's background in nursing, human development, experimental psychology, and education led her to use a holistic nursing perspective, social psychology, and learning theory as the foundations for the HPM. The HPM (Figure 21-1) integrates several constructs. Central to the HPM is the social learning theory of Albert Bandura (1977), which postulates the importance of cognitive processes in the changing of behavior. Social learning theory, now titled social cognitive theory, includes the following self-beliefs: self-attribution, self-evaluation, and self-efficacy. Self-efficacy is a central construct of the HPM (Pender, 1996; Pender et al.,

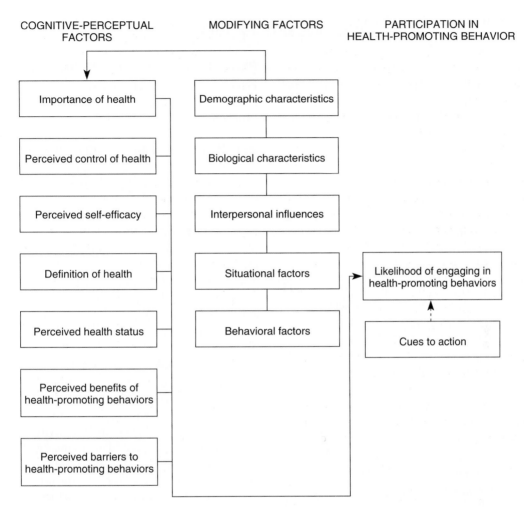

COGNITIVE-PERCEPTUAL FACTORS

MODIFYING FACTORS

PARTICIPATION IN HEALTH-PROMOTING BEHAVIOR

Importance of health

Perceived control of health

Perceived self-efficacy

Definition of health

Perceived health status

Perceived benefits of health-promoting behaviors

Perceived barriers to health-promoting behaviors

Demographic characteristics

Biological characteristics

Interpersonal influences

Situational factors

Behavioral factors

Likelihood of engaging in health-promoting behaviors

Cues to action

Figure **21-1** **Health Promotion Model.** (From Pender, N. J. [1987]. *Health promotion in nursing practice* [2nd ed., p. 58]. New York: Appleton & Lange. Copyright Pearson Education, Upper Saddle River, NJ.)

2002). In addition, the expectancy-value model of human motivation that Feather (1982) described, which supports that behavior is rational and economical, is important to the model's development.

The HPM is similar in construction to the health belief model (Becker, 1974) but is not limited to explaining disease-prevention behavior. The HPM differs from the health belief model in that the HPM does not include fear or threat as a source of motivation for health behavior. For this reason, the HPM expands to encompass behaviors for enhancing health and potentially applies across the life-span (Pender, 1996; Pender et al., 2002).

MAJOR CONCEPTS *&* DEFINITIONS

The major concepts and definitions presented are found in the revised HPM (N. Pender, personal interview, May 6, 2004). The following are individual characteristics and experiences that affect subsequent health actions (N. Pender, curriculum vitae, 2000).

PRIOR RELATED BEHAVIOR

Frequency of the same or similar behavior in the past. Direct and indirect effects on the likelihood of engaging in health-promoting behaviors.

PERSONAL FACTORS

Categorized as biological, psychological, and sociocultural. These factors are predictive of a given behavior and shaped by the nature of the target behavior being considered.

Personal Biological Factors

Included in these factors are variables such as age, gender, body mass index, pubertal status, menopausal status, aerobic capacity, strength, agility, or balance.

Personal Psychological Factors

These factors include variables such as self-esteem, self-motivation, personal competence, perceived health status, and definition of health.

Personal Sociocultural Factors

These factors include variables such as race, ethnicity, acculturation, education, and socioeconomic status.

The following are behavioral-specific cognitions and affect that are considered of major motivational significance, and these variables are modifiable through nursing actions (Pender, 1996).

PERCEIVED BENEFITS OF ACTION

Perceived benefits of action are anticipated positive outcomes that will occur from health behavior.

PERCEIVED BARRIERS TO ACTION

Perceived barriers to action are anticipated, imagined, or real blocks and personal costs of undertaking a given behavior.

PERCEIVED SELF-EFFICACY

Perceived self-efficacy is judgment of personal capability to organize and execute a health-promoting behavior. Perceived self-efficacy influences perceived barriers to action, so higher efficacy results in lowered perceptions of barriers to the performance of the behavior.

ACTIVITY-RELATED AFFECT

An activity-related affect describes subjective positive or negative feelings that occur before, during, and following behavior based on the stimulus properties of the behavior itself. Activity-related affect influences perceived self-efficacy, which means the more positive the subjective feeling, the greater the feeling of efficacy. In turn, increased feelings of efficacy can generate further positive affect.

INTERPERSONAL INFLUENCES

These influences are cognitions concerning behaviors, beliefs, or attitudes of others. Interpersonal influences include norms (expectations of significant others), social support (instrumental and emotional encouragement), and modeling (vicarious learning through observing others engaged in a particular behavior). Primary sources of interpersonal influences are families, peers, and health care providers.

MAJOR CONCEPTS & DEFINITIONS—cont'd

SITUATIONAL INFLUENCES

Situational influences are personal perceptions and cognitions of any given situation or context that can facilitate or impede behavior. They include perceptions of options available, demand characteristics, and aesthetic features of the environment in which given health-promoting behavior is proposed to take place. Situational influences may have direct or indirect influences on health behavior.

The following are immediate antecedents of behavior or behavioral outcomes. A behavioral event is initiated by a commitment to action unless there is a competing demand that cannot be avoided or a competing preference that cannot be resisted (N. Pender, personal interview, July 19, 2000).

COMMITMENT TO A PLAN OF ACTION

This commitment describes the concept of intention and identification of a planned strategy that leads to implementation of health behavior.

IMMEDIATE COMPETING DEMANDS AND PREFERENCES

Competing demands are alternative behaviors over which individuals have low control, because there are environmental contingencies such as work or family care responsibilities. Competing preferences are alternative behaviors over which individuals exert relatively high control, such as choice of ice cream or an apple for a snack.

HEALTH-PROMOTING BEHAVIOR

A health-promoting behavior is an end point or action outcome directed toward attaining positive health outcomes such as optimal well being, personal fulfillment, and productive living. Examples of health-promoting behavior are eating a healthy diet, exercising regularly, managing stress, gaining adequate rest and spiritual growth, and building positive relationships.

USE OF EMPIRICAL EVIDENCE

The HPM, as depicted in Figure 21-1, has served as a framework for research aimed at predicting overall health-promoting lifestyles and specific behaviors such as exercise and use of hearing protection (Pender, 1987). Pender and colleagues have conducted a program of research funded by the National Institute of Nursing Research to evaluate the HPM in the following four populations: (1) working adults, (2) older community-dwelling adults, (3) ambulatory patients with cancer, and (4) patients undergoing cardiac rehabilitation. The studies tested the validity of the HPM (N. Pender, personal interview, May 24, 2000). A summary of findings from earlier studies is listed in the 1996 edition of *Health Promotion in Nursing Practice*

(Pender, 1996). Additional studies testing the model are presented in the fourth edition of *Health Promotion in Nursing Practice* (Pender et al., 2002).

The rationale for revision of the HPM stemmed from the analyses of research studies. The process of refining the HPM, as published in 1987, led to several changes (see Figure 21-1) (Pender, 1996). First, importance of health, perceived control of health, and cues for action were deleted from the model. Second, definition of health, perceived health status, and demographic and biological characteristics were repositioned in the category of personal factors in the 1996 revision of the HPM (Pender, 1996) and are also displayed in the fourth edition of *Health Promotion in Nursing Practice* (Pender et al., 2002) (Figure 21-2). Last, the revised HPM (see Figure 21-2) adds the following three new

INDIVIDUAL
CHARACTERISTICS
AND EXPERIENCES

BEHAVIOR-SPECIFIC
COGNITIONS
AND AFFECT

BEHAVIORAL
OUTCOME

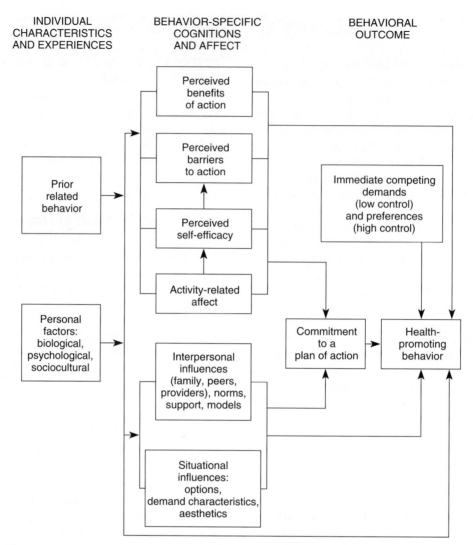

Figure **21-2 Revised Health Promotion Model.** (From Pender, N. J., Murdaugh, C. L., & Parsons, M. A. [2002]. *Health promotion in nursing practice* [4th ed., p. 60]. Upper Saddle River, NJ: Prentice-Hall. Copyright Pearson Education, Upper Saddle River, NJ.)

variables that serve to influence the individual to engage in health-promoting behaviors (Pender, 1996):

1. Activity-related affect
2. Commitment to a plan of action
3. Immediate competing demand and preferences

The revised HPM focuses upon 10 categories of determinants of health-promoting behavior. Currently being tested empirically, the revised model identifies concepts relevant to health-promoting behaviors and facilitates the generation of testable hypotheses (Pender et al., 2002).

The HPM provides a paradigm for the development of instruments. The Health Promoting Lifestyle Profile and the Exercise Benefits-Barriers Scale (EBBS) are two examples.* Both of these instruments serve to test the model and further model development.

The purpose of the Health Promotion Lifestyle Profile instrument is to measure health-promoting lifestyle (Pender, 1996). The Health Promotion Lifestyle Profile II (HPLP-II), a revision of the original instrument, is used in research.† The 52-item, four-point, Likert-styled instrument consists of the following six subscales: (1) health responsibility, (2) physical activity, (3) nutrition, (4) interpersonal relations, (5) spiritual growth, and (6) stress management. Means can be derived for each subscale or a total mean signifying overall health-promoting lifestyle (Walker, Sechrist, & Pender, 1987). The instrument provides an assessment of health-promoting lifestyle of individuals that is useful to nurses clinically in patient support and education.

The HPM identifies cognitive and perceptual factors as major determinants of health-promoting behavior. The EBBS measures the cognitive and perceptual factors of perceived benefits and perceived barriers to exercise (Sechrist, Walker, & Pender, 1987). The 43-item, four-point, Likert-styled instrument consists of a 29-item benefits scale and a 14-item barriers scale that may be scored separately or as a whole. The higher the overall score on the 43-item instrument, the more positively the individual perceives the benefits to exercise in relation to barriers to exercise (Sechrist, et al., 1987). The EBBS provides a clinically useful means for evaluating exercise perceptions.

MAJOR ASSUMPTIONS

The assumptions reflect the behavioral science perspective and emphasize the active role of the patient

*The EBBS can be obtained from the Health Promotion Research Program, Social Science Research Institute, Northern Illinois University, DeKalb, IL 60115.
†The HPLP-II can be obtained from Dr. Susan Noble Walker, Ed.D., R.N., at the College of Nursing, University of Nebraska Medical Center, 42nd and Dewey Avenue, Omaha, NE 68105-1065. Fax: (402) 559-6379; telephone (402) 559-6561.

for managing health behaviors by modifying the environmental context. In the third edition of her book, *Health Promotion in Nursing Practice,* Pender (1996) states the major assumptions of the HPM as follows:

1. Persons seek to create conditions of living through which they can express their unique human health potential.
2. Persons have the capacity for reflective self-awareness, including assessment of their own competencies.
3. Persons value growth in directions viewed as positive and attempt to achieve a personally acceptable balance between change and stability.
4. Individuals seek to actively regulate their own behavior.
5. Individuals in all their biopsychosocial complexity interact with the environment, progressively transforming the environment and being transformed over time.
6. Health professionals constitute a part of the interpersonal environment, which exerts influence on persons throughout their life-spans.
7. Self-initiated reconfiguration of person-environment interactive patterns is essential to behavioral change. (pp. 54-55)

THEORETICAL ASSERTIONS

The model is an attempt to depict the multifaceted natures of persons interacting with the environment as they pursue health. Unlike avoidance-oriented models that rely upon fear or threat to health as motivation for health behavior, the HPM has a competence or approach-oriented focus (Pender, 1996). Health promotion is motivated by the desire to increase well-being and actualize human potential (Pender, 1996). In her first book, *Health Promotion in Nursing Practice,* Pender (1982) asserts that complex biopsychosocial processes motivate individuals to engage in behaviors directed toward the enhancement of health. Fourteen theoretical assertions derived from the model appear in the fourth edition of the book, *Health Promotion in Nursing Practice* (Pender et al., 2002):

1. Prior behavior and inherited and acquired characteristics influence beliefs, affect, and enactment of health-promoting behavior.

2. Persons commit to engaging in behaviors from which they anticipate deriving personally valued benefits.

3. Perceived barriers can constrain commitment to action, mediator of behavior, and actual behavior.

4. Perceived competence or self-efficacy to execute a given behavior increases the likelihood of commitment to action and actual performance of behavior.

5. Greater perceived self-efficacy results in fewer perceived barriers to specific health behavior.

6. Positive affect toward a behavior results in greater perceived self-efficacy, which can, in turn, result in increased positive affect.

7. When positive emotions or affect are associated with a behavior, the probability of commitment and action are increased.

8. Persons are more likely to commit to and engage in health-promoting behaviors when significant others model the behavior, expect the behavior to occur, and provide assistance and support to enable the behavior.

9. Families, peers, and health care providers are important sources of interpersonal influence that can increase or decrease commitment to and engagement in health-promoting behavior.

10. Situational influences in the external environment can increase or decrease commitment to or participation in health-promoting behavior.

11. The greater the commitment to a specific plan of action, the more likely health-promoting behaviors are to be maintained over time.

12. Commitment to a plan of action is less likely to result in the desired behavior when competing demands over which persons have little control require immediate attention.

13. Commitment to a plan of action is less likely to result in the desired behavior when other actions are more attractive and thus preferred over the target behavior.

14. Persons can modify cognitions, affect, and the interpersonal and physical environments to create incentives for health actions. (pp. 63-64)

LOGICAL FORM

The HPM has been formulated through induction by use of existing research to form a pattern of knowledge about health behavior. Middle range theories commonly are generated through this approach. The HPM is a conceptual model that was formulated with the goal of integrating what is known about health-promoting behavior to generate questions for further testing. This model provides a framework for seeing how the results of previous research fit together more clearly and how concepts can be manipulated for further study.

ACCEPTANCE BY THE NURSING COMMUNITY
Practice

Wellness as a nursing specialty has grown in prominence during the past decade. Current state-of-the-art clinical practice includes health-promotion education. Nursing professionals find the HPM very relevant, because it applies across the life-span and is useful in a variety of settings (Pender, 1996; Pender et al., 2002).

The clinical interest in health behaviors represents a philosophical shift that emphasizes the quality of lives alongside the saving of lives. In addition, there are financial, human, and environmental burdens upon society when individuals do not engage in prevention and health promotion. The HPM contributes a nursing solution to health policy and health care reform by providing a means for understanding how consumers can be motivated to attain personal health. Future empirical findings will be of increasing importance to nurse planners of health care delivery and to those who provide the care.

Education

The HPM is used widely in graduate education and it is being used increasingly in undergraduate nursing education in the United States (N. Pender, personal interview, May 24, 2000). In the past, health promotion was being placed behind illness care, because clinical education was conducted primarily in acute care settings (Pender, Baraukas, Hayman, Rice, & Anderson, 1992). Increasingly, the HPM is incorporated in nursing curricula as an aspect of health assessment, community health nursing, and wellness-focused courses (N. Pender, personal interview, May 24, 2000). There are growing international efforts across a number of countries to integrate the HPM into nursing curricula (N. Pender, personal interview, May 6, 2004; Pender et al., 2002).

Research

The HPM is a tool for research. Pender's research agenda and other researchers test the empirical precision of the model. Many researchers report using the model as a frame of reference. The Health Promoting Lifestyle Profile, derived from the model, often serves as the operational definition for health-promoting behaviors. The model has implications for application by emphasizing the importance of individual assessment of the factors believed to influence health behavior changes.

FURTHER DEVELOPMENT

The model continues to be refined and tested for its power to explain the relationships among the factors believed to influence changes in a wide array of health behaviors. Sufficient empirical support for model variables now exists for some behaviors to warrant design and conduct of intervention studies to test model-based nursing interventions. Lusk and colleagues (Lusk, Hong, Ronis, Eakin, Kerr, & Early, 1999; Lusk, Kwee, Ronis, & Eakin, 1999) used important predictors of construction workers' use of hearing protection from the HPM (self-efficacy, barriers, interpersonal influences, and situational influences) to develop an interactive, video-based program to increase use. This large, multiple-site study found that the intervention increased use of workers' hearing protection by 20% compared with the group without intervention, a statistically significant improvement from baseline (Lusk, Hong et al., 1999). Further intervention studies represent the next step in the use of the model to build nursing science.

CRITIQUE
Simplicity

The HPM is simple to understand. The conceptual definitions provide clarity and lead to greater understanding of the complexity of health behavior phenomena. The various factors in each set are linked logically. The relationships are clarified in the theoretical assertions. The sets of factors, which are direct or indirect influences, are clearly set out in a visually simple diagram that displays their association. Factors are seen as independent, but the sets have an interactive effect that results in action.

Generality

The model is middle range in scope. It is highly generalizable to adult populations. The research used to derive the model was based on male, female, young, old, well, and ill samples. The research agenda includes application in a variety of settings. A research program is testing the applicability of the model to children aged 10 to 16 years old (N. Pender, personal interview, May 6, 2004). Cultural and diversity considerations support model testing in diverse populations.

Empirical Precision

The model has been supported through testing by Pender and others as a framework for explaining health promotion. The model continues to evolve through planned programs of research. Continued empirical research, especially intervention studies, will further refine the model. The Health Promoting Lifestyle Profile has emerged as an instrument to assess health-promoting behaviors (Pender et al., 2002).

Derivable Consequences

Pender has identified health promotion as a goal for the twenty-first century, just as disease prevention was a task of the twentieth century. The model potentially can influence the interaction between the nurse and the consumer. Pender has responded to the political, social, and personal environment of her time to clarify nursing's role in delivering health promotion services to persons of all ages.

SUMMARY

The movement to greater responsibility and accountability for successful personal health practices requires the support of the nursing profession through development of evidence-based practice. The HPM evolved from a substantive research program and continues to provide direction for better health practices. The model guides further research in various populations. Dr. Pender's visionary leadership continues to influence health promotion–related education, research, and policy.

Case Study

Thomas, a 26-year-old graduate student of Cuban descent, comes to the college health clinic to discuss his perceived weight problem. He tells you that he wants a more businesslike look and wants to have more energy. He says that he is tired of having his belly fall over his belt. In your physical assessment you find that Thomas is 5'11", weighs 260 pounds, and has mild hypertension, 132/90 mm Hg. His mother has a history of diabetes mellitus, and he tells you that high blood pressure runs in the family. His 64-year-old father had a heart attack 1 year ago. His electrocardiogram demonstrates normal sinus rhythm. He does not smoke. He says that his stress level is high, because he is working on his master's thesis. Thomas leaves to have some screening blood work and makes an appointment to see you next week. In the meantime, you begin some preliminary planning.

1. What online state-of-the-science resources would you use to help you in planning disease prevention and health promotion?
   - The Agency for Healthcare Research and Quality provides a Guide to Clinical Preventive Services that lists the latest available recommendations on preventive

interventions: screening tests, counseling, immunizations, and medication regimens for more than 80 conditions. Age-specific periodic screenings based on gender and individual risk factors are available from the Web site (*http://www.ahrq.gov/clinic/prevnew.htm*). The consumer section for downloadable files for your personal digital assistant is another resource.
   - Go to *http://www.ahrq.gov/clinic/cps3dix.htm*. Look under the Clinical Category: Metabolic, Nutritional, and Endocrine Conditions to find Obesity in Adults: Screening.
   - *Healthy People 2010* presents a comprehensive set of disease prevention and health promotion objectives developed to improve the health of all people in the United States during the first decade of the twenty-first century (*http://www.healthypeople.gov*).
   - The U.S. Department of Health and Human Services Web site contains information about safety and wellness and more (*http://www.hhs.gov*).

2. What were some of the emotional and behavioral cues provided that Thomas is ready for a weight loss management plan?
   - Thomas demonstrated self-direction, because he came to the clinic on his own.
   - He told you that he wants a more businesslike look and wants to have more energy.
   - He stated that he is tired of having his belly fall over his belt.
   - He stated that his stress level is high.

3. In establishing a behavior change plan with Thomas, what are some of the interpersonal facilitators and potential barriers to change?
   - *Facilitators:* self-direction, motivation by family medical history, desire for change
   - *Potential barriers:* graduate students may have limited financial resources; stress level is high and Thomas may view self with limited time for physical activity, possibly using eating

as a coping mechanism. (Additional assessment is indicated to validate barriers.)

4. List some alternatives in the behavior change plan that you will discuss with Thomas at your next meeting. In general, discuss diet, physical activity, and stress management.
   - Complete a behavioral contract as a commitment to a plan of action. In the plan, establish a long-term weight loss goal and short-term progress goals.
     - Review kinds of foods he enjoys, assessing dietary concerns, if any.
     - Discuss ways to increase physical activity, which of the activities he intends to carry out, and establish a calendar.
     - Provide a referral to the campus physical activity trainer.
     - Discuss stress management.
   - Establish follow-up.
     - Schedule weight checks every week.
     - Begin reward-reinforcement planning.

CRITICAL THINKING *Activities*

1. Choose one health-promoting behavior in which you do not engage. Identify factors, as defined in the HPM, which contribute to your decision not to participate. Include immediate competing alternatives.

2. Analyze the factors in your life that contribute to your participation in any health-promoting activity in which you currently engage. Place each factor under the appropriate label from the HPM.

3. Prepare your own description of wellness. Ask three friends, three family members, and three co-workers to describe what wellness means to them. Compare the descriptions given by individuals with different ages and backgrounds. How are they alike? Is absence of disease more prominent than positive, active statements of health?

4. Anticipate the health-promoting behaviors important at various stages of development across the life-span. In light of the nurse as a health educator, what health-promotion topics would you include in your practice?

5. Consider the changes made in health care delivery during the last century related to advances in disease prevention and cure. What changes can you predict for the nurse of 2050 if health promotion becomes the primary focus of health care? Include potential locations for the work of nursing, possible new tools, and how the shift in emphasis would affect the demand for nurses.

REFERENCES

Bandura, A. (1977). Self-efficacy: Toward a unifying theory of behavioral change. *Psychology Review, 84*(2), 191-215.

Becker, M. H. (1974). *The health belief model and personal behavior.* Thorofare, NJ: Charles B. Slack.

Dunn, H. L. (1961). *High-level wellness.* Arlington, VA: Beatty.

Feather, N. T. (1982). *Expectations and actions: Expectancy-value models in psychology.* Hillsdale, NJ: Lawrence Erlbaum Associates.

Lusk, S. L., Hong, O. S., Ronis, S. L., Eakin, B. L., Kerr, M. J., & Early, M. R. (1999). Effectiveness of an intervention to increase construction worker's use of hearing protection. *Human Factors, 41*(3), 487-494.

Lusk, S. L., Kwee, M. J., Ronis, D. L., & Eakin, B. L. (1999). Applying the health promotion model to development of a worksite intervention. *American Journal of Health Promotion, 13*(4), 219-226.

Pender, N. J. (1970). A developmental study of conceptual, semantic differential, and acoustical dimensions as encoding categories in short-term memory (Doctoral dissertation Northwestern University, 1970). *Dissertation Abstracts International, A, 30*(10), 4283.

Pender, N. J. (1975). A conceptual model for preventive health behavior. *Nursing Outlook, 23*(6), 385-390.

Pender, N. J. (1982). *Health promotion in nursing practice.* New York: Appleton-Century-Crofts.

Pender, N. J. (1987). *Health promotion in nursing practice* (2nd ed.). New York: Appleton & Lange.

Pender, N. J. (1996). *Health promotion in nursing practice* (3rd ed.). Stamford, CT: Appleton & Lange.

Pender, N. J. (1997a). *Health promotion in nursing practice* (3rd ed.). Stamford, CT: Appleton & Lange. [Japanese translation].

Pender, N. J. (1997b). *Health promotion in nursing practice* (3rd ed.). Stamford, CT: Appleton & Lange. [Korean translation].

Pender, N. J. (2000). *Biographic sketch* (Online). Ann Arbor, MI: University of Michigan. Retrieved May 5, 2004, from *http://www.nursing.umich.edu/faculty/pender/pender_bio.html*.

Pender, N. J., Baraukas, V. H., Hayman, L., Rice, V. H., & Anderson, E. T. (1992). Health promotion and disease prevention: Toward excellence in nursing practice and education. *Nursing Outlook, 40*(3), 106-120.

Pender, N. J., Murdaugh, C. L., & Parsons, M. A. (2002). *Health promotion in nursing practice* (4th ed.). Upper Saddle River, NJ: Prentice-Hall.

Pender, N. J., Walker, S. N., Sechrist, K. R., & Stromborg, M. F. (1988). Development and testing of the health promotion model. *Cardiovascular Nursing, 24*(6), 41-43.

Sechrist, K. R., Walker, S. N., & Pender, N. J. (1987). Development and psychometric evaluation of the exercise/barriers scale. *Research in Nursing and Health, 10,* 357-365.

Walker, S. N., Sechrist, K. R., & Pender, N. J. (1987). The health-promoting lifestyle profile: Development and psychometric characteristics. *Nursing Research, 36*(2), 76-80.

BIBLIOGRAPHY
Primary Sources
Books

Pender, N. J. (1982). *Health promotion in nursing practice.* New York: Appleton-Century-Crofts.

Pender, N. J. (1987). *Health promotion in nursing practice* (2nd ed.). New York: Appleton & Lange.

Pender, N. J. (1996). *Health promotion in nursing practice* (3rd ed.). Stamford, CT: Appleton & Lange.

Pender, N. J., Murdaugh, C. L., & Parsons, M. A. (2002). *Health promotion in nursing practice* (4th ed.). Upper Saddle River, NJ: Prentice Hall.

Book Chapters

Pender, N. J. (1984). Health promotion and illness prevention. In H. Werley & J. Fitzpatrick (Eds.), *Annual review of nursing research* (pp. 83-105). New York: Springer.

Pender, N. J. (1985). Self modification. In G. Bulechek & J. McCloskey (Eds.), *Interventions: Treatments for nursing diagnosis* (pp. 80-91). Philadelphia: Saunders.

Pender, N. J. (1986). Health promotion: Implementing strategies. In B. Logan & C. Dawkins (Eds.), *Family-centered nursing in the community* (pp. 295-334). Menlo Park, CA: Addison-Wesley.

Pender, N. J. (1987). Health and health promotion: The conceptual dilemmas. In M. E. Duffy & N. J. Pender (Eds.), *Conceptual issues in health promotion: Report of proceedings of a wingspread conference* (pp. 7-23). Indianapolis: Sigma Theta Tau International.

Pender, N. J. (1989). Languaging a health perspective for NANDA taxonomy on research and theory. In R. M. Carroll-Johnson (Ed.), *Classification of nursing diagnoses* (pp. 31-36). Philadelphia: Lippincott.

Pender, N. J. (1989). The pursuit of happiness, stress, and health. In S. Wald (Ed.), *Community health nursing: Issues and topics* (pp. 145-175). Englewood Cliffs, NJ: Prentice-Hall.

Pender, N. J. (1998). Motivation for physical activity among children and adolescents. In J. Fitzpatrick & J. S. Stevenson (Eds.), *Annual review of nursing research* (Vol. 16, pp. 139-172). New York: Springer.

Pender, N. J., & Pender, A. R. (1989). Attitudes, subjective norms, and intentions to engage in health behaviors. In C. A. Tanner (Ed.), *Using nursing research* (NLN Pub. No. 15-2232, pp. 466-472). New York: National League for Nursing Publications.

Pender, N. J., & Sallis, J. (1995). Exercise counseling by health professionals. In R. Dishman (Ed.), *Exercise adherence* (2nd ed.). Champaign, IL: Human Kinetics.

Dissertation

Pender, N. J. (1970). A developmental study of conceptual, semantic differential, and acoustical dimensions as encoding categories in short-term memory (Doctoral dissertation Northwestern University, 1970). *Dissertation Abstracts International, A, 30*(10), 4283.

International Journal Articles

Garcia, A. W., Broda, M. A., Frenn, M., Coviak, C., Pender, N. J., & Ronis, D. L. (1997). Gender and developmental differences in exercise beliefs among youth and prediction of their exercise behavior [Japanese translation]. *The Japanese Journal of Nursing Research, 30*(3), 51-61.

Garcia, A. W., George, T. R., Coviack, C., & Pender, N. J. (1997). Development of the child/adolescent activity log: A comprehensive and feasible measure of leisure-time physical activity. *International Journal of Behavioral Medicine, 4*(4), 323-338.

Wu, T. Y., Pender, N., & Noureddine, S. (2003). Gender differences in the psychosocial and cognitive correlates of physical activity among Taiwanese adolescents: A structural equation modeling approach. *International Journal of Behavioral Medicine, 10*(2), 93-105.

Journal Articles

Brimmer, P. F., Skoner, M., Pender, N. J., Williams, C. A., Fleming, J. W., & Werley, H. H. (1983). Nurses with doctoral degrees: Education and employment characteristics. *Research in Nursing and Health, 6,* 157-165.

Eden, K. B., Orleans, C. T., Mulrow, C. D., Pender, N. J., & Teutsch, S. M. (2002). Does counseling by clinicians improve physical activity? A summary of the evidence for the U.S. Preventive Services Task Force, *Annals of Internal Medicine, 137*(3), E208-E215.

Educating APHs for implementing the guidelines for adolescents in bright futures: Guidelines of health supervision of infants, children, and adolescents. *Nursing Outlook, 45*(6), 252-257.

Frank-Stromborg, M., Pender, N. J., Walker, S. N., & Sechrist, K. R. (1990). Determinants of health-promoting lifestyle in ambulatory cancer patients. *Social Science and Medicine, 31*(10), 1159-1168.

Garcia, A. W., Broda, M. A. N., Frenn, M., Coviak, C., Pender, N. J., & Ronis, D. L. (1995). Gender and developmental differences in exercise beliefs among youth and prediction of their exercise behavior. *Journal of School Health, 65*(6), 213-219.

Garcia, A. W., Broda, M. A. N., Frenn, M., Coviak, C., Pender, N. J., & Ronis, D. L. (1997). Gender differences: Exercise beliefs among youth. *Reflections, 23*(1), 21-22.

Garcia, A. W., Pender, N. J., Antonakos, C. L., Ronis, D. L. (1998). Changes in physical activity beliefs and behaviors of boys and girls across the transition to junior high school. *Journal of Adolescent Health, 5,* 394-402.

Pender, N. J. (1967). The debate as a teaching and learning tool. *Nursing Outlook, 15,* 42-43.

Pender, N. J. (1971). Students who choose nursing: Are they success oriented? *Nursing Forum, 16*(1), 64-71.

Pender, N. J. (1974). Patient identification of health information received during hospitalization. *Nursing Research, 23*(3), 262-267.

Pender, N. J. (1975). A conceptual model for preventive health behavior. *Nursing Outlook, 23*(6), 385-390.

Pender, N. J. (1984). Physiologic responses of clients with essential hypertension to progressive muscle relaxation training. *Research in Nursing and Health, 7,* 197-203.

Pender, N. J. (1985). Effects of progressive muscle relaxation training on anxiety and health locus of control among hypertensive adults. *Research in Nursing and Health, 8,* 67-72.

Pender, N. J. (1987). Interview: James Michael McGinnis, MD, MPP. *Family and Community Health, 10*(2), 59-65.

Pender, N. J. (1988). Research agenda: Identifying research ideas and priorities. *American Journal of Health Promotion, 2*(4), 42-51.

Pender, N. J. (1988). Research agenda: The influences of health policy on an evolving research agenda. *American Journal of Health Promotion, 2*(3), 51-54.

Pender, N. J. (1989). Health promotion in the workplace: Suggested directions for research. *American Journal of Health Promotion, 3*(3), 38-43.

Pender, N. J. (1990). Expressing health through lifestyle patterns. *Nursing Science Quarterly, 3*(3), 115-122.

Pender, N. J. (1990). Research agenda: A revised research agenda model. *American Journal of Health Promotion, 4*(3), 220-222.

Pender, N. J. (1992). Making a difference in health policy . . . from AAN president. *Nursing Outlook, 40*(3), 104-105.

Pender, N. J. (1992). Reforming health care: Future direction . . . from AAN president. *Nursing Outlook, 40*(1), 8-9.

Pender, N. J. (1992). The NIH strategic plan: How will it affect the future of nursing science and practice? *Nursing Outlook, 40*(2), 55-56.

Pender, N. J. (1993). Creating change through partnerships . . . from AAN president. *Nursing Outlook, 41*(1), 8-9.

Pender, N. J. (1993). Health care reform: One view of the future . . . from AAN president. *Nursing Outlook, 41*(2), 56-57.

Pender, N. J. (1993). Reaching out . . . from AAN president. *Nursing Outlook, 41*(3), 103-104.

Pender, N. J., Barkaukas, V. H., Hayman, L., Rice, V. H., & Anderson, E. T. (1992). Health promotion and disease prevention: Toward excellence in nursing practice and education. *Nursing Outlook, 40*(3), 106-112, 120.

Pender, N. J., Bar-Or, O., Wilk, B., & Mitchell, S. (2002). Self-efficacy and perceived exertion of girls during exercise. *Nursing Research, 51*(2), 86-91.

Pender, N. J., & Pender, A. R. (1980). Illness prevention and health promotion services provided by nurse practitioners: Predicting potential consumers. *American Journal of Public Health, 70*(8), 798-803.

Pender, N. J., & Pender, A. R. (1986). Attitudes, subjective norms, and intentions to engage in health behaviors. *Nursing Research, 35*(1), 15-18.

Pender, N. J., Sechrist, K. R., Stromborg, M., & Walker, S. N. (1987). Collaboration in developing a research program grant. *Image: The Journal of Nursing Scholarship, 19*(2), 75-77.

Pender, N. J., Smith, L. C., & Vernof, J. A. (1987). Building better workers. *American Association of Occupational Health Nurses Journal, 35*(9), 386-390.

Pender, N. J., Walker, S. N., Frank-Stromborg, M., & Sechrist, K. R. (1990). Predicting health-promoting lifestyles in the workplace. *Nursing Research, 39*(6), 326-332.

Pender, N. J., Walker, S. N., Sechrist, K. R., & Frank-Stromborg, M. (1988). Development and testing of the health promotion model. *Cardiovascular Nursing, 24*(6), 41-43.

Pignone, M. P., Ammerman, A., Fernandez, L., Orleans, C. T., Pender, N., Woolf, S., et al. (2003). Counseling to promote a healthy diet in adults: A summary of the evidence for the U.S. Preventive Services Task Force. *American Journal of Preventive Medicine, 24*(1), 75-92.

Porter, C. P., Pender, N. J., Hayman, L. L., Armstrong, M. L., Riesch, S. K., & Lewis, M. A. (1997). Educating APNs for implementing the guidelines for adolescents in bright futures: Guidelines of health supervision of infants, children, and adolescents. *Nursing Outlook, 45*(6), 252-257.

Robbins, L. B, Pender, N. J, Conn, V. S., Frenn, M. D., Neuberger, G. B., Nies, M. A., et al. (2001). Physical activity research in nursing. *Journal of Nursing Scholarship, 33*(4), 315-321.

Sechrist, K. R., Walker, S. N., & Pender, N. J. (1987). Development and psychometric evaluation of the exercise benefits/barriers scale. *Research in Nursing and Health, 10,* 357-365.

Shin, Y., Jang, H., & Pender, N. J. (2001). Psychometric evaluation of the Exercise Self-Efficacy Scale among Korean adults with chronic diseases. *Research in Nursing & Health, 24*(1), 68-76.

Walker, S. N., Kerr, M. J., Pender, N. J., & Sechrist, K. R. (1990). A Spanish language version of the health promoting lifestyle profile. *Nursing Research, 39*(5), 268-273.

Walker, S. N., Sechrist, K. R., & Pender, N. J. (1987). The health-promoting lifestyle profile: Development and psychometric characteristics. *Nursing Research, 36*(2), 76-81.

Walker, S. N., Volkan, K., Sechrist, K. R., & Pender, N. J. (1988). Health-promoting life styles of older adults: Comparisons with young and middle-aged adults, correlates and patterns. *ANS Advances in Nursing Science, 11*(1), 76-90.

Whitlock, E. P., Orleans, C. T., Pender, N., & Allan, J. (2002). Evaluating primary care behavioral counseling interventions: An evidence-based approach. *American Journal of Preventive Medicine, 22*(4), 267-284.

Wu, T. Y., & Pender, N. (2002). Determinants of physical activity among Taiwanese adolescents: An application of the health promotional model. *Research in Nursing & Health, 25*(1), 25-36.

Wu, T. Y., Pender, N., & Yang, K. P. (2002). Promoting physical activity among Taiwanese and American adolescents. *The Journal of Nursing Research: JNR, 10*(1), 57-64.

Wu, T. Y., Ronis, D. L., Pender, N., & Jwo, J. (2002). Development of questionnaires to measure physical activity cognitions among Taiwanese adolescents. *Preventive Medicine, 35*(1), 54-64.

Report

Pender, N. J., Walker, S. N., Frank-Stromberg, M., & Sechrist, K. R. (1990). *The health promotion model: Refinement and validation.* Final report to the National Center for Nursing Research, National Institutes of Health (Grant No. NR01121). DeKalb, IL: Northern Illinois University Press.

Videotapes

Pender, N. J. (1986, Oct.). *Enhancing wellness through nursing research* (Videotape). Recorded at the Nursing Conference, October 16-17, Memphis, TN. Available through University of Tennessee, Memphis, School of Nursing.

Pender, N. J. (1989, May). *Expressing health through beliefs and actions* (Videotape). Recorded live at Discovery International, Inc.'s Nurse Theorist Conference, May 11-12, Pittsburgh. Available through Meetings Internationale, Louisville, KY.

Secondary Sources
Dissertations and Theses

Al-Obeisat, S. M. (1999). Prenatal care utilization among Jordanian women (health care utilization, health promotion model). *Dissertation Abstracts International, 60-04B,* 1525.

Anthony, J. S. (1999). Mental health correlates of self-advocacy in health care decision-making among elderly African-Americans (Doctoral dissertation, George Mason University, 1999). *Dissertation Abstracts International, 59-12B,* 6259.

Bagwell, M. M. (1988). *Wellness in two developmental phases of employed adults.* Unpublished doctoral dissertation, Texas Woman's University, Houston.

Baker, O. G. (2003). Relationship of parental tobacco use, peer influence, self-esteem, and tobacco use among Yemeni American adolescents: Mid-range theory testing. *Dissertation Abstracts International, 64-03B,* 1175. (University Microfilms No. AAT3086416)

Barnett, F. C. (1989). *The relationship of selected cognitive-perceptual factors to health-promoting behaviors of adolescents.* Unpublished doctoral dissertation, University of Texas at Austin.

Beunting, J. A. (1990). *Psychosocial variables and gender as factors in wellness promotion.* Unpublished doctoral dissertation, State University of New York at Buffalo.

Bilderback, L. K. (1990). Health-promoting behaviors and perceived health status of rural families: A descriptive-correlational study. *Masters Abstracts International, 29-01,* 0089.

Bolio, S. M. (1999). Reported health-promoting behaviors of incarcerated males (prisoner health, family support). *Dissertation Abstracts International, 60-02B,* 0575.

Bond-Kinkade, M. A. (1999). The relationship of locus of control and participation in health-promoting behaviors among kidney transplant recipients. *Masters Abstracts International, 37-06,* 1815.

Bruna, A. C. (1998). Health promoting behaviors of rural Kansas women throughout the lifespan. *Masters Abstracts International, 37-01,* 234.

Burrill, E. B. (1998). Health conception, family health work and health promoting lifestyle practices in Latin American Mennonite families. *Masters Abstracts International, 37-01,* 239.

Butler, M. R. (1995). *Self-esteem and health-promoting lifestyle as predictors of health-risk behavior among older adolescents.* Unpublished doctoral dissertation, Texas Woman's University, Houston.

Carroll, S. A. (1995). The relationship of choice of infant feeding method and influencing factors among Hispanic mothers of the Permian basin. *Masters Abstracts International, 34-03,* 1147.

Carter, L. M. (1990). *Functional wellness among older adults: The interface of motivation, lifestyle, and capability.* Unpublished doctoral dissertation, Texas Woman's University, Houston.

Chandrasekhar, R. (1999). Cues to action which influence engagement in health-promoting behaviors among nursing students. *Masters Abstracts International, 37-02,* 0587.

Chen, C. (1995). *Physical exercise and sense of well-being among Chinese elderly in Taiwan.* Unpublished doctoral dissertation, University of Texas at Austin.

Cunningham, G. D. (1989). Health promoting self care behaviors in an older adult community. *Dissertation Abstracts International, 50-11B,* 4968.

Dunham, K. L. (1992). Health promoting lifestyles of nursing faculty. *Masters Abstracts International, 31-02,* 0760.

Easom, L. R. (2003). Determinants of participation in health promotion activities in rural elderly caregivers. *Dissertation Abstracts International, 64-02B,* 636. (University Microfilms No. AAT3081342)

Ellis, J. R. (1990). *Health status, health behavior, multidimensional health locus-of-control and factors in the development of personal control in individuals with rheumatoid arthritis.* Unpublished doctoral dissertation, University of Texas at Austin.

Fehir, J. S. (1988). Motivation, and selected demographics as determinants of health-promoting lifestyle behavior in men 35 to 64 years old: A nursing investigation. *Dissertation Abstracts International, 50-05B,* 1851.

Gasalberti, D. (1999). Early detection of breast cancer by self-examination: The influence of perceived barriers and health conception (cancer detection). *Dissertation Abstracts International, 60-01B,* 0129.

Gava, M. Z. (1996). *The AIDS crisis: Examining factors that influence use of condoms by young adult Zimbabwean males.* Unpublished doctoral dissertation, University of Michigan, Ann Arbor.

Gerard, M. S. (1993). *Factors related to long-term physical activity following coronary artery bypass graft surgery.* Unpublished doctoral dissertation, Rush University College of Nursing, Chicago.

Gillis, A. J. (1993). *The relationship of definition of health, perceived health status, self-efficacy, parental health-promoting lifestyle, and selected demographics to health-promoting lifestyle in adolescent females.* Unpublished doctoral dissertation, University of Texas at Austin.

Grabowski, B. J. (1997). Determinants of health promotion behavior in active duty Air Force personnel. *Masters Abstracts International, 36-01,* 0156.

Harms, J. M. (1995). Health-promoting behaviors in exercising and nonexercising seniors: A comparison. *Masters Abstracts International, 34-02,* 0719.

Harrison, R. L. (1993). *The relationship among hope, perceived health status, and health-promoting lifestyle among HIV seropositive men.* Unpublished doctoral dissertation, New York University, New York.

Hatmaker, D. D. (1993). *The effects of individual factors and health promotion during pregnancy on maternal-child health.* Unpublished doctoral dissertation, Medical College of Georgia, Augusta.

Haus, C. S. (2003). Medication management strategies used by community-dwelling older adults living alone. *Dissertation Abstracts International, 64-07B,* 3188. (University Microfilms No. AAT3097641)

Hemstron, M. M. (1993). *Relationships and differences in definition of health, perceived personal competence, perceived health status and health-promoting lifestyle profile in three elderly cohorts.* Unpublished doctoral dissertation, Rush University College of Nursing, Chicago.

Hubbard, A. B. (2002). The impact of curriculum design on health promoting behaviors at a community college in south Florida. *Dissertation Abstracts International, 63-06,* 2112.

Hubbard, D. (1987). The patterns of family interaction that promote positive child health behaviors. *Masters Abstracts International, 26-04,* 0419.

Hudak, J. W. (1988). A comparative study of the health beliefs and health-promoting behaviors of normal weight and overweight male Army personnel. *Dissertation Abstracts International, 50-06B,* 2337.

Jones, C. J. (1991). *Relationship of participation in health promotion behaviors to health-related hardiness and other selected factors in older adults.* Unpublished doctoral dissertation, Texas Woman's University, Houston.

Kalampakorn, S. (2000). Stages of constructions workers' use of hearing protection. *Dissertation Abstracts International, 61-07B,* 3508.

Kerr, M. J. (1994). Factors related to Mexican-American workers' use of hearing protection (noise). *Dissertation Abstracts International, 50-08B,* 3238.

Kurtz, A. C. (1996). *Correlates of health-promoting lifestyles among women with rheumatoid arthritis.* Unpublished doctoral dissertation, Columbia University Teachers College, New York.

Lee, N. (1987). Health knowledge and health-promoting behavior in Chinese students. *Masters Abstracts International, 27-01,* 0086.

Lewallen, L. P. (1995). *Barriers to prenatal care in low-income women.* Unpublished doctoral dissertation, University of North Carolina at Chapel Hill.

Luther, C. H. (2003). Living the coming of osteoporosis: Health promotion behaviors of women at risk for osteoporosis in Mississippi. *Dissertation Abstracts International, 64-08B,* 3746. (University Microfilms No. AAT3101544)

Martinelli, A. M. (1996). *A study of health locus of control, self-efficacy, health promotion behaviors, and environmental factors related to the self-report of the avoidance of environmental smoke in young adults.* Unpublished doctoral dissertation, Catholic University of America, Washington, DC.

McCullagh, M. C. (1999). Factors affecting hearing protector use among farmers. *Dissertation Abstracts International, 61-02B,* 780.

McKeon, F. M. (1997). Health-promoting behaviors: Predictors of early vs. late initiation to prenatal care. *Masters Abstracts International, 35-05,* 1390.

McMemamin, C. A. (2002). Parental perception concerning the use of peak flow meters in the child with asthma. *Masters Abstracts International, 41-05,* 1420.

Medcalf, P. L. (1988). Value placed on health and number of health promoting behaviors of adults. *Masters Abstracts International, 27-04,* 0492.

Merren, V. A. (1991). Determinants of health promotion in the elderly. *Masters Abstracts International, 29-04,* 0648.

Mitchell, M. L. (1993). *Effects of a self-efficacy intervention on adherence to antihypertensive regimens.* Unpublished doctoral dissertation, University of Rochester, Rochester, NY.

Moore, E. J. (1992). *The relationship among self-efficacy, health knowledge, self-rated health status, and selected demographics as determinants of health promoting behavior of older adults.* Unpublished doctoral dissertation, University of Akron, Akron, OH.

Oh, H. (1993). Health promoting behaviors and quality of life of Korean women with arthritis. *Dissertation Abstracts International, 54-08B,* 4083.

Phillips, P. S. (1993). Health promoting behaviors of adults attending a worksite health fair. *Masters Abstracts International, 32-05,* 1375.

Rothschild, S. L. (1996). *Mental health representations of attachment: Implications for health-promoting behavior and perceived stress.* Unpublished doctoral dissertation, Ohio State University, Columbus.

Rummel, C. B. (1991). *The relationship of health value and hardiness to health-promoting behavior in nurses.* Unpublished doctoral dissertation, New York University, New York.

Sakraida, T. J. (2002). Divorce transition, coping responses, and health promoting behavior of midlife women. *Dissertation Abstracts International, 62-12B,* 5646. (University Microfilms No. AAT3037817)

Sallee, A. M. (1996). The relationship of health locus of control and participation in health-promoting behaviors among older hypertensive persons. *Masters Abstracts International, 34-18,* 2349.

Sapp, C. J. (2003). Adolescents with asthma: Effects of personal characteristics and health-promoting lifestyle behaviors on health-related quality of life. *Dissertation Abstracts International, 64-05B,* 2131. (University Microfilms No. AAT3092071)

Smith Hendricks, C. K. (1992). *Perceptual determinants of early adolescent health promoting behaviors in one Alabama black belt country.* Unpublished doctoral dissertation, Boston College, Boston.

Stone, S. A. (1990). The relationship between self-esteem and health promoting behaviors in working women. *Masters Abstracts International, 30-04,* 1326.

Stutts, W. C. (1997). *Use of the health promotion model to predict physical activity in adults.* Unpublished doctoral dissertation, University of North Carolina at Chapel Hill.

Suwonnaroop, N. (1999). Health-promoting behaviors in older adults: The effect of social support, perceived health status, and personal factors. *Dissertation Abstracts International, 60-08B,* 3854.

Tapler, D. A. (1996). *The relationship between health value, self-efficacy, health barriers, and health behavior practices in mothers.* Unpublished doctoral dissertation, Texas Woman's University, Houston.

Tashiro, J. (1996). Health promoting lifestyle behaviors of college women in Japan: An exploratory study. *Dissertation Abstracts International, 57-04B,* 2486.

Thompson, E. M. (1995). *A descriptive study of women who successfully quit smoking.* Unpublished doctoral dissertation, Georgia State University, Atlanta.

Turner, S. J. (1989). Health protective behavior and the elderly: Hemoccult testing for early colorectal cancer detection. *Masters Abstracts International, 28-02,* 0277.

Vines, W. R. (1991). *Psychological stress reaction, coping strategies, and health promotion lifestyles among hospital nurses.* Unpublished doctoral dissertation, University of Alabama at Birmingham.

Warner, K. D. (2000). Health-related lifestyle behaviors of twins: Interpersonal and situational influences. *Dissertation Abstracts International, 61-03B,* 1331.

Warren, M. T. (1993). *The relationships of self-motivation and perceived personal competence to engaging in a health-promoting lifestyle for men in cardiac rehabilitation programs.* Unpublished doctoral dissertation, New York University, New York.

White, D. A. (1994). The relationship of intrinsic motivation and health beliefs on positive health behavior in pregnant adolescents. *Masters Abstracts International, 34-02*, 0730.

White, J. L. (1996). *Outcomes of an individualized health promotion program for homebound older community residents.* Unpublished doctoral dissertation, Texas Woman's University, Houston.

Willis, J. L. (2001). The effect of multiple roles in the health promotion activities of college women. *Masters Abstracts International, 39-05*, 1382.

Wilson, A. H. (1991). Health promoting behaviors among married and unmarried mothers. *Dissertation Abstracts International, 52-06B*, 2999.

Wisnewski, C. A. (1996). *A study of the health-promoting behavioral effects of an exercise educational intervention in adult diabetics.* Unpublished doctoral dissertation, Texas Woman's University, Houston.

Yue, S. P. (1998). Assessing the needs of the post-cardiac event population in a rural southeastern New Mexico community. *Masters Abstracts International, 36-06*, 1594.

Yuhos, J. L. (1997). Health patterns of nurses who smoke. *Masters Abstracts International, 36-01*, 0166.

Journal Articles

Agazio, J. G., Ephraim, P. M., Flaherty, N. B., & Gurney, C. A. (2002). Health promotion in active-duty military women with children. *Women & Health, 35*(1), 65-82.

Bonin, J. (1999). Psychosocial determinants for lithium compliance in bipolar disorder [French]. *Canadian Journal of Nursing Research, 31*(2), 25-40.

Burns, C. M. (1998). A retrospective theoretical model of the pathway to chemical dependency in nurses. *Archives of Psychiatric Nursing, 12*(1), 59-65.

Campbell, J., & Kreidler, M. (1994). Older adults' perceptions about wellness. *Journal of Holistic Nursing, 12*(4), 437-447.

Capik, L. K. (1998). The health promotion model applied to family-centered perinatal education. *Journal of Perinatal Education, 7*(1), 9-17.

Clement, M., Bouchard, L., Jankowski, L. W., & Perreault, M. (1995). Health promotion behaviors in first-year undergraduate nursing students: A pilot study [French]. *Canadian Journal of Nursing Research, 27*(4), 111-131.

Coppens, M. N., & McCabe, B. M. (1995). Promoting children's use of bicycle helmets. *Journal of Pediatric Health Care, 9*(2), 51-58.

Duffy, M. E. (1988). Determinants of health promotion in midlife women. *Nursing Research, 37*(6), 358-362.

Duffy, M. E. (1988). Health promotion in the family: Current findings and directives for nursing research. *Journal of Advanced Nursing, 13*(1), 109-117.

Duffy, M. E. (1989). Determinants of health status in employed women. *Health Values: Achieving High Level Wellness, 13*(2), 50-57.

Duffy, M. E. (1993). Determinants of health-promoting lifestyles of older persons. *Image: The Journal of Nursing Scholarship, 25*(1), 23-28.

Duffy, M. E. (1997). Determinants of reported health promotion behaviors in employed Mexican American women. *Health Care for Women International, 18*(2), 149-163.

Felton, G. M. (1996). Female adolescent contraceptive use or nonuse at first and most recent coitus. *Public Health Nursing, 13*(3), 223-230.

Flowers, J. S., & McLean, J. E. (1996). Psychometric studies of the Flowers midlife questionnaire (FMHQ) for women. *Journal of Nursing Science, 1*(3/4), 115-126.

Foster, M. F. (1992). Health promotion and life satisfaction in elderly Black adults . . . including commentary by Hess, P., Foxall, M. J., Roberson, M. H. B., and author response. *Western Journal of Nursing Research, 14*(4), 444-463.

Gillis, A. J. (1993). Determinants of a health-promoting lifestyle: An integrative review. *Journal of Advanced Nursing, 18*(3), 345-353.

Gillis, A. J. (1994). Determinants of health-promoting lifestyles in adolescent females. *Canadian Journal of Nursing Research, 26*(2), 13-28.

Gillis, A., & Perry, A. (1991). The relationships between physical activity and health-promoting behaviours in mid-life women. *Journal of Advanced Nursing, 16*(3), 299-310.

Haddad, L. G, Al-Ma'aitah, R. M., Cameron, S. J., & Armstrong-Stassen, M. (1998). An Arabic language version of the health promotion lifestyle profile. *Public Health Nursing, 15*(2), 74-81.

Harrison, L. L. (1990). A health promotion model for wellness education. *American Journal of Maternal/Child Nursing, 15*(3), 191.

Hui, W. H. (2002). The health-promoting lifestyles of undergraduate nurses in Hong Kong. *Journal of Professional Nursing, 18*(2), 101-111.

Jackson, C. P. (1995). The association between childbirth education, infant birthweight, and health promotion behaviors. *Journal of Perinatal Education, 4*(1), 27-33.

Johnson, J. L., Ratner, P. A., Botteroff, J. L., & Hayduk, L. A. (1993). An exploration of Pender's health promotion model using LISREL. *Nursing Research, 42*(3), 132-138.

Jones, M., & Nies, M. A. (1996). The relationship of perceived benefits of and barriers to reported exercise in older African American women. *Public Health Nursing, 13*(2), 151-158.

Kerr, M. J., Lusk, S. L., & Ronis, D. L. (2002). Explaining Mexican American workers' hearing protection use with the health promotion model. *Nursing Research, 51*(2), 100-109.

Lannon, S. L. (1997). Using a health promotion model to enhance medication compliance. *Journal of Neuroscience Nursing, 29*(3), 170-178.

Lohse, J. L. (2003). A bicycle safety education program for parents of young children. *Journal of School Nursing, 19*(2), 100-110.

Lookinland, S., & Harms, J. (1996). Comparison of health-promotive behaviours among seniors: Exercisers versus nonexercisers. *Social Sciences in Health: International Journal of Research and Practice, 2*(3), 147-161.

Lucas, J. A., Orshan, S. A., & Cook, F. (2000). Determinants of health-promoting behavior among women ages 65 and above living in the community. *Scholarly Inquiry for Nursing Practice, 14*(1), 77-100.

Lusk, S. L., Hong, O. S., Ronis, S. L., Eakin, B. L., Kerr, M. J., & Early, M. R. (1999). Effectiveness of an intervention to increase construction worker's use of hearing protection. *Human Factors, 41*(3), 487-494.

Lusk, S. L., & Kelemen, M. J. (1993). Predicting use of hearing protection: A preliminary study. *Public Health Nursing, 10*(3), 189-196.

Lusk, S. L., Kwee, M. J., Ronis, D. L., & Eakin, B. L. (1999). Applying the health promotion model to development of a worksite intervention. *American Journal of Health Promotion, 13*(4), 219-226.

Lusk, S. L., Ronis, D. L., & Baer, L. M. (1997). Gender differences in blue collar worker's use of hearing protection. *Women and Health, 25*(4), 69-89.

Lusk, S. L., Ronis, D. L., & Hogan, M. M. (1997). Test of the health promotion model as a causal model of construction worker's use of hearing protection. *Research in Nursing and Health, 20*(3), 183-194.

Lusk, S. L., Ronis, D. L., Kerr, M. J., & Atwood, J. R. (1994). Test of the health promotion model as a causal model of worker's use of hearing protection. *Nursing Research, 43*(3), 151-157.

MacDonald, M. B., Laing, G. B., & Faulkner, R. A. (1994). The relationship of health-promoting behaviour to health locus of control: Analysis of one baccalaureate nursing class. *Canadian Journal of Cardiovascular Nursing, 5*(2), 11-18.

Martinelli, A. M. (1999). An explanatory model of variables influencing health promotion behaviors in smoking and nonsmoking college students. *Public Health Nursing, 16*(4), 263-269.

McCabe, B. W., Walker, S. N., & Clark, K. A. (1997). Health promotion in long term care facilities. *Journal of Nursing Science, 2*(1-6), 153-167.

McCleary-Jones, V. (1996). Health promotion practices of smoking and non-smoking black women. *Association of Black Nursing Faculty Journal, 7*(1), 7-10.

McCullagh, M., Lusk, S. L., & Ronis, D. L. (2002). Factors influencing use of hearing protection among farmers: A test of the Pender health promotion model. *Nursing Research, 51*(1),33-39.

Montgomery, K. S. (2002). Health promotion with adolescents: Examining theoretical perspectives to guide research. *Research & Theory for Nursing Practice, 16*(2), 119-134.

Moylan, J. P. (1993). The achievement of dietary goals in patients with documented CAD: A test of Nola Pender's health promotion model. *Nursing Scan in Research, 6*(6), 3-4.

Neuberger, G. B., Kasal, S., Smith, K. V., Hassanein, R., & DeViney, S. (1994). Determinants of exercise and aerobic fitness in outpatients with arthritis. *Nursing Research, 43*(1), 11-17.

O'Quinn, J. L. (1995). Worksite wellness programs and lifestyle behaviors. *Journal of Holistic Nursing, 13*(4), 346-360.

Padula, C. A. (1997). Predictors of participation in health promotion activities by elderly couples. *Journal of Family Nursing, 3*(1), 88-106.

Palank, C. L. (1991). Determinants of health-promotive behavior: A review of current research. *Nursing Clinics of North America, 26*(4), 815-832.

Piazza, J., Conrad, K., & Wilbur, J. (2001). Exercise behavior among female occupational health nurses. Influence of self efficacy, perceived health control, and age. *AAOHN Journal, 49*(2),79-86.

Ratner, P. A., Bottorff, J. L., Johnson, J. L., & Hayduk, L. A. (1994). The interaction effects of gender within the health promotion model. *Research in Nursing and Health, 17*(5), 341-350.

Ratner, P. A., Bottorff, J. L., Johnson, J. L., & Hayduk, L. A. (1996). Using multiple indicators to test the dimensionality of concepts in the health promotion model. *Research in Nursing and Health, 19*(3), 237-247.

Riffle, K. L., Yoho, J., & Sams, J. (1989). Health-promoting behaviors, perceived social support, and self-reported health of Appalachian elderly. *Public Health Nursing, 6*(4), 204-211.

Sisk, R. J. (2000). Caregiver burden and health promotion. *International Journal of Nursing Studies, 37*(1), 37-43.

Speake, D. L., Cowart, M. E., & Pellet, K. (1989). Health perceptions and lifestyles of the elderly. *Research in Nursing and Health, 12*(2), 93-100.

Speake, D. L., Cowart, M. E., & Stephens, R. (1991). Healthy lifestyle practices of rural and urban elderly. *Health Values: Achieving High Level Wellness, 15*(1), 45-51.

Stegbauer, C. C. (1995). Smoking cessation in women: Findings from qualitative research. *Nurse Practitioner: American Journal of Primary Health Care, 20*(11), 80, 83-86.

Stuifbergen, A. K., & Becker, H. A. (1994). Predictors of health-promoting lifestyles in persons with disabilities. *Research in Nursing and Health, 17*(1), 3-13.

Telleen, T. M. (1993). Health promotion practices of pregnant and nonpregnant women. *Journal of Holistic Nursing, 11*(3), 237-245.

Volden, C., Langemo, D., Adamson, M., & Oechsle, L. (1990). The relationship of age, gender, and exercise practices to measures of health, lifestyle, and self-esteem. *Applied Nursing Research, 3*(1), 20-26.

Wang, H. H. (1999). Predictors of health promotion lifestyle among three ethnic groups of elderly rural women in Taiwan. *Public Health Nursing, 16*(5), 321-328.

Wang, H. H. (2001). A comparison of two models of health-promoting lifestyle in rural elderly Taiwanese women. *Public Health Nursing, 18*(3), 204-211.

Weitzel, M. H. (1989). A test of the health promotion model with blue collar workers. *Nursing Research, 38*(2), 99-104.

Web Site

Nola J. Pender University of Michigan faculty profile. Accessed December 20, 2004: *http://www.nursing.umich.edu/faculty/pender_nola.html*

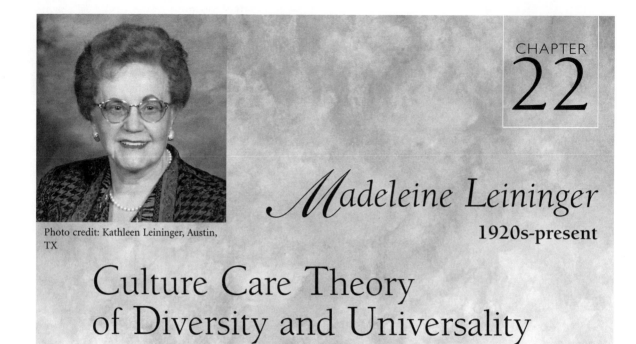

Photo credit: Kathleen Leininger, Austin, TX

CHAPTER

22

*M*adeleine Leininger
1920s-present

Culture Care Theory of Diversity and Universality

Marilyn McFarland

CREDENTIALS AND BACKGROUND OF THE THEORIST

Madeleine M. Leininger is the founder of transcultural nursing and a leader in transcultural nursing and human care theory. She is the first professional nurse with graduate preparation in nursing to hold a Ph.D. in cultural and social anthropology. She was born in Sutton, Nebraska, and began her nursing career after graduating from the diploma program at St. Anthony's School of Nursing in Denver, Colorado. She was in the U.S. Army Nurse Corps while pursuing the basic nursing program. In 1950, she obtained a bachelor's degree in biological science from Benedictine College in Atchison, Kansas, with a minor in philosophy and humanistic studies. After graduation, she served as an instructor, staff nurse, and head nurse on a medical-surgical

unit and opened a new psychiatric unit while director of the nursing service at St. Joseph's Hospital in Omaha, Nebraska. During this time, she pursued advanced study in nursing, nursing administration, teaching and curriculum in nursing, and tests and measurements at Creighton University in Omaha (Leininger, 1995c, 1996b).

In 1954, Leininger obtained a master's degree in psychiatric nursing from Catholic University of America in Washington, D.C. She was then employed at the College of Health at the University of Cincinnati, Ohio, where she began the first master's level–clinical specialist program in child psychiatric nursing in the world. She also initiated and directed the first graduate nursing program in psychiatric nursing at the University of Cincinnati and the Therapeutic Psychiatric Nursing Center at the University Hospital. During this time, she wrote one of the first basic psychiatric nursing texts with Hofling entitled *Basic Psychiatric Concepts in Nursing*, which was published in 1960 in 11 languages and used worldwide (Hofling & Leininger, 1960).

While working at a child guidance home in the mid-1950s in Cincinnati, Leininger discovered the staff lacked understanding of cultural factors influencing the behavior of children. Among these children of diverse cultural backgrounds, she observed differences in the care and psychiatric treatments that deeply concerned her. Psychoanalytical theories and therapy strategies did not seem to reach children who were of different cultural backgrounds and needs. She became increasingly concerned that her nursing decisions and actions, and those of other staff, did not appear to help these children adequately. Leininger posed many questions to herself and the staff about cultural differences among children and therapy outcomes. She found few staff members who were interested or knowledgeable about cultural factors in the diagnosis and treatment of clients. A short time later, Margaret Mead became a visiting professor in the Department of Psychiatry, University of Cincinnati, and Leininger discussed the potential interrelationships between nursing and anthropology with Mead. Although she did not get any direct help, encouragement, or solutions from Mead, Leininger decided to pursue her interests with doctoral focus on cultural, social, and psychological anthropology at the University of Washington, Seattle.

As a doctoral student, Leininger studied many cultures. She found anthropology fascinating and believed it was an area that should be of interest to all nurses. She focused on the Gadsup people of the Eastern Highlands of New Guinea, where she lived alone with the indigenous people for nearly 2 years and undertook an ethnographical and ethnonursing study of two villages (Leininger, 1995c, 1996b). Not only was she able to observe unique features of the culture, she also observed a number of marked differences between Western and non-Western cultures related to caring health and well-being practices. From her in-depth study and first-hand experiences with the Gadsup, she continued to develop her Theory of Culture Care and the ethnonursing

method (Leininger, 1978, 1981, 1991b, 1995c). Her research and theory have helped nursing students understand cultural differences in human care, health, and illness. She has been the major nurse leader to encourage many students and faculty to pursue graduate education and practice. Her enthusiasm and deep interests in developing this field of transcultural nursing with a human care focus has sustained her for more than 5 decades.

During the 1950s and 1960s, Leininger (1970, 1978) identified several common areas of knowledge and theoretical research interests between nursing and anthropology, formulating transcultural nursing concepts, theory, principles, and practices. The book *Nursing and Anthropology: Two Worlds to Blend* (1970) laid the foundation for developing the field of transcultural nursing, the Theory of Culture Care, and culturally based health care. Her next book, *Transcultural Nursing: Concepts, Theories, and Practice* (1978), identified major concepts, theoretical ideas, and practices in transcultural nursing and was the first definitive publication on transcultural nursing. During the past 50 years, Leininger has established, explicated, and used the Theory of Culture Care to study many cultures within the United States and worldwide. She developed the ethnonursing qualitative research method to fit the theory and to discover the insider or emic view of cultures (Leininger, 1991b, 1995c). The ethnonursing research method was the first nursing research method developed for nurses to examine complex care and cultural phenomena. During the past 5 decades, approximately 50 nurses with doctoral degrees and many master's and baccalaureate students have been prepared in transcultural nursing and have used Leininger's Theory of Culture Care (Leininger, 1990a, 1991b; Leininger & McFarland, 2002a; Leininger & Watson, 1990).

The first course offered in transcultural nursing was in 1966 at the University of Colorado, where Leininger was a professor of nursing and anthropology. This marked the first joint appointment in the United States of a professor of nursing with another discipline. Leininger also initiated and served as the director of the first nurse scientist program (Ph.D.) in the United States. In 1969 she was appointed Dean and Professor of Nursing and Lecturer in Anthropology at the University of Washington, Seattle. There she established the first academic nursing department on comparative nursing care systems to support master's and doctoral programs in transcultural nursing. Under her leadership, the Research Facilitation Office was established in 1968 and 1969. She initiated several transcultural nursing courses and guided the first nurses in a special Ph.D. program in transcultural nursing. She initiated the Committee on Nursing and Anthropology with the American Anthropological Association in 1968.

In 1974, Leininger was appointed Dean and Professor of Nursing at the College of Nursing and Adjunct Professor of Anthropology at the University of Utah in Salt Lake City. At this institution, she initiated the first master's and doctoral programs in transcultural nursing and established the first doctoral program offerings at this institution (Leininger, 1978). These programs were the first with substantive courses in the world focused specifically on transcultural nursing.

She also initiated and was director of a new research facilitation office at the University of Utah.

In 1981, Leininger was recruited to Wayne State University in Detroit, where she was Professor of Nursing and Adjunct Professor of Anthropology and Director of Transcultural Nursing Offerings until her semi-retirement in 1995. She was also Director of the Center for Health Research at this university for 5 years. While at Wayne State, she again developed several courses and seminars in transcultural nursing, caring, and qualitative research methods for baccalaureate, master's, doctoral, and postdoctoral nursing and nonnursing students. In addition to directing the transcultural course offerings at Wayne State University, Dr. Leininger taught and mentored many students and nurses in field research in transcultural nursing. One of the first nurse leaders to use qualitative research methods during the early 1960s, she has continued to teach these methods at various universities within the United States and worldwide. To date, she has studied 14 cultures and continues to consult for many research projects and institutions, especially those that are using her Theory of Culture Care.

With the growing interest in transcultural nursing and health care, Leininger (personal communication, 1996) has delivered keynote addresses annually and conducted workshops and conferences both nationally and internationally since 1965. Her academic vitae records nearly 600 conferences, keynote addresses, workshops, and consultant services in the United States, Canada, Europe, Pacific island nations, Asia, Africa, Australia, and the Nordic countries. Educational and service organizations continue to request her consultation on transcultural nursing, humanistic caring, ethnonursing research, the Theory of Culture Care, and futuristic trends in health care worldwide.

As the first professional nurse to complete a doctoral degree in anthropology and to initiate several master's and doctoral nursing educational programs, Leininger has many areas of expertise and interests. She has studied 14 major cultures in depth and has had experience with many other diverse cultures. In addition to transcultural nursing with care as a central focus, her areas of interest are comparative education and administration, nursing theories, politics, ethical dilemmas of nursing and health care, qualitative research methods, the future of nursing and health care, and nursing leadership. Her Theory of Culture Care is now used worldwide and is growing in relevance and importance in the discovery of data from diverse cultures.

In 1974, Leininger initiated the National Transcultural Nursing Society and has been an active leader since its inception. She also established the National Research Care Conference in 1978 to help nurses focus on the study of human care phenomena (Leininger, 1981, 1984a, 1988a, 1990a, 1991b; Leininger & Watson, 1990). She initiated the *Journal of Transcultural Nursing* in 1989 and served as its editor through 1995.

Dr. Leininger has gained international recognition in nursing and related fields through her transcultural nursing and care writings, theory, research, consultation, courses, and dynamic addresses. She has worked enthusiastically to persuade nursing educators and practitioners to incorporate transcultural nursing and culture-specific care concepts based upon research findings into nursing curricula and clinical practices as the new and futuristic direction of all aspects of nursing (Leininger, 1991b, 1995c; Leininger & McFarland, 2002a; Leininger & Watson, 1990). She has found time to give lectures to anthropologists, physicians, social workers, pharmacists, and educators, and to do research with colleagues. She is one of the few nurses who has kept active in two disciplines and has continued to contribute to both nursing and anthropology in national and international transcultural conferences and association meetings. Currently, Dr. Leininger resides in Omaha, Nebraska, and is semi-retired but still active in consulting, writing, and lecturing. Her present interest is to establish transcultural nursing institutes to educate and to conduct and facilitate research on transcultural nursing and health phenomena.

Leininger has written or edited more than 27 books. Some of her books include *Nursing and Anthropology: Two Worlds to Blend* (1970), *Transcultural Nursing: Concepts, Theories, Research, and Practice* (1978; Leininger & McFarland, 2002a), *Caring: An Essential Human Need* (Leininger, 1981), *Care: The Essence of Nursing and Health* (1984a), *Qualitative Research Methods in Nursing* (1985a), *Ethical and Moral Dimensions of Care: Chapters from Conference on the Ethics and Morality of Caring* (1990a), *The Caring Imperative in Education* (Leininger & Watson, 1990), and *Culture Care Diversity and Universality: A Theory of Nursing* (1991b; Leininger & McFarland, 2005), which is a full account of her theory with the method. She has published more than 200 articles and 45 book chapters plus numerous films, videos, and research reports focused on transcultural nursing, human care and health phenomena, the future of nursing, and related topics relevant in nursing and anthropology. She serves on eight editorial boards and several refereed publications. She is known as one of the most creative, productive, innovative, and futuristic authors in nursing, always providing new and substantive research-based transcultural nursing content and ideas to advance nursing as a discipline and profession.

Leininger has received many awards and honors for her lifetime professional and academic accomplishments. She is in *Who's Who of American Women, Who's Who in Health Care, Who's Who in Community Leaders, Who's Who of Women in Education, International Who's Who in Community Service, Who's Who in International Women,* and other such listings. Her name appears on the *National Register of Prominent Americans and International Notables, International Women,* and the *National Register of Prominent Community Leaders.* She has received several honorary degrees, such as an L.H.D. from Benedictine College in Atchison, Kansas, a Ph.D. from the University of Kuopio, Finland, and a D.S. from the University of Indiana, Indianapolis. In 1976 and 1995, she was recognized for her unique and significant contribution to the American Association of Colleges of Nursing as its first full-time president. Leininger received the Russell Sage Outstanding Leadership Award in 1995. Leininger is a fellow in the American Academy of Nursing, a fellow of the American Anthropology Society, and a fellow of the Society for Applied Anthropology. Other affiliations include Sigma Theta Tau, the national honor society for nursing; Delta Kappa Gamma, the national honor society in education; and the Scandinavian College of Caring Science in Stockholm, Sweden. She has served as a distinguished visiting scholar and lecturer at 85 universities in the United States and worldwide and has been a visiting professor at numerous foreign universities, including schools in Sweden, Wales, Japan, China, Australia, Finland, New Zealand, and the Philippines. While at Wayne State University, she received the Board of Regents' Distinguished Faculty Award, Distinguished Research Award, the President's Excellence in Teaching, and the Outstanding Graduate Faculty Mentor Award. In 1996, Madonna University, Livonia, Michigan honored her with the dedication of the Leininger Book Collection and a special Leininger Reading Room for her outstanding contributions to nursing and the social sciences and humanities.

THEORETICAL SOURCES

Leininger's theory is derived from the disciplines of anthropology and nursing (Leininger, 1991b, 1995c;

Leininger & McFarland 2002b, 2005). She has defined transcultural nursing as a major area of nursing that focuses on the comparative study and analysis of diverse cultures and subcultures in the world with respect to their caring values, expressions, and health-illness beliefs and patterns of behavior.

The purpose of the theory was to discover human care diversities and universalities in relation to worldview, social structure, and other dimensions cited, and then to discover ways to provide culturally congruent care to people of different or similar cultures in order to maintain or regain their well-being, health, or face death in a culturally appropriate way (Leininger, 1985b, 1988b, 1988c, 1988d; as cited in 1991b).

The goal of the theory is to improve and to provide culturally congruent care to people that is beneficial, will fit with, and will be useful to the client, family, or culture group healthy lifeways (Leininger, 1991b).

Transcultural nursing goes beyond an awareness state to that of using culture care nursing knowledge to practice culturally congruent and responsible care (Leininger, 1991b, 1995c). Leininger has stated that in time, there will be a new kind of nursing practice that reflects different nursing practices that are culturally defined, grounded, and specific to guide nursing care to individuals, families, groups, and institutions. She contends that because culture and care knowledge are the broadest and most holistic means to conceptualize and understand people, they are central to and imperative to nursing education and practice (Leininger, 1991b, 1995c; Leininger & McFarland, 2002a, 2005). In addition, she states that transcultural nursing has become one of the most important, relevant, and highly promising areas of formal study, research, and practice because people live in a multicultural world (Leininger, 1984a, 1988a, 1995c; Leininger & McFarland, 2002a, 2005). Leininger predicts that for nursing to be meaningful and relevant to clients and other nurses in the world, transcultural nursing knowledge and competencies will be imperative to guide all nursing decisions and actions for effective and successful outcomes (Leininger, 1991b, 1995c, 1996a, 1996b; Leininger & McFarland, 2002a, 2005).

Leininger (2002a) makes a distinction between transcultural nursing and cross-cultural nursing. The former refers to nurses prepared in transcultural nursing who are prepared and committed to develop knowledge and practice in transcultural nursing, whereas cross-cultural nursing refers to nurses using applied or medical anthropological concepts, with many nurses not committed to developing transcultural nursing theory and research-based practices (Leininger, 1995c; Leininger & McFarland, 2002a). She also identifies that international nursing and transcultural nursing are different. International nursing focuses on nurses functioning between two cultures; however, transcultural nursing focuses on several cultures with a comparative theoretical and practice base (Leininger, 1995c; Leininger & McFarland, 2002a).

Leininger describes the transcultural nurse generalist as a nurse prepared at the baccalaureate level who is able to apply transcultural nursing concepts, principles, and practices that are generated by transcultural nurse specialists (Leininger, 1989a, 1989b, 1991c, 1995c; Leininger & McFarland, 2002a). The transcultural nurse specialist prepared in graduate programs receives in-depth preparation and mentorship in transcultural nursing knowledge and practice. This specialist has acquired competency skills through postbaccalaureate education. "This specialist has studied selected cultures in sufficient depth (values, beliefs, and lifeways) and is highly knowledgeable and theoretically based about care, health, and environmental factors related to transcultural nursing perspectives" (Leininger, 1984b, p. 252). The transcultural nurse specialist serves as an expert field practitioner, teacher, researcher, and consultant with respect to select cultures. This individual also values and uses nursing theory to develop and advance knowledge within the discipline of transcultural nursing, the field Leininger (1995c, 2001) predicts must be the focus of all nursing education and practice.

Leininger (1996b) holds and promotes a new and different theory from traditional theories in nursing, which usually define theory as a set of logically interrelated concepts and hypothetical propositions that can be tested for the purpose of explaining or predicting an event, phenomenon, or situation. Instead, Leininger defines theory as the systematic and creative discovery of knowledge about a domain of interest or a phenomenon that appears important to understand or to account for some unknown phenomenon. She believes that nursing theory must take into account the creative discovery about individuals, families, and groups, and their caring, values, expressions, beliefs, and actions or practices based on their cultural lifeways to provide effective, satisfying, and culturally congruent care. If nursing practices fail to recognize the cultural aspects of human needs, there will be signs of less beneficial or efficacious nursing care practices and even evidence of dissatisfaction with nursing services, which limits healing and well-being (Leininger, 1991b, 1995a, 1995c; Leininger & McFarland, 2002a, 2005).

Leininger (1991b) developed her Theory of Culture Care Diversity and Universality, which is based on the belief that people of different cultures can inform and are capable of guiding professionals to receive the kind of care they desire or need from others. Culture is the patterned and valued lifeways of people that influence their decisions and actions; therefore, the theory is directed toward nurses to discover and document the world of the client and to use their emic viewpoints, knowledge, and practices with appropriate etic (professional knowledge), as bases for making culturally congruent professional care actions and decisions (Leininger, 1991b, 1995c). Indeed, culture care is the broadest holistic nursing theory, because it takes into account the totality and holistic perspective of human life and existence over time, including the social structure factors, worldview, cultural history and values, environmental context (Leininger, 1981), language expressions, and folk (generic) and professional patterns. These are some of the critical and essential bases for the discovery of grounded care knowledge that as the essence of nursing that can lead to the health and well-being of clients and guide therapeutic nursing practice. The Theory of Culture Care can be inductive and deductive, derived from emic (insider) and etic (outsider) knowledge. However,

Leininger encourages obtaining grounded emic knowledge from the people or culture because such knowledge is most credible (1991b).

The theory is neither middle range nor macro theory but must be viewed holistically with specific domains of interest. Leininger believes the terms *middle* range and *macro* are outdated in theory development and usage (1991b, 1995c; Leininger & McFarland, 2002a, 2005).

Unique Features of the Theory

According to Leininger (2002c), the Theory of Culture Care Diversity and Universality has several distinct features, different from those of other nursing theories. It is the only theory that is focused explicitly on discovering holistic and comprehensive culture care, and it is a theory that can be used in Western and non-Western cultures because of the inclusion of multiple holistic factors universally found in cultures. It is the only theory focused on discovering comprehensive factors influencing human care such as worldview, social structure factors, language, generic and professional care, ethnohistory, and the environmental context. The theory has both abstract and practice dimensions that can be examined systematically to arrive at culturally congruent care outcomes. It is the only theory in nursing explicitly focused on culture and care of diverse cultures, with three theoretical practice modalities to arrive at culturally congruent care decisions and actions to support well-being, health, and satisfactory lifeways for people. The theory is designed to ultimately discover care—what is diverse and what is universal related to care and health—and has a comparative focus to identify different or contrasting transcultural nursing care practices with specific care constructs. The theory with the ethnonursing method (the first nursing research method designed to fit a theory) has enablers designed to tease out in-depth informant emic data, and these enablers can also be used for cultural health care assessments. The theory can generate new knowledge in nursing and health care to arrive at culturally congruent, safe, and responsible care.

MAJOR CONCEPTS & DEFINITIONS

Leininger has developed many terms relevant to the theory. The major ones are defined here. The reader can study her full theory from her definitive works (Leininger, 1991b, 1995c; Leininger & McFarland, 2002a, 2005).

HUMAN CARE AND CARING

The concept of human care and caring refers to the abstract and manifest phenomena with expressions of assistive, supportive, enabling, and facilitating ways to help self or others with evident or anticipated needs to improve health, a human condition, or a lifeway, or to face disabilities or dying.

CULTURE

Culture refers to patterned lifeways, values, beliefs, norms, symbols, and practices of individuals, groups, or institutions that are learned, shared, and usually transmitted from one generation to another.

CULTURE CARE

Culture care refers to the synthesized and culturally constituted assistive, supportive, enabling, or facilitative caring acts toward self or others focused on evident or anticipated needs for the client's health or well-being, or to face disabilities, death, or other human conditions.

CULTURE CARE DIVERSITY

Culture care diversity refers to cultural variability or differences in care beliefs, meanings, patterns, values, symbols, and lifeways within and between cultures and human beings.

CULTURE CARE UNIVERSALITY

Culture care universality refers to commonalities or similar culturally based care meanings ("truths"), patterns, values, symbols, and lifeways reflecting care as a universal humanity.

WORLDVIEW

Worldview refers to the way an individual or group looks out on and understands the world about them as a value, stance, picture, or perspective about life and the world.

CULTURAL AND SOCIAL STRUCTURE DIMENSIONS

Cultural and social structure dimensions refer to the dynamic, holistic, and interrelated patterns of structured features of a culture (or subculture), including religion (or spirituality), kinship (social), political characteristics (legal), economics, education, technology, cultural values, philosophy, history, and language.

ENVIRONMENTAL CONTEXT

Environmental context refers to the totality of an environment (physical, geographic, and sociocultural), situation, or event with related experiences that give interpretative meanings to guide human expressions and decisions with reference to a particular environment or situation.

ETHNOHISTORY

Ethnohistory refers to the sequence of facts, events, or developments over time as known, witnessed, or documented about a designated people of a culture.

EMIC

Emic refers to the local, indigenous, or insider's views and values about a phenomenon.

ETIC

Etic refers to the outsider's or more universal views and values about a phenomenon.

MAJOR CONCEPTS *&* DEFINITIONS—cont'd

HEALTH

Health refers to a state of well-being or restorative state that is culturally constituted, defined, valued, and practiced by individuals or groups that enables them to function in their daily lives.

TRANSCULTURAL NURSING

Transcultural nursing refers to a formal area of humanistic and scientific knowledge and practices focused on holistic culture care (caring) phenomena and competencies to assist individuals or groups to maintain or regain their health (or well-being) and to deal with disabilities, dying, or other human conditions in culturally congruent and beneficial ways.

CULTURE CARE PRESERVATION OR MAINTENANCE

Culture care preservation or maintenance refers to those assistive, supportive, facilitative, or enabling professional actions and decisions that help people of a particular culture to retain or maintain meaningful care values and lifeways for their well-being, to recover from illness, or to deal with handicaps or dying.

CULTURE CARE ACCOMMODATION OR NEGOTIATION

Culture care accommodation or negotiation refers to those assistive, supportive, facilitative, or enabling professional actions and decisions that help people of a designated culture (or subculture) to adapt to or to negotiate with others for meaningful, beneficial, and congruent health outcomes.

CULTURE CARE REPATTERNING OR RESTRUCTURING

Culture care repatterning or restructuring refers to the assistive, supportive facilitative, or enabling professional actions and decisions that help clients reorder, change, or modify their lifeways for new, different, and beneficial health outcomes.

CULTURALLY COMPETENT NURSING CARE

Culturally competent nursing care refers to the explicit use of culturally based care and health knowledge in sensitive, creative, and meaningful ways to fit the general lifeways and needs of individuals or groups for beneficial and meaningful health and well-being or to face illness, disabilities, or death.

USE OF EMPIRICAL EVIDENCE

For more than 5 decades, Leininger has held that care is the essence of nursing and the dominant, distinctive, and unifying feature of nursing (1970, 1981, 1988a, 1991b; Leininger & McFarland, 2002a, 2005). She states that care is complex, elusive, and often embedded in social structure and other aspects of culture (1991b; Leininger & McFarland, 2005). She holds that different forms, expressions, and patterns of care are diverse, and some are universal (Leininger, 1991b; Leininger & McFarland, 2002a, 2005). Leininger (1985a, 1990b) favors qualitative ethnomethods, especially ethnonursing, to study care. These methods are directed toward discovering the people-truths, views, beliefs, and patterned lifeways of people. During the 1960s, Leininger developed the ethnonursing method to study transcultural nursing phenomena specifically and systematically. The method focuses on the classification of care beliefs, values, and practices as cognitively or subjectively known by a designated culture (or cultural representatives) through their local emic people-centered language, experiences, beliefs, and value systems about actual or potential nursing phenomena such as care, health, and environmental factors (Leininger, 1991b, 1995c; Leininger & McFarland, 2002a, 2005). Although nursing has used the words *care* and *caring* for more than a century, the definitions and usage have been vague and used as clichés, without specific meanings to the culture of the client or nurse (Leininger, 1981, 1984a). "Indeed, the concepts about caring have been some of the least understood and studied of all human knowledge and research areas within and outside of nursing" (Leininger, 1978, p. 33). With the transcultural care theory and ethnonursing method based on emic (insider views) beliefs, a person gets close to the discovery of people-based care, because data come directly from the people and are not derived from the etic (outsider views) beliefs and practices of the researcher. An important purpose of the theory is to document, know, predict, and explain systematically through field data what is diverse and universal about generic and professional care of the cultures being studied (Leininger, 1991b).

Leininger (1984a, 1988a) holds that detailed and culturally based caring knowledge and practices should distinguish nursing's contributions from those of other disciplines. The first reason for studying care theory is that the construct of care has been critical to human growth, development, and survival for human beings from the beginning of human species (Leininger, 1981, 1984a). The second reason is to explicate and fully understand cultural knowledge and the roles of caregivers and care recipients in different cultures to provide culturally congruent care (Leininger, 1991b, 1995c, 2002a, 2002b, 2002c). Third, care knowledge is discovered and can be used as essential to promote the healing and well-being of clients, to face death, or to ensure the survival of human cultures over time (Leininger, 1981, 1984a, 1991b). Fourth, the nursing profession needs to systematically study care from a broad and holistic cultural perspective to discover the expressions and meanings of care, health, illness, and well-being as nursing knowledge (Leininger, 1991b, 1995c, 2002a, 2002b, 2002c). Leininger (1991b, 1995c, 2002a, 2002b, 2002c) finds that care is largely an elusive

phenomenon often embedded in cultural lifeways and values. However, this knowledge is a sound basis for nurses to guide their practice for culturally congruent care and specific therapeutic ways to maintain health, prevent illness, heal, or help people face death (Leininger, 1994). A central thesis of the theory is that if the meaning of care can be fully grasped, the well-being or health care of individuals, families, and groups can be predicted and culturally congruent care can be provided (Leininger, 1991b). Leininger (1991b) views care as one of the most powerful constructs and the central phenomena of nursing. However, such care constructs and patterns must be fully documented, understood, and used to ensure that culturally based care becomes the major guide to transcultural nursing therapy and is used to explain or predict nursing practices (Leininger, 1991b).

To date, Leininger has studied several cultures in depth and has studied many cultures with undergraduate and graduate students and faculty using qualitative research methods. She has extensively explicated care constructs throughout many cultures in which each culture has different meanings, cultural experiences, and uses by the people of diverse and similar cultures (Leininger, 1991b, 1995c; Leininger & McFarland, 2002a, 2005). A new body of knowledge continues to be discovered by transcultural nurses in the development of transcultural care practices with diverse and similar cultures. In time, Leininger (1991b) believes, both diverse and universal features of care and health will be documented as the essence of nursing knowledge and practice.

Leininger stated that the goal of the care theory is to provide culturally congruent care (1991b, 1995c, 2002a, 2002b, 2002c; Leininger & McFarland, 2005). She believes nurses must work toward explicating care use and meanings so that culture care, values, beliefs, and lifeways can provide accurate and reliable bases for planning and effectively implementing culture-specific care and for identifying any universal or common features about care. She maintains that nurses cannot separate worldviews, social structures, and cultural beliefs (folk and professional) from health, wellness, illness, or care when working with cultures, because these factors are closely linked. Social structure factors such as religion, politics, culture, economics, and kinship are significant forces affecting care and influencing illness patterns and well-being. She also emphasizes the importance of discovering generic (folk, local, and indigenous) care from the cultures and comparing it with professional care (Leininger, 1991b).

Leininger has found that cultural blindness, shock, imposition, and ethnocentrism by present-day nurses continues to greatly reduce the quality of care to clients of different cultures (Leininger, 1991a, 1994, 1995c; Leininger & McFarland, 2002a, 2005). Moreover, nursing diagnoses and medical diagnoses that are not culturally based and known create serious problems for cultures that lead to unfavorable and sometimes serious outcomes (Leininger, 1990c). Culturally congruent care is what makes clients satisfied that they have received good care; it is a powerful healing force for quality health care. Quality care is what clients seek most when they come for services from nurses, and it can be realized only when culturally derived care is known and used.

MAJOR ASSUMPTIONS

Major assumptions to support Leininger's Culture Care Theory of Diversity and Universality follow. The definitions were derived from Leininger's definitive works on the theory (Leininger, 1991b; Leininger & McFarland, 2002a, 2005).

1. Care is the essence of nursing and a distinct, dominant, central, and unifying focus.
2. Culturally based care (caring) is essential for well-being, health, growth and survival, and to face handicaps or death.
3. Culturally based care is the most comprehensive and holistic means to know, explain, interpret, and predict nursing care phenomena and to guide nursing decisions and actions.
4. Transcultural nursing is a humanistic and scientific care discipline and profession with the central purpose to serve individuals, groups, communities, societies, and institutions.

5. Culturally based caring is essential to curing and healing, for there can be no curing without caring, but caring can exist without curing.
6. Culture care concepts, meanings, expressions, patterns, processes, and structural forms of care vary transculturally with diversities (differences) and some universalities (commonalities).
7. Every human culture has generic (lay, folk, or indigenous) care knowledge and practices and usually professional care knowledge and practices, which vary transculturally and individually.
8. Culture care values, beliefs, and practices are influenced by and tend to be embedded in the worldview, language, philosophy, religion (and spirituality), kinship, social, political, legal, educational, economic, technological, ethnohistorical, and environmental context of cultures.
9. Beneficial, healthy, and satisfying culturally based care influences the health and well-being of individuals, families, groups, and communities within their environmental contexts.
10. Culturally congruent and beneficial nursing care can occur only when care values, expressions, or patterns are known and used explicitly for appropriate, safe, and meaningful care.
11. Culture care differences and similarities exist between professional and client-generic care in human cultures worldwide.
12. Cultural conflicts, cultural impositions practices, cultural stresses, and cultural pain reflect the lack of culture care knowledge to provide culturally congruent, responsible, safe, and sensitive care.
13. The ethnonursing qualitative research method provides an important means to accurately discover and interpret emic and etic embedded, complex, and diverse culture care data. (Leininger, 1991b, pp. 44-45)

The universality of care reveals the common nature of human beings and humanity, whereas diversity of care reveals the variability and selected, unique features of human beings.

THEORETICAL ASSERTIONS

Tenets are the position one holds or are givens that the theorist uses with a theory. In developing the theory, the following four major tenets were conceptualized and formulated with the Theory of Culture Care (Leininger, 2002c):

1. Culture care expressions, meaning, patterns, and practices are diverse, and yet there are shared commonalities and some universal attributes.
2. The worldview consists of multiple social structure factors, such as religion, economics, cultural values, ethnohistory, environmental context, language, and generic and professional care, that are critical influencers of cultural care patterns to predict health, well-being, illness, healing, and ways people face disabilities and death.
3. Generic emic (folk) and professional etic care in different environmental contexts can greatly influence health and illness outcomes.
4. From an analysis of the previously listed influencers, three major actions and decision guides were predicted to provide ways to give culturally congruent, safe, and meaningful health care to cultures. The three culturally based action and decision modes were the following: (1) culture care preservation or maintenance, (2) culture care accommodation or negotiation, and (3) culture care repatterning or restructuring. Decision and action modes based on culture care were predicted as key factors to arrive at congruent, safe, and meaningful care.

In conceptualizing the theory, the first major and central theoretical tenet was, "care diversities (differences) and universalities (commonalities) existed among and between cultures in the world" (Leininger, 2002c, p. 78). However, Leininger asserted that culture care meanings and uses had to be discovered to establish a body of transcultural knowledge. A second major theoretical tenet was "[that the] worldview, social structure factors such as religion, economics, education, technology, politics, kinship (social), ethnohistory, environment, language, and generic and professional care factors would greatly influence culture care meanings, expressions, and patterns in different cultures" (Leininger, 2002c, p. 78).

Leininger has maintained that these factors needed to be documented in order to provide meaningful and satisfying care to people and are predicted to be powerful influencers on culturally based care.

These factors also needed to be discovered directly from the informants as influencing factors related to health, well-being, illness, and death. The third major theoretical tenet was, "both generic (emic) and professional (etic) care needs to be taught, researched, and brought together into care practices for satisfying care for clients which lead to their health and wellbeing" (Leininger, 2002c).

The fourth major theoretical tenet was the conceptualization of the "three major care actions and decisions, to arrive at culturally congruent care for the general health and wellbeing of clients, or to help them face death or disabilities" (Leininger, 2002c, p. 78). These modes are culture care preservation or maintenance; culture care accommodation, negotiation; and culture care repatterning or restructuring. The researcher draws upon findings from the social structure, generic and professional practices, and other influencing factors while studying culturally based care for individuals, families, and groups. These factors would need to be studied, assessed and responded to in a dynamic and participatory nurse-client relationship (Leininger 1991a, 1991b, 2002b; Leininger & McFarland, 2002a).

LOGICAL FORM

Leininger's theory (1995c) is derived from anthropology and nursing but is reformulated to become transcultural nursing with human care perspective. She developed the ethnonursing research method and has emphasized the importance of studying people from their emic or local knowledge and experiences and later contrasting them with the etic (outsider) beliefs and practices. Her book, *Qualitative Research Methods in Nursing* (Leininger, 1985a), and related publications (Leininger, 1990b, 1995c, 2002c) provide substantive knowledge about qualitative methods in nursing.

In her own words, Leininger is skilled in using ethnonursing, ethnography, life histories, life stories, photography, and phenomenological methods that provide a holistic approach to study cultural behavior in diverse environmental contexts. With these qualitative methods, the researcher moves with the people in their daily living activities to grasp their world. The nurse researcher inductively obtains data of documented descriptive and interpretative accounts from informants through observations and participation or in other ways explicating care as a major challenge within the method. The qualitative approach is important to develop basic and substantive grounded data-based knowledge about cultural care to guide nurses in their work. From the beginning, ethnonursing has been grounded primarily in data from the cultures under study, which is different from the grounded theory of Glasser and Strauss (1967).

Although other methods of research such as hypothesis testing and experimental quantitative methods can be used to study transcultural care, the method of choice depends upon the researcher's purposes, the goals of the study, and the phenomena to be studied. Creativity and the willingness of the nurse researcher to use different research methods to discover nursing knowledge are encouraged. However, Leininger holds that qualitative methods are important to establish meanings and accurate cultural knowledge. Quantitative methods generally have been of limited value to study cultures and care. Combining both qualitative and quantitative methods tends to obscure the findings and is a misuse of both paradigms (Leininger, 1991b, 1995c).

Leininger developed the Sunrise Enabler (Figure 22-1) in the 1970s to depict the essential components of the theory. She has refined the sunrise to the present and thus the evolved enabler is more definitive and valuable to study accurately the diverse elements or the components of the theory and to make culturally congruent clinical assessments. This enabler and the complete theory of cultural care diversity and universality are not fully addressed here. Only selected ideas are offered to introduce the reader to Leininger's pioneering and creative work of evolving theory over time. The sunrise enabler symbolizes the rising of the sun (care) (Leininger, 1991b, 1995c; Leininger & McFarland, 2002a, 2005). The upper half of the circle depicts components of the social structure and worldview factors that influence care and health through language, ethnohistory, and environmental

context. These factors also influence the folk, professional, and nursing system(s), which are the middle part of the model. The two halves together form a full sun, which represents the universe that nurses must consider to appreciate human care and health (Leininger, 1991b, 1995c; Leininger & McFarland, 2002a, 2005). According to Leininger, nursing acts as a bridge between folk (generic) and the professional system. Three kinds of nursing care and decisions and actions are predicted in the theory: culture care preservation or maintenance, culture care accommodation or negotiation, and culture care repatterning or restructuring (Leininger, 1991b, 1995c; Leininger & McFarland, 2002a, 2005).

The Sunrise Enabler depicts human beings as inseparable from their cultural background and social structure, worldview, history, and environmental context as a basic tenet of Leininger's theory (Leininger, 1991b, 1995c; Leininger & McFarland, 2002a, 2005). Gender, race, age, and class are embedded in social structure factors and are studied. Biological, emotional, and other dimensions are studied from a holistic view and not fragmented or separate. Theory generation from this model may occur at multiple levels from the micro range (small-scale specific individuals) or to study groups, families, communities, or large-scale phenomena (several cultures). Leininger has also developed several enablers to facilitate studying phenomena using the four phases of qualitative data analysis. Most importantly, the qualitative criteria are used to analyze the data; they are credibility, confirmability, meaning in context, saturation, repatterning, and transferability (Leininger, 1995c, 2002c). Quantitative criteria should not be used with qualitative methods, because the former have specific criteria to measure outcomes.

Leininger also developed four other enablers to assist nurse researchers in their use of the ethnonursing method. "Enablers sharply contrast with mechanistic devices such as tools, scales, measurement instruments, and other impersonal objective distancing tools generally used in quantitative studies. These tools are often viewed as unnatural and frightening to cultural informants" (Leininger, 2002c, p. 89).

CULTURE CARE

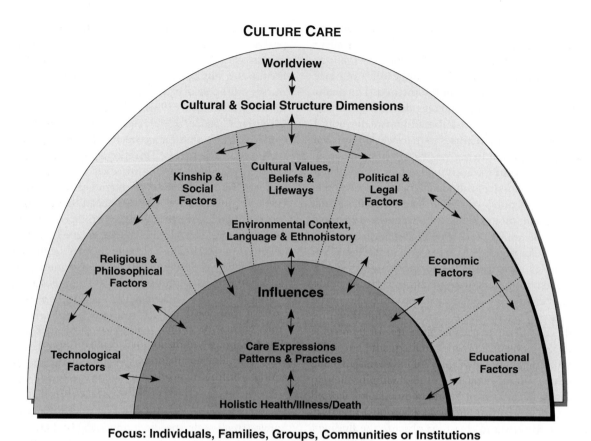

Focus: Individuals, Families, Groups, Communities or Institutions in Diverse Health Contexts of

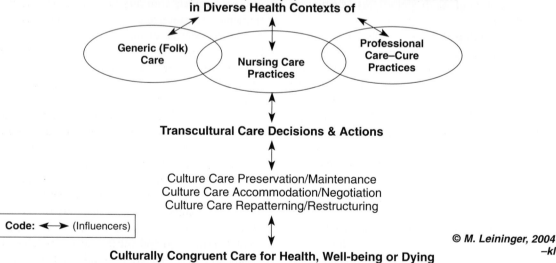

Transcultural Care Decisions & Actions

Culture Care Preservation/Maintenance
Culture Care Accommodation/Negotiation
Culture Care Repatterning/Restructuring

Code: ◄——► (Influencers)

© *M. Leininger, 2004*
—kl

Culturally Congruent Care for Health, Well-being or Dying

Figure 22-1 Leininger's Sunrise Enabler to depict the Theory of Culture Care Diversity and Universality. (Copyright Madeleine Leininger. Modified by Madeleine Leininger and received in October 2004 via personal correspondence.)

The observation participation reflection enabler is used to facilitate the researcher in entering and remaining with informants in their familiar or natural context during the study. The researcher gradually moves from the role of observer and listener, transitioning to that of participant and reflector with the informants. By moving slowly and politely with permission, the researcher does not disrupt and therefore is able to observe what is naturally occurring in the environment or with the people.

With the stranger to trusted friend enabler, the nurse researcher is able to learn much about oneself and the people and culture being studied. The goal with this guide is to become a trusted friend as one moves from distrusted stranger to trusted friend and different attitudes, behaviors, and expectations can be identified. This process is essential for the researcher to become trusted such that honest, credible, and in-depth data may be discovered from informants.

The domain of inquiry enabler is used by nurse researchers for each study to clearly establish the researcher's interest and area of focus. The domain of inquiry is a "succinct tailor made statement focused directly and specifically on culture care and health phenomena" (Leininger, 2002c, p. 92), stating questions or ideas related to the focus of the study, its purpose, and goals.

The acculturation health assessment enabler is another important guide used with the method. It is essential when studying cultures to assess the extent of the informants' acculturation as to whether they are more "traditionally or non-traditionally oriented in their values, beliefs, and general lifeways" (Leininger, 2002c, p. 92). This enabler is used for both cultural assessments and ethnonursing research studies.

ACCEPTANCE BY THE NURSING COMMUNITY

Practice

Leininger identifies several factors related to the slowness of nurses to recognize and value transcultural nursing and cultural factors in nursing practices and education (Leininger, 1991b; Leininger & McFarland, 2005). First, the theory was conceptualized during the 1950s, when virtually no nurses were prepared in anthropology or cultural knowledge to understand transcultural concepts, models, or theory. In the early days, most nurses had no knowledge of the nature of anthropology and how anthropological knowledge might contribute to human care and health behaviors or serve as background knowledge to understand nursing phenomena or problems. Second, although people had longstanding and inherent cultural needs, many clients were reluctant to push health personnel to meet their cultural needs and therefore did not demand that their cultural and social needs be recognized or met (Leininger, 1970, 1978, 1995c; Leininger & McFarland, 2002a). Third, until the past decade, transcultural nursing articles submitted for publication were often rejected because editors did not know, value, or understand the relevance of cultural knowledge to transcultural nursing or as essential to nursing. Fourth, the concept of care was of limited interest to nurses until the late 1970s, when Leininger began promoting the importance of nurses studying human care, obtaining background knowledge in anthropology, and obtaining graduate preparation in transcultural nursing, research, and practice. Fifth, Leininger contends that nursing tends to remain too ethnocentric and far too involved in following medicine's interest and directions. Sixth, nursing has been slow to make substantive progress in the development of a distinct body of knowledge, because many nurse researchers have been far too dependent on quantitative research methods to obtain measurable outcomes rather than qualitative data outcomes. The recent acceptance and use of qualitative research methods in nursing will provide new insights and knowledge related to nursing and transcultural nursing (Leininger, 1991b, 1995c; Leininger & McFarland, 2002a). There is growing interest in using transcultural nursing knowledge, research, and practice by nurses worldwide.

Nurses are now realizing the importance of transcultural nursing, human care, and qualitative methods. Leininger (personal communication, April 2002) has stated:

> We are entering a new phase of nursing as we value and use transcultural nursing knowledge with a focus on human caring, health, and illness behaviors. With the migration of many cultural groups and the rise of the consumer cultural identity, and demands in culturally based care, nurses are realizing the need for culturally sensitive and competent practices. Most countries and communities of the world are multicultural today, and so health personnel are expected to understand and respond to clients of diverse and similar cultures. Immigrants and people from unfamiliar cultures expect nurses to respect and respond to values, beliefs, lifeways, and needs. No longer can nurses practice unicultural nursing.

As the world becomes more culturally diverse, nurses will find the urgent need to be prepared to provide culturally competent care. Some nurses are experiencing culture shock, conflict, and clashes as they move from one area to another and from rural to urban communities without transcultural nursing preparation. As cultural conflicts arise, families are less satisfied with nursing and medical services (Leininger, 1991b). Nurses who travel and seek employment in foreign lands are experiencing cultural stresses. Transcultural nursing education has become imperative for all nurses worldwide. Certification of transcultural nurses by the Transcultural Nursing Society has provided a major step toward protecting the public from unsafe and culturally incompetent nursing practices (Leininger, 1991a, 2001). Accordingly, more nurses are seeking transcultural certification to protect themselves and their clients. The *Journal of Transcultural Nursing* has also provided research and theoretical perspectives of over 100 cultures worldwide to guide transcultural nurses in their practices.

Education

The inclusion of culture and comparative care in nursing curricula began in 1966 at the University of Colorado, where Leininger was professor of nursing and anthropology. Awareness of the importance of culture care to nursing gradually began to appear during the late 1960s, but very few nurse educators were prepared adequately to teach courses about transcultural nursing. Since the world's first master's and doctoral programs in transcultural nursing were approved and implemented in 1977 at the University of Utah, more nurses have been prepared specifically in transcultural nursing. Today, with the heightened public awareness of health care costs, different cultures, and human rights, there is much greater demand for comprehensive, holistic, and transcultural people care to protect and provide quality-based care and to prevent legal suits related to improper care. Leininger's demand for culture-specific care based on theoretical insights has been critical for the discovery of diverse and universal aspects of care (Leininger, 1995c, 1996a, 1996b; Leininger & McFarland, 2002b). A critical need remains for nurses to be educated in transcultural nursing in undergraduate and graduate programs. There is also a need for well-qualified faculty prepared in transcultural nursing to teach and to guide research in nursing schools within the United States and in other countries (Leininger, 1995c, 1996b; Tom-Orne, 2002).

Since 1980 an increasing number of nursing curricula are emphasizing transcultural nursing and human care. One of the early programs to focus on care was at Cuesta College in California during the 1970s, where they developed an undergraduate nursing program with care as a central theme. Course titles included Caring Concepts I & II, Caring of Families, and Professional Self Care (Leininger, 1984a). During the late 1980s, four master's and four doctoral programs in the United States offered transcultural nursing courses, research experiences, and guided field study experiences (Leininger, 1995c). Leininger continues to receive numerous requests to give courses, lectures, and workshops on human care and transcultural nursing in the United States and other countries. The demand for transcultural nurses far exceeds available faculty, money, and other resources. Therefore, in 1996, Leininger put out a call for schools of nursing to offer transcultural programs to meet the worldwide demand for many nurses and cultures

(Leininger, 1995a, 1995b, 1996b). These nursing programs are needed urgently for practice and preparation for certification of transcultural nurses. They are also needed for research and for worldwide consultation. At this time, there are still inadequate research funds to study transcultural nursing education and practice. Although the societal demand for transcultural nurses is evident, the educational preparation remains weak and limited for many nurses worldwide. There are still graduate nursing faculty members who do not understand transcultural nursing and the Theory of Culture Care and, consequently, will not permit students to study or research the phenomena, which causes great distress to nursing students (Leininger, 2002d).

Research

Many nurses today are using Leininger's culture care theory worldwide. The theory is the only one in nursing focused specifically on culture care and with a research method (ethnonursing) to examine the theory (Leininger, 1991b, 1995c; Leininger & McFarland, 2002a, 2005). Approximately 100 cultures and subcultures have been studied as of 1995, and more are in progress (Leininger, 1991b, 1995c, 1996a; Leininger & McFarland, 2002a). Funds to support transcultural nursing are meager and limited in most societies, because biomedical and technical research funds head the priority list. Very few nursing schools in the United States receive federal support for nursing or transcultural nursing research unless they have a quantitative, objective (measurement) focus. Transcultural nurses and other nurses interested in transcultural nursing research are continuing their research despite limited or nonexistent funds. These nurses are leaders in sharing their research at conferences and instructional programs related to transcultural nursing. They have been instrumental in opening doors to transcultural nursing in many organizations. Despite societal demands for culturally competent, sensitive, responsible care, national and international organizations began to support transcultural nursing only in the 1990s. Through

persistent efforts and exacting competencies of transcultural nurse specialists, progress has been forthcoming. Transcultural nurses have stimulated many other nurses to pursue research and to discover some entirely new knowledge in nursing. This knowledge will greatly reshape and transform nursing in the future.

CLINICAL APPLICATION OF THEORY TO PRACTICE

The ethnonursing study by McFarland (1995, 2002), that covered 2 years starting in the late 1980s, compared Anglo-American and African-American groups living in a residence home for the elderly in one large Midwestern United States city. The research was another in-depth emic and etic culture care investigation that revealed several significant findings and the importance of using the three action and decision modes of the theory when caring for the elderly. The culturally congruent care findings were as follows:

- Anglo-American and African-American elderly expect culture care preservation and maintenance of their lifelong generic or folk care patterns.
- Doing for other residents rather than having a self-care focus was a major care maintenance value for both cultures and was a dominant finding.
- Protective care was more important to African-American than Anglo-American elders, but nursing staff provided protective care and practiced culture care accommodation for both groups of elders, such as accompanying them when they desired to go for walks in the surrounding inner city neighborhood.
- African-American nurses practiced culture accommodation when they linked their emic care with generic care values and practices.

Culture care maintenance-preservation and culture care accommodation-negotiation were new ways for nurses to provide culturally congruent and safe lifeways care practices for the elderly of both cultures. Based on the findings of this study, several institutional culture care policies were developed to guide professional elderly care.

FURTHER DEVELOPMENT

Leininger predicts that all professional nurses in the world must be prepared in transcultural nursing and must demonstrate competencies in transcultural nursing (Leininger, 1981, 1995c; Leininger & McFarland, 2002a, 2005). Transcultural nursing must become an integral part of education and practice for nurses to be relevant in the twenty-first century. Currently, the demand for prepared transcultural nurses far exceeds the number of nurses, faculty, and clinical specialists in the world. Far more transcultural nurse theorists, researchers, and scholars are urgently needed to continue to develop a new body of transcultural knowledge and to transform nursing education and practice. By the year 2010, all nurses will need to have a basic knowledge about diverse cultures in the world and in-depth knowledge of at least two or three cultures (Leininger, 1995c, 1996a). Leininger believes transcultural nursing research has already begun to lead to some highly promising and different ways to advance nursing education and practice (Leininger & McFarland, 2002a, 2005). All health disciplines, including medicine, pharmacy, and social work, gradually will incorporate transcultural health knowledge and practice into their programs of study in the near future. This trend will increase the demand for competent faculty in transcultural health care. Leininger (1995c) believes that the development of transcultural institutes will be essential to fill the growing need for transcultural nurses prepared to work with other disciplines.

Present and future theories and studies in transcultural nursing will be essential to meet the needs of culturally diverse people. The Theory of Culture Care will grow in importance worldwide. Both universal and diverse care knowledge will be extremely important to establish a substantive body of transcultural nursing knowledge and to make nursing a transcultural profession and discipline. Leininger's theory has already gained worldwide interest and use because it is holistic, relevant, and futuristic and deals with specific, yet abstract, care knowledge. The sunrise enabler remains invaluable as a dominant image and guide to study and assess people of diverse and similar cultural needs.

CRITIQUE

Simplicity

Transcultural nursing theory is really a broad, holistic, comprehensive perspective of human groups, populations, and species. This theory continues to generate many domains of inquiry for nurse researchers to pursue for scientific and humanistic knowledge. The theory challenges nurses to seek both universal and diverse culturally based care phenomena by diverse cultures, the culture of nursing, and the cultures of social unsteadiness worldwide. The theory is truly transcultural and global in scope; it is both complex and practical. It requires transcultural nursing knowledge and appropriate research methods to explicate the phenomena. Leininger's culture care theory is relevant worldwide to help guide nurse researchers in conceptualizing the theory and research approaches and to guide practice. It is holistic and comprehensive in nature; therefore, several concepts and constructs related to social structure, environment, and language are extremely important to discover and obtain culturally based knowledge or knowledge grounded in the people's world. The theory shows multiple interrelationships of concepts and diversity of key concepts and relationships, especially to social structure factors. It requires some basic anthropological knowledge, but also considerable transcultural nursing knowledge, to be used in an accurate and scholarly fashion. Once the theory has been fully conceptualized, Leininger finds that undergraduate and graduate nursing students are excited to use the theory and discover how practical, relevant, and useful it is in their work. The use of the sunrise enabler becomes imprinted on their minds as a way of knowing.

Generality

The transcultural nursing theory does demonstrate the criterion of generality because it is a qualitatively oriented theory that is broad, comprehensive, and worldwide in scope. Transcultural nursing theory addresses nursing care from a multicultural and worldview perspective. It is useful and applicable to both groups and individuals with the goal of rendering culture-specific nursing care. The broad or generic concepts are well organized and defined for study in specific cultures. The research had led to a vast amount of expert knowledge largely unknown in the past. Many aspects of culture, care, and health are being identified, because these factors have an impact on nursing. Even more research is needed for comparative purposes from both culture-specific data and some universal care knowledge. More of the world's cultural groups need to be studied and compared to validate the caring constructs in the future. The theory is most helpful as a guide for the study of any culture and for the comparative study of several cultures. Findings from the theory are being used presently in client care in a variety of health and community settings worldwide to transform nursing education and service. It is being valued especially in developing a new and different approach to the traditional community nursing perspective.

Empirical Precision

The transcultural nursing theory is researchable, and qualitative research has been the primary paradigm to discover largely unknown phenomena of care and health in diverse cultures. This qualitative approach differs from the traditional quantitative research method, which renders measurement the goal of research. However, the ethnonursing research method is extremely rigorous and linguistically exacting in nature and outcomes. One hundred thirty-five care constructs have been identified and more are being discovered each day, with a wealth of other transcultural nursing knowledge. The important attribute is that the accuracy of grounded data derived with the use of ethnomethods or from an emic or people's viewpoint is leading to high credibility, confirmability, and a wealth of empirical data. Ongoing and future research will

lead to additional care and health findings and implications for ethnonursing practices and education to fit specific cultures and universal features. The qualitative criteria of credibility and confirmability from in-depth studies of informants and their contexts are becoming clearly evident. Unequivocally, the body of transcultural nursing knowledge that has been established over the past decade has had a great impact on nursing and many health care systems (Leininger, 1995c; Leininger & McFarland 2002a, 2005).

Derivable Consequences

Transcultural nursing theory has important outcomes for nursing. Rendering culture-specific care is a necessary and essential new goal in nursing. It places the transcultural nursing theory central to the domain of nursing knowledge acquisition and use. The theory is highly useful, applicable, and essential to nursing practice, education, and research. The concept of care as the primary focus of nursing and the base of nursing knowledge and practice is long overdue and essential to advance nursing knowledge and practices. Leininger (1991a) notes that, although nursing has always made claims to the concept of care, rigorous research on care has been limited until the past 3 decades. This theory could be the means to establish a sound and defensible discipline and profession, guiding practice to meet a multicultural world.

SUMMARY

In this chapter the nature, importance, and major features of the Theory of Culture Care were discussed. The ethnonursing research method and the enablers were presented to show the fit between the theory and the method. Knowledge of both the theory and the method are needed before launching an ethnonursing study. Fully understanding the theory and method (with the enablers) leads to credible and meaningful study findings. Through complete understanding, the research becomes meaningful, exciting, and rewarding to do, and the researcher develops confidence and competence in the use of the theory and method.

As a premier theory in nursing, culture care is greatly valued worldwide. Other disciplines have found the theory and method very helpful and valuable. Nurses who use the theory and method frequently communicate how valuable and important it is to discover culturally based ways to know and practice nursing and health care. Practicing nurses now have holistic, culturally based research findings for use in caring for clients of diverse and similar cultures or subcultures in different countries. The theory is not difficult to use once the researcher understands it and method and has mentor guidance. Newcomers to the theory and method can benefit from experienced, expert mentors in addition to studying transcultural research conducted using the theory and method. Most importantly, nurses often express that this theory and method are the only ones that it makes sense to use in nursing. They contend it is very natural to nursing and helps one to gain fresh new insights about care, health, and well-being. Unquestionably, it is the theory of today and tomorrow and one which will grow in use in the future in our growing and increasingly multicultural world. The research and theory provide a new pathway to advance the profession of nursing and the body of transcultural knowledge for application in nursing practice, education, research, and clinical consultation worldwide.

Case Study

An elderly Arab-American Muslim man who spoke little English was admitted to the hospital for increasing pain at rest in his left foot. His foot was cool and pale and he had a history of vascular surgical procedures. He had many chronic health problems including type II diabetes, hypertension, and chronic obstructive pulmonary disease. He also had had a myocardial infarction and several cerebral vascular accidents. While in the hospital, he developed abdominal pain and underwent a cholecystectomy. This elderly grandfather had a large family, including a wife, nine children, and many grandchildren. His wife insisted that all family members visit him every day while he was in the hospital. The family wanted the man's face turned toward Mecca (toward the east) while they prayed with him. They brought taped passages from the Koran, which they played at his bedside. Other families who were visiting their sick relatives complained to the nurses that the Arab family was taking up the entire waiting room and there was no place for any one else to sit.

As a nurse, how might you use the three modes from the Theory of Culture Care to provide culturally congruent care for this elderly man and his family, as well as for the other clients and their families in the critical care unit?

CRITICAL THINKING *Activities*

1. Select four research studies reported in the *Journal of Transcultural Nursing* that used Leininger's Theory of Culture Care Diversity and Universality. Each of the studies selected should represent different cultures, different research settings, and cultures different from the student's culture.
   a. each of the studies and identify the relationship of the theory to domain of inquiry, purpose, assumptions, definitions, methods, research design, data analysis, nursing decisions, and conclusions.
   b. Provide evidence that the findings from the studies confirm the findings of the theory in relation to the domain of inquiry, theory tenets, and derivable consequences.

2. Discuss the usefulness of the Theory of Culture Care Diversity and Universality in the twenty-first century to discover nursing knowledge and provide culturally congruent care. Take into consideration the current trends of consumers of health care, cultural diversity factors, and changes in medical and nursing school curricula. Following are some examples of trends and changes you may want to consider in your discussion:

a. The importance of transcultural nursing knowledge in an increasingly diverse world

b. Growth of lay support groups to provide information and sharing of experiences and support for clients, families, and groups experiencing chronic, terminal, or life-threatening illnesses or treatment modalities from diverse or similar (common) cultures

c. Use of cultural values, beliefs, health practices, and research knowledge in undergraduate and graduate nursing curricula across the life-span

d. Inclusion of alternative or generic care in nursing curricula, such as medicine men (Native American healers, curers, and herbalists in the Southwest) and selected substantiated Chinese methods shown to be effective for the treatment of chronic diseases

e. Use of cultural caring research knowledge as the new and future direction of nursing in the twenty-first century

f. The increased number of books, audiotapes, and videotapes published on health maintenance, alternative medicine, herbs, vitamins, minerals, and other over-the-counter medications and preparations, which demands a transcultural knowledge base

g. Spiraling health care costs, forced use of health maintenance organizations, lack of health insurance, increased reliance on self diagnosis, treatment, and care, and increased availability of diagnostic kits for acquired immunodeficiency syndrome testing, glucose monitoring, cholesterol screening, ovulation and pregnancy tests, fecal occult blood tests, and the like

h. Problems related to cultural conflicts, stress, pain, and cultural imposition practices

3. Arrange for several observation and interview experiences at a local university student health center or public health department with people of diverse cultures. Ascertain the following:

a. Identify the cultures represented by the clientele with the use of Leininger's theory and the sunrise enabler.

b. What is the cultural mix of the staff (physicians, nurses, social workers, and clerics) of the center or health department? How does the cultural background of the staff differ from that of the clientele?

c. Arrange a conference with the nursing staff and ascertain their culture-based attitudes, values, and beliefs, and those that are reflected in the clients using the center or department. Compare and contrast the values, attitudes, and beliefs of the staff with those of the clients. What are the cultural similarities and differences?

d. Arrange an interview with the director of the center or department and ascertain the economic, political, legal, and other factors from Leininger's sunrise enabler that affect the clients' use of the center or department.

e. Survey the printed materials available in the waiting and examination rooms and classrooms and identify what cultures and languages are depicted by the visual aids, artifacts, and paintings.

f. On the basis of data obtained from these exercises, how can the Theory of Culture Care Diversity and Universality be used to provide culturally sensitive and congruent care to the clients using the center or department and increase the satisfaction with care received?

4. Discuss the type of prerequisite knowledge, experiences, attitudes, and skills needed to effectively use the Theory of Culture Care Diversity and Universality.

5. Discuss the relevancy of the Theory of Culture Care Diversity and Universality to nurses working in different practice settings and roles.

REFERENCES

Glasser, B. G., & Strauss, A. L. (1967). *The discovery of grounded theories: Strategies for qualitative research.* Chicago: Aldine.

Hofling, C. K., & Leininger, M. (1960). *Basic psychiatric concepts in nursing.* Philadelphia: J. B. Lippincott.

Leininger, M. (1970). *Nursing and anthropology: Two worlds to blend.* New York: John Wiley & Sons.

Leininger, M. (Ed.). (1978). *Transcultural nursing: Concepts, theories, and practice.* New York: John Wiley & Sons.

Leininger, M. (Ed.). (1981). *Caring: An essential human need.* Thorofare, NJ: Charles B. Slack.

Leininger, M. (Ed.). (1984a). *Care: The essence of nursing and health.* Thorofare, NJ: Charles B. Slack.

Leininger, M. (1984b). *Reference sources for transcultural health and nursing for teaching, curriculum, and clinical-field practice.* Thorofare, NJ: Charles B. Slack.

Leininger, M. (Ed.). (1985a). *Qualitative research methods in nursing.* New York: Grune & Stratton.

Leininger, M. (1985b). Transcultural care diversity and universality: A theory of nursing. *Nursing and Health Care, 6*(4), 202-212.

Leininger, M. (1988a). *Care: Discovery and uses in clinical and community nursing.* Detroit: Wayne State University Press.

Leininger, M. (Ed.). (1988b). *Care: The essence of nursing and health.* Detroit: Wayne State University Press.

Leininger, M. (Ed.). (1988c). *Caring: An essential human need.* Detroit: Wayne State University Press.

Leininger, M. (Ed.). (1988d). Leininger's theory of nursing: Cultural diversity and universality. *Nursing Science Quarterly, 2*(4), 11-20.

Leininger, M. (1989a). Transcultural nurse specialists and generalists: New practitioners in nursing. *Journal of Transcultural Nursing, 1,* 4-16.

Leininger, M. (1989b). Transcultural nurse specialists and generalists: Imperative in today's world. *Nursing and Health Care, 10*(5), 250-256.

Leininger, M. (1990a). *Ethical and moral dimensions of care: Chapters from conference on the ethics and morality of caring.* Detroit: Wayne State University Press.

Leininger, M. (1990b). Ethnomethods: The philosophic and epistemic bases to explicate transcultural nursing knowledge. *Journal of Transcultural Nursing, 1*(2), 40-51.

Leininger, M. (1990c). Issues, questions, and concerns related to the nursing diagnosis cultural movement from transcultural nursing perspective. *Journal of Transcultural Nursing, 2*(1), 23-32.

Leininger, M. (1991a). Becoming aware of types of health practitioners and cultural imposition. *Journal of Transcultural Nursing, 2*(2), 32-49.

Leininger, M. (1991b). *Culture care diversity and universality: A theory of nursing.* New York: National League for Nursing Press.

Leininger, M. (1991c). The transcultural nurse specialist: Imperative in today's world. *Perspective in Family and Community Health, 17,* 137-144.

Leininger, M. (1994). Quality of life from a transcultural nursing perspective. *Nursing Science Quarterly, 7*(1), 22-28.

Leininger, M. (1995a). Culture care theory, research, and practice. *Nursing Science Quarterly, 9*(20), 71-78.

Leininger, M. (1995b). Editorial: Teaching transcultural nursing to transform nursing for the 21st century. *Journal of Transcultural Nursing, 6*(2), 2-3.

Leininger, M. (1995c). *Transcultural nursing: Concepts, theories, and practice* (2nd ed.). Columbus, OH: McGraw-Hill College Custom Series.

Leininger, M. (1996a). Major directions for transcultural nursing: A journey into the 21st century. *Journal of Transcultural Nursing, 7*(2), 37-40.

Leininger, M. (1996b). Future directions for transcultural nursing in the 21st century. *International Nursing Review, 44*(1), 19-23.

Leininger, M. (2001). Founder's focus: Certification of transcultural nurses for quality and safe consumer care. *Journal of Transcultural Nursing, 12*(3), 242.

Leininger, M. (2002a). Transcultural nursing and globalization of health care: Importance, focus, and historical aspects. In M. Leininger & M. R. McFarland (Eds.), *Transcultural nursing: Concepts, theories, research, & practice* (3rd ed., pp. 3-43). New York: McGraw-Hill Medical Publishing Division.

Leininger, M. (2002b). Essential transcultural nursing concepts, principles, examples, and policy statements. In M. Leininger & M. R. McFarland (Eds.), *Transcultural nursing: Concepts, theories, research, & practice* (3rd ed., pp. 45-69). New York: McGraw-Hill Medical Publishing Division.

Leininger, M. (2002c). Part I. The theory of culture care and the ethnonursing research method. In M. Leininger & M. R. McFarland (Eds.), *Transcultural nursing: Concepts, theories, research, & practice* (3rd ed., pp. 71-98). New York: McGraw-Hill Medical Publishing Division.

Leininger, M. (2002d). The future of transcultural nursing: A global perspective. In M. Leininger & M. R. McFarland (Eds.), *Transcultural nursing: Concepts, theories, research, & practice* (3rd ed., pp. 577-595). New York: McGraw-Hill Medical Publishing Division.

Leininger, M., & McFarland, M. R. (2002a). *Transcultural nursing: Concepts, theories, research, & practice* (3rd ed.). New York: McGraw-Hill Medical Publishing Division.

Leininger, M., & McFarland, M. R. (2002b). Transcultural nursing: Curricular concepts, principles, and teaching and learning activities for the 21st century. In M. Leininger & M. R. McFarland (Eds.). *Transcultural* nursing: Concepts, theories, research, & practice (3rd ed., pp. 527-561). New York: McGraw-Hill Medical Publishing Division.

Leininger, M. M., & McFarland, M. R. (Eds.). (2005). *Culture care diversity and universality: A worldwide theory of nursing* (2nd ed.). Sudbury, MA: Jones and Bartlett.

Leininger, M., & Watson, J. (Eds.). (1990). *The caring imperative in education*. New York: National League for Nursing Press.

McFarland, M. R. (1995). *Cultural care of Anglo and African American elderly residents within the environmental context of a long term care institution*. Detroit: Wayne State University Press.

McFarland, M. R. (2002). Part II: Selected research findings from the culture care theory. In M. Leininger & M. R. McFarland (Eds.), *Transcultural nursing: Concepts, theories, research, & practice* (3rd ed., pp. 99-116). New York: McGraw-Hill Medical Publishing Division.

Tom-Orne, L. (2002). Transcultural nursing and health care among Native American peoples. In M. M. Leininger & M. R. McFarland (Eds.), *Transcultural nursing: Concepts, theories, research, & practice* (3rd ed., pp. 429-440). New York: McGraw-Hill Medical Publishing Division.

BIBLIOGRAPHY
Primary Sources
Books

Gaut, D., & Leininger, M. (1991). *Caring: The compassionate healer*. New York: National League for Nursing Press.

Hofling, C. K., & Leininger, M. (1960). *Basic psychiatric concepts in nursing*. Philadelphia: J. B. Lippincott.

Leininger, M. (1970). *Nursing and anthropology: Two worlds to blend*. New York: John Wiley & Sons.

Leininger, M. (1973). *Contemporary issues in mental health nursing*. Boston: Little, Brown & Co.

Leininger, M. (Ed.). (1978). *Transcultural nursing care of the elderly*. Salt Lake City, UT: University of Utah, College of Nursing.

Leininger, M. (Ed.). (1979). *Transcultural nursing care of the adolescent and middle age adult*. Salt Lake City, UT: University of Utah, College of Nursing.

Leininger, M. (Ed.). (1979). *Transcultural nursing: Proceedings from four transcultural nursing conferences*. New York: Masson.

Leininger, M. (Ed.). (1981). *Caring: An essential and human need*. Thorofare, NJ: Charles B. Slack.

Leininger, M. (Ed.). (1984). *Caring: The essence of nursing and health*. Thorofare, NJ: Charles B. Slack.

Leininger, M. (Ed.). (1984). *Reference sources for transcultural health and nursing for teaching, curriculum, and clinical-field practice*. Thorofare, NJ: Charles B. Slack.

Leininger, M. (Ed.). (1985). *Qualitative research methods in nursing*. New York: Grune & Stratton.

Leininger, M. (Ed.). (1988). *Care: Discovery and uses in clinical and community nursing*. Detroit: Wayne State University Press.

Leininger, M. (1990). *Ethical and moral dimensions of care: Chapters from conference on the ethics and morality of caring*. Detroit: Wayne State University Press.

Leininger, M. (1991). *Culture care universality and diversity: A theory of nursing*. New York: National League for Nursing Press.

Leininger, M. (1995). *Transcultural Nursing: Concepts, theories, and practice* (2nd ed.). Columbus, OH: McGraw-Hill College Custom Series.

Leininger, M., & McFarland, M. R. (2002). *Transcultural Nursing: Concepts, theories, research, & practice* (3rd ed.). New York: McGraw-Hill Medical Publishing Division.

Leininger, M., & Watson, J. (Eds.). (1990). *The caring imperative in education*. New York: National League for Nursing Press.

Leininger, M. M., & McFarland, M. R. (Eds.). (2005). *Culture diversity & universality: A worldwide nursing theory* (2nd ed.). Sudbury, MA: Jones and Bartlett.

Book Chapters

Leininger, M. (1988). Culture care and nursing administration. In B. Henry, C. Arndt, M. DiVincenti, & A. Marriner Tomey (Eds.), *Dimensions of nursing administration*. Boston: Blackwell Scientific.

Leininger, M. (1990). Introduction: Care: The imperative of nursing education and service. In M. Leininger & J. Watson (Eds.), *The caring imperative in education*. New York: NLN Publication, Center for Human Caring.

Leininger, M. (1992). Reflections on Nightingale with a focus on human care theory and leadership. In F. Nightingale & B. S. Barnum (Eds.), *Nightingale: Notes on nursing: What it is, and what it is not*. Philadelphia: J. B. Lippincott.

Leininger, M. (1992). Theory of culture care and uses in clinical and community contexts. In M. Parker (Ed.), *Theories on nursing* (pp. 345-372). New York: National League for Nursing Press.

Leininger, M. (1992). Transcultural mental health nursing assessment of children and adolescents. In P. West & C. Sieloff Evans (Eds.), *Psychiatric and mental health nursing with children and adolescents* (pp. 53-58). Gaithersburg, MD: Aspen Publications.

Leininger, M. (1993). Culture care theory: The comparative global theory to advance human care nursing knowledge and practice. In D. Gaut (Ed.), *A global agenda for caring* (pp. 3-18). New York: National League for Nursing.

Leininger, M. (1993). Evaluation criteria and critique of qualitative research studies. In J. Morse (Ed.),

Qualitative nursing research: A contemporary dialogue (pp. 393-414). Newbury Park, CA: Sage Publications.

Leininger, M. (2002). Essential transcultural nursing concepts, principles, examples, and policy statements. In M. Leininger & M. R. McFarland (Eds.), *Transcultural nursing: Concepts, theories, research, & practice* (3rd ed., pp. 45-69). New York: McGraw-Hill Medical Publishing Division.

Leininger, M. (2002). Part I. The theory of culture care and the ethnonursing research method. In M. Leininger & M. R. McFarland (Eds.), *Transcultural nursing: Concepts, theories, research, & practice* (3rd ed., pp. 71-98). New York: McGraw-Hill Medical Publishing Division.

Leininger, M. (2002). The future of transcultural nursing: A global perspective. In M. Leininger & M. R. McFarland (Eds.), *Transcultural nursing: Concepts, theories, research, & practice* (3rd ed., pp. 577-595). New York: McGraw-Hill Medical Publishing Division.

Leininger, M. (2002). Transcultural nursing and globalization of health care: Importance, focus, and historical aspects. In M. Leininger & M. R. McFarland (Eds.), *Transcultural nursing: Concepts, theories, research, & practice* (3rd ed., pp. 3-43). New York: McGraw-Hill Medical Publishing Division.

McFarland, M., Hall, B., Buckwalter, K., Dumas, R., Haack, M., Leininger, M., et al. (1990). Group IV: Behavior problems/mental illness/addictions. In J. S. Stevens (Ed.), *Knowledge about care and caring: State of the art and future developments* (G-177, pp. 135-139). New York: ANA Publications, American Academy of Nursing.

Book Prefaces and Foreword

Leininger, M. (1978). Foreword. In J. Watson, *Nursing: The philosophy and science of caring.* Boston: Little, Brown & Co.

Leininger, M. (1983). Preface. In M. Leininger (Ed.), *Care: The essence of nursing and health.* Thorofare, NJ: Charles B. Slack.

Leininger, M. (1984). Preface. In M. Leininger, *Reference sources for transcultural health and nursing for teaching, curriculum, and clinical-field practice.* Thorofare, NJ: Charles B. Slack.

Journal Articles

Leininger, M. (1988). Leininger's theory of nursing: Cultural care diversity and universality. *Nursing Science Quarterly, 1*(4), 152-160.

Leininger, M. (1992). Transcultural nursing care values, beliefs, and practices of American (USA) gypsies. *Journal of Transcultural Nursing, 4*(1), 17-28.

Leininger, M. (1994). Nursing's agenda of health reform: Regressive or advanced—Discipline status. *Nursing Science Quarterly, 7*(2), 93-94.

Leininger, M. (1994). Reflections: Culturally congruent care: Visible and invisible. *Journal of Transcultural Nursing, 6*(1), 23-25.

Leininger, M. (1995). Culture care theory, research, and practice. *Nursing Science Quarterly, 9*(2), 71-78.

Leininger, M. (1995). Founder's focus: Nursing theories and cultures: Fit or misfit. *Journal of Transcultural Nursing, 7*(1), 41-42.

Leininger, M. (1995). Founder's focus: Transcultural nurses and consumers tell their stories. *Journal of Transcultural Nursing, 7*(2), 37-40.

Leininger, M., & Cummings, S. H. (1996). Nursing's new paradigm is transcultural nursing: An interview with Madeleine Leininger. *Advanced Nursing Practice Quarterly, 2*(2), 62-70.

Leininger, M. M. (1983). Creativity and challenges for nurse researchers in this economic recession: Part 2. *Nurse Educator, 8*(1), 13-14.

Leininger, M. M. (1984). Qualitative research methods—to document and discover nursing knowledge. *Western Journal of Nursing Research, 6*(2), 151-152.

Leininger, M. M. (1987). Importance and uses of ethnomethods: Ethnography and ethnonursing research. *Recent Advances in Nursing, 17,* 12-36.

Leininger, M. M. (1988). Leininger's theory of nursing: Cultural care diversity and universality. *Nursing Science Quarterly, 1*(4), 152-160.

Leininger, M. M. (1989). The Journal of Transcultural Nursing has become a reality. *Journal of Transcultural Nursing, 1*(1), 1-2.

Leininger, M. M. (1989). The transcultural nurse specialist: Imperative in today's world. *Nursing and Health Care, 10*(5), 250-256.

Leininger, M. M. (1989). Transcultural nurse specialists and generalists: New practitioners in nursing. *Journal of Transcultural Nursing, 1*(1), 4-16.

Leininger, M. M., (1989). Transcultural nursing: Quo vadis (where goeth the field)? *Journal of Transcultural Nursing, 1*(1), 33-45.

Leininger, M. M. (1990). A new and changing decade ahead: Are nurses prepared? *Journal of Transcultural Nursing, 1*(2), 1.

Leininger, M. M. (1990). Ethnomethods: The philosophic and epistemic bases to explicate transcultural nursing knowledge. *Journal of Transcultural Nursing, 1*(2), 40-51.

Leininger, M. M. (1990). Issues, questions, and concerns related to the nursing diagnosis cultural movement from a transcultural nursing perspective. *Journal of Transcultural Nursing, 2*(1), 23-32.

Leininger, M. M. (1990). Leininger clarifies transcultural nursing (Letter to the Editor). *International Nursing Review, 36*(6), 356.

Leininger, M. M. (1990). The significance of cultural concepts in nursing. 1966. *Journal of Transcultural Nursing, 2*(1), 52-59.

Leininger, M. M. (1991). Second reflection: Comparative care as central to transcultural nursing. *Journal of Transcultural Nursing, 3*(1), 2.

Leininger, M. M. (1991). Transcultural care principles, human rights, and ethical considerations. *Journal of Transcultural Nursing, 3*(1), 21-23.

Leininger, M. M. (1991). Transcultural nursing goals and challenges for 1991 and beyond. *Journal of Transcultural Nursing, 2*(2), 1-2.

Secondary Sources
Journal Articles

Berry, A. (1999). Mexican American women's expressions of the meaning of culturally congruent prenatal care. *Journal of Transcultural Nursing, 10*(3), 203-212.

Bialoskurski, M., Cox, C. L., & Hayes, J. A. (1999). The nature of attachment in a neonatal intensive care unit. *Journal of Perinatal and Neonatal Nursing, 10*(3), 66-77.

Brooke, D., & Omeri, A. (1999). Beliefs about childhood immunization among Lebanese Muslim immigrants in Australia. *Journal of Transcultural Nursing, 10*(3), 229-236.

George, T. (2000). Defining care in the culture of the chronically mentally ill living in the community. *Journal of Transcultural Nursing, 11*(2), 102-110.

Higgins, B. (2000). Puerto Rican cultural beliefs: Influence on infant feeding practices in western New York. *Journal of Transcultural Nursing, 11*(1), 19-30.

Lumberg, P. (2000). Culture care of Thai immigrants in Uppsala: A study of transcultural nursing in Sweden. *Journal of Transcultural Nursing, 11*(4), 274-280.

McFarland, M. R. (1997). Use of the culture care theory with Anglo- and African Americans in a long-term care setting. *Nursing Science Quarterly, 10*(4), 186-192.

Nahas, V., & Amasheh, N. (1999). Cultural care meanings and experiences of postpartum depression among Jordanian Australian women: A transcultural study. *Journal of Transcultural Nursing, 10*(1), 37-45.

Omeri, A. (1997). Culture care of Iranian immigrants in New South Wales, Australia: Sharing transcultural nursing knowledge. *Journal of Transcultural Nursing, 8*(2), 5-16.

Sellers, S. C., Poduska, M. D., Propp, L. H., & White, S. I. (1999). The health care meanings, values, and practices of Anglo American males in the rural Midwest. *Journal of Transcultural Nursing, 10*(4), 320-330.

Dissertations Mentored by Leininger

Berry, A. (1995). *Culture care statements, meanings, and expressions of Mexican American women within Leininger's culture care theory.* Unpublished doctoral dissertation, Wayne State University, Detroit.

Cameron, C. (1990). *An ethnonursing study of health status of elderly Anglo Canadian wives providing extended care-giving to their disabled husbands.* Unpublished doctoral dissertation, Wayne State University, Detroit.

Curtis, M. (1997). *Cultural care by private practice APRNs in community contexts.* Unpublished doctoral dissertation, Wayne State University, Detroit.

Ehrmin, J. (1998). *Culture care meanings and statements, and experiences of care of African American women residing in an inner city transitional home for substance abuse.* Unpublished doctoral dissertation, Wayne State University, Detroit.

Finn, J. (1993). *Professional nurse and generic caregiving of childbearing women conceptualized with Leininger's theory of culture care theory.* Unpublished doctoral dissertation, Wayne State University, Detroit.

Gates, M. (1988). *Care and meanings, experiences and orientations of persons dying in hospitals and hospital settings.* Unpublished doctoral dissertation, Wayne State University, Detroit.

Gelazis, R. (1994). *Lithuanian care: Meanings and experiences with humor using Leininger's culture care theory.* Unpublished doctoral dissertation, Wayne State University, Detroit.

George, T. (1998). *Meanings and statements and experiences of care of chronically mentally ill in a day treatment center using Leininger's culture care theory.* Unpublished doctoral dissertation, Wayne State University, Detroit.

Horton, G. (1998). *Culture care by private practice APRN in a community context.* Unpublished doctoral dissertation, Wayne State University, Detroit.

Lamp, J. (1998). *Generic and professional care meanings and practices of Finnish women in birth within Leininger's theory of culture care diversity and universality.* Unpublished doctoral dissertation, Wayne State University, Detroit.

Luna, L. (1989). *Care and cultural context of Lebanese Muslims in an urban US community within Leininger's culture care theory.* Unpublished doctoral dissertation, Wayne State University, Detroit.

MacNeil, J. (1994). *Cultural care: Meanings, patterns, and expressions for Baganda women as AIDS caregivers within Leininger's theory.* Unpublished doctoral dissertation, Wayne State University, Detroit.

McFarland, M. R. (1995). *Cultural care of Anglo and African American elderly residents within the environmental context of a long term care institution.* Unpublished doctoral dissertation, Wayne State University, Detroit.

Miller, J. E. (1996). *Politics and care: A study of Czech Americans within Leininger's theory of culture care diversity and universality.* Unpublished doctoral dissertation, Wayne State University, Detroit.

Morgan, M. (1994). *African American neonatal care in northern and southern contexts using Leininger's culture care theory.* Unpublished doctoral dissertation, Wayne State University, Detroit.

Morris, E. (2004). *Culture care values, meanings, and experiences of African American adolescent gang members.* Unpublished doctoral dissertation, Wayne State University, Detroit.

Omeri, A. S. (1996). *Transcultural nursing care values, beliefs, and practices of Iranian immigrants in New South Wales, Australia.* Unpublished doctoral dissertation, University of Sydney, Sydney, Australia.

Rosenbaum, J. (1990). *Cultural care, culture health and grief phenomena related to older Greek Canadian widows with Leininger's theory of culture care.* Unpublished doctoral dissertation, Wayne State University, Detroit.

Spangler, Z. (1991). *Nursing care values and practices of Philippine American and Anglo American nurses.* Unpublished doctoral dissertation, Wayne State University, Detroit.

Stitzlein, D. (1999). *The phenomenon of moral care/caring conceptualized within Leininger's theory of culture care diversity and universality.* Unpublished doctoral dissertation, Wayne State University, Detroit.

Thompson, T. (1990). *A qualitative investigation of rehabilitation nursing care in an inpatient rehabilitation unit using Leininger's theory.* Unpublished doctoral dissertation, Wayne State University, Detroit.

Villarruel, A. (1993). *Mexican American cultural meanings, expressions: Self care and dependent care actions associated with experiences of pain.* Unpublished doctoral dissertation, Wayne State University, Detroit.

Welch, A. (1987). *Concepts of health, illness, caring, aging, and problems of adjustment among elderly Filipinas residing in Hampton Roads, Virginia.* Unpublished doctoral dissertation, University of Utah, Salt Lake City.

Wenger, A. F. (1988). *The phenomenon of care of old order Amish: A high context culture.* Unpublished doctoral dissertation, Wayne State University, Detroit.

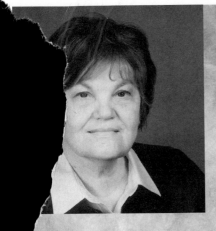

$\mathcal{M}$argaret A. Newman

1933-present

Health as Expanding Consciousness

Janet Witucki Brown

CREDENTIALS AND BACKGROUND OF THE THEORIST

Margaret A. Newman was born on October 10, 1933, in Memphis, Tennessee. She earned her first bachelor's degree in home economics and English from Baylor University in Waco, Texas, in 1954, and she earned her second bachelor's degree in nursing from the University of Tennessee in Memphis in 1962 (M. Newman, curriculum vitae, 1996).

Newman received her master's degree in medical-surgical nursing and teaching from the University of California, San Francisco, in 1964. She earned her

Previous authors: Snehlata Desai, M. Jan Keffer, DeAnn M. Hensley, Kimberly A. Kilgore-Keever, Jill Vass Langfitt, and LaPhyllis Peterson.
The author wishes to thank Margaret A. Newman for her contributions to the chapter.

Ph.D. in nursing science and rehabilitation nursing in 1971 from New York University in New York City.

Newman progressed through the academic ranks at the University of Tennessee, New York University, and Pennsylvania State University and was a professor at the University of Minnesota in Minneapolis until her retirement in 1996. She has been Professor Emeritus at the University of Minnesota since 1996 (M. Newman, curriculum vitae, 2000). In addition, she has been the Director of Nursing for the Clinical Research Center at the University of Tennessee, the Acting Director of the Ph.D. program in the Division of Nursing at New York University, and Professor-in-Charge of the Graduate Program and Research in Nursing at Pennsylvania State University.

Newman was admitted to the American Academy of Nursing in 1976. She received the Outstanding Alumnus Award from the University of Tennessee

College of Nursing in Memphis in both 1975 and 2002, the Distinguished Alumnus Award from the Division of Nursing at New York University in 1984, and she was admitted to the hall of fame at the University of Mississippi School of Nursing in 1988 (M. Newman, curriculum vitae, 2000; personal correspondence, 2004). She was a Latin-American teaching fellow in 1976 and 1977 and an *American Journal of Nursing* scholar in 1979. She was Distinguished Faculty at the Seventh International Conference on Human Functioning at Wichita, Kansas, in 1983, and she received the E. Louis Grant Award for Nursing Excellence from the University of Minnesota in 1996. She is listed in *Who's Who in American Women, Who's Who in America,* and *Who's Who in American Nursing.* Newman was included as one of the featured nursing theorists in the videotape series sponsored by Helene Fuld Health Trust in 1990 (M. Newman, curriculum vitae, 2000). She was a Distinguished Resident at Westminster College in Salt Lake City, Utah, in 1991. She received the Distinguished Scholar in Nursing Award, New York University Division of Nursing in 1992, the Sigma Theta Tau Founders Elizabeth McWilliams Miller Award for Excellence in Research in 1993, and the Nurse Scholar Award at Saint Xavier University School of Nursing in 1994 (M. Newman, personal correspondence, 1996; curriculum vitae, 2000).

In 1978, Newman presented her ideas on a theory of health for the first time at a conference on nursing theory in New York. During that time, she was also pursuing research on the relationship of movement, time, and consciousness and was expanding development of the theory of health as expanding consciousness.

In 1985, as a traveling research fellow, Newman conducted workshops in four locations in New Zealand (M. Newman, personal correspondence, 1988). At the University of Tampere, Finland, in 1985, Newman was the major speaker for a week-long conference on the theory of consciousness as it related to nursing (M. Newman, personal correspondence, 1988).

Newman has presented many papers on topics pertaining to her theory of health as expanding consciousness. She published *Theory Development in Nursing* (1979), *Health as Expanding Consciousness* (1986, 1994), and *A Developing Discipline: Selected Works of Margaret Newman* (1995a). written numerous journal articles and book chapters. In 1986, she did a case study analysis of practice in three sites within the Minneapolis area in which she discussed the background of the health care system, findings within each site, and conclusions concerning the changes necessary in hospital nursing practice (Newman & Autio,). From 1986 to 1997, Newman investigated sequential patterns of persons with heart disease and cancer in relation to the theory of health as expanding consciousness (Newman, 1995c; Newman & Moch, 1991). Her more recent publications reflect her passion for integration of nursing theory, practice, and research. Her evolving viewpoints on trends in philosophy of nursing, analysis of theoretical models of nursing practice, and nursing research are noteworthy (Newman, 1992, 1997b, 1999, 2003).

During 1989 and 1990, Newman was the principal investigator of a project that explored the theory and structure of a professional model of nursing practice. This research was conducted at Carondelet St. Mary's Community Hospitals and Health Centers in Tucson, Arizona (Newman, 1990c; Newman, Lamb, & Michaels, 1991).

In addition to her research and teaching, Newman is sought for consultation regarding the expansion of her theory of health in more than 40 states and Australia, Brazil, Canada, Finland, Germany, Japan, New Zealand, and the United Kingdom (M. Newman, curriculum vitae, 1992). Newman has served on several editorial review panels, including those of *Nursing Research, Western Journal of Nursing Research, Nursing and Health Care, Advances in Nursing Science,* and *Nursing Science Quarterly* (M. Newman, curriculum , 1992). She is currently on the advisory board of *Advances in Nursing Science* (M. Newman, correspondence, 2004). She also participated member of the nurse theorist task force to 1982 with the North American Nursing sis Association (NANDA).

RELATIONSHIP TO METAPARADIGM CONCEPTS

Newman has designated "caring in the human health experience" (M. Newman, personal correspondence 2004; Newman, Sime, & Corcoran-Perry, 1991, p. 3) as the focus of the nursing discipline and has specified this focus as the metaparadigm of the discipline. She asserts that the interrelated concepts of nursing, person, health, and environment are inherent in this focus (M. Newman, personal correspondence, 2004). Coming from a unitary, transformative paradigm of the discipline, Newman does not see these concepts in isolation. Therefore, she does not discuss them separately in her books, but she has elaborated on some of these dimensions, particularly nursing and health, in explications of her position. In the following paragraphs, implicit definitions from Newman's work are used to discuss the four components.

Nursing

From the Newman perspective, the role of the nurse is to help clients get in touch with the meaning of their lives by identification of their patterns of relating (M. Newman, personal correspondence, 2004). Intervention is a form of nonintervention whereby the nurse's presence assists clients to recognize their own patterns of interacting with the environment (M. Newman, telephone interview, 2000). Insight into these patterns provides clients with illumination of action possibilities, which then opens the way for transformation (Newman, 1990a).

The nurse facilitates pattern recognition in clients by forming relationships with them at critical points in their lives and connecting with them in an authentic way. The nurse-client relationship is characterized by "a rhythmic coming together and moving apart as clients encounter disruption of their organized, predictable state" (Newman, 1999, p. 228). She further states that the nurse will continue to connect with clients as they move through the period of disorganization and unpredictability to arrive at a higher, organized state (Newman, 1999). The nurse comes together with clients at these critical choice points in their lives and participates with them in the process of expanding consciousness. The relationship is one of rhythmicity and timing, with the nurse letting go of the need to direct the relationship or fix things. As the nurse relinquishes the need to manipulate or control, there is a greater ability to enter into this fluctuating, rhythmic partnership with the client (Newman, 1999).

Nurses are seen as partners in the process of expanding consciousness. The nurse can connect with the person when an understanding of changing circumstances is sought (M. Newman, telephone interview, 2000). As a facilitator, the nurse helps an individual, family, or community focus on patterns of relating (M. Newman, telephone interview, 2004). The nursing process is one of pattern recognition.

Newman's early suggestion (Newman, 1995b) was that the NANDA health assessment framework, based on unitary person-environment patterns of interaction, be used to facilitate clients' pattern recognition. These nine patterns of interaction consist of dimensions of the following: (1) choosing, (2) communicating, (3) exchanging, (4) feeling, (5) knowing, (6) moving, (7) perceiving, (8) relating, and (9) valuing (Roy, Rogers, Fitzpatrick, Neuman, & Orem, 1982). At the time, the patterns were intended to guide nurses to make holistic observations of "person-environment behaviors that together depict a very specific pattern of the whole for each person" (Newman, 1995b, p. 261). Newman has since emphasized concentrating on what is most meaningful to clients in their own stories and patterns of relating (M. Newman, telephone interview, 2000). Descriptions of the evolving pattern of the person are presented as sequential patterns over time (Newman, 1990b).

"Pattern recognition comes from within the observer" (Newman, 1987b, p. 38). The nurse perceives the patterns in the patient's stories or sequence of events and the pattern of the individual changes with the new information. The process of pattern recognition first involves an attempt to view the pattern of a person as "sequential patterns over time" (Newman, 1987b, p. 38). Follow-up interviews are conducted to share the nurse's perspective with the client. The nurse can use this process to facilitate the client's pattern recognition insight regarding action possibilities (Newman, 1987b).

Person

Throughout Newman's work, the terms *client, patient, person, individual,* and *human being* are used interchangeably. Persons as individuals are identified by their individual patterns of consciousness (Newman, 1986). Persons are further defined as "centers of consciousness within an overall pattern of expanding consciousness" (Newman, 1986, p. 31). The definition of persons has also been expanded to include family and community (Newman, 1986, 1994).

Environment

Environment is not explicitly defined but is described as being the larger whole, which is beyond the consciousness of the individual. The pattern of consciousness that is the person interacts within the pattern of consciousness that is the family and within the pattern of community interactions (Newman, 1986). A major assumption is that "consciousness is coextensive in the universe and resides in all matter" (Newman, 1986, p. 33).

Newman identifies interactions between person and environment as a key process that creates unique configurations for each individual. Patterns of person-environment evolve to higher levels of consciousness of the self. The assumption is that all matter in the universe-environment possesses consciousness, but at different levels. Interpretation of Newman's view clarifies that health is the interaction pattern of a person with the environment. Disease in a human energy field is a manifestation of a unique pattern of person-environment interaction (Figure 23-1).

Health

Health is the major concept of Newman's theory of expanding consciousness. A fusion of disease and nondisease creates a synthesis that is regarded as health (Newman, 1978, 1979, 1991, 1992). Disease and nondisease are each reflections of the larger whole; therefore, a new concept, "pattern of the whole," is formed (Newman, 1986, p. 12). Newman (1999) has further elaborated her view of health by stating that "health is the pattern of the whole, and wholeness *is*" (p. 228). Further, this wholeness cannot be gained or lost. Within this perspective, becoming ill does not diminish wholeness, but wholeness takes on a different form. Newman (1986) has stated that pattern recognition is the essence of the emerging of health. "Manifest health, encompassing disease and non-disease can be regarded as the explication of the underlying pattern of person-environment" (Newman, 1994, p. 11). Therefore, health and the evolving pattern of consciousness are the same (Newman, 1994).

THEORETICAL SOURCES

The theory of health as expanding consciousness stems from Rogers' (1980) science of unitary human beings. Rogers' assumptions regarding wholeness, pattern, and unidirectionality are the foundation of Newman's theory (M. Newman, personal correspondence, 2004). Hegel's process of the fusion of opposites (Acton, 1967) helped Newman to conceptualize the fusion of health and illness into a new concept of health. Bentov's (1977) explication of life as the process of expanding consciousness prompted Newman to assert that this new concept of health is the process of expanding consciousness (M. Newman, personal correspondence, 2004).

Bohm's (1980) theory of implicate order supports Newman's postulate that disease is a manifestation of the pattern of health. Newman (1994) stated she began to comprehend "the underlying, unseen pattern that manifests itself in varying forms, including disease, and the interconnectedness and omnipresence of all that there is" (p. xxvi). Young's (1976) theory of human evolution pinpointed the role of pattern recognition for Newman. She explained that Young's ideas provided the impetus for her efforts to integrate the basic

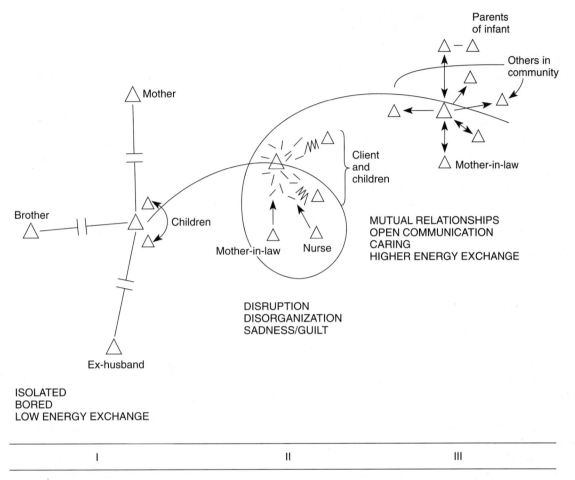

Figure **23-1** Sequential patterns of person-environment relations. (From Newman, M. A. [1987]. Nursing's emerging paradigm: The diagnosis of pattern. In A. M. McLane [Ed.], *Classification of nursing diagnoses: Proceedings of the seventh conference.* St. Louis: Mosby.)

concepts of her new theory, movement, space, time, and consciousness, into a dynamic portrayal of life and health (Newman, 1994). Further, Moss' (1981) experience of love as the highest level of consciousness was important to Newman in providing affirmation and elaboration of her intuition regarding the nature of health (Newman, 1994). Newman also incorporated Prigogine's (1976) theory of dissipative structures as an explanation for the timing of nursing presence as the patient fluctuates from one level of organization to a higher level (M. Newman, personal correspondence, 2004).

Although Newman (1997a) acknowledges the contributions of these theories to her theory, she has stated that her theory "was enriched by them, but was not based on them" (p. 23). She emphasizes that her theory emerged from a new science of unitary human beings.

MAJOR CONCEPTS & DEFINITIONS

HEALTH

Health encompasses disease and nondisease. Health can be regarded as the evolving pattern of the person and the environment (Newman, 1986). Health is viewed as a process of developing awareness of self and environment together with an increasing ability to perceive alternatives and respond in a variety of ways (Newman, 1978). Health is viewed as the "pattern of the whole" of a person and is further described as including disease as a meaningful manifestation of the pattern of the whole, based on the premise that life is an ongoing process of expanding consciousness (Newman, 1986).

Using Hegel's dialectical fusion of opposites, Newman explained how the concept disease fuses with its opposite, nondisease or absence of disease, to create a new concept, health. She explained that this new paradigm of health is relational and is "patterned, emergent, unpredictable, unitary, intuitive, and innovative," whereas the traditional paradigm is linear, "causal, predictive, dichotomous, rational, and controlling" (Newman, 1994, p. 13). However, she appears to take the characteristics of the old paradigm of health as special cases of the new holistic paradigm to find patterns and new meaning. To her, health and the evolving pattern of consciousness are the same. The essence of the emerging paradigm of health is recognition of pattern. Newman (1994) sees the life process as a progression toward higher levels of consciousness.

PATTERN

Pattern is seen as information that depicts the whole, and understanding of the meaning of all of the relationships at once (M. Newman, personal correspondence, 2004). It is conceptualized as a fundamental attribute of all there is, and Newman (1986) sees it as giving unity in diversity. Pattern is what identifies an individual as a particular person. An example of explicit manifestations of

the underlying pattern of a person would be the genetic pattern that contains information that directs becoming, the voice pattern, and the movement pattern (Newman, 1986). Characteristics of pattern include movement, diversity, and rhythm. Pattern is further conceptualized as being somehow intimately involved in both energy exchange and transformation (Newman, 1986). According to Newman (1987b), "*Whatever* manifests itself in a person's life is the explication of the underlying implicate pattern . . . the phenomenon we call health is the manifestation of that evolving pattern" (p. 37).

In *Health as Expanding Consciousness,* Newman (1986, 1994) developed pattern as a major concept that was used to understand the individual as a whole being. Newman described a paradigm shift that was occurring in the field of health care. The shift was from treatment of symptoms of a disease to the search for patterns and the meaning of those patterns. Newman (1986) stated that the patterns of interaction of person-environment constitute health. Embedded within the concepts of movement, time, and space is the idea that an event such as a disease occurrence is part of a larger process. By interacting with the event, no matter how destructive the force might seem to be, its energy augments the person's own energy and enhances his or her own power in the situation. To see this, it is necessary to grasp the pattern of the whole (Newman, 1986).

CONSCIOUSNESS

Consciousness is defined as both the informational capacity of the system and the ability of the system to interact with its environment (Newman, 1986). Newman asserted that an understanding of her definition of consciousness is essential to understanding the theory. Consciousness includes not only cognitive and affective awareness, but also the "interconnectedness of the entire living system which includes physicochemical maintenance and growth processes as well as the immune system" (Newman, 1990a, p. 38). In 1978, Newman identified three correlates of consciousness (time, movement, and space) as explanations for the changing pattern of the whole and major concepts in the theory of health.

The life process was seen as a progression toward higher levels of consciousness. Newman (1971) viewed the expansion of consciousness as what life, and therefore health, was all about. She referred to the sense of time as a factor altered in the changing level of consciousness.

Bentov (1977) defined absolute consciousness as "a state in which contrasting concepts become reconciled and fused. Movement and rest fuse into one" (p. 67). The last stage of absolute consciousness is equated with love, where all opposites are reconciled and all experiences are accepted equally

and unconditionally, such as love and hate, pain and pleasure, and disease and nondisease.

Reed (1996) concurred that Newman's theory described the phase of evolutionary development at which the person moves beyond a focus on self as limited by time, space, and physical concerns. Transcendence is a process through which the person moves to a high level of consciousness.

MOVEMENT-SPACE-TIME

Newman states that it is important to examine movement-space-time as dimensions of emerging patterns of consciousness, not in isolation as separate concepts of the theory, like in the old paradigm (M. Newman, personal correspondence, 2004). Therefore, movement, space, and time, are no longer considered major concepts of the theory as they were in earlier works.

USE OF EMPIRICAL EVIDENCE

Evidence for the theory of health as expanding consciousness emanated from Newman's early personal family experiences. Her mother's struggle with amyotrophic lateral sclerosis, a chronic illness, and her dependence on Newman, then a young college graduate, sparked an interest in nursing. From that experience evolved the idea that "illness reflected the life patterns of the person and that what was needed was the recognition of that pattern and acceptance of it for what it meant to that person" (Newman, 1986, p. 3).

Throughout Newman's writing (1986), terms are used such as *call to nursing, growing conscience-like feeling, fear, power, meaning of life and health, belief of life after death, rituals of health,* and *love.* The terms provide a clue concerning Newman's endeavors to make a disturbing life experience logical. The life experience triggered her beginning maturation toward theory development in nursing. Within

her philosophical framework, Newman began to develop a synthesis of disease-nondisease-health as recognition of the total patterning of a person.

Research has been conducted on the theoretical sources (Newman, 1987b). In 1979, Newman wrote that in order for nursing research to have meaning in terms of theory development, it must have three components. These components are as follows: (1) having as its purpose the testing of theory, (2) making explicit the theoretical framework upon which the testing relies, and (3) reexamining the theoretical underpinnings in light of the findings (Newman, 1979). She believed that if health is considered an individual personal process, research should focus on studies that explore changes and similarities in personal meaning and patterns.

MAJOR ASSUMPTIONS

The foundation for Newman's assumptions (M. Newman, telephone interview, 2000) is her definition of health, which is grounded in Rogers' 1970 model for nursing, specifically the focus on wholeness, pattern, and unidirectionality. From this, Newman (1979) developed the following assumptions:

1. Health encompasses conditions heretofore described as illness or, in medical terms, pathology . . .
2. These "pathological" conditions can be considered a manifestation of the total pattern of the individual . . .
3. The pattern of the individual that eventually manifests itself as pathology is primary and exists prior to structural or functional changes . . .
4. Removal of the pathology in itself will not change the pattern of the individual . . .
5. If becoming "ill" is the only way an individual's pattern can manifest itself, then that is health for that person . . .
6. Health is the expansion of consciousness . . . (pp. 57-58)

Newman's implicit assumptions about human nature include being unitary, being an open system, being in continuous interconnectedness with the open system of the universe, and being continuously engaged in an evolving pattern of the whole (M. Newman, telephone interview, 2000). Newman (1971) developed her central premise and assumption, "Health is the expansion of consciousness" (p. 58). Unfolding consciousness is a process that will occur regardless of what actions nurses perform. Nurses can assist clients in getting in touch with what is going on and, in that way, facilitate the process (Newman, 1994).

THEORETICAL ASSERTIONS AND DEVELOPMENT
Early Designation of Concepts and Propositions

Early definition of concepts and propositions focused heavily on the concepts of movement, space, time, and consciousness. In *Theory Development in Nursing*, Newman, (1979) delineated the relationships between movement, space, time, and consciousness. One proposition was that there was a complimentary relationship between time and space (Newman, 1979, 1983). Newman gave examples of this relationship at the macrocosmic, microcosmic, and humanistic (everyday) levels. She stated that, at the humanistic level, highly mobile individuals live in a world of expanded space and compartmentalized time. There is an inverse relationship between space and time in that when a person's life space is decreased, such as by either physical or social immobility, that person's time is increased (Newman, 1979).

Movement is said to be a "means whereby space and time become a reality" (Newman, 1979, p. 60; 1983, p. 165). Humankind is in a constant state of motion and is constantly changing. This occurs both internally (at the cellular level) and externally (through body movement and interaction with the environment). This movement through time and space is what gives humankind a unique perception of reality. Movement brings change and enables the individual to experience the world (Newman, 1979).

Movement is also referred to as a "reflection of consciousness" (Newman, 1979, p. 60; 1983, p. 165). Movement is the means of experiencing reality and also the means by which an individual expresses thoughts and feelings about the reality of experiences. An individual conveys his or her awareness of self through the movement involved in language, posture, and body movement (Newman, 1979). An indication of the internal organization of a person and that person's perception of the world can be found in the rhythm and pattern of the person's movement. Movement patterns provide additional communication beyond that which language can convey (Newman, 1979).

The concept of time is seen as a function of movement (Newman, 1979). This assertion is supported by Newman's (1972) previous studies regarding the experience of time as related to movement and gait tempo. Newman's research showed that the slower an individual walks, the less subjective time he or she experiences. However, when compared with clock time, time seems to "fly." Although the individual who is moving quickly subjectively feels that he or she is "beating the clock," the individual finds that time seems to be dragging when checking a clock (Newman, 1971, 1979).

Time is also conceptualized as a measure of consciousness (Newman, 1979). Bentov (1977), who measured consciousness with a ratio of subjective to objective time, first proposed this assertion. Newman applied this measure of consciousness to the subjective and objective data compiled in her research. She found that the consciousness index increased with age. Some of her research has also supported the finding of "increasing consciousness with age" (Newman, 1982, p. 293). Newman cited this evidence as support for her position that the life process evolves toward consciousness expansion. However, she asserted that certain moods, such as depression, might be accompanied by a diminished sense of time (Newman & Gaudiano, 1984).

Synthesis of Patterns of Movement, Space-Time, and Consciousness

As the theory evolved, Newman developed a synthesis of pattern movement, space, time, and consciousness (M. Newman, personal correspondence, 2004). Time in the theory of health as expanding consciousness was not merely conceptualized as either subjective or objective, but was also viewed in a holographic sense (M. Newman, telephone interview, 2000). According to Newman (1994), "Each moment has an explicate order and also enfolds all others, meaning that each moment of our lives contains all others of all time" (p. 62).

Newman (1986) used excellent examples to illustrate the centrality of space-time, one of which is as follows:

> Mrs. V. made repeated attempts to *move* away from her husband and to *move* into an educational program to become more independent. She felt she had no *space* for herself, and she tried to distance herself (space) from her husband. She felt she had no *time* for leisure (self), was overworked, and was constantly meeting other people's needs. She was submissive to the demands and criticism of her husband. (p. 56)

Space, time, and movement later became linked with Newman's (1986) assertion that the intersection of movement-space-time represented the person as a center of consciousness. Further, this varied from person to person, place to place, and time to time. Newman (1986) also emphasized that the crucial task of nursing is to be able to see the concepts of movement-space-and time relational to each other, and all at once, recognizing patterns of evolving consciousness.

In *Health as Expanding Consciousness* (Newman, 1986, 1994), Newman's theory encompassed the work of Young's spectrum of consciousness (Young, 1976). She saw Young's central theme as being that self, or universe, were of the same nature. This essential nature could not be defined but was characterized by complete freedom and unrestricted choice at both the beginning and the end (Newman, 1986).

Newman established a corollary between her model of health as expanding consciousness and Young's conception of the evolution of human beings (Figure 23-2). She explained that individuals came into being from a state of consciousness, they were bound in time, found their identity in space, and through movement they learned the "law" of the way that things worked and then made choices that ultimately took them beyond space and time to a state of absolute consciousness (Newman, 1986).

Newman (1986) also stated that restrictions in movement-space-time have the effect of forcing an awareness that extends beyond the physical self. When natural movement is altered, space and time are also altered. When movement is restricted (physical or social), it is necessary for an individual to move beyond self, thereby making movement an important choice point in the process of evolving human consciousness (Newman, 1994). She assumed that the awareness corresponded to the "inward, self-generated reformation that Young [spoke] of as the turning point of the process" (Newman, 1994, p. 46). When a person progresses to the sixth state, which is timelessness, there is increasing freedom from time (Newman, 1986). Finally, the last stage is absolute consciousness, which Newman asserted is equated with love (Newman, 1986).

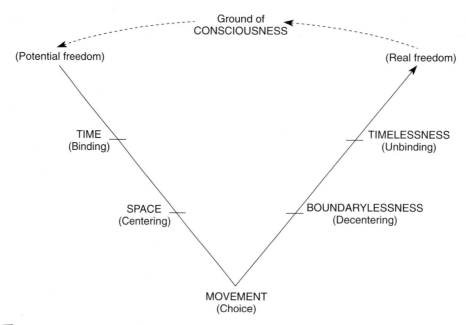

Figure 23-2 Parallel between Newman's theory of expanding consciousness and Young's stages of human evolution. (From Newman, M. A. [1990]. Newman's theory of health as praxis. *Nursing Science Quarterly, 3*[1], 37-41.)

Emphasis on Experiential Process of Nurse-Client

As Newman realized that the early research testing of propositional statements stemmed from a mechanistic view of movement-space-time-consciousness and failed to honor the basic assumptions of her theory, she shifted the focus of the research to authentic involvement of the nurse researcher as a participant with the client in the unfolding pattern of expanding consciousness (M. Newman, personal correspondence, 2004). The unitary, transformative paradigm demanded that the research honor and reveal the mutuality of interaction between nurse and client, the uniqueness and wholeness of pattern in each client situation, and movement of the life process toward higher consciousness.

The protocol for this research was first started in 1994, and variations of this guide continue to be implemented in current praxis research. Litchfield (1999) explicated this process as "practice wisdom"

in her work with families of hospitalized children, and Endo (1998) analyzed the phases of the process in her work with women with ovarian cancer. The data of this praxis research reveal evidence of expanding consciousness in the quality and connectedness of the client's relationships and support the importance of the nurse's creative presence in the participant's insight (M. Newman, personal correspondence, 2004).

LOGICAL FORM

In the early development of the theory, Newman used both inductive and deductive logic. Inductive logic is based on observing particular instances and then relating those instances to form a whole. Newman's theory development was derived from her earlier research on time perception and gait tempo. Time and movement, with space and consciousness, were used subsequently as central components in her early conceptual framework. These concepts helped explain "the phenomena of the life process and therefore of health" (Newman, 1979, p. 59). Newman (1997b) has described the evolution of the theory as it moved from linear explication and testing of concepts of time, space, and movement to an elaboration of interacting patterns as manifestations of expanding consciousness. Illumination of the theory of health as expanding consciousness as a process of evolving, in conjunction with the research, progressed through several stages (Newman, 1997a, 1997b). These stages included testing the relationships of the concepts of movement, space, and time, identifying sequential person-environmental patterns, and recognizing the centrality of nurse-client relationships or dialogue in the clients' evolving insight and accompanying potential for action. The process actually became cyclical as the original concepts of movement-space-time emerged as dimensions in the unitary evolving process of consciousness (Newman, 1997a).

ACCEPTANCE BY THE NURSING COMMUNITY

Practice

In Newman's view, the responsibility of professional nursing practice is to establish a primary relationship with the client for the purpose of identifying meaningful patterns and facilitating the client's action potential and decision-making ability (M. Newman, personal correspondence, 2004). Communication and collaboration with other nurses, associates, and health care professionals are essential (Newman, 1989). Maintenance of a direct, ongoing relationship so long as nursing consultation and services are required is the structure of the practice. Such primary care providers, focusing directly and completely, relate to her view of the role of professional nursing, which Newman (Newman, Lamb, & Michaels, 1991) referred to as *nursing clinician–case manager,* which is the sine qua non of the integrative model.

Relating her theory of health as expanding consciousness and acknowledging the contemporary and radical shift in philosophy of nursing that views health as a unitary human field dynamic embedded in a larger unitary field, Newman (1979) believes that "the goal of nursing is not to make people well, or to prevent their getting sick, but to assist people to utilize the power that is within them as they evolve toward higher levels of consciousness" (p. 67). She stated that the task of nursing is not to try to change the pattern of another person, but to recognize it as information that depicts the whole and relate to it as it unfolds (Newman, 1994).

Newman's more recent works have elaborated on the role of nursing practice in the theory. From the Newman perspective, nursing is the study of "caring in the human health experience" (Newman, Sime, & Corcoran-Perry, 1991, p. 3). Within this framework, the role of the nurse in this experience is to help clients recognize their own patterns, which results in the illumination of action possibilities that open the way for transformation to occur (M. Newman, personal correspondence, 1990).

At first, Newman's theory of health was useful in the practice of nursing because it contained concepts used by the nursing profession. Movement and time are an intrinsic part of nursing intervention, such as range-of-motion and ambulation (Newman, 1987a). During the 1980s, Barbara Doberneck (telephone interview, 1985) used Newman's theory to work with caregivers of chronically ill people. Doberneck (telephone interview, 1985) believed Newman's theory addressed issues intrinsic to caring that other theories omitted, such as unconditionally being with another person and noncommitment to specific predetermined outcomes.

Also during the 1980s, Joanne Marchione, within the context of health as expanding consciousness, investigated and reported the meaning of disabling events in families (J. Marchione, telephone interview, 1986). She presented a case study in which an additional person became part of the nuclear family for an extended period. The addition was a disruptive event for the family and created disturbances in time, space, movement, and consciousness. Analysis of the case study of the family suggested that Newman's work with patterns could be used to understand family interactions (J. Marchione, telephone interview, 1985; Marchione, 1986). Marchione has also advocated application of the theory to practice with communities (J. Marchione, telephone interview, 1985).

Kalb applied Newman's theory of health in the clinical management of pregnant women hospitalized for complications of maternal-fetal health. The pregnant woman is the conduit through which care can be delivered to the unborn child; therefore, she becomes the choice maker for the care of the child (Kalb, 1990).

Gustafson found that practice as a parish nurse supported Newman's theory of health as demonstration of pattern recognition. Patient needs were based on communication, decisions, and actions in the process of development of pattern recognition (Gustafson, 1990).

More recently, the theory has been used in practice with various client populations. Endo has studied pattern recognition as nursing intervention with adults with cancer (Endo, 1998; Endo et al., 2000). Litchfield (1993) described the patterning of nurse-client relationships in families with frequent illnesses and hospitalizations of toddlers. Additionally, Magan, Gibbon, and Mrozek (1990) reported on implementation of the theory, as one of several theories, in the care of the mentally ill. Weingourt (1998) reported on use of Newman's theory of health with elderly nursing home residents.

Quinn's (1992) reconceptualization of therapeutic touch described a shared consciousness. Schubert (1989) viewed the nurse-client relationship as progressing from trusting, through joining, to bonding, and Lamb and Stempel (1994) described the role of the nurse as an insider-expert. Newman, Lamb, and Michaels (1991) described the role of the nurse case manager at St. Mary's as emanating from a philosophical and theoretical base agreeing with the unitary-transformative paradigm and exemplifying an integrated stage of professional nursing. Further, the theory of health as expanding consciousness has been proposed as beneficial for the school nurse and the adolescent with insulin-dependent diabetes (Schlotzhauer & Farnham, 1997). Finally, Flannagan and colleagues reported

on the use of the theory in development of a preadmission nursing practice model and its use at Massachusetts General Hospital (Flannagan, 2002; Flannagan et al., 2000).

From the inception of Newman's theory in 1971 until the present, numerous nurse practitioners and scientists have used the theory either to incorporate the concepts in their nursing practice or to elaborate the theory in research. Newman advocates a convergence of nursing theories as the basis of the discipline (Newman, 2003). She sees health as expanding consciousness as emerging from a Rogerian perspective, incorporating theories of caring, and projecting a transformative process (Newman, 2005).

Newman has consulted with faculty and students from numerous universities. Graduate students at various institutions continue to conduct research based on her theory.

Newman's theory of pattern recognition provides the basis for the process of nurse-client interaction. Newman (1986) suggested that the task in intervention is pattern recognition accomplished by the health professional becoming aware of the pattern of the other person by becoming in touch with their own pattern. Newman (1986) suggested that the professional should focus on the pattern of the other person, acting as the "reference beam in a hologram" (p. 70). The holographic model of intervention is described by "imagining the emanating waves that appear when two pebbles are thrown into water. As the waves radiate ... they meet and interact ... [forming] an interference pattern" (Newman, 1986, p. 70) (Figure 23-3).

Education

Newman (1986) stated that a new role is needed for the nurse to function in the paradigm of the evolving consciousness of the whole. "Nurses need to be free to relate to patients in an ongoing partnership that is not limited to a particular place or time " (p. 89). Newman (1986) suggested that nursing education should revolve around pattern as a concept, substance, process, and method. Education by this method would enable nursing to be an important resource for the continued development of health

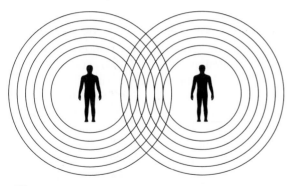

Figure **23-3** Interaction pattern of two persons—a holographic model of intervention. (From Newman, M. [1994]. *Health as expanding consciousness* [2nd ed., p. 106]. New York: National League for Nursing Press and Sudbury, MA: Jones and Bartlett.)

care. Newman (1986) stated that nursing is at the intersection of the focus of the health care industry; therefore, "nursing is in position to bring about the fluctuation within the system that will shift the system to a new higher order of functioning" (p. 90).

Examining pragmatic adequacy of Newman's theory in relation to nursing education reveals that teaching the research method associated with the theory also teaches the students a practice method that is congruent with the theory. Newman sees the theory, the practice, and the research as a process rather than a separate domain of nursing discipline. Teaching the theory of health as expanding consciousness would necessitate a shift in thinking from the existing view of health to a newer and synthesized view that accepts disease as a manifestation of health. Not only that, learning to let go of the professional's control and respecting the client's choices are an integral part of practice within this framework. Students and practicing nurses who plan to use Newman's theory will face personal transformation in learning to recognize pattern by acting as a participant-observer of phenomena related to health. An individual's personal experience will be the core of not just teaching and practice, but research as well. Newman (1994) explained that

the nurse would need to sense his or her own pattern of relating as an indication of the nurse-client interacting pattern. She emphasized that there needs to be a study or sense of the process of the relationship with clients from within, giving attention to the "we" in the nurse-client relationship (Newman, 1997b).

Newman's theory has also been used in nursing education to provide some content into a model called the *healing web*. This model was designed to integrate nursing education and nursing service together with private and public education programs for baccalaureate and associate nursing degree programs in South Dakota (Bunkers et al., 1992). Jacono and Jacono (1996) suggested that student creativity could be enhanced if nursing faculty apply the theory by recognizing that all experience has the potential for expanding the creativity (consciousness) of individuals. Additionally, Picard and Mariolis (2002) described the application of the health as expanding consciousness theory to teaching psychiatric nursing.

Research

Research has a dual role, to test theory and to establish a knowledge base from which to practice professional nursing. Early research with the theory manipulated the early basic theory concepts of space, time, and movement. In addition to Newman, several researchers have undertaken research about time, space, or movement. Newman and Gaudiano (1984) focused on the occurrence of depression in the elderly and decreased subjective time. Mentzer and Schorr (1986) used Newman's model of duration of time as an index to consciousness in a study of institutionalized elderly. Engle (1986) addressed the relationship between movement, time, and assessment of health. Schorr and Schroeder (1989) studied differences in consciousness with regard to time and movement, with results supporting the concept of expanding consciousness. In another study by Schorr and Schroeder (1991), relationships among type A behavior, temporal orientation, and death anxiety were examined as manifestations of consciousness, with mixed results.

However, with evolution of the theory, research was also viewed as practice having a function of assisting clients in pattern recognition (Newman, 1990a). Schorr, Farnham, and Ervin (1991) investigated the health patterns in 60 aging women, using the theory of health as the theoretical framework. The phenomenon of powerlessness was assumed to be operative for the subjects, but it was rejected in favor of high levels of perceived situational control or powerfulness. A study of music and pattern change in chronic pain by Schorr (1993) also supported Newman's theory of health as expanding consciousness. Fryback's (1991) dissertation revealed that persons with acquired immunodeficiency syndrome (AIDS) and human immunodeficiency virus (HIV) infection did, in fact, describe health within physical, health promotion, and spiritual domains and was consistent with Newman's theory.

Other studies investigating patterns of expanding consciousness included Smith's (1995) work with the health of rural African-American women and Yamashita's (1995, 1999) work with Japanese and Canadian family caregivers. Several studies have focused on patterns of persons with rheumatoid arthritis (Brauer, 2001; Neill, 2002; Schmidt, Brauer, & Peden-McAlpine, 2003). A number of research studies have been conducted with the theory focusing on patterns of patients with cancer as a meaningful part of health (Barron, 2000; Bruce-Barrett, 1998; Endo, 1998; Endo, et al., 2000; Karian, Jankowski, & Beal, 1998; Kiser-Larson, 1999, 2002; Moch, 1990; Newman, 1995c; Roux, 1994; Utley, 1999). Other studies include studies of life patterns of persons with coronary heart disease (Newman & Moch, 1991), patterns of persons with chronic obstructive pulmonary disease (Jonsdottir, 1998; Noveletsky-Rosenthal, 1996), life patterns of people with hepatitis C (Thomas, 2002), and patterns of expanding consciousness in persons with HIV and AIDS (Lamendola & Newman, 1994).

Additional research includes studies that involved recognizing health patterns in persons with multiple sclerosis (Gulick & Bugg, 1992; Neill, 2002, 2005), help-seeking patterns in older wife caregivers of husbands with dementia (Brown & Alligood, 2004;

Witucki, 2000), patterns in adolescent males incarcerated for murder (Pharris, 1999, 2002), and giving and re-ceiving social support by spouse caregivers and their spouses (Schmitt, 1991). Further studies have included studies of life patterns of women who successfully lose weight and maintain the loss (Berry, 2002), of victimizing sexuality and healing patterns (Smith, 1996, 1997), of the meaning of the death of an adult child to an elder (Weed, 2004), of the experience of family members living through sudden death of a child (Picard, 2002), of nurse facilitation of health as expanding consciousness in families of children with special health care needs (Falkenstern, 2003), and of the use of health as expanding consciousness to conceptualize adaptation in burn patients (Casper, 1999). Newman's research as praxis has also been used to describe the lived experience of life passing in middle-adolescent females (Shanahan, 1993), to describe patterns of expanding consciousness in women in midlife (Picard, 2000), to explore pain reduction with music therapy (Schorr, 1993), with pattern recognition of high-risk pregnant women (Schroeder, 1993) and low-risk pregnant women (Batty, 1999), and to explore the nature of nursing practice with families of young children (Litchfield, 1997) and patterns of families of medically fragile children (Tommet, 1997, 2003). Lastly, health as expanding consciousness was used as a framework to analyze patterns for evidence of empowerment in community health care workers by Walls (1999).

Newman states that her research over time assisted not only clients who participated, but also herself and fellow researchers, in gaining a better understanding of self as a nurse researcher and understanding the limitations of previous methods used. Newman (1986) further stated that research should center around investigations that are participatory and in which client-subjects are partners and co-researchers in the search for health patterns. This method of inquiry is called *cooperative inquiry* or *interactive, integrative participation*. Newman (1989, 1990a) has developed a method to describe pattern as unfolding and evolving over time. She used the method of interviewing a subject regarding different time frames to establish a pattern for that subject (Newman 1987b). Newman (1990a) stated that during the development of a methodology to test the theory of health, "sharing our (researcher's) perception of the person's pattern with the person was meaningful to the participants and stimulated new insights regarding their lives" (p. 37). The process made a difference in the researchers' lives and the participants' lives. Newman (1990a) asserted that the research process took on the form of nursing practice. In 1994, she described a protocol for the research and has labeled it *hermeneutic dialectic*. This method allows the pattern of person-environment to reveal itself without disturbing the unity of the pattern (M. Newman, personal correspondence, 2000). A Web site is maintained at the University of Minnesota for disseminating research information pertaining to the theory.

FURTHER DEVELOPMENT

Previously discussed research studies have supported the theory of health as expanding consciousness, illuminating the importance of pattern recognition in the process of expanding consciousness. The theory has been used extensively in exploring and understanding the experience of health within illness, supporting a basic premise of the theory that disruptive situations may provide a catalytic effect and facilitate movement to higher levels of consciousness.

CRITIQUE
Clarity

Semantic clarity is evident in the definitions, descriptions, and dimensions of the concepts of the theory.

Simplicity

The deeper meaning of the theory of health as expanding consciousness is complex. The theory as a whole must be understood, not just the isolated concepts. If an individual wanted to use a positivist approach, Newman's original propositions would serve as guides for hypothesis development.

However, researchers who have tried that approach have concluded that it is inadequate to study the theory. As Newman has advocated in the 1994 edition of her book, *Health As Expanding Consciousness,* the holistic approach of the hermeneutic dialectic method is consistent with the theory and requires a high level of understanding of the theory on the part of the researcher to extend the theory in praxis research (M. Newman, telephone interview, 1996).

Generality

The concepts in Newman's theory are broad in scope because they all relate to health. The theory has been applied in several different cultures and is applicable across the spectrum of nursing care situations (M. Newman, personal correspondence, 2004). This renders her theory generalizable. The broad scope provides a focus for future theory development.

Empirical Precision

In the early stages of development, aspects of the theory were operationalized and tested within a traditional scientific mode. However, quantitative methods are inadequate in capturing the dynamic, changing nature of this theory. A hermeneutic dialectic approach has been developed for a full explication of its meaning and application.

Derivable Consequences

The focus of Newman's theory of health as expanding consciousness provides an evolving guide for all health-related disciplines. In the quest for understanding the phenomenon of health, this unique view of health challenges nurses to make a difference in nursing practice by the application of this theory.

SUMMARY

Although Newman (1997a) started with a rational, empirical approach that was both inductive and deductive, she found it restrictive and "not consistent with the paradigm from which the theory was drawn" (p. 23). Little by little, she relinquished some of the experimental control, and her work evolved to a more interactive, integrative approach that continued to be objective and controlled. When that still did not work, she gave up the research paradigm with its objectivity and control and allowed the principles of her theoretical paradigm to guide her research. Then she began to see the core of pattern and process as nursing practice. She saw the evolving pattern as meaning in process that required an approach of mutual process, not just objective observation. Patterns showed that expanding consciousness was related to quality and connectedness of relationships. The nurse researcher's creative presence was important to the participant's insight. Newman (1986) concluded that individuals experience a theory in living it. She labeled her research as hermeneutic dialectic. The theory of health as expanding consciousness, along with the research as praxis method, has been used extensively in nursing practice with a variety of client and family situations, nursing education in several settings, and nursing research in the United States and several other countries. Newman continues to write, consult, and lecture, advancing her work.

Case Study

Alice is an 81-year-old widow who has lived alone in a low-income apartment complex in a small rural, Appalachian town since her husband's death 8 years ago. She has one surviving family member, a granddaughter, who lives 30 miles away. Alice has never learned to drive and depends on her granddaughter for all transportation to physician appointments, shopping, and getting medications. Her income is $824 monthly, and she requires several expensive prescriptions for arthritis, hypertension, and cardiac problems. She has osteoarthritis in her knees and requires a quad cane for support and safety when getting around her apartment. A visiting nurse stops by weekly to check her blood pressure and give her an injection for her arthritis. The visiting nurse notes that Alice's blood pressure is elevated, and Alice states that she has been unable to get her

medication because her granddaughter's car is broken. Alice also mentions that she is running low on food in the apartment because she can't get out to shop.

Alice admits that she hardly knows or speaks to her neighbors despite having lived there for 8 years, and she still feels like a stranger and doesn't want to "push myself in." She says that she hates to bother people and "won't hardly unless I just have to." She says she sometimes gets lonely for "her people" who are all deceased.

The visiting nurse, in working with Alice, recognizes the current situation as a choice point, with potential for increased interaction with others and increased consciousness. The old ways no longer work for Alice and new ways of relating are necessary. The nurse incorporates the elements of Newman's method to assist Alice in pattern recognition for the purpose of discovering new potentials for action. As the nurse has Alice relate her story, through dialogue and interacting with Alice, she helps Alice recognize past patterns of relating and how present circumstances have changed those patterns. Alice talks about how she and her husband lived for 56 years in a rural mountain cabin with few neighbors except for two sisters and their sole daughter. They were very self sufficient, grew large gardens, had their own livestock, and rarely went into town. All these family members are now deceased except the granddaughter, who insisted that Alice leave the cabin and move into town after the death of her husband. It is apparent that Alice's past patterns have been those of independence and limiting social contact to mainly family members.

The nurse shares her perceptions with Alice who confirms and verifies the pattern identification. Alice states, "I just don't know how long I am going to manage by myself anymore." The nurse helps her explore sources of help, besides the granddaughter, that will help Alice remain in her apartment as independently as possible. Alice relates that there is one man, a few doors away who has stopped several times to ask if she needed anything from the grocery store, but she hasn't asked him because she hates to bother him and doesn't want "to be beholden." After further discussion, she decides that she will ask him to pick up staples and medications for her and pay him back by baking him some bread saying, "I just love to bake anyway and haven't had anyone much to bake for."

In subsequent weekly visits, Alice and the nurse explore the possibility of getting medications at a reduced price through the local nurse-managed clinic. Alice states that she might try getting to know some of her neighbors. The nurse helps Alice make arrangements to be picked up by the Senior Van for physician appointments. As Alice begins to build her own support system, she finds that she relies on the nurse less for help with maintaining her independence, and they resume their previous pattern of simply checking her blood pressure and giving her injections weekly.

CRITICAL THINKING *Activities*

1. What is the worldview of nursing? What is the nurse scientist view of nursing?

2. How does that worldview dictate or direct knowledge development for nursing?

3. What dictates the change in paradigms of health, health care practice, and nursing practice? Examine Newman's view about it.

4. How is the process of health as expanding consciousness different from the process of self-actualization? Compare and contrast the characteristics of both processes and phenomena.

5. Where and how does Newman accept or depart from the Rogerian unitary man theory?

6. How does Newman relate her theory of health with contemporary and future nursing practice, education, and research?

7. How do you agree or disagree with her claims and explanations regarding relatedness of her theory with the pragmatic expectations of the nursing profession?

REFERENCES

Acton, H. B. (1967). George Wilhelm Freidrich Hegel 1770-1831. In P. Edwards (Ed.), *The encyclopedia of philosophy* (Vols. 3 & 4). New York: Macmillan & Free Press.

Barron, A. (2000). Life meanings and the experience of cancer: Application of Newman's research method and phenomenological analysis (Doctoral dissertation, Boston College, 2000). *Dissertation Abstracts International, 62,* 1313.

Batty, M. L. E. (1999). Pattern identification and expanding consciousness during the transition of "low risk" pregnancy. A study embodying Newman's health as expanding consciousness (Margaret Newman) (Master's thesis, The University of New Brunswick, Canada, 1999). *Masters Abstracts International, 39,* 826.

Bentov, I. (1977). *Stalking the wild pendulum.* New York: E. P. Dutton.

Berry, D. C. (2002). Newman's theory of health as expanding consciousness in women maintaining weight loss (Doctoral dissertation, Boston College, 2002). *Dissertation Abstracts International, 63,* 2300.

Bohm, D. (1980). *Wholeness and the implicate order.* London: Routledge and Kegan Paul.

Brauer, D. J. (2001). Common patterns of person-environment interaction in persons with rheumatoid arthritis. *Western Journal of Nursing Research, 23,* 414-430.

Brown, J. W., & Alligood, M. R. (2004). Realizing wrongness: Stories of older wife caregivers. *Journal of Applied Gerontology, 23*(2), 104-119.

Bruce-Barrett, C. A. (1998). Patterns of health and healing: Peer support and prostate cancer (Master's thesis, D'Youville College, 1998). *Masters Abstracts International, 37,* 0233.

Bunkers, S. S., Bendtro, M., Holmes, P. K., Howell, J., Johnson, S., Koerner, J., et al. (1992). The healing web: A transformative model for nursing. *Nursing and Health Care, 13,* 68-73.

Casper, S. A. (1999). Psychological adaptation as a dimension of health as expanding consciousness: Effectiveness of burn survivors support groups (Master's thesis, D'Youville College, 1999). *Masters Abstracts International, 37,* 1433.

Endo, E. (1998). Pattern recognition as a nursing intervention with Japanese women with ovarian cancer. *ANS Advances in Nursing Science, 20*(4), 49-61.

Endo, E., Nitta, N., Inayoshi, M., Saito, R., Takemura, K., Minegishi, H., et al. (2000). Pattern recognition as a caring partnership in families with cancer. *Journal of Advanced Nursing, 32,* 603-610.

Engle, V. (1986). The relationship of movement and time to older adults' functional health. *Research in Nursing and Health, 9,* 123-129.

Falkenstern, S. K. (2003). *Nursing facilitation of health as expanding consciousness in families who have a child with special health care needs*. Unpublished doctoral dissertation, Pennsylvania State University, University Park, PA.

Flannagan, J., Farrell, C., Zelano, P., Morrison, H., Quigley, J. D., & Braccio, J. (2000). *The nursing theory and practice link: Creating a healing environment*. Proceedings of the International Conference on Emerging Nursing Knowledge, Boston.

Flannagan, J. M. (2002). Nurse and patient perceptions of the pre-admission nursing practice model: Linking theory to practice (Doctoral dissertation, Boston College). *Dissertation Abstracts International, 63,* 2304.

Fryback, P. B. (1991). Perceptions of health by persons with a terminal disease: Implications for nursing. *Dissertation Abstracts International, 52,* 1951.

Gulick, E. E., & Bugg, A. (1992). Holistic health patterning in multiple sclerosis. *Research in Nursing and Health, 15,* 175-185.

Gustafson, W. (1990). Application of Newman's theory of health: Pattern recognition as nursing practice. In M. Parker (Ed.), *Nursing theories in practice* (pp. 141-161). New York: National League for Nursing.

Jacono, B. J., & Jacono, J. J. (1996). The benefits of Newman and Parse in helping nurse teachers determine methods to enhance student creativity. *Nurse Education Today, 16,* 356-362.

Jonsdottir, H. (1998). Life patterns of people with chronic obstructive pulmonary disease: Isolation and being closed in. *Nursing Science Quarterly, 11,* 160-166.

Kalb, K. A. (1990). The gift: Applying Newman's theory of health in nursing practice. In M. Parker (Ed.), *Nursing theories in practice* (pp. 163-186). New York: National League for Nursing.

Karian, V. E., Jankowski, S. M, & Beal, J. A. (1998). Exploring the lived experience of childhood cancer survivors. *Journal of Pediatric Oncology, 15,* 153-162.

Kiser-Larson, N. (2002). Life pattern of native women experiencing breast cancer. *International Journal for Human Caring, 6*(2), 61-68.

Kiser-Larson, N. K. (1999). Life patterns of Native American women experiencing breast cancer (Doctoral dissertation, University of Minnesota). *Dissertation Abstracts International, 60,* 2062.

Lamb, G. S., & Stempel, J. E. (1994). Nurse case management from the client's view: Growing as insider-expert. *Nursing Outlook, 42,* 7-13.

Lamendola, F. P., & Newman, M. A. (1994). The paradox of HIV/AIDS as expanding consciousness. *ANS Advances in Nursing Science, 16*(3), 13-21.

Litchfield, M. (1999). Practice wisdom. *ANS Advances in Nursing Science, 22*(2), 62-73.

Litchfield, M. C. (1993). *The process of health patterning in families with young children who have been repeatedly*

hospitalized. Unpublished master's thesis, University of Minnesota, Rochester.

Litchfield, M. C. (1997). The process of nursing partnership in family health (Doctoral dissertation, University of Minnesota). *Dissertation Abstracts International, 59,* 1802.

Magan, S. J., Gibbon, E. J., & Mrozek, R. (1990). Nursing theory application: A practice model. *Issues in Mental Health Nursing, 11,* 297-312.

Marchione, J. M. (1986). Pattern as methodology for assessing family health: Newman's theory of health. In P. Winstead-Fry (Ed.), *Case studies in nursing theory.* New York: National League for Nursing.

Mentzer, C., & Schorr, J. A. (1986). Perceived situational control and perceived duration of time: Expressions of life patterns. *ANS Advances in Nursing Science, 9*(1), 13-20.

Moch, S. D. (1990). Health within the experience of breast cancer. *Journal of Advanced Nursing, 15,* 1426-1435.

Moss, R. (1981). *The I that is we.* Millbrae, CA: Celestial Arts.

Neill, J. (2002). Transcendence and transformation in the life patterns of women living with rheumatoid arthritis. *ANS Advances in Nursing Science, 24*(4), 27-47.

Neill, J. (2005). Recognizing pattern in the lives of women with multiple sclerosis. In C. Picard & D. Jones (Eds.), *Giving voice to what we know* (pp. 153-165). Sudbury. MA: Jones and Bartlett.

Newman, M. A. (1971). *An investigation of the relationship between gait tempo and time perception.* Unpublished doctoral dissertation, New York University, New York.

Newman, M. A. (1972). Time estimation in relation to gait tempo. *Perceptual and Motor Skills, 34,* 359-366.

Newman, M. A. (1978). *Second annual nurse educator's conference* (Audiotape). New York: Teach 'em, Inc. Available through Teach 'em, Inc., 160 E. Illinois Street, Chicago, IL 60611.

Newman, M. A. (1979). *Theory development in nursing.* Philadelphia: F. A. Davis.

Newman, M. A. (1982). Time as an index of expanding consciousness with age. *Nursing Research, 31,* 290-293.

Newman, M. A. (1983). Newman's health theory. In I. W. Clements & F. B. Roberts (Eds.), *Family health: A theoretical approach to nursing care.* New York: John Wiley & Sons.

Newman, M. A. (1986). *Health as expanding consciousness.* St. Louis: Mosby.

Newman, M. A. (1987a). Aging as increasing complexity. *Journal of Gerontological Nursing, 13*(9), 16-18.

Newman, M. A. (1987b). Patterning. In M. Duffy & N. J. Pender (Eds.), *Conceptual issues in health promotion.* A report of proceedings of a wingspread conference, Racine, WI, April 13-15, 1987. Indianapolis: Sigma Theta Tau.

Newman, M. A. (1989). The spirit of nursing. *Holistic Nursing Practice, 3*(3), 1-6.

Newman, M. A. (1990a). Newman's theory of health as praxis. *Nursing Science Quarterly, 3*, 37-41.

Newman, M. A. (1990b). Nursing paradigms and realities. In N. L. Chaska (Ed.), *The nursing profession: Turning points* (pp. 230-235). St. Louis: Mosby.

Newman, M. A. (1990c). Shifting to higher consciousness. In M. Parker (Ed.), *Nursing theories in practice* (pp. 129-139). New York: National League for Nursing.

Newman, M. A. (1991). Health conceptualizations. In J. J. Fitzpatrick, R. L. Taunton, & A. K. Jacox (Eds.), *Annual review of nursing research* (Vol. 9). New York: Springer.

Newman, M. A. (1992). Nightingale's vision of nursing theory and health. In Nightingale, F., *Notes on nursing: What it is, and what it is not* (commemorative edition, pp. 44-47). Philadelphia: Lippincott.

Newman, M. A. (1994). *Health as expanding consciousness* (2nd ed.). New York: National League for Nursing Press.

Newman, M. A. (1995a). *A developing discipline: Selected works of Margaret Newman.* New York: National League for Nursing Press.

Newman, M. A. (1995b). Dialogue: Margaret Newman and the rhetoric of nursing theory. *Image: The Journal of Nursing Scholarship, 27*, 261.

Newman, M. A. (1995c). Recognizing a pattern of expanding consciousness in persons with cancer. In M. A. Newman (Ed.), *A developing discipline: Selected works of Margaret Newman* (pp. 159-171). New York: National League for Nursing Press.

Newman, M. A. (1997a). Evolution of the theory of health as expanding consciousness. *Nursing Science Quarterly, 10*, 22-25.

Newman, M. A. (1997b). Experiencing the whole. *ANS Advances in Nursing Science, 20*, 34-39.

Newman, M. A. (1999). The rhythm of relating in a paradigm of wholeness. *Image: The Journal of Nursing Scholarship, 31*, 227-230.

Newman, M. A. (2003). A world of no boundaries. *ANS Advances in Nursing Science, 26*(4), 240-245.

Newman, M. A. (2005). Foreword. In C. Picard & D. Jones (Eds.), *Giving voice to what we know: Margaret Newman's theory of health as expanding consciousness* (pp. xii-xv). Sudbury, MA: Jones and Bartlett.

Newman, M. A., & Autio, S. (1986). *Nursing in a prospective payment system health care environment.* Minneapolis: University of Minnesota.

Newman, M. A., & Gaudiano, J. K. (1984). Depression as an explanation for decreased subjective time in the elderly. *Nursing Research, 33*, 137-139.

Newman, M. A., Lamb, G. S., & Michaels, C. (1991). Nurse case management: The coming together of theory and practice. *Nursing and Health Care, 12*, 404-408.

Newman, M. A., & Moch, S. D. (1991). Life patterns of persons with coronary heart disease. *Nursing Science Quarterly, 4*, 161-167.

Newman, M. A., Sime, M. A., & Corcoran-Perry, S. A. (1991). The focus of the discipline of nursing. *ANS Advances in Nursing Science, 14*, 1-6.

Noveletsky-Rosenthal, H. T. (1996). Pattern recognition in older adults living with chronic illness (Doctoral dissertation, Boston College). *Dissertation Abstracts International, 57*, 6180.

Pharris, M. D. (1999). The process of pattern recognition as a nursing intervention with adolescent males incarcerated for murder (Doctoral dissertation, University of Minnesota). *Dissertation Abstracts International, 60*, 5436.

Pharris, M. D. (2002). Coming to know ourselves as community through a nursing partnership with adolescents convicted of murder. *ANS Advances in Nursing Science, 24*(3), 21-42.

Picard, C. (2002). Family reflections on living through sudden death of a child. *Nursing Science Quarterly, 15*, 242-250.

Picard, C. A. (2000). Pattern of expanding consciousness in mid-life women: Creative movement and the narrative as modes of expression. *Nursing Science Quarterly, 13*, 150-158.

Picard, C., & Mariolis, T. (2002). Teaching-learning process. Praxis as a mirroring process: Teaching psychiatric nursing grounded in Newman's health as expanding consciousness. *Nursing Science Quarterly, 15*, 118-122.

Prigogine, I. (1976). Order through fluctuation: Self-organization and social system. In E. Jantsch & C. H. Waddington (Eds.), *Evolution and consciousness* (pp. 93-133). Reading, MA: Addison-Wesley.

Quinn, J. F. (1992). Holding sacred space: The nurse as healing environment. *Holistic Nursing Practice, 6*(4), 26-36.

Reed, P. G. (1996). Transcendence: Formulating nursing perspectives. *Nursing Science Quarterly, 9*, 2-4.

Rogers, M. E. (1980). Nursing, a science of unitary man. In J. P. Riehl & C. Roy (Eds.), *Conceptual models for nursing practice.* New York: Appleton-Century-Crofts.

Roux, G. M. (1994). *Phenomenologic study: Inner strength in women with breast cancer.* Unpublished doctoral dissertation, Texas Women's University, Denton, TX.

Roy, C., Rogers, M. C., Fitzpatrick, J. J., Neuman, M., & Orem, D. E. (1982). Nursing diagnosis and nursing theory. In M. J. King & D. A. Moritz (Eds.), *Classification of nursing diagnosis* (pp. 215-231). New York: McGraw Hill.

Schlotzhauer, M., & Farnham, R. (1997). Newman's theory and insulin dependent diabetes mellitus in adolescence. *Journal of School Nursing, 13*(3), 20-23.

Schmidt, B. J., Brauer, D. J., & Peden-McAlpine, C. (2003). Experiencing health in the context of rheumatoid arthritis. *Nursing Science Quarterly, 16,* 155-162.

Schmitt, N. (1991). *Caregiving couples: The experience of giving and receiving social support.* Unpublished doctoral dissertation, University of Minnesota, Rochester.

Schorr, J. A. (1993). Music and pattern change in chronic pain. *ANS Advances in Nursing Science, 15*(4), 27-36.

Schorr, J. A., Farnham, R. C., & Ervin, S. M. (1991). Health patterns in aging women as expanding consciousness. *ANS Advances in Nursing Science, 13*(4), 52-63.

Schorr, J. A., & Schroeder, C. A. (1989). Consciousness as a dissipative structure: An extension of the Newman model. *Nursing Science Quarterly, 2,* 183-193.

Schorr, J. A., & Schroeder, C. A. (1991). Movement and time: Exertion and perceived duration. *Science Quarterly, 4,* 104-112.

Schroeder, C. A. (1993) Perceived duration of time and bedrest in high risk pregnancy: An exploration of the Newman model. *Dissertation Abstracts International, 54,* 1984.

Schubert, P. E. (1989). *Mutual connectedness: Holistic nursing practice under varying conditions of intimacy.* Unpublished doctoral dissertation, University of California, San Francisco.

Shanahan, S. M. (1993). The lived experience of life-passing in middle adolescent females. *Masters Abstracts International, 32,* 1376.

Smith, C. A. (1995). The lived experience of staying healthy in rural African American families. *Nursing Science Quarterly, 8,* 17-21.

Smith, S. K. (1996). Women's experiences of victimizing sexualization and healing (Doctoral dissertation, University of Minnesota). *Dissertation Abstracts International, 57,* 3659.

Smith, S. K. (1997). Women's experiences of victimizing socialization. Part I: Responses related to abuse and home and family environment. *Issues in Mental Health Nursing, 18,* 395-416.

Thomas, J. A. (2002). What are the life patterns of people with hepatitis C? (Doctoral dissertation, University of Nevada, Reno). *Dissertation Abstracts International, 41,* 194.

Tommet, P. A. (1997). Nurse-parent dialogue: Illuminating the pattern of families with children who are medically fragile (Doctoral dissertation, University of Minnesota). *Dissertation Abstracts International, 58,* 2359.

Tommet, P. A. (2003). Nurse-parent dialogue: Illuminating the evolving pattern of families of children who are medically fragile. *Nursing Science Quarterly, 16*(3), 239-246.

Utley, R. (1999). The evolving meaning of cancer for long-term survivors of breast cancer. *Oncology Nursing Forum, 26,* 1519-1523.

Walls, P. W. (1999). Community participation in primary health care: A qualitative study of empowerment of health care workers (Doctoral dissertation, Loyola University of Chicago). *Dissertation Abstracts International, 60,* 2065.

Weed, L. D. (2004). *The meaning of the death of an adult child to an elder: A phenomenological investigation.* Unpublished doctoral dissertation, University of Tennessee, Knoxville.

Weingourt, R. (1998). Using Margaret A. Newman's theory of health with elderly nursing home residents. *Perspectives in Psychiatric Care, 34*(3), 25-30.

Witucki, J. (2000). Help-seeking by older wife caregivers of demented husbands: A grounded theory approach (Doctoral dissertation, University of Tennessee, Knoxville). *Dissertation Abstracts International, 61,* 2996.

Yamashita, M. (1995). *Family coping with mental illness: An application of Newman's research as praxis.* Paper presented at the Midwest Nursing Research Society 19th Annual Conference, Kansas City, MO.

Yamashita, M. (1999). Newman's theory of health applied to family caregiving in Canada. *Nursing Science Quarterly, 12,* 73-79.

Young, A. M. (1976). *The reflexive universe: Evolution of consciousness.* San Francisco: Robert Briggs.

BIBLIOGRAPHY
Primary Sources
Books

Newman, M. A. (1979). *Theory development in nursing.* Philadelphia: F. A. Davis. [Japanese rights assigned to Gendasha Publishing Company, Tokyo, 1986.]

Newman, M. A. (1986). *Health as expanding consciousness.* St. Louis: Mosby. [Japanese translation, 1995; Korean translation, 1996.]

Newman, M. A. (1994). *Health as expanding consciousness* (2nd ed.). New York: National League for Nursing Press. [Japanese translation, 1995; Korean translation, 1996.]

Newman, M. A. (1995). *A developing discipline: Selected work of Margaret Newman.* New York: National League for Nursing Press.

Book Chapters

Newman, M. A. (1981). The meaning of health. In G. E. Laskar (Ed.), *Applied systems research and cybernetics: Vol. 4. Systems research in health care, biocybernetics and ecology* (pp. 1739-1743). New York: Pergamon.

Newman, M. A. (1983). Newman's health theory. In I. Clements & F. Roberts (Eds.), *Family health: A theoretical approach to nursing care* (pp. 161-175). New York: John Wiley & Sons.

Newman, M. A. (1987). Nursing's emerging paradigm: The diagnosis of pattern. In A. M. McLane (Ed.),

Classification of nursing diagnoses. Proceedings of the seventh conference, North American nursing diagnosis association (pp. 53-60). St. Louis: Mosby.

Newman, M. A. (1987). Patterning. In M. Duffy & N. J. Pender (Eds.), *Conceptual issues in health promotion: A report of proceedings of a wingspread conference, Racine, WI* (pp. 36-50). Indianapolis: Sigma Theta Tau.

Newman, M. A. (1990). Shifting to higher consciousness. In M. Parker (Ed.), *Nursing theories in practice* (pp. 129-139). New York: National League for Nursing.

Newman, M. A. (1995). Recognizing a pattern of expanding consciousness in persons with cancer. In M. A. Newman (Ed.), *A developing discipline: Selected works of Margaret Newman* (pp. 159-171). New York: National League for Nursing Press.

Newman, M. A. (1996). Prevailing paradigms in nursing. In J. W. Kenney (Ed.), *Philosophical and theoretical perspectives for advanced nursing practice* (pp. 302-307). Sudbury, MA: Jones and Bartlett.

Newman, M. A. (1996). Theory of the nurse-client partnership. In E. Cohen (Ed.), *Nurse case management in the 21st century* (pp. 119-123). St. Louis: Mosby.

Newman, M. A. (1997). A dialogue with Martha Rogers and David Bohm about the science of unitary human beings. In M. Madrid (Ed.), *Patterns of Rogerian knowing* (pp. 3-10). New York: National League for Nursing Press.

Newman, M. A. (2004). Foreword. In C. Picard & D. Jones (Eds.), *Giving voice to what we know: Margaret Newman's theory of health as expanding consciousness in practice, research, and education.* Sudbury, MA: Jones and Bartlett.

Newman, M. A., Sime, A. M., & Corcoran-Perry, S. A. (1996). The focus of the discipline of nursing. In J. W. Kenney (Ed.), *Philosophical and theoretical perspectives for advanced nursing practice* (pp. 297-301). Sudbury, MA: Jones and Bartlett.

Dissertation

Newman, M. A. (1971). *An investigation of the relationship between gait tempo and time perception.* Unpublished doctoral dissertation, New York University School of Education, New York.

Journal Articles

Allender, C. D., Egan, E. C., & Newman, M. A. (1995). An instrument for measuring differentiated nursing practice. *Nursing Management, 26*(4), 42-44.

Lamendola, F. P., & Newman, M. A. (1994). The paradox of HIV/AIDS as expanding consciousness. *ANS Advances in Nursing Science, 16*(3), 13-21.

Newman, M. A. (1982). Time as an index of expanding consciousness with age. *Nursing Research, 31,* 290-293.

Newman, M. A. (1989). The spirit of nursing. *Holistic Nursing Practice, 3*(3), 1-6.

Newman, M. A. (1990). Newman's theory of health as praxis. *Nursing Science Quarterly, 3,* 37-41.

Newman, M. A. (1994). Theory for nursing practice. *Nursing Science Quarterly, 7,* 153-157.

Newman, M. A. (1995). Dialogue: Margaret Newman and the rhetoric of nursing theory. *Image: The Journal of Nursing Scholarship, 27,* 261.

Newman, M. A. (1997). Evolution of the theory of health as expanding consciousness. *Nursing Science Quarterly, 10,* 22-25.

Newman, M. A. (1997). Experiencing the whole. *ANS Advances in Nursing Science, 20,* 34-39.

Newman, M. A. (1997). The professional doctorate in nursing: A position paper. *Image: The Journal of Nursing Scholarship, 29,* 361-362.

Newman, M. A. (1999). Letters to the editor . . . a commentary on Newman's theory of health as expanding consciousness. *ANS Advances in Nursing Science, 21*(3), viii-ix.

Newman, M. A. (1999). The rhythm of relating in a paradigm of wholeness. *Image: The Journal of Nursing Scholarship, 31,* 227-230.

Newman, M. A. (2001). Response to "Conversation across paradigms: Unitary-transformative and critical feminist perspectives." *Scholarly Inquiry for Nursing Practice, 15,* 367-370.

Newman, M. A. (2002). Caring in the human health experience. *International Journal for Human Caring, 6*(2), 8-12.

Newman, M. A. (2003). A world of no boundaries. *ANS Advances in Nursing Science, 26*(4), 240-245.

Newman, M. A. (2003). The immediate applicability of nursing praxis. *Quality Nursing: The Japanese Journal of Nursing Education and Nursing Research, 9*(5), 4-6.

Newman, M. A., & Moch, S. D. (1991). Life patterns of persons with coronary heart disease. *Nursing Science Quarterly, 4,* 161-167.

Newman, M. A., Sime, A. M., & Corcoran-Perry, S. A. (1991). The focus of the discipline of nursing. *ANS Advances in Nursing Science, 14,* 1-6.

Other Media

Margaret Newman, nurse theorists: Portraits of excellence (Videotape). (1990). Produced by Helene Fuld Health Trust. Oakland, CA: Studio Three Production.

Newman, M. A. (1997). *Margaret Newman: Health as expanding consciousness* (CD-ROM). Available through Fuld Institute for Technology in Nursing Education, 5 Depot Street, Athens, OH 45701, (800) 691-8480.

Selected Paper Presentations From 1995 to Present

Newman, M. A. (1995, Oct.). *Dialogue on theory underlying practice.* Paper presented at First National Healing Web Partners Conference, Park City, UT.

Newman, M. A. (1996, June). *A dialogue with Martha Rogers and David Bohm.* Paper presented at Society of Rogerian Scholars, New York.

Newman, M. A. (1996, June). *The rhythm of relating.* Paper presented at American Holistic Nurses Association, St. Louis.

Newman, M. A. (1996, Oct.). *Process as content.* Paper presented at Knowledge Conference 1996: Developing Knowledge for Nursing Practice, Boston College of Nursing and Eastern Nursing Research Society Theory Interest Group, Boston.

Newman, M. A. (1998, April). *Dialogue with Margaret Newman: Health, nursing theory and research as praxis.* Paper presented at keynote address, Ann Berdahl Lecture Series and Zeta Zeta Research Day, Augustana College, Sioux Falls, SD.

Newman, M. A. (1998, May). *Dialogue with Margaret Newman and panel.* Paper presented at Sixth Nurse Theorist Conference, Augsburg College, Minneapolis.

Newman, M. A. (1999, May). *The science of nursing practice: Philosophy in the nurse's world.* Paper presented at Pursuit of Nursing Science: Contemporary Issues and Controversies, for Philosophical Nursing Research, University of Alberta, The Banff Centre, Banff, Alberta, Canada.

Newman, M. A. (2000, June). *The science of nursing practice.* Revealing Meaning for Nursing and Health II: A Conference on Phenomenology and Hermeneutics, University of Minnesota and Sigma Theta Tau Zeta Chapter, Minneapolis.

Newman, M. A. (2002, May). *Caring in the human health experience.* Keynote address, 24th International Association for Human Caring Conference, Boston.

Newman, M. A. (2002, October). *No boundaries.* Keynote address, Conference of the Society of Rogerian Scholars, Richmond, VA.

Newman, M. A. (2004, June). *A dialogue with Margaret Newman.* Ninth Martha E. Rogers Conference, New York.

Secondary Sources
Book Reviews

[Review of the book *Health as expanding consciousness*]. (1995, Feb.). *Journal of Advanced Nursing, 21*(2), 407-408.

[Review of the book *Health as expanding consciousness*]. (1995, Summer). *Image: The Journal of Nursing Scholarship, 27*(2), 163.

Gold, C. R. (1996). [Review of the book *Health as expanding consciousness*]. *Nursing Science Quarterly, 9*(3), 136-137.

Matas, K. E. (1995). [Review of the book *Health as expanding consciousness*]. *Image: The Journal of Nursing Scholarship, 27*(2), 163.

Yamashita, M. (1997). [Review of the book *A developing discipline*]. *Image: The Journal of Nursing Scholarship, 29*(4), 391.

Books

Chinn, P. L., & Kramer, M. K. (1995). *Theory and nursing: A systematic approach* (4th ed.). St. Louis: Mosby.

Marchione, J. (1993). *Margaret Newman: Health as expanding consciousness.* Newbury Park, CA: Sage.

Parker, M. (2001). *Nursing theories and nursing practice.* Philadelphia: F. A. Davis.

Picard, C., & Jones, D. (2004 in press). *Giving voice to what we know: Margaret Newman's theory of health as expanding consciousness in practice, research, and education.* Sudbury, MA: Jones and Bartlett.

Book Chapters

Desai, S. M., Keffer, J., Hensley, D. M., Kilgore-Keever, K. A., Langfitt, J. V., & Peterson, L. (1998). Margaret A. Newman: Model of health. In A. M. Tomey & M. R. Alligood (Eds.), *Nursing theorists and their work* (4th ed.). St. Louis: Mosby.

Hichman, J. S. (1995). An introduction to nursing theory. In J. B. George (Ed.), *Nursing theories: The base for professional nursing practice* (4th ed., pp. 1-12). Norwalk, CT: Appleton & Lange.

Witucki, J. (2002). Margaret A. Newman: Model of health. In A. M. Tomey & M. R. Alligood (Eds.), *Nursing theorists and their work* (5th ed). St. Louis: Mosby.

Witucki, J. (2002). Newman's theory of health and nursing practice. In M. R. Alligood & A. M. Tomey (Eds.), *Nursing theory: Utilization & application* (2nd ed.). St. Louis: Mosby.

Dissertations

Barron, A. (2000). Life meanings and the experience of cancer: Application of Newman's research method and phenomenological analysis (Doctoral dissertation, Boston College, 2000). *Dissertation Abstracts International, 62,* 1313.

Berry, D. C. (2002). Newman's theory of health as expanding consciousness in women maintaining weight loss (Doctoral dissertation, Boston College, 2002). *Dissertation Abstracts International, 63,* 2300.

Endo, E. (1996). Pattern recognition as a nursing intervention with adults with cancer (Doctoral dissertation, University of Minnesota, 1996). *Dissertation Abstracts International, 57,* 3653.

Falkenstern, S. K. (2003). *Nursing facilitation of health as expanding consciousness in families who have a child with special health care needs.* Unpublished doctoral dissertation, Pennsylvania State University, University Park, PA.

Flannagan, J. M. (2002). Nurse and patient perceptions of the pre-admission nursing practice model: Linking theory to practice (Doctoral dissertation, Boston College, 2002). *Dissertation Abstracts International, 63,* 2304.

Geddes, N. J. (1999). The experience of personal transformation in healing touch (HT) practitioners: A heuristic inquiry (Doctoral dissertation, Virginia Commonwealth University, 1999). *Dissertation Abstracts International, 60,* 2607.

Gross, S. W. (1995). The impact of a nursing intervention of relaxation with guided imagery on breast cancer patients' stress and health as expanding consciousness (Doctoral dissertation, University of Texas at Austin, 1995). *Dissertation Abstracts International, 56,* 5416.

Kiser-Larson, N. K. (1999). Life patterns of Native American women experiencing breast cancer (Doctoral dissertation, University of Minnesota, 1999). *Dissertation Abstracts International, 60,* 2062.

Lamendola, F. P. (1998). Patterns of the caregiving experience of selected nurses in hospice and HIV/AIDS care (Doctoral dissertation, University of Minnesota, 1999). *Dissertation Abstracts International, 59,* 1048.

Litchfield, M. C. (1997). The process of nursing partnership in family health (Doctoral dissertation, University of Minnesota, 1997). *Dissertation Abstracts International, 59,* 1802.

Neill, J. (2001). *Broken into wholeness: Life patterns of women living with multiple sclerosis or rheumatoid arthritis.* Unpublished doctoral dissertation, School of Nursing and Midwifery, Flanders University, Adelaide, Australia.

Noveletsky-Rosenthal, H. T. (1996). Pattern recognition in older adults living with chronic illness (Doctoral dissertation, Boston College, 1996). *Dissertation Abstracts International, 57,* 6180.

Pharris, M. D. (1999). The process of pattern recognition as a nursing intervention with adolescent incarcerated for murder (Doctoral dissertation, University of Minnesota, 1999). *Dissertation Abstracts International, 60,* 5436.

Picard, C. A. (1998). Uncovering pattern of expanding consciousness in mid-life women: Creative movement and the narrative as modes of expression (Doctoral dissertation, Boston College, 1998). *Dissertation Abstracts International, 59-03B,* 1049.

Smith, S. K. (1996). Women's experiences of victimizing sexualization (Doctoral dissertation, University of Minnesota, 1996). *Dissertation Abstracts International, 57,* 3659.

Thomas, J. A. (2002). What are the life patterns of people with hepatitis C? (Doctoral dissertation, University of

Nevada, Reno, 2002). *Dissertation Abstracts International, 41,* 194.

Tommet, P. A. (1997). Nurse-parent dialogue: Illuminating the pattern of families with children who are medically fragile (Doctoral dissertation, University of Minnesota, 1997). *Dissertation Abstracts International, 58,* 2359.

Utley, R. (1997). Life patterns of older women who have survived breast cancer (Doctoral dissertation, Wayne State University, 1997). *Dissertation Abstracts International, 58,* 5892.

Walls, P. W. (1999). Community participation in primary health care: A qualitative study of empowerment of health care workers (Doctoral dissertation, Loyola University of Chicago, 1999). *Dissertation Abstracts International, 60,* 2065.

Weed, L. D. (2004). *The meaning of the death of an adult child to an elder: A phenomenological investigation.* Unpublished doctoral dissertation, University of Tennessee, Knoxville.

Witucki, J. (2000). Help-seeking by older wife caregivers of demented husbands: A grounded theory approach (Doctoral dissertation, University of Tennessee, Knoxville, 2000). *Dissertation Abstracts International, 61,* 2996.

Journal Articles

Ammende, M. (1996). Change of paradigm in nursing. Part 1: Theory of Martha Rogers [German]. *Pflege, 9,* 5-11.

Ammende, M. (1996). Change of paradigm in nursing. Part 2: Elizabeth Barrett's "Theory of power" [German]. *Pflege, 9,* 98-104.

Brauer, D. J. (2001). Common patterns of person-environment interaction in persons with rheumatoid arthritis. *Western Journal of Nursing Research, 23,* 414-430.

Brown, J. W., & Alligood, M. R. (2004). Realizing wrongness: Stories of older wife caregivers. *Journal of Applied Gerontology, 23*(2), 104-119.

Bunkers, S. S. (2000). Teaching-learning process. The nurse scholar of the 21st century. *Nursing Science Quarterly, 13,* 116-123.

Bunkers, S. S., Michaels, C., & Ethridge, P. (1997) Advanced practice nursing in community: Nursing's opportunity. *Advanced Practice Nursing Quarterly, 2*(4), 79-84.

Capasso, V. A. (1998). The theory is the practice: An exemplar. *Clinical Nurse Specialist, 12,* 226-229.

Connor, M. J. (1998). Expanding the dialogue on praxis in nursing research and practice. *Nursing Science Quarterly, 11,* 51-55.

Dean, P. J. (2002). Aesthetic expression. A poem dedicated to the nursing theories of Martha Rogers and Margaret

Newman. *International Journal for Human Caring, 6,* 70.

Endo, E. (1998). Pattern recognition as a nursing intervention with Japanese women with ovarian cancer. *ANS Advances in Nursing Science, 20*(4), 49-61.

Endo, E. (1999). Letters to the editor . . . a commentary on Newman's theory of health as expanding consciousness. *ANS Advances in Nursing Science, 21*(3), vii-viii.

Endo, E., Nitta, N., Inayoshi, M., Saito, R., Takemura, K., Minegishi, H., et al. (2000). Pattern recognition as a caring partnership in families with cancer. *Journal of Advanced Nursing, 32,* 603-610.

Ford-Gilboe, M. V. (1994). A comparison of two nursing models: Allen's developmental health model and Newman's theory of health as expanding consciousness. *Nursing Science Quarterly, 7,* 113-118.

Freshwater, D. (1999). Polarity and unity in caring: The healing power of symptoms. *Complementary Therapies in Nursing and Midwifery, 5,* 136-139.

Haggman, L. A. (1997). Health as an individual's way of existence. *Journal of Advanced Nursing, 25,* 45-53.

Hall, E. O. C. (1996). Husserlian phenomenology and nursing in a unitary-transformative paradigm. Vard I. Norden. *Nursing Science and Research in the Nordic Countries, 16*(3), 4-8.

Jacono, B. J., & Jacono, J. J. (1996). The benefits of Newman and Parse in helping nurse teachers determine methods to enhance student creativity. *Nurse Education Today, 16,* 356-362.

Jan, R., & Smith, C. A. (1998). Staying healthy in immigrant Pakistani families living in the United States. *Image: Journal of Nursing Scholarship, 30,* 157-159.

Jonsdottir, H. (1998). Life patterns of people with chronic obstructive pulmonary disease: Isolation and being closed in. *Nursing Science Quarterly, 11,* 160-166.

Jonsdottir, H., Litchfield, M., & Pharris, M. D. (2003). Partnership in practice. *Research and Theory for Nursing Practice, 17,* 51-63.

Karian, V. E., Jankowski, S. M., & Beal, J. A. (1998). Exploring the lived-experience of childhood cancer survivors. *Journal of Pediatric Oncology Nursing, 15,* 153-162.

Kendall, J. (1996). Human association as a factor influencing wellness in homosexual men with human immunodeficiency virus disease. *Applied Nursing Research, 9,* 195-203.

Kiser-Larson, N. (2000). The concepts of caring and story viewed from three nursing paradigms. *International Journal for Human Caring, 4*(2), 26-32.

Kiser-Larson, N. (2002). Life pattern of native women experiencing breast cancer. *International Journal for Human Caring, 6*(2), 61-68.

Litchfield, M. (1999). Practice wisdom. *ANS Advances in Nursing Science, 22,* 62-73.

Martsolf, D. S., & Mickley, J. R. (1998). The concept of spirituality in nursing theories: Differing world-views and extent of focus. *Journal of Advanced Nursing, 27,* 294-303.

Michaels, C. (2000). Becoming a bard: A journey to self. *Nursing Science Quarterly, 13,* 28-30.

Moch, S. D. (1998). Health-within-illness: Concept development through research and practice. *Journal of Advanced Nursing, 28,* 305-310.

Neill, J. (2002). From practice to caring praxis through Newman's theory of health as expanding consciousness: A personal journey. *International Journal for Human Caring, 6*(2), 48-54.

Neill, J. (2002). Transcendence and transformation in the life patterns of women living with rheumatoid arthritis. *ANS Advances in Nursing Science, 24*(4), 27-47.

Nelson, M. L., Howell, J. K., Larson, J. C., & Karpiuk, K. L. (2001). Student outcomes of the healing web: Evaluation of a transformative model for nursing education. *Journal of Nursing Education, 40,* 404-413.

Pharris, M. D. (2002). Coming to know ourselves as community through nursing partnership with adolescents convicted of murder. *ANS Advances in Nursing Science, 24*(3), 21-42.

Picard, C. (1997). Embodied soul: The focus for nursing praxis. *Journal of Holistic Nursing, 15,* 41-53.

Picard, C. (2000). Pattern of expanding consciousness in mid-life women: Creative movement and the narrative as modes of expression. *Nursing Quarterly, 13*(1), 150-158.

Picard, C. (2002). Family reflections on living through sudden death of a child. *Nursing Science Quarterly, 15,* 242-250.

Picard, C., & Mariolis, T. (2002). Teaching-learning process. Praxis as a mirroring process: Teaching psychiatric nursing grounded in Newman's health as expanding consciousness. *Nursing Science Quarterly, 15,* 118-122.

Picard, C., Sickul, C., & Natale, S. (1998). Healing reflections: The transformative mirror. The narrative as modes of expression. *Nursing Science Quarterly, 13,* 150-158.

Reed, P. G. (1996). Theoretical concerns. Transcendence: Formulating nursing perspectives. *Nursing Science Quarterly, 9,* 2-4.

Roux, G., Bush, H. A., & Dingley, C. E. (2001). Inner strength in women with breast cancer. *Journal of Theory Construction and Testing, 5*(1), 19-27.

Schlotzhauser, M., & Farnham, R. (1997). Newman's theory and insulin dependent diabetes mellitus in adolescence. *Journal of School Nursing, 13*(3), 20-23.

Schmidt, B. J., Brauer, D. J., & Peden-McAlpine, C. (2003). Experiencing health in the context of rheumatoid arthritis. *Nursing Science Quarterly, 16,* 155-162.

Smith, C. A. (1995). The lived experience of staying healthy in rural African American families. *Nursing Science Quarterly, 8,* 17-21.

Smith, S. K. (1997). Women's experience of victimizing sexualization. Part I: Responses related to abuse and home and family environment. *Issues in Mental Health Nursing, 18,* 395-416.

Smith, S. K. (1997). Women's experience of victimizing sexualization. Part II: Community and longer term personal impacts. *Issues in Mental Health Nursing, 18,* 417-435.

Sohl-Krieger, R., Lagaard, M. W., & Scherrer, J. (1996). Nursing case management—relationships as a strategy to improve care. *Clinical Nurse Specialist, 10,* 107-113.

Solari-Twadell, P., Bunkers, S., Wang, C., & Snyder, D. (1995). The pinwheel model of bereavement. *Image: Journal of Nursing Scholarship, 27,* 323-326.

Tommet, P. A. (2003). Nurse-parent dialogue: Illuminating the evolving pattern of families of children who are medically fragile. *Nursing Science Quarterly, 16,* 239-246.

Utley, R. (1999). The evolving meaning of cancer for long-term survivors of breast cancer. *Oncology Nursing Forum, 26,* 1519-1523.

Wade, G. H. (1998). A concept analysis of personal transformation. *Journal of Advanced Nursing, 28,* 713-719.

Weingourt, R. (1998). Using Margaret A. Newman's theory of health with elderly nursing home residents. *Perspectives in Psychiatric Care, Journal of Nurse Psychotherapists, 34*(3), 25-30.

Wendler, M. C. (1996). Understanding healing: A conceptual analysis. *Journal of Advanced Nursing, 24,* 836-842.

Yamashita, M. (1997). Family caregiving: Application of Newman's and Peplau's theories. *Journal of Psychiatric and Mental Health Nursing, 4,* 401-405.

Yamashita, M. (1998). Family coping with mental illness: A comparative study. *Journal of Psychiatric and Mental Health Nursing, 5,* 515-523.

Yamashita, M. (1998). Newman's theory of health as expanding consciousness: Research on family caregiving in mental illness in Japan. *Nursing Science Quarterly, 11,* 110-115.

Yamashita, M. (1999). Newman's theory of health applied in family caregiving in Canada. *Nursing Science Quarterly, 12,* 73-79.

Yamashita, M., & Forsyth, D. M. (1998). Family coping with mental illness: An aggregate from two studies, Canada and the United States. *Journal of the American Psychiatric Nurses Association, 4,* 1-8.

Yamashita, M., Jensen, E., & Tall, F. (1998). Therapeutic touch: Applying Newman's theoretic approach. *Nursing Science Quarterly, 11,* 49-50.

Yamashita, M., & Tall, F. D. (1998). A commentary on Newman's theory of health as expanding consciousness. *ANS Advances in Nursing Science, 21,* 65-75.

Yamashita, M., & Tall, F. D. (1999). Letters to the editor . . . a commentary on Newman: Theory of health as expanding consciousness. *ANS Advances in Nursing Science, 22*(1), vi-viii.

Zahourek, R. P. (2002). Intentionality: A view through a Rogerian and a Newman lens—lightly. *International Journal for Human Caring, 6*(2), 29-37.

Listings

Who's Who of American Women. (1983-1985). New Providence, NJ: Reed Reference Publishing.

Who's Who in America. (1996). New Providence, NJ: Reed Reference Publishing.

Who's Who in American Nursing. (1996-2004). New Providence, NJ: Reed Reference Publishing.

Theses

Batty, M. L. E. (1999). Pattern identification and expanding consciousness during the transition of "low risk" pregnancy. A study embodying Newman's health as expanding consciousness (Master's thesis, University of New Brunswick, Canada, 1999). *Masters Abstracts International, 39,* 826.

Bruce-Barrett, C. A. (1998). Patterns of health and healing: Peer support and prostate cancer (Master's thesis, D'Youville College). *Masters Abstracts International, 37,* 0233.

Casper, S. A. (1999). Psychosocial adaptation as a dimension of health as expanding consciousness: Effectiveness of burn survivors support groups (Master's thesis, D'Youville College). *Masters Abstracts International, 37,* 1433.

Web Site

Health as Expanding Consciousness. Accessed December 31, 2004: *http://www.healthasexpandingconsciousness.org*

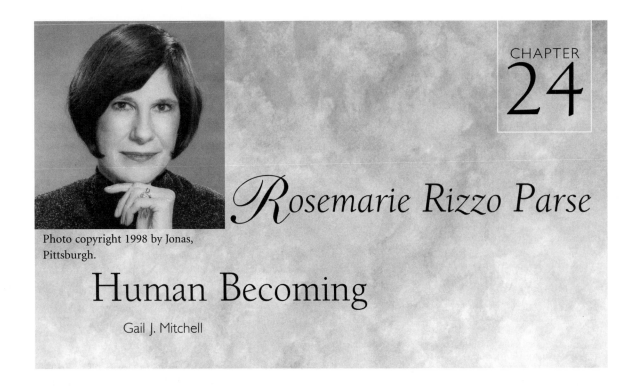

Photo copyright 1998 by Jonas,
Pittsburgh.

Rosemarie Rizzo Parse

Human Becoming

Gail J. Mitchell

CREDENTIALS AND BACKGROUND OF THE THEORIST

Rosemarie Rizzo Parse is a graduate of Duquesne University in Pittsburgh and received her master's and doctorate degrees from the University of Pittsburgh. She was a faculty member at the University of Pittsburgh, dean of the Nursing School at Duquesne University and, from 1983 to 1993, she was professor and coordinator of the Center for Nursing Research at Hunter College of the City University of New York. She has consulted throughout the world with doctoral programs in nursing and with health care organizations that have selected her theory as a guide to research, practice, administration, education, and regulation.

Previous authors: Kathleen D. Pickrell, Rickard E. Lee, Larry P. Schumacher, and Prudence Twigg.
The author wishes to thank Dr. Rosemarie Rizzo Parse for reviewing the chapter.

Parse is a professor and holds the Niehoff Chair at the Marcella Niehoff School of Nursing, Loyola University, Chicago. She is founder and editor of *Nursing Science Quarterly,* president of Discovery International Incorporated, which sponsors international nursing theory conferences, and founder of the Institute of Human Becoming, where she teaches the ontological, epistemological, and methodological aspects of the human becoming school of thought (Parse, 1981, 1992, 1996, 1998). Parse has authored many articles and books, including *Nursing Fundamentals* (1974), *Man-Living-Health: A Theory of Nursing* (1981), *Nursing Science: Major Paradigms, Theories, and Critiques* (1987), *Illuminations: The Human Becoming Theory in Practice and Research* (1995), *The Human Becoming School of Thought: A Perspective for Nurses and Other Health Professionals* (1998), *Hope: An International Human Becoming Perspective* (1999), *Qualitative Inquiry: The Path of Sciencing* (2001a), and *Community: A*

Human Becoming Perspective (2003a). Some of her works have been published in Danish, Finnish, French, German, Japanese, and Korean. In addition, *The Human Becoming School of Thought: A Perspective for Nurses and Other Health Professionals* (Parse, 1998) was selected for Sigma Theta Tau and Doody Publishing's Best Picks list in the nursing theory book category in 1998. *Hope: An International Human Becoming Perspective* (Parse, 1999) was selected for the same list in 1999.

Parse's multiple research projects and interests are focused on lived experiences of health and human becoming. She has developed basic and applied science research methodologies congruent with the ontology of human becoming and has conducted and published numerous investigations on a wide variety of phenomena, including laughter, health, aging, quality of life, joy-sorrow, contentment, feeling very tired, and hope. The hope study, for which she was the principle investigator, included participants and co-investigators from nine countries (Parse, 1999). Parse's research methodologies are used as methods of inquiry by nurse scholars in Australia, Canada, Denmark, Finland, Greece, Italy, Japan, South Korea, Sweden, the United Kingdom, and the United States. Her theory guides practice in various health care settings in Canada, Finland, South Korea, Sweden, the United Kingdom, and the United States. Human becoming is also used as a guide for education, administration, and regulation in several settings in North America.

THEORETICAL SOURCES

The human becoming school of thought is grounded in the human sciences as espoused by Dilthey and others over the past century (Cody & Mitchell, 2002; Mitchell & Cody, 1992; Parse, 1981, 1987, 1998). The human becoming school of thought is "consistent with Martha E. Rogers' principles and postulates about unitary human beings and it is consistent with major tenets and concepts from existential-phenomenological thought, but it is a new product, a different conceptual system" (Parse, 1998, p. 4). At the time she was developing

her theory, Parse was working at Duquesne University in Pittsburgh. While she was there (during the 1960s and 1970s), Duquesne was regarded as the center of the existential-phenomenological movement in the United States. Dialogues she had with scholars in this school of thought, such as van Kaam and Giorgi, stimulated and focused her thinking on the lived experiences of human beings and their situated freedom and participation in life.

By synthesizing the science of unitary human beings, developed by Martha E. Rogers (1970, 1992), with the fundamental tenets from existential-phenomenological thought, as articulated by Heidegger, Sartre, and Merleau-Ponty, Parse secured nursing as a human science. Parse contends that humans cannot be reduced to component systems or parts and still be understood. Persons are living beings who are more than and different from any schemata that divides them. Parse challenges the traditional medical view of nursing and distinguishes the discipline of nursing as a unique, basic science. Parse supports the notion that nurses require a unique knowledge base that informs their practice and research and this knowledge (of the human-universe-health process) is essential for nurses to fulfill their commitment to humankind (Parse, 1981, 1987, 1993).

In developing her theory, Parse was especially influenced by Rogers' principles of helicy, integrality, and resonancy and by her postulates (energy field, openness, pattern, and pandimensionality) (Parse, 1981; Rogers, 1970, 1992). These ideas underpin Parse's notions about persons as open beings who relate at multiple realms with the universe and who are irreducible, ever changing, and recognized by patterns (Parse, 1981, 1998).

From existential-phenomenological thought, Parse drew on the tenets of intentionality and human subjectivity and the corresponding concepts of coconstitution, coexistence, and situated freedom (Parse, 1981, 1998). Parse uses the prefix *co* on many of her words to denote the participative nature of persons. *Co* means *together with* and for Parse, humans can never be separated from their relationships with the universe. Relationships with the universe include all the linkages humans have with other people and with ideas, projects, predecessors, history, and culture (Parse, 1981, 1998).

From Parse's perspective, humans are intentional beings. By this she means that human beings have an open and meaningful stance with the universe and the people, projects, and ideas that constitute lived experience. Human beings are intentional in that their involvements are not random but chosen for reasons known and not known. Parse says that being human is being intentional and present, open, and knowing with the world. Intentionality is also about purpose and how persons choose direction and ways of thinking and acting toward projects and people. People choose attitudes and next actions from a realm of possibilities (Parse, 1981, 1998).

The basic tenet, human subjectivity, means viewing human beings not as things or objects but as beings that are unitary and as beings that are a mystery of being with nonbeing. Human beings live what was, is, and will be in the now moments of their intersubjective relationships with the universe. Parse posits that the human's presence and relationship with the world is subjectivity and humans assign meaning to their lives and their projects in the process of becoming who they are. As people choose meanings and projects, according to their value priorities, they coparticipate with the world at multiple realms (Parse, 1981, 1998). Every person, although inseparable from the world and from others, crafts a unique relationship with the universe. Human beings have a personal relationship with the universe that is open to new possibilities and directions. The personal relationship is the person's becoming and becoming is complex, multilayered, and full of explicit-implicit meanings (Parse, 1981, 1998).

Coconstitution is the idea that the meaning of any moment or situation is linked with the particulars that contribute to the moment or situation (Parse, 1981, 1998). Human beings choose and assign meaning as they see and evaluate the particular constituents of day-to-day life. Life happens, events unfold in expected and unexpected ways, and the human being engages these constituents and contributes personal meaning and significance. This engaging and assigning of meaning is how coconstitution emerges day to day, and coconstitution surfaces both opportunities and limitations for human

beings as they live their presence with the world and as they make choices about what things mean and how to proceed. The term *coconstitution* also links to the ways people create different meanings from the same situations. People change and are changed through their personal interpretations of life situations. Various ways of thinking and acting unite familiar patterns with the newly emerging as people proceed with crafting their unique realities.

The term *coexistence* means that "the human is not alone in any dimension of becoming" (Parse, 1998, p. 17). Human beings are always with the world of things, ideas, language, unfolding events, and cherished traditions and they are also always with others—not only contemporaries, but also predecessors and successors. There is no individual in Parse's human becoming theory. There is the personal and there is the intersubjective, and even the way one knows self as a human being is linked intimately to the ways others think and act around persons. Indeed, Parse posits that "without others, one would not know that one is a being" (Parse, 1998, p. 17). Persons think about themselves in relation to how they are with others and how they might be with their plans and dreams. Coexistence links with the notion of mutual process and the unity of lived experience. No objective-subjective dualities or cause-effect relationships can represent human becoming. Linked to the assumption of freedom, Parse describes an abiding respect for human change and possibility.

Finally, situated freedom means that human beings emerge in the context of a time and history, a culture and language, physicality and potentiality. Parse suggests that human freedom means "reflectively and prereflectively one participates in choosing the situations in which one finds oneself as well as one's attitude toward the situations" (Parse, 1998, p. 17). Humans are always choosing. Persons decide what is important in their lives. They decide how to approach situations and what projects and people to pay attention to. Day-to-day living represents people choosing and acting on their value priorities, and value priorities shift as life unfolds. Sometimes being able to act on beliefs is as important as achieving the desired outcome. Personal integrity is linked intimately to the notion of situated freedom.

MAJOR CONCEPTS & DEFINITIONS

The three principles, which constitute the human becoming theory, flow from the themes (Parse, 1981, 1998). Each principle contains three concepts that require thoughtful exploration to understand the depth of the human becoming theory. The principles are as follows:

1. Structuring meaning multidimensionally is cocreating reality through the languaging of valuing and imaging.
2. Cocreating rhythmical patterns of relating is living the paradoxical unity of revealing-concealing and enabling-limiting while connecting-separating.
3. Cotranscending with the possibles is powering unique ways of originating in the process of transforming.

PRINCIPLE I: STRUCTURING

The first principle proposes that persons structure, or choose, the meaning of their realities, and this choosing happens at realms that are not always known explicitly. Sometimes questions are not answerable, because people may not know why they think or feel one way or another. The first principle suggests that the way people see the world, their imaging of it, is their reality, and they create this reality with others, and they show or language their reality in the ways they speak and remain silent and in the ways they move and stay still. When people language their realities, they also language their value priorities and meanings (according to the first principle). The first principle has three concepts as follows: (1) imaging, (2) valuing, and (3) languaging.

Imaging

Imaging is an individual's view of reality. It is the shaping of personal knowledge in explicit and tacit ways (Parse, 1981, 1998). For Parse, people are inherently curious and seek to find answers and figure things out. The answers to questions emerge as persons explore meaning in light of reality and their view of things. Imaging is a personal interpretation of meaning, possibility, and consequence. Nurses cannot completely know another's imaging, but they can explore, respect, and bear witness as people struggle with the processes of shaping, exploring, integrating, rejecting, and interpreting.

Valuing

Valuing is the second concept of the first principle. This concept is about how persons confirm and do not confirm beliefs in light of a personal perspective or worldview (Parse, 1981, 1998). Persons are continuously confirming–not confirming beliefs as they are making choices about how to think, act, and feel, and these choices may be consistent with prior choices or they may be radically different and require a shifting of value priorities. Sometimes people may think about anticipated choices and, once the choice arrives, they change their thinking and direction in life. Values reflect what is important in life to a person or a family. For Parse, living value priorities is how an individual expresses health and human becoming. Nurses learn about persons' perspectives by asking them what is most important.

Languaging

Languaging is a concept that relates to how human beings symbolize and express their imaged realities and their value priorities. Languaging is visible in the way people speak and remain silent and in the way they move and remain still. Languaging is lived multidimensionally when people picture themselves in situations that have been or in situations that are only possibilities. When languaging is visible to others, it often is expressed in patterns that are shared with those who are close. Family members or close friends often share similar patterns, such as speaking, moving, and being quiet (Parse, 1981, 1998). People disclose things about themselves when they language, even when they are silent and remain still. Nurses can witness

Continued

MAJOR CONCEPTS *&* DEFINITIONS—cont'd

some of the languaging that people show, but they cannot know the meaning of the languaging. To understand languaging, nurses must ask people what their words, actions, and gestures mean. It is possible that the person does not yet know the meaning of their languaging, in which case the nurse respects the process of coming to understand the meaning of a situation. Explicating meaning can take time, and people know when it is right to illuminate the meaning and significance of an event or happening.

PRINCIPLE 2: COCREATING

The second principle of human becoming is "cocreating rhythmical patterns of relating is living the paradoxical unity of revealing-concealing and enabling-limiting while connecting-separating" (Parse, 1981, p. 41). This principle means that human beings create patterns in day-to-day life and these patterns tell about personal meanings and values. In the patterns of relating that people create, many freedoms and restrictions surface with choices; all patterns involve complex engagements and disengagements with people, ideas, and preferences. The second principle has three concepts as follows: (1) revealing-concealing, (2) enabling-limiting, and (3) connecting-separating.

Revealing-Concealing

Revealing-concealing is the way persons disclose and keep hidden, all-at-once, the persons they are becoming (Parse, 1981, 1998). There is always more to tell and more to know about ourselves and others. Parse identifies the notion of mystery as central to understanding this paradoxical concept. It is mysterious how people choose to give and withhold messages about who they are and what they think and know. Sometimes people know what they want to say and they deliver messages with great clarity and, at other times, people may surprise themselves with the messages they

give. Some layers of reality and experience remain concealed. People also reveal-conceal differently in different situations and with different people. Further, patterns of revealing-concealing are cocreated and intimately linked to the mutual process of the moment and to the intentions of those persons present. In choosing how to be with others, nurses cocreate what happens in the nurse-person process.

Enabling-Limiting

Enabling-limiting represents the freedoms and opportunities that surface with the restrictions and obstacles of everyday living. Every choice, even those made at prereflective realms, surface opportunities and restrictions. It is not possible to know all the consequences of any given choice; therefore, people make choices amid the reality of ambiguity. Every choice is pregnant with possibility in both opportunity and restriction. This is verified in practice daily when patients and families say things like, "This is the worst thing that could have happened to our family, but it has helped us in many ways." Enabling-limiting is about choosing from the possibilities and living with the consequences of those choices. Nurses can be helpful to others as they contemplate the options and anticipated consequences of difficult choices.

Connecting-Separating

Connecting-separating is the third concept of the second principle. This concept has layers of paradoxical meaning. The concept relates to the ways persons create patterns of connecting and separating with people and projects. The patterns created reveal value priorities. Connecting-separating is about the paradox communion-aloneness and the ways people separate from some to join with others. Connecting-separating also explains the way two people can be very close and yet maintain separateness between the two. Sometimes

MAJOR CONCEPTS *&* DEFINITIONS—cont'd

there is connecting when people are separating because persons can dwell with an absent presence with great intimacy, especially when grieving for another (Bournes, 2000a; Cody, 1995b; Pilkington, 1993). Nurses learn about persons' patterns of connecting-separating by asking about their important relationships and projects.

PRINCIPLE 3: COTRANSCENDING

Cotranscending is the third theme of the human becoming theory. "Cotranscending with the possibles is powering unique ways of originating in the process of transforming" (Parse, 1981, p. 41). The meaning of this principle is that persons are always engaging with and choosing from infinite possibilities about how to be, what attitude or approach to have, who to relate with, what interests or concerns to be bothered with. The choices reflect the persons' ways of moving and changing in the process of becoming. The three concepts of this principle are as follows: (1) powering, (2) originating, and (3) transforming.

Powering

Powering is a concept that conveys meaning about struggle and life and the will to go on despite hardship and threat. Parse (1981, 1998) describes powering as a pushing-resisting process that is always happening and that affirms our being in light of the possibility of nonbeing. People constantly engage being and nonbeing. Nonbeing is about loss and the risk of death and rejection. Powering is the force exerted, the pushing to act and live with purpose amid possibilities for affirming and holding what is cherished, while simultaneously living with loss and threat of nonbeing. There is always resistance with the pushing force of powering, because persons live with others who are also powering toward different possibilities. Conflict, according to Parse (1981, 1998), presents opportunities to clarify meanings and values and nurses can enhance this process by being present with persons who are exploring issues, conflicts, and options.

Originating

Originating is a concept about human uniqueness and holds the following two paradoxes: (1) conforming–not conforming and (2) certainty-uncertainty. People strive to be like others, and yet they also strive to be unique. Choices about originating occur with the reality of certainty-uncertainty. It is not possible to know all that may come from choosing to be different or from choosing to be like others. For some, there is greater danger in being too much like others; some may say the greater danger is in being different. Each person defines and lives originating in light of their worldview and values. Originating and creating anew is a pattern that coexists with constancy and conformity (Parse, 1981, 1998). Humans craft their unique patterns of originating as they engage the possibilities of everyday life. Nurses witness originating with persons who are in the process of choosing how they are going to be with their changing health patterns.

Transforming

Transforming, the third concept of the third principle, is about deliberate change and the shifting views that people have about their lives. People are always struggling to integrate the unfamiliar with the familiar in the living of everydayness. When new discoveries are made, people change their understanding and, sometimes, life patterns and worldviews can shift with the mystery of an insight that illuminates a familiar situation in a new light. Transforming is the ongoing change characteristic of mutual process and human ingenuity as people find ways to change in the direction of their cherished hopes and dreams (Parse, 1981, 1998). Nurses, in the way they are present with others, help or hinder persons' efforts to clarify their hopes, dreams, and desired directions.

USE OF EMPIRICAL EVIDENCE

Research guided by the human becoming theory is meant to enhance the theoretical foundation, or the knowledge contained in the principles and concepts of the human becoming theory. Research is not used to test Parse's theory. Nurses do not set out to test if people have unique meanings of life situations, or if persons have situated freedom, or if humans are unitary beings, or if persons relate with others and the universe in paradoxical patterns. To test these beliefs would be comparable to testing the assumption that humans are spiritual beings or that people are composed of complex systems. These statements are abstract beliefs based on experience, observation, and beliefs about the nature of reality. The statements are value laden and, as noted earlier, a nurse either has an attraction and commitment to these foundational beliefs or not. The idea of a unitary human being in mutual process is an assumption that is either believable or not. Assumptions about human beings are theoretical, not factual. A student or nurse relates to one notion of human being or another. According to Parse, this is why there is a need for multiple views; the discipline of nursing can and does accommodate different views and different theories about the human-universe-health process. In agreement with Hall, Parse (1993) stated the following when discussing the issue of testing the human becoming theory:

> The human becoming theory does not lend itself to testing, since it is not a predictive theory and is not based on a cause-effect view of the human-universe process. The purpose of the research is not to verify the theory or test it but, rather, the focus is on uncovering the essences of lived phenomena to gain further understanding of universal human experiences. This understanding evolves from connecting the descriptions given by people to the theory, thus making more explicit the essences of being human. (p. 12)

Research with Parse's theory expands understanding about the human-universe-health process and inquiry builds new knowledge about human becoming. Knowledge of human becoming contributes to the substantive knowledge of the nursing discipline. Disciplinary knowledge is different than the practical or technical knowledge that nurses use in various health care settings. Disciplinary knowledge is theoretical and identifies the phenomenon of concern for nurses—for Parse, human becoming. According to Parse (1998), "Scholarly research is formal inquiry leading to the discovery of new knowledge with the enhancement of theory" (p. 59). This idea of new knowledge with enhancement of theory requires additional attention to clarify the distinctions among different ways of thinking.

Research guided by the human becoming theory explores universal lived experiences with people as they live them in day-to-day life. Parse contends that there are universal human experiences, such as hope, joy, sorrow, grief, anticipation, fear, confidence, and contemplation. Further, persons experience the what was, the what is, and the what will be—all at once. This means that research guided by human becoming theory explores lived experiences as people are living them in the moment. People live in the moment, and what is remembered and what is hoped for are always viewed within the reality of the now. Further, universal experiences cannot be reduced to linear time frames because lived experience is unitary and multidimensional. A nurse researcher conducting a Parse method study invites persons to speak about a particular universal experience. For instance, a researcher might invite a participant to talk about his or her experience of grieving (Cody, 1995a, 2000; Pilkington, 1993). The researcher would not ask the participant to speak about grieving while in the hospital, for example, because lived experience is not compartmentalized. Rather, lived experience is multidimensional and people speak from the way they know universal experiences in the context of their own lives. The researcher guided by human becoming knows that the person's reality encompasses the what was, is, and the will be as it is appearing in the moment. The researcher also assumes that the person knows his or her experience and can offer an account of the experience as he or she lives it.

In 1987, Parse first developed a specific research method consistent with the human becoming theory; since then, the human becoming herme-neutic method has been articulated (Cody, 1995c; Parse, 2001a). A third method, an applied science method (qualitative descriptive preproject-process-postproject) has been articulated (Parse, 2001a). For details of all these methods, please see *The Human Becoming School of Thought: A Perspective for Nurses and Other Health Professionals* (Parse, 1998) and *Qualitative Inquiry: The Path of Sciencing* (Parse, 2001a). The Parse research method records accounts of personal experiences and systematically examines those accounts to identify the aspects of lived experiences that are shared across participants. The core concepts, or ideas shared across all participants, form a structure of the phenomenon under study. The structure as defined by Parse (1999) is the "paradoxical living of the remembered, the now-moment, and the not-yet, all-at-once" (p. 5). New knowledge is embedded in the core concepts and, once discovered, the new knowledge enhances theory and understanding in ways that go beyond the particular study. The weaving of the new knowledge with the theoretical concepts expands the content of the human becoming theory, and that is how the new knowledge with enhancement develops disciplinary and interdisciplinary thinking and dialogue.

A metaphor of panning for gold may help describe the Parse method. The researcher gathers description from participants like a person panning for gold gathers up the earth. The extraction-synthesis processes of the Parse method can be imagined to be like the gathering, sifting, swirling, seeking, and separating that happens when panning for gold. Researchers following the Parse method work to separate particular context from core ideas. The gathering and discovering happen over and over as context and earth are separated from the core ideas or nuggets that eventually stand out from the surrounding context or earth. Panning for gold is thought of as back-breaking work, and the Parse research method is also arduous. Both processes include excitement and anticipation of what is to be discovered. The extraction-synthesis processes of the Parse method separate the core ideas that are present in all the participant descriptions. The core ideas, like gold nuggets, can be isolated but are not yet refined to a form that will make them meaningful in the world at large. Gold nuggets get refined into coins or jewelry. Core ideas get refined by being abstracted to the language of human becoming and nursing science so that other nurses can see not only the gold nuggets, which are the newly discovered ideas, but also the meaningfulness of the ideas in light of a language of nursing science. Because all research is theory driven, research findings require interpretation in light of the guiding frame of reference in order to advance disciplinary knowledge.

MAJOR ASSUMPTIONS

Parse (1998) synthesized "principles, tenets, and concepts from Rogers, Heidegger, Merleau-Ponty, and Sartre . . . in the creation of the assumptions about the human and becoming, underpinning a view of nursing grounded in the human sciences. Each assumption is unique and represents a synthesis of three of the postulates and concepts drawn from Rogers' work and from existential phenomenology" (p. 19). This underscores just how firmly Parse's theoretical sources underpin her development of the human becoming school of thought. Parse draws upon the work of other theorists to build a solid foundation for a new nursing science. Accordingly, the assumptions underpinning the human becoming theory focus on beliefs about humans and about their becoming, which is health. Parse does not specify separate assumptions about the universe, because her belief is that the universe is multidimensional and in mutual process with the human and not separate from the human. This is evident in the following assumptions about human beings and human becoming:

- The human is coexisting while coconstituting rhythmical patterns with the universe (coexistence, coconstitution, and pattern).
- The human is open, freely choosing meaning in situation, bearing responsibility for decisions (situated freedom, openness, and energy field).
- The human is unitary, continuously coconstituting patterns of relating (energy field, pattern, and coconstitution).

- The human is transcending multidimensionally with the possibles (pandimensionality, openness, and situated freedom).
- Becoming is unitary human-living-health (openness, situated freedom, and coconstitution).
- Becoming is a rhythmically coconstituting human-universe process (coconstitution, pattern, and pandimensionality).
- Becoming is the human's patterns of relating value priorities (situated freedom, pattern, and openness).
- Becoming is an intersubjective process of transcending with the possibles (openness, situated freedom, and coexistence).
- Becoming is unitary human's emerging (coexistence, energy field, and pandimensionality). (Parse, 1998, pp. 19-20, 28)

Parse (1998) synthesized the original nine assumptions about humans and becoming into three assumptions about human becoming, as follows:

1. Human becoming is freely choosing personal meaning in situation in the intersubjective process of living value priorities.
2. Human becoming is cocreating rhythmical patterns of relating in mutual process with the universe.
3. Human becoming is cotranscending multidimensionally with emerging possibilities. (p. 29)

Three themes linked to the assumptions of the human becoming theory are as follows: (1) meaning, (2) rhythmicity, and (3) cotranscendence (Parse, 1998). Meaning is borne in the messages that persons give and take with others in speaking, acting, silence, and stillness. Meaning indicates the significance of something and significance is chosen by people. Outsiders cannot decide the meaning or significance of something for another person. Nurses cannot know what it will mean for a family to hear news of an unexpected illness or change in health until they learn the meaning it holds from the family's perspective. Sometimes people may not know the significance of something until meaning is explored and possibilities examined. Personal meanings are shared with others

when people express their views, concerns, hopes, and dreams. According to Parse (1998), meaning surfaces or comes to light in the human-universe process, and meaning is linked with the moments of day-to-day living as well as to the meaning or purpose of life itself.

Rhythmicity is about patterns, paradox, and possibility. Parse (1981) suggests that people live unrepeatable patterns that are their priorities and that these patterns are changing constantly as people integrate new experiences and ideas. Lived experience is inherently paradoxical, from Parse's view, and according to Mitchell (1993), "living paradox is experiencing the contradiction of opposites" (p. 47). For Parse, people are recognized by their unique patterns that signify both consistency and change. People change their patterns when they integrate new priorities, ideas, and dreams and they show consistent patterns that continue like threads of familiarity and sameness throughout life.

Cotranscendence is the third major theme of the human becoming school of thought. Cotranscendence is about change and possibility, the infinite possibility that is human becoming. "The possibilities arise with the human-universe process as options from which to choose personal ways of becoming" (Parse, 1998, p. 30). To believe one thing or another, to go in one direction or another, to be persistent or to let go, to struggle or acquiesce, to hope or despair—all these options surface in day-to-day living. Considering and choosing from these options is cotranscending with the possibles.

Nursing

Consistent with her beliefs, Parse does not describe or write about nursing as a concept in the metaparadigm of the discipline. However, she has written extensively about her beliefs concerning nursing as a basic science. Parse (2000) wrote, "It is the hope of many nurses that nursing as a discipline will enjoy the recognition of having a unique knowledge base and the profession will be sufficiently distinct from medicine that people will actually seek nurses for nursing care, not medical diagnoses" (p. 3). For more than 30 years, Parse has been advancing the belief that nursing is a basic science and that nurses require theories that are different from other disciplines. Parse believes that nursing is a unique service to humankind. This does not mean that nurses do not benefit from and employ knowledge from other disciplines and fields of study. It means that nurses primarily rely on and value the knowledge of nursing in their practice and research activities. Parse (1992) has articulated clearly that she believes "nursing is a science, the practice of which is a performing art" (p. 35). From this view, nursing is a learned discipline and nursing theories guide practice and research. The belief that nursing is a unique discipline requiring its own theories is not the predominant view and, hopefully, debates about this issue will continue to clarify the opportunities nurses have for creating the future of nursing science.

The practice of nursing for nurses choosing Parse's theory is guided by a specific methodology that emerges directly from the human becoming ontology. The practice dimensions and processes are illuminating meaning through explicating, synchronizing rhythms through dwelling, and mobilizing transcendence through moving beyond. For details of practice methodology, see *The Human Becoming School of Thought: A Perspective for Nurses and Other Health Professionals* (Parse, 1998). "Nurses who value the human becoming belief system live the theory in true presence with others" (Parse, 1993, p. 12). Parse (1993) describes practice in the following way:

> The nurse is in true presence with the individual (or family) as the individual (or family) uncovers the personal meaning of the situation and makes choices to move forward in the now moment with cherished hopes and dreams. The focus is on the meaning of the lived experience for the person (or family) unfolding "there with" the presence of the nurse. . . . The living of the theory in practice is indeed what makes a difference to the people touched by it. (p. 12)

Nursing, for Parse, is a science, and the performing art of nursing is practiced in relationships with persons (individuals, groups, and communities) in

their processes of becoming. Parse (1989a) offers the following set of fundamentals that she believes are essential for practicing the art of nursing:

- Know and use nursing frameworks and theories.
- Be available to others.
- Value the other as a human presence.
- Respect differences in view.
- Own what you believe and be accountable for your actions.
- Move on to the new and untested.
- Connect with others.
- Take pride in self.
- Like what you do.
- Recognize the moments of joy in the struggles of living.
- Appreciate mystery and be open to new discoveries.
- Be competent in your chosen area.
- Rest and begin anew. (p. 11)

Human-Universe-Health Process

Parse views the concepts human, universe, and health as inseparable and irreducible. Parse (1990, 1996, 1998) speaks of the human-universe-health process and, although each can be described, they are intimately linked in mutual process. For Parse, health is human becoming. Health is structuring meaning, cocreating rhythmical patterns of relating, and cotranscending with the possibles. Parse (1990) also speaks of health as a personal commitment, which means "an individual's way of becoming is cocreated by that individual, incarnating his or her own value priorities" (p. 136). For Parse (1990), health is a flowing process, a personal creation, and a personal responsibility. As such, personal health can be changed by changing commitment, which "can include creative imagining, affirming self, and spontaneous glimpsing of the paradoxical" (Parse, 1990, p. 138).

Human beings come into the world through others and live life in patterns of communion-aloneness. Persons change and are changed with the universe. Persons influence and are influenced by others. People become known and understood as they coexist with the universe through their patterns of relating with people, ideas, culture, history,

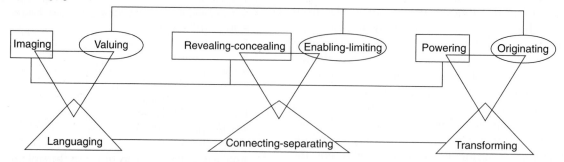

Principle 1: Structuring meaning multidimensionally is cocreating reality through the languaging of valuing and imaging.

Principle 2: Cocreating rhythmical patterns of relating is living the paradoxical unity of revealing-concealing and enabling-limiting while connecting-separating.

Principle 3: Cotranscending with the possibles is powering unique ways of originating in the process of transforming.

Relationship of the concepts in the squares: *Powering* is a way of *revealing and concealing imaging.*
Relationship of the concepts in the ovals: *Originating* is a manifestation of *enabling and limiting valuing.*
Relationship of the concepts in the triangles: *Transforming* unfolds in the *languaging of connecting and separating.*

Figure **24-1** Relationship of principles, concepts, and theoretical structures of the **human becoming theory.** (From Parse, R. R. [1981]. *Man-living-health: A theory of nursing* [p. 69]. New York: John Wiley & Sons.)

meanings, and hopes. To understand human life and human beings, an individual must start from the premise that all people are interconnected with predecessors, contemporaries, and even people who are not yet present in the world. Parents may imagine and have a relationship with a child long before the child is conceived and long after a child is lost through death (Pilkington, 1993). Experience has shown that many people at various times have relationships with their parents, and other loved ones, who are no longer in this world. These are examples of ways that people relate with the universe at multidimensional realms and these ways demonstrate the complex mutual process of human becoming.

THEORETICAL ASSERTIONS

Parse's (1981, 1998) principles are the assertions of the human becoming theory. Each principle interrelates the following nine concepts of human becoming: (1) languaging, (2) valuing, (3) imaging, (4) revealing-concealing, (5) enabling-limiting, (6) connecting-separating, (7) powering, (8) originating, and (9) transforming (Figure 24-1). Research projects generate structures that further specify relationships among the theoretical concepts. For example, Wang (1999) studied hope for persons living with leprosy in Taiwan, and she presented the following theoretical structure: the lived experience of hope is imaging the connecting-separating in originating valuing. Theoretical structures can be used to enhance understanding of specific phenomena as readers consider the detailed participant descriptions that are linked to the concepts of human becoming theory.

LOGICAL FORM

The inductive-deductive process was central to the creation of the human becoming theory. The theory originated from Parse's personal experiences with her readings and in nursing practice. She deductively-inductively crafted major components of human becoming from Rogers' Science of Unitary

Human Beings and existential-phenomenological thought. With her intuitive sense, Parse methodically derived the assumptions, concepts, principles, and practice and research methodologies of the human becoming school of thought. Figure 24-1 shows how the principles, concepts, and theoretical structures can be linked. The figure shows the most abstract view of human becoming—the simplicity and complexity of the theory are evident. Abstraction and complexity create possibility for growth, scholarship, and sustainability.

ACCEPTANCE BY THE NURSING COMMUNITY

Practice

The following bibliography demonstrates the broad scope of acceptance by the nursing community. A strong and influential group of nursing scholars is advancing human becoming in practice, research, and education. As shown in Box 24-1, the theory has made a difference to nurses and to persons (patients) who experience human becoming practice. The theory informs nurses who work with older persons and with children. The theory guides practice for nurses who work with families with persons in hospital settings, clinics, and community settings. A community-based health action model, for instance, has been developed and is receiving support from the local community and other funding agencies (Crane, Josephson, & Letcher, 1999). The theory of human becoming has also helped to generate controversy and scholarly dialogue about nursing as an evolving discipline and distinct human science (see Box 24-1). Interestingly, the theory of human becoming provides a set of beliefs that can be lived by nurses who have opportunities to be with human beings. It is not a question of whether or not the theory works in any particular setting. The theory has been lived by nurses in the operating theater, in parishes, in shelters, in acute care hospitals, and in other long-term and community settings. A more important question for nurses may be: what settings consistently provide opportunities for nurses to have relationships with persons and families?

Education

The human becoming school of thought and the philosophical assumptions and theoretical beliefs specified by Parse have helped fuel many scholarly dialogues and comparisons about outcomes in practice, research, and education when different theories guide professional activities (see examples in Box 24-1). In *Nursing Science Quarterly* and other journals, nurses informed by the human becoming theory have advanced dialogue and debate about the role of theory in nursing practice, the limitations and contributions of the medical model, the ethics of nursing diagnoses and the nurse-person relationship, paternalism and health care, the knowledge of advanced nursing practice, paradigmatic issues in nursing, the limitations of evidence-based nursing, the possibilities and politics of human science, freedom and choice, the focus of community-based nursing, the nature of truth, leadership and nursing theory, and the scope of mis-takes in nursing.

Teachers in academic and practice settings have contributed new understanding and new processes of teaching-learning (see Box 24-1), and Parse's theory has been used as a model for explicating pros and cons of teleapprenticeship (Norris, 2002). The human becoming school of thought also informs nursing courses at the undergraduate and graduate level in many schools of nursing.

In the text, *Man-Living-Health: A Theory of Nursing,* Parse (1981) presented a sample master's in nursing curriculum that incorporated the assumptions, principles, concepts, and theoretical structures of human becoming theory. She outlined this process-based curriculum in detail, including course descriptions and course sequencing. The curriculum plan was updated in the 1998 text, *The Human Becoming School of Thought: a Perspective for Nurses and Other Health Professionals,* in which Parse outlined a program philosophy and goals, a conceptual framework with themes for the curriculum, program indicators, course culture content, and the evaluation process and provided a sample curriculum plan consistent with human becoming.

Text continued on p. 540

Box 24-1

Abridged List of Publications of Human Becoming Theory Related to Practice, Research, Education, Critique, and Scholarly Dialogue

PRACTICE AND HUMAN BECOMING

Nurses' Experiences

Melnechenko, K. L. (2003). To make a difference: Nursing presence. *Nursing Forum, 38,* 18-24.

Mitchell, G. J., & Bournes, D. A. (1998). *Finding the way: A video guide to patient focused care* (Videotape). Toronto, Ontario, Canada: Sunnybrook & Women's Health Science Centre.

Mitchell, G. J., & Lawton, C. (2000). Living with the consequences of personal choices for persons with diabetes: Implications for educators and practitioners. *Canadian Journal of Diabetes Care, 24*(2), 23-31.

Quiquero, A., Knights, D., & Meo, C. O. (1991). Theory as a guide to practice: Staff nurses choose Parse's theory. *Canadian Journal of Nursing Administration, 4*(1), 14-16.

Rasmusson, D. L., Jonas, C. M., & Mitchell, G. J. (1991). The eye of the beholder: Applying Parse's theory with homeless individuals. *Clinical Nurse Specialist Journal, 5*(3), 139-143.

Stanley, G. D., & Meghani, S. H. (2001). Reflections on using Parse's theory of human becoming in a palliative care setting in Pakistan. *Canadian Nurse, 97,* 23-25.

Patient Perspectives

Mitchell, G. J., Bernardo, A., & Bournes, D. (1997). Nursing guided by Parse's theory: Patient views at Sunnybrook. *Nursing Science Quarterly, 10,* 55-56.

Williamson, G. J. (2000). The test of a nursing theory: A personal view. *Nursing Science Quarterly, 13,* 124-128.

Practice With Older Persons

Baumann, S. (1997). Contrasting two approaches in a community-based nursing practice with older adults: The medical model and Parse's nursing theory. *Nursing Science Quarterly, 10,* 124-130.

Mitchell, G. J. (1986). Utilizing Parse's theory of man-living-health in Mrs. M's neighborhood. *Perspectives, 10*(4), 5-7.

Mitchell, G. J. (1988). Man-living-health: The theory in practice. *Nursing Science Quarterly, 1,* 120-127.

Practice With Children

Baumann, S. L., & Carroll, K. (2001). Human becoming practice with children. *Nursing Science Quarterly, 14,* 120-125.

Cody, W. K., Hudepohl, J. H., & Brinkman, K. S. (1995). True presence with a child and his family. In R. R. Parse (Ed.), *Illuminations: The human becoming theory in practice and research* (pp. 135-146). New York: National League for Nursing Press.

Santopinto, M. D. A., & Smith, M. C. (1995). Evaluation of the human becoming theory in practice with adults and children. In R. R. Parse (Ed.), *Illuminations: The human becoming theory in practice and research* (pp. 309-346). New York: National League for Nursing Press.

Practice With Families

Butler, M. J. (1988). Family transformation: Parse's theory in practice. *Nursing Science Quarterly, 1,* 68-74.

Cody, W. K. (1995). True presence with families living with HIV disease. In R. R. Parse (Ed.), *Illuminations: The human becoming theory in practice and research* (pp. 115-133). New York: National League for Nursing Press.

Cody, W. K. (2000). Parse's human becoming school of thought and families. *Nursing Science Quarterly, 13,* 281-284.

Cody, W. K., Hudepohl, J. H., & Brinkman, K. S. (1995). True presence with a child and his

Box 24-1

Abridged List of Publications of Human Becoming Theory Related to Practice, Research, Education, Critique, and Scholarly Dialogue—cont'd

family. In R. R. Parse (Ed.), *Illuminations: The human becoming theory in practice and research* (pp. 135-146). New York: National League for Nursing Press.

Practice in Hospital Settings

Mitchell, G. J. (1998). Living with diabetes: How understanding expands theory for professional practice. *Canadian Journal of Diabetes Care, 22*(1), 30-37.

Mitchell, G. J., & Cody, W. K. (1999). Human becoming theory: A complement to medical science. *Nursing Science Quarterly, 12,* 304-310.

Mitchell, G. J., Closson, T., Coulis, N., Flint, F., & Gray, B. (2000). Patient-focused care and human becoming thought: Connecting the right stuff. *Nursing Science Quarterly, 13,* 216-224.

Mitchell, G. J., & Copplestone, C. (1990). Applying Parse's theory to perioperative nursing: A nontraditional approach. *AORN Journal, 51,* 787-798.

Mitchell, G. J., & Pilkington, B. (1990). Theoretical approaches in nursing practice: A comparison of Roy and Parse. *Nursing Science Quarterly, 3,* 81-87.

Nelligan, P., Grinspun, D., Jonas-Simpson, C., et al. (2002, Summer). Client centred care: Making the ideal real. *Hospital Quarterly, 5*(4), 70-76.

Practice in Clinics and With Community

Bunkers, S. S. (1998). A nursing theory–guided model of health ministry: Human becoming in parish nursing. *Nursing Science Quarterly, 11,* 7-8.

Bunkers, S. S., Michaels, C., & Ethridge, P. (1997). Advanced practice nursing in community: Nursing's opportunity. *Advanced Practice Nursing Quarterly, 2*(4), 79-84.

Crane, J., Josephson, D., & Letcher, D. (1999, Nov.). *The human becoming health action model in community.* Paper presented at The Seventh Annual International Colloquium on Human Becoming, Loyola University, Chicago.

Huch, M. H., & Bournes, D. A. (2003). Community dwellers' perspectives on the experience of feeling tired. *Nursing Science Quarterly, 16,* 334-339.

Jonas, C. M. (1995). Evaluation of the human becoming theory in family practice. In R. R. Parse (Ed.), *Illuminations: The human becoming theory in practice and research* (pp. 347-366). New York: National League for Nursing Press.

Kelley, L. S. (1995). Parse's theory in practice with a group in the community. *Nursing Science Quarterly, 8,* 127-132.

Milton, C. L., & Buseman, J. (2002). Cocreating anew in public health nursing. *Nursing Science Quarterly, 15,* 113-116.

SCHOLARLY DIALOGUES

Nursing: A Unique Discipline and Human Science

Arrigo, B., & Cody, W. K. (2004). A dialogue on existential-phenomenological thought in psychology and in nursing. *Nursing Science Quarterly, 17,* 6-11.

Baumann, S. L., & Englert, R. (2003). A comparison of three views of spirituality in oncology nursing. *Nursing Science Quarterly, 16,* 52-59.

Cody, W. K. (2003). Diversity and becoming: Implications of human existence as coexistence. *Nursing Science Quarterly, 16,* 195-200.

Cody, W. K., & Mitchell, G. J. (2002). Nursing knowledge and human science revisited: Practical and political considerations. *Nursing Science Quarterly, 15,* 4-13.

Continued

Box 24-1

Abridged List of Publications of Human Becoming Theory Related to Practice, Research, Education, Critique, and Scholarly Dialogue—cont'd

Mitchell, G. J. (1991). Diagnosis: Clarifying or obscuring the nature of nursing. *Nursing Science Quarterly, 4,* 52.

Mitchell, G. J. (1999). Evidence-based practice: Critique and alternative view. *Nursing Science Quarterly, 12,* 30-35.

Mitchell, G. J., & Cody, W. K. (1992). Nursing knowledge and human science: Ontological and epistemological considerations. *Nursing Science Quarterly, 5,* 54-61.

Mitchell, G. J., & Cody, W. K. (1999). Human becoming theory: A complement to medical science. *Nursing Science Quarterly, 12,* 304-310.

Mitchell, G. J., & Cody, W. K. (2002). Ambiguous opportunity: Toiling for truth of nursing art and science. *Nursing Science Quarterly, 15,* 71-79.

Paille, M., & Pilkington, F. B. (2002). The global context of nursing: A human becoming perspective. *Nursing Science Quarterly, 15,* 165-170.

Parse, R. R. (1993). Scholarly dialogue: Theory guides research and practice. *Nursing Science Quarterly, 6,* 12.

Comparison of Outcomes in Practice, Research, and Education

Baumann, S. L., & Englert, R. (2003). A comparison of three views of spirituality in oncology nursing. *Nursing Science Quarterly, 16,* 52-59.

Bournes, D. (2000). A commitment to honouring people's choices. *Nursing Science Quarterly, 13,* 18-23.

Bournes, D. A., & Flint, F. (2003). Mis-takes: Mistakes in the nurse-person process. *Nursing Science Quarterly, 16,* 127-130.

Bunkers, S. S. (2003). Understanding the stranger. *Nursing Science Quarterly, 16,* 305-309.

Cody, W. K. (2003). Paternalism in nursing and healthcare: Central issues and their relation to theory. *Nursing Science Quarterly, 16,* 288-296.

Cody, W. K., & Mitchell, G. J. (1992). Parse's theory as a model for practice: The cutting edge. *ANS Advances in Nursing Science, 15*(2), 52-65.

Damgaard, G., & Bunkers, S. S. (1998). Nursing science–guided practice and education: A state board of nursing perspective. *Nursing Science Quarterly, 11,* 142-144.

Huchings, D. (2002). Parallels in practice: Palliative nursing practice and Parse's theory of human becoming. *American Journal of Hospice and Palliative Care, 19,* 408-414.

Mitchell, G. J. (1998). Standards of nursing and the winds of change. *Nursing Science Quarterly, 11,* 97-98.

Mitchell, G. J. (2001). Policy, procedure, and routine: Matters of moral influence. *Nursing Science Quarterly, 14,* 109-114.

Mitchell, G. J. (2002). Self-serving and other-serving: Matters of trust and intent. *Nursing Science Quarterly, 15*(4), 288-293.

Mitchell, G. J., & Bournes, D. A. (2000). Nurse as patient advocate? In search of straight thinking. *Nursing Science Quarterly, 13,* 204-209.

Mitchell, G. J., & Bunkers, S. S. (2003). Engaging the abyss: A mis-take of opportunity? *Nursing Science Quarterly, 16,* 121-125.

Mitchell, G. J., Closson, T., Coulis, N., Flint, F., & Gray, B. (2000). Patient-focused care and human becoming thought: Connecting the right stuff. *Nursing Science Quarterly, 13,* 216-224.

Pilkington, F. B. (2004). Exploring ethical implications for acting faithfully in professional relationships. *Nursing Science Quarterly, 17,* 27-32.

Box **24-1**

Abridged List of Publications of Human Becoming Theory Related to Practice, Research, Education, Critique, and Scholarly Dialogue—cont'd

Saltmarche, A., Kolodny, V., & Mitchell, G. J. (1998). An educational approach for patient-focused care: Shifting attitudes and practice. *Journal of Nursing Staff Development, 14*(2), 81-86.

Role of Nursing Theory in Practice

Hall, B. A. (1993). Commentary: The inherent value of practice theories. *Nursing Science Quarterly, 6,* 10-11.

Hansen-Ketchum, P. (2004). Parse's theory in practice. *Journal of Holistic Nursing, 22,* 57-72.

Jonas-Simpson, C. (1997). Living the art of the human becoming theory. *Nursing Science Quarterly, 10,* 175-179.

Lee, O. J., & Pilkington, F. B. (1999). Practice with persons living their dying: A human becoming perspective. *Nursing Science Quarterly, 12,* 324-328.

Mitchell, G. J. (2003). Abstractions and particulars: Learning theory for practice. *Nursing Science Quarterly, 16,* 310-314.

Limitations and Contributions of Medical Science

Baumann, S. (1997). Contrasting two approaches in a community-based nursing practice with older adults: The medical model and Parse's nursing theory. *Nursing Science Quarterly, 10,* 124-130.

Linscott, J., Spee, R., Flint, F., & Fisher, A. (1999). Creating a culture of patient-focused care through a learner-centered philosophy. *Canadian Journal of Nursing Leadership, 12*(4), 5-10.

Mitchell, G. J., & Cody, W. K. (1999). Human becoming theory: A complement to medical science. *Nursing Science Quarterly, 12,* 304-310.

Ethical Issues in Practice

Bournes, D. (2000a). A commitment to honouring people's choices. *Nursing Science Quarterly, 13,* 18-23.

Cody, W. K. (2003b). Paternalism in nursing and healthcare: Central issues and their relation to theory. *Nursing Science Quarterly, 16,* 288-296.

Cody, W. K., & Mitchell, G. J. (2002). Nursing knowledge and human science revisited: Practical and political considerations. *Nursing Science Quarterly, 15,* 4-13.

Milton, C. L. (2003b). The American Nurses Association Code of Ethics: A reflection on the ethics of respect and human dignity with nurse as expert. *Nursing Science Quarterly, 16,* 301-304.

Mitchell, G. J. (1991). Diagnosis: Clarifying or obscuring the nature of nursing. *Nursing Science Quarterly, 4,* 52.

Mitchell, G. J. (2001). Policy, procedure, and routine: Matters of moral influence. *Nursing Science Quarterly, 14,* 109-114.

Mitchell, G. J. (2002). Self-serving and other-serving: Matters of trust and intent. *Nursing Science Quarterly, 15*(4), 288-293.

Mitchell, G. J., & Bournes, D. A. (2000). Nurse as patient advocate? In search of straight thinking. *Nursing Science Quarterly, 13,* 204-209.

Pilkington, F. B. (2004). Exploring ethical implications for acting faithfully in professional relationships. *Nursing Science Quarterly, 17,* 27-32.

Advanced Practice and Evidence

Bunkers, S. S., Michaels, C., & Ethridge, P. (1997). Advanced practice nursing in community: Nursing's opportunity. *Advanced Practice Nursing Quarterly, 2*(4), 79-84.

Continued

Box **24-1**

Abridged List of Publications of Human Becoming Theory Related to Practice, Research, Education, Critique, and Scholarly Dialogue—cont'd

Jonas, C. M. (1995). True presence through music for persons living their dying. In R. R. Parse (Ed.), *Illuminations: The human becoming theory in practice* (pp. 97-104). New York: National League for Nursing Press.

Legault, F., & Ferguson-Paré, M. (1999). Advancing nursing practice: An evaluation study of Parse's theory of human becoming. *Canadian Journal of Nursing Leadership, 12*(1), 30-35.

Mitchell, G. J. (1999). Evidence-based practice: Critique and alternative view. *Nursing Science Quarterly, 12,* 30-35.

Noh, C. H. (2004). Meaning of quality of life for persons with serious mental illness: Human becoming practice with groups. *Nursing Science Quarterly, 17,* 220-225.

Parse, R. R., Bournes, D. A., Barrett, E. A., Malinski, V. M., & Phillips, J. R. (1999). A better way. *On Call, 2*(8), 14-17.

Parse, R. R., Coyne, B., & Smith, M. J. (1985). *Nursing research: Qualitative methods.* Bowie, MD: Brady.

Smith, M. K. (2002). Human becoming and women living with violence: The art of practice. *Nursing Science Quarterly, 15,* 302-307.

Wang, C. H. (1997). Quality of life and health for persons living with leprosy. *Nursing Science Quarterly, 10,* 144-145.

Mis-Takes in Nursing

Bournes, D. A., & Flint, F. (2003). Mis-takes: Mistakes in the nurse-person process. *Nursing Science Quarterly, 16,* 127-130.

Mitchell, G. J., & Bunkers, S. S. (2003). Engaging the abyss: A mis-take of opportunity? *Nursing Science Quarterly, 16,* 121-125.

Leadership and Nursing Theory

Bournes, D. A., & Das Gupta, T. L. (1997). Professional practice leader: A

transformational role that addresses human diversity. *Nursing Administration Quarterly, 21*(4), 61-68.

Linscott, J., Spee, R., Flint, F., & Fisher, A. (1999). Creating a culture of patient-focused care through a learner-centered philosophy. *Canadian Journal of Nursing Leadership, 12*(4), 5-10.

Parse, R. R. (1989b). Parse's man-living-health model and administration of nursing service. In B. Henry, C. Arndt, M. DiVincenti, & A. Marriner Tomey (Eds.), *Dimensions of nursing administration: Theory, research, education, and practice.* Cambridge, MA: Blackwell Scientific.

Teaching-Learning

Bunkers, S. S. (2002). Lifelong learning: A human becoming perspective. *Nursing Science Quarterly, 15,* 294-300.

Letcher, D. C., & Yancey, N. R. (2004). Witnessing change with aspiring nurses: A human becoming teaching-learning process in nursing education. *Nursing Science Quarterly, 17,* 36-41.

Milton, C. L. (2003). A graduate curriculum guided by human becoming: Journeying with the possible. *Nursing Science Quarterly, 16,* 214-218.

Parse, R. R. (2004). A human becoming teaching-learning model. *Nursing Science Quarterly, 17,* 33-35.

Saltmarche, A., Kolodny, V., & Mitchell, G. J. (1998). An educational approach for patient-focused care: Shifting attitudes and practice. *Journal of Nursing Staff Development, 14*(2), 81-86.

Woude, D. V., Damgaard, G., Hegge, M. J., Soholt, D., & Bunkers, S. S. (2003). The unfolding: Scenario planning in nursing. *Nursing Science Quarterly, 16,* 27-35.

Box 24-1

Abridged List of Publications of Human Becoming Theory Related to Practice, Research, Education, Critique, and Scholarly Dialogue—cont'd

Evaluations and Critique of Human Becoming Theory

Cowling, W. R. (1989). Parse's theory of nursing. In J. J. Fitzpatrick & A. L. Wall (Eds.), *Conceptual models of nursing: Analysis and application* (2nd ed., pp. 385-399). Norwalk, CT: Appleton & Lange.

Fawcett, J. (2001). The nurse theorists: 21st-century updates—Rosemarie Rizzo Parse. *Nursing Science Quarterly, 14*, 126-131.

Huch, M. H. (2002). Response to: Critical review of R. R. Parse's "The human becoming school of thought. A perspective for nurses and other health professionals." *Journal of Advanced Nursing, 37*, 217.

Phillips, J. R. (1987). A critique of Parse's man-living-health theory. In R. R. Parse (Ed.), *Nursing science: Major paradigms, theories, and critiques* (pp. 181-204). Philadelphia: W. B. Saunders.

Smith, M. C., & Hudepohl, J. H. (1988). Analysis and evaluation of Parse's theory of man-living-health. *The Canadian Journal of Nursing Research: Nursing Papers, 20*(4), 43-58.

Winkler, S. J. (1983). Parse's theory of nursing. In J. Fitzpatrick & A. Wall (Eds.), *Conceptual models of nursing: Analysis and application* (pp. 275-294). Bowie, MD: Robert J. Brady.

Research Guided by Human Becoming Theory

Baumann, S. L. (2000). The lived experience of feeling loved: A study of mothers in a parolee program. *Nursing Science Quarterly, 13*, 332-338.

Baumann, S. L. (2003). The lived experience of feeling very tired: A study of adolescent girls. *Nursing Science Quarterly, 16*, 326-333.

Bournes, D. A. (2000). Concepts inventing: A process for creating a unitary definition of having courage. *Nursing Science Quarterly, 13*, 143-149.

Bournes, D. A. (2002). Having courage: A lived experience of human becoming. *Nursing Science Quarterly, 15*, 220-229.

Bournes, D. A., & Mitchell, G. J. (2002). Waiting: The experience of persons in a critical care waiting room. *Research in Nursing & Health, 25*, 58-67.

Bunkers, S. S. (2003). Comparison of three Parse method studies on feeling very tired. *Nursing Science Quarterly, 16*, 340-344.

Bunkers, S. S. (2004). The lived experience of feeling cared for: A human becoming perspective. *Nursing Science Quarterly, 17*, 63-71.

Cody, W. K. (1995). Of life immense in passion, pulse, and power: Dialoguing with Whitman and Parse. A hermeneutic study. In R. R. Parse (Ed.), *Illuminations: The human becoming theory in practice and research* (pp. 269-308). New York: National League for Nursing Press.

Cody, W. K. (1995). The lived experience of grieving for families living with AIDS: Family-centered research using Parse's method. In R. R. Parse (Ed.), *Illuminations: The human becoming theory in practice and research* (pp. 197-242). New York: National League for Nursing Press.

Cody, W. K. (1995). The meaning of grieving for families living with AIDS. *Nursing Science Quarterly, 8*, 104-114.

Cody, W. K. (2000). The lived experience of grieving for persons living with HIV who have used injection drugs. *Journal of the Association of Nurses in AIDS Care, 11*, 82-92.

Continued

Box **24-1**

Abridged List of Publications of Human Becoming Theory Related to Practice, Research, Education, Critique, and Scholarly Dialogue—cont'd

Gates, K. M. (2000). The experience of caring for a loved one: A phenomenological study. *Nursing Science Quarterly, 13,* 54-59.

Jonas-Simpson, C. M. (2001). Feeling understood: A melody of human becoming. *Nursing Science Quarterly, 14,* 222-230.

Jonas-Simpson, C. M. (2003). The experience of being listened to: A human becoming study with music. *Nursing Science Quarterly, 16,* 232-238.

Mitchell, G. J. (1998). Living with diabetes: How understanding expands theory for professional practice. *Canadian Journal of Diabetes Care, 22*(1), 30-37.

Mitchell, G. J., & Lawton, C. (2000). Living with the consequences of personal choices for persons with diabetes: Implications for educators and practitioners. *Canadian Journal of Diabetes Care, 24*(2), 23-31.

Norris, J. R. (2002). One-to-one teleapprenticeship as a means for nurses teaching and learning Parse's theory of human becoming. *Nursing Science Quarterly, 15,* 143-149.

Northrup, D. T. (2002). Time passing: A Parse research method study. *Nursing Science Quarterly, 15,* 318-326.

Ortiz, M. R. (2003). Lingering presence: A study using the human becoming hermeneutic method. *Nursing Science Quarterly, 16,* 146-154.

Parse, R. R. (1999). *Hope: An international human becoming perspective.* Sudbury, MA: Jones and Bartlett.

Parse, R. R. (2001). The lived experience of contentment: A study using the Parse research method. *Nursing Science Quarterly, 14,* 330-338.

Parse, R. R. (2003). The lived experience of feeling very tired: A study using the Parse research method. *Nursing Science Quarterly, 16,* 319-325.

Pilkington, F. B. (1993). The lived experience of grieving the loss of an important other. *Nursing Science Quarterly, 6,* 130-139.

Pilkington, F. B. (2000). Persisting while wanting to change: Women's lived experiences. *Health Care for Women International, 21,* 501-516.

Pilkington, F. B., & Mitchell, G. J. (2004). Quality of life for women living with a gynecological cancer. *Nursing Science Quarterly, 17,* 147-155.

Thornburg, P. (2002). "Waiting" as experienced by women hospitalized during the antepartum period. *MCN, American Journal of Maternal Child Nursing, 27,* 245-248.

Wang, C. E. (1999). He-bung: Hope for persons living with leprosy in Taiwan. In R. R. Parse (Ed.), *Hope: An international human becoming perspective* (pp. 143-162). Sudbury, MA: Jones and Bartlett.

A master's degree of nursing curriculum consistent with human becoming has been developed at Olivet Nazarene University in Kankakee, Illinois (Milton, 2003a). Many schools of nursing offer students some learning of human becoming theory. To date, most students who study the human becoming theory and who are guided by the theory in their prac-tice and research activities were introduced to Parse's work at the master's level. Parse's ideas and the human becoming theory are increasingly being integrated in undergraduate programs, which will help to expand options for students being taught that nursing is an art and a science that supports multiple perspectives.

Research

Human becoming theory has guided research studies in many different countries about numerous lived experiences, including feeling loved, feeling very tired, having courage, waiting, feeling cared for, grieving, caring for a loved one, persisting while wanting to change, feeling understood, being listened to, time passing, quality of life, health, lingering presence, hope, and contentment (see Box 24-1 for examples). The Parse and hermeneutic methods underpinned by the human becoming school of thought generate new knowledge about universal lived experiences (Cody, 1995b, 1995c; Parse, 2001b). For instance, research findings have helped to promote understanding about how people experience hope while imaging new possibilities and how people create moments of respite amid the anguish of grieving a loss. Research findings are woven with the theory so that findings can inform thinking beyond any particular study.

For instance, in several of the grieving and loss studies, researchers described a rhythm of engaging and disengaging with the one lost and with others who remind the one grieving about the absent presence (Cody, 1995a; Pilkington, 1993). Women who had a miscarriage already had a relationship with their babies, and the anguish of losing the child was so intense that women invented ways to distance themselves from the reality of the lost child. When they were alone, the pain was unbearable, and when they were with others the anguish was both eased and intensified as consoling expressions mingled with words acknowledging the reality of the lost child (Pilkington, 1993). Women described rhythms of engaging-disengaging with the lost child, close others, pain, and respite. Linking the rhythm to the theoretical concept connecting-separating means that readers can think about and be present with others' expressions of engaging-disengaging as they surface in discussions about grieving and loss. How do families in palliative care express their engaging and distancing from the one who is moving toward death? How do parents losing adult children engage and disengage with the absent children? Additional research studies about loss and grieving may further

enhance understanding about the connecting-separating concept and other concepts of human becoming.

The Parse (2001a) research method continues to be refined. For example, in the text, *Qualitative Inquiry: The Path of Sciencing*, Parse introduced a process in which the researcher constructs each participant's story, including core ideas of the phenomenon under study. Most recently, Parse changed the name of the participant proposition to language art, and she added a process that requires the researcher to select or create an artistic expression that shows how the researcher was transfigured through the research process (R. Parse, personal communication, May 29, 2004). The artistic expression enhances understanding of what was learned about the phenomenon under study.

CRITIQUE

Human becoming is an abstract and complex theory. It is a theory, not a model, because its concepts and interrelationships are defined in principles that are written at an abstract level of discourse—the language of science. Readers can study various critiques of human becoming that help clarify the issues and diverse views of reviewers (see Box 24-1). Ultimately, the theory's meaning and usefulness to the discipline of nursing will be decided by the nurses who choose to live it and by the historians who will comment on its place in the evolution of knowledge and of health care practices, research activities, ethics, and policies. The theory has penetrated deeply the foundation of traditional nursing and health care in general. The penetration may be limited to cracklike fissures, or the streams of activity may yet dramatically expand op-portunities to advance thinking about the knowledge required to inform nurses so that they might have more comfort about how to be with people in ways that are helpful and that enhance quality of life.

Simplicity

In keeping with the theoretical discourse, the major concepts of human becoming are defined in highly abstract and philosophical terms. The abstract language has been a source of comfort and discomfort for nurses (Mitchell & Bournes, 2000). Discomfort with the language is sometimes linked more with unfamiliar beliefs and assumptions about human beings and how they relate with the universe than with abstract concepts. Also, discomfiting for some are the nondirectional statements that do not specify causal or predictive relationships about the human-universe process.

The concepts of human becoming often resonate with people when considered at the level of lived experience. For instance, the concept of valuing when discussed at the level of lived experience focuses on the ways persons choose and act on what is important in their lives. This idea should be inherently familiar, as should the idea that people sometimes disclose intimate details about their lives and sometimes they keep secrets from others (revealing-concealing). Pickrell, Lee, Schumacher, and Twigg (1998) noted that a first-time reader might be tempted to dismiss the concepts as too simple to convey the complexity inherent in the theory, but the authors caution that to do so would be a mistake. Parse's principles describe a complex and realistic picture of human becoming, and the picture provides a meaningful framework for understanding the human-universe-health interrelationship.

Generality

The human becoming school of thought has been chosen as a theoretical guide by nurses and other health professionals in many different settings, including acute care, long-term care, and community (see examples in Box 24-1). The theory has helped nurses be with individuals, families, and groups. The theory has been evaluated in practice settings and patients have commented on the difference it makes (Jonas, 1995a; Mitchell, Bernardo, & Bournes, 1997; Northrup & Cody, 1998; Williamson, 2000). Human becoming has helped leaders to create beneficial change in organizational culture, and it has informed development of stan-

dards of care (Mitchell, 1998b; Mitchell & Bournes, 1998) and best-practice guidelines (Nelligan et al., 2002; Registered Nurses Association of Ontario, 2002). The theory of human becoming changes what professionals see when they engage with persons in practice and research. The theory changes the thinking, acting, attitudes, and approaches that professionals rely on to fulfill their intentions with others. Indeed, the human becoming theory changes the intentions and purposes of professionals and there is no limit to how this learning can contribute to meaningful practices and approaches for all professional activities linked with research, education, and leadership.

Empirical Precision

Empirical precision, as discussed by Marriner Tomey (1998), relates to the testability, relevance, and usefulness of a theory. The questions asked are as follows:

- Does evidence (taken here to mean does reality) support the theory?
- Do the principles and concepts of the human becoming theory make sense to nurses when they are with people in practice?
- Does the human becoming theory help nurses to be with persons in ways that are helpful and that make a difference from the patient's perspective?
- Is the theory useful for administrators and researchers? Do research findings expand knowledge and enhance the theoretical base?

The answer to these questions is, clearly, an enthusiastic "yes." The theory is useful because it provides a meaningful foundation that is helpful for nurses who want to live certain values in practice and research. Usefulness is a personal notion, and nurses given the opportunity to study human becoming thought will decide its usefulness for themselves.

A nurse learning the theory might ask the following questions:

- What is the human becoming theory saying about people and do I believe in the ideas as they are presented?

- Am I comfortable with the basic beliefs espoused in the human becoming theory?

The answers to the initial questions about evidence or congruence with reality often lead to a decision to pursue the more difficult task of studying the theory. A commitment to learn more requires some attraction to the basic underlying values and assumptions Parse makes about the human-universe-health process. Additional questions that may be useful for nurses interested in the human becoming theory include the following:

- In my experience of reality, do different people have their own unique views about life and their health situations?
- Do people speak about what things mean on a personal level?
- Do people live their value priorities and pursue what is important to them?
- Do people make their own choices?
- Do people speak about paradoxical thoughts and feelings?
- Have I ever heard a person say something like, "On the one hand I think this way, but on the other hand I think something else" or "I know I said I feel such and such, but as soon as I said it, I realized I also feel different than that"?
- What is my experience of how people change? Do I believe that people make choices that help them move in the direction of their own hopes and dreams?

Derivable Consequences

Parse calls nursing a human science and, as such, it represents particular beliefs that have been around for more than 100 years. The human becoming theory has taken human science beliefs into service and knowledge development in new and important ways. The human becoming research and practice methodologies are generating transformations in care and a renewed sense of professional purpose. For example, a team of human becoming researchers, practitioners, artistic writers, actors, and consumers are currently in the process of translating research findings into a dramatic performance about living with Alzheimer's disease (Ivonoffski, Mitchell, & Jonas-Simpson, 2004). A new framework for critiquing human becoming research has been developed and is expanding options for critics engaging unitary nursing science (Mitchell, 2004).

The human becoming theory is providing meaningful options for nurses in the twenty-first century. The consumer movement, technology, and the global transfer of knowledge on the Internet invite new approaches in health care. A team of researchers, clinicians, engineers, consumers, and others are constructing a Web-based suite of tools that has a program for enabling self-care for persons living with diabetes. The suite of tools is based on research findings generated with the human becoming theory and includes processes that enhance self-care and decision making for quality of life. Other functions in the suite of Web-based tools include a virtual spa, an art gallery, and video clip visits (Mitchell, Nagle, & Mason, in progress). Funding for developing the prototype of this technology was provided by the Richard Ivy Foundation, in conjunction with Mount Sinai Hospital in Toronto, Canada.

There are convincing indications that the human becoming theory is a fitting guide for practitioners who want to create respectful partnerships with people seeking assistance with health and quality of life. More than a decade ago, Phillips (1987) suggested that Parse's work would transform the knowledge base and the practice of nursing from a unitary perspective. Indeed, the human becoming theory is transforming practice in numerous settings, and evaluations of the change are positive (Jonas, 1995a; Legault & Ferguson-Paré, 1999). The human becoming theory directs attention to the persons' meanings of health and quality of life and to their wishes, needs, concerns, and preferences for information and care. The future of health care is based on the development of theories and practices that truly honor and respect people as partners and experts about life experience and health. At least four of the largest teaching hospitals in Canada have supported nurses piloting and implementing standards of practice that are explicitly informed by the human becoming theory. University Health Network, the largest teaching hospital affiliated with the University of Toronto, is currently supporting nurses from one surgical unit with 20% of their time paid to participate in a 2-year-long pilot study to evaluate changes with human becoming patient-centered care.

SUMMARY

Work with the human becoming theory will continue to evolve, as will the theory itself. Important developments happened in 1998 when Parse extended thinking about human becoming beyond the notion of theory to the idea of the human becoming school of thought and with the introduction of the text, *Community: A Human Becoming Perspective* (2003a), which offered new concepts about change in community. Ongoing research will expand understanding and illuminate new relationships among theoretical concepts. As schools of nursing continue to introduce and teach the human becoming school of thought, more nurses will try the theory in practice. Learning the theory requires formal study, a reverence for quiet contemplation, and creative synthesis. As more nurses use the theory in practice and research, there will be more scholarly dialogue and advancement of the nursing discipline.

The theory of human becoming continues to be a theory for the future. As more and more nurses question how they are relating with others in the world, and as more nurses question the knowledge base of their discipline, the human becoming theory will provide a perspective and a field of possibilities for change and growth. Persons who engage nurses and other health care professionals are continuing to speak and to clarify not only what they want from professionals but also how they want professionals to work with them. The dominance of the mechanistic model, along with its aligned practices of assessing and diagnosing, will continue to lose appeal for health care professionals who have a mandate to work with people, human beings, as they live with health and illness, hope and no hope, joy and sorrow, life and death. The human becoming theory provides one alternative to the mechanistic model; there are other alternatives, and there will be more to come as humankind evolves.

Case Study

Mrs. Brown, a 48-year-old woman, is living with a diagnosis of breast cancer. She has just come into the oncology clinic for her third round of chemotherapy. When asked how she is doing, Mrs. Brown starts speaking about how tired she is and how she is feeling burdened with keeping secrets from her daughter. Mrs. Brown has not told her daughter about her cancer diagnosis because she is afraid of how her daughter might react. Mrs. Brown says she is just barely holding on to things at this time and she cannot take much more. She is also concerned about the chemotherapy and what she can expect, because the side effects are getting more intense.

CRITICAL THINKING *Activities*

1. Describe how different theoretical beliefs make a difference in practice. Think about Parse's (1987) practice methodology—illuminating meaning through explicating, synchronizing rhythms through dwelling with, and mobilizing transcendence through moving beyond. Nurses live true presence with persons, and this means centering and preparing to bear witness to Mrs. Brown's reality. In order to invite Mrs. Brown to speak, the nurse may initially ask her to say more about her situation. In the cadence of speech, Mrs. Brown may pause, giving the nurse an opening to pose questions that assist Mrs. Brown's exploration of how she is feeling. The nurse may ask: What is the burden about? What does it mean? What does Mrs. Brown think will happen if her daughter gets upset? Thinking about and picturing an anticipated event is, according

to Parse, an opportunity to rehearse and to clarify how best to be in light of anticipated consequences. In this way the person is helped with decisions about how best to go forward or how to change the situation. The practice dimensions and processes happen all at once as nurses honor the other's unfolding meanings, rhythms, and ways of moving forward.

2. Articulate the judgments that are called for in the human becoming theory. The nurse refrains from summarizing, comparing, judging, or labeling Mrs. Brown as she struggles with the possibilities and choices in her situation. The unconditional regard called for by the human becoming theory is extremely challenging. It can be much easier to give advice or to try to teach, but the outcomes in the nurse-person process, the opportunities for Mrs. Brown to see her situation differently, will vary according to different nursing words and actions.

3. Where does experience lie for nurses guided by the human becoming theory? The nurse guided by human becoming theory believes that Mrs. Brown knows the best way to proceed—the nurse cannot possibly know the way for another person's quality of life. Mrs. Brown said she cannot take much more in her life and yet she is burdened with her secret. This struggle is hers to wrestle with and choose a way to move on. The mother knows her daughter and she also knows how much upset she can take in her life. The nurse's true presence and theory-guided questions can help Mrs. Brown to figure out how to be in light of her value priorities in the moment. The nurse also knows that Mrs. Brown's value priorities may change at any time, leading to a different course of action. The nurse may have expertise in other areas, based on her knowledge and experience, and trusts that persons will seek information when ready.

4. Think of several questions that help individuals speak about their realities. Mrs. Brown spoke about being tired. The nurse might explore this further. How does the tiredness show itself? What does Mrs. Brown find helpful? What would she like to do about it? Until these things are known, the nurse cannot know how to proceed. The nurse may discover helpful suggestions to offer. The nurse guided by human becoming offers information as people indicate their readiness to hear it. The nurse believes that providing information or suggestions as persons seek it in the flow of dialogue and listening is the most respectful and meaningful way of teaching.

5. Specify three benefits for humanity when nurses follow the human becoming theory. Human becoming practice is consistent with what people say they want from health professionals. Persons have indicated in numerous reports and publications that they want to be listened to, respected, involved in their care, and provided with meaningful information—when they want and need it. People want competent professionals, but if respect for the client's reality is not the foundation of the nurse-person process, it does not matter how expert or knowledgeable the professional. People do not want to be judged or labeled when it comes to their choices or ways of living. Persons want to be believed, understood, and respected. Human becoming theory provides a guide for nurses who want to practice in ways that clients want. It has been shown that nurses guided by the human becoming perspective are more vigilant, more inclined to act on client concerns, and more likely to involve

clients and families in their care (Mitchell & Bournes, 1998).

REFERENCES

Baumann, S. (1997). Contrasting two approaches in a community-based nursing practice with older adults: The medical model and Parse's nursing theory. *Nursing Science Quarterly, 10*, 124-130.

Baumann, S. L. (2000). The lived experience of feeling loved: A study of mothers in a parolee program. *Nursing Science Quarterly, 13*, 332-338.

Baumann, S. L. (2003). The lived experience of feeling very tired: A study of adolescent girls. *Nursing Science Quarterly, 16*, 326-333.

Baumann, S. L., & Englert, R. (2003). A comparison of three views of spirituality in oncology nursing. *Nursing Science Quarterly, 16*, 52-59.

Bournes, D. (2000a). A commitment to honouring people's choices. *Nursing Science Quarterly, 13*, 18-23.

Bournes, D. A. (2000b). Concept inventing: A process for creating a unitary definition of having courage. *Nursing Science Quarterly, 13*, 143-149.

Bournes, D. A. (2002). Having courage: A lived experience of human becoming. *Nursing Science Quarterly, 15*, 220-229.

Bournes, D. A., & Das Gupta, T. L. (1997). Professional practice leader: A transformational role that addresses human diversity. *Nursing Administration Quarterly, 21*(4), 61-68.

Bournes, D. A., & Flint, F. (2003). Mis-takes: Mistakes in the nurse-person process. *Nursing Science Quarterly, 16*, 127-130.

Bournes, D. A., & Mitchell, G. J. (2002). Waiting: The experience of persons in a critical care waiting room. *Research in Nursing & Health, 25*, 58-67.

Bunkers, S. S. (1998). A nursing theory–guided model of health ministry: Human becoming in parish nursing. *Nursing Science Quarterly, 11*, 7-8.

Bunkers, S. S. (2002). Lifelong learning: A human becoming perspective. *Nursing Science Quarterly, 15*, 294-300.

Bunkers, S. S. (2003a). Understanding the stranger. *Nursing Science Quarterly, 16*, 305-309.

Bunkers, S. S. (2003b). Comparison of three Parse method studies on feeling very tired. *Nursing Science Quarterly, 16*, 340-344.

Bunkers, S. S. (2004). The lived experience of feeling cared for: A human becoming perspective. *Nursing Science Quarterly, 17*, 63-71.

Bunkers, S. S., Michaels, C., & Ethridge, P. (1997). Advanced practice nursing in community: Nursing's opportunity. *Advanced Practice Nursing Quarterly, 2*(4), 79-84.

Cody, W. K. (1995a). The lived experience of grieving for families living with AIDS: Family-centered research using Parse's method. In R. R. Parse (Ed.), *Illuminations: The human becoming theory in practice and research* (pp. 197-242). New York: National League for Nursing Press.

Cody, W. K. (1995b). The meaning of grieving for families living with AIDS. *Nursing Science Quarterly, 8*, 104-114.

Cody, W. K. (1995c). Of life immense in passion, pulse, and power: Dialoguing with Whitman and Parse. A hermeneutic study. In R. R. Parse (Ed.), *Illuminations: The human becoming theory in practice and research* (pp. 269-308). New York: National League for Nursing Press.

Cody, W. K. (1995d). True presence with families living with HIV disease. In R. R. Parse (Ed.), *Illuminations: The human becoming theory in practice and research* (pp. 115-133). New York: National League for Nursing Press.

Cody, W. K. (2000). The lived experience of grieving for persons living with HIV who have used injection drugs. *Journal of the Association of Nurses in AIDS Care, 11*, 82-92.

Cody, W. K., & Mitchell, G. J. (1992). Parse's theory as a model for practice: The cutting edge. *ANS Advances in Nursing Science, 15*(2), 52-65.

Cody, W. K., & Mitchell, G. J. (2002). Nursing knowledge and human science revisited: Practical and political considerations. *Nursing Science Quarterly, 15*, 4-13.

Cowling, W. R. (1989). Parse's theory of nursing. In J. J. Fitzpatrick & A. L. Whall (Eds.), *Conceptual models of nursing: Analysis and application* (2nd ed., pp. 385-399). Norwalk, CT: Appleton & Lange.

Crane, J., Josephson, D., & Letcher, D. (1999, Nov.). *The human becoming health action model in community.* Paper presented at The Seventh Annual International Colloquium on Human Becoming. Loyola University, Chicago.

Damgaard, G., & Bunkers, S. S. (1998). Nursing science-guided practice and education: A state board of nursing perspective. *Nursing Science Quarterly, 11*, 142-144.

Fawcett, J. (2001). The nurse theorists: 21st-century updates—Rosemarie Rizzo Parse. *Nursing Science Quarterly, 14*, 126-131.

Gates, K. M. (2000). The experience of caring for a loved one: A phenomenological study. *Nursing Science Quarterly, 13*, 54-59.

Hall, B. A. (1993). Commentary: The inherent value of practice theories. *Nursing Science Quarterly, 6*, 10-11.

Hansen-Ketchum, P. (2004). Parse's theory in practice. *Journal of Holistic Nursing, 22*, 57-72.

Huch, M. H. (2002). Response to: Critical review of R. R. Parse's "The human becoming school of thought. A perspective for nurses and other health professionals." *Journal of Advanced Nursing, 37*, 217.

Huchings, D. (2002). Parallels in practice: Palliative nursing practice and Parse's theory of human becoming. *American Journal of Hospice and Palliative Care, 19,* 408-414.

Jonas, C. M. (1995a). Evaluation of the human becoming theory in family practice. In R. R. Parse (Ed.), *Illuminations: The human becoming theory in practice and research* (pp. 347-366). New York: National League for Nursing Press.

Jonas, C. M. (1995b). True presence through music for persons living their dying. In R. R. Parse (Ed.), *Illuminations: The human becoming theory in practice and research* (pp. 97-104). New York: National League for Nursing Press.

Jonas-Simpson, C. (1997). Living the art of the human becoming theory. *Nursing Science Quarterly, 10,* 175-179.

Jonas-Simpson, C. M. (2001). Feeling understood: A melody of human becoming. *Nursing Science Quarterly, 14,* 222-230.

Jonas-Simpson, C. M. (2003). The experience of being listened to: A human becoming study with music. *Nursing Science Quarterly, 16,* 232-238.

Lee, O. J., & Pilkington, F. B. (1999). Practice with persons living their dying: A human becoming perspective. *Nursing Science Quarterly, 12,* 324-328.

Legault, F., & Ferguson-Paré, M. (1999). Advancing nursing practice: An evaluation study of Parse's theory of human becoming. *Canadian Journal of Nursing Leadership, 12*(1), 30-35.

Letcher, D. C., & Yancey, N. R. (2004). Witnessing change with aspiring nurses: A human becoming teaching-learning process in nursing education. *Nursing Science Quarterly, 17,* 36-41.

Linscott, J., Spee, R., Flint, F., & Fisher, A. (1999). Creating a culture of patient-focused care through a learner-centered philosophy. *Canadian Journal of Nursing Leadership, 12*(4), 5-10.

Marriner Tomey, A. (1998). Introduction to analysis of nursing theories. In A. M. Tomey & M. R. Alligood (Eds.), *Nursing theorists and their work* (4th ed., pp. 3-15). St. Louis: Mosby.

Milton, C. L. (2003a). A graduate curriculum guided by human becoming: Journeying with the possible. *Nursing Science Quarterly, 16,* 214-218.

Milton, C. L. (2003b). The American Nurses Association Code of Ethics: A reflection on the ethics of respect and human dignity with nurse as expert. *Nursing Science Quarterly, 16,* 301-304.

Mitchell, G. J. (1991). Diagnosis: Clarifying or obscuring the nature of nursing. *Nursing Science Quarterly, 4,* 52.

Mitchell, G. J. (1993). Living paradox in Parse's theory. *Nursing Science Quarterly, 6,* 44-51.

Mitchell, G. J. (1998a). Living with diabetes: How understanding expands theory for professional practice. *Canadian Journal of Diabetes Care, 22*(1), 30-37.

Mitchell, G. J. (1998b). Standards of nursing and the winds of change. *Nursing Science Quarterly, 11,* 97-98.

Mitchell, G. J. (1999). Evidence-based practice: Critique and alternative view. *Nursing Science Quarterly, 12,* 30-35.

Mitchell, G. J. (2001). Policy, procedure, and routine: Matters of moral influence. *Nursing Science Quarterly, 14,* 109-114.

Mitchell, G. J. (2002). Self-serving and other-serving: Matters of trust and intent. *Nursing Science Quarterly, 15*(4), 288-293.

Mitchell, G. J. (2003). Abstractions and particulars: Learning theory for practice. *Nursing Science Quarterly, 16,* 310-314.

Mitchell, G. J. (2004). An emerging framework for human becoming criticism. *Nursing Science Quarterly, 17,* 103-109.

Mitchell, G. J., Bernardo, A., & Bournes, D. (1997). Nursing guided by Parse's theory: Patient views at Sunnybrook. *Nursing Science Quarterly, 10,* 55-56.

Mitchell, G. J., & Bournes, D. A. (1998). *Finding the way: A video guide to patient focused care* (Videotape). Toronto, Ontario, Canada: Sunnybrook & Women's Health Science Centre.

Mitchell, G. J., & Bournes, D. A. (2000). Nurse as patient advocate? In search of straight thinking. *Nursing Science Quarterly, 13,* 204-209.

Mitchell, G. J., & Bunkers, S. S. (2003). Engaging the abyss: A mis-take of opportunity? *Nursing Science Quarterly, 16,* 121-125.

Mitchell, G. J., Closson, T., Coulis, N., Flint, F., & Gray, B. (2000). Patient-focused care and human becoming thought: Connecting the right stuff. *Nursing Science Quarterly, 13,* 216-224.

Mitchell, G. J., & Cody, W. K. (1992). Nursing knowledge and human science: Ontological and epistemological considerations. *Nursing Science Quarterly, 5,* 54-61.

Mitchell, G. J., & Cody, W. K. (1999). Human becoming theory: A complement to medical science. *Nursing Science Quarterly, 12,* 304-310.

Mitchell, G. J., & Cody, W. K. (2002). Ambiguous opportunity: Toiling for truth of nursing art and science. *Nursing Science Quarterly, 15,* 71-79.

Mitchell, G. J., & Lawton, C. (2000). Living with the consequences of personal choices for persons with diabetes: Implications for educators and practitioners. *Canadian Journal of Diabetes Care, 24*(2), 23-31.

Nelligan, P., Grinspun, D., Jonas-Simpson, C., McConnell, H., Peter, E., Pilkington, B. (2002, Summer). Client centered care: Making the ideal real. *Hospital Quarterly, 5*(4), 70-76.

Noh, C. H. (2004). Meaning of quality of life for persons with serious mental illness: Human becoming practice with groups. *Nursing Science Quarterly, 17,* 220-225.

Norris, J. R. (2002). One-to-one teleapprenticeship as a means for nurses teaching and learning Parse's theory of human becoming. *Nursing Science Quarterly, 15,* 143-149.

Northrup, D. T. (2002). Time passing: A Parse research method study. *Nursing Science Quarterly, 15,* 318-326.

Northrup, D. T., & Cody, W. K. (1998). Evaluation of the human becoming theory in practice in an acute care psychiatric setting. *Nursing Science Quarterly, 11,* 23-30.

Ortiz, M. R. (2003). Lingering presence: A study using the human becoming hermeneutic method. *Nursing Science Quarterly, 16,* 146-154.

Paille, M., & Pilkington, F. B. (2002). The global context of nursing: A human becoming perspective. *Nursing Science Quarterly, 15,* 165-170.

Parse, R. R. (1974). *Nursing fundamentals.* Flushing, NY: Medical Examination.

Parse, R. R. (1981). *Man-living-health: A theory of nursing.* New York: Wiley.

Parse, R. R. (1987). *Nursing science: Major paradigms, theories, and critiques.* Philadelphia: W. B. Saunders.

Parse, R. R. (1989a). Essentials for practicing the art of nursing. *Nursing Science Quarterly, 2,* 111.

Parse, R. R. (1989b). Parse's man-living-health model and administration of nursing service. In B. Henry, C. Arndt, M. DiVincenti, & A. Marriner Tomey (Eds.), *Dimensions of nursing administration: Theory, research, education, and practice.* Cambridge, MA: Blackwell Scientific.

Parse, R. R. (1990). Health: A personal commitment. *Nursing Science Quarterly, 3,* 136-140.

Parse, R. R. (1992). Human becoming: Parse's theory of nursing. *Nursing Science Quarterly, 5,* 35-42.

Parse, R. R. (1993). Scholarly dialogue: Theory guides research and practice. *Nursing Science Quarterly, 6,* 12.

Parse, R. R. (1996). The human becoming theory: Challenges in practice and research. *Nursing Science Quarterly, 9,* 55-60.

Parse, R. R. (1998). *The human becoming school of thought: A perspective for nurses and other health professionals.* Thousand Oaks, CA: Sage.

Parse, R. R. (1999). *Hope: An international human becoming perspective.* Sudbury, MA: Jones and Bartlett.

Parse, R. R. (2000). Into the new millennium. *Nursing Science Quarterly, 13,* 3.

Parse, R. R. (2001a). *Qualitative inquiry: The path of sciencing.* Boston: Jones and Bartlett.

Parse, R. R. (2001b). The lived experience of contentment: A study using the Parse research method. *Nursing Science Quarterly, 14,* 330-338.

Parse, R. R. (2003a). *Community: A human becoming perspective.* Sudbury, MA: Jones and Bartlett.

Parse, R. R. (2003b). The lived experience of feeling very tired: A study using the Parse research method. *Nursing Science Quarterly, 16,* 319-325.

Parse, R. R. (2004). A human becoming teaching-learning model. *Nursing Science Quarterly, 17,* 33-35.

Parse, R. R., Bournes, D. A., Barrett, E. A., Malinski, V. M., & Phillips, J. R. (1999). A better way. *On Call, 2*(8), 14-17.

Parse, R. R., Coyne, B., & Smith, M. J. (1985). *Nursing research: Qualitative methods.* Bowie, MD: Brady.

Parse, R. R. (Ed.). (1995). *Illuminations: The human becoming theory in practice and research.* New York: National League for Nursing Press.

Phillips, J. R. (1987). A critique of Parse's man-living-health theory. In R. R. Parse (Ed.), *Nursing science: Major paradigms, theories, and critiques* (pp. 181-204). Philadelphia: W. B. Saunders.

Pickrell, K. D., Lee, R. E., Schumacher, L. P., & Twigg, P. (1998). Rosemarie Rizzo Parse: Human becoming. In A. M. Tomey & M. R. Alligood (Eds.), *Nursing theorists and their work* (4th ed., pp. 463-481). St. Louis: Mosby.

Pilkington, F. B. (1993). The lived experience of grieving the loss of an important other. *Nursing Science Quarterly, 6,* 130-139.

Pilkington, F. B. (2000). Persisting while wanting to change: Women's lived experiences. *Health Care for Women International, 21,* 501-516.

Pilkington, F. B. (2004). Exploring ethical implications for acting faithfully in professional relationships. *Nursing Science Quarterly, 17,* 27-32.

Pilkington, F. B., & Mitchell, G. J. (2004). Quality of life for women living with a gynecological cancer. *Nursing Science Quarterly, 17,* 147-155.

Registered Nurses Association of Ontario. (2002). *Client centered care: Nursing best practice guideline.* Toronto, Ontario, Canada: Registered Nurses Association of Ontario.

Rogers, M. (1992). Nursing science and the space age. *Nursing Science Quarterly, 5,* 27-34.

Rogers, M. E. (1970). *An introduction to the theoretical basis of nursing.* Philadelphia: F. A. Davis.

Saltmarche, A., Kolodny, V., & Mitchell, G. J. (1998). An educational approach for patient-focused care: Shifting attitudes and practice. *Journal of Nursing Staff Development, 14*(2), 81-86.

Santopinto, M. D. A., & Smith, M. C. (1995). Evaluation of the human becoming theory in practice with adults and children. In R. R. Parse (Ed.), *Illuminations: The human becoming theory in practice and research* (pp. 309-346). New York: National League for Nursing Press.

Smith, M. C., & Hudepohl, J. H. (1988). Analysis and evaluation of Parse's theory of man-living-health. *The Canadian Journal of Nursing Research: Nursing Papers, 20*(4), 43-58.

Smith, M. K. (2002). Human becoming and women living with violence: The art of practice. *Nursing Science Quarterly, 15,* 302-307.

Stanley, G. D., & Meghani, S. H. (2001). Reflections on using Parse's theory of human becoming in a palliative care setting in Pakistan. *Canadian Nurse, 97,* 23-25.

Thornburg, P. (2002). "Waiting" as experienced by women hospitalized during the antepartum period. *MCN, American Journal of Maternal Child Nursing, 27,* 245-248.

Wang, C. E. (1999). He-bung: Hope for persons living with leprosy in Taiwan. In R. R. Parse (Ed.), *Hope: An international human becoming perspective* (pp. 143-162). Sudbury, MA: Jones and Bartlett.

Wang, C. H. (1997). Quality of life and health for persons living with leprosy. *Nursing Science Quarterly, 10,* 144-145.

Williamson, G. J. (2000). The test of a nursing theory: A personal view. *Nursing Science Quarterly, 13,* 124-128.

Winkler, S. J. (1983). Parse's theory of nursing. In J. Fitzpatrick & A. Whall (Eds.), *Conceptual models of nursing: Analysis and application* (pp. 275-294). Bowie, MD: Robert J. Brady.

Woude, D. V., Damgaard, G., Hegge, M. J., Soholt, D., & Bunkers, S. S. (2003). The unfolding: Scenario planning in nursing. *Nursing Science Quarterly, 16,* 27-35.

BIBLIOGRAPHY
Primary Sources
Books

Parse, R. R. (1974). *Nursing fundamentals.* Flushing, NY: Medical Examination.

Parse, R. R. (1981). *Man-living-health: A theory of nursing.* New York: Wiley.

Parse, R. R. (1987). *Nursing science: Major paradigms, theories, and critiques.* Philadelphia: W. B. Saunders.

Parse, R. R. (Ed.). (1995). *Illuminations: The human becoming theory in practice and research.* New York: National League for Nursing Press.

Parse, R. R. (1998). *The human becoming school of thought: A perspective for nurses and other health professionals.* Thousand Oaks, CA: Sage.

Parse, R. R. (1999). *Hope: An international human becoming perspective.* Sudbury, MA: Jones and Bartlett.

Parse, R. R. (2001). *Qualitative inquiry: The path of sciencing.* Boston: Jones and Bartlett.

Parse, R. R. (2003). *Community: A human becoming perspective.* Sudbury, MA: Jones and Bartlett.

Parse, R. R., Coyne, A. B., & Smith, M. J. (1985). *Nursing research: Qualitative methods.* Bowie, MD: Brady.

Book Chapters

Parse, R. R. (1978). Rights of medical patients. In C. T. Fischer & S. L. Brodsky (Eds.), *Client participation in human services.* New Brunswick, NJ: Transaction.

Parse, R. R. (1981). Caring from a human science perspective. In M. M. Leininger (Ed.), *Caring: An essential human need* (pp. 129-132). Thorofare, NJ: Slack.

Parse, R. R. (1989). Man-living-health: A theory of nursing. In J. Riehl-Sisca (Ed.), *Conceptual models for nursing practice* (3rd ed.). Norwalk, CT: Appleton & Lange.

Parse, R. R. (1989). Parse's man-living-health model and administration of nursing service. In B. Henry, C. Arndt, M. DiVincenti, & A. M. Tomey (Eds.), *Dimensions of nursing administration: Theory, research, education, and practice.* Cambridge, MA: Blackwell Scientific.

Parse, R. R. (1989). The phenomenological research method: Its value for management science. In B. Henry, C. Arndt, M. DiVincenti, & A. M. Tomey (Eds.), *Dimensions of nursing administration: Theory, research, education, and practice.* Cambridge, MA: Blackwell Scientific.

Parse, R. R. (1991). Parse's theory of human becoming. In I. E. Goertzen (Ed.), *Differentiating nursing practice: Into the twenty-first century* (pp. 51-53). Kansas City, MO: American Academy of Nursing.

Parse, R. R. (1993). Parse's human becoming theory: Its research and practice implications. In M. E. Parker (Ed.), *Patterns of nursing theories in practice* (pp. 49-61). New York: National League for Nursing Press.

Parse, R. R. (1995). Foreword. In M. A. Frey & C. L. Sieloff (Eds.), *Advancing King's systems framework and theory of nursing.* Thousand Oaks, CA: Sage.

Parse, R. R. (1995). Man-living-health. A theory of nursing. In M. Mischo-Kelling & K. Wittneben (Eds.), *Auffassungen von pflege in theorie und praxis* (pp. 114-132). Munchen: Urban & Schwarzenberg.

Parse, R. R. (1997). The human becoming theory and its research and practice methodologies. In J. Osterbrink (Ed.), *Pflegetheorien—eine zusammenfassung der 1st international conference.* Freiburg, Germany: Verlag Hans Huber.

Parse, R. R. (1997). The language of nursing knowledge: Saying what we mean. In J. Fawcett & I. M. King (Eds.), *The language of nursing theory and metatheory* (pp. 73-77). Indianapolis: Sigma Theta Tau Monograph.

Parse, R. R. (1999). The lived experience of hope for family members of persons living in a Canadian chronic care facility. In R. R. Parse (Ed.), *Hope: An international human becoming perspective* (pp. 63-77). Sudbury, MA: Jones and Bartlett.

Parse, R. R. (2001). The human becoming school of thought in research. In M. Parker (Ed.), *Nursing theo-*

ries and nursing practice (pp. 227-238). Philadelphia: F. A. Davis.

Book Reviews

Parse, R. R. (1996). [Review of the book *Martha E. Rogers: Her life and her work*]. *Visions: The Journal of Rogerian Science, 2,* 52-53.

Parse, R. R. (1997). [Review of the book *Quality of life in behavioral medicine*]. *Women and Health, 25*(3), 83-86.

Doctoral Dissertation

Parse, R. R. (1969). An instructional model for the teaching of nursing, interrelating objectives and media (Doctoral dissertation, Dusquesne University, 1969). *Dissertation Abstracts International, 31,* 180A.

Journal Articles

Parse, R. R. (1967, Aug.). Advantages and disadvantages of associate degree nursing programs. *Journal of Nursing Education, 6*(15), 5-8.

Parse, R. R. (1988). Beginnings. *Nursing Science Quarterly, 1*(1), 1-2.

Parse, R. R. (1988). Creating traditions: The art of putting it together. *Nursing Science Quarterly, 1*(2), 45.

Parse, R. R. (1988). Scholarly dialogue: The fire of refinement. *Nursing Science Quarterly, 1*(4), 141.

Parse, R. R. (1988). The mainstream of science: Framing the issue. *Nursing Science Quarterly, 1*(3), 93.

Parse, R. R. (1989). Essentials for practicing the art of nursing. *Nursing Science Quarterly, 2*(3), 111.

Parse, R. R. (1989). Making more out of less. *Nursing Science Quarterly, 2*(4), 155.

Parse, R. R. (1989). Martha E. Rogers: A birthday celebration. *Nursing Science Quarterly, 2*(2), 55.

Parse, R. R. (1989). Qualitative research: Publishing and funding. *Nursing Science Quarterly, 2*(1), 1-2.

Parse, R. R. (1990). A time for reflection and projection. *Nursing Science Quarterly, 3*(4), 143.

Parse, R. R. (1990). Health: A personal commitment. *Nursing Science Quarterly, 3*(3), 136-140.

Parse, R. R. (1990). Nursing theory–based practice: A challenge for the 90s. *Nursing Science Quarterly, 3*(2), 53.

Parse, R. R. (1990). Parse's research methodology with an illustration of the lived experience of hope. *Nursing Science Quarterly, 3*(1), 9-17.

Parse, R. R. (1990). Promotion and prevention: Two distinct cosmologies. *Nursing Science Quarterly, 3*(3), 101.

Parse, R. R. (1991). Electronic publishing: Beyond browsing. *Nursing Science Quarterly, 4*(1), 1.

Parse, R. R. (1991). Growing the discipline of nursing. *Nursing Science Quarterly, 4*(4), 139.

Parse, R. R. (1991). Mysteries of health and healing: Two perspectives. *Nursing Science Quarterly, 4*(3), 93.

Parse, R. R. (1991). Phenomenology and nursing. *Japanese Journal of Nursing, 17*(2), 261-269.

Parse, R. R. (1991). The right soil, the right stuff. *Nursing Science Quarterly, 4*(2), 47.

Parse, R. R. (1992). Human becoming: Parse's theory of nursing. *Nursing Science Quarterly, 5*(1), 35-42.

Parse, R. R. (1992). Moving beyond the barrier reef. *Nursing Science Quarterly, 5*(3), 97.

Parse, R. R. (1992). Nursing knowledge for the 21st century: An international commitment. *Nursing Science Quarterly, 5*(1), 8-12.

Parse, R. R. (1992). The performing art of nursing. *Nursing Science Quarterly, 5*(4), 147.

Parse, R. R. (1992). The unsung shapers of nursing science. *Nursing Science Quarterly, 5*(2), 47.

Parse, R. R. (1993). Cartoons: Glimpsing paradoxical moments. *Nursing Science Quarterly, 6*(1), 1.

Parse, R. R. (1993). Critical appraisal: Risking to challenge. *Nursing Science Quarterly, 6*(4), 163.

Parse, R. R. (1993). Nursing and medicine: Two different disciplines. *Nursing Science Quarterly, 6*(3), 109.

Parse, R. R. (1993). Plant now; reap later. *Nursing Science Quarterly, 6*(2), 55.

Parse, R. R. (1993). Scholarly dialogue: Theory guides research and practice. *Nursing Science Quarterly, 6*(1), 12.

Parse, R. R. (1993). The experience of laughter: A phenomenological study. *Nursing Science Quarterly, 6*(1), 39-43.

Parse, R. R. (1994). Charley Potatoes or mashed potatoes? *Nursing Science Quarterly, 7*(3), 97.

Parse, R. R. (1994). Laughing and health: A study using Parse's research method. *Nursing Science Quarterly, 7*(2), 55-64.

Parse, R. R. (1994). Martha E. Rogers: Her voice will not be silenced. *Nursing Science Quarterly, 7*(2), 47.

Parse, R. R. (1994). Quality of life: Sciencing and living the art of human becoming. *Nursing Science Quarterly, 7*(1), 16-21.

Parse, R. R. (1994). Scholarship: Three essential processes. *Nursing Science Quarterly, 7*(4), 143.

Parse, R. R. (1995). Again: What is nursing? *Nursing Science Quarterly, 8*(4), 143.

Parse, R. R. (1995). Building the realm of nursing knowledge. *Nursing Science Quarterly, 8*(2), 51.

Parse, R. R. (1995). Commentary: Parse's theory of human becoming: An alternative to nursing practice for pediatric oncology nurses. *Journal of Pediatric Oncology Nursing, 12*(3), 128.

Parse, R. R. (1995). Nursing theories and frameworks: The essence of advanced practice nursing. *Nursing Science Quarterly, 8*(1), 1.

Parse, R. R. (1995). Nursing theory based research and practice. A conference coming to Japan. Tokyo, Japan: Igacu Shoin. *Medical News Weekly.*

Parse, R. R. (1996). Building knowledge through qualitative research: The road less traveled. *Nursing Science Quarterly, 9*(1), 10-16.

Parse, R. R. (1996). Critical thinking: What is it? *Nursing Science Quarterly, 9*(3), 138.

Parse, R. R. (1996). Hear ye, hear ye: Novice and seasoned authors! *Nursing Science Quarterly, 9*(1), 1.

Parse, R. R. (1996). Nursing theories: An original path. *Nursing Science Quarterly, 9*(2), 85.

Parse, R. R. (1996). Quality of life for persons living with Alzheimer's disease: A human becoming perspective. *Nursing Science Quarterly, 9*(3), 126-133.

Parse, R. R. (1996). Reality: A seamless symphony of becoming. *Nursing Science Quarterly, 9*(4), 181-183.

Parse, R. R. (1996). The human becoming theory: Challenges in practice and research. *Nursing Science Quarterly, 9*(1), 55-60.

Parse, R. R. (1997). Concept inventing: Unitary creations. *Nursing Science Quarterly, 10*(2), 63-64.

Parse, R. R. (1997). Investing the legacy: Martha E. Rogers' voice will not be silenced. *Visions: The Journal of Rogerian Science, 5*, 7-11.

Parse, R. R. (1997). Joy-sorrow: A study using the Parse research method. *Nursing Science Quarterly, 10*(2), 80-87.

Parse, R. R. (1997). Leadership: The essentials. *Nursing Science Quarterly, 10*(3), 109.

Parse, R. R. (1997). New beginnings in a quiet revolution. *Nursing Science Quarterly, 10*(1), 1.

Parse, R. R. (1997). The human becoming theory: The was, is, and will be. *Nursing Science Quarterly, 10*(1), 32-38.

Parse, R. R. (1997). Transforming research and practice with the human becoming theory. *Nursing Science Quarterly, 10*(4), 171-174.

Parse, R. R. (1998). Moving on. *Nursing Science Quarterly, 11*(4), 135.

Parse, R. R. (1998). The art of criticism. *Nursing Science Quarterly, 11*(2), 43.

Parse, R. R. (1998). Will nursing exist tomorrow? A reprise. *Nursing Science Quarterly, 11*(1), 1.

Parse, R. R. (1999). Authorship: Whose responsibility? *Nursing Science Quarterly, 12*(2), 99.

Parse, R. R. (1999). Community: An alternative view. *Nursing Science Quarterly, 12*(2), 119-124.

Parse, R. R. (1999). Expanding the vision: Tilling the field of nursing knowledge. *Nursing Science Quarterly, 12*(1), 3.

Parse, R. R. (1999). Integrity and the advancement of nursing knowledge. *Nursing Science Quarterly, 12*(3), 187.

Parse, R. R. (1999). Nursing science: The transformation of practice. *Journal of Advanced Nursing, 30*(6), 1383-1387.

Parse, R. R. (1999). Nursing: The discipline and the profession. *Nursing Science Quarterly, 12*(4), 275.

Parse, R. R. (1999). Witnessing as true presence. *Illuminations: Newsletter for the International Consortium of Parse Scholars, 8*(3), 1.

Parse, R. R. (2000). Into the new millennium. *Nursing Science Quarterly, 13*(1), 3.

Parse, R. R. (2000). Language: Words reflect and cocreate meaning. *Nursing Science Quarterly, 13*(3), 187.

Parse, R. R. (2000). Obfuscating: The persistent practice of misnaming. *Nursing Science Quarterly, 13*(2), 91-92.

Parse, R. R. (2000). Paradigms: A reprise. *Nursing Science Quarterly, 13*(4), 275-276.

Parse, R. R. (2001). Contributions to the discipline. *Nursing Science Quarterly, 14*(1), 5.

Parse, R. R. (2001). Nursing: Still in the shadow of medicine. *Nursing Science Quarterly, 14*(3), 181.

Parse, R. R. (2001). The lived experience of contentment: A study using the Parse research method. *Nursing Science Quarterly, 14*, 330-338.

Parse, R. R. (2001). The universe is flat. *Nursing Science Quarterly, 14*(2), 93.

Parse. R. R. (2002). 15th anniversary celebration. *Nursing Science Quarterly, 15*, 3.

Parse, R. R. (2002). Aha! a! hha! Discovery, wonder, laughter. *Nursing Science Quarterly, 15*, 273.

Parse, R. R. (2002). Mentoring moments. *Nursing Science Quarterly, 15*, 97.

Parse, R. R. (2002). Transforming healthcare with a unitary view of human. *Nursing Science Quarterly, 15*, 46-50.

Parse, R. R. (2002). Words, words, words: Meanings, meanings, meanings! *Nursing Science Quarterly, 15*, 183.

Parse, R. R. (2003). A call for dignity in nursing. *Nursing Science Quarterly, 16*, 193.

Parse, R. R. (2003). Research approaches: Likenesses and differences. *Nursing Science Quarterly, 16*, 5.

Parse, R. R. (2003). Silos and schools of thought. *Nursing Science Quarterly, 16*, 101.

Parse, R. R. (2003). The lived experience of feeling very tired: A study using the Parse research method. *Nursing Science Quarterly, 16*, 319-325.

Parse, R. R. (2003). What constitutes nursing research? *Nursing Science Quarterly, 16*, 287.

Parse, R. R. (2004). A human becoming teaching-learning model. *Nursing Science Quarterly, 17*, 33-35.

Parse, R. R. (2004). New directions. *Nursing Science Quarterly, 17*, 5.

Parse, R. R. (2004). Power in position. *Nursing Science Quarterly, 17*, 101.

Parse, R. R., Bournes, D. A., Barrett, E. A. M., Malinski, V. M., & Phillips, J. R. (1999). A better way: 10 things health professionals can do to move toward a more personal and meaningful system. *On Call: A Magazine for Nurses and Healthcare Professionals, 2*(8), 14-17.

Proceedings of a Conference

Parse, R. R. (1993). *Critique of critical phenomena of nursing science suggested by O'Brien, Reed, and Stevenson* (pp. 71-81). Proceedings of the 1993 Annual Forum on Doctoral Nursing Education: A Call for Substance: Preparing Leaders for Global Health. St. Paul, MN: University of Minnesota School of Nursing.

Secondary Sources
Book Chapters About Parse's Theory

Allchin-Petardi, L. (1999). Hope for American women with children. In R. R. Parse (Ed.), *Hope: An international human becoming perspective* (pp. 273-285). Sudbury, MA: Jones and Bartlett.

Banonis, B. C. (1995). Metaphors in the practice of the human becoming theory. In R. R. Parse (Ed.), *Illuminations: The human becoming theory in practice and research* (pp. 87-95). New York: National League for Nursing Press.

Baumann, S. L. (1999). The lived experience of hope: Children in families struggling to make a home. In R. R. Parse (Ed.), *Hope: An international human becoming perspective* (pp. 191-210). Sudbury, MA: Jones and Bartlett.

Bunkers, S. S. (1999). The lived experience of hope for those working with homeless persons. In R. R. Parse (Ed.), *Hope: An international human becoming perspective* (pp. 227-250). Sudbury, MA: Jones and Bartlett.

Bunkers, S. S. (1999). Translating nursing conceptual frameworks and theory for nursing practice. In A. Solari-Twadell & M. A. McDermott (Eds.), *Parish nursing: Promoting whole person health within faith communities* (pp. 205-214). Thousand Oaks, CA: Sage.

Bunkers, S. S., & Daly, J. (1999). The lived experience of hope for Australian families living with coronary disease. In R. R. Parse (Ed.), *Hope: An international human becoming perspective* (pp. 45-61). Sudbury, MA: Jones and Bartlett.

Cody, W. K. (1995). Of life immense in passion, pulse, and power: Dialoguing with Whitman and Parse. A hermeneutic study. In R. R. Parse (Ed.), *Illuminations: The human becoming theory in practice and research* (pp. 269-307). New York: National League for Nursing Press.

Cody, W. K. (1995). The lived experience of grieving for families living with AIDS: Family-centered research using Parse's method. In R. R. Parse (Ed.), *Illuminations: The human becoming theory in practice and research* (pp. 197-242). New York: National League for Nursing Press.

Cody, W. K. (1995). The view of the family within the human becoming theory. In R. R. Parse (Ed.), *Illuminations: The human becoming theory in practice and research* (pp. 9-26). New York: National League for Nursing Press.

Cody, W. K. (1995). True presence with families living with HIV disease. In R. R. Parse (Ed.), *Illuminations: The human becoming theory in practice and research* (pp. 115-133). New York: National League for Nursing Press.

Cody, W. K., & Filler, J. E. (1999). The lived experience of hope for women residing in a shelter. In R. R. Parse (Ed.), *Hope: An international human becoming perspective* (pp. 211-225). Sudbury, MA: Jones and Bartlett.

Cody, W. K., Hudepohl, J. H., & Brinkman, K. S. (1995). True presence with a child and his family. In R. R. Parse (Ed.), *Illuminations: The human becoming theory in practice and research* (pp. 135-146). New York: National League for Nursing Press.

Daly, J. (1995). The lived experience of suffering. In R. R. Parse (Ed.), *Illuminations: The human becoming theory in practice and research* (pp. 253-268). New York: National League for Nursing Press.

Daly, J. (1995). The view of suffering within the human becoming theory. In R. R. Parse (Ed.), *Illuminations: The human becoming theory in practice and research* (pp. 45-59). New York: National League for Nursing Press.

Daly, J., & Watson, J. (1996). Parse's human becoming theory of nursing. In J. Greenwood (Ed.), *Nursing theory in Australia: Development and application* (pp. 177-200). Pymble, NSW, Australia: Harper Educational Publishers.

Jonas, C. M. (1995). Evaluation of the human becoming theory in family practice. In R. R. Parse (Ed.), *Illuminations: The human becoming theory in practice and research* (pp. 347-366). New York: National League for Nursing Press.

Jonas, C. M. (1995). True presence through music for persons living their dying. In R. R. Parse (Ed.), *Illuminations: The human becoming theory in practice* (pp. 97-104). New York: National League for Nursing Press.

Kelley, L. S. (1995). The house-garden-wilderness metaphor: Caring frameworks and the human becoming theory. In R. R. Parse (Ed.), *Illuminations: The human becoming theory in practice and research* (pp. 61-76). New York: National League for Nursing Press.

Kelley, L. S. (1999). Hope as lived by Native Americans. In R. R. Parse (Ed.), *Hope: An international human becoming perspective* (pp. 251-272). Sudbury, MA: Jones and Bartlett.

Mitchell, G. J. (1991). Distinguishing practice with Parse's theory. In I. E. Goertzen (Ed.), *Differentiating nursing practice into the twenty-first century* (pp. 55-58). New York: American Nurses Association Publication.

Mitchell, G. J. (1993). Parse's theory in practice. In M. E. Parker (Ed.), *Patterns of nursing theories in practice* (pp. 62-80). New York: National League for Nursing Press.

Mitchell, G. J. (1995). Evaluation of the human becoming theory in practice in an acute care setting. In R. R. Parse (Ed.), *Illuminations: The human becoming theory in practice and research* (pp. 367-399). New York: National League for Nursing Press.

Mitchell, G. J. (1995). The lived experience of restriction-freedom in later life. In R. R. Parse (Ed.), *Illuminations: The human becoming theory in practice and research* (pp. 159-195). New York: National League for Nursing Press.

Mitchell, G. J. (1995). The view of freedom within the human becoming theory. In R. R. Parse (Ed.), *Illumination: The human becoming theory in practice and research* (pp. 27-43). New York: National League for Nursing Press.

Pickrell, K. D., Lee, R. E., Schumacher, L. P., & Twigg, P. (1998). Rosemarie Rizzo Parse: Human becoming. In A. M. Tomey & M. R. Alligood (Eds.), *Nursing theorists and their work* (4th ed.). St. Louis: Mosby.

Pilkington, F. B., & Millar, B. (1999). The lived experience of hope with persons from Wales, UK. In R. R. Parse (Ed.), *Hope: An international human becoming perspective* (pp. 163-189). Sudbury, MA: Jones and Bartlett.

Rasmusson, D. L. (1995). True presence with homeless persons. In R. R. Parse (Ed.), *Illuminations: The human becoming theory in practice and research* (pp. 105-113). New York: National League for Nursing Press.

Santopinto, M. D. A., & Smith, M. C. (1995). Evaluation of the human becoming theory in practice with adults and children. In R. R. Parse (Ed.), *Illuminations: The human becoming theory in practice and research* (pp. 309-346). New York: National League for Nursing Press.

Smith, M. J. (1989). Research and practice application related to man-living-health. In J. Riehl-Sisca (Ed.), *Conceptual models for nursing practice* (3rd ed., pp. 267-276). Norwalk, CT: Appleton & Lange.

Takahashi, T. (1999). Kibou: Hope for persons in Japan. In R. R. Parse (Ed.), *Hope: An international human becoming perspective* (pp. 115-128). Sudbury, MA: Jones and Bartlett.

Toikkanen, T., & Muurinen, E. (1999). Toivo: Hope for persons in Finland. In R. R. Parse (Ed.), *Hope: An international human becoming perspective* (pp. 79-96). Sudbury, MA: Jones and Bartlett.

Wang, C. E. H. (1999). He-Bung: Hope for persons living with leprosy in Taiwan. In R. R. Parse (Ed.), *Hope: An international human becoming perspective* (pp. 45-61). Sudbury, MA: Jones and Bartlett.

Willman, A. (1999). Hopp: The lived experience for Swedish elders. In R. R. Parse (Ed.), *Hope: An international human becoming perspective* (pp. 129-142). Sudbury, MA: Jones and Bartlett.

Zanotti, R., & Bournes, D. A. (1999). Speranza: A study of the lived experience of hope with persons from Italy. In R. R. Parse (Ed.), *Hope: An international human becoming perspective* (pp. 97-114). Sudbury, MA: Jones and Bartlett.

Journal Articles About Parse's Theory

Allchin-Petardi, L. (1998). Weathering the storm: Persevering through a difficult time. *Nursing Science Quarterly, 11*(4), 172-177.

Andrus, K. (1995). Parse's nursing theory and the practice of perioperative nursing. *Canadian Operating Room Nursing Journal, 13*(3), 19-22.

Arndt, M. J. (1995). Parse's theory of human becoming in practice with hospitalized adolescents. *Nursing Science Quarterly, 8*(2), 86-90.

Arrigo, B., & Cody, W. K. (2004). A dialogue on existential-phenomenological thought in psychology and in nursing. *Nursing Science Quarterly, 17*, 6-11.

Banonis, B. C. (1989). The lived experience of recovering from addiction: A phenomenological study. *Nursing Science Quarterly, 2*(1), 37-43.

Baumann, S. (1994). No place of their own: An exploratory study. *Nursing Science Quarterly, 7*(4), 162-169.

Baumann, S. (1995). Two views of children's art: Psychoanalysis and Parse's human becoming theory. *Nursing Science Quarterly, 8*(2), 65-70.

Baumann, S. (1996). Feeling uncomfortable: Children in families with no place of their own. *Nursing Science Quarterly, 9*(4), 152-159.

Baumann, S. (1996). Parse's research methodology and the nurse-researcher-child process. *Nursing Science Quarterly, 9*(1), 27-32.

Baumann, S. (1997). Contrasting two approaches in a community-based nursing practice with older adults: The medical model and Parse's nursing theory. *Nursing Science Quarterly, 10*(3), 124-130.

Baumann, S., & Braddick, M. (1999). Out of their element: Fathers of children who are "not the same." *Journal of Pediatric Nursing, 14*(6), 269-278.

Baumann, S. L. (1997). Qualitative research with children as participants. *Nursing Science Quarterly, 10*(2), 68-69.

Baumann, S. L. (1999). Art as a path of inquiry. *Nursing Science Quarterly, 12*(2), 106-110.

Baumann, S. L. (2003). The lived experience of feeling very tired: A study of adolescent girls. *Nursing Science Quarterly, 16*, 326-333.

Baumann, S. L., & Englert, R. (2003). A comparison of three views of spirituality in oncology nursing. *Nursing Science Quarterly, 16*, 52-59.

Benedict, L. L., Bunkers, S. S., Damgaard, G. A., Duffy, C. E., Hohman, M. L., & Vander Woude, D. L. (2000). The

South Dakota board of nursing theory–based regulatory decisioning model. *Nursing Science Quarterly, 13*(2), 167-171.

Bernardo, A. (1998). Technology and true presence in nursing. *Holistic Nursing Practice, 12*(4), 40-49.

Bournes, D. A. (2000). A commitment to honoring people's choices. *Nursing Science Quarterly, 13*(1), 18-23.

Bournes, D. A. (2000). Concept inventing: A process for creating a unitary definition of having courage. *Nursing Science Quarterly, 13*(2), 143-149.

Bournes, D. A. (2002). Having courage: A lived experience of human becoming. *Nursing Science Quarterly, 15,* 220-229.

Bournes, D. A., & Das Gupta, T. L. (1997). Professional practice leader: A transformational role that addresses human diversity. *Nursing Administration Quarterly, 21*(4), 61-68.

Bournes, D. A., & Flint, F. (2003). Mis-takes: Mistakes in the nurse-person process. *Nursing Science Quarterly, 16,* 127-130.

Bournes, D. A., & Linscott, J. (1998). Patient-focused care: A process of discovery. *Theoria, 7*(4), 3-5.

Bournes, D. A., & Mitchell, G. J. (2002). Waiting: The experience of persons in a critical care waiting room. *Research in Nursing & Health, 25,* 58-67.

Bunkers, S. S. (1998). A nursing theory–guided model of health ministry: Human becoming in parish nursing. *Nursing Science Quarterly, 11*(1), 7-8.

Bunkers, S. S. (1998). Considering tomorrow: Parse's theory-guided research. *Nursing Science Quarterly, 11*(2), 56-63.

Bunkers, S. S. (1999). Commentary on Parse's view of community. *Nursing Science Quarterly, 12*(2), 121-124.

Bunkers, S. S. (1999). Emerging discoveries and possibilities in nursing. *Nursing Science Quarterly, 12*(1), 26-29.

Bunkers, S. S. (1999). Learning to be still. *Nursing Science Quarterly, 12,* 172-173.

Bunkers, S. S. (1999). The meaning of new age: The judging and misjudging of values and beliefs. *Nursing Science Quarterly, 12*(2), 100-105.

Bunkers, S. S. (1999). The teaching-learning process and the theory of human becoming. *Nursing Science Quarterly, 12*(3), 227-232.

Bunkers, S. S. (2002). Lifelong learning: A human becoming perspective. *Nursing Science Quarterly, 15,* 294-300.

Bunkers, S. S. (2003). Comparison of three Parse method studies on feeling very tired. *Nursing Science Quarterly, 16,* 340-344.

Bunkers, S. S. (2003). Understanding the stranger. *Nursing Science Quarterly, 16,* 305-309.

Bunkers, S. S. (2004). The lived experience of feeling cared for: A human becoming perspective. *Nursing Science Quarterly, 17,* 63-71.

Bunkers, S. S., Michaels, C., & Ethridge, P. (1997). Advanced practice nursing in community: Nursing's opportunity. *Advanced Practice Nursing Quarterly, 2*(4), 79-84.

Butler, M. J. (1988). Family transformation: Parse's theory in practice. *Nursing Science Quarterly, 1*(2), 68-74.

Butler, M. J., & Snodgrass, F. G. (1991). Beyond abuse: Parse's theory in practice. *Nursing Science Quarterly, 4*(2), 76-82.

Carson, M. G., & Mitchell, G. J. (1998). The experience of living with persistent pain. *Journal of Advanced Nursing, 28*(6), 1242-1248.

Chapman, J. S., Mitchell, G. J., & Forchuk, C. (1994). A glimpse of nursing theory-based practice in Canada. *Nursing Science Quarterly, 7*(3), 104-112.

Cody, W. K. (1991). Grieving a personal loss. *Nursing Science Quarterly, 4,* 61-68.

Cody, W. K. (1991). Multidimensionality: Its meaning and significance. *Nursing Science Quarterly, 4,* 140-141.

Cody, W. K. (1993). Norms and nursing science: A question of values. *Nursing Science Quarterly, 6*(3), 110-112.

Cody, W. K. (1994). Meaning and mystery in nursing science and art. *Nursing Science Quarterly, 7*(2), 48-51.

Cody, W. K. (1994). Nursing theory–guided practice: What it is and what it is not. *Nursing Science Quarterly, 7*(4), 144-145.

Cody, W. K. (1994). Radical health care reform: The person as case manager. *Nursing Science Quarterly, 7*(4), 180-182.

Cody, W. K. (1995). All those paradigms: Many in the universe, two in nursing. *Nursing Science Quarterly, 8*(4), 144-147.

Cody, W. K. (1995). The meaning of grieving for families living with AIDS. *Nursing Science Quarterly, 8*(3), 104-114.

Cody, W. K. (1996). Drowning in eclecticism. *Nursing Science Quarterly, 9,* 86-88.

Cody, W. K. (1996). Occult reductionism in the discourse of theory development. *Nursing Science Quarterly, 9*(4), 140-142.

Cody, W. K. (1997). The many faces of change: Discomfort with the new. *Nursing Science Quarterly, 10*(2), 65-67.

Cody, W. K. (1998). Critical theory and nursing science: Freedom in theory and practice. *Nursing Science Quarterly, 11*(2), 44-46.

Cody, W. K. (1999). Affirming reflection. *Nursing Science Quarterly, 12*(1), 4-6.

Cody, W. K. (1999). Middle-range theories: Do they foster the development of nursing science? *Nursing Science Quarterly, 12*(1), 9-14.

Cody, W. K. (2000). Paradigm shift or paradigm drift? A meditation on commitment and transcendence. *Nursing Science Quarterly, 13*(2), 93-102.

Cody, W. K. (2000). The challenge of unitary conceptualizations: An exemplar. *Nursing Science Quarterly, 13*(1), 4.

Cody, W. K. (2003). Diversity and becoming: Implications of human existence as coexistence. *Nursing Science Quarterly, 16*, 195-200.

Cody, W. K., & Mitchell, G. J. (1992). Parse's theory as a model for practice: The cutting edge. *ANS Advances in Nursing Science, 15*(2), 52-65.

Costello-Nickitas, D. M. (1994). Choosing life goals: A phenomenological study. *Nursing Science Quarterly, 7*(2), 87-92.

Daly, J., & Jackson, D. (1999). On the use of nursing theory in nursing education, nursing practice, and nursing research in Australia. *Nursing Science Quarterly, 12*(4), 342-345.

Daly, J., Mitchell, G. J., & Jonas-Simpson, C. M. (1996). Quality of life and the human becoming theory: Exploring discipline-specific contributions. *Nursing Science Quarterly, 9*(4), 170-174.

Damgaard, G., & Bunkers, S. S. (1998). Nursing science–guided practice and education: A state board of nursing perspective. *Nursing Science Quarterly, 11*(4), 142-144.

Davis, C., & Cannava, E. (1995). The meaning of retirement for communally-living retired performing artists. *Nursing Science Quarterly, 8*(1), 8-16.

Fawcett, J. (2001). The nurse theorists: 21st-century updates—Rosemarie Rizzo Parse. *Nursing Science Quarterly, 14*, 126-131.

Fisher, M. A., & Mitchell, G. J. (1998). Patients' views of quality of life: Transforming the knowledge base of nursing. *Clinical Nurse Specialist, 12*(3), 99-105.

Futrell, M., Wondolowski, C., & Mitchell, G. J. (1994). Aging in the oldest old living in Scotland: A phenomenological study. *Nursing Science Quarterly, 6*(4), 189-194.

Gates, K. M. (2000). The experience of caring for a loved one: A phenomenological study. *Nursing Science Quarterly, 13*(1), 54-59.

Hamalis, P. (1999). Reaching out. *Nursing Science Quarterly, 12*(4), 346.

Hansen-Ketchum, P. (2004). Parse's theory in practice. *Journal of Holistic Nursing, 22*, 57-72.

Heine, C. (1991). Development of gerontological nursing theory: Applying man-living-health theory of nursing. *Nursing and Health Care, 12*, 184-188.

Hodges, H. F., Keeley, A. C., & Grier, E. C. (2001). Masterworks of art and chronic illness experiences in the elderly. *Journal of Advanced Nursing, 36*, 389-398.

Huch, M. H. (2002). Response to: Critical review of R. R. Parse's "The human becoming school of thought. A perspective for nurses and other health professionals." *Journal of Advanced Nursing, 37*, 217.

Huchings, D. (2002). Parallels in practice: Palliative nursing practice and Parse's theory of human becoming. *American Journal of Hospice and Palliative Care, 19*, 408-414.

Huch, M. H., & Bournes, D. A. (2003). Community dwellers' perspectives on the experience of feeling very tired. *Nursing Science Quarterly, 16*, 334-339.

International Consortium of Parse Scholars. (1999). A nursing position on global healthcare: Our commitment to humankind. *Nursing Science Quarterly, 12*(4), 347.

Jacono, B. J., & Jacono, J. J. (1996). The benefits of Newman and Parse in helping nurse teachers determine methods to enhance student creativity. *Nursing Education Today, 16*, 356-362.

Janes, N. M., & Wells, D. L. (1997). Elderly patients' experiences with nurses guided by Parse's theory of human becoming. *Clinical Nursing Research, 6*, 205-224.

Jonas, C. M. (1992). The meaning of being an elder in Nepal. *Nursing Science Quarterly, 5*(4), 171-175.

Jonas-Simpson, C. M. (1996). The patient-focused care journey: Where patients and families guide the way. *Nursing Science Quarterly, 9*(4), 145-146.

Jonas-Simpson, C. (1997). Living the art of the human becoming theory. *Nursing Science Quarterly, 10*(4), 175-179.

Jonas-Simpson, C. M. (1997). The Parse research method through music. *Nursing Science Quarterly, 10*(3), 112-114.

Jonas-Simpson, C. M. (2001). Feeling understood: A melody of human becoming. *Nursing Science Quarterly, 14*, 222-230.

Jonas-Simpson, C. M. (2003). The experience of being listened to: A human becoming study with music. *Nursing Science Quarterly, 16*, 232-238.

Kelley, L. S. (1991). Struggling with going along when you do not believe. *Nursing Science Quarterly, 4*(3), 123-129.

Kelley, L. S. (1995). Parse's theory in practice with a group in the community. *Nursing Science Quarterly, 8*(3), 127-132.

Kelley, L. S. (1999). Evaluating change in quality of life from the perspective of the person: Advanced practice nursing and Parse's goal of nursing. *Holistic Nursing Practice, 13*(4), 61-70.

Kim, M. S., Shin, K. R., & Shin, S. R. (1998). Korean adolescents' experiences of smoking cessation: A prelude to research with the human becoming perspective. *Nursing Science Quarterly, 11*(3), 105-109.

Kruse, B. G. (1999). The lived experience of serenity: Using Parse's research method. *Nursing Science Quarterly, 12*(2), 143-150.

Lee, O. J., & Pilkington, F. B. (1999). Practice with persons living their dying: A human becoming perspective. *Nursing Science Quarterly, 12*(4), 324-328.

Legault, F., & Ferguson-Paré, M. (1999). Advancing nursing practice: An evaluation study of Parse's theory of human becoming. *Canadian Journal of Nursing Leadership, 12*(1), 30-35.

Letcher, D. C., & Yancey, N. R. (2004). Witnessing change with aspiring nurses: A human becoming teaching-learning process in nursing education. *Nursing Science Quarterly, 17,* 36-41.

Liehr, P. R. (1989). The core of true presence: A loving center. *Nursing Science Quarterly, 2*(1), 7-8.

Linscott, J., Spee, R., Flint, F., & Fisher, A. (1999). Creating a culture of patient-focused care through a learner-centered philosophy. *Canadian Journal of Nursing Leadership, 12*(4), 5-10.

Liu, S. L. (1994). The lived experience of health for hospitalized older women in Taiwan. *Journal of National Taipei College of Nursing, 1,* 1-84.

Markovic, M. (1997). From theory to perioperative practice with Parse. *Canadian Operating Room Nursing Journal, 15*(1), 13-16.

Mattice, M. (1991). Parse's theory of nursing in practice: A manager's perspective. *Canadian Journal of Nursing Administration, 4*(1), 11-13.

Mattice, M., & Mitchell, G. J. (1990). Caring for confused elders. *The Canadian Nurse, 86*(11), 16-18.

Melnechenko, K. L. (2003). To make a difference: Nursing presence. *Nursing Forum, 38,* 18-24.

Milton, C. L. (2000). Beneficence: Honoring the commitment. *Nursing Science Quarterly, 13*(2), 111-115.

Milton, C. L. (2003). A graduate curriculum guided by human becoming: Journeying with the possible. *Nursing Science Quarterly, 16,* 214-218.

Milton, C. L. (2003). The American Nurses Association Code of Ethics: A reflection on the ethics of respect and human dignity with nurse as expert. *Nursing Science Quarterly, 16,* 301-304.

Milton, C. L., & Buseman, J. (2002). Cocreating anew in public health nursing. *Nursing Science Quarterly, 15,* 113-116.

Mitchell, G. J. (1986). Utilizing Parse's theory of man-living-health in Mrs. M's neighborhood. *Perspectives, 10*(4), 5-7.

Mitchell, G. J. (1988). Man-living-health: The theory in practice. *Nursing Science Quarterly, 1*(3), 120-127.

Mitchell, G. J. (1990). Struggling in change: From the traditional approach to Parse's theory-based practice. *Nursing Science Quarterly, 3*(4), 170-176.

Mitchell, G. J. (1990). The lived experience of taking life day-by-day in later life: Research guided by Parse's emergent method. *Nursing Science Quarterly, 3*(1), 29-36.

Mitchell, G. J. (1991). Diagnosis: Clarifying or obscuring the nature of nursing. *Nursing Science Quarterly, 4*(2), 52-53.

Mitchell, G. J. (1991). Human subjectivity: The cocreation of self. *Nursing Science Quarterly, 4*(3), 144-145.

Mitchell, G. J. (1991). Nursing diagnosis: An ethical analysis. *Image: The Journal of Nursing Scholarship, 23*(2), 99-103.

Mitchell, G. J. (1992). Parse's theory and the multidisciplinary team: Clarifying scientific values. *Nursing Science Quarterly, 5*(3), 104-106.

Mitchell, G. J. (1993). Living paradox in Parse's theory. *Nursing Science Quarterly, 6*(1), 44-51.

Mitchell, G. J. (1993). The same-thing-yet-different phenomenon: A way of coming to know—Or not? *Nursing Science Quarterly, 6*(2), 61-62.

Mitchell, G. J. (1993). Time and a waning moon: Seniors describe the meaning to later life. *The Canadian Journal of Nursing Research, 25*(1), 51-66.

Mitchell, G. J. (1994). Discipline-specific inquiry: The hermeneutics of theory-guided nursing research. *Nursing Outlook, 42*(5), 224-228.

Mitchell, G. J. (1994). The meaning of being a senior: A phenomenological study and interpretation with Parse's theory of nursing. *Nursing Science Quarterly, 7,* 70-79.

Mitchell, G. J. (1996). Clarifying contributions of qualitative research findings. *Nursing Science Quarterly, 9*(4), 143-144.

Mitchell, G. J. (1996). Pretending: A way to get through the day. *Nursing Science Quarterly, 9*(2), 92-93.

Mitchell, G. J. (1997). Retrospective and prospective of practice applications: Views in the fog. *Nursing Science Quarterly, 10*(1), 8-9.

Mitchell, G. J. (1997). Theory and practice in long term care: The acorn doesn't fall far from the tree. *Long Term Care, 7*(4), 31-34.

Mitchell, G. J. (1998). Living with diabetes: How understanding expands theory for professional practice. *Canadian Journal of Diabetes Care, 22*(1), 30-37.

Mitchell, G. J. (1998). Standards of nursing and the winds of change. *Nursing Science Quarterly, 11*(3), 97-98.

Mitchell, G. J. (2003). Abstractions and particulars: Learning theory for practice. *Nursing Science Quarterly, 16,* 310-314.

Mitchell, G. J. (2004). An emerging framework for human becoming criticism. *Nursing Science Quarterly, 17,* 103-109.

Mitchell, G. J., Bernardo, A., & Bournes, D. (1997). Nursing guided by Parse's theory: Patient views at Sunnybrook. *Nursing Science Quarterly, 10*(1), 55-56.

Mitchell, G. J., & Bunkers, S. S. (2003). Engaging the abyss: A mis-take of opportunity? *Nursing Science Quarterly, 16,* 121-125.

Mitchell, G. J., & Cody, W. K. (1993). The role of theory in qualitative research. *Nursing Science Quarterly, 6*(4), 170-178.

Mitchell, G. J., & Cody, W. K. (1999). Human becoming theory: A complement to medical science. *Nursing Science Quarterly, 12*(4), 304-310.

Mitchell, G. J., & Cody, W. K. (1992). Nursing knowledge and human science: Ontological and epistemological considerations. *Nursing Science Quarterly, 5*(2), 54-61.

Mitchell, G. J., & Cody, W. K. (2002). Ambiguous opportunity: Toiling for truth of nursing art and science. *Nursing Science Quarterly, 15*, 71-79.

Mitchell, G. J., & Copplestone, C. (1990). Applying Parse's theory to perioperative nursing: A nontraditional approach. *AORN Journal, 51*(3), 787-798.

Mitchell, G. J., & Heidt, P. (1994). The lived experience of wanting to help another. *Nursing Science Quarterly, 7*(3), 119-127.

Mitchell, G. J., & Lawton, C. (2000). Living with the consequences of personal choices for person with diabetes: Implications for educators and practitioners. *Canadian Journal of Diabetes Care, 24*(2), 23-31.

Mitchell, G. J., & Pilkington, F. B. (1990). Theoretical approaches in nursing practice: A comparison of Roy and Parse. *Nursing Science Quarterly, 3*(2), 81-87.

Mitchell, G. J., & Pilkington, F. B. (1999). A dialogue on the comparability of research paradigms—And other theoretical things. *Nursing Science Quarterly, 12*(4), 283-289.

Mitchell, G. J., & Pilkington, F. B. (2000). Comfort-discomfort with ambiguity: Flight and freedom in nursing practice. *Nursing Science Quarterly, 13*(1), 31-36.

Mitchell, G. J., & Santopinto, M. D. A. (1988). An alternative to nursing diagnosis. *The Canadian Nurse, 84*(10), 25-28.

Mitchell, G. J., & Santopinto, M. D. A. (1988). The expanded role nurse: A dissenting viewpoint. *Canadian Journal of Nursing Administration, 4*(1), 8-14.

Mitchell, M. G. (2002). Patient-focused care on a complex continuing care dialysis unit: Rose's story. *CAANT Journal—Canadian Association of Nephrology Nurses & Technicians, 12*, 48-49.

Nokes, K. M., & Carver, K. (1991). The meaning of living with AIDS: A study using Parse's theory of man-living-health. *Nursing Science Quarterly, 4*(4), 175-179.

Norris, J. R. (2002). One-to-one teleapprenticeship as a means for nurses teaching and learning Parse's theory of human becoming. *Nursing Science Quarterly, 15*, 143-149.

Northrup, D. T. (2002). Time passing: A Parse research method study. *Nursing Science Quarterly, 15*, 318-326.

Northrup, D. T., & Cody, W. K. (1998). Evaluation of the human becoming theory in practice in an acute care psychiatric setting. *Nursing Science Quarterly, 11*(1), 23-30.

Ortiz, M. R. (2003). Lingering presence: A study using the human becoming hermeneutic method. *Nursing Science Quarterly, 16*, 146-154.

Paille, M., & Pilkington, F. B. (2002). The global context of nursing: A human becoming perspective. *Nursing Science Quarterly, 15*, 165-170.

Pilkington, F. B. (1993). The lived experience of grieving the loss of an important other. *Nursing Science Quarterly, 6*(3), 130-139.

Pilkington, F. B. (1999). An ethical framework for nursing practice: Parse's human becoming theory. *Nursing Science Quarterly, 12*(1), 21-25.

Pilkington, F. B. (1999). A qualitative study of life after stroke. *Journal of Neuroscience Nursing, 31*(6), 336-347.

Pilkington, F. B. (2000). A unitary view of persistence-change. *Nursing Science Quarterly, 13*(1), 5-11.

Pilkington, F. B. (2004). Exploring ethical implications for acting faithfully in professional relationships. *Nursing Science Quarterly, 17*, 27-32.

Pilkington, F. B., & Mitchell, G. J. (2004). Quality of life for women living with a gynecological cancer. *Nursing Science Quarterly, 17*, 147-155.

Profile: Rosemarie Rizzo Parse. (1991). *The Japanese Journal of Nursing, 55*(8), 744.

Quiquero, A., Knights, D., & Meo, C. O. (1991). Theory as a guide to practice: Staff nurses choose Parse's theory. *Canadian Journal of Nursing Administration, 4*(1), 14-16.

Rasmusson, D. L., Jonas, C. M., & Mitchell, G. J. (1991). The eye of the beholder: Applying Parse's theory with homeless individuals. *Clinical Nurse Specialist Journal, 5*(3), 139-143.

Rendon, D. C., Sales, R., Leal, I., & Pique, J. (1995). The lived experience of aging in community-dwelling elders in Valencia, Spain: A phenomenological study. *Nursing Science Quarterly, 8*(4), 152-157.

Ross, J. R. L. (1997). A paradigm shift: What a difference a day makes. *Perspectives, 21*(4), 2-6.

Saltmarche, A., Kolodny, V., & Mitchell, G. J. (1998). An educational approach for patient-focused care: Shifting attitudes and practice. *Journal of Nursing Staff Development, 14*(2), 81-86.

Santopinto, M. D. A. (1989). The relentless drive to be ever thinner: A study using the phenomenological method. *Nursing Science Quarterly, 2*(1), 29-36.

Smith, M. C. (1990). Struggling through a difficult time for unemployed persons. *Nursing Science Quarterly, 3*(1), 18-28.

Smith, M. K. (2002). Human becoming and women living with violence: The art of practice. *Nursing Science Quarterly, 15*, 302-307.

Spenceley, S. M. (1995). The CNS in multidisciplinary pulmonary rehabilitation: A nursing science perspective. *Clinical Nurse Specialist, 9*, 192-198.

Stanley, G. D., & Meghani, S. H. (2001). Reflections on using Parse's theory of human becoming in a palliative care setting in Pakistan. *Canadian Nurse, 97,* 23-25.

Thornburg, P. (2002). "Waiting" as experienced by women hospitalized during the antepartum period. *MCN, American Journal of Maternal Child Nursing, 27,* 245-248.

Vander Woude, D. (1998). Nursing theory–based regulatory decisioning model in South Dakota. *Issues, 19*(3), 14.

Walker, C. A. (1996). Coalescing the theories of two nurse visionaries: Parse and Watson. *Journal of Advanced Nursing, 24,* 988-996.

Wang, C. E. (2000). Developing a concept of hope from a human science perspective. *Nursing Science Quarterly, 13,* 248-251.

Wang, C. H. (1997). Quality of life and health for persons living with leprosy. *Nursing Science Quarterly, 10*(3), 144-145.

Williamson, G. J. (2000). The test of a nursing theory: A personal view. *Nursing Science Quarterly, 13*(2), 124-128.

Wimpenny, P. (1993). The paradox of Parse's theory. *Senior Nurse, 13*(5), 10-13.

Wing, D. M. (1999). The aesthetics of caring: Where folk healers and nurse theorists converge. *Nursing Science Quarterly, 12*(13), 256-262.

Wondolowski, C., & Davis, D. K. (1988). The lived experience of aging in the oldest old: A phenomenological study. *The American Journal of Psychoanalysis, 48,* 261-270.

Wondolowski, C., & Davis, D. K. (1991). The lived experience of health in the oldest old: A phenomenological study. *Nursing Science Quarterly, 4*(3), 113-118.

Woude, D. V., Damgaard, G., Hegge, M. J., Soholt, D., & Bunkers, S. S. (2003). The unfolding: Scenario planning in nursing. *Nursing Science Quarterly, 16,* 27-35.

Book Chapters and Journal Articles by Others Critiquing Parse's Theory

Cowling, W. R. (1989). Parse's theory of nursing. In J. J. Fitzpatrick & A. L. Whall (Eds.), *Conceptual models of nursing: Analysis and application* (2nd ed., pp. 385-399). Norwalk, CT: Appleton & Lange.

Hickman, J. S. (1990). Rosemarie Rizzo Parse. In J. B. George (Ed.), *Nursing theories: The base for professional nursing practice* (3rd ed., pp. 311-332). Norwalk, CT: Appleton & Lange.

Lee, R. E., & Schumacher, L. P. (1989). Rosemarie Rizzo Parse: Man-living-health. In A. Marriner Tomey (Ed.), *Nurse theorists and their work* (2nd ed., pp. 174-186). St. Louis: Mosby.

Phillips, J. (1987). A critique of Parse's man-living-health theory. In R. R. Parse (Ed.), *Nursing science: Major paradigms, theories, and critiques* (pp. 181-204). Philadelphia: W. B. Saunders.

Pugliese, L. (1989). The theory of man-living-health: An analysis. In J. Riehl-Sisca (Ed.), *Conceptual models for nursing practice* (3rd ed., pp. 259-265). Norwalk, CT: Appleton & Lange.

Smith, M. C., & Hudepohl, J. H. (1988). Analysis and evaluation of Parse's theory of man-living-health. *The Canadian Journal of Nursing Research: Nursing Papers, 20*(4), 43-58.

Winkler, S. J. (1983). Parse's theory of nursing. In J. J. Fitzpatrick & A. L. Whall (Eds.), *Conceptual models of nursing: Analysis and application* (pp. 275-294). Bowie, MD: Brady.

Directories and Biographical Sources

AAN directory: Fellows of the American academy of nursing. (1989). Kansas City, MO: American Academy of Nursing.

Directory of nurse researchers (2nd ed.). (1987). Indianapolis: Sigma Theta Tau.

Reviews of Parse's Books

[Review of the book *Man-living-health: A theory of nursing*]. (1981). *International Journal of Rehabilitation Research, 4,* 449.

Clarke, P. N. (1996). [Review of the book *Illuminations: The human becoming theory in practice and research*]. *Nursing Science Quarterly, 9*(2), 81-82.

Fawcett, J. (1996). [Review of the book *Illuminations: The human becoming theory in practice and research*]. *Nursing Science Quarterly, 9*(2), 82-83.

Fawcett, J., & Phillips, J. R. (1999). [Review of the book *The human becoming school of thought: A perspective for nurses and other health professionals*]. *Nursing Science Quarterly, 12*(1), 85-89.

Jacobs-Kramer, M. K., Levine, M. E., & Menke, E. M. (1988). Three perspectives on a scholarly work [Review of the book *Nursing science: Major paradigms, theories, and critiques*]. *Nursing Science Quarterly, 1*(4), 182-186.

Jonas-Simpson, C. (2004). *Community: A human becoming perspective* [Reviewed by K. Egenes, S. H. Gueldner, & L. S. Kelley]. *Nursing Science Quarterly, 17,* 177-182.

Limandri, B. J. (1982). [Review of the book *Man-living-health: A theory of nursing*]. *Western Journal of Nursing Research, 4*(1), 105-106.

Rawnsley, M. M. (1988). Quest for quality: A comparative review [Review of the book *Nursing research: Qualitative methods*]. *Nursing Science Quarterly, 1*(1), 40-41.

Web Sites

International Consortium of Parse Scholars. Accessed December 28, 2004: *http://www.humanbecoming.org*

Discovery International and the Institute of Human Becoming. Accessed December 28, 2004: *http://www.discoveryinternationalonline.com*

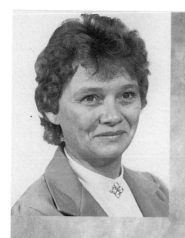

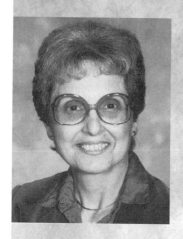

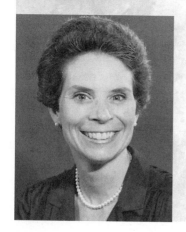

Helen C. Erickson
1937-present

Evelyn M. Tomlin
1929-present

Mary Ann P. Swain
1941-present

560

Modeling and Role-Modeling

Margaret E. Erickson

CREDENTIALS AND BACKGROUND OF THE THEORISTS

Helen C. Erickson

Helen C. Erickson received a diploma from Saginaw General Hospital, Saginaw, Michigan, in 1957. Her degrees include a baccalaureate in nursing in 1974, a master's degree in psychiatric nursing and in medical-surgical nursing in 1976, and a Doctor of Educational Psychology in 1984, all from the University of Michigan.

Erickson's professional experience began in the emergency room of the Midland Community Hospital in Midland, Texas, where she was the head nurse for 2 years. She then worked in Mount Pleasant, Michigan, as night supervisor of nursing in the Michigan State Home for the Mentally Impaired and Handicapped. Thereafter, she moved to Puerto Rico with her husband and assumed the position of Director of Health Services at the Inter-American University in San German, Puerto Rico, from 1960 to 1964. On her return to the United States, she worked as a staff nurse at both St. Joseph's Hospital and University Hospital in Ann Arbor, Michigan. Erickson later served as a psychiatric nurse consul-

Previous authors: Margaret E. Erickson, Jane A. Caldwell-Gwin, Lisa A. Carr, Brenda Kay Harmon, Karen Hartman, Connie Rae Jarlsberg, Judy McCormick, and Kathryn W. Noone.
The authors wish to express appreciation to Helen C. Erickson, Evelyn M. Tomlin, and Mary Ann P. Swain for critiquing earlier editions of this chapter.

tant to the Pediatric Nurse Practitioner Program at the University of Michigan and the University of Michigan Hospitals–Adult Care.

Her academic career began as an assistant instructor in the RN Studies Program at the University of Michigan School of Nursing, where she later served as chairperson of the undergraduate program and Dean for Undergraduate Studies. Erickson was an assistant professor of nursing at the University of Michigan from 1978 to 1986. In 1986, she left Michigan to go to the University of South Carolina College of Nursing. Initially, she served as an associate professor and assistant dean for academic programs; later she held the position of Associate Dean for Academic Affairs. In 1988, she moved to Austin, Texas, and served as a professor of nursing and chair of Adult Health at the University of Texas at Austin School of Nursing. In addition, she served as Special Assistant to the Dean, Graduate Programs. Since 1997 she has been an emeritus professor at the University of Texas at Austin. Erickson has maintained an independent nursing practice since 1976.

Erickson is a member of the American Nurses Association, American Nurses Foundation, the Charter Club, American Holistic Nurses Association, Texas Nurses Association, Sigma Theta Tau, and the Institute for the Advancement of Health. In addition, she served as President of the Society for the Advancement of Modeling and Role-Modeling from 1986 to 1990. She was the chairperson of the First National Symposium on Modeling and

Role-Modeling in 1986 and served on the planning committee for the second, third, fourth, fifth, sixth, seventh, eighth, and ninth national conferences in 1988, 1990, 1992, 1994, 1996, 1998, 2000, 2002, and 2004, respectively.

Erickson has been listed in *Who's Who Among University Students* and is a member of Phi Kappa Phi. She received the Sigma Theta Tau Rho Chapter Award of Excellence in Nursing in 1980, the Amoco Foundation Good Teaching Award in 1982, and was accepted into ADARA (a University of Michigan honor society for women in leadership) in 1982. In 1990, she received the Faculty Teaching Award, University of Texas at Austin, School of Nursing. She received a founders award from the Sigma Theta Tau International Honor Society in Nursing, Excellence in Education Award by the Epsilon Theta Chapter in 1993; she received the Graduate Faculty Teaching Award, University of Texas at Austin School of Nursing in 1995; and she was inducted as a fellow in the American Academy of Nursing in 1996. The Helen Erickson Endowed Lectureship in Holistic Health Nursing was established in her honor in 1997 at the University of Texas at Austin. She received the Distinguished Faculty citation from Humboldt State University in California in 2001.

Erickson continues to research actively the Modeling and Role-Modeling Theory and has presented numerous seminars, conferences, and papers on various aspects of the theory, both nationally and internationally. She has served as a consultant in the implementation of the theory in clinical practice at the University of Michigan Medical Center in the surgical area, at Brigham and Women's Hospital, Boston, and at the University of Pittsburgh hospitals. She has consulted with faculty members who have adopted the theory into their curricula and practice in various schools of nursing and service agencies. Humboldt University School of Nursing in Arcata, California, was the first school to use the Modeling and Role-Modeling Theory as its conceptual base. Metropolitan State University at St. Paul, Minnesota, has adopted the Modeling and Role-Modeling Theory for its R.N. and baccalaureate and master's in nursing programs. St. Catherine's College, St. Paul, Minnesota, has also adopted it for the associate degree in nursing program. The Uni-

versity of Texas at Austin has adopted concepts as a foundation for the alternative entry program, and the University of Texas at Galveston has adopted core concepts for the academic and service model at the University of Texas Medical Branch in Galveston (H. Erickson, personal correspondence, July 1992).

Erickson has been an invited speaker at many national and international conferences. She has participated in numerous workshops, including several congresses on Ericksonian approaches to hypnosis sponsored by the Erickson Foundation and in several conferences sponsored by the National Institute for the Clinical Application of Behavioral Medicine. She has also been involved in activities sponsored by the American Holistic Nurses' Association. She served as a content expert for certification curricula and was included in a book featuring nurse healers (H. Erickson, personal correspondence, July 1992). Although retired from the University of Texas at Austin, Erickson continues to be actively involved in the promotion of holistic nursing. She became chairman for the board of directors of the American Holistic Nurses' Certification Corporation in 2002, provides consultation and educational programs, and is actively involved in the Society for the Advancement of Modeling and Role-Modeling (H. Erickson, personal correspondence, June 10, 2000).

Evelyn M. Tomlin

Evelyn M. Tomlin's nursing education began in Southern California. She attended Pasadena City College, Los Angeles County General Hospital School of Nursing, and the University of Southern California, where she received her Bachelor of Science in Nursing. She received a Master of Science in Psychiatric Nursing from the University of Michigan in 1976.

Tomlin's professional experiences are varied. She began as a clinical instructor at Los Angeles County General Hospital School of Nursing in surgical nursing and maternal and premature infant nursing. She later lived in Kabul, Afghanistan, where she taught English at the Afghan Institute of Technology. She then served as a school nurse and practiced family nursing in the overseas American and European communities where she lived, a role that included participating in more than 46 home deliveries with a certified nurse midwife. After the establishment of medical services at the United States Embassy Hospital, she functioned as a relief staff nurse. Upon her return to the United States, she was employed by the Visiting Nurse Association (VNA) as a staff nurse in Ann Arbor, Michigan. At the VNA she acted as the coordinator and clinical instructor for student practical nurses. In addition, she was a staff nurse in a coronary care unit for 5 years, worked in the respiratory intensive care unit, and was the head nurse of the emergency department at St. Joseph's Mercy Hospital in Ann Arbor. For the next 8 years, she taught the fundamentals of nursing as an assistant professor of nursing in the RN Studies Program at the University of Michigan School of Nursing. During that time, she also served as the mental health consultant to the pediatric nurse practitioner program at the University of Michigan.

Tomlin was among the first 16 nurses in the United States to be certified by the American Association of Critical Care Nurses. With several colleagues, she opened one of the first offices for independent nursing practice in Michigan. She continued her independent practice until 1993.

She is a member of Sigma Theta Tau Rho Chapter, the California Scholarship Federation, and the Philomathian Society. She has presented programs incorporating a variety of nursing topics based on the Modeling and Role-Modeling Theory and paradigm, with an emphasis on clinical applications.

In 1985, she moved to Big Rock, Illinois, where she enjoyed teaching small community and nursing groups and working with a community shelter serving the women and children of Fox Valley. Later she moved to Geneva, Illinois, where she currently resides with her husband. Tomlin has had inquiries from staff nurses for help in integrating the framework into practice. She believes that elements of the theory and paradigm can be introduced easily in many settings and can be very valuable for practicing nurses (E. Tomlin, telephone interview, 1992). She was first editor for the newsletter of the Society for the Advancement of Modeling and Role-Modeling (E. Tomlin, curriculum vitae, 1992).

Tomlin identifies herself as a Christian in retirement from nursing for pay, but not from nursing practice. She is pursuing her interest in the practice of healing prayer, stating that she has always been interested in the interface of the Modeling and Role-Modeling Theory and Judeo-Christian principles. She is on the board of directors and works as a volunteer at Wayside Cross Ministries in Aurora, Illinois, where she teaches and counsels homeless women, most of whom are single mothers. She is semiretired but continues to help them develop skills necessary to live healthier, happier lives (E. Tomlin, telephone interview, July 10, 1996).

Mary Ann P. Swain

Mary Ann P. Swain's educational background is in psychology. She received her bachelor of arts degree in psychology from DePauw University in Greencastle, Indiana, and her master of science and doctoral degrees from the University of Michigan, both in the field of psychology.

Swain taught psychology, research methods, and statistics as a teaching assistant at DePauw University and later as a lecturer and a professor of psychology and nursing research at the University of Michigan. She became the Director of the Doctoral Program in Nursing in 1975 and served in that capacity for 1 year. She was Chairperson of Nursing Research from 1977 to 1982. In 1983, she became Associate Vice President for Academic Affairs at the University of Michigan (M. Swain, curriculum vitae, February 1988).

She is a member of the American Psychological Association and an associate member of the Michigan Nurses Association. She developed and taught classes in psychology, research, and nursing research methods. She also collaborated with nurse researchers on various projects, including health promotion among diabetics and influencing compliance among patients with hypertension. She helped Erickson publish a model that assessed an individual's potential to mobilize resources and adapt to stress, which is significant to the Modeling and Role-Modeling Theory.

Swain received the Alpha Lambda Delta, Psi Chi, Mortar Board, and Phi Beta Kappa awards while at DePauw University. In 1981, she was recognized by the Rho Chapter of Sigma Theta Tau for Contributions to Nursing and, in 1983, became an honorary member of Sigma Theta Tau. In 1994 she moved to Appalachia, New York, with her husband when she accepted the position of provost for the New York State University system.

THEORETICAL SOURCES

The theory and paradigm modeling and role-modeling was developed using a retroductive process. The original model was derived inductively from the primary author's clinical and personal life experiences. The works of Maslow, Erikson, Piaget, Engel, Selye, and M. Erickson were then integrated and synthesized into the original model to label, further articulate, and refine a holistic theory and paradigm for nursing. Erickson (1976) argued that people have mind-body relations and have an identifiable resource potential that predicts their ability to contend with stress. She also articulated a relationship between needs status and developmental processes, satisfaction with needs and attachment objects, loss and illness, and health and need satisfaction. Tomlin and Swain validated and affirmed Erickson's practice model and helped to expand and articulate labeled phenomena, concepts, and theoretical relationships.

The authors used Maslow's theory of human needs to label and articulate their personal observations that "all people want to be the best that they can possibly be; unmet basic needs interfere with holistic growth whereas satisfied needs promote growth" (Erickson, Tomlin, & Swain, 2002, p. 56; Jensen, 1995). The authors further integrated the model to state that unmet basic needs create need deficits, which can lead to initiation or aggravation of physical or mental distress or illness. At the same time, need satisfaction creates assets that provide resources needed to contend with stress and promote health, growth, and development.

Piaget's theory of cognitive development provides a framework for understanding the development of thinking. On the other hand, integration of Erik Erikson's work on the stages of psychosocial development through the life span provides a theoretical basis for understanding the psychosocial evolution of the individual. Each of his eight stages represents developmental tasks. As an individual resolves each task, he or she gains strengths that contribute to character development and health. Furthermore, as an outcome of each stage, people develop a sense of their own worth and, therefore, a projection of themselves into the future. "The utility of Erikson's theory is the freedom we may take to view aspects of people's problems as uncompleted tasks. This perspective provides a hopeful expectation for the individual's future since it connotes something still in progress" (Erickson et al., 2002, pp. 62-63).

The works of Winnicott, Klein, Mahler, and Bowlby on object attachment were integrated with the original model to develop and articulate the concept of affiliated-individuation (AI). Object relations theory proposes that an infant initially forms an attachment to his or her caregiver after having repeated positive contacts. As the child grows and begins to move toward a more separate and individuated state, a sense of autonomy develops. During this time, he or she usually transfers some attachment to an inanimate object such as a cuddly blanket or a teddy bear. Later, the child may attach to a favorite baseball glove, doll, or pet and finally onto more abstract things in adulthood, such as an educational degree, professional role, or relationship. On the basis of the work of these individuals, a theoretical relationship was identified between object attachment and need satisfaction. According to the theorists, when an object repeatedly meets an individual's basic needs, attachment or connectedness to that object occurs. After further synthesis of these theoretical linkages and research findings, the authors identified a new concept, AI. They defined AI as the inherent need to be connected with significant others at the same time that there is a sense of separateness from them that enhances their uniqueness. AI runs across the life-span from birth to death. Research supports that AI and object attachment are essential to need satisfaction, adaptive coping, and healthy growth and development.

The authors further state that "object loss results in basic need deficits" (Erickson et al., 2002, p. 88).

Loss is real, threatened, or perceived; it may be a normal part of the developmental process, or it may be situational. Loss always results in grief; normal grief is resolved in approximately 1 year. When only inadequate or inappropriate objects are available to meet needs, morbid grief results. Morbid grief interferes with the individual's ability to grow and develop to maximal potential. The work of Selye and Engel, as cited by Erickson, Tomlin, and Swain (1983), provided additional conceptual basis for the beliefs the theorists hold regarding loss and an individual's stress response to that loss or losses. Selye's theory pertains to an individual's biophysical responses to stress, whereas Engel's work explores the psychosocial responses to stressors.

The synthesis of these theories, with the integration of the primary author's clinical observations and lived experiences, resulted in the development of the Adaptive Potential Assessment Model (APAM). The APAM focuses on the individual's ability to mobilize resources when confronted with stressors, rather than the adaptation process. This model was first developed by Erickson (1976) and later described in publication by Erickson and Swain (1982).

Erickson credits Milton H. Erickson with influencing her clinical practice and providing inspiration and direction in the development of this theory. Initially, he articulated the formulation of the Modeling and Role-Modeling Theory when he urged Erickson to "model the client's world, understand it as they do, then role-model the picture the client has drawn, building a healthy world for them" (H. Erickson, telephone interview, November 1984).

MAJOR CONCEPTS *&* DEFINITIONS

The theory and paradigm modeling and role-modeling contains multiple concepts.

MODELING

The act of Modeling, then, is the process the nurse uses as she develops an image and understanding of the client's world—an image and understanding developed within the client's framework and from the client's perspective. . . . The art of Modeling is the development of a mirror image of the situation from the client's perspective. . . . The science of Modeling is the scientific aggregation and analysis of data collected about the client's model. (Erickson et al., 2002, p. 95)

Modeling occurs as the nurse accepts and understands her client. (Erickson et al., 2002, p. 96)

ROLE-MODELING

The art of Role-Modeling occurs when the nurse plans and implements interventions that are unique for the client. The science of Role-Mod-

eling occurs as the nurse plans interventions with respect to her theoretical base for the practice of nursing. . . . Role-Modeling is . . . the essence of nurturance. . . . Role-Modeling requires an unconditional acceptance of the person as the person is while gently encouraging the facilitating growth and development at the person's own pace and within the person's own model. (Erickson et al., 2002, p. 95)

Role-Modeling starts the second the nurse moves from the analysis phase of the nursing process to the planning of nursing interventions. (Erickson et al., 2002, p. 95)

NURSING

Nursing is the holistic helping of persons with their self-care activities in relation to their health. This is an interactive, interpersonal process that nurtures strengths to enable development, release, and channeling of resources for coping with one's circumstances and environment. The goal is to achieve a state of perceived optimum health and contentment. (Erickson et al., 2002, p. 49)

Continued

MAJOR CONCEPTS *&* DEFINITIONS—cont'd

NURTURANCE

Nurturance fuses and integrates cognitive, physiological and affective processes, with the aim of assisting a client to move toward holistic health. Nurturance implies that the nurse seeks to know and understand the client's personal model of his or her world and to appreciate its value and significance for that client from the client's perspective. (Erickson et al., 2002, p. 48)

UNCONDITIONAL ACCEPTANCE

Being accepted as a unique, worthwhile, important individual—with no strings attached—is imperative if the individual is to be facilitated in developing his or her own potential. The nurse's use of empathy helps the individual learn that the nurse accepts and respects him or her as is. The acceptance will facilitate the mobilization of resources needed as this individual strives for adaptive equilibrium. (Erickson et al., 2002, p. 49)

PERSON

People are alike because they have holism, lifetime growth and development, and their need for AI. They are different because they have inherent endowment, adaptation, and self-care knowledge (Erickson et al., 1983).

HOW PEOPLE ARE ALIKE

Holism

Human beings are holistic persons who have multiple interacting subsystems. Permeating all subsystems are the inherent bases. These include genetic makeup and spiritual drive. Body, mind, emotion, and spirit are a total unit and they act together. They affect and control one another interactively. The interaction of the multiple subsystems and the inherent bases creates holism: Holism implies that the whole is greater than the sum of the parts. (Erickson et al., 2002, pp. 44-45)

Basic Needs

All human beings have basic needs that can be satisfied, but only from within the framework of the individual. (Erickson, et al., 2002, p. 58)

Basic needs are only met when the individual perceives that they are met. (Erickson et al., 2002, p. 57)

Lifetime Development

Lifetime development evolves through psychological and cognitive stages, as follows:

- Psychological Stages:
  Each stage represents a developmental task or decisive encounter resulting in a turning point, a moment of decision between alternative basic attitudes (for example, trust versus mistrust or autonomy versus shame and doubt). As a maturing individual negotiates or resolves each age-specific crisis or task, the individual gains enduring strengths and attitudes that contribute to the character and health of the individual's personality in his or her culture. (Erickson et al., 2002, p. 61)

- Cognitive Stages:
  Consider how thinking develops rather than what happens in psychosocial or affective development. . . . Piaget believed that cognitive learning develops in a sequential manner and he has identified several periods in this process. Essentially, there are four periods: sensorimotor, preoperational, concrete operations, and formal operations. (Erickson et al., 2002, pp. 63-64)

Affiliated-Individuation

Individuals have an instinctual need for affiliated-individuation. They need to be able to be dependent on support systems while simultaneously maintaining independence from these support systems. They need to feel a deep sense of both the "I" and the "we" states of being and to perceive freedom and acceptance in both states. (Erickson et al., 2002, p. 47)

MAJOR CONCEPTS *&* DEFINITIONS—cont'd

HOW PEOPLE ARE DIFFERENT

Inherent Endowment

Each individual is born with a set of genes that will to some extent predetermine appearance, growth, development, and responses to life events.... Clearly, both genetic makeup and inherited characteristics influence growth and development. They might influence how one perceives oneself and one's world. They make individuals different from one another, each unique in his or her own way. (Erickson et al., 2002, pp. 74-75)

Adaptation

Adaptation occurs as the individual responds to external and internal stressors in a health-directed and growth-directed manner. Adaptation involves mobilizing internal and external coping resources. No subsystem is left in jeopardy when adaptation occurs (Erickson et al., 2002).

The individual's ability to mobilize resources is depicted by the APAM. The APAM identifies three different coping potential states: (1) arousal, (2) equilibrium (adaptive and maladaptive), and (3) impoverishment. Each of these states represents a different potential to mobilize self-care resources. "Movement among the states is influenced by one's ability to cope [with ongoing stressors] and the presence of new stressors" (Erickson et al., 2002, pp. 80-81).

Nurses can use this model to predict an individual's potential to mobilize self-care resources in response to stress.

Mind-Body Relationships

We are all biophysical, psychosocial beings who want to develop our potential, this is, to be the best we can be. (Erickson et al., 2002, p. 70)

Self-Care

Self-care involves the use of knowledge, resources, and action, as follows:

- Self-Care Knowledge:
  At some level a person knows what has made him or her sick, lessened his or her effectiveness, or interfered with his or her growth. The person also knows what will make him or her well, optimize his or her effectiveness or fulfillment (given circumstances), or promote his or her growth. (Erickson et al., 2002, p. 48)
- Self-Care Resources:
Self-care resources are "the internal resources, as well as additional resources, mobilized through self-care action that help gain, maintain, and promote an optimum level of holistic health" (Erickson et al., 2002, pp. 254-255).
- Self-Care Action:
  Self-care action is "the development and utilization of self-care knowledge and self-care resources" (Erickson et al., 2002, p. 254).

USE OF EMPIRICAL EVIDENCE

Several studies have provided initial evidence for philosophical premises and theoretical linkages implied in the original book by Erickson, Tomlin, and Swain (1983) and later specified by Erickson (1990b). The APAM (Figures 25-1 and 25-2) has been tested as a classification model (Barnfather, 1987; Erickson, 1976; Kleinbeck, 1977), as a

predictor for health status (Barnfather, 1990b), for length of hospital stay (Erickson & Swain, 1982), and as it relates to basic need status (Barnfather, 1993). Findings from these studies provide beginning evidence for the proposed three-state model across populations, a relationship between health and ability to mobilize resources, and ability to mobilize resources and needs status. Two other studies have shown relationships among stressors

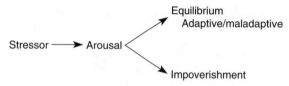

Figure **25-1 Adaptive Potential Assessment Model.** (From Erickson, H. C., Tomlin, E. M., & Swain, M. A. P. [1983]. *Modeling and role-modeling: A theory and paradigm for nursing.* Englewood Cliffs, NJ: Prentice Hall.)

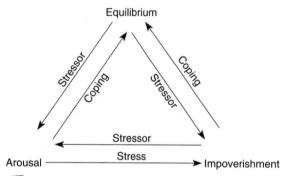

Figure **25-2 Dynamic relationship among the states of the Adaptive Potential Assessment Model.** (From Erickson, H. C., Tomlin, E. M., & Swain, M. A. P. [1983]. *Modeling and role-modeling: A theory and paradigm for nursing.* Englewood Cliffs, NJ: Prentice Hall.)

(measured as life events) and propensity for accidents (Babcock & Mueller, 1980) and resource state and ability to take in and use new information (Clementino & Lapinske, 1980). Finally, Benson (2003) has studied the APAM as applied to small groups.

Relationships among self-care knowledge, resources, and activities have been demonstrated in several studies (Acton, 1993; Baas, 1992; Irvin, 1993; Jensen, 1995; Miller, 1994). The self-care knowledge construct, first studied by Erickson (1985) was replicated and found to be significantly associated with perceived control (Cain & Perzynski, 1986). Self-directedness, need for harmony (affiliation), and need for autonomy (individuation) were found when multidimensional scaling was used to explore relationships among self-care knowledge, resources, and actions. The author concluded that a positive attitude was a major factor when health-directed self-care actions were assessed (Rosenow, 1991). Physical activity in patients after myocardial infarction was shown to be affected by life satisfaction (not physical condition); life satisfaction was predicted by availability of self-care resources and resources needed. Furthermore, resources needed served as a suppressor for resources available (Baas, 1992). In a sample of caregivers, social support predicted for stress level and self-worth and had an indirect effect on hope through self-worth (Irvin, 1993), whereas persons with diabetes with spiritual well-being were better able to cope (Landis, 1991).

When the Modeling and Role-Modeling Theory was used as a guideline, interviews were used to determine the client's model of the world. The following seven themes emerged (Erickson, 1990a):

1. Cause of the problem, which was unique to the individual
2. Related factors, also unique to the individual
3. Expectations for the future
4. Types of perceived control
5. Affiliation
6. Lack of affiliation
7. Trust in the caregiver

Each model was unique and each warranted individualized interventions. Other qualitative studies on self-care knowledge showed that acutely ill patients perceived monitoring, caring, presence, touch, and voice tones as comforting (Kennedy, 1991), healthy adults sought need satisfaction from the nurse practitioner in primary care (Boodley, 1990), and hospice patients benefited from nurse empathy (Raudonis, 1991). Studies also showed relationships among mistrust and length of stay in hospitalized subjects (Finch, 1990), perceived enactment of autonomy, self-care, and holistic health in the elderly (Anschutz, 2000; Hertz & Anschutz, 2002), perceived support, control, and well being in the elderly (Chen, 1996), and loss, morbid grief, and onset of symptoms of Alzheimer's disease (Erickson, Kinney et al., 1994; Irvin & Acton, 1996).

Other studies addressed linkages between role-modeled interventions and outcomes (Erickson, et al., 1994; Hertz, 1991; Irvin, 1993; Jensen, 1995; Kennedy, 1991). College-level students who perceived need satisfaction were more successful in school. Seven nursing students who perceived that they were supported were more able to attain their goals for advanced education (Smith, 1980), the elderly who felt supported reported higher need satisfaction and were better able to cope (Keck, 1989), adolescent mothers who felt supported and perceived need satisfaction had a more positive maternal-infant attachment (Erickson, 1996), those with a strong social network reported better health (Doornbos, 1983), and persons convicted of sexual offenses and then provided with support to remodel their worlds were able to develop new behaviors and move on with their lives (Scheela, 1991). Families and post–myocardial infarction patients who were able to participate in planning their own care through contracting had less anxiety and more perceived control and perceived support (Holl, 1992), and caregivers of adults with dementia who experienced theory-based nursing using the Modeling and Role-Modeling Theory perceived that their needs were met and that they were healthier (Hopkins, 1995). They also reported feeling that they were encouraged, which helped them accept the situation and transcend the experience of caregiving (Hopkins, 1995). Self-care resources, measured as needs, are related to perceived support and coping in women with breast cancer (Keck, 1989), physical well-being in persons with chronic obstructive pulmonary disease (Kline, 1988), and anxiety in hospitalized patients who have had cardiac surgery and their families (Holl, 1992). Finally, when AI was tested as a buffer between stress and well being, a mediation effect was found (Irvin, 1993).

Other studies operationalizing self-care resources by measuring developmental residuals have shown that identity resolution in adolescents with facial disfiguration can be predicted by previous developmental residual (Miller, 1986). Chen (1996) found that feelings of control over one's health (health control orientation) status in elderly individuals with hypertension correlated highly with self-efficacy and self-care. In addition, her work supported that health control orientation, self-efficacy, and self-care were associated with well-being. Other researchers found that trust predicts for adolescent clients' involvement in the prescribed medical regimen (Finch, 1987), perceived support and adaptation are related to developmental residual in families with newborn infants (Darling-Fisher & Leidy, 1988), mistrust predicts length of hospital stay, and positive residual serves as a buffer (Finch, 1987). Positive residual in the intimacy stage of healthy adults predicts for health behaviors (MacLean, 1987), developmental residual predicts for hope, trust-mistrust residual predicts for generalized hope, autonomy-shame and doubt residual predicts for particularized hope in the elderly (Curl, 1992), and negative residual is related to speed and impatience behaviors in a healthy sample of military personnel (Kinney, 1992). Case study methods have been used to show relationships among needs, attachment, and developmental residual (Kinney, 1990, 1992; Kinney & Erickson, 1990) and needs and coping (Jensen, 1995), and two unpublished studies have shown relationships between healthy adults and need status (Erickson, Kinney, Stone, & Acton, 1990).

Studies have also been used to explore self-care knowledge in informants in the hospital (Erickson, 1985), perceived enactment of autonomy and life satisfaction in the elderly (Anschutz, 2000), the experience of persons 85 and older as they manage their health (Beltz, 1999), perceptions of hope in elementary school children (Baldwin, 1996), the experiential meaning of well-being and the lived experience in employed mothers (Weber, 1995, 1999), developmental growth in adults with heart failure (Baas, Beery, Fontana, & Wagoner, 1999), the individual's ability to mobilize coping resources and basic needs (Barnfather, 1990a), the relationship between basic need satisfaction and emotionally motivated eating (Timmerman & Acton, 2001), relations among hostility, self-esteem, self-concept, and psychosocial residual in persons with coronary heart disease (Sofhauser, 1996), and the human-environment relationship when healing from an episodic illness (Bowman, 1998).

Tools that have been developed to test the Modeling and Role-Modeling Theory include the Basic Needs Satisfaction Inventory (Kline, 1988), the Erikson Psychosocial Stage Inventory (Darling-Fisher & Leidy, 1988), the Perceived Enactment of Autonomy tool designed to measure a prerequisite to self-care actions in the elderly (Hertz, 1991, 1999; Hertz & Anschutz, 2002), the Self-Care Resource Inventory (Baas, 1992), the Robinson Self-Appraisal Inventory designed to measure denial (the first stage in the grief process) in patients after myocardial infarction (Robinson, 1992), the Erikson Maternal Bonding-Attachment Tool designed to measure self-care knowledge as motivational style (deficit or being motivation) and self-care resource (Erickson, 1996), a theory-based nursing assessment (Finch, 1990), and the Hopkins Clinical Assessment of the APAM (Hopkins, 1995).

MAJOR ASSUMPTIONS
Nursing

"The nurse is a facilitator, not an effector. Our nurse-client relationship is an interactive, interpersonal process that aids the individual to identify, mobilize, and develop his or her own strengths to achieve a perceived optimal state of health and well-being" (H. Erickson, personal correspondence, 2004). Rogers (1996) has defined this relationship as facilitative-affiliation. The five aims of nursing interventions are to build trust, affirm and promote client strengths, promote positive orientation, facilitate perceived control, and set health-directed mutual goals (Erickson et al., 2002).

Person

A differentiation is made between patients and clients in this theory. A patient is given treatment and instruction; a client participates in his or her own care. "Our goal is for nurses to work with clients" (Erickson et al., 2002, p. 21). "A client is one who is considered to be a legitimate member of the decision-making team, who always has some control over the planned regimen, and who is incorporated into the planning and implementation of his or her own care as much as possible" (Erickson, et al., 1990, p. 20; Erickson et al., 2002, p. 253).

Health

"Health is a state of physical, mental, and social well-being, not merely the absence of disease or infirmity. It connotes a state of dynamic equilibrium among the various subsystems [of a holistic person]" (Erickson et al., 2002, p. 46).

Environment

"Environment is not identified in the theory as an entity of its own. The theorists see environment in the social subsystems as the interaction between self and others both cultural and individual. Biophysical stressors are seen as part of the environment" (H. Erickson, telephone interview, March 30, 1988).

THEORETICAL ASSERTIONS

The theoretical assertions of the Modeling and Role-Modeling Theory are based on the linkages between completion of developmental tasks and basic need satisfaction; among basic need satisfaction, object attachment and loss, and developmental tasks; and between the ability to mobilize coping resources and need satisfaction. Three generic theoretical assertions that constitute several theoretical linkages implied in the theory, but are delineated less specifically, are as follows:

1. "The degree to which developmental tasks are resolved is dependent on the degree to which human needs are satisfied" (Erickson et al., 2002, p. 87).
2. "The degree to which needs are satisfied by object attachment depends on the availability of those objects and the degree to which they provide comfort and security as opposed to threat and anxiety" (Erickson et al., 1983, p. 90).
3. "An individual's potential for mobilizing resources, the person's state of coping according to the APAM is directly associated with the

person's need satisfaction level" (Erickson et al., 2002, p. 91).

LOGICAL FORM

The Modeling and Role-Modeling Theory was formulated by the use of retroductive thinking. The theorists went through four levels of theory development and then recycled from inductive to deductive to inductive to deductive reasoning (H. Erickson, telephone interview, March 30, 1988). Theoretical sources were used to validate clinical observations. Clinical observations were tested in light of the theoretical bases. These sources were synthesized with their observations, which enabled Erickson, Tomlin, and Swain to develop a "multidimensional new theory and paradigm—modeling and role-modeling" (H. Erickson, telephone interview, November 1984).

The theorists label modeling and role-modeling as a theory and a paradigm. The Modeling and Role-Modeling Theory meets the following five functions of a paradigm as identified by Merton (1968), who said that paradigms "provide a compact arrangement of central concepts and their interrelations that are utilized for description and analysis" (p. 70):

1. The theorists provide a clear presentation of their central concepts and build on the relationships as they described them.
2. "Paradigms lessen the likelihood of inadvertently introducing hidden assumptions and concepts, for each new assumption and concept must be either logically derived from previous components or explicitly introduced into it" (Merton, 1968, p. 71). Erickson, Tomlin, and Swain build on previous components as their paradigm is developed, each component being logically derived from clinical observations or based in theory.
3. Paradigms provide a foundation for the continued advancement of theoretical interpretation (Merton, 1968). The assumptions and concepts of this theory allow for interpretation in multiple clinical and research situations in which the concepts may be applied, thereby expanding the theory base of nursing.
4. Paradigms facilitate analysis rather than focusing on and describing factual, concrete details (Merton, 1968). The Modeling and Role-Modeling Theory promotes analysis of significant concepts. The interrelationships among the concepts can be examined empirically because they have broad applicability and lend themselves to research questions.
5. Paradigms provide a logical method for codification of qualitative analysis (Merton, 1968). Erickson states that a qualitative approach has been used to form concepts. On the basis of that approach, scales were built with deductive logic to test those concepts (H. Erickson, telephone interview, November 1984). The methods used are available for replication of studies as they are published.

ACCEPTANCE BY THE NURSING COMMUNITY
Practice

The book, *Modeling and Role-Modeling: A Theory and Paradigm for Nursing* (Erickson et al., 2002), chapters in several nursing theory books, and research studies based on the theory have exposed practicing nurses to this theory. Nurses on surgical units at the University of Michigan Medical Center are using an assessment tool based on the Modeling and Role-Modeling Theory. The tool is used to gather information to identify the client's need assets, deficits, developmental residual, attachment-loss and grief status, and potential therapeutic interventions (see Appendix at the end of this chapter) (Bowman, 1998; H. Erickson, personal correspondence, 1988).

Helen Erickson has lectured extensively on their theory and has held one-on-one consultations that exposed nurses (nationally and internationally) from various practice and educational backgrounds to the theory. Nurses in adult health, case management, community health, critical and intensive care, infant, adolescent and family health, gerontology, mental health, emergency rooms, and hospices are using the theory. Erickson noted that what seemed to be a revolutionary idea as recently as 1972 (calling for the client to be the head of the health care team) gained acceptance, as has the notion that nurses can practice independently (H. Erickson, telephone interview, November 1984). According to Erickson, negative responses to the theory came from individuals who cannot accept the idea of listening to the client first or who do not take the concept of holism seriously (H. Erickson, telephone interview, November 1984).

Brigham and Women's Hospital in Boston has used the Modeling and Role-Modeling Theory as a theoretical basis for the professional practice model for the past several years. The nurses use the theory as a framework to structure care planning and conduct case conferences. Jenny James, the former vice president for nursing, stated that "consistency of language, the way care is talked about and planned" is one of the major advantages of using this theoretical basis (J. James, telephone interview, July 6, 1992). The basic fundamentals of the theory are easy to apply in practice and, with a small amount of knowledge, an individual can begin to apply the theory. Nurses at Brigham and Women's Hospital use an adaptation of the assessment tool developed at the University of Michigan Medical Center. At the Fourth National Conference on Modeling and Role-Modeling held in Boston in October 1992, information on the implementation of the professional practice model at Brigham and Women's Hospital and case studies were presented by staff nurses (J. James, telephone interview, July 6, 1992). Nurses at the University of Pittsburgh Medical Center, Children's Hospital of the University of Wisconsin at Madison, and other hospitals and state agencies across the United States have also adopted the Modeling and Role-Modeling Theory as a foundation for their professional practice model.

Education

The Modeling and Role-Modeling Theory is introduced into the curriculum during the sophomore year at the University of Michigan School of Nursing and is required for returning registered nursing students, as well. Faculty members at several nursing schools have contacted Erickson regarding the use of the theory in their curricula. Many use the theory for specific courses. Others, such as those at Humboldt State University at Arcata, California, selected modeling and role-modeling as a conceptual framework for their curriculum. Students are taught theory-based practice throughout the program. Other nursing programs that use the Modeling and Role-Modeling Theory as a basis for curriculum include Metropolitan State University at St. Paul, Minnesota; St. Catherine's University in St. Paul, Minnesota; the Alternate Entry Master's Nursing program at the University of Texas at Austin; and Foo Yin College of Nursing and Medical Technology in Taiwan.

Research

Nurses throughout the world continue to study and research the theory of modeling and role-modeling. Research activity continues to support and validate the self-care knowledge construct and the importance of support and control. The initial study provided evidence that psychosocial factors are significantly related to physical health problems (Erickson, 1976). A follow-up study in 1988 conducted by Erickson, Lock, and Swain (H. Erickson, curriculum vitae, February 1988) supported these findings, and subsequent research has provided for expansion and enrichment of the concepts. Key concepts include perceived support, perceived control, hope for the future, and satisfaction with daily life. The theorists identified several other research projects that have tested the theory. Several master's and doctoral students at the University of Michigan School of Nursing, the University of Texas at Austin, and other universities have pursed various research questions based on this theory. Campbell, Finch, Allport, Erickson, and Swain (1985) conducted a research study at the University of Michigan Medical Center and hypothesized that the length of hospital stay correlated with stages of development. They used a nursing assessment tool adapted from the assessment model to measure a patient's psychosocial development and to relate developmental status to the length of hospitalization and the number of health problems identified during hospitalization.

Results indicated that the balance of trust-mistrust accounts for a large percentage of the variance in the length of hospitalization. No significant relationship was evident between psychosocial coping skills and the number of health problems identified.

Erickson was the principal investigator of a research project, Modeling and Role-Modeling with Alzheimer's Patients, funded by the National Institutes of Health, National Center for Nursing Research. This research project included 10 other investigators. Results supported the constructs of self-care knowledge and affiliated individuation (H. Erickson, personal correspondence, July 1, 1992).

Numerous graduate students have used the Modeling and Role-Modeling Theory as a basis for their theses and dissertations. In addition, extensive work has been published that substantiates many of the major constructs and theoretical linkages of the theory (Erickson, 1990a). Hertz, Baas, Curl, and Robinson (1994) conducted an integrative review of research from 1982 to 1992 using modeling and role-modeling as a theoretical basis. Empirical evidence has provided bases for validation, refinement, and revision of the theory. Research will continue to expand the Modeling and Role-Modeling Theory.

FURTHER DEVELOPMENT

As this theory is practiced, explored, examined, and researched, much potential exists for further development. The theory continues to gain national and international attention. One reason for this increased attention is the founding of the Society for the Advancement of Modeling and Role-Modeling. The society was formed to develop a network of colleagues who could advance the development and application of the Modeling and Role-Modeling Theory. One of the society's goals is to promote continued research related to the theory. The society held its first national symposium in 1986 and has met biennially thereafter. At the 1988 conference, held at Hilton Head, South Carolina, the membership chair announced that society members came from 12 states (H. Erickson, personal correspondence, 1988). By the 1990 conference in Austin, Texas, members represented more than 33 states (H.

Erickson, personal correspondence, July 1, 1992). These conferences provide a forum for researchers, educators, and practitioners to disseminate knowledge pertaining to the Modeling and Role-Modeling Theory and paradigm (H. Erickson, personal correspondence, 1988).

The Fourth National Conference on Modeling and Role-Modeling Theory and Paradigm for Professionals, held in Boston in October 1992, demonstrated the breadth and depth of the use and research for the Modeling and Role-Modeling Theory. Presentations included studies based in critical care units and community-based practice, in multiple types of educational settings, and across the age span. The biennial conferences held throughout the country continue to provide an opportunity for nurses to discuss interrelationships among nursing practice, theory, research, and education. The tenth national conference was held in Galveston, Texas, in May 2004. The 2006 conference will be in Portland, Oregon.

Much of the research data related to the theory are yet to be published. Erickson stated, "Every part of it [the theory] needs further development.... There are a thousand research questions in that book....You can take any one statement we make and ask a research question about it.... Modeling and Role-Modeling has only begun" (H. Erickson, telephone interview, November 1984).

CRITIQUE
Clarity

Erickson, Tomlin, and Swain present their theory clearly. Definitions in the theory are denotative, with the concepts explicitly defined. They use everyday language and offer many examples to illustrate their meaning. Their definitions and assumptions are consistent and there is a logical progression from assumptions to assertions.

Simplicity

The theory appears simple at first. However, on closer inspection it appears complex. It is based on biological and psychological theories and several of the theorists' own assumptions. The interactions among the major concepts, assumptions, and assertions add depth to the theory and increase its complexity.

Generality

Major assumptions that deal with developmental tasks, basic needs satisfaction, object attachment and loss, and adaptive potential are broad enough to be applicable in diverse nursing situations; therefore, the theory is generalizable to all nursing and patient situations. The theorists cite numerous examples of the applicability of their concepts in the educational setting, clinical practice, and research. It may be argued that the theory lacks applicability in nonverbal or comatose populations. However, the theorists believe that the theory is also applicable in these situations, although it may require creativity of the clinician. The Modeling and Role-Modeling Theory is generalizable to all aspects and settings of professional nursing practice.

Empirical Precision

Empirical precision is increased if the theory has operationally defined concepts, identifiable subconcepts, and denotative definitions. The major concepts, modeling and role-modeling, are reality based, which makes them more empirical than general. Definitions in the theory are denotative, making it possible to test the concepts identified empirically. The theorists provide an outline for collecting, analyzing, and synthesizing data and guidelines for implementing their theory based on the client's model. These explicit guidelines increase the empirical precision of the theory by allowing any practitioner to test the theory using these tools.

Chinn and Jacobs (1983) state, "Empirical precision is necessarily increased with research testing" (p. 42). Data reflecting research testing of the theory continue to support the theory. The Modeling and Role-Modeling Theory will gain more empirical precision as new and ongoing data become available for critical analysis. The theorists recognize the need for further research of their theory and encourage practicing nurses to do it.

Derivable Consequences

One of the many challenges facing the profession of nursing is the development of a unique, scientific knowledge base. One aid in this process is the use of nursing theory as a basis for professional practice. The Modeling and Role-Modeling Theory can provide the stimulus to accomplish this goal. Although this theory is relatively young, it is gaining recognition in the nursing community. As interest grows, additional research supporting its theoretical statements will be generated. Numerous nurses have engaged in research based on this theory. Further publication of the findings will continue to lend more credence to the theoretical propositions.

Chinn and Jacobs (1983) state that a theory should be evaluated in terms of its derivable consequences. The derivable consequences can be determined by examining whether the theory guides research, directs practice, generates new ideas, and differentiates the focus of nursing from other professions. In terms of these criteria, this theory does appear to possess inherent value, and research supports that it has a wide, extensive scope.

SUMMARY

Nurses have the opportunity to share in important, intimate life experiences with their clients. We have the ability and responsibility to facilitate healing and achieving our clients' perceived maximal state of health and well-being. The Modeling and Role-Modeling Theory provides nurses with a practice-based theoretical framework that allows them to attain these goals, in any setting, with any population. Data from numerous research studies as well as ongoing scientific work provide empirical support for this nursing theory. As the theory matures, the extent of its merit and worth will become evident.

Case Study

Robert, a 75-year-old rancher with a history of chronic obstructive pulmonary disease (COPD), is admitted with shortness of breath, angina, and nausea (unmet physiological needs). It is his fourth admission in 6 months (he is having difficulty adapting to stressors in his life). The nurse introduces herself in a quiet, calm voice and tells him she will be his primary nurse during his stay (interventions designed to establish trust, a sense of safety and security and facilitate a sense of connectedness). She asks him why he came in (he is the primary source of data). He states "I can't breath and my chest hurts." After he is stabilized (physiological needs are met so the nurse can focus on his other needs), she says" I notice that you have had multiple admissions in the last few months. Why do you think you are here today?" (the nurse seeks information from the client who is the primary data source and facilitates a sense of client control). He replies "my wife of 49 years died a few months ago; she took care of me and my heart is broken. My life no longer has meaning" (he is experiencing unmet needs, is having problems with the developmental stage of generativity, and is grieving the loss of his wife).

During her assessment, the nurse discovers that Robert lives on a ranch by himself, his nearest neighbor is 4 miles away, his son lives out of state, he has no help with his daily living activities, he is housebound because he no longer can drive, he has no support system, and he feels unable to get on with his life without his wife. The nurse asks him what he needs to feel better and help him get through the next few weeks (promoting positive future orientation). He replies "I need to be closer to my friends and the hospital. I am so lonely and afraid out there by myself" (unmet love and belonging and safety and security needs).

After a lengthy discussion, they decide together to implement a plan of care (the nurse is facilitating client control, affirming his strengths and his self-care knowledge that he knows what will make him heal). Robert calls and speaks to his son who plans to come and visit (this action facilitates his sense of perceived support and AI). His minister is called and grief counseling is arranged (support is perceived, facilitation of grief resolution is initiated, client is facilitated in being future focused). A social worker visits, and Robert decides that he will move to town into a senior citizen apartment that provides meals and other services. This will help him feel safer and more secure, because he will be closer to the hospital and other people if he needs them. His love and belonging needs can be met, because he can choose when to visit with friends or participate in social activities that are offered at the complex (facilitates client's sense of control). He can also receive assistance with basic physiological needs when needed (meals, housekeeping services). The nurse provides him with her phone number so he can call if he needs anything or if he just wants to check in (support and love and belonging needs are met). This action facilitates the client's trust and AI. His control is maintained, and his strengths and self-care knowledge are affirmed (he will know and be able to call when he needs assistance or to be connected to the nurse). Arrangements are made for him to have help with the moving process. Finally, the nurse schedules regular phone calls (based on the client's schedule) to check in on him to see how he is doing and address any concerns or questions he has. This action facilitates trust, and his safety and security and love and belonging needs are met.

CRITICAL THINKING *Activities*

1. Interview a client and use the theory to interpret the data. Identify nursing diagnoses based on the interpretations.

2. Given the findings, propose a nursing plan of care. Identify what predictions can be made if the care is not given.

3. Assuming that the goal is to promote the client's health and development, predict the outcome on the basis of the proposed nursing plan of care.

4. Assess the client from primary, secondary, and tertiary sources. Compare for congruency among the three types of sources.

REFERENCES

Acton, G. (1993). *Relationships among stressors, stress, affiliated-individuation, burden, and well-being in caregivers of adults with dementia: A test of the theory and paradigm for nursing, modeling and role-modeling.* Unpublished doctoral dissertation, University of Texas, Austin.

Anschutz, C. A. (2000). *Perceived enactment of autonomy and life satisfaction: An elderly perspective.* Unpublished master's thesis, Fort Hays State University, Hays, KS.

Baas, L. C., Beery, T. A., Fontana, J. A., & Wagoner, L. E. (1999). An exploratory study of developmental growth in adults with heart failure. *Journal of Holistic Nursing, 17*(2), 117-138.

Baas, L. S. (1992). The relationships among self-care knowledge, self-care resources, activity level and life satisfaction in persons three to six months after a myocardial infarction. *Dissertation Abstracts International, 53,* 1780B.

Babcock, M., & Mueller, P. (1980). *Accidents and life stress.* Unpublished master's thesis, University of Michigan, Ann Arbor, MI.

Baldwin, C. M. (1996). Perceptions of hope: Lived experiences of elementary school children in an urban setting. *The Journal of Multicultural Nursing & Health, 2*(3), 41-45.

Barnfather, J. S. (1987). Mobilizing coping resources related to basic need status in healthy, young adults. *Dissertation Abstracts International, 49/02-B,* 0360.

Barnfather, J. S. (1990a). An overview of the ability to mobilize coping resources related to basic needs. In H. Erickson & C. Kinney (Eds.), *Modeling and role-modeling: Theory, practice and research* (Vol. 1). Austin, TX: Society for the Advancement of Modeling and Role-Modeling.

Barnfather, J. S. (1990b). Mobilizing coping resources related to basic need status. In H. Erickson & C. Kinney (Eds.), *Modeling and role-modeling: Theory, practice and research* (Vol. 1). Austin, TX: Society for the Advancement of Modeling and Role-Modeling.

Barnfather, J. (1993). Testing a theoretical proposition for modeling and role-modeling: A basic need and adaptive potential status. *Issues in Mental Health Nursing, 13,* 1-18.

Beltz, S. (1999). *How persons 85 years and older, living in congregate housing, experience managing their health: Preservation of self.* Unpublished doctoral dissertation, University of Texas, Austin, TX.

Benson, D. (2003). *Adaptive potential assessment model as applied to small groups.* Unpublished doctoral dissertation, University of LaVerne, LaVerne CA.

Boodley, C. A. (1990). The experience of having a healthy examination. In H. Erickson & C. Kinney (Eds.), *Modeling and role-modeling: Theory, practice and research* (Vol. 1). Austin, TX: Society for the Advancement of Modeling and Role-Modeling.

Bowman, S. S. (1998). *The human-environment relationship in self-care when healing from episodic illness.* Unpublished doctoral dissertation, University of Texas, Austin, TX.

Cain, E., & Perzynski, K. (1986). *Utilization of the self-care knowledge model with wife caregivers.* Unpublished master's thesis, University of Michigan, Ann Arbor, MI.

Campbell, J., Finch, D., Allport, C., Erickson, H. C., & Swain, M. A. (1985). A theoretical approach to nursing assessment. *Journal of Advanced Nursing, 10,* 111-115.

Chen, Y. (1996). *Relationships among health control orientation, self-efficacy, self-care, and subjective well-being in the elderly with hypertension.* Unpublished doctoral dissertation, University of Texas, Austin, TX.

Chinn, P. L., & Jacobs, M. K. (1983). *Theory and nursing: A systematic approach.* St. Louis: Mosby.

Clementino, D., & Lapinske, M. (1980). *The effects of different preparatory messages on distress from a bronchoscopy.* Unpublished master's thesis, University of Michigan, Ann Arbor, MI.

Curl, E. D. (1992). Hope in the elderly: Exploring the relationship between psychosocial developmental residual and hope. *Dissertation Abstracts International, 47,* 992B.

Darling-Fisher, C., & Leidy, N. (1988). Measuring Eriksonian development of the adult: The modified Erikson psychosocial stage inventory. *Psychological Reports, 62,* 747-754.

Doornbos, M. (1983). *The relationship of the social network to emotional health in the aged.* Unpublished master's thesis, University of Michigan, Ann Arbor, MI.

Erickson, H. (1985). Self-care knowledge: Relations among the concepts support, hope, control, satisfaction with life, and physical health. In Sigma Theta Tau International Proceedings, *Social support and health: New directions for theory development and research.* Rochester, NY: University of Rochester.

Erickson, H. (1990a). Modeling and role-modeling with psychophysiological problems. In J. K. Zeig & S. Gilligan (Eds.), *Brief therapy: Myths, methods, and metaphors.* New York: Brunner/Mazel.

Erickson, H. (1990b). Theory based nursing. In H. Erickson & C. Kinney (Eds.), *Modeling and role-modeling: Theory, practice and research* (Vol. 1). Austin, TX: Society for the Advancement of Modeling and Role-Modeling.

Erickson, H. C. (1976). *Identification of states of coping utilization physiological and psychological data.* Unpublished master's thesis, University of Michigan, Ann Arbor, MI.

Erickson, H. C., Kinney, C., Becker, H., Acton, G., Irvin, B., Hopkins, R., et al. (1994). *Modeling and role-modeling with Alzheimer's patients* (National Institutes of Health funded grant). Unpublished manuscript, University of Texas, Austin, TX.

Erickson, H. C., Kinney, C., Stone, D., & Acton, G. (1990). *Self-care activities, knowledge, and resources related to physical health.* Unpublished manuscript, University of Texas, Austin, TX.

Erickson, H. C., & Swain, M. A. (1982). A model for assessing potential adaptation to stress. *Research in Nursing and Health, 5,* 93-101.

Erickson, H. C., Tomlin, E. M., & Swain, M. A. P. (1983). *Modeling and role-modeling: A theory and paradigm for nursing.* Englewood Cliffs, NJ: Prentice Hall.

Erickson, H., Tomlin, E., & Swain, M. (2002). *Modeling and role-modeling: A theory and paradigm for nursing.* Cedar Park, TX: Est. Co.

Erickson, M. (1996). *Relationships among support, needs satisfaction, and maternal attachment in the adolescent mother.* Unpublished doctoral dissertation, University of Texas, Austin, TX.

Finch, D. (1987). *Testing a theoretically based nursing assessment.* Unpublished doctoral dissertation, University of Michigan, Ann Arbor, MI.

Finch, D. A. (1990). Testing a theoretically based nursing assessment. In H. Erickson & C. Kinney (Eds.), *Modeling and role-modeling: Theory, practice and research* (Vol. 1). Austin, TX: Society for the Advancement of Modeling and Role-Modeling.

Hertz, J. E. (1999). Testing two self-care measures in elderly home care clients. In S. H. Gueldner & L. W. Poon (Eds.), *Gerontological nursing issues for the 21st century* (pp. 195-205). Indianapolis: Center Nursing Press.

Hertz, J., Baas, L., Curl, E., & Robinson, K. (1994). *An integrative review of research for modeling and role-modeling theory: 1982-1992.* Unpublished manuscript, University of Illinois at Urbana-Champaign, Champaign, IL.

Hertz, J. E., & Anschutz, C. A. (2002). Relationships among perceived enactment of autonomy, self-care, and holistic health in community-dwelling older adults. *Journal of Holistic Nursing, 20*(2), 166-186.

Hertz, J. E. G. (1991). The perceived enactment of autonomy scale: Measuring the potential for self-care action in the elderly. *Dissertation Abstracts International, 52,* 1953B.

Holl, R. M. (1992). The effect of role-modeled visiting in comparison to restricted visiting on the well-being of clients who had open heart surgery and their significant family members in the critical care unit. *Dissertation Abstracts International, 53,* 4030B.

Hopkins, B. A. (1995). *Adaptive potential of caregivers of adults with dementia.* Paper presented at the meeting of Sigma Theta Tau International, Detroit.

Irvin, B. L. (1993). Social support, self-worth and hope as self-care resources for coping with caregiver stress. *Dissertation Abstracts International, 54*(06), B2995.

Irvin, B. L., & Acton, G. (1996). Stress mediation in caregivers of cognitively impaired adults: Theoretical model testing. *Nursing Research, 45*(3), 160-166.

Jensen, B. (1995). *Caregiver responses to a theoretically based intervention program: Case study analysis.* Unpublished doctoral dissertation, University of Texas, Austin, TX.

Keck, V. E. (1989). Perceived social support, basic needs satisfaction, and coping strategies of the chronically ill. *Dissertation Abstracts International, 50,* 3921B.

Kennedy, G. T. (1991). A nursing investigation of comfort and comforting care of the acutely ill patient. *Dissertation Abstracts International, 52,* 6318B.

Kinney, C. (1992). *Psychosocial developmental correlates of coronary prone behavior in healthy adults.* Unpublished manuscript, University of Texas at Austin, Austin, TX.

Kinney, C., & Erickson, H. (1990). Modeling the client's world: A way to holistic care. *Issues in Mental Health Nursing, 11,* 93-108.

Kinney, C. K. (1990). Facilitating growth and development: A paradigm case for modeling and role-modeling. *Issues in Mental Health Nursing, 11,* 375-395.

Kleinbeck, S. (1977). *Coping states of stress.* Unpublished master's thesis, University of Michigan, Ann Arbor, MI.

Kline, N. W. (1988). Psychophysiological processes of stress in people with a chronic physical illness. *Dissertation Abstracts International, 49,* 2129B.

Landis, B. J. (1991). Uncertainty, spiritual well-being, and psychosocial adjustment to chronic illness. *Dissertation Abstracts International, 52,* 4124B.

MacLean, T. T. (1987). Erikson's development and stressors as factors in healthy lifestyle. *Dissertation Abstracts International, 48,* 1710A.

Merton, R. K. (1968). *Social theory and social structure.* New York: The Free Press.

Miller, E. W. (1994). *The meaning of encouragement and its connection to the inner-spirit as perceived by caregivers of the cognitively impaired.* Unpublished doctoral dissertation, University of Texas, Austin, TX.

Miller, S. H. (1986). The relationship between psychosocial development and coping ability among disabled teenagers. *Dissertation Abstracts International, 47,* 4113B.

Raudonis, B. (1991). *A nursing study of empathy from the hospice patient's perspective.* Unpublished doctoral dissertation, University of Texas, Austin, TX.

Robinson, K. R. (1992). Developing a scale to measure responses of clients with actual or potential myocardial infarctions. *Dissertation Abstracts International, 53,* 6226B.

Rogers, S. (1996). Facilitative affiliation: Nurse-client interactions that enhance healing. *Issues in Mental Health Nursing, 17,* 171-184.

Rosenow, D. J. (1991). Multidimensional scaling analysis of self-care actions for reintegrating holistic health after a myocardial infarction: Implications for nursing. *Dissertation Abstracts International, 53*, 1789B.

Scheela, R. (1991). *The remodeling process: A grounded study of adult male incest offenders' perceptions of the treatment process.* Unpublished doctoral dissertation, University of Texas, Austin, TX.

Sofhauser, C. (1996). The relations among hostility, self-esteem, self-concept, psychosocial residual in persons with coronary heart disease. *Dissertations Abstracts International 5B/01-B.*

Smith, K. (1980). *Relationship between social support and goal attainment.* Unpublished master's thesis, University of Michigan, Ann Arbor, MI.

Timmerman, G., & Acton, G. (2001). The relationship between basic need satisfaction and emotional eating. *Issues in Mental Health Nursing, 22*(7), 691-701.

Weber, G. J. (1999). The experiential meaning of well-being for employed mothers. *Western Journal of Nursing Research, 21*(6), 785-795.

Weber, G. J. T. (1995) Employed mothers with pre-school-aged children: An exploration of their lived experiences and the nature of their well-being. *Dissertation Abstracts International, 56-06(B)*, 3131.

BIBLIOGRAPHY
Primary Sources
Books

Erickson, H. (1986). *Synthesizing clinical experiences: A step in theory development.* Ann Arbor, MI: Biomedical Communications.

Erickson, H. C., Tomlin, E. M., & Swain, M. A. (2002). *Modeling and role-modeling: A theory and paradigm for nursing.* Cedar Park, TX: Est. Co. (Originally work published 1983, Englewood Cliffs, NJ: Prentice-Hall.)

Erickson, H., & Kinney, C. (Eds.). (1990). *Modeling and role-modeling: Theory, practice and research* (Vol. 1). Austin, TX: Society for the Advancement of Modeling and Role-Modeling.

Book Chapters

Erickson, H. (1977). Communication in nursing. In H. Erickson (Ed.), *Professional nursing matrix: A workbook* (pp. 1-150). Ann Arbor, MI: Media Library, University of Michigan.

Erickson, H. (1985). Modeling and role-modeling: Ericksonian approaches with physiological problems. In J. Zeig & S. Langton (Eds.), *Ericksonian psychotherapy: The state of the art.* New York: Brunner/Mazel.

Erickson, H. (1990). Modeling and role-modeling with psychophysiological problems. In J. K. Zeig & S. Gilligan (Eds.), *Brief therapy: Myths, methods, and metaphors* (pp. 473-491). New York: Brunner/Mazel.

Erickson, H. (1990). Self-care knowledge: An exploratory study. In C. Kinney & H. Erickson (Eds.), *Modeling and role-modeling: Theory, practice and research* (Vol. 1, pp. 178-202). Austin, TX: Society for the Advancement of Modeling and Role-Modeling.

Erickson, H. (1990). Theory based nursing. In C. Kinney & H. Erickson (Eds.), *Modeling and role-modeling: Theory, practice and research* (Vol. 1, pp. 1-27). Austin, TX: Society for the Advancement of Modeling and Role-Modeling.

Journal Articles

Barnfather, J., Swain, M. A., & Erickson, H. (1989). Construct validity of an aspect of the coping process: Potential adaptation to stress. *Issues in Mental Health Nursing, 10*, 23-40.

Barnfather, J., Swain, M. A., & Erickson, H. (1989). Evaluation of two assessment techniques. *Nursing Science Quarterly, 4*, 172-182.

Campbell, J., Finch, D., Allport, C., Erickson, H., & Swain, M. (1985). A theoretical approach to nursing assessment. *Journal of Advanced Nursing, 10*, 111-115.

Erickson, H. (1983, March). Coping with new systems. *Journal of Nursing Education, 22*(3), 132-135.

Erickson, H. (1991). Modeling y role-modeling con psychophysiological problemas. *Rapport: Hipnosis de Milton H. Erickson—Revista del Instituto Milton H. Erickson de Buenos Aires* (Argentina), *1*(1), 41-53.

Erickson, H., & Swain, M. A. (1982). A model for assessing potential adaptation to stress. *Research in Nursing and Health, 5*, 93-101.

Erickson, H., & Swain, M. A. (1990). Mobilizing self-care resources: A nursing intervention for hypertension. *Issues in Mental Health Nursing, 11*, 217-236.

Erickson, M. (1996). Factors that influence the mother-infant dyad relationships and infant well-being. *Issues in Mental Health Nursing, 17*, 185-200.

Abstracts

Erickson, H. (1985). Self-care knowledge: Relations among the concepts support, hope, control, satisfaction with life, and physical health (Abstract). In Sigma Theta Tau International Proceedings, *Social support and health: New directions for theory development and research* (pp. 208-212). Rochester, NY: University of Rochester.

Erickson, H. (1989). *Mind-body relationships as a factor in the care of people with diabetes* (Abstract, p. 47). Third Annual Conference of the Southern Nursing Research Society, Austin, TX.

Erickson, H. (1989). *Study of the self-care knowledge construct* (Abstract, p. 10). Third Annual Conference of the Southern Nursing Research Society, Austin, TX.

Erickson, H. (1990). *The McKennell model: using qualitative methods to guide instrument development* (Abstract, p. 115). Fourth Annual Conference of the Southern Nursing Research Society, Orlando, FL.

Erickson, H. (1991). *The relationships among self-care knowledge, self-care resources and physical health* (Abstract). Proceedings of the Fifth Annual Conference of the Southern Nursing Research Society, Orlando, FL.

Erickson, H. (1993). *Intervention research with cognitively impaired persons and their caregivers. Nursing's challenge: Leadership in changing times* (Abstract). Sigma Theta Tau International 32nd Biennial Convention, Indianapolis.

Erickson, H. (1995). *Caring, comforting and healing* (Abstract). Proceedings of the Sixth National American Journal of Nursing Conference on Medical-Surgical and Geriatric Nursing, Chicago.

Erickson, H., & Kennedy, G. (1992). *Viewing the world through the patient's eyes. Proceedings: Celebrating partnerships* (Abstract). American Association of Critical Care Nursing National Technology Institute, New Orleans.

Erickson, H., Kinney, C., Acton, G., Becker, H., Irvin, B., Jensen, B., et al. (1994). *An intervention study: Persons with Alzheimer's disease and their caregivers* (Abstract). Proceedings of the Fifth National Conference for the Theory of Modeling and Role-Modeling, Arcata, CA.

Erickson, H., Lock, S., & Swain, M. (1989). *Continuation of the study of the self-care knowledge construct in the modeling and role-modeling theory. Advances in international nursing scholarship. Sigma Theta Tau International Research Congress* (Abstract, p. 84). Taipei, Taiwan: Sigma Theta Tau International Honor Society.

Erickson, H. C., & Swain, M. A. (1977). The utilization of a nursing care model for treatment of essential hypertension (Abstract). *Circulation, 56*(Suppl III), 145.

Secondary Sources
Books

Bowlby, J. (1969). *Attachment.* New York: Basic Books.

Bowlby, J. (1973). *Separation.* New York: Basic Books.

Bowlby, J. (1980). *Loss.* New York: Basic Books.

Chinn, P. L., & Kramer, M. K. (1994). *Theory and nursing: A systematic approach* (3rd ed.). St. Louis: Mosby.

Engel, G. S. (1962). *Psychological development in health and disease.* Philadelphia: W. B. Saunders.

Erikson, E. (1963). *Childhood and society.* New York: W. W. Norton.

Haley, J. (1973). *Uncommon therapy: The psychiatric techniques of Milton H. Erickson, M.D.* New York: W. W. Norton.

Mahler, M. S., & Furer, M. (1968). *On human symbiosis and the vicissitudes of individuation* (Vol. I). *Infantile psychosis.* New York: International Universities Press.

Maslow, A. H. (1968). *Toward a psychology of being* (2nd ed.). New York: D. Von Nostrand.

Maslow, A. H. (1970). *Motivation and personality* (2nd ed.). New York: Harper & Row.

Merton, R. K. (1968). *Social theory and social structure.* New York: The Free Press.

Piaget, J. (1952). *The origins of intelligence in children.* New York: International Universities Press.

Piaget, J., & Inhelder, B. (1969). *The psychology of the child.* New York: Basic Books.

Rossi, E. (1986). *The psychobiology of mind-body healing.* New York: W. W. Norton.

Selye, H. (1974). *Stress without distress.* Philadelphia: J. B. Lippincott.

Selye, H. (1976). *The stress of life* (2nd ed.). New York: McGraw-Hill.

Book Chapters

Barnfather, J. (1990). An overview of the ability to mobilize coping resources related to basic needs. In H. Erickson & C. Kinney (Eds.), *Modeling and role-modeling: Theory, practice and research* (Vol. 1, pp. 156-169). Austin, TX: Society for the Advancement of Modeling and Role-Modeling.

Bowlby, J. (1960). Child care and the growth of love. In M. Haimowitz & N. Haimowitz (Eds.), *Human development* (2nd ed., pp. 155-166). New York: Thomas Y. Crowell.

Erikson, E. (1960). Identity versus self-diffusion. In M. Haimowitz & N. Haimowitz (Eds.), *Human development* (2nd ed., pp. 766-770). New York: Thomas Y. Crowell.

Erikson, E. (1960). The case of Peter. In M. Haimowitz & N. Haimowitz, *Human development* (2nd ed., pp. 355-359). New York: Thomas Y. Crowell.

Hassan, A., & Hassan, B. M. (1987). Interpersonal development across the life span: Communion and its interaction with agency in psychosocial development. In L. A. Meachem (Ed.), *Contributions to human development* (Vol. 18, pp. 102-127). Basel: Werner Druck AG.

Klein, M. (1952). Some theoretical conclusions regarding the emotional life of the infant. In J. Riviere (Ed.), *Developments in psychoanalysis* (pp. 198-236). London: Hogarth Press.

Piaget, J. (1974). The pathway between subjects' recent life changes and their near-future illness reports: Representative results and methodological issues. In B. S. Dohrenwend & B. P. Dohrenwend (Eds.), *Stressful life events: Their nature and effects* (pp. 73-86). New York: John Wiley & Sons.

Winnicott, D. W. (1965). The theory of the parent-infant relationship. In D. W. Winnicott (Ed.), *The maturational processes and the facilitating environment.* London: Hogarth Press.

Journal Articles

Acton, G., & Miller, E. (1996). Affiliated-individuation in caregivers of adults with dementia. *Issues in Mental Health Nursing, 17,* 245-260.

Adamson, J., & Schmale, A. (1965). Object loss, giving up, and the onset of psychiatric disease. *Psychosomatic Medicine, 27*(6), 557-576.

Baas, L. S., Fontana, J. A., & Bhat, G. (1997). Relationships between self-care resources and the quality of life of persons with heart failure: A comparison of treatment groups. *Progress in Cardiovascular Nursing, 12*(1), 25-38.

Barnfather, J. (1993). Testing a theoretical proposition for modeling and role-modeling: A basic need and adaptive potential status. *Issues in Mental Health Nursing, 13,* 1-18.

Bartholomew, K. (1990). Avoidance of intimacy: An attachment perspective. *Journal of Social and Personal Relationships, 7,* 147-178.

Beery, T., & Baas, L. (1996). Medical devices and attachment: Holistic healing in the age of invasive technology. *Issues in Mental Health Nursing, 17,* 233-243.

Bowlby, J. (1958). The nature of the child's tie to his mother. *International Journal of Psychoanalysis, 39,* 89-97.

Bowlby, J. (1961). Childhood mourning and its explications for psychiatry. *American Journal of Psychiatry, 118,* 481-498.

Bowlby, J. (1961). Process of mourning. *International Journal of Psychoanalysis, 42,* 317-340.

Bowlby, J., Robertson, J., & Rosenbluth, D. (1952). A two-year-old goes to the hospital. *Psychoanalytic Study of the Child, 7,* 89-94.

Engel, G. (1968). A life setting conducive to illness: The giving-up–given-up complex. *Annuals of Internal Medicine, 69*(2), 293-300.

Hertz, J. (1996). Conceptualization of perceived enactment of autonomy in the elderly. *Issues in Mental Health Nursing, 17,* 261-273.

Irvin, B., & Acton, G. (1996). Stress mediation in caregivers of cognitively impaired adults: Theoretical model testing. *Nursing Research, 45*(3), 160-166.

Irvin, B., & Acton, G. (1997). Stress, hope and well-being of women caring for family members with Alzheimer's disease. *Holistic Nursing Practice, 11*(2), 69-79.

Kinney, C. (1996). Transcending breast cancer: Reconstructing one's self. *Issues in Mental Health Nursing, 17,* 201-216.

Landis, B. J. (1996). Uncertainty, spiritual well-being, and psychosocial adjustment to chronic illness. *Issues in Mental Health Nursing, 17,* 217-231.

Leidy, N. (1994). Operationalizing Maslow's theory: Development and testing of the Basic Needs Satisfaction Inventory. *Issues in Mental Health Nursing, 15,* 277-295.

Leidy, N. K., & Traver, G. A. (1995). Psychophysiological factors contribution to functional performance in people with COPD: Are there gender differences? *Research in Nursing and Health, 18,* 535-546.

Miller, E. W. (1995). Encouraging Alzheimer's caregivers. *Journal of Christian Nursing, 12*(4), 7-12.

Mahler, M. S. (1967). On human symbiosis and the vicissitudes of individuation. *Journal of the American Psychoanalytic Association, 15,* 740-763.

Maslow, A. H. (1936). The need to know and the fear of knowing. *Journal of General Psychology, 68,* 111-125.

Robinson, K. R. (1994). Developing a scale to measure denial levels of clients with actual or potential myocardial infarctions. *Heart and Lung, 23,* 36-44.

Rogers, S. (1996). Facilitative affiliation: Nurse-client interactions that enhance healing. *Issues in Mental Health Nursing, 17,* 171-184.

Sappington, J., & Kelley, J. H. (1996). Modeling and role-modeling theory: A case study of holistic care. *Journal of Holistic Nursing, 14*(2), 130-141.

Selye, H. (1979). Further thoughts on stress without distress. *Resident and Staff Physician, 25,* 125-134.

Stoddard, J., & Stoddard, H. J. (1985). Affectional bonding and the impact of bereavement. *Advances: Institute for the Advancement of Health, 2*(2), 19-28.

Walsh, K. K., Vanden Bosch, T. M., & Boehm, S. (1989). Modeling and role-modeling: Integrating nursing theory into practice. *Journal of Advanced Nursing, 14,* 755-761.

Winnicott, D. W. (1953). Transitional objects and transitional phenomena: A study of the first not-me possession. *International Journal of Psychoanalysis, 34,* 89-97.

Theses

Kirk, L. (1996). *A descriptive study of level of hope in cancer patients.* Unpublished master's thesis, University of Texas, San Antonio, TX.

Kleinbeck, S. (1977). *Coping states of stress.* Unpublished master's thesis, University of Michigan, Ann Arbor, MI.

Dissertations

Acton, G. (1993). *Relationships among stressors, stress, affiliated-individuation, burden, and well-being in caregivers of adults with dementia: A test of the theory and paradigm for nursing, modeling and role-modeling.* Unpublished doctoral dissertation, University of Texas, Austin, TX.

Baas, L. S. (1992). The relationships among self-care knowledge, self-care resources, activity level and life satisfaction in persons three to six months after a myocardial infarction. *Dissertation Abstracts International, 53,* 1780B.

Barnfather, J. S. (1987). Mobilizing coping resources related to basic need status in healthy, young adults. *Dissertation Abstracts International, 49,* 360B.

Beltz, S. (1999). *How persons 85 years and older, living in congregate housing, experience managing their health:*

Preservation of self. Unpublished doctoral dissertation, University of Texas, Austin, TX.

Benson, D. (2003). *Adaptive potential assessment model as applied to small groups.* Unpublished doctoral dissertation, The University of LaVerne, LaVerne, CA.

Chen, Y. (1996). *Relationships among health control orientation, self-efficacy, self-care, and subjective well-being in the elderly with hypertension.* Unpublished doctoral dissertation, University of Texas, Austin, TX.

Curl, E. D. (1992). Hope in the elderly: Exploring the relationship between psychosocial developmental residual and hope. *Dissertation Abstracts International, 47,* 992B.

Daniels, R. (1994). *Exploring the self-care variables that explains a wellness lifestyle in spinal cord injured wheelchair basketball athletes.* Unpublished doctoral dissertation, University of Texas, Austin, TX.

Darling-Fisher, C. S. (1987). The relationship between mothers' and fathers' Eriksonian psychosocial attributes, perceptions of family support, and adaptation to parenthood. *Dissertation Abstracts International, 48,* 1640B.

Erickson, M. (1996). *Relationships among support, needs satisfaction, and maternal attachment in the adolescent mother.* Unpublished doctoral dissertation, University of Texas, Austin, TX.

Hertz, J. E. G. (1991). The perceived enactment of autonomy scale: Measuring the potential for self-care action in the elderly. *Dissertation Abstracts International, 52,* 1953B.

Hopkins, B. (1994). *Assessment of adaptive potential.* Unpublished doctoral dissertation, University of Texas, Austin, TX.

Irvin, B. L. (1993). Social support, self-worth and hope as self-care resources for coping with caregiver stress. *Dissertation Abstracts International, 54*(06), B2995.

Jensen, B. (1995). *Caregiver responses to a theoretically based intervention program: Case study analysis.* Unpublished doctoral dissertation, University of Texas, Austin, TX.

Kline, N. W. (1988). Psychophysiological processes of stress in people with a chronic physical illness. *Dissertation Abstracts International, 49,* 2129B.

Landis, B. J. (1991). Uncertainty, spiritual well-being, and psychosocial adjustment to chronic illness. *Dissertation Abstracts International, 52,* 4124B.

MacLean, T. T. (1987). Erikson's development and stressors as factors in healthy lifestyle. *Dissertation Abstracts International, 48,* 1710A.

Miller, E. W. (1994). *The meaning of encouragement and its connection to the inner-spirit as perceived by caregivers of the cognitively impaired.* Unpublished doctoral dissertation, University of Texas, Austin, TX.

Nash, K. (2003). *Evaluation of a holistic peer support and education program aimed at facilitating self-care resources in adolescents* (Unpublished doctoral dissertation). The University of Texas at Galveston, Galveston, TX.

Raudonis, B. (1991). *A nursing study of empathy from the hospice patient's perspective.* Unpublished doctoral dissertation, University of Texas, Austin, TX.

Robinson, K. R. (1992). Developing a scale to measure responses of client with actual or potential myocardial infarctions. *Dissertation Abstracts International, 53,* 6226B.

Sofhauser, C. (1996). The relations among hostility, self-esteem, self-concept, psychosocial residual in persons with coronary heart disease. *Dissertation Abstracts International* 5B/01-B.

Weber, G. (1995). Employed mothers with pre-school-aged children: An exploration of their lived experiences and the nature of their well-being. *Dissertation Abstracts International* 56/06-B3/31.

Web Site

Modeling and Role-Modeling (MRM) Nursing Theory Page. Accessed December 29, 2004: *http://www.mrmnursingtheory.org/*

APPENDIX

ASSESSMENT TOOL BASED ON MODELING AND ROLE-MODELING*

I. Description of the situation
   A. Overview of the situation
   B. Etiology
      1. Eustressors
      2. Stressors
      3. Distressors
   C. Therapeutic needs
II. Expectations
   A. Immediate
   B. Long term
III. Resource potential
   A. External
      1. Social network
      2. Support system
      3. Health care system
   B. Internal
      1. Strengths
      2. Adaptive potential
         a. Feeling states
         b. Physiological parameters
IV. Goals and life tasks
   A. Current
   B. Future

DATA INTERPRETATION TOOL BASED ON MODELING AND ROLE-MODELING†

I. Interpret data for ability to mobilize resources (APAM)

II. Interpret data for needs status (assets and deficits related to type of need), attachment objects, loss, grief (normal or morbid), life tasks (developmental: actual and chronological)

DATA ANALYSIS TOOL BASED ON MODELING AND ROLE-MODELING‡

I. Step one
   A. Articulate relationships between stressors and needs status
   B. Articulate relationships between needs status and ability to mobilize resources
   C. Articulate relationships between needs status and loss of attachment
   D. Articulate relationships between loss and type of grief response
   E. Articulate relationships between type of need assets and deficits and developmental residual
   F. Articulate relationships between chronological developmental task and developmental residual
II. Step two
   A. Articulate relationships among stressors, resource potential, needs status, loss, grief status, developmental residual, chronological task, and attachment potential

---

*Interview questions and thoughts that guide critical thinking are suggested in Erickson, H. C., Tomlin, E. M., & Swain, M. A. (1983). *Modeling and role-modeling: A theory and paradigm for nursing* (pp. 116-168). Englewood Cliffs, NJ: Prentice-Hall. Suggestions for interviewing techniques are found in Erickson, H. C. (1990). Self-care knowledge. In H. C. Erickson & C. Kinney (Eds.), *Modeling and role-modeling: Theory, practice and research* (Vol. 1). Austin, TX: Society for the Advancement of Modeling and Role-Modeling.

†Critical thinking guidelines for data interpretation are suggested in Erickson, H. C., Tomlin, E. M., & Swain, M. A. (1983). *Modeling and role-modeling: A theory and paradigm for nursing* (pp. 148-166). Englewood Cliffs, NJ: Prentice-Hall; and Erickson, H. C. (1990). Theory based nursing. In H. C. Erickson & C. Kinney (Eds.), *Modeling and role-modeling: Theory, practice and research* (Vol. 1). Austin, TX: Society for the Advancement of Modeling and Role-Modeling.

‡Critical thinking guidelines for data analysis are suggested in Erickson, H. C., Tomlin, E. M., & Swain, M. A. (1983). *Modeling and role-modeling: A theory and paradigm for nursing* (pp. 148-166). Englewood Cliffs, NJ: Prentice-Hall; and Erickson, H. C. (1990). Theory-based nursing. In H. C. Erickson & C. Kinney (Eds.), *Modeling and role-modeling: Theory, practice and research* (Vol. 1). Austin, TX: Society for the Advancement of Modeling and Role-Modeling.

APAM, Adaptive Potential Assessment Model.

APPENDIX—cont'd

B. Articulate relationships among needs, status, potential resources, developmental residual, and personal goals

PLANNING TOOL BASED ON MODELING AND ROLE-MODELING[§]

I. Aims of interventions
  A. Build trust
  B. Promote positive orientation
  C. Promote client control
  D. Promote strengths
  E. Set health-directed goals
II. Intervention goals

A. Develop a trusting and functional relationship between yourself and your client
B. Facilitate a self-projection that is futuristic and positive
C. Promote AI with the minimal degree of ambivalence possible
D. Promote a dynamic, adaptive, and holistic state of health
E. Promote and nurture a coping mechanism that satisfies basic needs and permits growth-need satisfaction
F. Facilitate congruent actual and chronological developmental stages

[§]Critical thinking guidelines for planning are suggested in Erickson, H. C., Tomlin, E. M., & Swain, M.A. (1983). *Modeling and role-modeling: A theory and paradigm for nursing* (pp. 169-220). Englewood Cliffs, NJ: Prentice-Hall; and Erickson, H. C. (1990). Theory-based nursing. In H. C. Erickson & C. Kinney (Eds.), *Modeling and role-modeling: Theory, practice and research* (Vol. 1). Austin, TX: Society for the Advancement of Modeling and Role-Modeling.
AI, Affiliated-individuation.

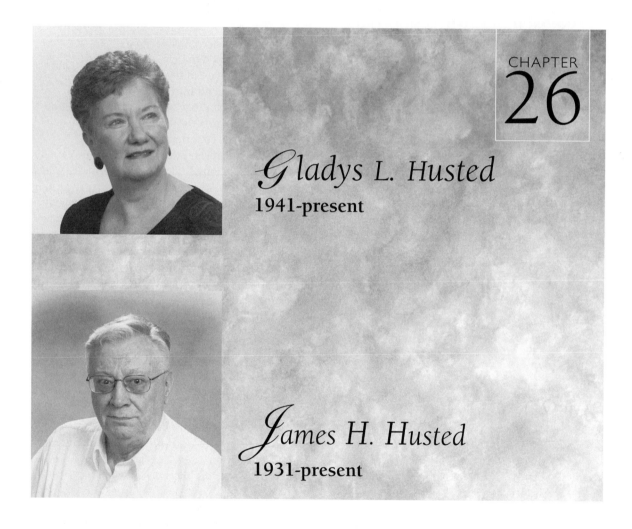

CHAPTER
26

Gladys L. Husted
1941-present

James H. Husted
1931-present

Symphonological Bioethical Theory

Carrie Scotto

CREDENTIALS AND BACKGROUND OF THE THEORISTS

Gladys Husted was born in Pittsburgh, where her life, practice, education, and teaching continue to influence the nursing profession. Husted received a Bachelor of Science in Nursing degree from University of Pittsburgh in 1962 and began practice in public health and acute in-patient medical-surgical care. Observations of interactions between nurses and patients initiated her interest in ethical issues. In 1968, she earned a master's degree in nursing education while teaching at the Louise Suyden School of Nursing at St. Margaret's Memorial Hospital in Pittsburgh. Her love of teaching prompted doctoral study that resulted in a terminal degree from the University of Pittsburgh Department of Curriculum and Supervision.

G. Husted is currently a professor at Duquesne University School of Nursing, where in 1998 she was awarded the title of School of Nursing Distinguished Professor. The school has also recognized her teaching excellence at all levels of the curriculum through the Duquesne University School of Nursing Recognition Award for Excellence 1990/1991 and the Faculty Award for Excellence in Teaching 1994/1995. The Medical College of Ohio chose Husted as the Distinguished Lecturer in 2000. She is a member of Sigma Theta Tau International, Phi Kappa Phi, and National League for Nursing.

G. Husted served as a consultant for Western Pennsylvania Hospital Nursing Division regarding the development of an ethics committee, including education of staff and management, and providing guidance for the newly formed committee. She also provided consultation for the Allegheny General Medical Center for staff development and the National Nursing Ethics Advisory Group for the Department of Veterans' Affairs. Most recently she served as curriculum consultant for Heritage Valley School of Nursing in Sewickley, Pennsylvania, to review and revise the curriculum for submission to the state board. In addition, G. Husted presented The Ethics of Teaching at the 2003 National League for Nursing Education Summit.

James Husted was born in Kingston, Pennsylvania, and has had a lifelong interest in philosophy. He studied voice for many years and performed with the American Opera Guild prior to joining the Army in 1950. While in the Army in Germany, he became interested in ethics, particularly the work of Benedict Spinoza, through conversations with a former ethics professor.

His post-Army career focused on sales and later in hiring and training agents for health insurance companies. He published many articles in insurance journals and won numerous awards for sales. However, he continued to read and develop his philosophical and ethical ideas. During the 1980s, J. Husted joined the high-IQ societies, Mensa and

Intertel, serving as a philosophy expert for Mensa and a regional director for Intertel. While active in these organizations, he wrote articles for their publications related to philosophy, ethics, and the theories of beauty and music. He is currently a member of many philosophical societies and has presented papers for the American Catholic Philosophical Society and the West Virginia Philosophical Society.

The theorists met and were married in 1974, establishing and cultivating a dialogue that brought about the theory of symphonology. They are coauthors of several editions of *Ethical Decision Making in Nursing*. Their book was selected by Nursing and Health Care's Notable Books of 1991, 1995a, and 2001. It also won the Nursing Society Award in 2001. Their regular column, "A Practice Based Bioethic," appeared in *Advanced Practice Nursing Quarterly* 1997-1998. In addition to publishing books, book chapters, and journal articles, they have presented their ethical theory at conferences and workshops.

The Husteds reside in Pittsburgh and continue to develop and disseminate their work through teaching, writing, and presenting at conferences and workshops.

THEORETICAL SOURCES

The authors define symphonology as "a system of interpersonal ethics based on the terms and presuppositions of an agreement," specifically the health care professional–patient agreement (Husted & Husted, 2001, p. 297). The agreement is based on the nature of the relationship between the parties involved. In its ethical dimensions it outlines the commitments and obligations of each. Although the theory developed from the observation of nurses and nursing practice, it later expanded to include all health care professionals (HCPs). The development of this theory has led to the construction of a practice-based decision-making model that assists in determining when and what actions are appropriate for HCPs and patients. The name of the theory is derived from the Greek word for agreement, *symphonia*.

Ethics is "a system of standards to motivate, determine, and justify actions directed to the pursuit

of vital and fundamental goals" (Husted & Husted, 2001, p. 289). Ethics examines what ought to be done, within the realm of what can be done, to preserve and enhance human life. The Husteds, therefore, described ethics as the science of living well.

Bioethics is concerned with the ethics of interactions between a patient and an HCP, what ought to be done to preserve and enhance human life within the health care arena. Within the past century, the expanding knowledge base and growth of technology altered existing health care practice. There arose threatening and confusing circumstances not previously encountered. Increasing numbers and types of treatment options allowed patients to survive conditions they would not have in the past. However, the morbidity of the survivors brought new questions: Who should receive treatment? What is the appropriateness of treatments under particular circumstances? Who should decide what treatments are appropriate? In this way, bioethics became a central issue in what previously had been a prescriptive environment. It became essential to consider ethical concerns, as well as scientific solutions, to questions of health (Jecker, Jonsen, & Pearlman, 1997). Through personal experience and observation of nurses, the Husteds recognized the increasingly complex nature of bioethical dilemmas and the failure of the health care system to adequately address the problem.

To clarify the reasons for the deficiency of the health care system in addressing the issue of delivering ethical care, the Husteds examined traditional ideas and concepts used to guide ethical behavior. These ideas include deontology, utilitarianism, emotivism, and social relativism. Deontology is a duty-based ethic in which the consequences of one's actions are irrelevant. One acts in accordance with preset standards regardless of the outcome. The inappropriateness of this type of guideline is obvious in relation to HCPs, because they are responsible for foreseeing the effects of their actions and acting only in ways that benefit a patient. Utilitarian thought would have HCPs acting to bring about the greatest good for the greatest number of people. This is inconsistent with the practice of HCPs who act as agents for individual patients.

Emotivism promotes ethical actions in accordance with the emotions of those involved. Rational thought has no place in emotive choices, making this type of decision-making process inappropriate in the health care arena. Social relativism imposes the beliefs of a society onto the individual. This approach is absurd when one considers the diversity of our emerging global society. The authors recognized that the inappropriateness of traditional methods of ethical reasoning brought about the failure of the health care system to successfully address bioethical issues.

Because traditional models proved inadequate to guide ethical behavior for HCPs, the Husteds began to conceive and develop a method by which HCPs might determine appropriate ethical actions. The theory was based on logical thinking, emphasizing the provision of holistic, individualized care. They drew from the work of Aristotle, Benedict Spinoza, and Michael Polanyi. These philosophers adhere to rational thought and value persons as individuals. Aristotle was a student of Plato who advanced his teacher's work by recognizing that there is more to understanding phenomena than simple rationality. He believed that one must develop insight and perception to recognize how principles can be applied to each situation (McKeon, 1941).

The Dutch philosopher, Spinoza, examined the nature of humans and human knowledge. He recognized that, although the process and outcomes of reasoning may be comparable for each person, intuitive and discerning thought is unique to each. Spinoza believed that reason must be coupled with intuitive thought for true understanding (Lloyd, 1996). Spinoza was noted for taking well-worn philosophical concepts and transforming them into new and engaging ideas. This is true of the Husteds' development of symphonology, particularly in the evolution of the meaning of the bioethical standards.

Polanyi proposed that understanding is derived from awareness of the entirety of a phenomenon, that the lived experience is greater than separate, observable parts. Tacit knowledge, that which is implied, is necessary to understand and interpret that which is explicit (Polanyi, 1964). These concepts, the uniqueness of the individual and the extension of reason and rationality with insight and discernment to create true understanding, are the foundations of symphonological method.

MAJOR CONCEPTS & DEFINITIONS

AGENCY

Agency is the capacity of an agent to initiate action toward a chosen goal. The shared goal of a nurse and a patient is to restore the patient's agency (Husted & Husted, 2001).

CONTEXT

The "context is the interweaving of the relevant facts of a situation" (Husted & Husted, 2001, p. 20). There are two interrelated elements of context, the context of the situation and the context of knowledge. The context of the situation includes all aspects of the situation that provide understanding of the situation and promote the ability to act effectively within it. The context of knowledge is an agent's preexisting knowledge and present awareness of the relevant aspects of the situation.

ENVIRONMENT-AGREEMENT

The environment established by symphonology is formed by agreement. Agreement is a shared state of awareness on the basis of which interaction occurs (Husted & Husted, 2001). Agreement creates the realm in which nursing and all other human interactions occur. Every agreement is aimed toward a final value to be attained through interactions made possible by understanding.

The HCP-patient agreement is formed by a meeting of the professional's and the patient's

Continued

MAJOR CONCEPTS & DEFINITIONS—cont'd

needs. Their agreement is one in which the needs and desires of the patient are central. The professional's commitment is defined in terms of the patient's needs. Without this agreement, there would be no context for interaction between the two; the relationship would be unintelligible to both (Husted & Husted, 1999).

HEALTH

Health is a concept applicable to every potential of a person's life. Health involves not only thriving of the physical body, but also happiness. Happiness is realized as individuals pursue and progress toward the goals of their chosen life plan (Husted & Husted, 2001). Health is evident when individuals experience, express, and engage in the fundamental bioethical standards.

NURSING

A nurse acts as the agent of the patient, doing for her patient what he would do for himself if he were able (Husted & Husted, 2001). The nurse's ethical responsibility is to encourage and strengthen those qualities in the patient that serve life, health, and well-being through their interaction (Fedorka & Husted, 2001).

PERSON-PATIENT

A person is an individual with a unique character structure, possessing the right to pursue vital goals as he chooses (Husted & Husted, 2001). Vital goals are related to survival and the enhancement of life. A person takes on the role of patient when he has lost or experienced a decrease in agency resulting in his inability to take the actions required for survival or happiness (Husted & Husted, 1998).

RIGHTS

The product of an implicit agreement among rational beings, by virtue of their rationality, not to obtain actions or the product of actions from others except through voluntary consent, objectively gained (Husted & Husted, 2001). The term *rights* is a singular term that represents the critical agreement of nonaggression among rational people (Husted & Husted, 1997b).

USE OF EMPIRICAL EVIDENCE

Study and dialogue between the two theorists, coupled with experience of the overall evolution of health care and observation of individual nurse-patient relationships, provided the impetus to develop symphonology theory. G. Husted's dissertation focused on the effect of teaching ethical principles on a student's ability to use these in practical ways through case studies. J. Husted was very instrumental in the selection of the dissertation topic and was used as a consultant during the process. Further development of G. Husted's doctoral work led to numerous publications and presentations before the first edition of the book *Ethical Decision Making in Nursing* was published in 1991. This first edition

presented their work as a conceptual model only. As they continued to develop their ideas, incorporating feedback from graduate students, the symphonological theory emerged. Before publication of the second edition, the Husteds (1995a) continued to clarify the theoretical concepts and developed the model for practice.

Beginning in 1990, Duquesne University offered a course devoted to this bioethical theory. The authors continued to seek critique and examples about their work from students, practitioners, and other experts. The third edition of the book, *Ethical Decision Making in Nursing and Healthcare: The Symphonological Approach* (Husted & Husted, 2001), offered a clarified description of the theory with advanced concepts separated from the basic concepts. In addition, the model was redrawn to better represent the nonlinear nature of the theory in practice. At present, testing of the theory by the authors and others is under way.

As the theory emerged, the need for an emphasis on the individual became apparent and essential. In recent years, it has become accepted practice in the literature to designate patients and nurses as he/she, or simply use the plural form, referring to nurses and their patients. The authors recognized that these awkward and anonymous terms distract readers from thinking in terms of real people within the context of a particular situation. Therefore, they chose to refer to individuals as *he,* in the case of patients, and *she,* in the case of HCPs in particular situations and examples. This chapter will continue with this practice.

MAJOR ASSUMPTIONS

The assumptions from this theory arise from the practical reasoning and discernment of the authors. The model is meant to provide nurses and other HCPs with a logical method of determining appropriate ethical actions (see the Major Concepts & Definitions box). Although many of the terms are familiar to nurses and HCPs, some have been redefined to support the reality of human interaction and ethical delivery of health care.

Nursing

Symphonology holds that a nurse or any other HCP acts as the agent of the patient. Using her education and experience, a nurse does for her patient what he would do for himself if he were able. Nursing cannot occur without both nurse and patient. "A nurse takes no actions that are not interactions" (Husted & Husted, 2001, p. 37). The nurse's ethical responsibility is to encourage and strengthen those qualities in the patient that serve life, health, and well-being through their interaction (Fedorka & Husted, 2001).

Agency is the capacity of an agent to initiate action toward a chosen goal. A nurse as agent takes action for a patient, one who cannot act on his own behalf. The shared goal of a nurse and a patient is to restore the patient's agency. The nurse acts with and for the patient toward this end.

Person or Patient

The Husteds define a person as an individual with a unique character structure possessing the right to pursue vital goals as he chooses (Husted & Husted, 2001). Vital goals are concerned with survival and the enhancement of life. A person takes on the role of patient when he has lost or experienced a decrease in agency resulting in his inability to take the actions required for survival or happiness. The inability to take action may result from physical or mental problems, or from a lack of knowledge or experience (Husted & Husted, 1998).

Health

The authors do not address or define health directly. The entire theory is driven by the concept of health in the broadest, most holistic sense. Health is a concept applicable to every potential of a person's life. Health involves not only thriving of the physical body, but also happiness. Happiness is realized as individuals pursue and progress toward the goals of their chosen life plan (Husted & Husted, 2001). Health is evident when individuals experience, express, and engage in the fundamental bioethical standards.

Environment-Agreement

The environment established by symphonology is formed by agreement. "Agreement is a shared state of awareness on the basis of which interaction occurs" (Husted & Husted, 2001, p. 61). Agreement creates the realm in which nursing and all other human interactions occur. Every agreement is aimed toward a final value to be attained through interactions made possible by understanding.

The HCP-patient agreement is formed by a meeting of the professional's and the patient's needs. Their agreement is one in which the needs and desires of the patient are central. The professional's commitment is defined in terms of the patient's needs. Without this agreement, there would be no context for interaction between the two. The relationship would be unintelligible to both (Husted & Husted, 1999).

Symphonology theory is not a compilation of traditional cultural platitudes. It is a method of determining what is practical and justifiable in the ethical dimensions of professional practice. Symphonology recognizes that what is possible and desirable in the agreement is dependent on the context.

The "context is the interweaving of the relevant facts of a situation—the facts that are necessary to act upon to bring about a desired result and the knowledge one has of how to most effectively deal with these facts" (Husted & Husted, 2001, p. 20). There are two interrelated elements of context, the context of the situation and the context of knowledge. The context of the situation includes all aspects of the situation that provide understanding of the situation and promote the ability to act effectively within it. The context of knowledge is an agent's preexisting knowledge and present awareness of the relevant aspects of the situation. A practice-based ethical system must allow for this.

THEORETICAL ASSERTIONS

Symphonology is classified as a grand theory because of its broad scope. Grand theories explicate a world view related to a specific discipline (Walker & Avant, 1995). Grand theories are developed through astute, perceptive, discerning consideration of existing ideas in regard to a general discipline (Fawcett, 1995). The authors developed symphonology theory not from natural progression of other work, but from the recognition of a need for theoretical guidelines related to the ethical delivery of health care. The understanding and use of this theory is based on a fundamental ethical element that describes the rational relationship between human beings: human rights.

Rights

The Husteds describe rights as the fundamental ethical element. Traditionally, rights are viewed as a list of options to which one is entitled, such as a list of items or actions to which one has a just claim. Symphonology holds rights as a singular concept. It is the implicit, species-wide, agreement that one will not force another to act, or take by force the products of another's actions. Rights is the critical agreement among rational people, the agreement of nonaggression (Husted & Husted, 1997a). This agreement emerged as humans became rational and developed a civilized social structure. A nonaggression agreement is preconditional to all human interaction. It serves as a foundation on which all other agreements rest. The formal definition is as follows: "the product of an implicit agreement among rational beings, held by virtue of their rationality, not to obtain actions or the products of actions from others except through voluntary consent, objectively gained" (Husted & Husted, 2001, p. 4). The operation of this is evident in human interaction.

According to the Husteds, symphonology theory can ensure ethical action in the provision of health care. Agreement is the foundation of symphonology. Agreements can occur based on the implicit understanding of human rights. The understanding of nonaggression that exists among rational persons constitutes human rights. This understanding makes negotiation and cooperation among individuals possible.

Ethical Standards

Ethical standards have been the benchmarks of ethical behavior. The standards include terms familiar to HCPs such as benevolence, autonomy, and confidentiality. However, the authors have conceived new meanings for ethical standards that correspond to the foundational concepts of symphonology: the person as a unique individual and the use of insight and discernment in addition to reason and rationality in order to achieve true understanding.

Traditionally, bioethical concepts have been used to guide ethical action by mandating concrete directives for action. For instance, the concept of beneficence conventionally maintains that one must see that no harm comes to a patient. However, it is not always possible to predict how and when harm will occur, making adherence to this directive an unrealistic goal. The concept of beneficence, viewed as a mandate, could also imply that defending yourself against a physical attack is unethical. Similarly, veracity, or truth telling, holds that one must always speak the truth regardless of the consequences. Therefore, it is unethical to withhold potentially harmful information, regardless of the consequences. Adhering to veracity may interfere with one's commitment to beneficence. Clearly, ethical standards taken as concrete directives do not allow for the consideration of context.

The authors have redefined the ethical standards, not as concrete rules, but as human qualities or character structures that can and must be recognized and respected in the individual (Husted & Husted, 1995b). For example, in symphonological terms, beneficence includes the idea of acting in the patient's best interest, but it begins with the patient's evaluation of what is beneficial. In this way, ethical standards are presuppositions in the HCP-patient agreement and ethical guides to decision making. The participants work together with the implicit understanding that each is possessed of human characteristics. The description and names of the bioethical standards have changed over time based on feedback from practitioners. Symphonological theory holds that patients have a right to receive the benefits specified in the bioethical standards. Box 26-1 provides definitions and examples of bioethical standards.

Just as the bioethical standards are not to be considered as concrete directives, so too, they are not distinct entities. Each standard blends with the others as representative of the unique character structure of the individual (J. Husted, personal communication, March 5, 2004). As stated earlier, recognition of these standards is preconditional to the implicit patient-HCP agreement. When recognized and respected in each individual, these human qualities and capabilities form the basis for ethical interaction. When they are disregarded, the context of the situation is lost. Interaction is then based on whatever is served by concrete directives or on the whim of the participants.

Box 26-1

Bioethical Standards

AUTONOMY

Autonomy is the uniqueness of the individual, the singular character structure of the individual. Every person has the right to act on his or her unique and independent purposes.

BENEFICENCE

Beneficence is the capability to act to acquire desired benefits and necessary life requirements. Each person may act to obtain those things he or she needs and prefers.

FIDELITY

Fidelity is an individual's faithfulness to his or her own uniqueness. Each person manages, maintains, and sustains his unique life. For the HCP, fidelity in agreement means the commitment to the obligations accepted in the professional role.

FREEDOM

Freedom is the capability and right to take action based on the agent's own evaluation of the situation. Every person may choose his or her course of action.

OBJECTIVITY

Objectivity is the right to achieve and sustain the exercise of objective awareness. Every person has an awareness and understanding of the universe outside himself or herself. Every person has the right to manage, maintain, and sustain that understanding as he or she chooses.

SELF-ASSERTION

Self-assertion is the right and capability to control one's time and effort. Each person has the right to pursue chosen courses of action without interference.

Certainty

There are circumstances in health care when a patient is unable to communicate his unique character structure, as in the case of an infant or a comatose patient. HCPs also interact with individuals from different cultures for whom a common language is lacking. In these cases, the bioethical standards can provide a measure of certainty when knowledge of an individual's unique character is unobtainable.

> If you know nothing whatever about an individual's uniqueness, then you are justified in acting on the basis that, as a member of the human species, he shares much in common with every other individual. (Fedorka & Husted, 2001, p. 58)

These commonalities are the bioethical standards. Each person needs the power to sustain his unique nature, the power to be objectively aware of his surroundings, the power to control his time and effort, to pursue benefit, and to avoid harm. Lacking other information, nurses and HCPs are justified to do all they can to restore the power to the individual.

Decision-Making Model

Figure 26-1 demonstrates the way the concepts of the theory interact with direct decision making. The elements of ethical decision making interact in the following way:

- A person is a rational being with a unique character structure. Each person has the right to choose and pursue, without interference, a course of action in accordance with his needs and desires.
- Agreements between individuals are demonstrated by a shared state of awareness directed toward a goal.
- The HCP-patient agreement is directed toward preserving and enhancing the life of the patient.
- Context is the basis for determining what actions are ethical within the HCP-patient agreement. Context consists of an interweaving of the facts of the patient situation and the knowledge and experience of the HCP as they apply to the situation. The specifics of the context indicate that which is ethically justifiable for each person. In this way, there are no universal ethical principles.
- Ethical decisions are the result of reasoning from the context of a situation to a decision rather than applying a decision or principle to a situation without regard for the context.

The Husteds described the ultimate application and practice of these assumptions by HCPs in the following way. The professional will come to understand and work from the philosophy that:

> My patient's virtues (autonomy) are such that he is moving (self-assertion) toward his goal (freedom) in these circumstances (objectivity) for this reason (beneficence). My virtues (autonomy) are such that I must act with him (interactive self-assertion) to assist him (his freedom) within the possibilities (of beneficence) in his circumstances to achieve every possible benefit that can be discovered (by objective awareness). (Husted & Husted, 2001, p. 154)

LOGICAL FORM

Abductive reasoning, like induction and deduction, follows a pattern:

- A is a collection of data (the process of discerning ethical action)
- B (if true) explains A (symphonology)
- No other hypothesis explains A as well as B does (traditional methods)
- Therefore B is probably correct.

The strength of an abductive conclusion depends on how solidly B can stand by itself, how clearly B exceeds alternatives, how comprehensive was the search for alternatives, the cost of B being wrong and the benefits of being right, and how strong the need is to come to a conclusion at all (Josephson & Josephson, 1994).

The abductive method is evident in the inception and evolution of symphonology. The strength of this theory is evident, as well. The concepts of symphonology clearly can be observed not only in health care but in all walks of life. It is clear that ethical action based on the context of an individual's particular circumstances is far superior to the impo-

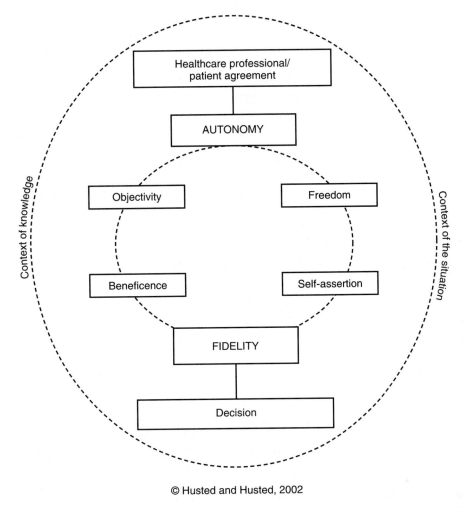

© Husted and Husted, 2002

Figure **26-1 Husteds' Symphonological Ethical Decision-Making Guide.** (Copyright Gladys L. Husted and James H. Husted, 2002, Pittsburgh.)

sition of concrete directives that often contradict each other or have little relationship to the situation at hand. The authors' extensive study of the philosophy of knowledge, science, and the human condition attests to the comprehensive search for alternative answers. The cost of symphonology being wrong would be no greater than any other inadequate method we now use to make ethical decisions. The benefit to patients and HCPs of receiving practice-based ethical care would be immeasurable. Finally, the need to address the problem of how to achieve ethical action in health care could not be more critical.

Since the initial development of symphonology, inductive reasoning based on observation and feedback from practitioners has provided for refinement of the concepts and clarification of the relationships among concepts. Research studies using inductive methods are under way to validate the theory.

ACCEPTANCE BY THE NURSING COMMUNITY

Practice

The Husted symphonological model for ethical decision making (Husted & Husted, 2001 p. 201) was developed as a practice model for applying the concepts of symphonology. This model, stressing the centrality of the individual and the necessity of reason directed by context, is vital in existing and emerging health care systems. The model provides a philosophical framework to ensure ethical care delivery by nurses and all other disciplines of health care. Unlike traditional models, the symphonological model provides for logically justifiable ethical decision making.

The call to care in nursing is central to the profession. Hartman (1998) asserted that caring is demonstrated when nurses recognize that the bioethical standards are so intertwined with caring that together they provide a perfect circle of ethical justification. Symphonology offers a practice-based approach to care, as follows:

> A practice-based approach is derived from, and therefore is intended to be appropriate to, the situation of a patient, the purpose of the health care setting, and the role of the nurse. The more an ethical system restricts practice based on abstract principles the more nurse and patient become alienated from each other. (Husted & Husted, 1997b, p. 14)

Many nurses practice within systems bound by protocols and critical pathways. Using a symphonological approach can ensure that nursing practice remains ethical and does not become prescriptive.

Offering culturally sensitive care is essential as our health care systems change in response to a global society. Although cultural factors can be helpful in directing caring for a patient, nurses must also consider the individual's personal commitment to the traditions and beliefs of that culture. In this way, a nurse provides care for the patient rather than the culture (Zoucha & Husted, 2000). Using the Husted model, care is directed within the context of the individual's circumstances. Imposition of a false context, cultural or otherwise, is avoided.

Brown (2001b) advocated the use of symphonology theory to direct discussion and education of patients regarding advance directives. Bioethical standards are used to guide discussion about what types of treatment an individual would or would not want given particular circumstances.

The emergence of health care teams as a method of delivering comprehensive care brings many disciplines together to serve patients' needs. Overlapping roles and disparate goals can cause confusion among team members. Symphonological theory, with its patient-centered focus, can serve as common ground to initiate and promote collaboration among HCPs of all disciplines.

Education

As symphonology is disseminated, it is easy to envision its use in nursing education. Currently, ethics is often addressed in nursing curricula as a topic separate from nursing. Frequently, the study and application of ethical concepts is reserved for advanced students. The broad applicability for symphonology makes it an excellent framework for nursing curricula. Beginning students can easily grasp and apply the theoretical concepts. Using this theory as a basis for nursing interactions would direct the student in ethical practice from the beginning of learning and practice. The concept of context can be used as the basis for assessment. The bioethical standards will direct the student in choosing appropriate approaches, timing, and type of interventions for each patient. Because of the holistic approach and central concern for the patient, symphonology can be incorporated easily in existing nursing curricula.

Brown (2001a) addressed the importance of ethical interaction between nurse educator and student. The agreement in this case is more explicit, because both parties are more aware of the commitments and responsibilities. Recognizing the bioethical standards in both the educator and the student serves to direct ethical actions between them. Above all, the educator and student recall that the educator-student-patient agreement is central to the learning process.

Steckler (1998) agreed with Brown's application of symphonology in the educational process and recommended incorporating the theory in continuing education. The Husted model not only identifies and organizes professional values and ethical principles for learners, but helps the educator to develop a consistent professional ethical orientation.

Administration

Health care administrators make decisions at several levels. They have responsibility to the following:

1. The community at large and the financial viability of the institution within the community
2. Employees, interpersonal relations, and approaches to care delivery
3. Patients, those receiving care

Hardt and Hopey (2001) described how administrators can use the principles of symphonology to guide their decision making to produce ethically justifiable outcomes.

With regard to issues at the community and institutional level, one considers the needed services provided by the institution. In cases in which the services needed would not be feasible for the institution, resources within the community can be shared and supported by the institution so that needed services are available with the least amount of loss to the institution. At the employee level, the administrators are concerned with care delivery as well as interpersonal relations. Symphonology guides decision making into equitable rather than equal solutions. For example, an employer may choose to forego use of a harsh sanction for absenteeism when the employee is able to show extenuating circumstances that prevented his attendance. This is also true for the development of policy regarding employees' behavior. Ethical policy provides guidelines for examining situations rather than prescribed rules with concrete directives for action. With regard to individual patients, administrators act as role models and consultants when addressing ethical issues.

Hardt and Hopey (2001) also described the problematic situations that occur within managed care systems. Difficulties that have been identified include the refusal of the organization to provide care deemed appropriate by HCPs and the inappropriate demands of patients and families. Using the principles of symphonology, HCPs can examine the context and determine appropriate ethical actions within the implicit and explicit agreements.

Research

The use of symphonology in research is useful in relation to the researcher-subject agreement. The HCP-patient relationship is to some extent implicit, but the relationship between a researcher and subject must be thoroughly explicit. Brown (2001c) suggested using the bioethical standards to develop ethical informed consent protocol. Particularly in cases where the research involves vulnerable populations, the consent of surrogates is made more acceptable and obtained more easily if the good of the individual is made central by using the bioethical standards.

Several research studies testing symphonology theory are under way and will be discussed in the next section.

FURTHER DEVELOPMENT

Initial testing of symphonological theory included three phases. First, a qualitative study examined the perceptions and satisfaction of nurses and patients and their significant others as they engaged in ethical decision making for health care issues (Husted, 2001). The themes that emerged from this study were used to develop visual analog tools to measure these feelings in nurses and patients. In the second phase, a pilot study to test the tool was completed. The Cronbach α for the nurse's tool was reported as 0.74, and 0.82 for the patient's tool (Husted, 2004). The third phase, a triangulated study, was conducted to determine the extent to which the theory can explain patients' experiences of being involved in health care decision making, as well as the utility of the theory when used as the foundation of a decision support counseling intervention with patients.

Irwin (2004) used a sample of 30 participants involved in a variety of decisions about health care and treatment during hospitalization in an acute care setting. The study included a decision support intervention for patients to determine the following: (1) whether key concepts of symphonological theory describe the experience of individuals making health care decisions and (2) whether application of the decision-making framework will enable nurses and patients to make ethically justifiable decisions. Results confirmed that patients expressed all the concepts of symphonology when discussing their experiences with health care decision making. Statistical analysis of pretest and posttest Bioethical Decision Making Preference Scale for Patients scores demonstrated that subjects had a more positive experience of being involved in decision making ($p = 0.02$) and felt more sufficiency of knowledge ($p = 0.013$), less frustration ($p = 0.014$), and more sense of power ($p = 0.009$) after the intervention. These findings support the validity of symphonology theory. The theory can be used to describe the experience of being involved in decision making, and symphonology has utility as a model for assisting patients through the decision-making process.

Further testing of this theory is being conducted by doctoral students. One study will determine if symphonology theory improves the experience of decision making for nurses and patients (Hardt, 2004). Another former graduate student used the nursing visual analog tool to discover how nurses felt when dealing with disclosure issues with patients. The Cronbach α for that study was 0.82 (Bavier, 2003). Further results are pending.

CRITIQUE
Clarity

In *Ethical Decision Making in Nursing* (Husted & Husted, 1995a), the authors presented the emerging concepts of symphonology and the relationships among the concepts. The book, in some parts, is a difficult read because the deeper concepts, meant for advanced practitioners, are presented along with the basics. The third edition, *Ethical Decision Making in Nursing and Healthcare: The Symphonological Approach,* begins with the basic concepts for understanding and using the theory, moving more advanced concepts to later sections (Husted & Husted, 2001). Along with this improved organization, the third edition also shows the emergence of increasing clarity for all concepts, the bioethical standards in particular.

This work challenges traditional methods of thought and requires the reader to develop a new understanding of familiar concepts. Storytelling and examples provide the opportunity to recognize and understand the importance of alternative and extended meanings for familiar terms. The conversational tone of the writing is appealing and creates a comfortable atmosphere for a complex subject.

Simplicity

The authors first challenge the truth and efficacy of traditional ideas about ethical behavior and decision making. This is a simple matter if the reader is willing to make the effort to be open-minded. Once the reader is beyond the challenge, the simplicity of the theory is evident. There are few concepts, and the relational statements flow logically from the definitions. The model clearly demonstrates the elements of the process of ethical reasoning and the manner in which those elements interact.

Generality

Symphonology is applicable at all levels of nursing practice and in all areas of the health care field. These principles can be applied between nurse and patient, researcher and subject, manager and employee, and educator and student. HCPs of all types can use this method to determine appropriate ethical behaviors in practice. This theory can also be applied to the process of establishing health care policy that is ethical in nature. Indeed, these principles can be applied in all walks of life, depending on the nature of the agreement between the parties involved.

Empirical Precision

Complex theories lend themselves more easily to producing empirical evidence. The research projects in progress will likely add to the reported findings that support this theory. Symphonology is a theory based in reality. Although evidence is gathered to support the theory, the reality of the usefulness of the theory in practice is evident. Nurses and other HCPs can easily understand the concepts and apply them in all situations. The result of using the symphonological model is a patient-centered, ethically justifiable decision.

Derivable Consequences

Being able to identify ethical actions in health care is of vital importance to patients, HCPs, and the health care industry itself. Before a nurse or any HCP takes action, regardless of how effective that action has proved in the past, the action must be justified as ethical with regard to the particular patient at hand. Reliance on concrete directives to guide action serves the directives, but only by chance serves the patient. Therefore, the pursuit of a practice-based ethical theory is essential for all of health care.

SUMMARY

The Husteds recognized that traditional methods of decision making were insufficient to address the bioethical problems emerging in the evolving health care system. They developed a theory of ethics and a decision-making model based on rational thought combined with insight and understanding. The theory is founded on the singular concept of human rights, the essential agreement of nonaggression among rational people that forms the foundation of all human interaction. Upon that foundation, HCPs and patients enter into an agreement to act to achieve the patient's goals. Preconditional to that agreement are recognition and respect for each person's unique character structure and the attendant properties of that structure: freedom, objectivity, beneficence, self-assertion, and fidelity. Ethical decisions are established within the context of a particular situation, using knowledge pertaining to the situation. Symphonological theory and the model for practice ensure ethically justifiable, individualized decisions.

Case Study

Alvin, 66, has been in the hospital for 12 weeks with multiple trauma following a motor vehicle accident. His condition worsens each day, and his prognosis is very grave. He is not alert, but he grimaces and withdraws from stimulation. Prior to his injury, Alvin signed a living will and discussed with his family his desire not to be kept alive in the event he was ill or injured and recovery was not possible. The health care team tells his family that, despite aggressive treatment, many of Alvin's body systems are failing. Even if Alvin survives, there is no hope he will be able to live without a ventilator because of extensive lung damage. The team suggests supportive care for Alvin and a do-not-resuscitate order. Most of the family members express the desire to ensure Alvin's comfort. Two family members believe Alvin will survive and recover. They refuse the team's suggestion and demand that Alvin receive every available treatment to keep him alive.

Analysis

Autonomy: Alvin's desires should be given priority over his family members' desires.

Freedom: Not to honor Alvin's wishes is a violation of his freedom.

Objectivity: The subjective feelings of two family members are in conflict with objective reality. Only the patient's subjective feelings are considered in ethical decisions.

Self-assertion: It is not justifiable to substitute family members' values for the patient's.

Beneficence: The patient's goals can not be obtained by aggressive treatment; however, aggressive treatment may well cause the patient further harm.

Fidelity: The HCP's agreement with Alvin was to act as his agent in pursuing goals that are possible to attain.

CRITICAL THINKING *Activities*

Using the Husted model, analyze this situation and those that follow from an ethical perspective.

1. Christina, 46, has been in the hospital for 2 weeks following a traumatic injury. Her condition was very grave, but she is beginning to show signs of recovery. The health care team suggests that a blood transfusion will provide the necessary support to continue her improvement. Christina and her family practice a religious faith that does not permit blood transfusions. Christina's husband and religious leader insist she not be given the transfusion regardless of the consequences. When the visitors leave, Christina tells the nurse that she would like to receive the transfusion, but only if it could be kept secret from her family. What should the nurse do?

2. Angela, 34, is dying of lung cancer. Despite counseling and support, she is very frightened. When her death is imminent, she screams over and over, "Don't let me die! Don't let me die!" Despite all efforts, Angela succumbs before her husband arrives. He asks, "How was she? Was she afraid?" What should the nurse say?

3. Johnny, 7, is a psychiatric in-patient with a diagnosis of trichlomania (hair pulling). His parents are very concerned about stopping his destructive behavior and have developed a series of punishments for incidents of hair pulling. Johnny has been seen pulling his hair out several times during the day. His parents arrive and ask how many times Johnny pulled his hair. What should the nurse say?

4. Eugene, 47, has several chronic illnesses. Despite education and support, Eugene declines to adhere to prescribed health care practices. Mark, a home health care nurse, has been seeing Eugene for several months and has made no progress in helping Eugene to improve his health. While discussing the situation, Eugene tells Mark he has no intention of changing any of his behaviors. Is Mark justified in asking the physician to discontinue home health visits?

5. Agnes is a nurse on a busy medical nursing unit. Mr. Brown frequently asks Agnes to interrupt her work to answer questions and perform nonemergent tasks for him. Agnes' other patients complain of neglect. What should Agnes do and how can she justify her actions?

6. Burt, 34, has a diagnosis of manic depression. He lives in a group home with several others like himself. Several times a year, Burt stops taking his medication and disappears for weeks at a time. Occasionally Burt is arrested for vagrancy, but he has never been violent with himself or others. He states he enjoys his "vacations" because his medicine makes his life seem boring, dull, and difficult. Burt's family calls the director of the group home and insists that Burt be required to take his medicine each morning under supervision. What should the director say and how could he justify various courses of action?

REFERENCES

Bavier, A. (2003). *Types of disclosure discussion between oncology nurses and their patients/families: An exploratory study.* Unpublished manuscript, Duquesne University, Pittsburgh.

Brown, B. (2001a). The educator student/patient agreement. In G. L. Husted & J. H. Husted, *Ethical decision making in nursing and healthcare: The symphonological approach* (3rd ed., pp. 215-217). New York: Springer.

Brown, B. (2001b). The professional/patient agreement and advanced directives. In G. L. Husted & J. H. Husted

(Eds.), *Ethical decision making in nursing and health-care: The symphonological approach* (3rd ed., pp. 233-237). New York: Springer.

Brown, B. (2001c). The researcher/subject agreement. In G. L. Husted & J. H. Husted (Eds.), *Ethical decision making in nursing and healthcare: The symphonological approach* (3rd ed., pp. 229-231). New York: Springer.

Fawcett, J. (1995). *Analysis and evaluation of conceptual models of nursing* (3rd ed.). Philadelphia: F. A. Davis.

Fedorka, P., & Husted, G. L. (2001). Ethical decision making in clinical emergencies. *Topics in Emergency Medicine, 26,* 52-60.

Hardt, M. (2004). *Efficacy of a symphonological intervention in promoting a positive experience for nurses and patients experiencing bioethical dilemmas.* Unpublished manuscript, Duquesne University, Pittsburgh.

Hardt, M., & Hopey, K. (2001). The administrator/health professional/patient agreement. In G. L. Husted & J. H. Husted (Eds.), *Ethical decision making in nursing and healthcare: The symphonological approach* (3rd ed., pp. 219-227). New York: Springer.

Hartman, R. (1998). Revisiting the call to care: An ethical perspective. *Advanced Practice Nursing Quarterly, 4*(2), 14-18.

Husted, G. L. (2001). The feelings nurses and patients/families experience when faced with the need to make bioethical decisions. *Nursing Administration Quarterly, 25*(3), 1-9.

Husted, G. L. (2004). *The feelings of nurses and patients/families involved in the bioethical decision making process: The psychometric testing of two instruments.* Unpublished manuscript, Duquesne University, Pittsburgh.

Husted, G. L., & Husted, J. H. (1991). *Ethical decision making in nursing.* St. Louis: Mosby.

Husted, G. L., & Husted, J. H. (1995a). *Ethical decision making in nursing* (2nd ed.). St. Louis: Mosby.

Husted, G. L., & Husted, J. H. (1995b). The bioethical standards: The analysis of dilemmas through the analysis of persons. *Advanced Practice Nursing Quarterly, 1*(2), 69-76.

Husted, G. L., & Husted, J. H. (1997a). An ethical defense against the plague of cloning. *Advanced Practice Nursing Quarterly, 3*(2), 82-84.

Husted, G. L., & Husted, J. H. (1997b). Is a return to a caring perspective desirable? *Advanced Practice Nursing Quarterly, 3*(1), 14-17.

Husted, G. L., & Husted, J. H. (2001). *Ethical decision making in nursing and healthcare: The symphonological approach* (3rd ed.). New York: Springer.

Husted, J. H., & Husted, G. L. (1998). The role of the nurse in ethical decision making. In G. DeLoughery (Ed.), *Issues and trends in nursing* (pp. 216-242). St. Louis: Mosby.

Husted, J. H., & Husted, G. L. (1999). Agreement: The origin of ethical action. *Critical Care Nursing, 22*(3), 12-18.

Irwin, M. (2004). *Effect of symphonology on patients' experience of involvement in health care decision making: A qualitative and quantitative study.* Unpublished manuscript, Duquesne University, Pittsburgh.

Jecker, N., Jonsen, A., & Pearlman, R. (1997). *Bioethics: An introduction to the history, methods and practice.* Sudbury, MA: Jones and Bartlett.

Josephson, J., & Josephson, S. (1994). *Abductive inference: Computation, philosophy, technology.* New York: Cambridge University Press.

Lloyd, G. (1996). *Spinoza and the ethics.* New York: Routledge.

McKeon, R. (Ed.). (1941). *The basic works of Aristotle.* New York: Random House.

Polanyi, M. (1964). *Personal knowledge.* New York: Harper & Row.

Steckler, J. (1998). Examination of ethical practice in nursing continuing education using the Husted model. *Advanced Practice Nursing Quarterly, 4*(2), 59-64.

Walker, L., & Avant, K. (1995). *Strategies of theory construction in nursing* (3rd ed.). Norwalk, CT: Appleton & Lange.

Zoucha, R., & Husted, G. (2000). The ethical dimensions of delivering cultural congruent nursing and health care. *Issues in Mental Health Nursing, 21,* 325-340.

BIBLIOGRAPHY
Primary Sources
Books

Husted, G. L., & Husted, J. H. (1991). *Ethical decision making in nursing.* St. Louis: Mosby.

Husted, G. L., & Husted, J. H. (1995). *Ethical decision making in nursing* (2nd ed.). St. Louis: Mosby.

Husted, G. L., & Husted, J. H. (2001). *Ethical decision making in nursing and healthcare: The symphonological approach* (3rd ed.). New York: Springer.

Book Chapters

Husted, G. L., & Husted, J. H. (1999). Strength of character through the ethics of nursing. In S. Osgood (Ed.), *Essential readings in nursing managed care* (pp. 102-106). Gaithersburg, MD: Aspen.

Husted, G. L., & Husted, J. H. (2004). Ethics and the advanced practice nurse. In L. A. Joel (Ed.), *Advanced practice nursing* (pp. 639-661). Philadelphia: F. A. Davis.

Husted, G. L., & Husted, J. H. (2005). The ethical experience of caring for vulnerable populations: The symphonological approach. In M. DeChesnay (Ed.), *Caring for vulnerable populations* (pp. 71-79). St Louis: Mosby.

Husted, J. H., & Husted, G. L. (1998). The role of the nurse in ethical decision making. In G. DeLoughery (Ed.),

Issues and trends in nursing (pp. 216-242). St Louis: Mosby.

Journal and Other Articles

Fedorka, P., & Husted, G. L. (2001). Ethical decision making in clinical emergencies. *Topics in Emergency Medicine, 26,* 52-60.

Husted, G. L. (2001). The feelings nurses and patients/families experience when faced with the need to make bioethical decisions. *Nursing Administration Quarterly, 25*(3), 1-9.

Husted, G. L. (submitted). The feelings of nurses and patients/families involved in the bioethical decision making process: The psychometric testing of two instruments.

Husted, G. L., & Husted, J. H. (1995). The bioethical standards: The analysis of dilemmas through the analysis of persons. *Advanced Practice Nursing Quarterly, 1*(2), 69-76.

Husted, G. L., & Husted, J. H. (1996). Ethical dilemmas: Time and fidelity. *American Journal of Nursing, 96*(11), 74.

Husted, G. L., & Husted, J. H. (1997). A modest proposal concerning policies. *Advanced Practice Nursing Quarterly, 3*(3), 17-19.

Husted, G. L., & Husted, J. H. (1997). An ethical defense against the plague of cloning. *Advanced Practice Nursing Quarterly, 3*(2), 82-84.

Husted, G. L., & Husted, J. H. (1997). An ethical examination of in-vitro fertilization and cloning. *AORN, 65*(6), 1-2.

Husted, G. L., & Husted, J. H. (1997). Is a return to a caring perspective desirable? *Advanced Practice Nursing Quarterly, 3*(1), 14-17.

Husted, G. L., & Husted, J. H. (1997). Is cloning moral? *Nursing and Health Care: Perspectives on Community, 18,* 168-169.

Husted, G. L., & Husted, J. H. (1998). Ethical balance versus ethical anomaly. *Advanced Practice Nursing Quarterly, 4*(1), 51-53.

Husted, G. L., & Husted, J. H. (1998). Strength of character through the ethics of nursing. *Advanced Practice Nursing Quarterly, 3*(4), 23-25.

Husted, G. L., & Husted, J. H. (1998). With the ethical agreement: Where are you now? *Advanced Practice Nursing Quarterly, 4*(2), 34-35.

Husted, J. H., & Husted, G. L. (1999). Agreement: The origin of ethical action. *Critical Care Nursing, 22*(3), 12-18.

Husted, J. H., & Husted, G. L. (2000). When is a health care system not an ethical health care system?: Suspending the do-not-resuscitate order in the operating room. *Critical Care Nursing Clinics of North America, 12,* 157-163.

Husted, G. L., Miller, M. C., & Brown, B. (1999). Test of an educational brochure on advance directives designed for the well-elderly. *Journal of Gerontological Nursing, 25*(1), 34-40.

Husted, G. L., Miller, M. C., Zaremba, J. A., Clutter, S. L., Jennings, K. R., & Stainbrook, D. (1997). Advance directives and what attracts elderly people to particular brochures. *Journal of Gerontological Nursing, 23*(2), 41-45.

Zoucha, R. D., & Husted, G. L. (2002). The ethical dimensions of delivering culturally congruent nursing and health care. *Review Series Psychiatry, Sweden, 3,* 10-11.

Zoucha, R., & Husted, G. L. (2000). Is delivering culturally congruent psychosocial healthcare ethical? *Issues in Mental Health Nursing, 21,* 325-340.

Secondary Sources
Books

Burkhardt, M. A., & Nathaniel, A. K. (2002). *Ethics and issues in contemporary nursing* (2nd ed.). Clifton Park, NJ: Delmar.

Lauritzen, P. (Ed.). (2001). *Cloning and the future of human embryo research.* London: Oxford University Press.

Lipe, S. K., & Beasley, S. (2004). *Critical thinking in nursing: A cognitive skills workbook.* Philadelphia: Lippincott Williams & Wilkins.

Spencer, E. M. (Ed.). (2000). *Organizational ethics in health care.* London: Oxford University Press.

Thomson Learning Series. (2001). *Surgical technology for surgical technologists: A positive care approach.* Clifton Park, NJ: Delmar.

Journal and Other Articles

Anderson, J., Biba, S., & Hartman, R. L. (1996). Ethical case comment. To tell or not to tell . . . the case . . . ethical analysis. *DCCN-Dimensions of Critical Care Nursing, 15*(6), 318-323.

Bavier, A. (2003). *Types of disclosure discussion between oncology nurses and their patients/families: An exploratory study.* Unpublished manuscript, Duquesne University, Pittsburgh.

Best, J. T. (2001). Effective teaching for the elderly: Back to basics. *Orthopedic Nursing, 20*(3), 46-52.

Bridger, J. C. (1997). A study of nurses' views about the prevention of nosocomial urinary tract infections. *Journal of Clinical Nursing, 6*(5), 379-387.

Burcham, J. L. R. (2002). Cultural competence: An evolutionary perspective. *Nursing Forum, 37*(4), 5-15.

Claassen, M. (2000). A handful of questions: supporting parental decision making. *Clinical Nurse Specialist, 14*(4), 189-195.

Greipp, M. E. (1995). A survey of ethical decision making models in nursing. *Journal of Nursing Science, 1*(1/2), 51-60.

Hardt, M. (2004). *Efficacy of a symphonological intervention in promoting a positive experience for nurses and patients experiencing bioethical dilemmas.* Unpublished manuscript, Duquesne University, Pittsburgh.

Irwin, M. (2004). *Effect of symphonology on patients' experience of involvement in health care decision making: A qualitative and quantitative study.* Unpublished manuscript, Duquesne University, Pittsburgh.

Johnson, J. E. (2002). Six steps to ethical leadership in health care. *Patient Care Management, 18*(2), 5-9.

Kinion, E. S., Jonke, N. L., & Paradise, N. (1995). Descriptive ethics and neuroleptic dose reduction. *Perspectives in Psychiatric Care, 31*(2), 11-14.

Mariano, C. (2001). Holistic ethics. *American Journal of Nursing, 101*(1 part 1), Hospital Extra: 24A-C.

McFadden, E. A. (1996). Moral development and reproductive health decisions. *Journal of Obsteric, Gynecologic, & Neonatal Nursing, 25*(6), 507-512.

Oberle, K., & Tenove, S. (2000). Ethical issues in public health nursing. *Nursing Ethics: An International Journal for Health Care Professionals, 7*(5), 425-438.

Oddi, L. F., Cassidy, V. R., & Fisher, C. (1995). Nurses' sensitivity to the ethical aspects of clinical practice. *Nursing Ethics: An International Journal for Health Care Professionals, 2*(3), 197-209.

Reveillere, C., Pham, T., Masclet, G., Nandrino, J. L., & Beaune, D. (2000). The relationship between burn-out and personality in care-givers in a palliative care unit. *Annals Medico Psychologiques, 158*(9), 716-721.

Rice, V. H., Beck, C., & Stevenson, J. S. (1997). Ethical issues relative to autonomy and personal control in independent and cognitive impaired elders. *Nursing Outlook, 45*(1), 27-34.

Saulo, M. (1996). How good case managers make tough choices: Ethics and mediation . . . part I. *Journal of Care Management, 2*(1), 8, 10, 12 passim.

Scotto, C. (2003). A new view of caring. *Journal of Nursing Education, 42*(7), 289-291.

Simko, L. (1999). Adults with congenital heart disease: Utilizing quality of life and Husted's nursing theory as a conceptual framework. *Critical Care Nursing Quarterly, 22*(3), 1-11.

Steckler, J. (1998). Examination of ethical practices in nursing continuing education using the Husted model. *Advanced Practice Nursing Quarterly, 4*(2), 59-64.

Thompson, L. W. (1998). Nursing ethics: The ANA code for nurses. *Tennessee Nurse, 61*(6), 23, 25-29.

Troskie, R. (1998). Ethical decision making in a transcultural context. *Health SA Gesondheid, 3*(1), 3-8.

Von Post, I. (1996). Exploring ethical dilemmas in perioperative nursing practice through critical incidents. *Nursing Ethics: An International Journal for Health Care Professionals, 3*(3), 236-249.

Weiner, C., Tabak, N., & Bergman, R. (2001). The use of physical restraints for patients suffering from dementia. *Nursing Ethics, 56*(2), 148-152.

Wilmot, S. (2000). Nurses and whistleblowing: The ethical issues. *Journal of Advanced Nursing, 32*(5), 1051-1057.

Wilson, D. M. (1998). Administrative decision making in response to sudden health care agency funding reductions: Is there a role for ethics? *Nursing Ethics: an International Journal for Health Care Professionals, 5*(4), 319-329.

Wurzbach, M. E. (1999). Acute care nurses' experiences of moral certainty. *Journal of Advanced Nursing, 30*(2), 287-293.

Middle Range Theories

- Middle range theories are a set of related concepts that focus on a limited dimension of the reality of nursing and can be depicted in a model.

- Middle range theories can describe a phenomenon, explain the relationship between phenomena, predict the effects of one phenomenon on another, and be used to control a limited dimension of nursing.

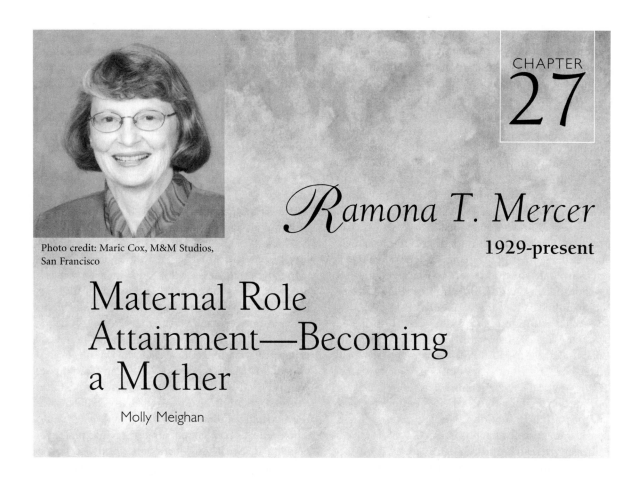

Photo credit: Maric Cox, M&M Studios,
San Francisco

$\mathcal{R}$amona T. Mercer

1929-present

Maternal Role Attainment—Becoming a Mother

Molly Meighan

CREDENTIALS AND BACKGROUND OF THE THEORIST

Ramona T. Mercer began her nursing career in 1950 when she received her diploma from St. Margaret's School of Nursing in Montgomery, Alabama. She graduated with the L.L. Hill Award for Highest Scholastic Standing. She returned to school in 1960 after working as a staff nurse, head nurse, and instructor in the areas of pediatrics, obstetrics, and contagious diseases. She completed a bachelor's degree in nursing in 1962, graduating with distinction from the University of New Mexico, Albuquerque. She went on to earn a master's degree in maternal-child nursing from Emory University in

Previous authors: Mary M. (Molly) Meighan, Alberta M. Bee, Denise Legge, and Stephanie Oetting.

1964 and completed a Ph.D. in maternity nursing at the University of Pittsburgh in 1973.

After receiving a Ph.D., Mercer moved to California and accepted the position of assistant professor in the Department of Family Health Care Nursing at the University of California, San Francisco. She was promoted to associate professor in 1977, and in 1983 she was promoted to professor. She remained in that role until her retirement in 1987. Currently, Dr. Mercer is Professor Emeritus in Family Health Nursing at the University of California, San Francisco. Today, she is active in writing and consultations (R. Mercer, curriculum vitae, 2002; R. Mercer, personal communication, April 5, 2004).

Mercer has received awards throughout her career. In 1963, while working and pursuing studies in nursing, she received the Department of Health, Education, and Welfare Public Health Service Nurse Trainee Award at Emory University and was inducted into Sigma Theta Tau. She received this award again during her years at the University of Pittsburgh. She also received the Bixler Scholarship for Nursing Education and Research, Southern Regional Board, for doctoral study. In 1982, she received the Maternal Child Health Nurse of the Year Award by the National Foundation of the March of Dimes and American Nurses Association, Division of Maternal Child Health Practice. She was presented with the Fourth Annual Helen Nahm Lecturer Award at the University of California, San Francisco, School of Nursing in 1984. Mercer's research awards include the American Society for Psychoprophylaxis in Obstetrics (ASPO)/Lamaze National Research Award in 1987; the Distinguished Research Lectureship Award, Western Institute of Nursing, Western Society for Research in Nursing in 1988; and the American Nurses Foundation's Distinguished Contribution to Nursing Science Award in 1990 (R. Mercer, curriculum vitae, 2000). Mercer has authored numerous articles, editorials, and commentaries. In addition, she has published six books and six book chapters.

In early research efforts, Mercer focused on the behaviors and needs of breast-feeding mothers, mothers with postpartum illness, mothers bearing infants with defects, and teenage mothers. Her first book, *Nursing Care for Parents at Risk* (1977), received an *American Journal of Nursing* Book of the Year Award in 1978. Her study of teenage mothers over the first year of motherhood resulted in the 1979 book, *Perspectives on Adolescent Health Care*, which also received an *American Journal of Nursing* Book of the Year Award in 1980. Preceding research led Mercer to study family relationships, antepartal stress as related to familial relationships and the maternal role, and mothers of various ages. In 1986, Mercer's research on three age groups of mothers was drawn together in her third book, *First-Time Motherhood: Experiences From Teens to Forties*. Mercer's fifth book, *Parents at Risk*, published in 1990, also received an *American Journal of Nursing* Book of the Year Award. *Parents at Risk* (1990)

focused on strategies for facilitating early parent-infant interactions and promoting parental competence in relation to specific risk situations. Mercer's sixth book, *Becoming a Mother: Research on Maternal Identity From Rubin to the Present,* was published by Springer Publishing Company of New York in 1995. This book contains a more complete description of Mercer's Theory of Maternal Role Attainment and her framework for studying variables that impact the maternal role.

Since her first publication in 1968, Mercer has written numerous articles for both nursing and nonnursing journals and continues to write for *Nurseweek.* Some of her most recent writing is found on the Internet at the *Nurseweek* site (*http://www.nurseweek.com*) and includes several online courses: Adolescent Sexuality and Childbearing, Transitions to Parenthood, and Helping Parents when the Unexpected Occurs.

Mercer has maintained membership in several professional organizations, including the American Nurses Association and the American Academy of Nursing, and has been an active member on many national committees. From 1983 to 1990, she was the associate editor of *Health Care for Women International.* She has served on the review panel for *Nursing Research* and *Western Journal of Nursing Research,* the editorial board of the *Journal of Adolescent Health Care,* and was on the executive advisory board of *Nurseweek.* She has also served as a reviewer for numerous grant proposals. Additionally, she has been actively involved with regional, national, and international scientific and professional meetings and workshops (R. Mercer, curriculum vitae, 2000). She was honored as a Living Legend by the American Academy of Nursing during the Annual Meeting and Conference in Carlsbad, California, in November 2003.

THEORETICAL SOURCES

Mercer's Theory of Maternal Role Attainment was based on her extensive research on the topic beginning in the late 1960s. Mercer's professor and mentor, Reva Rubin at the University of Pittsburgh, was a major stimulus for both research and theory development. Rubin (1977, 1984) is well known for her work in defining and describing maternal role attainment as a process of binding-in, or being attached, to the child and achieving a maternal role identity or seeing oneself in the role and having a sense of comfort about it. Mercer's framework and study variables clearly reflect many of Rubin's concepts.

In addition to Rubin's work, Mercer based her research on both role and developmental theories. She relied heavily on an interactionist approach to role theory, using Mead's (1934) theory on role enactment and Turner's (1978) theory on the core self. In addition, Thornton and Nardi's (1975) role acquisition process also helped shape Mercer's

theory, as did the work of Burr, Leigh, Day, and Constantine (1979). Werner's (1957) developmental process theories also contributed. In addition, Mercer's work was influenced by von Bertalanffy's (1968) general system theory. Her model of maternal role attainment depicted in Figure 27-1 uses Bronfenbrenner's (1979) concepts of nested circles as a means of portraying interactional environmental influences on the maternal role. The complexity of her research interest led Mercer to rely on several theoretical sources to identify and study variables that affect maternal role attainment. Although much of her work involved testing and extending Rubin's theories, she has consistently looked to the research of others in the development and expansion of her theory.

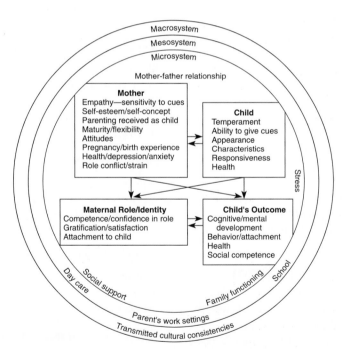

Figure **27-1 Model of Maternal Role Attainment.** (Modified from Mercer, R. T. [1991]. *Maternal role: Models and consequences.* Paper presented at the International Research Conference sponsored by the Council of Nurse Researchers and the American Nurses Association, Los Angeles, CA. Copyright Ramona T. Mercer, 1991. NOTE: This figure has been modified based on personal communication with R. T. Mercer [January 4, 2000]. The word *exosystem* was replaced with the word *mesosystem* to be more consistent with Bronfenbrenner's [1979] model on which it is based.)

MAJOR CONCEPTS & DEFINITIONS

Mercer uses the concepts outlined below in her theory.

MATERNAL ROLE ATTAINMENT

Maternal role attainment is an interactional and developmental process occurring over time in which the mother becomes attached to her infant, acquires competence in the caretaking tasks involved in the role, and expresses pleasure and gratification in the role (Mercer, 1986a). "The movement to the personal state in which the mother experiences a sense of harmony, confidence, and competence in how she performs the role is the end point of maternal role attainment—maternal identity" (Mercer, 1981, p. 74).

MATERNAL IDENTITY

Maternal identify is defined as having an internalized view of the self as a mother (Mercer, 1995).

PERCEPTION OF BIRTH EXPERIENCE

A woman's perception of her performance during labor and birth is her perception of the birth experience (Mercer, 1990).

SELF-ESTEEM

Mercer, May, Ferketich and DeJoseph (1986) describe self-esteem as "an individual's perception of how others view one and self-acceptance of the perceptions" (p. 341).

SELF-CONCEPT (SELF-REGARD)

Mercer (1986a) outlines self-concept, or self-regard, as "The overall perception of self that includes self-satisfaction, self-acceptance, self-esteem, and congruence or discrepancy between self and ideal self" (p. 18).

FLEXIBILITY

Roles are not rigidly fixed; therefore, who fills the roles is not important (Mercer, 1990). "Flexibility of childrearing attitudes increases with increased development. . . . Older mothers have the potential to respond less rigidly to their infants and to view each situation in respect to the unique nuances" (Mercer, 1986a, p. 43; 1990, p. 12).

CHILDREARING ATTITUDES

Childrearing attitudes are maternal attitudes or beliefs about childrearing (Mercer, 1986a).

HEALTH STATUS

Health status is defined as "The mother's and father's perception of their prior health, current health, health outlook, resistance-susceptibility to illness, health worry concern, sickness orientation, and rejection of the sick role" (Mercer, et al., 1986, p. 342).

ANXIETY

Mercer and colleagues (1986) describe anxiety as "a trait in which there is specific proneness to perceive stressful situations as dangerous or threatening, and as situation-specific state" (p. 342).

DEPRESSION

According to Mercer and colleagues (1986), depression is "having a group of depressive symptoms, and in particular the affective component of the depressed mood" (p. 342).

ROLE STRAIN–ROLE CONFLICT

Role strain is the conflict and difficulty felt by the woman in fulfilling the maternal role obligation (Mercer, 1985a).

GRATIFICATION-SATISFACTION

Mercer (1985b) describes gratification as "the satisfaction, enjoyment, reward, or pleasure that a woman experiences in interacting with her infant, and in fulfilling the usual tasks inherent in mothering."

MAJOR CONCEPTS *&* DEFINITIONS—cont'd

ATTACHMENT

Attachment is a component of the parental role and identity. It is viewed as a process in which an enduring affectional and emotional commitment to an individual is formed (Mercer, 1990).

INFANT TEMPERAMENT

An easy versus a difficult temperament is related to whether the infant sends hard-to-read cues, leading to feelings of incompetence and frustration in the mother (Mercer, 1986a).

INFANT HEALTH STATUS

Infant health status is illness causing maternal-infant separation, interfering with the attachment process (Mercer, 1986a).

INFANT CHARACTERISTICS

Characteristics include infant temperament, appearance, and health status (Mercer, 1981).

INFANT CUES

Infant cues are infant behaviors that elicit a response from the mother (R. Mercer, personal communication, September 3, 2003).

FAMILY

Mercer and colleagues (1986) define family as "a dynamic system which includes subsystems—individuals (mother, father, fetus/infant) and dyads (mother-father, mother-fetus/infant, and father-fetus/infant) within the overall family system" (p. 339).

FAMILY FUNCTIONING

Family functioning is the individual's view of the activities and relationships between the family and its subsystems and broader social units (Mercer & Ferketich, 1995).

FATHER OR INTIMATE PARTNER

The father or intimate partner contributes to the process of maternal role attainment in a way that cannot be duplicated by any other person (R. T. Mercer, personal communication, January 4, 2000). The father's interactions help diffuse tension and facilitate maternal role attainment (Donley, 1993; Mercer, 1995).

STRESS

Stress is made up of positively and negatively perceived life events and environmental variables (Mercer, 1990).

SOCIAL SUPPORT

According to Mercer and colleagues (1986), social support is "the amount of help actually received, satisfaction with that help, and the persons (network) providing that help" (p. 341).

Four areas of social support are as follows:

1. *Emotional support:* "Feeling loved, cared for, trusted, and understood" (Mercer, 1986a, p. 14)
2. *Informational support:* "Helps the individual help herself by providing information that is useful in dealing with the problem and/or situation" (Mercer, 1986a, p. 14)
3. *Physical support:* A direct kind of help (Mercer, Hackley, & Bostrom, 1984)
4. *Appraisal support:* "A support that tells the role taker how she is performing in the role; it enables the individual to evaluate herself in relationship to others' performance in the role" (Mercer, 1986a, p. 14)

MOTHER-FATHER RELATIONSHIP

The mother-father relationship is the perception of the mate relationship that includes intended and actual values, goals, and agreements between the two (Mercer, 1986b). The maternal attachment to the infant develops within the emotional field of the parent's relationship (Donley, 1993; Mercer, 1995).

USE OF EMPIRICAL EVIDENCE

Mercer selected both maternal and infant variables for her studies on the basis of her review of the literature and findings of researchers in several disciplines. She found that many factors may have a direct or indirect influence on the maternal role, adding to the complexity of her studies. Maternal factors in Mercer's research included age at first birth, birth experience, early separation from the infant, social stress, social support, personality traits, self-concept, childrearing attitudes, and health. She included the infant variables of temperament, appearance, responsiveness, health status, and ability to give cues. Mercer (1995) and Ferketich and Mercer (1995a, 1995b, 1995c) also noted the importance of the father's role and applied many of Mercer's previous findings in studying the paternal response to parenthood. Her research required numerous instruments to measure the variables of interest.

Mercer has studied the influence of these variables on parental attachment and competence over several intervals, including the immediate postpartum period and 1 month, 4 months, 8 months, and 1 year following birth (Mercer & Ferketich, 1990a, 1990b). In addition, she has included adolescents, older mothers, ill mothers, mothers dealing with congenital defects, families experiencing antepartal stress, parents at high risk, mothers who had cesarean deliveries, and fathers in her research (Mercer, 1989; Mercer & Ferketich, 1994, 1995; Mercer, Ferketich, & DeJoseph, 1993). As a recent step, she compared her findings and the basis for her original theory with current research. As a result, Mercer (2004) has proposed that the term *maternal role attainment* be replaced with *becoming a mother,* because this more accurately describes the continued evolution of the role across the woman's lifespan. In addition, she proposes using more recent nursing research findings to describe the stages and process of becoming a mother.

MAJOR ASSUMPTIONS

For maternal role attainment, Mercer (1981, 1986a, 1995) stated the following assumptions:

- A relatively stable core self, acquired through lifelong socialization, determines how a mother defines and perceives events; her perceptions of her infant's and others' responses to her mothering, with her life situation, are the real world to which she responds (Mercer, 1986a).
- In addition to the mother's socialization, her developmental level and innate personality characteristics also influence her behavioral responses (Mercer, 1986a).
- The mother's role partner, her infant, will reflect the mother's competence in the mothering role through growth and development (Mercer, 1986a).
- The infant is considered an active partner in the maternal role-taking process, affecting and being affected by the role enactment (Mercer, 1981).
- The father or mother's intimate partner contributes to role attainment in a way that cannot be duplicated by any other supportive person (Mercer, 1995).
- Maternal identity develops concurrently with maternal attachment and each depends on the other (Mercer, 1995; Rubin, 1977).

Nursing

Mercer (1995) stated that, "Nurses are the health professionals having the most sustained and intense interaction with women in the maternity cycle" (p. xii). Nurses are responsible for promoting the health of families and children; nurses are pioneers in developing and sharing assessment strategies for these patients, she explained. Her definition of nursing provided in a personal communication is as follows:

Nursing is a dynamic profession with three major foci: health promotion and prevention of illness, providing care for those who need professional assistance to achieve their optimal level of health and functioning, and research to enhance the knowledge base for providing excellent nursing care. Nurses provide health care for individuals, families, and communities. Following assessment of the client's situation and environment, the nurse identifies goals with the client, provides assistance to the client through teaching, supporting, providing care the client is unable to provide for self, and interfacing with the environment and the client. (R. Mercer, personal communication, March 21, 2004)

In her writing, Mercer (1995) refers to the importance of nursing care. Although she does not specifically mention nursing care, in her book, *Becoming a Mother: Research on Maternal Identity From Rubin to the Present,* Mercer emphasizes that the kind of help or care a woman receives during pregnancy and over the first year following birth can have long-term effects for her and her child. Nurses in maternal-child settings play a sizable role in providing both care and information during this period.

Person

Mercer (1985a) does not specifically define person, but refers to the self or core self. She views the self as separate from the roles that are played. Through maternal individuation, a woman may regain her own personhood as she extrapolates her self from the mother-infant dyad (Mercer, 1985b). The core self evolves from a cultural context and determines how situations are defined and shaped (Mercer, 1985a). The concepts of self-esteem and self-confidence are important in attainment of the maternal role. The mother as a separate person interacts with her infant and with the father or her significant other. She is both influential and is influenced by both of them (Mercer, 1995).

Health

In her theory, Mercer defines health status as the mother's and father's perception of their prior health, current health, health outlook, resistance-susceptibility to illness, health worry or concern, sickness orientation, and rejection of the sick role. Health status of the newborn is the extent of disease present and infant health status by parental rating of overall health (Mercer, 1986b). The health status of a family is affected negatively by antepartum stress (Mercer, Ferketich, DeJoseph, May, & Sollid, 1988; Mercer, May, Ferketich, & DeJoseph, 1986). Health

status is an important indirect influence on satisfaction with relationships in childbearing families. Health is also viewed as a desired outcome for the child. It is influenced by both maternal and infant variables. Mercer (1995) stresses the importance of health care during the childbearing and childrearing processes.

Environment

Mercer conceptualized the environment from Bronfenbrenner's definition of the ecological environment and based her earliest model in Figure 27-1 on it (Mercer, 1995; R. Mercer, personal communication, June 24, 2000). This model illustrates the ecological interacting environments in which maternal role attainment develops. During a personal communication on January 4, 2000, Mercer explained, "Development of a role/person cannot be considered apart from the environment; there is a mutual accommodation between the developing person and the changing properties of the immediate settings, relationships between the settings, and the larger contexts in which the settings are embedded." Stresses and social support within the environment influence both maternal and paternal role attainment and the developing child.

THEORETICAL ASSERTIONS

Mercer's original Theory and Model of Maternal Role Attainment were first introduced in 1991 during a symposium at the International Research Conference sponsored by the Council of Nursing Research and American Nurses Association in Los Angeles, California (Mercer, 1995). It was refined and was presented more clearly in her 1995 book, *Becoming a Mother: Research on Maternal Identity From Rubin to the Present* (see Figure 27-1).

Mercer's (2004) more recent revision of her theory focuses on the woman's transition in becoming a mother. It involves an extensive change in her life space that requires her ongoing development. According to Mercer, becoming a mother is more extensive than just assuming a role. It is unending and continuously evolving. Therefore she recommends that the term *maternal role attainment* be retired.

Maternal Role Attainment: Mercer's Original Model

Mercer's Model of Maternal Role Attainment was placed within Bronfenbrenner's (1979) nested circles of the microsystem, mesosystem, and macrosystem (see Figure 27-1). The original model proposed by Mercer was altered in 2000, changing the term *exosystem* originally found in the second circle and replacing it with the term *mesosystem.* Mercer (personal communication, January 4, 2000) explained that this change made the model more consistent with Bronfenbrenner's terminology, as follows:

1. The microsystem is the immediate environment in which maternal role attainment occurs. It includes factors such as family functioning, mother-father relationships, social support, economic status, family values, and stressors. The variables contained within this immediate environment interact with one or more of the other variables in affecting the transition to motherhood. The infant as an individual is embedded within the family system. The family is viewed as a semi-closed system maintaining boundaries and control over interchange between the family system and other social systems (Mercer, 1990).

   The microsystem is the most influential on maternal role attainment (Mercer, 1995; R. Mercer, personal communication, January 4, 2000). In 1995, Mercer expanded her earlier concepts and model to emphasize the importance of the father on role attainment, stating that he helps "diffuse tension developing within the mother-infant dyad" (p. 15). Maternal role attainment is achieved through the interactions of father, mother, and infant. Figure 27-2, first introduced in Mercer's (1995) sixth book, *Becoming a Mother: Research on Maternal Identity From Rubin to the Present,* depicts this interaction. The layers *a* through *d* represent the stages of maternal role attainment from anticipatory to personal (role identity) and the

infant's growth and developmental stages (Mercer, 1995).

2. The mesosystem encompasses, influences, and interacts with persons in the microsystem. Mesosystem interactions may influence what happens to the developing maternal role and the child. The mesosystem includes day care, school, work setting, places of worship, and other entities within the immediate community.

3. The macrosystem refers to the general prototypes existing in a particular culture or transmitted cultural consistencies. The macrosystem includes the social, political, and cultural influences on the other two systems. The health care environment and the current health care system policies that affect maternal role attainment originate in this system (Mercer, 1995). National laws regarding women and children and health priorities that influence maternal role attainment are within the macrosystem.

Maternal role attainment is a process that follows four stages of role acquisition; these stages have been adapted from Thornton and Nardi's 1975 research. The following stages are indicated in Figure 27-2 as the layers *a* through *d*:

a. *Anticipatory:* The anticipatory stage begins during pregnancy and includes the initial social and psychological adjustments to pregnancy. The mother learns the expectations of the role,

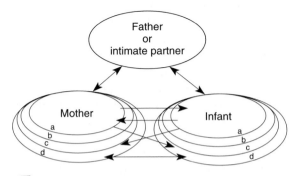

Figure **27-2 A microsystem within the evolving model of maternal role attainment.** (From Mercer, R. T. [1995]. *Becoming a mother: Research on maternal identity from Rubin to the present.* New York: Springer Used by permission.)

fantasizes about the role, relates to the fetus in utero, and begins role play.

b. *Formal:* The formal stage begins with the birth of the infant and includes learning and taking on the role of mother. Role behaviors are guided by formal, consensual expectations of others in the mother's social system.

c. *Informal:* Begins as the mother develops unique ways of dealing with the role not conveyed by the social system. The woman makes her new role fit within her existing lifestyle based on past experiences and future goals.

d. *Personal:* The personal or role-identity stage occurs as the woman internalizes her role. The mother experiences a sense of harmony, confidence, and competence in the way she performs the role and the maternal role is achieved.

Stages of role attainment overlap and are altered as the infant grows and develops. A maternal role identity may be achieved in a month, or it can take several months (Mercer, 1995). The stages are influenced by social support, stress, family functioning, and the relationship between mother and father or significant other.

Traits and behaviors of both the mother and the infant may influence maternal role identity and child outcome. Maternal traits and behaviors included in Mercer's model are empathy, sensitivity to infant cues, self-esteem and self-concept, parenting received as a child, maturity and flexibility, attitudes, pregnancy and birth experience, health, depression, and role conflict. Infant traits having an impact on maternal role identity include temperament, ability to send cues, appearance, general characteristics, responsiveness, and health. Examples of the infant's developmental responses that interact with mother's developing maternal identity—depicted as *a* through *d* in Figure 27-2—include the following:

a. Eye contact with the mother as she talks to her or him, grasp reflex

b. Smile reflex and quieting behavior in response to mother's care

c. Consistent interactive behaviors with mother

d. Eliciting responses from the mother; increasingly more mobile

According to Mercer (1995):

The personal role identity stage is reached when the mother has integrated the role into her self system with a congruence of self and other roles; she is secure in her identity as mother, is emotionally committed to her infant, and feels a sense of harmony, satisfaction, and competence in the role. (p. 14)

Using Burke and Tully's (1977) work, Mercer (1995) stated that a role identity has internal and external components: the identity is the internalized view of self (recognized maternal identity), and role is the external, behavioral component.

Becoming a Mother: A Revised Model

Mercer has continued to use both her own research and the research of others as building blocks for her theory. In 2003, she began reexamining the Theory of Maternal Role Attainment, proposing that the term *becoming a mother* more accurately reflects the process based on recent research. According to Mercer (2004), the concept of role attainment suggests an end point rather than an ongoing process and may not address the continued expansion of the self as a mother. Mercer's conclusions are based largely on current nursing research about the cognitive and behavioral dimensions of women becoming mothers. Walker, Crain, and Thompson's (1986a, 1986b) questions about maternal role attainment as a continuing process contributed to Mercer's reexamination of her theory. Koniak-Griffin (1993) also questioned the behavioral and cognitive dimensions of maternal role attainment. Hartrick (1997) reported that women in her study of mothers of children from 3 to 16 years old undergo a continual process of self-definition. McBride and Shore (2001) in their research on mothers and grandmothers suggested that there may be a need to retire the term *maternal role attainment* because "it implies a static situation rather than fluctuating process" (p. 79). Finally, in a synthesis of nine qualitative studies, Nelson (2003) described continued growth and transformation in women as they become mothers. Mercer (2004) acknowledged that new challenges in motherhood require making new connections to regain confidence in the self and proposes replacing the term *maternal role attainment* with *becoming a mother*.

Qualitative studies have identified stages of maternal role attainment using the descriptive terms of participants. A compilation of the results of several of these studies have led Mercer (2004) to the following proposed changes in the names of stages leading to maternal role identity:

- Commitment and preparation (pregnancy)
- Acquaintance, practice, and physical restoration (first 2 weeks)
- Approaching normalization (second week to 4 months)
- Integration of maternal identity (approximately 4 months)

These stages parallel the original stages in Mercer's theory, but they embrace the maternal experience more completely and use terminology derived from new mothers' descriptions of their experiences.

Theory-building, according to Mercer (personal communication, September 3, 2003), is a continual process as research provides evidence for clarifying concepts, additions, and deletions. Although many of the more recent studies support the findings of both Rubin and Mercer, Mercer (2004) recognized the evidence for needed changes in her original theory for greater clarity and consistency. It is with this insight that she proposed retiring the term *maternal role attainment*. Mercer (2004) acknowledges that becoming a mother, which connotes continued growth in mothering, is more descriptive of the process, which is much larger than a role. Although some roles may be terminated, motherhood is a life-long commitment.

Mercer has continued to use Bronfenbrenner's concept of interacting nested ecological environments. However, she renamed them to reflect the living environments: family and friends, community, and society at large (Figure 27-3). The new model places the interactions between mother, infant, and father at the center of the interacting, living environments (R. Mercer, personal communication, September 3, 2003). Variables within the family and friends environment include social support, family values, cultural guidelines for parenting, family functioning, and stressors. The community environment includes day care, places of worship, schools, work setting, hospitals, recreational facilities, and cultural centers. Within the society at large, influences come from laws affecting woman and children, evolving reproductive and neonatal science, transmitted cultural consistencies, and national health care programs.

LOGICAL FORM

Mercer used both deductive and inductive logic in developing the theoretical framework for studying factors that influence maternal role attainment during the first year of motherhood and in her theory. Deductive logic is demonstrated in Mercer's use of works from other researchers and disciplines. Role and developmental theories and the work of Rubin on maternal role attainment provided a base for the original framework. Mercer also used inductive logic in the development of her Theory of Maternal Role Attainment. Through practice and research, she observed adaptation to motherhood from a variety of circumstances. She noted that differences existed in adaptation to motherhood when maternal illness complicated the postpartum period, when a child with a defect was born, and when a teenager became a mother. These observations directed the research about those situations and the subsequent development of her theory. Proposed changes to her theory have been based on more recent research and deductive reasoning coupled with her belief in improving the clarity and usefulness of her theory.

ACCEPTANCE BY THE NURSING COMMUNITY
Practice

Mercer's theory is highly practice oriented. The concepts in her theory have been cited in many obstetrical textbooks and have been used in practice by

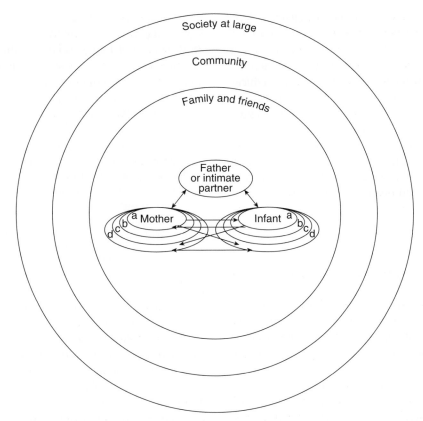

Figure **27-3** **Becoming a Mother: A revised model.** (From R. T. Mercer, personal communication, September 3, 2003.)

nurses and those in other disciplines. Both the theory and the model are capable of serving as a framework for assessment, planning, implementing, and evaluating nursing care of new mothers and their infants. The utility of Mercer's theory and its relationship to practice is described by Meighan (2001) in the second edition of *Nursing Theory: Utilization & Application* by Alligood and Marriner Tomey. Mercer's theory is useful to practicing nurses across many maternal-child settings. Mercer (1986a, 1986b) linked her research findings with nursing practice at each interval from birth through the first year, making her theory applicable in a variety of pediatric settings.

In addition, Mercer's theory has been used in organizing patient care. Concepts in the research conducted by Neeson, Patterson, Mercer, and May (1983), "Pregnancy Outcome for Adolescents Receiving Prenatal Care by Nurse Practitioners in Extended Roles," were used in setting up a clinical practice. Clark, Rapkin, Busen, and Vasquez (2001) used Mercer's theory to establish and test a parent education curriculum for substance-abusing women in a residential treatment facility.

Education

Mercer's work has appeared extensively in both maternity and pediatric nursing texts, but not only as it relates to maternal role attainment; each piece of research is used and valued. Many of the current concepts in maternal-child nursing are based on

Mercer's research. Her theory and model help simplify the very complex process of becoming a parent. The Theory of Maternal Role Attainment is credited with enhancing understanding and making Mercer's contribution extremely valuable to nursing education. The Theory of Maternal Role Attainment provides a framework for students as they learn to plan and provide care for parents in a wide variety of settings. Mercer's theory and research have also been used in other disciplines as they relate to parenting and maternal role attainment. It has been shown to be helpful to students in psychology, sociology, and education.

Research

Mercer has advocated the involvement of students in faculty research. During her tenure at the University of California, San Francisco, she chaired committees and was a committee member for numerous graduate theses and dissertations. Her work has been used as the basis for several graduate students' topics of research. Collaborative research with a graduate student and junior faculty member in 1977 and 1978 led to the development of a highly reliable, valid instrument to measure mothers' attitudes about the labor and delivery experience. Numerous researchers have requested permission to use the instrument.

Mercer's many research and scholarly achievements are evidence of her great contribution to nursing research. Her work has served as a springboard for other researchers. Mercer's theoretical framework for a correlational study exploring differences between three age groups of first-time mothers (ages 15 to 19, 20 to 29, and 30 to 42) has been tested in part by others, including Walker and colleagues (1986a, 1986b). Sank (1991) used Mercer's theory in her doctoral dissertation research at the University of Texas, Austin, entitled *Factors in the Prenatal Period That Affect Parental Role Attainment During the Postpartum Period in Black American Mothers and Fathers*. Mercer's Theory of Maternal Role Attainment also served as the framework for Washington's (1997) dissertation, *Learning Needs of Adolescent Mothers When Identifying Fever and Illnesses in Infants Less Than Twelve Months of Age* at the University of Miami. Bacon (2001), a student at the Chicago School of Professional Psychology, used Mercer's theory in her dissertation, Maternal Role Attainment *and* Maternal *Identity in Mothers of Premature Infants.*

McBride (1984) wrote the following:

> Maternal role attainment has been a fundamental concern of nursing since the pioneering work of Mercer's mentor, Rubin, almost two decades ago. It is now becoming the research-based, theoretically sound construct that nurse researchers have been searching for in their analysis of the experience of new mothers. (p. 72)

FURTHER DEVELOPMENT

Mercer used her initial research as a building block for other studies. In later research, Mercer aimed at identifying predictors of maternal-infant attachment on the basis of maternal experience with childbirth and maternal risk status. She also examined paternal competence on the basis of experience with childbirth and pregnancy risk status. In another study, she developed and tested a causal model to predict partner relationships in high-risk and low-risk pregnancy. More work and refinement of the original model and theory have taken place during the past few years, as described earlier. She included the importance of the father in maternal role attainment, adding this to her model and theory in a section of her 1995 book, *Becoming a Mother: Research on Maternal Identity From Rubin to the Present.*

In her book, *First-Time Motherhood: Experiences From Teens to Forties,* Mercer (1986a) presented a model of the following four phases occurring in the process of maternal role attainment during the first year of motherhood:

1. The physical recovery phase, occurring from birth to 1 month
2. The achievement phase, from 2 to 4 or 5 months
3. The disruptions phase, occurring from 6 to 8 months
4. The reorganization phase, from after the eighth month and still in process at 1 year

Additionally, adaptation to the maternal role was proposed to occur at three levels (biological, psychological, and social), which are interacting and interdependent throughout the phases. These phases and levels of adaptation were described briefly and were applied to her research. In 2003, additional changes to the theory were proposed by Mercer (2004), including abandoning maternal role attainment for the term *becoming a mother*. Changes to the model and adoption of the following four more descriptive phases to the process of becoming a mother were also proposed:

1. Commitment and preparation (pregnancy)
2. Acquaintance, practice, and physical restoration (first 2 weeks)
3. Approaching normalization (second week to 4 months)
4. Integration of maternal identity (approximately 4 months)

These changes were based on the research studies of other nurses and are evidence of Mercer's continued scrutiny and critique of her own theory to improve its utility in practice and research.

According to Mercer, further research is needed in several areas. More testing and revision of the proposed causal model, developed to predict partner relationships, are needed (Mercer et al., 1988; Mercer & Ferketich, 1990a, 1995). In addition, more information is needed about the antecedents and mediators of partner relationships when pregnancy is at high risk (Mercer & Ferketich, 1990b, 1994, 1995). Mercer also emphasized the need for more research into sources of stress and anxiety that potentially interfere with maternal-infant attachment and role competence (Ferketich & Mercer, 1995a, 1995b).

In paternal-infant attachment and paternal role competence studies, Mercer noted higher rates of depression among inexperienced fathers (Ferketich & Mercer, 1995a, 1995c). She stresses the need for further research to develop interventions for depression among first-time fathers during the first year (Ferketich & Mercer, 1995b). Continued testing of the application of Mercer's framework in a variety of perinatal situations, including multiple gestation, would be useful, and investigation of theory beyond the first year is also warranted.

Mercer's concern for the utility and applicability of her theory is evident in her continued work toward clarity and usefulness. Her revisions to her theory in 2003, although based on nursing research, have not been tested in other studies. Mercer's (2004) proposal of abandoning maternal role attainment for the term *becoming a mother* is argued logically but has not been put to use in practice or research. Although qualitative research to describe the phases of becoming a mother uses the exact words of women experiencing this transition, these phases have not been confirmed among women in other cultures or in different circumstances.

CRITIQUE
Clarity

The concepts, variables, and relationships have not always been defined explicitly, but they were described and implied in Mercer's earlier work. However, the concepts were defined theoretically and operationalized consistently. Work toward improving clarity is evident. Concepts, assumptions, and goals have been organized into a logical and coherent whole, so that understanding the interrelationships among the concepts is relatively easy. Some interchanging of terms and labels used to identify concepts, such as adaptation and attainment, social support, and support network, are potentially confusing for the reader. Additionally, maternal role attainment has not been defined consistently, which can obstruct clarity. Maternal identity, a term that Mercer defines as the final stage of role attainment (personal or role identity stage), is sometimes substituted for maternal role attainment. According to Mercer (1995), when the maternal role has been attained, the mother has achieved a maternal identity, the internalized role of mother. However, the terms *attainment* and *role identity* are sometimes confusing.

Mercer has continued to work toward greater clarity. She has proposed using terms derived from nursing researchers that would be understood more clearly by users of her theory. She has questioned the use of the term *maternal role attainment,* because it connotes a static state rather than the continuously evolving role as a mother. She has also examined qualitative research containing the exact words of women experiencing motherhood and has favored using these words to describe the stages of becoming a mother.

Simplicity

Despite numerous concepts and relationships, the theoretical framework for maternal role attainment or becoming a mother organizes a rather complex phenomenon into an easily understood and useful form. The theory is predictive in nature and readily lends itself to guide practice. Concepts are not specific to time and place and are abstract, but they are described and operationalized to the extent that meanings are not easily misinterpreted. However, it should be noted that the research to define and support the theoretical relationships was very complex, which was due largely to the great number of concepts. The process of becoming a mother is multifaceted and varies considerably according to the individual and to environmental influences. Mercer's theory provides a framework for understanding this complex, multidimensional process.

Generality

Mercer's theory is derived from and is specific to parent-child nursing but has been used by other disciplines concerned with mothering and parenting. The theory can be generalized to all women during pregnancy through the first year after birth, regardless of age, parity, or environment. It is among the few theories applicable to high-risk perinatal patients and their families. As previously mentioned, it can be applied to a variety of pediatric settings. Mercer (1995) has also respecified her theory to study and predict parental attachment, including that of the pregnant woman's partner. Therefore, it is useful in both studying and working with family members following birth. Mercer's work has done

much to broaden the range of application of previously existing theories on maternal role attainment, because her studies have spanned various developmental levels and situational contexts, a quality that many other studies do not share.

Empirical Precision

Mercer's work has evolved from extensive research efforts. The concepts, assumptions, and relationships are grounded predominantly in empirical observations and are congruent. The degree of concreteness and the completeness of operational definitions further increase the empirical precision. The theoretical framework for exploring differences among age groups of first-time mothers lends itself well to further testing and is being used by others for this purpose. The continued scrutiny by Mercer herself has continually improved her theory and solidified her concepts. Mercer's most recent proposed changes to improve clarity of concepts are based on research studies of others within the discipline of nursing.

Derivable Consequences

The theoretical framework for maternal role attainment during the first year has proved to be useful, practical, and valuable to nursing. Mercer's work is used repeatedly in research, practice, and education. The framework is also readily applicable to any discipline that works with mothers and children during the first year of motherhood. McBride (1984) wrote, "Dr. Mercer is the one who developed the most complete theoretical framework for studying one aspect of parental experience, namely, the factors that influence the attainment of the maternal role in the first year of motherhood" (p. 72).

Throughout her career, Mercer consistently has linked research to practice. Implications for nursing or nursing interventions are addressed and provide the bond between research and practice in most of her works. She believes that nursing research is the "bridge to excellence" in nursing practice (Mercer, 1984, p. 47).

SUMMARY

The Theory of Maternal Role Attainment has been shown to be useful in both research and practice for nurses, as well as other disciplines concerned with parenting. Mercer's continued devotion to improving the usefulness and clarity of her theory and model is evident and has served well those who use her theory. Mercer's use of both her own and the research of others strengthens her work. Her proposal to adopt the Theory of Becoming a Mother is based solidly on the research process. Motherhood and attainment of the parenting role is a very complex, multilevel process. Mercer's theory and her work make this process logical and understandable and provide a solid foundation for practice, education, and research.

Case Study

Susan, a 19-year-old woman, delivered her first infant prematurely 5 days ago. Although her postpartum course has been relatively uneventful, the infant has had difficulty and must remain hospitalized. Susan and her young husband visit the nursery every afternoon to be with the baby, but they ask very few questions. In talking with the couple, the nurse learns that the only living grandparents of the baby live a great distance away. Susan will not have any family or friends to turn to when she takes the baby home.

In this high-risk perinatal case, Mercer's framework should be useful for nursing assessment and intervention to facilitate maternal role attainment. How would you use it as a guide in planning care for Susan?

CRITICAL THINKING *Activities*

1. In your own practice, consider Mercer's Theory and Model of Maternal Role Attainment as a guide. In what ways is it useful?

2. High-risk families often continue to experience problems for years after the birth of a child with a congenital problem. Can Mercer's theory be adapted to help in assessment and intervention for these mothers and their families beyond the first year? What areas need further research and development?

3. Consider the current health care environment. Does the model proposed by Mercer adequately address current changes in health care delivery and the impact on the family? What changes in Mercer's model, if any, would you suggest?

4. Mercer has proposed changing her theory from Maternal Role Attainment to Becoming a Mother to address the evolving role of motherhood. Do you agree or disagree with this change? Would this alter the theory's use in the clinical setting in any way?

REFERENCES

Bacon, A. C. (2001). Maternal role attainment and maternal identity in mothers of premature infants (Doctoral dissertation, Chicago School of Professional Psychology, Chicago, 2001). *Dissertation Abstracts International, 61,* 8-B. (University Microfilms No. 2001-95004-447)

Bronfenbrenner, U. (1979). *The ecology of human development: Experiment by nature and design.* Cambridge, MA: Harvard University Press.

Burke, P. J., & Tully, J. C. (1977). The measurement of role identity. *Social Forces, 55,* 881-897.

Burr, W. R., Leigh, G. K., Day, R. D., & Constantine, J. (1979). Symbolic interaction and the family. In W. R. Burr, R. Hill, F. I. Nye, & I. L. Reiss (Eds.), *Contemporary theories about the family* (Vol. 2, pp. 42-111). New York: Free Press.

Clark, B. S., Rapkin, D., Busen, N. H., & Vasquez, E. (2001). Nurse practitioners and parent education: A partnership for health. *Journal of the American Academy of Nurse Practitioners, 13*(7), 310-316.

Donley, M. G. (1993). Attachment and the emotional unit. *Family Process, 32,* 3-20.

Ferketich, S. L., & Mercer, R. T. (1995a). Paternal-infant attachment of experienced and inexperienced fathers during infancy. *Nursing Research, 44,* 31-37.

Ferketich, S. L., & Mercer, R. T. (1995b). Predictors of paternal role competence by risk status. *Nursing Research, 43,* 80-85.

Ferketich, S. L., & Mercer, R. T. (1995c). Predictors of role competence for experienced and inexperienced fathers. *Nursing Research, 44,* 89-95.

Hartrick, G. A. (1997). Women who are mothers: The experience of defining self. *Health Care for Women International, 18,* 263-277.

Koniak-Griffin, D. (1993). Maternal role attainment. *Image: The Journal of Nursing Scholarship, 25,* 257-262.

McBride, A. B. (1984). The experience of being a parent. *Annual Review of Nursing Research, 2,* 63-81.

McBride, A. B., & Shore, C. P. (2001). Women as mothers and grandmothers. *Annual Review of Nursing Research, 19,* 63-85.

Mead, G. H. (1934). *Mind, self and society.* Chicago: University of Chicago Press.

Meighan, M. (2001). Mercer's maternal role theory and nursing practice. In M. R. Alligood & A. Marriner Tomey (Eds.), *Nursing theory: Utilization & application* (2nd ed., pp. 367-383). St. Louis: Mosby.

Mercer, R. T. (1977). *Nursing care for parents at risk.* Thorofare, NJ: Charles B. Slack.

Mercer, R. T. (1979). *Perspectives on adolescent health care.* Philadelphia: J. B. Lippincott.

Mercer, R. T. (1981). A theoretical framework for studying factors that impact on the maternal role. *Nursing Research, 30,* 73-77.

Mercer, R. T. (1984). Nursing research: The bridge to excellence in practice. *Image: The Journal of Nursing Scholarship, 16*(2), 47-51.

Mercer, R. T. (1985a). The process of maternal role attainment over the first years. *Nursing Research, 34,* 198-204.

Mercer, R. T. (1985b). The relationship of age and other variables to gratification in mothering. *Health Care for Women International, 6,* 295-308.

Mercer, R. T. (1986a). *First-time motherhood: Experiences from teens to forties.* New York: Springer.

Mercer, R. T. (1986b). The relationship of developmental variables to maternal behavior. *Research in Nursing Health, 9,* 25-33.

Mercer, R. T. (1989). Responses to life-span development: A review of theory and practice for families with chronically ill members. *Scholarly Inquiry for Nursing Practice: An International Journal, 3,* 23-26.

Mercer, R. T. (1990). *Parents at risk.* New York: Springer.

Mercer, R. T. (1995). *Becoming a mother: Research on maternal identity from Rubin to the present.* New York: Springer.

Mercer, R. T. (2004). Becoming a mother versus maternal role attainment. *Journal of Nursing Scholarship, 36*(3), 226-232.

Mercer, R. T., & Ferketich, S. L. (1990a). Predictors of family functioning eight months following birth. *Nursing Research, 39,* 76-82.

Mercer, R. T., & Ferketich, S. L. (1990b). Predictors of parental attachment during early parenthood. *Journal of Advanced Nursing, 15,* 268-280.

Mercer, R. T., & Ferketich, S. L. (1994). Maternal-infant attachment of experienced and inexperienced mothers during infancy. *Nursing Research, 43,* 344-350.

Mercer, R. T., & Ferketich, S. L. (1995). Experienced and inexperienced mothers' maternal competence during infancy. *Research in Nursing Health, 18,* 333-343.

Mercer, R. T., Ferketich, S. L., & DeJoseph, J. F. (1993). Predictors of partner relationships during pregnancy and infancy. *Research in Nursing Health, 16,* 45-56.

Mercer, R. T., Ferketich, S. L., DeJoseph, J., May, K. A., & Sollid, D. (1988). Effects of stress on family functioning during pregnancy. *Nursing Research, 37,* 268-275.

Mercer, R. T., Hackley, K. C., & Bostrom, A. (1984). Social support of teenage mothers. *Birth Defects: Original Article Series, 20*(5), 245-290.

Mercer, R. T., May, K. A., Ferketich, S., & DeJoseph, J. (1986). Theoretical models for studying the effect of antepartum stress on the family. *Nursing Research, 35,* 339-346.

Neeson, J. D., Patterson, K. A., Mercer, R. T., & May, K. A. (1983). Pregnancy outcome for adolescents receiving prenatal care by nurse practitioners in extended roles. *Journal of Adolescent Health Care, 4,* 94-99.

Nelson, A. M. (2003). Transition to motherhood. *Journal of Obstetric, Gynecologic, & Neonatal Nursing, 32,* 465-477.

Rubin, R. (1977). Binding-in in the postpartum period. *Maternal Child Nursing Journal, 6,* 67-75.

Rubin, R. (1984). *Maternal identity and the maternal experience.* New York: Springer.

Sank, J. C. (1991). Factors in the prenatal period that affect parental role attainment during the postpartum period in black American mothers and fathers (Doctoral dissertation, University of Texas, Austin, Texas, 1991). (University Microfilms No. 1993-155453)

Thornton, R., & Nardi, P. M. (1975). The dynamics of role acquisition. *American Journal of Sociology, 80,* 870-885.

Turner, J. H. (1978). *The structure of sociological theory* (Revised ed.). Homewood, IL: Dorsey Press.

von Bertalanffy, L. (1968). *General system theory.* New York: George Braziller.

Walker, L. O., Crain, H., & Thompson, E. (1986a). Maternal role attainment and identity in the postpartum period: Stability and change. *Nursing Research, 35*(2), 68-71.

Walker, L. O., Crain, H., & Thompson, E. (1986b). Mothering behavior and maternal role attainment during the postpartum period. *Nursing Research, 35*(6), 322-325.

Washington, L. J. (1997). Learning needs of adolescent mothers when identifying fever and illnesses in infants less than twelve months of age (Doctoral dissertation, University of Miami, Miami). *Dissertation Abstracts International, 57,* (12-B). (University Microfilms No. 1997-95012-208)

Werner, H. (1957). The concept of development from a comparative and organismic point of view. In D. H. Harris (Ed.), *The concept of development* (pp. 125-148). Minneapolis: University of Minnesota.

BIBLIOGRAPHY
Primary Sources
Books

Mercer, R. T. (1977). *Nursing care for parents at risk.* Thorofare, NJ: Charles B. Slack.

Mercer, R. T. (1979). *Perspectives on adolescent health care.* Philadelphia: J. B. Lippincott.

Mercer, R. T. (1986). *First-time motherhood: Experiences from teens to forties.* New York: Springer.

Mercer, R. T. (1990). *Parents at risk.* New York: Springer.

Mercer, R. T. (1995). *Becoming a mother: Research on maternal identity from Rubin to the present.* New York: Springer.

Journal Articles

Ferketich, S. L., & Mercer, R. T. (1995). Paternal-infant attachment of experienced and inexperienced fathers during infancy. *Nursing Research, 44,* 31-37.

Ferketich, S. L., & Mercer, R. T. (1995). Predictors of role competence for experienced and inexperienced fathers. *Nursing Research, 44,* 89-95.

Mercer, R. T. (1995). A tribute to Reva Rubin. *Maternal Child Nursing, 20,* 184.

Mercer, R. T. (1997). Chronically ill children: How families adjust. *Nurseweek, 10*(9), 14-15, 17.

Mercer, R. T. (1997). The employed mother's challenges. *Nurseweek, 10*(17), 10-11, 15.

Mercer, R. T. (2000). Response to "Life-span development: A review of theory and practice for families with chronically ill members." *Scholarly Inquiry for Nursing Practice, 14*(4), 375-378.

Mercer, R. T. (2004). Becoming a mother versus maternal role attainment. *Journal of Nursing Scholarship, 36*(3), 226-232.

Mercer, R. T., & Ferketich, S. L. (1995). Experienced and inexperienced mothers' maternal competence during infancy. *Research in Nursing Health, 18,* 333-343.

Continuing Education Courses

Mercer, R. T. (1998, 2000, 2004). Adolescent sexuality and childbearing (Online). *Nurseweek* Continuing Education Offering.

Mercer, R. T. (1998, 2000, 2004). Transitions to parenthood. A continuing education offering 6.0 hours (Online). *Nurseweek.* Accessed March 25, 2005: *www2.nurseweek.com/ce/self-study_modules/syllabus.html?=40b*

Mercer, R. T. (1991, 1997, 2001, 2003). Helping parents when the unexpected occurs (Online). *Nurseweek.* Accessed January 4, 2005: *www2.nurseweek.com/ce/self-study_modules/syllabus.html?ID=390*

Online Publications

Mercer, R. T. (1991). Chronically ill children: How families adjust (Online). *Nurseweek.* Accessed January 4, 2005: *http://nurseweek.com/ce/ce565a.html*

Mercer, R. T. (1997, 26 August). The employed mother's challenges (Online). *Nurseweek.* Accessed January 4, 2005: *http://nurseweek.com/ce/ce250a.html*

Secondary Sources
Web Sites

Cardinal Stritch University Library. (2004). *Model and theories of nursing. Ramona T. Mercer: Maternal role attainment.* Milwaukee, WI: Cardinal Stritch University. Accessed January 4, 2005: *http://library.stritch.edu/nursingtheroies/mercer.htm*

Hahn School of Nursing and Health Science. (2000). *Mid-range theories: Maternal role attainment.* San Diego, CA: University of San Diego. Accessed January 4, 2005: *http://www.sandiego.edu/nursing/theory/*

Nurses for Nurses Everywhere. (2004). *Nurse information: Ramona T. Mercer.* Melbourne, Australia: Nurses.info. Accessed January 4, 2005: *http://www.nurses.info/nursing_theory_midrange_theories_ramona_mercer.htm*

Nurses for Nurses Everywhere. (2004). *Nurse information: Reva Rubin.* Melbourne, Australia: Nurses.info.

Accessed January 4, 2005: *http://www.nurses.info/ nursing_theory_midrange_theories_reva_rubin.htm*

Sartore, A. T. (1996). Maternal role attainment in adolescent mothers: Foundations and implications. *Online Journal of Knowledge Synthesis for Nursing, 3*(11). Accessed January 4, 2005: *http://www.stti.iupui.edu/ library/ojksn/articles/030011.pdf.*

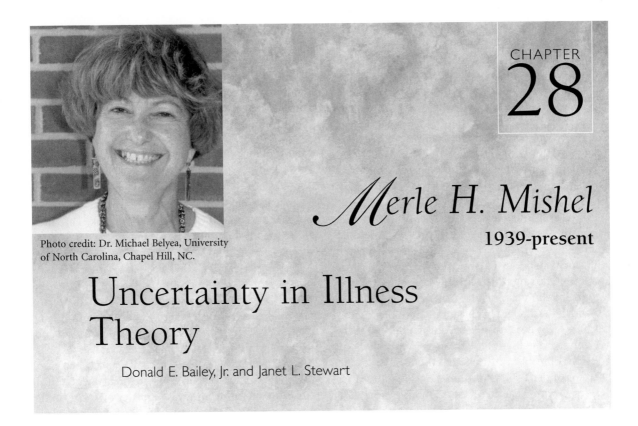

Photo credit: Dr. Michael Belyea, University of North Carolina, Chapel Hill, NC.

Merle H. Mishel

1939-present

Uncertainty in Illness Theory

Donald E. Bailey, Jr. and Janet L. Stewart

CREDENTIALS AND BACKGROUND OF THE THEORIST

Merle H. Mishel was born in Boston, Massachusetts. She graduated from Boston University with a B.A. in 1961 and received her M.S. in psychiatric nursing from the University of California in 1966. Mishel completed her M.A. and Ph.D. in social psychology at the Claremont Graduate School, Claremont, California, in 1976 and 1980, respectively. Her dissertation research, supported by an individual National Research Service Award, was the development and testing of the Perceived Ambiguity in Illness Scale, later renamed the Mishel Uncertainty in Illness Scale (MUIS-A). The original scale has been used as the basis for the following three additional scales:

The authors wish to think Dr. Merle Mishel for her review and input for this chapter.

1. A community version (MUIS-C) for chronically ill individuals who are not hospitalized or receiving active medical care
2. A measure of parents' perceptions of uncertainty (PPUS) with regard to their child's illness experience
3. A measure of uncertainty in spouses or other family members when another member of the family is acutely ill (PPUS-FM)

Early in her professional career, Mishel practiced as a psychiatric nurse in acute care and community settings. While persuing her doctorate, she was on faculty in the Department of Nursing at the California State University at Los Angeles, rising from assistant to full professor. In addition, she practiced as a nurse therapist in both community and private practice settings from 1973 to 1979. After completing her doctorate in social psychology, she relocated to the University of Arizona College of Nursing in

623

1981 as an associate professor and was promoted to professor in 1988. She served as Division Head of Mental Health Nursing from 1984 to 1991. While at the University of Arizona, Mishel received numerous intramural and extramural research grants that supported the continued development of the theoretical framework of uncertainty in illness. During this period, she continued practicing as a nurse therapist, working with the heart transplant program at the University Medical Center. She was inducted as a fellow in the American Academy of Nursing in 1990.

Mishel returned to the east coast in 1991 and joined the faculty as a professor in the School of Nursing, University of North Carolina at Chapel Hill, and was awarded the endowed Kenan Professor of Nursing Chair in 1994. Friends of the National Institute of Nursing Research presented her with a Research Merit Award in 1997 and invited her to present her research as an exemplar of federally funded nursing intervention studies at a Congressional Breakfast in 1999. In addition, she is the Director of the T-32 Institutional National Research Service Award Training Grant, Interventions for Preventing and Managing Chronic Illness. The T-32 awards predoctoral and postdoctoral fellowships to nurses interested in developing interventions for a variety of underserved chronically ill patients. Mishel also maintains a prolific program of nursing intervention research with several cancer populations. Of note is that Mishel's research program has been funded continually by the NIH since 1984, such that each research grant has built upon findings from prior studies in order to move systematically toward theoretically derived, scientifically tested nursing interventions.

In addition to the awards previously identified, Mishel was the recipient of a Sigma Theta Tau International Sigma Xi Chapter Nurse Research Predoctoral Fellowship from 1977 to 1979 and received the Mary Opal Wolanin Research Award in 1986. In 1987, Mishel was first alternate for the Fulbright Award. She has been a visiting scholar at many institutions throughout North America, including University of Nebraska, University of Texas at Houston, University of Tennessee at Knoxville, University of South Carolina, University of Rochester, Yale University, and McGill University. She served as doctoral program consultant for the University of Cincinnati College of Nursing from 1991 to 1992 and Rutgers University School of Nursing in 1993. Over the last 10 years, Mishel has presented more than 75 invited addresses at schools of nursing throughout the United States and Canada. Reflecting the growing international interest in her theory and measurement models, Mishel conducted an International Symposium on Uncertainty at Kyungpook National University in Daegu, South Korea, and served as a visiting scholar at Mahidol University in Bangkok, Thailand.

Mishel is a member of a number of professional organizations. They include the American Academy of Nursing, Sigma Theta Tau International, American Psychological Association, American Nurses Association, Society of Behavioral Medicine, Oncology Nursing Society, Southern Nursing Research Society, and the Society for Education and Research in Psychiatric Nursing. She has served as a grant reviewer for the National Cancer Institute, National Center for Nursing Research, and National Institute on Aging and was a charter member of the study section on human immunodeficiency virus (HIV) at the National Institute of Mental Health.

THEORETICAL SOURCES

When Mishel began her research into uncertainty, the concept had not previously been applied in the health and illness context. Her original Uncertainty in Illness Theory (Mishel, 1988) drew from existing information-processing models (Warburton, 1979) and personality research (Budner, 1962) from the psychology discipline, which characterized uncertainty as a cognitive state resulting from insufficient cues with which to form a cognitive schema or internal representation of a situation or event. Mishel attributes the underlying stress-appraisal-coping-adaptation framework in the original theory to the work of Lazarus and Folkman (1984). The unique aspect was her application of this framework to uncertainty as a stressor in the context of illness, which made the framework particularly meaningful for nursing.

With the reconceptualization of the theory, Mishel (1990) recognized that the Western approach to science supported a mechanistic view in its emphasis on control and predictability. By using critical social theory, Mishel recognized the bias inherent in the original theory, an orientation toward certainty and adaptation. Mishel then incorporated tenets from chaos theory which, because of its focus on open systems, allowed for a more accurate representation of how chronic illness creates disequilibrium and how people ultimately can incorporate continual uncertainty to find new meaning in illness.

MAJOR CONCEPTS & DEFINITIONS

UNCERTAINTY

Uncertainty is the inability to determine the meaning of illness-related events, occurring when the decision maker is unable to assign definite value to objects or events, or is unable to predict outcomes accurately (Mishel, 1988).

COGNITIVE SCHEMA

Cognitive schema is a person's subjective interpretation of illness, treatment, and hospitalization (Mishel, 1988).

STIMULI FRAME

Stimuli frame is the form, composition, and structure of the stimuli that a person perceives, which are then structured into a cognitive schema (Mishel, 1988).

Symptom Pattern

Symptom pattern is the degree to which symptoms occur with sufficient consistency to be perceived as having a pattern or configuration (Mishel, 1988).

Event Familiarity

Event familiarity is the degree to which a situation is habitual, repetitive, or contains recognized cues (Mishel, 1988).

Event Congruence

Event congruence refers to the consistency between the expected and the experienced in illness-related events (Mishel, 1988).

STRUCTURE PROVIDERS

Structure providers are the resources available to assist the person in the interpretation of the stimuli frame (Mishel, 1988).

Credible Authority

Credible authority is the degree of trust and confidence a person has in his or her health care providers (Mishel, 1988).

Social Supports

Social supports influence uncertainty by assisting the individual to interpret the meaning of events (Mishel, 1988).

COGNITIVE CAPACITIES

Cognitive capacities are the information-processing abilities of a person, reflecting both innate capabilities and situational constraints (Mishel, 1988).

INFERENCE

Inference refers to the evaluation of uncertainty using related, recalled experiences (Mishel, 1988).

ILLUSION

Illusion refers to beliefs constructed out of uncertainty (Mishel, 1988).

ADAPTATION

Adaptation reflects biopsychosocial behavior occurring within persons' individually defined range of usual behavior (Mishel, 1988).

Continued

MAJOR CONCEPTS *&* DEFINITIONS—cont'd

NEW VIEW OF LIFE

New view of life refers to the formulation of a new sense of order, resulting from the integration of continual uncertainty into one's self-structure, in which uncertainty is accepted as the natural rhythm of life (Mishel, 1988).

PROBABILISTIC THINKING

Probabilistic thinking refers to a belief in a conditional world in which the expectation of continual certainty and predictability is abandoned (Mishel, 1988).

USE OF EMPIRICAL EVIDENCE

The Uncertainty in Illness Theory grew out of Mishel's dissertation research with hospitalized patients, for which she used both qualitative and quantitative findings to generate the first conceptualization of uncertainty in the context of illness. Beginning with the publication of Mishel's Uncertainty in Illness Scale (Mishel, 1981), there has been extensive research into adults' experiences with uncertainty related to chronic and life-threatening illnesses. Considerable empirical evidence has accumulated to support Mishel's theoretical model in adults. Several recent integrative reviews of uncertainty research have comprehensively summarized and critiqued the current state of the science (Mast, 1995; Mishel, 1997a, 1999; Stewart & Mishel, 2000). The authors include studies here that directly support the elements of Mishel's uncertainty model.

Most empirical studies have focused predominantly on two of the antecedents of uncertainty, stimuli frame and structure providers, and the relationship between uncertainty and psychological outcomes. Mishel tested other elements of the model, such as the mediating roles of appraisal and coping, early in her program of research (Mishel & Braden, 1987; Mishel, Padilla, Grant, & Sorenson, 1991; Mishel & Sorenson, 1991), but these model elements, along with cognitive capacity as an antecedent to uncertainty, have generated less research attention.

Several studies have shown that objective or subjective indicators of the severity of life-threat or illness symptoms were associated positively with uncertainty (Braden, 1990; Grootenhuis & Last, 1997; Hinds, Birenbaum, Clarke-Steffen, Quargnenti, Kreissman et al., 1996; Janson-Bjerklie, Ferketich, & Benner, 1993; Tomlinson, Kirschbaum, Harbaugh, & Anderson, 1996). Across a sustained illness trajectory, unpredictability in symptom onset, duration, and intensity have been related to perceived uncertainty (Becker, Jason-Bjerklie, Benner, Slobin, & Ferketich, 1993; Brown & Powell-Cope, 1991; Jessop & Stein, 1985; Mishel & Braden, 1988; Murray, 1993). Similarly, the ambiguous nature of illness symptoms and the consequent difficulty in determining the significance of physical sensations frequently have been identified as sources of uncertainty (Cohen, 1993; Comaroff & Maguire, 1981; Hilton, 1988; Nelson, 1996; Weitz, 1989).

Mishel and Braden (1988) found that social support had a direct impact on uncertainty by reducing perceived complexity and an indirect impact through its effect on the predictability of symptom pattern. The perception of stigma associated with some conditions, particularly HIV infection (Regan-Kubinski & Sharts-Hopko, 1995; Weitz, 1989) and Down's syndrome (Van Riper & Selder, 1989), served to create uncertainty when families were unsure about how others would respond to the diagnosis. Family members have been shown consistently to experience high levels of uncertainty, as well, which may further reduce the amount of support experienced by the patient (Brown & Powell-Cope, 1991; Hilton, 1996; Wineman, O'Brien, Nealon, & Kaskel, 1993). In addition, uncertainty was heightened by interactions with health care providers in which patients and family members received unclear information or simplistic explanations that did not fit their experience, or perceived that care providers were not expert or responsive enough to help them manage the intricacies of the illness (Becker et al., 1993; Comaroff & Maguire, 1981; Mason, 1985; Sharkey, 1995).

Numerous studies have reported the negative impact of uncertainty on psychological outcomes, characterized variously as anxiety, depression, hopelessness, and psychological distress (Failla, Kuper, Nick, & Lee, 1996; Grootenhuis & Last, 1997; Jessop & Stein, 1985; Miles, Funk, & Kasper, 1992; Mishel & Sorenson, 1991; Schepp, 1991; Wineman, 1990). Uncertainty has also been shown to negatively impact quality of life (Braden, 1990; Padilla, Mishel, & Grant, 1992), satisfaction with family relationships (Wineman et al., 1993), satisfaction with health care services (Green & Murton, 1996; Turner, Tomlinson, & Harbaugh, 1990), and family caregivers' maintenance of their own self-care activities (Brett & Davies, 1988; Lang, 1987; O'Brien, Wineman, & Nealon, 1995).

Mishel reconceptualized the uncertainty theory in 1990 to accommodate responses to uncertainty over time in people with chronic conditions. The original theory was expanded to include the idea that uncertainty may not be resolved but may become part of an individual's reality. In this context, uncertainty is reappraised as an opportunity and prompts the formation of a new, probabilistic view of life. To adopt this new view of life, the patient must be able to rely on social resources and health care providers who themselves accept the idea of probabilistic thinking (Mishel, 1990). If uncertainty can be framed as a normal part of life, it can become a positive force for multiple opportunities with resulting positive mood states (Gelatt, 1989; Mishel, 1990).

Support for the reconceptualized Uncertainty in Illness Theory has been found in predominantly qualitative studies of people with a variety of chronic and life-threatening illnesses. The process of formulating a new view of life has been described by women with breast cancer and cardiac disease as a revised life perspective (Hilton, 1988), new life goals (Carter, 1993), new ways of being in the world

(Mast, 1998; Nelson, 1996), growth through uncertainty (Pelusi, 1997), and new levels of self-organization (Fleury, Kimbrell, & Kruszewski, 1995). In studies of predominantly men with chronic illness or their caregivers, the process has been described as transformed self-identity and new goals for living (Brown & Powell-Cope, 1991), a more positive perspective on life (Katz, 1996), reevaluating what is worthwhile (Nyhlin, 1990), contemplation and self-appraisal (Charmaz, 1995), uncertainty viewed as opportunity (Baier, 1995), and redefining normal and building new dreams (Mishel & Murdaugh, 1987).

MAJOR ASSUMPTIONS

Mishel's original Uncertainty in Illness Theory, first published in 1988, included several major assumptions (Figure 28-1). The first two reflect how uncertainty was conceptualized originally within the psychology discipline's information-processing models, as follows:

1. Uncertainty is a cognitive state, representing the inadequacy of an existing cognitive schema to support the interpretation of illness-related events.
2. Uncertainty is an inherently neutral experience, neither desirable nor aversive until it is appraised as such.

The next two assumptions reflect the uncertainty theory's roots in traditional stress and coping models, which posit a linear stress $\rightarrow$ coping $\rightarrow$ adaptation relationship, as follows:

3. Adaptation represents the continuity of an individual's usual biopsychosocial behavior and is the desired outcome of coping efforts to either reduce uncertainty appraised as danger or maintain uncertainty appraised as opportunity.
4. The relationships among illness events, uncertainty, appraisal, coping, and adaptation are linear and unidirectional, moving from situations promoting uncertainty toward adaptation.

Mishel herself challenged these last two assumptions in her reconceptualization of the theory, published in 1990. The reconceptualization came about as a result of contradictory findings when the theory

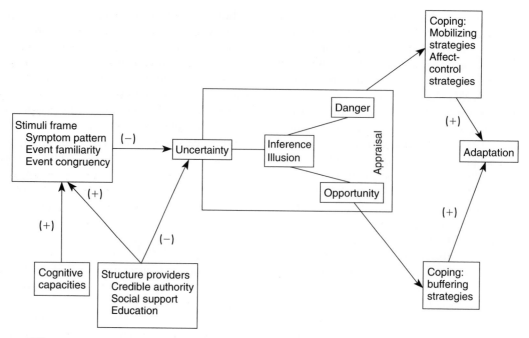

Figure **28-1 Model of perceived uncertainty in illness.** (From Mishel, M. H. [1988, Winter]. Uncertainty in illness. *Image: The Journal of Nursing Scholarship, 20,* 226.)

was applied to people with chronic illnesses. The original formulation of the theory held that uncertainty typically is appraised as an opportunity only in conditions that represent a known downward trajectory; in other words, uncertainty is appraised as opportunity when it is the alternative to negative certainty. Mishel and others found that people also appraised uncertainty as an opportunity in situations without a certain downward trajectory, particularly in long-term chronic illnesses, and that in this context people often developed a new view of life.

Dissatisfied with the traditional linear models that informed the original theory, Mishel turned to the more dynamic chaos theory to explain how prolonged uncertainty could function as a catalyst to change a person's perspective on life and illness. Chaos theory contributed two of the following theoretical assumptions, which replace the linear stress → coping → adaptation outcome portion of the model as follows:

1. People, as biopsychosocial systems, typically function in far-from-equilibrium states.
2. Major fluctuations in a far-from-equilibrium system enhance the system's receptivity to change.
3. Fluctuations result in repatterning, which is repeated at each level of the system.

In Mishel's reconceptualized model, neither the antecedents to uncertainty nor the process of cognitive appraisal of uncertainty as danger or opportunity changes. However, uncertainty over time, associated with a serious illness, functions as a catalyst for fluctuation in the system by threatening one's preexisting cognitive model of life as predictable and controllable. Because uncertainty pervades nearly every aspect of a person's life, its effects become concentrated and ultimately challenge the stability of the system. In response to the confusion and disorganization created by continued uncertainty, the system ultimately must change in order to survive.

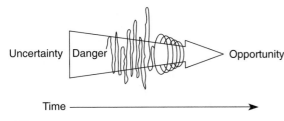

Figure **28-2** Reconceptualized model of uncertainty in chronic illness. (Copyright Merle Mishel, 1990.)

Ideally, under conditions of chronic uncertainty, a person gradually moves away from an evaluation of uncertainty as aversive to adopt a new view of life that accepts uncertainty as a part of reality (Figure 28-2). Thus uncertainty, especially in chronic or life-threatening illness, can result in a new level of organization and a new perspective on life, incorporating the growth and change that can result from uncertain experiences.

THEORETICAL ASSERTIONS

Mishel asserted the following (1988, 1990):

- Uncertainty occurs when a person cannot adequately structure or categorize an illness-related event because of the lack of sufficient cues.
- Uncertainty can take the form of ambiguity, complexity, lack of or inconsistent information, or unpredictability.
- As symptom pattern, event familiarity, and event congruence (stimuli frame) increase, uncertainty decreases.
- Structure providers (credible authority, social support, and education) decrease uncertainty directly by promoting interpretation of events, and indirectly by strengthening the stimuli frame.
- Uncertainty appraised as danger prompts coping efforts directed at reducing the uncertainty and managing the emotional arousal generated by it.
- Uncertainty appraised as opportunity prompts coping efforts directed at maintaining the uncertainty.

- The influence of uncertainty on psychological outcomes is mediated by the effectiveness of coping efforts to reduce uncertainty appraised as danger or to maintain uncertainty appraised as opportunity.
- When uncertainty appraised as danger cannot be reduced effectively, coping strategies can be employed to manage the emotional response.
- The longer uncertainty continues in the illness context, the more unstable the individual's previously accepted mode of functioning becomes.
- Under conditions of enduring uncertainty, individuals may develop a new, probabilistic perspective on life, which accepts uncertainty as a natural part of life.
- The process of integrating continual uncertainty into a new view of life can be blocked or prolonged by structure providers who do not support probabilistic thinking.
- Prolonged exposure to uncertainty appraised as danger can lead to intrusive thoughts, avoidance, and severe emotional distress.

LOGICAL FORM

As a middle range theory both derived from and applicable to clinical practice, Mishel's Uncertainty in Illness Theory is a classic example of the multiple steps required to develop theory with both heuristic and practical value. Neither purely inductive nor deductive, Mishel's theoretical work initially arose from asking questions about the nature of an important clinical problem, followed by systematic qualitative and quantitative inquiry and careful application of theoretical models borrowed from other disciplines. Since publication of the original theory in 1988, Mishel and others have carried out numerous empirical tests of the relationships among the major constructs in the model, applying and largely confirming the theory in many illness contexts. Mishel's reconceptualization of the theory in 1990 was deductive, in that it was generated from principles of chaos theory, and was confirmed by empirical evidence from qualitative studies that suggested that people's responses to uncertainty changed over time within the context of serious chronic illnesses. Thus Mishel's theory represents the bidirectional process by which theory both informs and is shaped by research.

ACCEPTANCE BY THE NURSING COMMUNITY

Practice

Mishel's theory describes a phenomenon experienced by acute and chronically ill individuals and their families. The theory has its beginning in Mishel's own experience with her father's battle with cancer. During his illness, he began to focus on events that seemed unimportant to those around him. When asked why he had chosen to focus on such events, he replied that when these activities were being done, he understood what was happening to him. Mishel believed this was her father's way of taking control and making sense out of an overwhelming situation. She knew early in the development of her concept and theory that nurses could identify the phenomenon from their experiences in caring for patients.

Several nurses have moved the theory from research to practice. Writing for an audience of critical care nurses, Hilton (1992) applied the theory in prescribing how to assess and intervene with patients experiencing uncertainty. Using examples of patients recovering from a cardiac event, Hilton explained how patients who misinterpret unclear physical symptoms may overprotect themselves by limiting physical activity that could be essential to their recovery. She further delineated how uncertainty can activate various types of coping to manage the situation, and described appropriate nursing interventions based on a thorough assessment of the patient's or family member's uncertainty.

Wurzbach (1992), writing for medical-surgical nurses, exemplified the experience of a woman hospitalized with a lump in her breast. Focusing on the woman's family history of breast cancer and no previous experience with hospitalization, Wurzbach counseled nurses to assess for certainty as well as uncertainty. Based on this assessment, management strategies in the form of nursing interventions were prescribed. Wurzbach cautioned nurses that intervention may not be appropriate in situations in which the patient experiences a moderate or optimal level of certainty-uncertainty. In these circumstances, patients may feel hopeful and may not require nursing intervention.

Mishel's Uncertainty in Illness Theory has also been applied to the practice of enterostomal therapy (ET) nursing. Righter (1995) described how trust in the ET nurse's knowledge and experiences helps patients develop a cognitive schema for the ostomy experience. Functioning as a credible authority, an antecedent of uncertainty, an ET nurse is able to intervene with patients to promote effective coping strategies.

Based on review of the database of the Managing Uncertainty in Illness Scale users (Mishel, 1997b), many are master's-prepared clinicians seeking to understand better the experience of uncertainty in a variety of clinical settings with different patient populations. The scale and theory have also been used by clinicians in eight countries outside of the United States.

Education

The Uncertainty in Illness Theory has been used widely by graduate students both nationally and internationally as the framework for theses and dissertations, as the topic of concept analysis, and for the critique of middle range nursing theory. Mishel also uses the theory as an exemplar of how theory guides the development of nursing interventions in her doctoral level courses. Mishel is frequently an invited guest at schools of nursing seminars and symposia nationally and internationally, presenting both her empirical findings and the process of theory development for audiences of faculty and students.

Research

As described above, a large body of knowledge has been generated by researchers using the Uncertainty in Illness Theory and scales. With her colleagues at the University of Arizona, Mishel tested and confirmed the major components of the theoretical model, predominantly in samples of women with cancer. Currently her program of research encompasses testing psychoeducational nursing interventions derived from the theoretical model, in samples of adults with breast and prostate cancer. The scales and theory have been used by nurse researchers as well as scientists from other disciplines to describe and explain the psychological responses of people experiencing uncertainty due to illness. The scales have been translated into 12 languages and applied in research throughout the world. Mishel (1997a, 1999) has reviewed the research conducted on uncertainty in both acute and chronic illness and coauthored a review of the research on uncertainty in childhood illness (Stewart & Mishel, 2000). However, she notes that although many investigators have used one of the scales derived from the theory, most studies have not used the uncertainty in illness framework to guide their research.

FURTHER DEVELOPMENT

Mishel and her colleagues have used the original theory as the framework for five federally funded nursing intervention studies. The intervention has proven effective in increasing cancer knowledge, reducing symptom burden, and improving quality of life in Mexican-American, white, and African-American women with breast cancer, and in African-American and white men with localized prostate cancer and their family members (Mishel, Belyea, Germino, Stewart, Bailey et al., 2002; Mishel, Germino, Belyea, Stewart, Bailey et al., 2003). Data analysis is underway for the continuation study that extended the intervention to African-American and white men with advanced or recurrent prostate cancer and their primary support persons. The applicability of the theory to the context of serious childhood illness has been supported in parents of children with HIV infection (Santacroce, Deatrick, & Ledlie, 2002) and in children undergoing treatment for cancer (Stewart, 2003).

From qualitative data supporting the reconceptualized theory, Mishel and Fleury (1994) developed the Growth Through Uncertainty Scale (GTUS) scale to measure the new view of life that can emerge from continual uncertainty. The reconceptualized theory has also been used by researchers to understand the uncertainty experience of long-term survivors of breast cancer (Mast, 1998) and individuals with schizophrenia and their family members (Baier, 1995). The reconceptualized theory serves as the foundation for Mishel and colleagues' most recent nursing intervention study with women facing the enduring uncertainties inherent in surviving breast cancer (Gil, Mishel, Belyea, Germino, Porter et al., 2004). Bailey and Mishel (1997) have used the theory, along with data from qualitative interviews with older men electing watchful waiting as treatment for their prostate cancer, to develop a nursing intervention helping men integrate uncertainty into their lives, view their lives in a positive perspective, and improve their quality of life. In the first trial of the Watchful Waiting Intervention, men did come to see their lives in a new and positive light, reported their quality of life as higher than did the control group, and expected it to be high in the future (Bailey, Mishel, Belyea, Stewart, & Mohler, 2004).

Mishel believes the most important product of her research program is the return of knowledge to practice. Toward that end, plans are underway to move the theoretically derived intervention into current practice, allowing nurses responsible for different types of patient populations to incorporate uncertainty assessment and intervention into their plans of care.

CRITIQUE
Clarity

Clarity refers to how well the theory is understood and how consistently the concepts are presented and conceptualized. Uncertainty is the primary concept of this theory and is defined as a cognitive state in which individuals are unable to determine the meaning of illness-related events (Mishel, 1988). The original theory postulates that managing uncertainty is critical to adaptation during illness and explains how individuals cognitively process illness-associated events and construct meaning from them.

The original theory's concepts are organized in a linear model around the following three major themes:

1. Antecedents of uncertainty
2. Process of uncertainty appraisal
3. Coping with uncertainty

The framework is easy to follow and is clear in all sections of the model. The antecedents of uncertainty include the stimuli frame, cognitive capacities, and structure providers. In the linear model these antecedent variables have both a direct and indirect inverse relationship with uncertainty.

The second conceptual component of the model is appraisal. Uncertainty is seen as a neutral state, neither positive nor negative until it has been appraised by the individual. Appraisal of uncertainty involves the following two processes: (1) inference and (2) illusion. Inference is constructed from the individual's personality disposition and includes learned resourcefulness, mastery, and locus of control. These characteristics contribute to an individual's confidence in the ability to handle life events. Illusion is defined as a belief constructed from uncertainty that considers the favorable aspects of a situation. Based on the appraisal process, uncertainty is viewed as either a danger or an opportunity. Uncertainty viewed as a danger results when the individual considers the possibility of a negative outcome. Uncertainty is viewed as an opportunity primarily through the use of illusion, but inference also can lead to the individual appraising the situation as having a positive outcome. In this situation, uncertainty is preferred and the individual remains hopeful.

Coping is the third theme of the original model of uncertainty. Coping occurs in two forms with the end result of adaptation. If uncertainty is appraised as a danger, then coping includes direct action, vigilance, and seeking information from mobilizing strategies, and it affects management using faith, disengagement, and cognitive support. If uncertainty is appraised as an opportunity, coping offers a buffer to maintain the uncertainty.

The original theory was reconceptualized in 1990 to incorporate the idea that chronic illness unfolds over time, possibly years, and with that, uncertainty is reappraised. The person is viewed as an open system exchanging energy within his or her environment and rather than seeking a return to a stable state, chronically ill individuals may move toward a complex world orientation, thus forming a new meaning for their lives. If uncertainty can be framed as a normal view of life, it can become a positive force for multiple opportunities with resulting positive mood states. To achieve this, the individual must develop probabilistic thinking, which allows one to examine a variety of possibilities and to consider numerous ways of achieving them. The individual envisions a variety of responses to situations and realizes that life can change from day to day.

Mishel described this process as a new view of life in which uncertainty shifts from being seen as a danger to being viewed as an opportunity. To adopt this new view of life, the patient must be able to rely on social resources and health care providers who accept probabilistic thinking. The relationship between the health care provider and the patient must focus on recognizing continual uncertainty and teaching the patient how to use the uncertainty to generate different explanations for events. Hence the importance of structure providers, introduced in the original theory, is maintained in the reconceptualized model.

Despite the complexity and dimensionality of the two models, they are presented clearly and conceptualized comprehensively. Mishel published her measurement model in 1981, her original theoretical model in 1988, and her reconceptualized theory in 1990, and these publications fully explicate the model so that it is applied easily in clinical and research contexts.

Simplicity

The two uncertainty in illness models contain concepts comprised of relationships that range from simple to complex and direct to indirect. Eleven major concepts are found in the three themes of the original theory, and several new concepts are introduced in the reconceptualized model. The antecedents of uncertainty are concise and their definitions are clear and simple. The appraisal component is complex because it considers cognitive processes along with beliefs and values held by the individual. The coping phase of the theory is also complex because it is dependent on the appraisal portion of the model and again involves different kinds of strategies targeted toward adaptation. The outcome portion of the model is differentiated into two conceptualizations of the theory, the first relating to patients with acute illness and the second representing an expansion of the model to accommodate patients with chronic illness. Although the models can hardly be called simple, overall the concept definitions and relationships are well operationalized and easily understood.

Generality

The theory explains how individuals construct meaning from illness-related events. It is broad and generalizable and can be used with individuals experiencing their own illnesses, as well as with spouses and parents of people experiencing illness-related uncertainty. The concept of credible authority can be applied to physicians, nurses, and other health care workers. The theory can be applied to many areas of nursing practice and has been used by clinicians for acute and chronic illnesses such as cancer, cardiac disease, and multiple sclerosis.

Empirical Precision

Mishel derived both theoretical models from her own program of research and that of others. Many of the concepts, assumptions, and relationships among variables draw support from empirical investigation. The concepts are well described and their relationships precisely constructed such that operational definitions have been written and tested. Testing of the theory has occurred in both research and clinical settings. The theory has allowed for development and testing of nursing interventions to manage uncertainty.

Derivable Consequences

Derivable consequences are determined by examining whether a theory guides research, informs practice, generates new ideas, and differentiates the focus of nursing from other professions. Mishel's work represents an exemplar of middle range theory which informs clinical practice within the encompassing context of acute and chronic illness. The theory has likewise generated considerable empirical research in adults dealing with their own illness or that of a family member and continue to stimulate new research directions, such as uncertainty in ill children, in older men electing watchful waiting as their treatment for prostate cancer, and in health care providers informing patients of treatment choices in conditions with uncertain prognoses. Mishel believes that by defining and conceptualizing an important clinical problem, her work supports and enriches nursing practice. The Uncertainty in Illness Theory and its reconceptualization represent frameworks derived from and for practice, a process which is essential to nursing as a practice discipline.

SUMMARY

The Uncertainty in Illness Theory provides a comprehensive framework within which to view the experience of acute and chronic illness and to organize nursing interventions to promote optimal adjustment. The theory helps explain the stresses associated with the diagnosis and treatment of a major illness or chronic condition, the processes by which individuals assess and respond to the uncertainty inherent in an illness experience, and the importance of professional caregivers in providing information and supporting individuals in understanding and managing uncertainty. The reconceptualized theory addresses the unique context of continual uncertainty and thereby expands the original theory to encompass the ongoing uncertain trajectory of many life-threatening and chronic illnesses. The original theory and its reconceptualization are well explicated, derive support from both sound theoretical foundations and extensive empirical confirmation, and can be applied in many illness contexts to support evidence-based nursing practice.

Case Study

Part 1: Original Theory

Rosie, a 45-year-old mother of three, has been diagnosed with stage III breast cancer. A mass was detected in her left breast during her annual gynecological appointment and she has undergone an extensive diagnostic workup, including mammography and sentinel node biopsy. She was referred by her primary physician to a comprehensive breast cancer program at a regional medical center 2 hours from her home. The multidisciplinary team has recommended that Rosie undergo preoperative chemotherapy, followed by partial mastectomy and reconstructive surgery. Rosie's husband has accompanied her to most of her medical encounters but was unable to attend the final conference in which the treatment recommendation was made.

Lily, the advanced practice nurse coordinating Rosie's care (structure provider–credible authority) directs her interventions toward addressing the many sources of uncertainty for Rosie and her family, including lack of information about treatment options and outcomes (event familiarity), unfamiliarity with the treatment environment (event familiarity), expectations for chemotherapy side effects and postoperative recovery (symptom pattern), impact of treatment on family relationships, and prognosis. In particular, Lily addresses Rosie's many questions about why her treatment plan is different from what her primary physician told her to expect (event congruence) and how she will manage her family life while undergoing treatment. Lily provides an audiotape of the treatment conference so that Rosie's husband (structure provider–social support) can hear what took place and support Rosie in asking questions and understanding the information provided. Lily's support for Rosie and her family continue throughout Rosie's treatment course, and she periodically reassesses the sources of uncertainty and the strategies Rosie and her family use to manage them.

Part 2: Reconceptualized Theory

Two years after her breast cancer diagnosis, Rosie returns to the center for a follow-up appointment. Lily asks Rosie to reflect on her cancer experience. Although Rosie describes the time of diagnosis and treatment as chaotic and dominated by uncertainty, and she wonders how she and her family got through it, she tells Lily that gradually she came to see the cancer experience as providing new meaning to her life and helping her set priorities. She left a job she was dissatisfied with and now directs her energy toward her relationships with her teen-age children. Rosie and her husband recently enjoyed a long-postponed second honeymoon trip to Hawaii. She tells Lily that she now embraces each day as an opportunity to live life and enrich the lives of her children.

CRITICAL THINKING *Activities*

1. Imagine you are interviewing a client new to your practice. Think about the kinds of questions you would ask to assess the level of uncertainty about the health issue that brought the client to you. What would you want to know about this person's perceptions of the current situation? Supportive relationships? Previous experiences with health and illness?

2. You are working with a young woman who has been living with multiple sclerosis for 6 years. During an exacerbation of her disease, she focuses not on her symptoms but on her plans for going to law school. One of your colleagues suggests that she may be in denial about the severity of her illness. How might you use the reconceptualized Uncertainty in Illness Theory to propose an alternative interpretation of her perspective?

REFERENCES

Baier, M. (1995). Uncertainty of illness for persons with schizophrenia. *Issues in Mental Health Nursing, 16,* 201-212.

Bailey, D. E., & Mishel, M. H. (1997). *Uncertainty and watchful waiting in men with prostate cancer: Findings from qualitative interviews.* Paper presented at the 11th Annual Meeting of the Southern Nursing Research Society, April 10-12, Norfolk, VA.

Bailey, D. E., Mishel, M. H., Belyea, M., Stewart, J. L., & Mohler, J. (2004). Uncertainty intervention for watchful waiting in prostate cancer. *Cancer Nursing, 27*(5), 339-346.

Becker, G., Jason-Bjerklie, S., Benner, P., Slobin, K., & Ferketich, S. (1993). The dilemma of seeking urgent care: Asthma episodes and emergency service use. *Social Science and Medicine, 37,* 305-313.

Braden, C. J. (1990). A test of the self-help model: Learned response to chronic illness experience. *Nursing Research, 39,* 42-47.

Brett, K. M., & Davies, E. M. B. (1988). "What does it mean?" Sibling and parental appraisals of childhood leukemia. *Cancer Nursing, 11,* 329-338.

Brown, M. A., & Powell-Cope, G. M. (1991). AIDS family caregiving: Transitions through uncertainty. *Nursing Research, 40,* 338-345.

Budner, S. (1962). Intolerance of ambiguity as a personality variable. *Journal of Personality, 30,* 29-50.

Carter, B. J. (1993). Long-term survivors of breast cancer. *Cancer Nursing, 16*(5), 354-361.

Charmaz, K. (1995). Identity dilemmas of chronically ill men. In D. Sobo & D. F. Gordon (Eds.), *Men's health and illness: Gender, power, and the body* (pp. 266-291). Thousand Oaks, CA: Sage.

Cohen, M. H. (1993). The unknown and the unknowable—Managing sustained uncertainty. *Western Journal of Nursing Research, 15,* 77-96.

Comaroff, J., & Maguire, P. (1981). Ambiguity and the search for meaning: Childhood leukaemia in the modern clinical context. *Social Science and Medicine, 15B,* 115-123.

Failla, S., Kuper, B. C., Nick, T. G., & Lee, F. A. (1996). Adjustment of women with systemic lupus erythematosus. *Applied Nursing Research, 9,* 87-96.

Fleury, J., Kimbrell, L. C., & Kruszewski, C. (1995). Life after cardiac event: Women's experience in healing. *Heart & Lung, 24,* 474-482.

Gelatt, H. B. (1989). Positive uncertainty: A new decision-making framework for counseling. *Journal of Consulting & Clinical Psychology, 36,* 252-256.

Gil, K. M., Mishel, M. H., Belyea, M., Germino, B., Porter, L. S., Stewart, J. L., et al. (2004). Triggers of uncertainty about recurrence and long term treatment side effects in older African American and Caucasian breast cancer survivors. *Oncology Nursing Forum, 31,* 633-639.

Green, J. M., & Murton, F. E. (1996). Diagnosis of Duchenne muscular dystrophy: Parents' experiences and satisfaction. *Child: Care, Health, and Development, 22,* 113-128.

Grootenhuis, M. A., & Last, B. L. (1997). Parents' emotional reactions related to different prospects for the survival of their children with cancer. *Journal of Psychosocial Oncology, 15,* 43-61.

Hilton, B. A. (1988). The phenomenon of uncertainty in women with breast cancer. *Issues in Mental Health Nursing, 9,* 217-238.

Hilton, B. A. (1992). Perceptions of uncertainty: Its relevance to life-threatening and chronic illness. *Critical Care Nurse, 12,* 70-73.

Hilton, B. A. (1996). Getting back to normal: The family experience during early stage breast cancer. *Oncology Nursing Forum, 23,* 605-614.

Hinds, P. S., Birenbaum, L. K., Clarke-Steffen, L., Quargnenti, A., Kreissman, S., Kazak, A., et al. (1996). Coming to terms: Parents' response to a first cancer recurrence in their child. *Nursing Research, 45,* 148-153.

Janson-Bjerklie, S., Ferketich, S., & Benner, P. (1993). Predicting the outcomes of living with asthma. *Research in Nursing and Health, 16,* 241-250.

Jessop, D. J., & Stein, R. E. K. (1985). Uncertainty and its relation to the psychological and social correlates of chronic illness in children. *Social Science and Medicine, 20,* 993-999.

Katz, A. (1996). Gaining a new perspective of life as a consequence of uncertainty in HIV infection. *JANAC, 7,* 51-60.

Lang, A. (1987). Nursing of families with an infant who requires home apnea monitoring. *Issues in Comprehensive Pediatric Nursing, 10,* 123-133.

Lazarus, R. S., & Folkman, S. (1984). *Stress, appraisal, and coping.* New York: Springer Publishing.

Mason, C. (1985). The production and effects of uncertainty with special reference to diabetes mellitus. *Social Science and Medicine, 21,* 1329-1334.

Mast, M. E. (1995). Adult uncertainty in illness: A critical review of the literature. *Scholarly Inquiry for Nursing Practice, 9,* 3-24.

Mast, M. E. (1998). Survivors of breast cancer: Illness uncertainty, positive reappraisal, and emotional distress. *Oncology Nursing Forum, 25,* 555-562.

Miles, M. S., Funk, S. G., & Kasper, M. A. (1992). The stress response of mothers and fathers of preterm infants. *Research in Nursing and Health, 15,* 261-269.

Mishel, M. H. (1981). The measurement of uncertainty in illness. *Nursing Research, 30,* 258-263.

Mishel, M. H. (1988). Uncertainty in illness. *Image: The Journal of Nursing Scholarship, 20,* 225-231.

Mishel, M. H. (1990). Reconceptualization of the uncertainty in illness theory. *Image: The Journal of Nursing Scholarship, 22,* 256-262.

Mishel, M. H. (1997a). Uncertainty in acute illness. *Annual Review of Nursing Research, 15,* 57-80.

Mishel, M. H. (1997b). *Uncertainty in illness scales manual.* Available upon request from the author at *http://nursing.unc.edu/music/instruments.html*

Mishel, M. H. (1999). Uncertainty in chronic illness. *Annual Review of Nursing Research, 17,* 269-294.

Mishel, M. H., Belyea, M., Germino, B. B., Stewart, J. L., Bailey, D. E., Robertson, C., et al. (2002). Helping patients with localized prostate carcinoma manage uncertainty and treatment side effects—Nurse-delivered psychoeducational intervention over the telephone. *Cancer, 94,* 1854-1866.

Mishel, M. H., & Braden, C. J. (1987). Uncertainty: A mediator between support and adjustment. *Western Journal of Nursing Research, 9,* 43-57.

Mishel, M. H., & Braden, C. J. (1988). Finding meaning: Antecedents of uncertainty in illness. *Nursing Research, 37,* 98-103.

Mishel, M. H., & Fleury, J. (1994). *Psychometric testing of the growth through uncertainty scale.* Unpublished data, University of North Carolina at Chapel Hill.

Mishel, M. H., Germino, B. B., Belyea, M., Stewart, J. L., Bailey, D. E., Mohler, J., et al. (2003). Moderators of an uncertainty management intervention for men with localized prostate cancer. *Nursing Research, 52,* 89-97.

Mishel, M. H., & Murdaugh, C. L. (1987). Family adjustment to heart transplantation: Redesigning the dream. *Nursing Research, 36,* 332-338.

Mishel, M. H., Padilla, G., Grant, M., & Sorenson, D. S. (1991). Uncertainty in illness theory: A replication of the mediating effects of mastery and coping. *Nursing Research, 40,* 236-240.

Mishel, M. H., & Sorenson, D. S. (1991). Coping with uncertainty in gynecological cancer: A test of the mediating function of mastery and coping. *Nursing Research, 40,* 167-171.

Murray, J. (1993). Coping with the uncertainty of uncontrolled epilepsy. *Seizure, 2,* 167-178.

Nelson, J. P. (1996). Struggling to gain meaning: Living with the uncertainty of breast cancer. *ANS Advances in Nursing Science, 18*(3), 59-76.

Nyhlin, K. T. (1990). Diabetic patients facing long-term complications: Coping with uncertainty. *Journal of Advanced Nursing, 15,* 1021-1029.

O'Brien, R. A., Wineman, N. M., & Nealon, N. R. (1995). Correlates of the caregiving process in multiple sclerosis. *Scholarly Inquiry for Nursing Practice, 9,* 323-342.

Padilla, G. V., Mishel, M. H., & Grant, M. M. (1992). Uncertainty, appraisal, and quality of life. *Quality of Life Research, 1,* 155-165.

Pelusi, J. (1997). The lived experience of surviving breast cancer. *Oncology Nursing Forum, 24,* 1343-1353.

Regan-Kubinski, M. J., Sharts-Hopko, N. (1995). Illness cognition of HIV-infected mothers. *Issues in Mental Health Nursing, 16,* 327-344.

Righter, B. M. (1995). Ostomy care: Uncertainty and the role of the credible authority during an ostomy experience. *Journal of Wound, Ostomy, and Continence Nurses Society, 22,* 100-104.

Santacroce, S. J., Deatrick, J. A., & Ledlie, S. W. (2002). Redefining treatment: How biological mothers manage their children's treatment for perinatally acquired HIV. *AIDS Care, 14,* 47-60.

Schepp, K. G. (1991). Factors influencing the coping effort of mothers of hospitalized children. *Nursing Research, 40,* 42-46.

Sharkey, T. (1995). The effects of uncertainty in families with children who are chronically ill. *Home Healthcare Nurse, 13*(4), 37-42.

Stewart, J. L. (2003). "Getting used to it": Children finding the ordinary and routine in the uncertain context of cancer. *Qualitative Health Research, 13,* 394-407.

Stewart, J. L., & Mishel, M. H. (2000). Uncertainty in childhood illness: A synthesis of the parent and child literature. *Scholarly Inquiry for Nursing Practice, 14,* 299-320.

Tomlinson, P. S., Kirschbaum, M., Harbaugh, B., & Anderson, K. H. (1996). The influence of illness severity and family resources on maternal uncertainty during critical pediatric hospitalization. *American Journal of Critical Care, 5,* 140-146.

Turner, M. A., Tomlinson, P. S., & Harbaugh, B. L. (1990). Parental uncertainty in critical care hospitalization of children. *Maternal Child Nursing Journal, 19,* 45-62.

Van Riper, M., & Selder, F. E. (1989). Parental responses to the birth of a child with Down syndrome. *Loss, Grief, & Care, 3*(3-4), 59-76.

Warburton, D. M. (1979). Physiological aspects of information processing and stress. In V. Hamilton & D. M. Warburton (Eds.), *Human stress and cognition: An information processing approach* (pp. 33-65). New York: John Wiley & Sons.

Weitz, R. (1989). Uncertainty and the lives of persons with AIDS. *Journal of Health and Social Behavior, 30,* 270-281.

Wineman, N. (1990). Adaptation to multiple sclerosis: The role of social support, functional disability, and perceived uncertainty. *Nursing Research, 39,* 294-299.

Wineman, N. M., O'Brien, R. A., Nealon, N. R., & Kaskel, B. (1993). Congruence in uncertainty between individuals with multiple sclerosis and their spouses. *Journal of Neuroscience Nursing, 25,* 356-361.

Wurzbach, M. E. (1992). Assessment and intervention for certainty and uncertainty. *Nursing Forum, 27,* 29-35.

BIBLIOGRAPHY
Primary Sources
Book Chapters

Mishel, M. H. (1993). Living with chronic illness: Living with uncertainty. In S. G. Funk, E. M. Tornquist, M. T. Champagne, & R. A. Weise (Eds.), *Key aspects of caring for the chronically ill, hospital and home* (pp. 46-58). New York: Springer.

Mishel, M. H. (1998). Methodological studies: Instrument development. In P. Brink & M. Woods (Eds.), *Advanced design in nursing research* (2nd ed., pp. 235-282). Beverly Hills, CA: Sage.

Mishel, M. H., Germino, B. G., Belyea, M., Harris, L., Stewart, J., Bailey, D. E. Jr., et al. (2001). Helping patients with localized prostate cancer: Managing after treatment. In S. G. Funk, E. M. Tornquist, J. Leeman, M. S. Miles, & J. S. Harrell (Eds.), *Key aspects of preventing and managing chronic illness* (pp. 235-246). New York: Springer.

Journal Articles

Badger, T. A., Braden, C. J., Longman, A. J., Mishel, M. H. (1999). Depression burden, self-help interventions, and social support in women receiving treatment for breast cancer. *Journal of Psychosocial Oncology, 17*(2), 17-35.

Badger, T. A., Braden, C. J., & Mishel, M. H. (2001). Depression burden, self-help interventions, and side effect experience in women receiving treatment for breast cancer. *Oncology Nursing Forum, 28,* 567-574.

Badger, T. A., Braden, C. J., Mishel, M. H., & Longman, A. (2004). Depression burden, psychological adjustment, and quality of life in women with breast cancer: Patterns over time. *Research in Nursing & Health, 27,* 19-28.

Braden, C. J., & Mishel, M. H. (2000). Highlights of the self-help intervention project (SHIP): Health-related quality of life during breast cancer treatment. *Innovations in Breast Cancer Care, 5,* 51-54.

Braden, C. J., Mishel, M. H., Longman, A. J., & Burns, L. R. (1998). Self-help intervention project: Women receiving treatment for breast cancer. *Cancer Practice, 6,* 87-98.

Germino, B. B., Mishel, M. H., Belyea, M., Harris, L., Ware, A., & Mohler, J. (1998). Uncertainty in prostate cancer: Ethnic and family patterns. *Cancer Practice, 6,* 107-113.

Gil, K. M., Mishel, M. H., Belyea, M., Germino, B., Porter, L. S., Stewart, J. L., et al. (2004). Triggers of uncertainty about recurrence and long term treatment side effects in older African American and Caucasian breast cancer survivors. *Oncology Nursing Forum, 31,* 633-639.

Longman, A., Braden, C. J., & Mishel, M. H. (1997). Pattern of association over time of side-effects burden, self-help and self-care in women with breast cancer. *Oncology Nursing Forum, 24,* 1555-1560.

Mishel, M. H. (1981). The measurement of uncertainty in illness. *Nursing Research, 30,* 258-263.

Mishel, M. H. (1983). Parents' perception of uncertainty concerning their hospitalized child: Reliability and validity of a scale. *Nursing Research, 32,* 324-330.

Mishel, M. H. (1988). Uncertainty in illness. *Image: The Journal of Nursing Scholarship, 20,* 225-232.

Mishel, M. H. (1990). Reconceptualization of the uncertainty in illness theory. *Image: The Journal of Nursing Scholarship, 22,* 256-262.

Mishel, M. H. (1997). Uncertainty in acute illness. *Annual Review of Nursing Research, 15,* 57-80.

Mishel, M. H. (1999). Uncertainty in chronic illness. *Annual Review of Nursing Research, 17,* 269-294.

Mishel, M. H., Belyea, M., Germino, B. B., Stewart, J. L., Bailey, D. E., Robertson, C., et al. (2002). Helping patients with localized prostate carcinoma manage uncertainty and treatment side effects—Nurse-delivered psychoeducational intervention over the telephone. *Cancer, 94,* 1854-1866.

Mishel, M. H., Germino, B. B., Belyea, M., Stewart, J. L., Bailey, D. E., Mohler, J., et al. (2003). Moderators of an uncertainty management intervention for men with localized prostate cancer. *Nursing Research, 52,* 89-97.

Stewart, J. L., & Mishel, M. H. (2000). Uncertainty in childhood illness: A synthesis of the parent and child literature. *Scholarly Inquiry for Nursing Practice, 14,* 299-320.

Proceedings of Conferences

Braden, C. J., Mishel, M. H., & Longman, A. (1995). *Efficacy of the self-help course for women receiving treatment for breast cancer.* Oncology Nursing Society 20th Annual Congress, April 26, Anaheim, CA.

Braden, C. J., Mishel, M. H., & Longman, A. (1995). *Efficacy of the self-help course/uncertainty management intervention for women receiving treatment for breast cancer.* 28th Annual Communicating Nursing Research Conference, Innovation and Collaboration: Responses to Health Care Needs, Western Society for Research in Nursing of the Western Institute of Nursing, May 4-6, San Diego.

Braden, C. J., Mishel, M. H., Longman, A., & Burns, R. (1995). *Ethnicity as a factor in breast cancer treatment experience.* The Second International and Interdisciplinary Health Research Symposium, School of Nursing, West Virginia University, Morgantown, WV.

Mishel, M. H. (1996). *Interventions sensitive to regional and cultural issues. Symposium on issues in the design and implementation of nursing interventions for underserved cancer patients.* 10th Annual Conference, Southern Nursing Research Society, February 8-10, Miami.

Mishel, M. H. (2001). *Symposium on how to identify who benefits from an intervention: The use of moderator effects*. 15th Annual Conference of the Southern Nursing Research Society, February 1-3, Baltimore.

Mishel, M. H., Germino, B., Belyea, M., & Braden, C. J. (1999). *Cultural beliefs of older African-American and Caucasian men treated for breast cancer.* 5th National Cancer Research Conference, February 11-13, Newport Beach, CA.

Mishel, M. H., Germino, B., Belyea, M., & Braden, C. J. (1999). *Cultural health beliefs of older African American and Caucasian women treated for breast cancer.* Pan American Congress of Psychosocial & Behavioral Oncology, October 20-23, New York.

Mishel, M. H., Germino, B., Belyea, M., Hamilton-Spruill, J., & Bailey, D. (1998). *Efficacy of an uncertainty management intervention on psychosocial outcomes in men treated for localized prostate cancer.* 4th International Congress of Psycho-Oncology, September 3-6, Hamburg, Germany.

Mishel, M. H., Germino, B., Belyea, M., Hamilton-Spruill, J., & Bailey, D. (1999). *Efficacy and moderators of efficacy of an uncertainty management intervention in men treated for localized prostate cancer.* Key Aspects of Interventions for the Prevention and Management of Chronic Illness, Chapel Hill, NC.

Mishel, M. H., Germino, B., Belyea, M., Hamilton-Spruill, J., & Bailey, D. (1999). *Efficacy of an uncertainty management intervention in men treated for localized prostate cancer.* 13th Annual Conference of the Southern Nursing Research Society, February 18-20, Charleston, SC.

Mishel, M. H., Germino, B., Harris, L., Hamilton-Spruill, J., & Ware, A. (1997). *Developing culturally sensitive nursing intervention research.* 11th Annual Conference of the Southern Nursing Research Society, April 10-12, Norfolk, VA.

Research Grant Awards

Braden, C. J. (P. I.), & Mishel, M. H. (Co-investigator). (1989 May/1994 June). *Nurse interventions promoting self help response to cancer* (R01 CA48450-01A1). Grant from National Cancer Institute, National Institutes of Health, Bethesda, MD.

Braden, C. J. (P. I.), & Mishel, M. H. (Co-P. I.). (1987-1988). *Antecedents of uncertainty, uncertainty appraisal and coping in patients with multiple sclerosis.* Biomedical research support grant from Division of Nursing, U. S. Department of Health and Human Services, Washington, DC, and University of Arizona, Tucson, AZ.

Braden, C. J. (P. I.), & Mishel, M. H. (Site P. I.). (1994 September/1998 September). *Self help in underserved women* (R01 CA64706-02). Grant from National Cancer Institute, National Institutes of Health, Bethesda, MD.

Harrel, J. S. (P. I.), & Mishel, M. H. (Center Investigator and Core Director). (1994 September/2004 September). *Preventing/managing chronic illness in vulnerable people* (P30 NRO3692). Grant from National Cancer Institute, National Institutes of Health, Bethesda, MD.

Kay, M. (P. I.), & Mishel, M. H. (Co-P. I.). (1987 April/1990 August). *Efficacy of support groups for Mexican-American widows* (RO1 MH41978-01A1). Grant from National Institute of Mental Health, National Institutes of Health, Bethesda, MD.

Mishel, M. H. (1976-1978). National Research Service Award, Nurse Research Predoctoral Fellowship (#1F31NU0504501). Awarded by Division of Nursing, Department of Health, Education and Welfare, Washington, DC.

Mishel, M. H. (1982-1983). *The impact of uncertainty and optimism upon adjustment in patients with gynecological cancer.* Grant from American Cancer Society, Atlanta, GA, and institutional research grant from University of Arizona, Tucson, AZ.

Mishel, M. H. (1983-1984). *Living with uncertainty in systemic lupus erythematosus.* Grant from American Lupus Society, Ventura, CA.

Mishel, M. H. (P. I.). (1982-1983). *Analysis of the reliability and validity of the parents' perception of uncertainty in illness scale* (Dean's Research Award). Grant from College of Nursing, University of Arizona, Tucson, AZ.

Mishel, M. H. (P. I.). (1983, Fall/1984). *A longitudinal investigation of psycho-social adjustment in patients with gynecological cancer.* Nurse research emphasis grant from Division of Nursing, U. S. Department of Health and Human Services, Washington, DC.

Mishel, M. H. (P. I.). (1984 August/1988 May). *Coping with uncertainty in gynecological cancer* (RO1 NU/CA01103-01). Grant from National Institutes of Health Center for Nursing Research, Bethesda, MD.

Mishel, M. H. (P. I.). (1984-1985). *The impact of cognitive style on perception of and response to uncertainty during a diagnostic procedure* (Dean's Research Award). Grant from College of Nursing, University of Arizona, Tucson, AZ.

Mishel, M. H. (P. I.). (1985-1986). *Maintaining hope and managing unpredictability: Scale development and testing.* Biomedical research support grant from Division of Nursing, U. S. Department of Health and Human Services, Washington, DC, and University of Arizona, Tucson, AZ.

Mishel, M. H. (P. I.). (1987 October/1988 September). *Depression awareness: A training program for nurses* (1T15MH18874-01). Grant from National Institute of Mental Health, National Institutes of Health, Bethesda, MD.

Mishel, M. H. (P. I.). (1993 September/1997 March). *Managing uncertainty in stage B prostate cancer* (R01 NR03782-01). Grant from National Institute for

Nursing Research, National Cancer Institute, National Institutes of Health, Bethesda, MD.

Mishel, M. H. (P. I.). (1993 September/1997 August). *Managing uncertainty: Self help in breast cancer* (R01 CA57764-01A2). Grant from National Cancer Institute, National Institutes of Health, Bethesda, MD.

Mishel, M. H. (P. I.). (1994 August/1995 July). *Managing uncertainty: Self help in breast cancer* (Suppl) (R01 CA55164). Grant from National Cancer Institute, National Institutes of Health, Bethesda, MD.

Mishel, M. H. (P. I.). (1995 October/1996 September). *Supplement: Managing uncertainty in stage B prostate cancer* (R01 NR/CA03781-03). Grant from National Institutes of Health Office for Research on Minority Health, Bethesda, MD.

Mishel, M. H. (P. I.). (1996 April/2006 June). *Interventions for preventing and managing chronic illness* (T32 NR07091-08). Grant from National Institute of Nursing Research, National Institutes of Health, Bethesda, MD.

Mishel, M. H. (P. I.). (1998 March/2002 August). *Managing uncertainty in advanced prostate cancer* (R01 NR03782-05). Grant from National Institute of Nursing Research, National Institutes of Health, Bethesda, MD.

Mishel, M. H. (P. I.). (1999 May/2004 February). *Managing uncertainty in older breast cancer survivors* (R01 CA78955-02). Grant from National Cancer Institute, National Institutes of Health, Bethesda, MD.

Mishel, M. H. (P. I.). (2002, September/2006 June). *Decision-making under uncertainty in prostate cancer* (RO1 NR08144-01). Grant from National Institute of Nursing Research, National Institutes of Health, Bethesda, MD.

Mishel, M. H. (Project Director). (1972-1973). *Integration of a nursing curriculum utilizing extended role and external degree concepts.* Nursing Department, California State University at Los Angeles (HEW grant #0347823). Grant from Division of Nursing, Department of Health, Education and Welfare, Washington, DC.

Mishel, M. H., Murdaugh, C., & Pergrin, J. (1986, Fall). *Mary Opal Wolanin Award for Excellence in Clinical Research,* University of Arizona.

Mishel, M. H., Murdaugh, C., & Pergrin, J. (Co-P. I. s). (1983-1984). *The impact of stress on caregivers of Alzheimer's disease victims* (Dean's Research Award). Grant from College of Nursing, University of Arizona, Tucson, AZ.

Murdaugh, C. (P. I.), & Mishel, M. H. (P. I.). (1988 April/1990 August). *Predictors of quality of life in heart transplantation.* Grant from National Institutes of Health Center for Nursing Research, Bethesda, MD.

Secondary Sources
Selected Publications Citing Mishel's Work

Afifi, W. A., & Burgoon, J. K. (1998). "We never talk about that": A comparison of cross-sex friendships and dating relationships on uncertainty and topic avoidance. *Personal Relationships, 5,* 255-272.

Akkasilpa, S., Minor, M., Goldman, D., Magder, L. S., & Petri, M. (2000). Association of coping responses with fibromyalgia tender points in patients with systemic lupus erythematosus. *Journal of Rheumatology, 27,* 671-674.

Andersson, S. I., & Albertsson, M. (2000). Stress and situationally related coping in cancer out-patients and their spouses. *Stress Medicine, 16*(4), 209-217.

Babrow, A. S., Kasch, C. R., & Ford, L. A. (1998). The many meanings of uncertainty in illness: Toward a systematic accounting. *Health Communication, 10,* 1-23.

Badger, T. A. (1996). Family members' experiences living with members with depression. *Western Journal of Nursing Research, 18,* 149-171.

Barroso, J. (1997). Social support and long-term survivors of AIDS. *Western Journal of Nursing Research, 19,* 554-573.

Bertero, C., Eriksson, B. E., & Ek, A. C. (1997). Explaining different profiles in quality of life experiences in acute and chronic leukemia. *Cancer Nursing, 20,* 100-104.

Bogart, L. M., & Helgeson, V. S. (2000). Social comparisons among women with breast cancer: A longitudinal investigation. *Journal of Applied Social Psychology, 30,* 547-575.

Bolse, K., Flemme, I., Ivarsson, A., Jinhage, B., Carroll, D., Edvardsson, N., et al. (2002). Life situation related to the ICD implantation; self-reported uncertainty and satisfaction in Swedish and U. S. samples. *European Journal of Cardiovascular Nursing, 1,* 243-251.

Boman, K., Lindahl, A., & Bjork, O. (2003). Disease-related distress in parents of children with cancer at various stages after the time of diagnosis. *Acta Oncologica, 42,* 137-146.

Boter, H., Mistiaen, P., & Groenewegen, I. (2000). A randomized trial of a Telephone Reassurance Programme for patients recently discharged from an ophthalmic unit. *Journal of Clinical Nursing, 9,* 199-206.

Brashers, D. E., Neidig, J. L., Russell, J. A., Cardillo, L. W., Haas, S. M., Dobbs, L. K., et al. (2003). The medical, personal, and social causes of uncertainty in HIV illness. *Issues in Mental Health Nursing, 24,* 497-522.

Bunzel, B., Laederach-Hofmann, K., & Schubert, M. T. (1999). Patients benefit—Partners suffer? The impact of heart transplantation on the partner relationship. *Transplant International, 12,* 33-41.

Canning, R. D., Dew, M. A., & Davidson, S. (1996). Psychological distress among caregivers to heart transplant recipients. *Social Science & Medicine, 42,* 599-608.

Carlsson, M. E., & Strang, P. M. (1998). Educational support programme for gynaecological cancer patients and their families. *Acta Oncologica, 37,* 269-275.

Carroll, D. L., Hamilton, G. A., & McGovern, B. A. (1999). Changes in health status and quality of life and the impact of uncertainty in patients who survive life-threatening arrhythmias. *Heart & Lung, 28,* 251-260.

Clark, M. S., & Smith, D. S. (1999). Changes in family functioning for stroke rehabilitation patients and their families. *International Journal of Rehabilitation Research, 22,* 171-179.

Clements, H., & Melby, V. (1998). An investigation into the information obtained by patients undergoing gastroscopy investigations. *Journal of Clinical Nursing, 7,* 333-342.

Collins, E. G., White-Williams, C., & Jalowiec, A. (1996). Spouse stressors while awaiting heart transplantation. *Heart & Lung, 25,* 4-13.

Cormier-Daigle, M., & Stewart, M. (1997). Support and coping of male hemodialysis-dependent patients. *International Journal of Nursing Studies, 34,* 420-430.

Cox, K. (1998). Investigating psychosocial aspects of participation in early anti-cancer drug trials: Towards a choice of methodology. *Journal of Advanced Nursing, 27,* 488-496.

Crigger, N. J. (1996). Testing an uncertainty model for women with multiple sclerosis. *ANS Advances in Nursing Science, 18,* 37-47.

Czuchta, D. M., & McCay, E. (2001). Help-seeking for parents of individuals experiencing a first episode of schizophrenia. *Archives of Psychiatric Nursing, 15,* 159-170.

Deane, K. A., & Degner, L. F. (1998). Information needs, uncertainty, and anxiety in women who had a breast biopsy with benign outcome. *Cancer Nursing, 21,* 117-126.

Delude, D., Wright, J., & Belanger, C. (2000). The effects of pregnancy complications on the parental adaptation process. *Journal of Reproductive and Infant Psychology, 18,* 5-20.

Dew, M. A., Roth, L. H., Schulberg, H. C., Simmons, R. G., Kormos, R. L., Trzepacz, P., et al. (1996). Prevalence and predictors of depression and anxiety-related disorders during the year after heart transplantation. *General Hospital Psychiatry, 18*(6 Suppl), 48S-61S.

Dias, L., & Lobel, M. (1997). Social comparison in medically high-risk pregnant women. *Journal of Applied Psychology, 27,* 1629-1649.

Dikken, C., & Sitzia, J. (1998). Patients' experiences of chemotherapy: Side-effects associated with 5-fluorouracil plus folinic acid in the treatment of colorectal cancer. *Journal of Clinical Nursing, 7,* 371-379.

Dirksen, S. R. (2000). Predicting well-being among breast cancer survivors. *Journal of Advanced Nursing, 32,* 937-943.

Dobratz, M. C. (2003). Putting the pieces together: Teaching undergraduate research from a theoretical perspective. *Journal of Advanced Nursing, 41,* 383-392.

Dulude, D., Wright, J., & Belanger, C. (2000). The effects of pregnancy complications on the parental adaptation

process. *Journal of Reproductive and Infant Psychology, 18,* 5-20.

Ehrenberger, H. E., Alligood, M. R., Thomas, S. P., Wallace, D. C., & Licavoli, C. M. (2002). Testing a theory of decision-making derived from King's systems framework in women eligible for a cancer clinical trial. *Nursing Science Quarterly, 15,* 156-163.

Failla, S., Kuper, B. C., Nick, T. G., & Lee, F. A. (1996). Adjustment of women with systemic lupus erythematosus. *Applied Nursing Research, 9,* 87-93.

Farnalls, S. L., & Rennick, J. (2003). Parents' caregiving approaches: Facing a new treatment alternative in severe intractable childhood epilepsy. *Seizure—European Journal of Epilepsy, 12,* 1-10.

Flemme, I., Bolse, K., Ivarsson, A., Jinhage, B., Sandstedt, B., Edvardsson, N., et al. (2001). Life situation of patients with an implantable cardioverter defibrillator: A descriptive longitudinal study. *Journal of Clinical Nursing, 10,* 563-572.

Ford, L. A., Babrow, A. S., & Stohl, C. (1996). Social support messages and the management of uncertainty in the experience of breast cancer: An application of problematic integration theory. *Communication Monographs, 63,* 189-207.

Fuemmeler, B. F., Mullins, L. L., & Marx, B. P. (2001). Post-traumatic stress and general distress among parents of children surviving a brain tumor. *Children's Health Care, 30,* 169-182.

Fukui, S., Kamiya, M., Koike, M., Kugaya, A., Okamura, H., Nakanishi, T., et al. (2000). Applicability of a Western-developed psychosocial group intervention for Japanese patients with primary breast cancer. *Psycho-Oncology, 9,* 169-177.

Galloway, S. C., & Graydon, J. E. (1996). Uncertainty, symptom distress, and information needs after surgery for cancer of the colon. *Cancer Nursing, 19,* 112-117.

Gold-Spink, E., Sher, T. G., & Theodos, V. (2000). Uncertainty in illness and optimism in couples with multiple sclerosis. *International Journal of Rehabilitation & Health, 5,* 157-164.

Gross, S. M., Ireys, H. T., & Kinsman, S. L. (2000). Young women with physical disabilities: Risk factors for symptoms of eating disorders. *Journal of Developmental and Behavioral Pediatrics, 21,* 87-96.

Heinrich, C. R. (2003). Enhancing the perceived health of HIV-seropositive men. *Western Journal of Nursing Research, 25,* 367-382.

Helgeson, V. S., Snyder, P., & Seltman, H. (2004). Psychological and physical adjustment to breast cancer over 4 years: Identifying distinct trajectories of change. *Health Psychology, 23,* 3-15.

Hoff, A. L., Mullins, L. L., Chaney, J. M., Hartman, V. L., & Domek, D. (2002). Illness uncertainty, perceived control, and psychological distress among adolescents with type 1 diabetes. *Research & Theory for Nursing Practice, 16,* 223-236.

Hommel, K. A., Chaney, J. M., Wagner, J. L., White, M. M., Hoff, A. L., & Mullins, L. L. (2003). Anxiety and depression in older adolescents with long-standing asthma: The role of illness uncertainty. *Children's Health Care, 32,* 51-63.

Horner, S. D. (1997). Uncertainty in mothers' care for their ill children. *Journal of Advanced Nursing, 26,* 658-663.

Hsu, T. H., Lu, M. S., Tsou, T. S., & Lin, C. C. (2003). The relationship of pain, uncertainty, and hope in Taiwanese lung cancer patients. *Journal of Pain and Symptom Management, 26,* 835-842.

Katz, P. P. (1998). The stresses of rheumatoid arthritis: Appraisals of perceived impact and coping efficacy. *Arthritis Care and Research, 11,* 9-22.

Kavanagh, T., Yacoub, M. H., Kennedy, J., & Austin, P. C. (1999). Return to work after heart transplantation: 12-year follow-up. *Journal of Heart and Lung Transplantation, 18,* 846-851.

Kendall, E., & Terry, D. J. (1996). Psychosocial adjustment following closed head injury: A model for understanding individual differences and predicting outcome. *Neuropsychological Rehabilitation, 6,* 101-132.

Konstam, V., Surman, O., Hizzazi, K. H., Fierstein, J., Konstam, M., Turbett, A., et al. (1998). Marital adjustment in heart transplantation patients and their spouses: A longitudinal perspective. *American Journal of Family Therapy, 26,* 147-158.

Kristensson-Hallstrom, I., Elander, G., & Malmfors, G. (1997). Increased parental participation in a paediatric surgical day-care unit. *Journal of Clinical Nursing, 6,* 297-302.

Kroencke, D. C., Denney, D. R., & Lynch, S. G. (2001). Depression during exacerbations in multiple sclerosis: The importance of uncertainty. *Multiple Sclerosis, 7,* 237-242.

Lauver, D. R., Kruse, K., & Baggot, A. (1999). Women's uncertainties, coping, and moods regarding abnormal Papanicolaou results. *Journal of Women's Health & Gender-Based Medicine, 8,* 1103-1112.

LeFort, S. M. (2000). A test of Braden's self-help model in adults with chronic pain. *Journal of Nursing Scholarship, 32,* 153-160.

Leith, B. A. (1999). Patients' and family members' perceptions of transfer from intensive care. *Heart & Lung, 28,* 210-218.

Lemaire, G. S. (2004). More than just menstrual cramps: Symptoms and uncertainty among women with endometriosis. *Journal of Obstetric Gynecologic and Neonatal Nursing, 33,* 71-79.

Lenz, E. R., Suppe, F., Gift, A. G., Pugh, L. C., & Milligan, R. A. (1995). Collaborative development of middle-range nursing theories. Toward a theory of unpleasant symptoms. *ANS Advances in Nursing Science, 17,* 1-13.

Lev, E. L., Paul, D., & Owen, S. V. (1999). Age, self-efficacy, and change in patients' adjustment to cancer. *Cancer Practice, 7,* 170-176.

Li, H. C. W., & Lam, H. Y. A. (2003). Paediatric day surgery: Impact on Hong Kong Chinese children and their parents. *Journal of Clinical Nursing, 12,* 882-887.

Liehr, P., & Smith, M. J. (1999). Middle range theory: Spinning research and practice to create knowledge for the new millennium. *ANS Advances in Nursing Science, 21,* 81-91.

LoBiondo-Wood, G., Williams, L., Wood, R. P., & Shaw, B. W. (1997). Impact of liver transplantation on quality of life: A longitudinal perspective. *Applied Nursing Research, 10,* 27-32.

Lok, P. (1996). Stressors, coping mechanisms and quality of life among dialysis patients in Australia. *Journal of Advanced Nursing, 23,* 873-881.

Lynch, S. G., Kroencke, D. C., & Denney, D. R. (2001). The relationship between disability and depression in multiple sclerosis: The role of uncertainty, coping, and hope. *Multiple Sclerosis, 7,* 411-416.

Margalith, I., & Shapiro, A. (1997). Anxiety and patient participation in clinical decision-making: The case of patients with ureteral calculi. *Social Science & Medicine, 45,* 419-427.

Mast, M. E. (1998). Survivors of breast cancer: Illness uncertainty, positive reappraisal, and emotional distress. *Oncology Nursing Forum, 25,* 555-562.

McCain, N. L., Munjas, B. A., Munro, C. L., Elswick, R. K., Robins, J. L. W., Ferreira-Gonzalez, A., et al. (2003). Effects of stress management on PNI-based outcomes in persons with HIV disease. *Research in Nursing & Health, 26,* 102-117.

Meiers, S. J., & Tomlinson, P. S. (2003). Family-nurse co-construction of meaning: A central phenomenon of family caring. *Scandinavian Journal of Caring Sciences, 17,* 193-201.

Melanson, P. M., & Downe-Wamboldt, B. (2003). Confronting life with rheumatoid arthritis. *Journal of Advanced Nursing, 42,* 125-133.

Molassiotis, A., Callaghan, P., Twinn, S. F., Lam, S. W., Chung, W. Y., & Li, C. K. (2002). A pilot study of the effects of cognitive-behavioral group therapy and peer support/counseling in decreasing psychologic distress and improving quality of life in Chinese patients with symptomatic HIV disease. *Aids Patient Care and Standards, 16,* 83-96.

Mu, P. F., Ma, F. C., Hwang, B., & Chao, Y. M. (2002). Families of children with cancer: The impact on anxiety experienced by fathers. *Cancer Nursing, 25,* 66-73.

Mu, P., Wong, T., Chang, K., & Kwan, S. (2001). Predictors of maternal depression for families having a child with epilepsy. *Journal of Nursing Research, 9,* 116-126.

Mullins, L. L., Chaney, J. M., Balderson, B., & Hommel, K. A. (2000). The relationship of illness uncertainty, illness intrusiveness, and asthma severity to depression in young adults with long-standing asthma. *International Journal of Rehabilitation & Health, 5,* 177-186.

Mullins, L. L., Cote, M. P., Fuemmeler, B. F., Jean, V. M., Beatty, W. W., & Paul, R. H. (2001). Illness intrusiveness, uncertainty, and distress in individuals with multiple sclerosis. *Rehabilitation Psychology, 46,* 139-153.

Northouse, L. L., Mood, D., Templin, T., Mellon, S., & George, T. (2000). Couples' patterns of adjustment to colon cancer. *Social Science & Medicine, 50,* 271-284.

Northouse, L., Templin, T., & Mood, D. (2001). Couples' adjustment to breast disease during the first year following diagnosis. *Journal of Behavioral Medicine, 24,* 115-136.

Northouse, L. L., Templin, T., Mood, D., & Oberst, M. (1998). Couples' adjustment to breast cancer and benign breast disease: A longitudinal analysis. *Psycho-Oncology, 7,* 37-48.

Parry, C. (2003). Embracing uncertainty: An exploration of the experiences of childhood cancer survivors. *Qualitative Health Research, 13,* 227-246.

Powell-Cope, G. M. (1995). The experiences of gay couples affected by HIV infection. *Qualitative Health Research, 5*(1), 36-62.

Sammarco, A. (2001). Perceived social support, uncertainty, and quality of life of younger breast cancer survivors. *Cancer Nursing, 24,* 212-219.

Sammarco, A. (2003). Quality of life among older survivors of breast cancer. *Cancer Nursing, 26,* 431-438.

Sanders-Dewey, N. E. J., Mullins, L. L., & Chaney, J. M. (2001). Coping style, perceived uncertainty in illness, and distress in individuals with Parkinson's disease and their caregivers. *Rehabilitation Psychology, 46,* 363-381.

Santacroce, S. J. (2003). Parental uncertainty and post-traumatic stress in serious childhood illness. *Journal of Nursing Scholarship, 35,* 45-51.

Siegel, K., Dean, L., & Schrimshaw, E. W. (1999). Symptom ambiguity among late-middle-aged and older adults with HIV. *Research on Aging, 21,* 595-618.

Steele, R. G., Tripp, G., Kotchick, B. A., Summers, P., & Forehand, R. (1997). Family members' uncertainty about parental chronic illness: The relationship of hemophilia and HIV infection to child functioning. *Journal of Pediatric Psychology, 22,* 577-591.

Stewart, J. L. (2003). "Getting used to it": Children finding the ordinary and routine in the uncertain context of cancer. *Qualitative Health Research, 13,* 394-407.

Swallow, V. M., & Jacoby, A. (2001). Mothers' coping in chronic childhood illness: The effect of presympto-matic diagnosis of vesicoureteric reflux. *Journal of Advanced Nursing, 33,* 69-78.

Sweet, L., Savoie, J. A., & Lemyre, L. (1999). Appraisals, coping, and stress in breast cancer screening: A longitudinal investigation of causal structure. *Canadian Journal of Behavioural Science, 31,* 240-253.

Taylor-Piliae, R. E., & Molassiotis, A. (2001). An exploration of the relationships between uncertainty, psychological distress and type of coping strategy among Chinese men after cardiac catheterization. *Journal of Advanced Nursing, 33,* 79-88.

Thomas, M. L. (1998). Quality of life and psychosocial adjustment in patients with myelodysplastic syndromes. *Leukemia Research, 22,* S41-S47.

Thompson, B. (2003). Lazarus phenomena: An exploratory study of gay men living with HIV. *Social Work in Health Care, 37,* 87-114.

Thorne, S. E. (1999). The science of meaning in chronic illness. *International Journal of Nursing Studies, 36,* 397-404.

Tomlinson, P. S., Thomlinson, E., Peden-McAlpine, C., & Kirschbaum, M. (2002). Clinical innovation for promoting family care in paediatric intensive care: Demonstration, role modeling and reflective practice. *Journal of Advanced Nursing, 38,* 161-170.

Tommet, P. A. (2003). Nurse-parent dialogue: Illuminating the evolving pattern of families with children who are medically fragile. *Nursing Science Quarterly, 16,* 239-246.

Wallace, M. (2003). Uncertainty and quality of life of older men who undergo watchful waiting for prostate cancer. *Oncology Nursing Forum, 30*(2 part 1), 303-309.

Webster, D. C. (1996). Sex, lies, and stereotypes: Women and interstitial cystitis. *Journal of Sex Research, 33,* 197-203.

Weiss, M. E., Saks, N. P., & Harris, S. (2002). Resolving the uncertainty of preterm symptoms: Women's experiences with the onset of preterm labor. *Journal of Obstetric, Gynecologic, & Neonatal Nursing, 31,* 66-76.

Wineman, N. M., Schwetz, K. M., Zeller, R., & Cyphert, J. (2003). Longitudinal analysis of illness uncertainty, coping, hopefulness, and mood during participation in a clinical drug trial. *Journal of Neuroscience Nursing, 35,* 100-106.

Wonghongkul, T., Moore, S. M., Musil, C., Schneider, S., & Deimling, G. (2000). The influence of uncertainty in illness, stress appraisal, and hope on coping in survivors of breast cancer. *Cancer Nursing, 23,* 422-429.

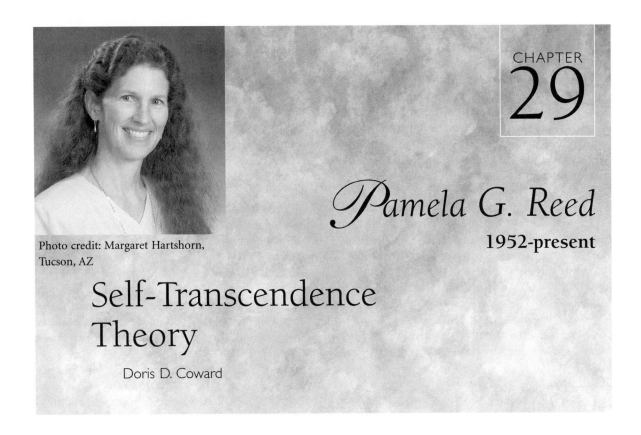

Photo credit: Margaret Hartshorn,
Tucson, AZ

Self-Transcendence Theory

Doris D. Coward

CREDENTIALS OF THE THEORIST

Pamela G. Reed was born in Detroit, Michigan, on June 13, 1952. She married her husband, Gary, in 1973, and they have two daughters. Reed graduated with her baccalaureate from Wayne State University in Detroit, Michigan, in 1974 and earned her M.S.N. in psychiatric-mental health of children and adolescents and in nursing education in 1976. She began doctoral study at that institution in 1979 and received her Ph.D. in 1982 with a concentration in nursing theory and research. Her dissertation research, directed by Joyce J. Fitzpatrick, focused on the relationship between well-being and spiritual perspectives on life and death in terminally ill and well individuals.

The author expresses her appreciation to Pamela G. Reed for her insights over the years and particularly for her support during the development of this chapter.

During her undergraduate and early graduate education at Wayne State, Reed was a research assistant for Jean E. Johnson. She also worked as a staff nurse at Mt. Sinai Hospital in Detroit and as an instructor at Oakland University School of Nursing in Rochester, Michigan. During her doctoral education, Reed was employed as a clinical nurse specialist at Lafayette Research and Psychiatric Clinic in Detroit. Since January 1983, Reed has taught, served in administrative positions, and conducted research at the University of Arizona College of Nursing in Tucson. She has received several awards for her teaching in psychiatric mental health nursing, nursing care in death and dying, nursing conceptual models, nursing theory, middle range theory, and metatheory courses. She was Acting Director of the Division of Mental Health Nursing at the College of Nursing in 1989 and 1991 to 1992, and served as Associate Dean for Academic Affairs from 1995 to

2002. Her major fields of research are spirituality, nursing philosophy, life-span development, aging, and mental health. Her research studies, financed by both intramural and extramural funding, were reported in many presentations and in scholarly nursing journals. Her current research examines the role of spirituality in self-transcendence as a developmental phenomenon related to well-being and health care decisions at end of life in patients and family caregivers.

Reed is a fellow in the American Academy of Nursing and is a member of a number of professional organizations including Sigma Theta Tau International, the American Nurses Association, and the International Society of Rogerian Scholars (board of directors). She is a manuscript reviewer for several journals, including *Western Journal of Nursing Research, Research in Nursing and Health, Nursing Philosophy, Alternative Therapies in Health and Medicine, Clinical Nursing Research,* and *Visions: Journal of Rogerian Nursing Science* and has served as an Editorial Review Board member for *Nursing Science Quarterly.*

Reed's influence is evident not only in her own research and publications. The impact of Reed's work is also reflected in the research of more than 50 students whose theses and dissertations she has directed and in the work of other scientists who have applied her theory or her measurement scales *(Self-Transcendence Scale* and *Spiritual Perspective Scale)* in their research. Her theoretical ideas have been supported and extended by the many nurses Reed has mentored.

THEORETICAL SOURCES

Reed (1991a) developed her theory of self-transcendence using the strategy of "deductive reformulation." This strategy, among other theory development approaches that deliberately utilize nursing models, originated with Reed's professors, notably Ann Whall and Joyce Fitzpatrick of Wayne State University. (See Fitzpatrick, Whall, Johnston, & Floyd, 1982; Shearer & Reed, 2004; and Whall, 1986 for applications of this strategy.) Deductive reformulation in constructing middle range theory

uses knowledge derived from nonnursing theory that is reformulated deductively from a nursing conceptual model. The primary nonnursing theory sources were life-span theories on adult social-cognitive and transpersonal development (e.g., Alexander & Langner, 1990; Commons, Richards, & Armon, 1984; Wilber, 1980, 1981, 1990). Principles from life-span theories were reformulated using the nursing perspective of Martha E. Rogers' conceptual system of unitary human beings (Rogers, 1970, 1980, 1990).

Reed describes her theory as originating from three sources (Reed, 2003). The first source was the new conceptualization of human development (Lerner, 2002) as a lifelong process that extended beyond the attainment of adulthood throughout the aging and dying processes. This emerging belief in the ongoing potential for development was a paradigm shift from previously held views that both physical growth and mental development ended at adolescence (Reed, 1983).

The second source for the theory was the early work of nursing theorist Martha E. Rogers (Rogers, 1970, 1980, 1990). Rogers' three principles of homeodynamics were congruent with the key principles of the evolving life-span developmental theory. Rogers' integrality principle identified development as a function of both human and contextual factors; it also identified disequilibrium between person and environment as an important trigger of development. Similarly, developmental theorist Riegel (1976) had proposed that asynchrony in development among physical, emotional, environmental, and social dimensions was necessary for developmental progress. Rogers' helicy principle characterized human development as innovative and unpredictable. This principle also was similar to life-span principles that identified development as nonlinear, continuous throughout the life-span, and evident in variability within and across individuals and groups. Rogers' resonancy principle described human development as a process of movement that, although unpredictable, had pattern and purpose. Life-span theorists also proposed that the process of development displayed patterns of complexity and organization. Thus knowledge gained from the nonnursing life-span developmental perspective could be reformulated, using an appropriate nursing conceptual system.

The third source for the theory was evidence from clinical experience and research that indicated that clinically depressed older persons reported fewer developmental resources to sustain their sense of well-being in the face of decreased physical and cognitive abilities than did a matched group of mentally healthy older adults (Reed, 1986b). In addition, development in elderly and in "oldest-old" adults was found not be a linear process of gain and subsequent loss, but a process of transforming old perspectives and behaviors, and integrating new views and activities (Reed, 1989, 1991b).

MAJOR CONCEPTS *&* DEFINITIONS

VULNERABILITY

Vulnerability is defined as one's awareness of personal mortality (Reed, 2003). In Reed's earlier work, the phrase "awareness of one's personal mortality" was the context for development or maturation in later adulthood or at the end of life. Self-transcendence was a pattern associated with advanced development within that context (Reed, 1991b). The concept of vulnerability broadens the awareness of personal mortality situations to include life crises such as disability, chronic illness, childbirth, and parenting.

SELF-TRANSCENDENCE

Self-transcendence initially was defined by Reed (1991b) as "expansion of self-conceptual boundaries multidimensionally: inwardly (e.g., through introspective experiences), outwardly (e.g., by reaching out to others), and temporally (whereby past and future are integrated into the present)" (p. 71). Reed (1997b) provided a more comprehensive definition, as follows, in a later publication:

> Self-transcendence refers to a fluctuation of perceived boundaries that extends the person (or self) beyond the immediate and constricted views of self and the world. This fluctuation is pandimensional, that is, outward (toward others and the environment), inward (toward greater awareness of one's own beliefs, values, and dreams), and temporal (toward integration of past and future in a way that enhances the relative present). (p. 192)

In 2003, another pattern of boundary expansion was incorporated so that self-transcendence is also the capacity to expand one's self-boundaries "transpersonally (to connect with dimensions beyond the typically discernible world)" (Reed, 2003, p. 147). Because self-transcendence is pandimensional, it is possible that other dimensions may be added to describe the capacities for boundary expansion. (P. Reed, personal communication, June 17, 2004).

WELL-BEING

Well-being is defined as "the sense of feeling whole and healthy, in accord with one's own criteria for wholeness and well-being" (Reed, 2003, p. 148). In her earlier work, Reed did not explicitly define well-being but linked the concept to mental health, which was dependent on salient issues of development within a given phase of life (Reed, 1989, 1991b). Reed also described the underlying mechanisms of well-being in a 1997 article. In that article, she proposed nursing to be "the study of the nursing processes of well being" (p. 76). Well-being as a nursing process, then, was described in terms of a synthesis of two kinds of change: changes in complexity in a life (i.e., the increasing frailness of advanced aging or the loss of a beloved spouse) tempered by changes in integration (i.e., constructing meaning from such life events) (Reed, 1997a).

Continued

MAJOR CONCEPTS & DEFINITIONS—cont'd

MODERATING-MEDIATING FACTORS

A wide variety of personal and contextual variables and their interactions may influence the process of self-transcendence as it contributes to well-being. Examples of such variables are age, gender, cognitive ability, life experiences, spiritual perspectives, social environment, and historical events. These personal and contextual variables may strengthen or weaken relationships between vulnerability and self-transcendence and between self-transcendence and well-being (Reed, 2003).

POINTS OF INTERVENTION

According to the self-transcendence theory, there are two points of intervention. Both points interface in some way with the process of self-transcendence. Nursing actions may focus directly on a person's inner resource for self-transcendence or focus on some of the personal and contextual factors that affect the relationships between vulnerability and self-transcendence and between self-transcendence and well-being (Reed, 2003).

USE OF EMPIRICAL EVIDENCE

Self-transcendence theory was grounded in belief in the developmental nature of older adults and the necessity of continued development to maintain mental health and a sense of well-being during the process of aging (Reed, 1983). Therefore, the initial research in theory building was conducted with older adults (Reed 1986b, 1989, 1991b).

In the first study, Reed (1986b) examined patterns of developmental resources and depression over time in 28 mentally healthy and 28 clinically depressed older adults (mean age 67.4 years). Levels of developmental resources were measured 3 times (6 weeks apart) with the 36-item Developmental Resources of Later Adulthood (DRLA) scale, previously developed and tested by Dr. Reed. The healthy adults perceived higher levels of resources across time than did the depressed adults. Scores on the Center for Epidemiological Studies Depression (CES-D) scale (Radloff, 1977) were significantly higher in depressed individuals across time than those of the mentally healthy. Strong relationships between DRLA scores and subsequent CES-D scores indicated that developmental resources influenced mental health outcomes in the healthy group; the reverse relationship was found in the depressed group, indicating that depression negatively influenced developmental resources in terms of the

ability to explore new outlooks on life, to share wisdom and experience with others, and to find spiritual meaning.

In the second study, Reed (1989) explored the degree to which key developmental resources of later adulthood were related to mental health in 30 hospitalized clinically depressed older adults (mean age 67 years). Participants completed the DRLA and CES-D measures and rated the importance in their current lives of each developmental resource reflected in the DRLA items. An inverse correlation was found between the level of resources and depression. Participants also reported that the resources represented by the DRLA items were highly important in their lives. In addition, key reasons given by participants for their psychiatric hospitalization were congruent with self-transcendence issues significant in later adulthood (e.g., physical health concerns, relationships with adult children, and questions about life and death).

During the initial DRLA instrument development and testing, a factor labeled *transcendence* had accounted for 45.2% of the variance in the DRLA scores. In the second study (Reed, 1989), the 15-item transcendence factor was also more highly correlated with the CES-D than was the entire DRLA. Therefore, a recommendation for future research was to examine further the psychometric properties of the instrument, with one goal being to shorten the DRLA to facilitate ease of administration in clinical settings.

A third study explored patterns of self-transcendence and mental health in 55 independent-living elders (ranging in age from 80 to 97 years) (Reed, 1991b). In this study, self-transcendence was defined as "the expansion of one's conceptual boundaries inwardly through introspective activities, outwardly through concerns about other's welfare, and temporally by integrating perceptions of one's past and future to enhance the present" (Reed, 1991b, p. 5). Self-transcendence was measured by the newly developed Self-Transcendence Scale (STS), derived from the previously identified 15-item transcendence factor in the original DRLA scale. The STS score was found to be inversely correlated with both CES-D and Langner scale of Mental Health Symptomatology (MHS) scores. The MHS is an index of general mental health on which higher scores indicate impairment in mental health in nonpsychiatric populations (Langner, 1962). The four patterns of self-transcendence identified by participants (generativity, introjectivity, temporal integration, and body-transcendence) were congruent with Reed's definition of the concept.

In summary, Reed's three studies provided evidence for the theoretical idea that self-transcendence views and behaviors were, in fact, present in older adults. Her data also indicated that such views and behaviors were related strongly to mental health. The findings thus supported a conceptualization of mental health in later adulthood that included the importance of resources that expanded self-concept boundaries beyond a preoccupation with the physical and cognitive declines of aging.

MAJOR ASSUMPTIONS

Early in her theoretical work, Reed (1986a, 1987) proposed a process model approach for constructing conceptual frameworks that would guide nurses and nursing education in clinical specialties. In that model, health was proposed as the central concept, or axis, around which revolved nursing activity, person, and environment. The assumption of the model was that the focus of the nursing discipline was on building and engaging knowledge to promote health processes.

Health

Health, in that early process model, was defined implicitly as a life process of both positive and negative experiences from which individuals create unique values and environments that promote well-being.

Nursing

The role of nursing activity was to assist persons (through interpersonal processes and therapeutic management of their environments) with the skills required for promoting health and well-being.

Person

Persons were conceived as developing over their life-span in interaction with other persons and within an environment of changing complexity and vibrancy that could both positively and negatively contribute to health and well-being.

Environment

Family, social networks, physical surroundings, and community resources were environments that significantly contributed to health processes that nurses influenced through "managing therapeutic interactions among people, objects, and [nursing] activities" (Reed, 1987, p. 26).

This metaparadigmatic approach to conceptual framework development for a nursing specialty was innovative and foundational to Reed's own future work with the concepts of spirituality and self-transcendence. Self-transcendence theory evolved from the perspective that self-transcendence is one of many processes related to health and that the overall goal of the theory was to provide nurses with another perspective on the human capacity for well-being.

In her initial explication of the emerging self-transcendence theory, Reed (1991a) identified one key assumption based on Rogers' conceptual system and influenced by life-span development theorists, psychiatric–mental health clinical knowledge, research findings, and personal experiences. This assumption was that persons were open systems who imposed conceptual boundaries upon themselves to define their reality and to provide a sense of wholeness and connectedness within themselves and their environment. Reed (2003) reaffirmed this assumption in a later publication, restating Rogers' basic assumption that "human beings are integral with their environment" (p. 146). Self-conceptual boundaries fluctuated in form across the life-span and were associated with human health and development. Self-transcendence was proposed as an important indicator of a person's conceptual self-boundaries that could be assessed at specific times.

A second assumption was identified in a later description of the theory wherein self-transcendence was assumed to be a developmental imperative (Reed, 2003). That is, self-transcendence must be expressed like any other developmental capacity in life for a person to realize a continuing sense of wholeness and connectedness. This assumption is congruent with Frankl's (1969) and Maslow's (1971) conceptualizations of self-transcendence as an innate human characteristic that, when actualized, gives purpose and meaning to a person's existence.

THEORETICAL ASSERTIONS

There are three basic concepts in the theory of self-transcendence: vulnerability, self-transcendence, and well-being (Reed, 2003). Vulnerability is the awareness of personal mortality that arises with aging and other life phases, or during health events and life crises (Reed, 2003). Although vulnerability is not explicated as a concept in Reed's earlier writings, it is not a new idea in her theory. The concept of vulnerability clarifies that the context within which self-transcendence is realized is not only in confronting end-of-own-life issues but includes life crises such as disability, chronic illness, childbirth, and parenting. Self-transcendence refers to the fluctuations in perceived boundaries that extend

persons beyond their immediate and constricted views of self and the world. The fluctuations are pandimensional: outward (toward awareness of others and the environment), inward (toward greater insight into one's own beliefs, values, and dreams), temporal (toward integration of past and future in a way that enhances the relative present), and transpersonal (toward awareness of dimensions beyond the typically discernible world) (Reed, 1997b, 2003). Well-being means "feeling whole and healthy, in accord with one's own criteria for wholeness and well-being" (Reed, 2003, p. 148).

Additional concepts in the theory are moderating-mediating factors and points of intervention. Moderating-mediating factors are personal and contextual variables such as age, gender, life experiences, and social environment that can influence the relationships between vulnerability and self-transcendence and between self-transcendence and well-being. Points of intervention are nursing activities that facilitate self-transcendence.

Three major propositions were developed using the three basic concepts of vulnerability, self-transcendence, and well-being. The first proposition of the theory is that self-transcendence is greater in persons facing end-of-own-life issues than in persons not facing such issues. End-of-own-life issues are interpreted broadly, as they arise with life events, illness, aging, and other experiences that increase awareness of personal mortality.

The second proposition of the theory is that conceptual boundaries are related to well-being (Reed, 1991a). Depending on their nature, fluctuations in conceptual boundaries influence well-being positively or negatively across the life-span. For example, an increase in self-transcendence views and behaviors is expected to be positively related to mental health as an indicator of well-being in persons confronting end-of-life issues. A specific example of a negative influence is that the inability to reach out for or to accept friendship would be expected to be related to depression as an indicator of mental health.

Given the key assumption about the person-environmental process (Reed, 1991a), a third set of propositions was identified by Reed in 2003. Personal and environmental factors function as correlates, moderators, or mediators of the relationships between vulnerability, self-transcendence, and well-being.

In summary, the 2003 model of the self-transcendence theory proposes the following three sets of relationships (Figure 29-1):

1. Increased vulnerability is related to increased self-transcendence.
2. Self-transcendence is positively related to well-being.
3. Personal and contextual factors may influence the relationship between vulnerability and self-transcendence and between self-transcendence and well-being.

LOGICAL FORM

Reed's empirical middle range theory was constructed using the strategy of deductive reformulation to enhance understanding of the end-of-life phenomenon of self-transcendence (Reed, 1991a). The logic used is primarily deduction, to ensure that the middle range theory was congruent with Rogerian and life-span principles. Analogical reasoning

was also used to work from other theories of life-span development, drawing comparisons between psychology and nursing about human development and potential for well-being at all phases of life. The key concepts of the theory are related in a clear and logical manner, while still allowing for creativity in the way the theory is applied, tested, and further developed. Reed's strategy of constructing a nursing theory—from nonnursing theories, a nursing conceptual model, research, and clinical and personal experiences—piqued nurses' interest in this phenomenon of developmental maturity and provided impetus for further theorizing and research into the variety of situations in which awareness of personal mortality occurs.

ACCEPTANCE BY THE NURSING COMMUNITY
Practice

Reed's (1986a, 1987) process model for clinical specialty education and psychiatric–mental health nursing practice articulated the relationships

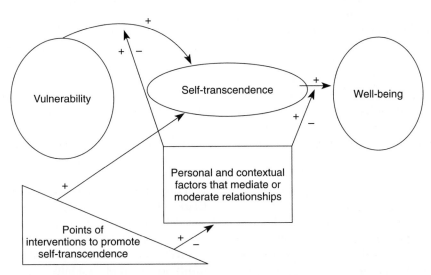

Figure **29-1 Model of self-transcendence theory.** (From Reed, P. G. [2003]. The theory of self-transcendence. In M. J. Smith & P. Liehr (Eds.), *Middle range theory for nursing* (p. 150). New York, Springer. Used by permission.)

between the metaparadigm constructs of health, persons and their environments, and nursing activity. Self-transcendence theory delineates specific concepts derived from the process model constructs of health (i.e., well-being), person (i.e., self-transcendence), and environment (i.e., vulnerability) and proposes relationships among those concepts to provide direction for nursing activities. Reed (1991a) and Coward and Reed (1996) suggested a variety of nursing activities that facilitate expansion of self-conceptual boundaries—journaling, meditation, life review, and religious expression, to name a few.

Self-transcendence may be integral to healing in many life situations. Nurse activities that promote the perspectives and activities of self-reflection, altruism, hope, and faith in vulnerable persons are associated with increased sense of well-being. Group psychotherapy (Young & Reed, 1995) and breast cancer support groups (Coward, 1998, 2003, 2004) are interventions nurse researchers have used to provide clients with opportunity for examining their values, for reaching out to share experience with and help similar others, and for finding meaning from their health situations. Others have suggested similar strategies to facilitate well-being in caregivers of persons with dementia (Acton & Wright, 2000) and in bereaved individuals (Joffrion & Douglas, 1994). Acton and Wright (2000) suggest arranging respite care for caregivers so that they have time and energy for transpersonal activities. McGee (2000) suggests that recovery in alcoholism involves a process of self-transcendence, as facilitated by a nurse-designed environment that supports the 12 steps and 12 traditions of Alcoholics Anonymous.

Education

Themes of self-transcendence are found in the writings of nurse theorists influential in nursing education. Sarter (1988) analyzed the philosophical roots of four contemporary nursing theories (Rogers' Science of Unitary Human Beings, 1970, 1980; Newman's theory of expanding consciousness, 1986; Watson's theory of caring, 1979, 1985; and Parse's

theory of man-living-health, 1981). These theories share a common view in identifying self-transcendence as an appropriate philosophical foundation for the discipline. Modeling and Role-Modeling Theory, which contains concepts similar to self-transcendence that are associated with development and health, guides the curricula of several undergraduate programs (Erickson, 2002; Erickson, Tomlin, & Swain, 1983).

Reed describes self-transcendence as "both a human capacity and a human struggle that can be facilitated by nursing" (Reed, 1997a, p. 3). Reed (1997a) went on to define nursing succinctly as "an inherent human process of well-being, manifested by complexity and integration" (p. 76), with self-transcendence as an important factor in the process of well-being. Given this link between well-being and self-transcendence, it is imperative that nurses be educated to promote self-transcendence views and behaviors in their clients. Self-transcendence is also a pathway for helping the healer, or healing the healer, so that nurses themselves maintain a healthy lifestyle as they care for others (Conti-O'Hare, 2002).

Research

A large number of research studies have provided evidence to support the association between self-transcendence and increased well-being in populations that typically are confronted with an awareness of their own personal mortality. The initial research studies relating self-transcendence to depression were conducted with elders (Reed, 1986b, 1989, 1991a). More recent research reported similar relationships in both depressed older adults (Klaas, 1998; Young & Reed, 1995) and middle-aged adults (Ellermann & Reed, 2001). Buchanan, Ferran, and Clark (1995) examined self-transcendence and suicidal thought in older adults. Upchurch (1993, 1999) explored the relationship between self-transcendence and activities of daily living in non-institutionalized older adults. Walton, Shultz, Beck, and Walls (1991) identified an inverse relationship between self-transcendence and loneliness in healthy older adults.

An impressive number of studies have demonstrated a positive relationship between self-transcendence and well-being or quality of life in persons with human immunodeficiency virus or acquired immunodeficiency syndrome (Coward, 1994, 1995; Coward & Lewis, 1993; McCormick, Holder, Wetsel, & Cawthon, 2001; Mellors, Erlen, Coontz, & Lucke, 2001; Mellors, Riley, & Erlen, 1997; Stevens, 1999). Several studies have described self-transcendence or related concepts in women with breast cancer (Carpenter, Brockopp, & Andrykowski, 1999; Coward, 1990a, 1990b, 1991, 2004; Coward & Kahn, 2004a, 2004b; Kamienski, 1997; Kinney, 1996; Matthews, 2000; Pelusi, 1997; Taylor, 2000). The positive effect of a self-transcendence theory–based cancer support group intervention on self-transcendence and well-being in newly diagnosed women also was documented by Coward (1998, 2003, 2004).

Self-transcendence in caregivers of persons with dementia was explored by Acton (2003) and Acton & Wright (2000) and was studied in caregivers of terminally ill patients who had died within the previous year (Enyert & Burman, 1999). Other populations studied include healthy middle-aged adults (Coward, 1996), elderly men with prostate cancer (Chin-A-Loy & Fernsler, 1998), female nursing students and faculty (Kilpatrick, 2002), homeless adults (Runquist, 2002), and liver transplant recipients (Wright, 2003). Other studies reported positive relationships between transcendence and transformation and finding meaning among elders (Klaas, 1998) and in women with rheumatoid arthritis (Neill, 2002).

In addition, Reed has mentored a number of master's and doctoral students in research on self-transcendence. Research results from these studies, some of which are cited above, provide additional empirical support for the theory. See the bibliography for a more complete listing.

FURTHER DEVELOPMENT

Reed's initial conceptualization of self-transcendence focused on later adulthood and identified the importance of personal resources that expand self-boundaries beyond the concerns generated by physical and cognitive decline. The more recent studies by Reed and others have extended the scope of the theory to include additional populations that have increased awareness of their own personal mortality.

Diverse personal and contextual variables may impact the relationship between self-transcendence and well-being. Although a number of studies have associated older age with increased self-transcendence, many younger research participants report self-transcendence views and behaviors and score high on self-transcendence measures. A variety of human experiences, such as childbirth and parenting, illness and disability, caregiving, creating a work of art or literature, and spiritual perspectives all may, over a long or short period in one's life, evoke the pandimensional views and behaviors indicative of self-transcendence. Continued research into these and other personal and contextual factors will increase understanding of the role they play in the theoretical propositions (Reed, 2003).

Further development of the theory also will include examination of points of intervention to facilitate self-transcendence perspectives and behaviors in persons who express a need for increased sense of wholeness and well-being. One such intervention, a self-transcendence theory–based support group, had a small positive effect on self-transcendence variables in women with newly diagnosed breast cancer (Coward, 2003, 2004). Young and Reed (1995) found group psychotherapy effective in facilitating self-transcendence in a small sample of elder adults. As the theory of self-transcendence evolves, nursing will learn more about new potentials for well-being in health experiences over the life-span.

Reed receives funding to study self-transcendence as it relates to end-of-life decisions and well-being in patients and their family caregivers. People facing the end of life represent some of the most vulnerable individuals to whom nurses may give care. Although an abundance of lay literature exists about the developmental and transcendent experiences of end of life and dying, there is a dearth of systematic research into this human experience. The theory of self-transcendence can guide initial questions and may undergo further refinement as this inquiry progresses.

Other forms of inquiry may also occur in reference to the theory, particularly in view of Reed's recent reconceptualization of nursing. Through her philosophical writings, Reed (1997a) has clarified a more foundational definition of nursing that shifted the source of nursing activity from that of external agent (i.e., the "nurse") to viewing nursing as an inner human process. Specifically, Reed defined nursing as a process of well-being that exists within and among human systems. The process of nursing is characterized by changing complexity and integration. From this, she presented self-transcendence as a nursing process. Further explorations into mechanisms of changing complexity and integration may help achieve new theoretical explanations about how self-transcendence emerges and functions in human lives.

CRITIQUE
Clarity and Consistency

Clarity and consistency are key criteria in the description of and critical reflection on a theory (Chinn & Kramer, 2004). Theory clarity is evaluated by how clearly defined are the concepts (semantic clarity) and by how understandable are the connections among the concepts and the reasoning within the theory (structural clarity). Semantic consistency is evaluated by how well the concepts are used in ways that are consistent with their definitions and the basic assumptions of the theory. Structural consistency evaluation involves assessing how congruent are the assumptions, theory purpose, concept definitions, and connections among the concepts.

Theoretical sources for development of the theory are described clearly in several publications (Reed, 1991b, 1996, 1997b, 2003). However, the definitions and assumptions about the concepts derived from life-span developmental theory and Rogers' Science of Unitary Human Beings have sometimes been difficult for nurses to grasp. In attempting to clarify concepts such as health and

self-transcendence, Reed has presented slightly varying definitions and numerous examples which, although theoretically consistent, may confuse some readers. In terms of structural clarity, some relationships in the schematic model of the theory (see Figure 29-1) are not yet fully defined and described in Reed's writings except in the publication in which that diagram appears (Reed, 2003). Structural consistency is good in that the identified relationships are logical and consistent.

It is not unusual to find these issues about clarity in definitions when a theory incorporates concepts that are somewhat abstract. In addition, some clarity and consistency may be challenged because theorizing is an ongoing process that develops over time, and theories may outgrow some of initial ideas of the theorist. Overall, however, Reed's theoretical thinking has remained congruent with the original Rogerian and life-span conceptual views and assumptions underlying her knowledge development, and she has conceptualized a theory that can be understood by both nurse clinicians and nurse researchers.

Simplicity

Simplicity, referring to having a minimal number of concepts and interrelationships (Chinn & Kramer, 2004), is valued in a middle range theory developed to guide nursing practice. Reed's theory is strong on simplicity, with three major concepts (vulnerability, self-transcendence, and well-being), along with two other concepts (personal and environmental factors, and points of intervention). The theory likely will increase in complexity somewhat as specific personal and environmental factors and their relationships to the major concepts are identified. Overall, the major concepts and the number of relationships generated by these concepts are minimal while still being meaningful and fairly comprehensive.

Generality

The scope and purpose of Reed's theory is such that the theory can be applied to a wide variety of human health situations. The purpose of the theory is to enhance nurses' understanding about well-being (Reed, 2003). When presented initially, Reed's work focused on developmental resources in persons confronted by challenges of later adulthood as related to indicators of mental health symptomatology (specifically, clinical depression) (Reed, 1983, 1986b, 1991a). In linking self-transcendence (an indicator of developmental maturity, but not necessarily associated with aging) to mental health (an indicator of overall well-being), the scope of the emerging theory was expanded to include persons other than elders who were facing end-of-own-life issues (Reed, 1991b). Further development and testing of the theory led to the specification of the additional concepts of vulnerability, points of intervention, and personal and contextual variables (Reed, 2003). The theory is now broader in scope and is more congruent with a life-span perspective, because the major concepts can be applied to anyone who is confronted with life events ranging from childbirth to life-threatening illness and dying. Broadening the scope and purpose of the theory from explaining mental health to explaining well-being increased its generality and resulted in a theory that is applicable in the many situations that involve both health and healing.

Empirical Precision

Empirical precision refers to how well the concepts are linked to observed or observable reality, particularly in contexts relevant to nursing practice. Chinn and Kramer (2004) refer to this criterion in terms of the accessibility of the theory. Although the theory's concepts are somewhat abstract (vulnerability, self-transcendence, and well-being), empirical indicators of subconcepts (e.g., the impact of life-threatening illness, reaching out to others, and depression, respectively) have been identified and studied by numerous researchers. In particular, measurement of self-transcendence has been honed through development and refinement of Reed's Self-Transcendence Scale. Well-being has been measured by a variety of empirical indicators.

Researchers may use different approaches and empirical indicators to measure self-transcendence because the concept lends itself to a variety of approaches and measures that fit the clinical nursing context of interest. Research findings that support a strong relationship among self-transcendence and various indicators of well-being, as hypothesized by the theory, also attest to the theory's empirical precision.

Derivable Consequences

Self-transcendence theory is a middle range theory that leads to valued goals in nursing education, practice, and research. The theory, grounded in nursing philosophy, research, and practice and tested in subsequent research, has led to new knowledge that can be useful in nursing practice. The theory provides insight into the developmental nature of humans as related to health situations relevant to nursing care. Nurses and patients often face events that challenge personal mortality; knowledge of developmental resources (i.e., self-transcendence) that can be engaged by or for the patient expands the nursing repertoire for facilitating well-being in times of increased vulnerability. The abstract yet definable nature of self-transcendence facilitates the development of many interventions that may be tested as strategies to promote self-transcendence in a variety of nurse-patient encounters.

SUMMARY

Self-transcendence theory was developed initially using the strategy of deductive reformulation from life-span developmental theories, Rogers' conceptual system of unitary human beings, empirical research, and clinical and personal experiences of the theorist. Although the theoretical concepts are abstract, more concrete subconcepts have been developed and studied extensively in a number of populations. Exploratory, descriptive correlational, and quasi-experimental studies have supported the hypothesized relationship between self-transcendence views and behaviors and indicators of well-being. Such research findings have increased nurses' understanding that, no matter how desperate a health situation, people retain a capacity for personal development that is associated with feelings of well-being.

Research findings also have suggested ways in which nurses can promote self-transcendence views and behaviors in themselves and in their clients. Further research will examine interventions to promote self-transcendence and study the personal and contextual factors that modify relationships among the theory concepts. In addition, qualitative research may assist in gaining further understanding of the concept of self-transcendence as a nursing process and as it expresses the depth and changing complexity and organization of human beings.

Case Study

Mr. Jones is a 65-year-old gentleman whose wife died 6 months ago after a long illness. The couple was married 45 years, and they were devoted to each other. They had three children who are now in their 30s. Two of the children live several hundred miles away, but one son lives with his wife and two preschool children less than a mile from the Jones' home.

Mr. Jones provided much of the care for his wife during her illness. Although her care was time consuming and fatiguing and kept him at home much of the time, he was grateful that he could care for her. He now is alone in their home, very lonely, uninterested in preparing meals or eating, and lacks energy to return to his former community and social activities or even interact with his son and family.

The hospice nurse contacted Mr. Jones for follow-up bereavement counseling. She told him that although he had "passed" a routine physical examination the week before, she was concerned about his continuing sadness and lack of energy. The nurse reassured him that it was not uncommon to grieve for many months after a major loss. She asked him if he thought his wife would have had a similar experience if he had been the first to die. His response was that his wife would have had an even more difficult time adjusting. The

nurse and Mr. Jones then spent some time reflecting on and talking about his response. The nurse's initial question and Mr. Jones' resulting insight that his grief was not as bad as his wife's would have been, helped him transcend his immediate experience of loss and to find some meaning in his grief.

This illustration is an example of an inward expansion of self-conceptual boundaries indicative of self-transcendence. Other expressions of self-transcendence might help Mr. Jones facilitate his own healing and regain a measure of well-being.

In terms of outward expansion, Mr. Jones, with some encouragement, might reach out to his son's family to begin to reconnect to the world outside himself. Walking to and from his home to theirs could expand his sensory world and provide opportunities to interact with other people and with nature along the way. Spending time with his grandchildren could be enlivening through the joy young children can bring to an older person, as could a sense of satisfaction derived from being helpful to his son and daughter-in-law.

Offering at a future time to use the skills he learned while caring for his wife through volunteering with hospice would be an example of transcending temporally. Integrating his memories of Mrs. Jones into his current life would be another example of temporal self-transcendence.

Transpersonal self-transcendence is another important experience for Mr. Jones. Although he was unable to attend church services for several years, he had in the past found worshiping with others a source of comfort. His spiritual life might even be expanded to consider new spiritual dimensions such as that found in the possibility of "being with" his wife again someday or in some way experiencing her presence in the present. Returning to church or to addressing spiritual dimensions outside of organized worship that relates Mr. Jones' understanding of death to some greater or divine design are other examples of transpersonal self-transcendence.

CRITICAL THINKING *Activities*

1. Considering the pandimensional aspect of self-transcendence, list a few examples of when you experienced expanded boundaries in your own life. Reflect on how this expanded awareness influenced your health or sense of well-being.

2. What are some personal and contextual factors in your life that are negatively or positively related to your own experience of self-transcendence?

3. What might you do to facilitate self-transcendence and a sense of wholeness in a woman with acquired immunodeficiency syndrome who is dying?

4. How could you apply the theory of self-transcendence to help a frail 95-year-old person living in a nursing home maintain or gain a sense of well-being?

REFERENCES

Acton, G. (2003). Self-transcendent views and behaviors: Exploring growth in caregivers of adults with dementia. *Journal of Gerontological Nursing, 28*(12), 22-30.

Acton, G., & Wright, K. (2000). Self-transcendence and family caregivers of adults with dementia. *Journal of Holistic Nursing, 18*(2), 143-158.

Alexander, C. N., & Langner, E. J. (1990). *Higher stages of human development: Perspectives on adult growth.* New York: Oxford University Press.

Buchanan, D., Ferran, C., & Clark, D. (1995). Suicidal thought and self-transcendence in older adults. *Journal of Psychosocial Nursing and Mental Health Services, 33*(10), 31-34, 42-43.

Carpenter, J. S., Brockopp, D., & Andrykowski, M. (1999). Self-transformation as a factor in the self-esteem and well-being of breast cancer survivors. *Journal of Advanced Nursing, 29*(6), 1042-1411.

Chin-A-Loy, S. S., & Fernsler, J. I. (1998). Self-transcendence in older men attending a prostate cancer support group. *Cancer Nursing, 21*(5), 358-363.

Chinn, P. L., & Kramer, M. K. (2004). *Integrated knowledge development in nursing* (6th ed.). St. Louis: Mosby.

Commons, M. L., Richards, F. A., & Armon, C. (Eds.). (1984). *Beyond formal operations: Late adolescent and adult cognitive development.* New York: Praeger.

Conti-O'Hare, M., (2002). *The nurse as wounded healer: From trauma to transcendence.* Sudbury, MA: Jones and Bartlett.

Coward, D. D. (1990a). The lived experience of self-transcendence in women with advanced breast cancer. *Nursing Science Quarterly, 3,* 162-169.

Coward, D. D. (1990b). Correlates of self-transcendence in women with advanced breast cancer. *Dissertation Abstracts International, B 52*(01). (University Microfilms No. 9108416)

Coward, D. D. (1991). Self-transcendence and emotional well-being in women with advanced breast cancer. *Oncology Nursing Forum, 18,* 857-863.

Coward, D. D. (1994). Meaning and purpose in the lives of persons with AIDS. *Public Health Nursing, 11*(5), 331-336.

Coward, D. D. (1995). Lived experience of self-transcendence in women with AIDS. *Journal of Obstetrics, Gynecologic, & Neonatal Nursing, 24,* 314-318.

Coward, D. D. (1996). Correlates of self-transcendence in a healthy population. *Nursing Research, 45*(2), 116-121.

Coward, D. D. (1998). Facilitation of self-transcendence in a breast cancer support group. *Oncology Nursing Forum, 25,* 75-84.

Coward, D. D. (2003). Facilitation of self-transcendence in a breast cancer support group II. *Oncology Nursing Forum, 30*(Part 1 of 2), 291-300.

Coward, D. D. (2004, May). *Self-transcendence in breast cancer support groups.* Poster session presented at the Oncology Nursing Society 28th Annual Congress, Santa Ana, CA.

Coward, D. D., & Kahn, D. L. (2004a). Resolution of spiritual disequilibrium in women newly diagnosed with breast cancer (Online exclusive). *Oncology Nursing Forum, 31*(2), E24-E31. Accessed January 4, 2004, at: *http://journals.ons.org/ONF/2004/march/E24-E31.pdf*

Coward, D. D., & Kahn, D. L. (2004b). Transcending breast cancer: Making meaning from diagnosis and treatment. *Journal of Holistic Nursing.*

Coward, D. D., & Lewis, F. M. (1993). The lived experience of self-transcendence in gay men with AIDS. *Oncology Nursing Forum, 20,* 1363-1369.

Coward, D. D., & Reed, P. G. (1996). Self-transcendence: A resource for healing at the end-of-life. *Issues in Mental Health Nursing, 17*(3), 275-288.

Ellermann, C. R., & Reed, P. G. (2001). Self-transcendence and depression in middle-aged adults. *Western Journal of Nursing Research, 23*(7), 698-713.

Enyert, G., & Burman, M. E. (1999). A qualitative study of self-transcendence in caregivers of terminally ill patients. *American Journal of Hospice and Palliative Care, 16*(2), 455-462.

Erickson, H. C., Tomlin, E. M., & Swain, M. A. P. (1983). *Modeling and role-modeling: A theory and paradigm for nursing.* Englewood Cliffs, NJ: Prentice-Hall.

Erickson, M. (2002). Modeling and role-modeling. In A. M. Tomey & M. R. Alligood (Eds.), *Nursing theorists and their work* (5th ed., pp. 443-464). St. Louis: Mosby.

Fitzpatrick, J. J., Whall, A. L., Johnston, R. L., & Floyd, J. A. (1982). *Nursing models and their psychiatric mental health applications.* Bowie, MD: Robert J. Brady.

Frankl, V. (1969). *The will to meaning.* New York: New American Library.

Joffrion, L. P., & Douglas, D. (1994). Grief resolution: Facilitating self-transcendence in the bereaved. *Journal of Psychosocial Nursing, 32*(3), 13-19.

Kamienski, M. C. (1997). An investigation of the relationship among suffering, self-transcendence, and social support in women with breast cancer. *Dissertation Abstracts International, B 58*(04). (University Microfilms No. ATT9729588)

Kilpatrick, J. A. W. (2002). Spiritual perspective, self-transcendence, and spiritual well-being in female nursing students and female nursing faculty. *Dissertation Abstracts International, B63*(02). (University Microfilms No. ATT 3044802)

Kinney, C. (1996). Transcending breast cancer: Reconstructing one's self. *Issues in Mental Health Nursing, 17*(3), 201-216.

Klaas, D. (1998). Testing two elements of spirituality in depressed and non-depressed elders. *The International Journal of Psychiatric Nursing Research, 4,* 452-462.

Langner, T. S. (1962). A twenty-two item screening score of psychiatric symptoms indicating impairment. *Journal of Health and Human Behavior, 3,* 269-276.

Lerner, R. (2002). *Concepts and theories of human development* (3rd ed.). Mahwah, NJ: Lawrence Erlbaum Associates.

Maslow, A. H. (1971). *Farther reaches of human nature.* New York: Viking Press.

Matthews, E. E. (2000). Optimism and emotional well-being in women with breast cancer: The role of mediators. *Dissertation Abstracts International, B61*(03). (University Microfilms No. 9967106)

McCormick, D. P., Holder, B., Wetsel, M., & Cawthon, T. (2001). Spirituality and HIV disease: An integrated perspective. *Journal of the Association of Nurses in AIDS care, 12*(3), 58-65.

McGee, E. (2000). Alcoholics Anonymous and nursing: Lessons in holism and spiritual care. *Journal of Holistic Nursing, 18*(1), 11-26.

Mellors M. P., Erlen, J. A., Coontz, P. D., & Lucke, K. T. (2001). Transcending the suffering of AIDS. *Journal of Community Health Nursing, 18*(4), 235-246.

Mellors, M. P., Riley, T. A., & Erlen, J. A. (1997). HIV, self-transcendence, and quality of life. *Journal of the Association of Nurses in AIDS Care, 8*(2), 59-69.

Newman, M. A. (1986). *Health as expanding consciousness.* St. Louis: Mosby.

Neill, J. (2002). Transcendence and transformation in life patterns of women living with rheumatoid arthritis. *ANS Advances in Nursing Science, 24*(2), 27-47.

Parse, R. R. (1981). *Man-living-health: A theory of nursing.* New York: John Wiley & Sons.

Pelusi, J. (1997). The lived experience of surviving breast cancer. *Oncology Nursing Forum, 24*(3), 1343-1353.

Radloff, L. S. (1977). The CES-D scale: A self-report depression scale for research in the general population. *Applied Psychological Measurement, 1,* 385-401.

Reed, P. G. (1983). Implications of the life span developmental framework for well-being in adulthood and aging. *ANS Advances in Nursing Science, 6*(1), 18-25.

Reed, P. G. (1986a). A model for constructing a conceptual framework for education in the clinical specialty. *Journal of Nursing Education, 25*(7), 295-299.

Reed, P. G. (1986b). Developmental resources and depression in the elderly. *Nursing Research, 35*(6), 368-374.

Reed, P. G. (1987). Constructing a conceptual framework for psychosocial nursing. *Journal of Psychosocial Nursing, 25*(2), 24-28.

Reed, P. G. (1989). Mental health of older adults. *Western Journal of Nursing Research, 11,* 143-163.

Reed, P. G. (1991a). Toward a nursing theory of self-transcendence: Deductive reformulation using developmental theories. *ANS Advances in Nursing Science, 13*(4), 64-77.

Reed, P. G. (1991b). Self-transcendence and mental health in the oldest-old adults. *Nursing Research, 40*(1), 5-11.

Reed, P. G. (1996). Transcendence: Formulating nursing perspectives. *Nursing Science Quarterly, 9*(1), 2-4.

Reed, P. G. (1997a). Nursing: The ontology of the discipline. *Nursing Science Quarterly, 10*(2), 76-79.

Reed, P. G. (1997b). The place of transcendence in nursing's science of unitary human beings: Theory and research. In M. Madrid (Ed.), *Patterns of Rogerian knowing* (pp. 187-196). New York: National League for Nursing.

Reed, P. G. (2003). The theory of self-transcendence. In M. J. Smith & P. R. Liehr (Eds.), *Middle range theory for nursing* (pp. 145-165). New York: Springer.

Riegel, K. (1976). The dialectics of human development. *American Psychologist, 31,* 689-699.

Rogers, M. E. (1970). *An introduction to the theoretical basis of nursing.* Philadelphia: F. A. Davis.

Rogers, M. E. (1980). A science of unitary man. In J. Riehl & C. Roy (Eds.), *Conceptual models for nursing practice* (2nd ed., pp. 329-338). New York: Appleton-Century-Crofts.

Rogers, M. E. (1990). Nursing: Science of unitary, irreducible, human beings: Update 1990. In E. A. M. Barrett (Ed.), *Visions of Rogers' science based nursing* (pp. 5-12). New York: National League for Nursing Press.

Runquist, J. J. (2002) Spirituality, self-transcendence, and health factors in homeless adults (Abstract). *Communicating Nursing Research, 35*(10), 262.

Sarter, B. (1988). Philosophical sources of nursing theory. *Nursing Science Quarterly, 1*(2), 52-59.

Shearer, N. B. C., & Reed, P. G. (2004). Empowerment: Reformulation of a non-Rogerian concept. *Nursing Science Quarterly, 17*(3), 253-259.

Stevens, D. D. (1999). Spirituality, self-transcendence and depression in young adults with AIDS (Immune deficiency). *Dissertation Abstracts International, B61*(02). (University Microfilms No. 9961253)

Taylor, E. J. (2000). Transformation of tragedy among women surviving breast cancer. *Oncology Nursing Forum, 27,* 781-788.

Upchurch, S. L. (1993). Self-transcendence, health status, and selected variables as determinants of the ability to perform activities of daily living in non-institutionalized adults. *Dissertation Abstracts International, B55*(01). (University Microfilms No. 9407736)

Upchurch, S. L. (1999). Self transcendence and activities of daily living: The woman with the pink slippers. *Journal of Holistic Nursing, 17*(3), 251-266.

Walton, C., Shultz, C., Beck, C., & Walls, R. (1991). Psychological correlates of loneliness in the older adult. *Archives of Psychiatric Nursing, 5*(3), 165-170.

Watson, J. (1979). *Nursing: The philosophy and science of caring.* Boston: Little, Brown & Co.

Watson, J. (1985). *Nursing: Human science and human care: A theory of nursing.* Norwalk, CT: Appleton-Century-Crofts.

Whall, A. L. (1986). *Family therapy theory for nursing: Four approaches.* East Norwalk, CT: Appleton-Century-Crofts.

Wilber, K. (1980). *The Atman project: A transpersonal view of human development.* Wheaton, IL: Quest.

Wilber, K. (1981). *Up from Eden: A transpersonal view of human evolution.* Garden City, NY: Theosophical Publishing House.

Wilber, K. (1990). *Eye to eye: The quest for the new paradigm* (2nd ed.). Boston: Shambhala.

Wright, K. (2003). Quality of life, self-transcendence, illness distress, and fatigue in liver transplant recipients. *Dissertation Abstracts International, B64*(12). (University Microfilms No. 3116238)

Young, C. A., & Reed, P. G. (1995). Elders' perceptions of the role group psychotherapy in fostering self-transcendence. *Archives of Psychiatric Nursing, 9*(6), 338-347.

BIBLIOGRAPHY
Primary Sources
Book

Reed, P. G., & Shearer, N. (Eds.) (2004). *Perspectives on nursing theory* (4th ed). New York: Lippincott Williams & Wilkins.

Book Chapters

Reed, P. G. (1985). Early and middle adulthood. In D. L. Critchley & J. T. Maurin (Eds.), *The clinical specialist in psychiatric–mental health nursing: Theory, research, and practice* (pp. 135-154). New York: John Wiley & Sons.

Reed, P. G. (1986). The developmental conceptual framework: Nursing reformulations and applications for family theory. In A. Whall (Ed.), *Family therapy theory for nursing: Four approaches* (pp. 69-92). New York: Appleton-Century-Crofts.

Reed, P. G. (1992). Nursing theorizing as an ethical endeavor. In L. Nicoll (Ed.), *Perspectives on nursing theory* (2nd ed., pp. 168-175). New York: Lippincott.

Reed, P. G. (1996). Peplau's interpersonal relations model. In J. J. Fitzpatrick & A. L. Whall (Eds.), *Conceptual models of nursing: Analysis and application* (3rd ed., pp. 55-76). Norwalk: Appleton & Lange.

Reed, P. G. (1997). The place of transcendence in nursing's science of unitary human beings: Theory and research. In M. Madrid (Ed.), *Patterns of Rogerian knowing* (pp. 187-196). New York: National League for Nursing Press.

Reed, P. G. (1998). Nursing theoretical models. In J. Fitzpatrick (Ed.), *Encyclopedia of nursing research* (pp. 385-387). New York: Springer.

Reed, P. G. (1998). The re-enchantment of health care: A paradigm of spirituality. In M. Cobb & V. Robshaw (Eds.), *The spiritual challenge of health care* (pp. 35-55). Edinburgh, Scotland: Churchill Livingstone.

Reed, P. G. (2003). The theory of self-transcendence. In M. J. Smith & P. Liehr (Eds.), *Middle range theory for nursing* (pp. 145-166). New York: Springer.

Reed, P. G. (2005). Peplau's nursing theory of interpersonal relations. In J. Fitzpatrick & A. L. Whall (Eds.), *Conceptual models of nursing: Analysis and application* (4th ed., pp. 46-67). Englewood Cliffs, NJ: Prentice Hall.

Reed, P. G., & Johnston, R. L. (1983). Peplau's model: The interpersonal process. In J. J. Fitzpatrick & A. Whall (Eds.), *Conceptual models of nursing: Analysis and application* (pp. 27-46). Bowie, MD: Brady.

Reed, P. G., & Johnston, R. L. (1989). Peplau's model: The interpersonal process. In J. J. Fitzpatrick & A. Whall (Eds.), *Conceptual models of nursing: Analysis and application* (2nd ed., pp. 49-68). Norwalk, CT: Appleton & Lange.

Reed, P. G., & Larson, C. (2005, in press). Spirituality. In J. J. Fitzpatrick & M. Wallace (Eds.), *Encyclopedia for nursing research* (2nd ed.). New York: Springer.

Reed, P. G., & Shearer, N. C. (in press). Peplau's theoretical model. In J. J. Fitzpatrick & M. Wallace (Eds.), *Encyclopedia for nursing research* (2nd ed.). New York: Springer.

Reed, P. G., & Zurakowski, T. (1983). Nightingale: A visionary model for nursing. In J. J. Fitzpatrick & A. Whall (Eds.), *Conceptual models of nursing: Analysis and application* (pp. 12-26). Bowie, MD: Brady.

Reed, P. G., & Zurakowski, T. (1989). Nightingale: A visionary model for nursing revisited. In J. J. Fitzpatrick & A. Whall (Eds.), *Conceptual models of nursing: Analysis and application* (2nd ed., pp. 33-48). Norwalk, CT: Appleton & Lange.

Reed, P. G., & Zurakowski, T. L. (1996). Florence Nightingale: Foundations of nursing theory, education, research, and practice. In J. J. Fitzpatrick & A. L. Whall (Eds.), *Conceptual models of nursing: Analysis and application* (3rd ed., pp. 27-54). Norwalk, CT: Appleton & Lange.

Shearer, N., & Reed, P. G. (1998). Peplau's theoretical model. In J. Fitzpatrick (Ed.), *Encyclopedia of nursing research*. New York: Springer.

Journal Articles

Coward, D. D., & Reed, P. G. (1996). Self-transcendence: A resource for healing at the end of life. *Issues in Mental Health Nursing, 17,* 275-288.

Ellermann, C., & Reed, P. G. (2001). Self-transcendence and depression in middle-aged adults. *Western Journal of Nursing Research, 23*(7), 698-713.

Felton, G., Reed, P. G., & Perla, S. (1981). Measurement of nursing students' and nurses' attitudes toward cancer. *Western Journal of Nursing Research, 3*(1), 62-75.

Fitzpatrick, J. J., & Reed, P. G. (1980). Stress in the crisis experience: Nursing intervention. *Occupational Health Nursing, 28*(12), 19-21.

Jesse, E., & Reed, P. G. (2004). Effects of spirituality and psychosocial well-being on health risk behaviors among pregnant women from Appalachia. *Journal of Obstetric, Gynecologic, & Neonatal Nursing, 33*(6), 739-747.

Moore, I. K., & Reed, P. G. (2000). Stress-response sequence model in pediatric oncology nurses: Theory critique and commentary. *Journal of Pediatric Oncology Nursing, 17*(2), 72-75.

Reed, P. G. (1982). On Smith's definition of health (Editorial). *ANS Advances in Nursing Science, 4,* ix-x.

Reed, P. G. (1983). Implications of the life-span developmental framework for well-being in adulthood and aging. *ANS Advances in Nursing Science, 6,* 18-25.

Reed, P. G. (1984). The developmental concept (Editorial). *ANS Advances in Nursing Science, 6,* vii.

Reed, P. G. (1985). Strategies for teaching nursing research: Theory and metatheory in an undergraduate course. *Western Journal of Nursing Research, 7,* 482-486.

Reed, P. G. (1986). A model for constructing a conceptual framework for education in the clinical specialty. *Journal of Nursing Education, 25*(7), 295-299.

Reed, P. G. (1986). Death perspectives and temporal variables in terminally ill and healthy adults. *Death Studies, 10,* 443-454.

Reed, P. G. (1986). Developmental resources and depression in the elderly: A longitudinal study. *Nursing Research, 35,* 368-374.

Reed, P. G. (1986). Religiousness among terminally ill and healthy adults. *Research in Nursing and Health, 9,* 35-42.

Reed, P. G. (1987). Constructing a conceptual framework for psychosocial nursing practice. *Journal of Psychosocial Nursing, 25*(2), 24-28.

Reed, P. G. (1987). Liberal arts and professional nursing education: Integration for knowledge and wisdom. *Nursing Educator, 12*(4), 37-40.

Reed, P. G. (1987). Spirituality and well-being in terminally ill hospitalized adults. *Research in Nursing and Health, 10*(5), 335-344.

Reed, P. G. (1988). Promoting research productivity in new faculty: A developmental perspective of the early postdoctoral years. *Journal of Professional Nursing, 4*(2), 119-125.

Reed, P. G. (1989). Mental health of older adults [includes commentaries and author's response]. *Western Journal of Nursing Research, 11*(2), 143-163.

Reed, P. G. (1989). Nursing theorizing as an ethical endeavor. *ANS Advances in Nursing Science, 11*(3), 1-9.

Reed, P. G. (1991). Preferences for spiritually-related nursing interventions among terminally ill and nonterminally ill hospitalized adults and well adults. *Applied Nursing Research, 4*(3), 122-128.

Reed, P. G. (1991). Response to "Serenity: Caring with perspective." *Scholarly Inquiry for Nursing Practice, 5*(2), 143-147.

Reed, P. G. (1991). Self-transcendence and mental health in oldest-old adults. *Nursing Research, 40,* 7-11.

Reed, P. G. (1991). Spirituality and mental health of older adults: Extant knowledge for nursing. *Family and Community Health, 14*(2), 14-25.

Reed, P. G. (1991). Toward a theory of self-transcendence: Deductive reformulation using developmental theories. *ANS Advances in Nursing Science, 13*(4), 64-77.

Reed, P. G. (1992). An emerging paradigm for the investigation of spirituality in nursing. *Research in Nursing and Health, 15,* 349-357.

Reed, P. G. (1994). The spirituality factor: Response to "The relationship between spiritual perspective, social support, and depression in care giving and non–care giving wives." *Scholarly Inquiry for Nursing Practice: An International Journal, 8*(4), 391-396.

Reed, P. G. (1995). A treatise on nursing knowledge development for the 21st century: Beyond postmodernism. *ANS Advances in Nursing Science, 17*(3), 70-84.

Reed, P. G. (1996). Transcendence: Formulating nursing perspectives. *Nursing Science Quarterly, 9*(1), 2-4.

Reed, P. G. (1996). Transforming knowledge into nursing knowledge through the scholarship of practice: A revisionist analysis of Peplau. *Image: The Journal of Nursing Scholarship, 28*(1), 29-33.

Reed, P. G. (1997). Nursing: The ontology of the discipline. *Nursing Science Quarterly, 10*(2), 76-79.

Reed, P. G. (1998). A holistic view of nursing concepts and theories in practice. *Journal of Holistic Nursing, 16*(4), 4415-4419.

Reed, P. G. (1998). Response to commentary on "The ontology of the discipline of nursing": Breaking through a breakdown in logic. *Nursing Science Quarterly, 11*(4), 146-148.

Reed, P. G. (1999). Commentary: Spirituality in older women who have osteoarthritis. *Graduate Research in Nursing* (Online publication), *1*(1). Retrieved November 12, 2004, from *http://www.graduateresearch.com/reed.htm*

Reed, P. G. (1999). Response to "Attentively-embracing story: A middle range theory with practice and research implications." *Scholarly Inquiry for Nursing Practice, 13*(2), 205-210.

Reed, P. G. (2000). Nursing reformation: Historical reflections and philosophic foundations. *Nursing Science Quarterly, 13*(2), 129-136.

Reed, P. G. (2001). Commentary: Spiritual care provided by parish nurses. *Western Journal of Nursing Research, 23*, 456-458.

Reed, P. G. (in press). Neomodernism and evidence-based nursing: Implications for the production of nursing knowledge. *Nursing Outlook, 53*(3).

Reed, P. G., & Leonard, V. E. (1989). An analysis of the concept of self-neglect. *ANS Advances in Nursing Science, 12*(1), 39-53.

Reed, P. G., & Verran, J. (1988). Cross-lag panel correlation analysis assumptions: Stationarity, synchronicity, stability. *Western Journal of Nursing Research, 10*(5), 671-676.

Shearer, N. B. C., & Reed, P. G. (2004). Empowerment: Reformulation of a non-Rogerian concept. *Nursing Science Quarterly, 17*(3), 253-259.

Young, C., & Reed, P. G. (1995). Elders' perceptions of the effectiveness of group psychotherapy in fostering self-transcendence. *Archives of Psychiatric Nursing, 9*(6), 338-347.

Book Reviews

Reed, P. G. (1999). *Nursing theorists and their work* by M. Tomey & M. Alligood. *Nursing Science Quarterly, 12*(3), 266-268.

Reed, P. G. (1999). *Theory and nursing: Integrated knowledge development* by P. Chinn & M. Kramer. *Nursing Leadership Forum, 4*(2), 2-3.

Reed, P. G. (2001). Nursing as a spiritual practice: A contemporary application of Florence Nightingale's views by Janet Macrae. *Nursing Leadership Forum, 6*(2), 90.

Reed, P. G. (2003). Nursing theories and nursing practice by Marilyn Parker. *Nursing Science Quarterly, 16*(2), 175-176.

Reed, P. G. (in press). Giving voice to what we know: Margaret Newman's Theory of Health as Expanding Consciousness in nursing practice, research, and education by Carol Picaro and Dorothy Jones. *Nursing Science Quarterly.*

Dissertation

Reed, P. G. (1982). *Well-being and perspectives on life and death among death-involved and non–death-involved individuals.* Unpublished doctoral dissertation, Wayne State University, Detroit.

Secondary Sources
Selected Book Chapters

Coward, D. D. (2000). Making meaning within the experience of life-threatening illness. In G. Reker & K. Chamberlain (Eds.), *Existential meaning: Optimizing human development across the life span* (pp. 157-170). Thousand Oaks, CA: Sage.

Haase, J., Britt, T., Coward, D., Kline Leidy, N., & Penn, P. (1993). Simultaneous concept analysis: A strategy for developing multiple interrelated concepts. In B. Rodgers & K. Knafl (Eds.), *Concept development in nursing: Foundations, techniques, and applications* (pp. 175-192). Philadelphia: W. B. Saunders.

Haase, J., Britt, T., Coward, D., Kline Leidy, N., & Penn, P. (2000). Simultaneous concept analysis: A strategy for developing multiple interrelated concepts. In B. Rodgers & K. Knafl (Eds.), *Concept development in nursing: Foundations, techniques, and applications* (2nd ed., pp. 209-229). Philadelphia: W. B. Saunders.

Selected Journal Articles

Acton, G. (2003). Self-transcendent views and behaviors: Exploring growth in caregivers of adults with dementia. *Journal of Gerontological Nursing, 28*(12), 22-30.

Acton, G., & Wright, K. (2000). Self-transcendence and family caregivers of adults with dementia. *Journal of Holistic Nursing, 18*(2), 143-158.

Bickerstaff, K., Grasser, C., McCabe, B. (2003). How elderly nursing home residents transcend losses of later life. *Holistic Nursing Practice, 17*(3), 159–165.

Buchanan, D., Ferran, C., & Clark, D. (1995). Suicidal thought and self-transcendence in older adults. *Journal of Psychosocial Nursing and Mental Health Services, 33*(10), 31-34, 42-43.

Budin, W. C. (2001). Birth and death: Opportunities for self-transcendence. *Journal of Perinatal Education, 10*(2), 38-42.

Chen, K., & Snyder, M. (1999). A research-based use of Tai Chi/movement therapy as a nursing intervention. *Journal of Holistic Nursing, 17*(3), 267-279.

Chin-A-Loy, S. S., & Fernsler, J. I. (1998). Self-transcendence in older men attending a prostate cancer support group. *Cancer Nursing, 21*(5), 358-363.

Chiu, L. (2000). Lived experience of spirituality in Taiwanese women with breast cancer. *Western Journal of Nursing Research, 22,* 29-53.

Chiu, L., Emblen, J., van Hofwegen, L., Sawatzky, R., & Meyerhoff, H. (2004). An integrative review of the concept of spirituality in the health sciences. *Western Journal of Nursing Research, 26*(4), 405-428.

Coward, D. D. (1990). The lived experience of self-transcendence in women with advanced breast cancer. *Nursing Science Quarterly, 3,* 162-169.

Coward, D. D. (1991). Self-transcendence and emotional well-being in women with advanced breast cancer. *Oncology Nursing Forum, 18,* 857-863.

Coward, D. D. (1994). Meaning and purpose in the lives of persons with AIDS. *Public Health Nursing, 11*(5), 331-336.

Coward, D. D. (1995). Lived experience of self-transcendence in women with AIDS. *Journal of Obstetrics, Gynecologic, & Neonatal Nursing, 24,* 314-318.

Coward, D. D. (1996). Correlates of self-transcendence in a healthy population. *Nursing Research, 45*(2), 116-121.

Coward, D. D. (1996). Self-transcendence: Making meaning from the cancer experience. *Quality of Life— A Nursing Challenge, 4*(2), 53-58.

Coward, D. D. (1998). Facilitation of self-transcendence in a breast cancer support group. *Oncology Nursing Forum, 25,* 75-84.

Coward, D. D. (2003). Facilitation of self-transcendence in a breast cancer support group II. *Oncology Nursing Forum, 3*(Part 1 of 2), 291-300.

Coward, D. D., & Kahn, D. L. (2004). Resolution of spiritual disequilibrium in women newly diagnosed with breast cancer (Online exclusive). *Oncology Nursing Forum, 31*(2), E24-E31. Accessed January 4, 2004, at: *http://journals.ons.org/xp6/ONS/Library.xml/ONS_Publications.xml/ONF/2004/march/E24-E31.pdf*

Coward, D. D., & Kahn, D. L. (in press). Transcending breast cancer: Making meaning from diagnosis and treatment. *Journal of Holistic Nursing.*

Coward, D. D., & Lewis, F. M. (1993). The lived experience of self-transcendence in gay men with AIDS. *Oncology Nursing Forum, 20,* 1363-1369.

Coward, D. D., & Reed, P. G. (1996). Self-transcendence: A resource for healing at the end-of-life. *Issues in Mental Health Nursing, 17*(3), 275-288.

Ellermann, C. R., & Reed, P. G. (2001). Self-transcendence and depression in middle-aged adults. *Western Journal of Nursing Research, 23*(7), 698-713.

Enyert, G., & Burman, M. E. (1999). A qualitative study of self-transcendence in caregivers of terminally ill patients. *American Journal of Hospice and Palliative Care, 16*(2), 455-462.

Haase, J. E., Britt, T., Coward, D. D., Leidy, N. K., & Penn, P. E. (1992). Simultaneous concept analysis of spiritual perspective, hope, acceptance, and self-transcendence. *Image: The Journal of Nursing Scholarship, 24*(2), 141-147.

Hall, B. (1997). Spirituality in terminal illness: An alternative view of theory. *Journal of Holistic Nursing, 15*(1), 82-96.

Joffrion, L. P., & Douglas, D. (1994). Grief resolution: Facilitating self-transcendence in the bereaved. *Journal of Psychosocial Nursing, 32*(3), 13-19.

Kinney, C. (1996). Transcending breast cancer: Reconstructing one's self. *Issues in Mental Health Nursing, 17*(3), 201-216.

Klaas, D. (1998). Testing two elements of spirituality in depressed and non-depressed elders. *The International Journal of Psychiatric Nursing Research, 4,* 452-462.

McCormick, D. P., Holder, B., Wetsel, M., & Cawthon, T. (2001). Spirituality and HIV disease: An integrated perspective. *Journal of the Association of Nurses in AIDS Care, 12*(3), 58-65.

McGee, E. (2000). Alcoholics Anonymous and nursing: Lessons in holism and spiritual care. *Journal of Holistic Nursing, 18*(1), 11-26.

Mellors, M. P., Erlen, J. A., Coontz, P. D., & Lucke, K. T. (2001). Transcending the suffering of AIDS. *Journal of Community Health Nursing, 18*(4), 235-246.

Mellors, M. P., Riley, T. A., & Erlen, J. A. (1997). HIV, self-transcendence, and quality of life. *Journal of the Association of Nurses in AIDS Care, 8*(2), 59-69.

Neill, J. (2002). Transcendence and transformation in life patterns of women living with rheumatoid arthritis. *ANS Advances in Nursing Science, 24*(2), 27-47.

Pelusi, J. (1997). The lived experience of surviving breast cancer. *Oncology Nursing Forum, 24*(3), 1343-1353.

Rawnsley, M. (2000). Response to Reed's nursing reformulation: Historical and philosophic foundations. *Nursing Science Quarterly, 13*(2), 134-136.

Reese, C. G., & Murray, R. B. (1996). Transcendence: The meaning of great-grandmothering. *Archives of Psychiatric Nursing, 10*(4), 245-251.

Runquist, J. J. (2002). Spirituality, self-transcendence, and health factors in homeless adults (Abstract). *Communicating Nursing Research, 35*(10), 262.

Sarter, B. (1988). Philosophical sources of nursing theory. *Nursing Science Quarterly, 1*(2), 52-59.

Shearer, N., & Reed, P. G. (2004). Empowerment: Reformulation of a non-Rogerian concept. *Nursing Science Quarterly, 17*(3), 253-259.

Taylor, E. J. (2000). Transformation of tragedy among women surviving breast cancer. *Oncology Nursing Forum, 27,* 781-788.

Thorne, S., & Paterson, B. (1998). Shifting images of chronic illness. *Image: The Journal of Nursing Scholarship, 30*(2), 173-178.

Upchurch, S. L. (1999). Self transcendence and activities of daily living: The woman with the pink slippers. *Journal of Holistic Nursing, 17*(3), 251-266.

Walton, C, Shultz, C., Beck, C., & Walls, R. (1991). Psychological correlates of loneliness in the older adult. *Archives of Psychiatric Nursing, 5*(3), 165-170.

Young, C. A., & Reed, P. G. (1995). Elders' perceptions of the role group psychotherapy in fostering self-transcendence. *Archives of Psychiatric Nursing, 9*(6), 338-347.

Selected Master's Theses and Dissertations

Billard, A. (2001). The impact of spiritual transcendence on the well-being of aging Catholic sisters. *Dissertation Abstracts International, B61*(12). (University Microfilms No. 9999061)

Bouwkamp, C. I. (1996). *The relationships among depression, quality of life, and spirituality in older adults.* Unpublished master's thesis, University of Arizona, Tucson, AZ.

Brauchler, D. S. (1992). *An empirical study of the relationship between spiritually-related variables and depression in hospitalized adults.* Unpublished master's thesis, University of Arizona, Tucson, AZ.

Britt, T. (1989). *The relationship of self-transcendence, spirituality, and hope to positive personal death perspectives in healthy older adults.* Unpublished master's thesis, University of Arizona, Tucson, AZ.

Brown, M. L. (1995). *The relationship of spirituality and self-transcendence to life satisfaction among chronically ill Euro-American and Mexican-American older adults.* Unpublished master's thesis, University of Arizona, Tucson, AZ.

Campesino-Flenniken, M. (2003). Voces de las madres: Traumatic bereavement after gang-related homicide. *Dissertation Abstracts International, B64*(09) (University Microfilms No. 3106975).

Cookman, C. A. (1992). Attachment structures of older adults. *Dissertation Abstracts International, B53*(07) (University Microfilms No. 9234901).

Coward, D. (1990). Correlates of self-transcendence in women with advanced breast cancer. *Dissertation Abstracts International, B52*(01) (University Microfilms No. 9108416).

Decker, I. (1998). Moral reasoning, self-transcendence, and end-of-life decisions in a group of community dwelling elders. *Dissertation Abstracts International, B59*(11) (University Microfilms No. 9912131).

Egan, S. R. (1996). *The relationship of meaning of death field patterns to well-being, spiritual perspective and perception of health in healthy older adults.* Unpublished master's thesis, University of Arizona, Tucson, AZ.

Ellermann, C. (1998). *Depression and self-transcendence in middle-aged adults.* Unpublished master's thesis, University of Arizona, Tucson, AZ.

Forbes, M. A. R. (1998). Testing a causal model of hope and its antecedents among chronically ill older adults. *Dissertation Abstracts International, B59*(08) (University Microfilms No. 9901665).

Gallup, J. R. (1985). *The relationship of death anxiety to developmental resources and perceived distance to personal death in later adulthood.* Unpublished master's thesis, University of Arizona, Tucson, AZ.

Gross, D. (1994). *Harvesting the wisdom of the elders: A study of the lives of seven exemplary aged women.* Unpublished doctoral dissertation, Institute of Transpersonal Psychology, Palo Alto, CA.

Jacobs, M. L. (1995). *Spiritual perspective and death acceptance as correlates of the aggressiveness of elders' end-of-life treatment choices.* Unpublished master's thesis, University of Arizona, Tucson, AZ.

Kamienski, M. C. (1997). An investigation of the relationship among suffering, self-transcendence, and social support in women with breast cancer. *Dissertation Abstracts International, B58*(04) (University Microfilms No. 9729588).

Kelley, M. G. (1999). *The lived experience of spiritual healing touch in older women with chronic pain.* Unpublished master's thesis, University of Arizona, Tucson, AZ.

Kilpatrick, J. A. W. (2002). Spiritual perspective, self-transcendence, and spiritual well-being in female nursing students and female nursing faculty. *Dissertation Abstracts International, B63*(02). (University Microfilms No. 3044802)

Klaas, D. J. K. (1996). The experience of depression, meaning in life and self-transcendence in two groups of elders. *Dissertation Abstracts International, B58*(02). (University Microfilms No. 9720690)

Larson, C. D. (1998). The relationship of spiritual perspective and functional status to morale in adults with chronic pulmonary disease. Unpublished master's thesis, University of Arizona, Tucson, AZ.

Larson, C. D. (2004). *Spiritual, psychosocial, and physical correlates of well-being across the breast cancer experience.* Unpublished doctoral dissertation, University of Arizona, Tucson, AZ.

Malcolm, J. D. (1989). *Self-transcendence, chronic illness and depression in later adulthood.* Unpublished master's thesis, Arizona State University, Tempe, AZ.

Matthews, E. E. (2000). Optimism and emotional well-being in women with breast cancer: The role of mediators. *Dissertation Abstracts International, B61*(03). (University Microfilms No. 9967106)

McGaffic, C. M. (1996). Patterns of spirituality and health. *Dissertation Abstracts International, B57*(03). (Unavailable from University Microfilms International). University of Arizona, Tucson, AZ.

McGee, E. M. (2004). *I'm better for having known you: An exploration of self-transcendence in nurses.* Unpublished doctoral dissertation, Boston College, Boston.

Nielson, S. T. P. (1992). *Life events as determinants of wisdom in older adults.* Unpublished doctoral dissertation, University of Arizona, Tucson, AZ.

Rieck, S. B. (2000). The relationship between the spiritual dimension of the nurse-patient relationship and patient well-being. *Dissertation Abstracts International, B61*(08). (University Microfilms No. 9983908)

Rosdahl, D. (2004). The effect of mindfulness meditation on tension headaches and secretory immunoglobulin A in saliva. *Dissertation Abstracts International, B65*(01). (University Microfilms No. 3119979)

Rose, S. S. (2003). Catastrophic injury and illness in the elderly. *Dissertation Abstracts International, B64*(05). (University Microfilms No. 3090018)

Sabre, L. K. (1997). *Perceived insomnia, life-events and self-transcendence in middle and older adults.* Unpublished master's thesis, University of Arizona, Tucson, AZ.

Scharpf, S. S. (1996). *Self-transcendence in older men with prostate cancer.* Unpublished master's thesis, University of Delaware, Newark.

Shearer, N. B. C. (2000). Facilitators of health empowerment in women. *Dissertation Abstracts International, B61*(03). (University Microfilms No. 9965911)

Stevens, D. D. (1999). Spirituality, self-transcendence and depression in young adults with AIDS (Immune deficiency). *Dissertation Abstracts International, B61*(02). (University Microfilms No. 9961253)

Suzuki, M. (1999). *The relationship of depression and self-transcendence among community-living Japanese elders.* Unpublished master's thesis, University of Arizona, Tucson, AZ.

Upchurch, S. L. (1993). Self-transcendence, health status, and selected variables as determinants of the ability to perform activities of daily living in non-institutionalized adults. *Dissertation Abstracts International, B55*(01). (University Microfilms No. 9407736)

Van Lent, D. (1988). *The relationship of spirituality, self-transcendence, and social support to morale in chronically ill elderly.* Unpublished master's thesis, University of Arizona, Tucson, AZ.

Walker, C. A. (2000). Aging among baby boomers. *Dissertation Abstracts International, B61*(11) (University Microfilms No. 9993966).

Wright, K. (2003). Quality of life, self-transcendence, illness distress, and fatigue in liver transplant recipients. *Dissertation Abstracts International, B64*(12) (University Microfilms No. 3116238).

Young, C. (1994). *Older adults group members' perceptions of the role of outpatient group psychotherapy in enhancing self-transcendence.* Unpublished master's thesis, University of Arizona, Tucson, AZ.

Selected Proceeding

Coward, D. D. (2004, May). *Self-transcendence in breast cancer support groups.* Poster session presented at the Oncology Nursing Society 28th Annual Congress, Santa Ana, CA (Proceedings not available.).

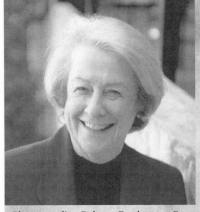

Photo credit: Robert Foothorap. From (2001). The UCSF School of Nursing annual Publication, *The Science of Caring, 13*(1): 7.

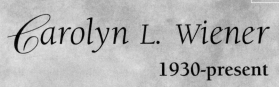

Carolyn L. Wiener

1930-present

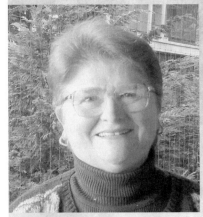

Photo credit: Craig Carlson.

Marylin J. Dodd

1946-present

Theory of Illness Trajectory

Janice Penrod and Chin-Fang Liu

CREDENTIALS OF THE THEORISTS

Carolyn L. Wiener

Carolyn L. Wiener was born in 1930 in San Francisco. She earned her bachelor's degree in interdisciplinary social science from San Francisco State University in 1972. Wiener received her master's degree in sociology from the University of California, San Francisco (UCSF) in 1975. She returned to UCSF to pursue her doctorate in sociology and completed her Ph.D. in 1978. After receiving a Ph.D., Wiener accepted the position of assistant research sociologist at UCSF.

Wiener is an adjunct professor and research sociologist in the Department of Physiological Nursing and the Department of Social and Behavioral Sciences at the School of Nursing at UCSF. Her research focuses on organization in health care institutions, chronic illness, and health policy. She teaches qualitative research methods and has conducted numerous seminars and workshops on the grounded theory method.

Throughout her career, Wiener's excellence has earned for her several meritorious awards and honors. Her intense collaborative relationship with the late Anselm Straus (co-originator of grounded theory methods) and prolific experience in grounded theory methods are evidenced by her invited presentations at the Celebration of the Life and Work of Anselm Strauss at UCSF in 1996

and at a conference entitled *Anselm Strauss, a Theoretician: The Impact of His Thinking on German and European Social Sciences* in Magdeburg, Germany, in 1999. She is highly sought as a methodological consultant to researchers and students from a variety of specialties.

Dissemination of research findings and methodological papers is a hallmark of Wiener's work. She has produced a steady stream of research and theory articles since the mid-1970s. In addition, she has authored or coauthored seven books (Fagerhaugh, Strauss, Suczek, & Wiener, 1987; Strauss, Corbin, Fagerhaugh, Glaser, Maines et al., 1984; Strauss, Fagerhaugh, Suczek, & Wiener, 1985; Wiener, 1981, 2000; Wiener & Strauss, 1997; Wiener & Wysmans, 1990). In her early efforts, Wiener focused on illness trajectories, biographies, and the evolving medical technology scene. From the late 1980s to 1990s, Wiener focused on coping, uncertainty, and accountability in hospitals. Then she completed a study examining the quality management and redesign efforts in hospitals and the interplay between agencies and hospitals around the issue of accountability (Wiener, 2004). All of this work is grounded in her strong methodological expertise and sociological perspective.

Marylin J. Dodd

Marylin J. Dodd was born in 1946 in Vancouver, Canada. She qualified as a registered nurse after studying at the Vancouver General Hospital, British Columbia, Canada. She continued her education, earning a bachelor's and a master's degree in nursing from the University of Washington in 1971 and 1973, respectively. Dodd worked as an instructor in nursing following graduation with her master's degree. By 1977, Dodd returned to academe and completed a Ph.D. in nursing from Wayne State University. She then accepted the position of assistant professor at UCSF. During her tenure there, Dodd has advanced to the rank of full professor, serving as the Associate Dean of Nursing and the acting director for the Center for Symptom Management at UCSF. In 2003 she was awarded the Sharon A. Lamb Endowed Chair in Symptom Management at the School of Nursing, UCSF.

Her exemplary program of research is focused in oncology nursing, specifically self-care and symptom management. Dodd's outstanding record of funded research provides evidence of the superiority and significance of her work. She has skillfully woven modest internal and external funding with numerous large federally funded projects to advance her research. Her research trajectory has advanced impeccably as she progressively utilized both descriptive studies and intervention studies employing randomized clinical trial methodologies to extend an understanding of complex phenomena in cancer care. The National Institutes of Health, National Cancer Institute, and National Institute of Nursing fund her current research, and additional projects are under review.

Dodd's research was designed to test self-care interventions (PRO-SELF Program) to manage the side effects of cancer treatment (mucositis) and symptoms of cancer (fatigue, pain). This research entitled The PRO-SELF: Pain Control Program— An Effective Approach for Cancer Pain Management was published in *Oncology Nursing Forum* (West, Dodd, Paul, Schumacher, Tripathy et al., 2003). Currently, she teaches in the Oncology Nursing Specialty, and in 2002 she instituted Biomarkers I & II, new courses which were developed by the Center for Symptom Management Faculty Group.

Dodd's illustrious career has merited several prestigious awards. Among these honors, she was recognized as a fellow of the American Academy of Nursing (1986). Her continued excellence and significant contributions to oncology nursing is evidenced by her having been awarded the Oncology Nursing Society/Schering Excellence in Research Award (1993, 1996), the Best Original Research Paper in *Cancer Nursing* (1994, 1996), Oncology Nursing Society Bristol-Meyers Distinguished Researcher Career Award (1997), and the Oncology Nursing Society/Chiron Excellence of Scholarship and Consistency of Contribution to the Oncology Nursing Literature Career Award (2000). This impressive partial listing of awards provides a sense of the magnitude of professional respect and admiration that Dodd has garnered throughout her career.

Dodd's record in research dissemination is equally illustrious. Her volume of original publications began in 1975. By the early 1980s, she was publishing multiple, focused articles each year, and that pace has only accelerated. During the first half of 2004, she has published five articles and has seven other manuscripts in review, thus ensuring that the productivity seen to date has no end in sight. She has authored or coauthored ten books (Brown, Dodd, Given, Grove, Hennessey et al., 1982; Cotanch & Dodd, 1990; Dodd, 1978, 1987, 1988, 1991, 1996, 2001; Miller, Dodd, Goodman, Pluth, & Ryan, 1984; Nielsen, Dodd, Green, Johnson, Longman et al., 1984), 20 book chapters, and numerous editorials, conference proceedings, and review papers. Her many presentations at scientific gatherings around the world accentuate this work. Dodd has been an invited speaker throughout North America, Australia, Asia, and Europe.

Her active service to the university, School of Nursing, Department of Physiological Nursing, and numerous professional and public organizations and journal review boards augments her outstanding record of service to the profession of nursing. Despite the breadth and volume of these activities, Dodd is an active teacher and mentor. She is the faculty member on record for several graduate courses and carries a significant advising load in the master's, doctoral, and postdoctoral options at UCSF. With this brief overview of but a few highlights in an illustrious career, it is clear that

Dodd is an exemplar of excellence in nursing scholarship.

THEORETICAL SOURCES

Being ill creates a disruption in normal life. Such disruption affects all aspects of life, including physiological functioning, social interactions, and the conceptions of self. Coping is the response to such disruption. Although coping with illness has been of interest to social scientists and nursing scholars for decades, Weiner and Dodd clearly explicate that formerly implicit theoretical assumptions have limited the utility of this body of work (Wiener & Dodd, 1993). Because the processes surrounding the disruption of illness are played out in the context of living, coping responses are inherently situated in sociological interactions with others and biographical processes of self. The complex interplay of physiological disruption, interactions with others, and the construction of biographical conceptions of the self warrant a more sophisticated perspective of coping than identifying a compendium of strategies used to manage the disruption, attempting to isolate specific responses to one event that is lived within the complexity of life context, or assigning value labels (e.g., good or bad) to the responsive behaviors that are described collectively as coping.

The Theory of Illness Trajectory* addresses these theoretical pitfalls by framing this phenomenon within a sociological perspective of a trajectory that emphasizes the experience of disruption related to illness within the changing contexts of interactional and sociological processes that ultimately influence the person's response to such disruption. This theoretical approach defines this theory's significant contribution to nursing: coping is not a simple stimulus-response phenomenon that can be isolated from the complex context of life. Because life is centered in the living body, the physiological disruptions of illness permeate other life contexts to create a new way of being, a new sense of self. Responses to the disruptions caused by illness are interwoven into the various contexts encountered in one's life and the interactions with other players in those life situations.

From this perspective, coping is best viewed as change over time that is highly variable in relation to biographical and sociological influences. The trajectory is this course of change, of variability, that cannot be confined to or modeled in linear phases or stages. Rather, the trajectory of illness organizes insights to better understand the dynamic interplay of the disruption of illness within the changing contexts of life.

Within this sociological framework, Wiener and Dodd address serious concerns regarding the conceptual overattribution of the role of uncertainty in the framework of understanding responses to living with the disruptions of illness (Wiener & Dodd, 1993). An old adage tells us that nothing in life is certain, except death and taxes. Living is fraught with uncertainty, yet illness (especially chronic illness) compounds this uncertainty in profound ways. Being chronically ill exaggerates the uncertainties of living within a being who is compromised (i.e., by illness) in his or her capability to respond to these uncertainties. Thus, although the concept of uncertainty provides a useful theoretical lens for understanding the illness trajectory, it cannot be theoretically positioned so as to overshadow conceptually the dynamic context of living with chronic illness.

In other words, the trajectory of illness is driven by the illness experience lived within contexts that are inherently uncertain and involve both the self and others. The dynamic flow of life contexts (both biographical and sociological) creates a dynamic flow of uncertainties that take on different forms, meanings, and combinations when living with chronic illness. Thus, tolerating uncertainty is a critical theoretical strand in the illness trajectory theory.

*The Theory of Illness Trajectory is used herein to refer to theoretical formulations regarding coping with uncertainty through the cancer illness trajectory. It is important to note that this work extends pre-existing theory on illness trajectories, biographies, and related concepts (identity, temporality, and body) that were developed through an extensive 4-year research project. Readers are advised to refer to the original works of Corbin, Fagerhaugh, Strauss, Suczek, and Wiener for further explication of the larger theory.

MAJOR CONCEPTS *&* DEFINITIONS

Life is situated in a biographical context. Conceptions of self are rooted in the physical body and are formulated based on the perceived capability to perform usual or expected activities to accomplish the objectives of varied roles. Interactions with others are a major influence on the establishment of the conception of self. As varied role behaviors are enacted, the person monitors reactions of others and a sense of self in an integrated process of establishing meaning. Identity, temporality, and body are key elements in the biographical context, as follows:

- *Identity*: the conception of self at a given time that unifies multiple aspects of self and is situated in the body
- *Temporality*: biographical time reflected in the continuous flow of the life course events; perceptions of the past, present, and possible future interwoven into the conception of self
- *Body*: activities of life and derived perceptions are based in the body

Illness, particularly cancer, disrupts the usual or everyday conception of self and is compounded by the perceived actions and reactions of others in the sociological context of life. This disruption permeates the interdependent elements of biography: identity, temporality, and body. This disruption or sense of disequilibrium is marked by a sense of a loss of control, resulting in states of uncertainty.

As life contexts continually unfold, dimensions of uncertainty are manifest, not in a linear sequence of stages or phases, but in an unsettling intermingling of perceptions of the uncertain body, uncertain temporality, and uncertain identity. The experience of illness always is placed within the biographical context; that is, illness is experienced in the continual flow of the life. The domains of illness-related uncertainty vary in dominance across the illness trajectory (Table 30-1) through a dynamic flow of perceptions of self and interactions with others.

The activities of life and of living with an illness are forms of work. The sphere of work includes the person and all others with whom he or she interacts, including family and health care providers. This network of players is called the *total organization*. The ill person (or patient) is the central worker; however, all work takes place within and is influenced by the total organization. Types of work are organized around the following four lines of trajectory work performed by patients and families:

1. *Illness-related work*: diagnostics, symptom management, care regimen, and crisis prevention
2. *Everyday-life work*: activities of daily living, keeping a household, maintaining an occupation, sustaining relationships, and recreation
3. *Biographical work*: the exchange of information, emotional expressions, and the division of tasks through interactions within the total organization
4. *Uncertainty abatement work*: activities enacted to lessen the impact of temporal, body, and identity uncertainty

The balance of these types of work is dynamically responsive, fluctuating across time, situations, perceptions, and varied players in the total organization in order to gain some sense of equilibrium (i.e., a sense of control). This interplay among the types of work creates a tension that is marked by shifts in the dominance of types of work across the trajectory. Recall, however, that the biographical context is rooted in the body. As the body changes through the course of illness and treatment, the capacity to perform certain types of work and, ultimately, one's identity are transformed.

A major contribution of this work was the delineation of types of uncertainty abate-

Continued

ment work (Table 30-2). These activities were enacted to lessen the impact of the varied states of uncertainty induced by undergoing cancer chemotherapy. These strategies were highly dynamic and responsive and occurred in varied combinations and configurations across the trajectory of illness for different players in the organization. Those enacting these strategies affected the conception of self as they monitored others' responses to the strategy as they attempted to manage living with illness.

Table **30-1**

Illness Trajectory: States of Uncertainty

DOMAIN	SOURCES OF UNCERTAINTY	DIMENSIONS OF UNCERTAINTY
UNCERTAIN TEMPORALITY Taken-for-granted expectations regarding the flow of life events are disrupted A temporal disjunction in the biography	Life is perceived to be in a constant state of flux related to illness and treatment The self of the past is viewed differently (e.g., the way it used to be) Expectations of the present self are distorted by illness and treatment Anticipation of the future self is altered	Loss of temporal predictability prompts concerns surrounding: • *Duration:* how long • *Pace:* how fast • *Frequency:* how often the experience of time is distorted (i.e., stretched out, constrained, or limitless)
UNCERTAIN BODY Changes related to illness and treatment centered in one's ability to perform usual activities, involving appearance, physiological functions, and response to treatment	Faith in the body is shaken (body failure) The conception of the former body (the way it used to be) commingles with the altered state of the body at present and the changed expectations for how the body may perform in the future	Ambiguity in reading body signs Concerns surrounding: • What is being done to the body • Jeopardized body resistance • Efficacy and risks of treatment • Disease recurrence
UNCERTAIN IDENTITY Interpretation of self is distorted as the body fails to perform in usual ways and expectations related to the flow of events (temporality) are altered by disease and treatment	Body failure and difficulty reading the new body upset the former conception of self Skewed temporality impairs the expected life course	Expected life course is shattered Evidence gleaned from reading the body is not interpretable within the usual frame of understanding Hope is sustained despite changing circumstances

Table **30-2**

Uncertainty Abatement Work	
TYPE OF ACTIVITY	**BEHAVIORAL MANIFESTATIONS**
Pacing	Resting or changing usual activities
Becoming "professional" patients	Using terminology related to illness and treatment
	Directing care
	Balancing expertise with super-medicalization
Seeking reinforcing comparisons	Comparing self with persons who are in worse condition to reassure self that it is not as bad as it could be
Engaging in reviews	Looking back to reinterpret emergent symptoms and interactions with others in the organization
Setting goals	Looking toward the future to achieve desired activities
Covering-up	Masking signs of illness or related emotions
	Bucking up to avoid stigma or to protect others
Finding a safe place to let down	Establishing a place where, or people with whom, true emotions and feelings could be expressed in a supportive atmosphere
Choosing a supportive network	Selective sharing with individuals deemed to be positive supporters
Taking charge	Asserting the right to determine the course of treatment

USE OF EMPIRICAL EVIDENCE

The Theory of Illness Trajectory was expanded through a secondary analysis of qualitative data collected during a prospective longitudinal study that examined family coping and self-care during 6 months of chemotherapy treatment. The sample for the larger study included 100 patients and their families. Each patient had been diagnosed with cancer (including breast, lung, colorectal, gynecological, or lymphoma) and was in the process of receiving chemotherapy for initial disease treatment or for recurrence. Subjects in the study designated at least one family member who was willing to participate in the study.

Although both quantitative and qualitative measures were used in data collection for the larger study, this theory was derived through analysis of the qualitative data. Interviews were structured around family coping and were conducted at three points during chemotherapeutic treatment. The patients and the family members were asked to recall the previous month and then discuss the most important problem or challenge with which they had to deal, the degree of distress created by that problem within the family, and their satisfaction with the management of that concern.

Meticulous attention was paid to consistency in data collection: family members were consistent and present for each interview, the interview guide was structured, and the same nurse-interviewer conducted each data collection point for a given family. Audiotaping the interview proceedings, verbatim transcription, and having a nurse-recorder present at each interview to note key phrases as the interview progressed further enhanced methodological rigor. The resultant data set consisted of 300 interviews (three interviews for each of 100 patient-family units) that were obtained at varied points in the course of chemotherapeutic treatment for cancer.

As the data for the larger study were analyzed, it became apparent to Dodd (principal investigator) that the qualitative interview data held significant insights that could further inform the study. Wiener, a renowned grounded theorist who collaborated with Anselm Strauss, one of the method's founders, was subsequently recruited to conduct a secondary analysis of interview data. It should be noted that traditional grounded theory methods typically involve a concurrent, reiterative process of data collection and analysis (Glaser, 1978; Glaser & Strauss, 1965). As theoretical insights are identified, sampling and the focus of subsequent data collection theoretically are driven to flesh out emergent concepts, dimensions, variations, and negative cases. However, in this project, the data were collected previously using a structured interview guide; this was a secondary analysis of an established data set.

Wiener's expertise in grounded theory methods permitted the adaptation of grounded theory methods for application to secondary data that proved successful. In essence, the principles undergirding analysis (i.e., the coding paradigm) were applied to the preexisting data set. The analytic inquiry proceeded inductively to reveal the core social-psychological process around which the theory is explicated: tolerating the uncertainty of living with cancer. Dimensions of the uncertainty, management processes, and consequences were further explicated to reveal the internal consistency of the theoretical perspective of illness trajectory.

When considering the authors' use of adapted grounded theory methods to analyze preexisting empirical evidence, several insights may be useful to support the integrity of this work. First, Wiener was certainly well prepared to advance new applications of the method by her training and experience as a grounded theorist. The methodological credibility of this researcher supports her extension of a traditional research method into a new application within her disciplinary perspective (sociology). Further, it is important to recall the size of this data set: 100 patients and families were interviewed 3 times each, for a total of 300 interviews. This is a very large data set for a qualitative inquiry. Oberst pointed out that given this volume of data, some semblance of theoretical sampling (within the full data set) would likely be permitted by the researchers (Oberst, 1993). But the sheer size of the data set does not tell the whole story.

Sampling patients who had a relatively wide range of types of cancers (ranging from gynecological cancers to lung cancer) and both patients undergoing initial chemotherapeutic treatment and those receiving treatment for recurrence contributed significantly to variation in the data set. These sampling strategies ultimately contributed to establishing an appropriate sample, especially for revealing a trajectory perspective of change over time. Finally, despite the structured format of the interview, it is important to note that the patients and families dialogued about the previous month's events in a form of "brainstorming" (Wiener & Dodd, 1993, p. 18). This technique would allow the subjects to introduce almost any topic that was of concern to them (regardless of the subsequent structure of the interview). The audiotaping and verbatim transcription of these dialogues contribute to the variation and appropriateness of the resultant data set. Given these insights, it may be concluded that the empirical evidence culled through the interviews conducted during the larger study provided adequate and appropriate data for a secondary analysis using expertly adapted grounded theory methods.

MAJOR ASSUMPTIONS

Wiener and Dodd's Theory of Illness Trajectory explicates major assumptions that reflect its derivation within a sociological perspective (Wiener & Dodd, 1993). Closer examination of each assumption reveals several related basic premises undergirding the theory. In contrast to other nursing theories, the constructs of nursing, person, health, and environment are not explicitly addressed; however, the following discussion of theoretical assumptions sheds some light on the theoretical interpretation of these constructs.

The trajectory model encompasses not only the physical components of the disease, but the "total organization of work done over the course of the disease" (Wiener & Dodd, 1993, p. 20). An illness trajectory is theoretically distinct from the course of an illness. In this theory, the illness trajectory is not limited to the person who suffers the illness. Rather, the total organization involves the person with the illness, family, and health care professionals who render health care.

Also, notice the use of the term *work*. "The varied players in the organization have different types of work; however, the patient is the "central worker" in the illness trajectory" (Wiener & Dodd, 1993, p. 20). This statement reaffirms an earlier assertion found in illness trajectory literature (Fagerhaugh et al., 1987; Strauss et al., 1985). The work of living with an illness produces certain consequences or impacts that permeate the lives of the people involved. In turn, consequences and reciprocal consequences ripple throughout the organization, enmeshing the total organization with the central worker (i.e., the patient) through the trajectory of living with the illness. The relationship among the workers in the trajectory is a critical attribute that "affects both the management of that course of illness, as well as the fate of the person who is ill" (Wiener & Dodd, 1993, p. 20).

THEORETICAL ASSERTIONS

The focus on the social context for work and the social relationships affecting the work of living with illness in the Theory of Illness Trajectory is based in the seminal work of Corbin and Strauss (1988). As the central worker, actions are undertaken by the person to manage the impact of living with illness within a range of contexts, including the biographical (conception of self) and the sociological (interactions with others). From this perspective, managing disruptions (or coping with uncertainty) involves interactions with the various players in the organization as well as external sociological conditions. Given the complexity of such interactions across multiple contexts and with the numerous players experienced throughout the trajectory of illness, coping is a highly variable and dynamic process.

Originally, it was anticipated that the trajectory of living with cancer had discernable phases or stages that could be identified by major shifts in reported problems, challenges, and activities. This was the rationale for collecting qualitative data at three points during the chemotherapy treatment. In fact, this conjecture did not hold true: the physical status of the patient with cancer and the social-psychological consequences of illness and treatment were the central themes at all points of measurement across the trajectory.

The authors conceptually equate uncertainty with loss of control, described as "the most problematic facet of living with cancer" (Wiener & Dodd, 1993, p. 18). This theoretical assertion is reflected further in the identification of the core social-psychological process of living with cancer, "tolerating the uncertainty that permeates the disease" (p. 19). Factors that influenced the degree of uncertainty expressed by the patient and family were based in the theoretical framework of the total organization and external sociological conditions, including the nature of family support, financial resources, and the quality of assistance from health care providers.

LOGICAL FORM

The primary logical form employed to produce this grounded theory was inductive reasoning. Analytic reading of the interviews provided insights that led to the identification of the core process that unifies the theoretical assertions: tolerating uncertainty. Systematic coding processes were applied to define further the dimensions of uncertainty and of management processes used to deal with the disease and its consequences. Then, given these insights, the findings were examined for their fit within extant theoretical writings to extend our understanding of the trajectory of illness. The resultant qualitatively derived theory was well grounded in the reported experiences of the participants and skillfully integrated with what was known of trajectories of illness to advance the state of the science.

ACCEPTANCE BY THE NURSING COMMUNITY
Practice

The importance of the Theory of Illness Trajectory for nursing practice is in providing a framework for understanding how cancer patients tolerate uncertainty manifested as a loss of control. The identification of types of uncertainty abatement work are especially useful in revealing the strategies commonly employed by oncology patients as they attempt to manage their lives as normally as possible in the wake of the uncertainty created by a diagnosis of cancer. Awareness of these themes of uncertainty and related management strategies faced by patients undergoing chemotherapy and their family members could have a significant impact on how nurses subsequently intervene with these compromised patient systems who are managing the work of their illness to "facilitate a less troubled trajectory course for some patients and their families" (Wiener & Dodd, 1993, p. 29). An example of such an intervention was described by Horner as she recommended that nurses explore family assumptions about health care experiences to open a dialogue about the work that surrounds the uncertainties faced in the illness trajectory (Horner, 1997).

Education

Wiener and Dodd are highly respected educators who share their ongoing work through international conferences, seminars, consultations, graduate thesis advising, and course offerings. Incorporation of this work into these presentations not only advances knowledge related to the utility of illness trajectory models but, perhaps more importantly, demonstrates how such data-based theoretical advancement contributes to an evolving program of research in cancer care (Dodd, 1997, 1999). The recent reprinting of the theory in a nursing text on research and theory in chronic illness will increase exposure of the work to nursing scholars (Wiener & Dodd, 2000).

Research

The theory has been referenced in a limited number of concept analyses or state-of-the-science papers addressing uncertainty (McCormick, 2002; Mishel, 1997; Parry, 2003). Mishel (1997) has praised the broad theoretical focus maintained through the

qualitative approach to theory derivation. Much of the work in coping with illness is constrained by the application of Lazarus and Folkman's framework of problem-based or emotion-based coping; however, in this study, inductive reasoning produced data-based theory that identifies a broad range of strategies related to tolerating and abating uncertainty (Lazarus & Folkman, 1984; Mishel, 1997). The variation and range of abatement strategies identified in this theory are a unique and significant contribution to the body of research in coping with the uncertainty of illness.

FURTHER DEVELOPMENT

In a response article to the original publication, Oberst (1993) took issue with the delimitation of the concept of uncertainty to loss of control. This criticism has been echoed by McCormick (2002), who theoretically positions loss of control as a component in the uncertainty cycle rather than as a manifestation of a state of uncertainty. Further research into the concept of control is warranted to untangle the conceptual boundaries and linkages between control and uncertainty throughout the illness trajectory.

Other researchers have criticized the implicit assertion that uncertainty (or loss of control) is always a negative event that requires some form of abatement (Oberst, 1993; Parry, 2003). Oberst (1993) suggests that further investigation is needed to differentiate work related to tolerating uncertainty from abatement work in order to reveal how effective strategies in each type of work affect the sense of uncertainty throughout the trajectory. Parry (2003) studied survivors of childhood cancer and revealed that although uncertain states may be a problematic stressor for some, a more universal theme of embracing uncertainty toward transformational growth was evident in these survivors.

These insights demonstrate an evolving body of research related to uncertainty, control, and the illness trajectory. A number of considerations for future research are revealed. Concept clarification, especially related to control and uncertainty, is critically needed. Inquiry must not be constrained by an assumption that uncertainty is necessarily a negative aspect of life; researchers must remain open to positive transformational outcomes of living through uncertainty. Wiener and Dodd's original recommendation to expand the scope of the illness trajectory framework remains salient (Wiener & Dodd, 1993). The illness trajectory theoretical framework would be especially useful for understanding variations in uncertainty and control across a fuller perspective of the illness trajectory in cancer and other conditions in which the significance of uncertainty and control may vary.

CRITIQUE
Clarity

One concern in the clarity in Wiener and Dodd's Theory of Illness Trajectory is the delimitation of the concept of uncertainty to a loss of control. This limited conceptual perspective of uncertainty is clearly set forth in the work; therefore, this issue does not create a significant or fatal flaw in the work. The theory is delineated clearly and well supported by previous work in illness trajectories. Propositional clarity is achieved in the logical presentation of relationships and the linkages between concepts discussed in the theory. The conceptual derivation of managing illness as work is well developed and provides unique insights into the meaning of living through chemotherapy during cancer treatment. The application of the trajectory model is used consistently to demonstrate the dynamic and fluctuations in coping, not in clearly demarcated stages or phases, but in situation-specific contexts of the work of managing illness. The dynamic flow of work contexts, players within the organization of work, and situation in cancer treatment make diagramming or modeling of the theory impractical.

Simplicity

This complex theory is interpreted in a highly accessible manner. The Theory of Illness Trajectory adopts a sociological framework that is applied to a phenomenon of concern to nursing: chemotherapeutic treatment of cancer patients and their families. The sense of understanding imparted by the theory is highly relevant to oncology nursing. The descriptions of patient and family behaviors and insights are congruent with clinical experiences. The theory presents an eloquent and parsimonious interpretation of the complexity of this phenomenon using key concepts with adequate definition; however, in order to comprehend fully the theoretical assertions of the theory, further study of previous work in trajectory models would be very helpful.

Generality

The authors have limited carefully the scope of this theory to patients and families progressing through chemotherapy for initial treatment or recurrence of cancer. The Theory of Illness Trajectory is well defined within this context. The integration of this middle range theory with other work in trajectories of illness and uncertainty theory indicates that there is an emergent fit with other models of illness trajectories and uncertainty. Further theory-building work may produce higher level theory of broader scope that may permit the application of these theoretical propositions in other contexts of illness trajectories.

Empirical Precision

Grounded theory methods rely on the dominance of inductive reasoning; that is, drawing abstractions or generalities from examples of specific situations. Thus, the derived theory is rooted in the experiences expressed in the hundreds of interviews with cancer patients and their families. The integration of data-based evidence (e.g., quotes) in the formal description of the theory supports the linkages between the theoretical abstractions and empirical observations. The empirical evidence is presented in a logical and consistent manner that rings true to clinical experiences. Thus, the theory is relevant and useful to clinicians and holds promise for further research application.

Derivable Consequences

The significance of the theoretical contributions made by this work, especially the types of work and uncertainty abatement strategies used during chemotherapy, has been established. The utility of this theory is apparent in cancer treatment and, with further theoretical development, the theory may be further generalizable to other contexts within cancer care or even other illness trajectories. Yet, there is limited evidence of directly derived consequences related to the application of the Theory of Illness Trajectory in practice-based studies in nursing.

This issue remains problematic. The sociological perspective reflected in the work should not inhibit nurse scholars. Applicability of this theory to phenomena of concern to nursing has been established by the authors' focus on cancer chemotherapy. The potential utility of the theory for guiding nursing practice is perhaps best demonstrated by the integration of the theory into Dodd's exemplary program of research in cancer care (Dodd, 1997, 1999).

SUMMARY

Wiener and Dodd's Theory of Illness Trajectory is at once complex, yet eloquently simple. The sociological perspective of defining the work of managing illness is especially relevant to the context of cancer care. The theory provides new ways of understanding how patients and families tolerate uncertainty and work strategically to abate uncertainty throughout a dynamic flow of illness events, treatment situations, and varied players who become involved in the organization of care. The theory is pragmatic and relevant to nursing. The merits of this work warrant further attention to use the theory to produce more direct practice implications that could change the way nurses interpret and facilitate the management of an illness.

Case Study

Mr. Miller is a 67-year-old man who has metastatic cancer. His primary caregiver is his wife, Mrs. Miller.

Early in the course of treatment in your outpatient cancer care center, the couple focused their questions on the course of the disease, treatment options, and potential side effects of varied treatment options. They were proud of their ability to maintain "normal life" as Mr. Miller continued to work throughout aggressive treatment, taking time off only when the discomforts of treatment were so debilitating that he was physically unable to get to his office. Mr. and Mrs. Miller expressed little emotion throughout the course of treatment; they frequently praised each other's strength and fortitude. During recent visits, Mrs. Miller has become extremely focused on laboratory values and test results, using highly technical language. She has also become adamant that certain staff members must perform certain tasks because "she does it better than anyone."

The Theory of Illness Trajectory helps the clinician to interpret these behaviors and to intervene to help ease transitions across this trajectory. For example, clinicians can identify easily with patients and families who have become "professional patients" as they learn to use complex technical jargon about their treatment, laboratory values, or illness (Wiener & Dodd, 1993). These "junior doctors" attempt to earn a modicum of control as they manage treatment by requesting particular staff members to perform specific tasks (Dodd, 1997, p. 988). Care providers have a tendency to view this behavior as a positive hallmark of assuming self-care and, therefore, often reinforce such behaviors.

Deeper consideration of the theoretical assertions of the Theory of Illness Trajectory reveals that these behavioral strategies are efforts to tolerate the uncertainty of the illness experience. The confidence built through these socially reinforced behaviors can be converted to guilt very quickly when situations beyond the expertise of the patient or family go awry. Given this perspective, the limitation of this management strategy becomes clear, and intervention is indicated: if patients and families are to manage care effectively, they must be educated proactively to do so (Dodd, 1997, 1999).

In proactively educating the patient-family system, consider the varied domains of uncertainty and the varied forms of uncertainty abatement work. To understand the patient-family trajectory, assessment data is critical. For example, although well-developed protocols for symptom management or palliation are available, such protocols are useless if patients or caregivers fail to describe the extent of symptoms because they perceive these "hassles" or "bothers" as trivial in the face of life-threatening disease. Compounding this issue, nurses may fall into a pattern of focusing on illness-related work, thereby diverting important attention from the other forms of work faced by these patients and their families. Understanding of the varied domains of uncertainty and forms of uncertainty abatement work facilitates a more open dialogue regarding these key areas of concern, allowing the nurse to encourage the patient and caregiver to share more about their experiences in an effort to help them through this difficult time.

CRITICAL THINKING *Activities*

1. How does a trajectory of illness differ from a course of illness? Differentiate how the application of each perspective may yield different foci for intervention for a selected health condition. Which perspective is most congruent with your paradigmatic views of nursing?

2. Considering your clinical experiences, give examples of how patients and their families have experienced health-related uncertainty. Is uncertainty always related to a loss of control? Are there different conditions under which health-related uncertainty is a perceived as a negative life event versus those in which the uncertainty is positioned as a growth-enhancing event?

3. As a clinician, you are intimately involved in the work of managing an illness. Based on your understanding of the work of illness

management espoused in the Theory of Illness Trajectory, what nursing behaviors may exacerbate feelings of loss of control or uncertainty in your patients? What factors (personal, environmental, or organizational) may contribute to these behaviors? What interventions would you suggest to create a less troubling trajectory for your patients and their families?

REFERENCES

Brown, J., Dodd, M. J., Given, B., Grove, M., Hennessey, S., Hausdorff, J., et al. (1982). *Outcome standards for cancer patient education.* Pittsburgh: Oncology Nursing Society.

Corbin, J., & Strauss, A. (1988). *Unending work and care.* San Francisco: Jossey Bass.

Cotanch, P., & Dodd, M. J. (1990). *Monograph of the advanced research sessions at the 14th Annual Oncology Nursing Society's Congress.* Pittsburgh: Oncology Nursing Society Press.

Dodd, M. J. (1978). *Oncology nursing case studies.* New York: Medical Publication Co.

Dodd, M. J. (1987). *Managing the side effects of chemotherapy and radiation therapy: A guide for patients and nurses.* Norwalk, CT: Appleton & Lange.

Dodd, M. J. (1988). *Monograph of the advanced research session at the 13th Annual Oncology Nursing Society's Congress.* Pittsburgh: Oncology Nursing Society Press.

Dodd, M. J. (1991). *Managing the side effects of chemotherapy and radiation: A guide for patients and their families* (2nd ed.). Englewood, NJ: Prentice-Hall.

Dodd, M. J. (1996). *Managing the side effects of chemotherapy and radiation therapy: A guide for patients and their families* (3rd ed.). San Francisco: UCSF School of Nursing Press.

Dodd, M. J. (1997). Self-care: Ready or not! *Oncology Nursing Forum, 24*(6), 981-990.

Dodd, M. J. (1999). Self-care: Not as simple as we hoped. *Communicating Nursing Research Conference Proceedings, 32*(7), 43-56. (Western Institute for Nursing, Denver.)

Dodd, M. J. (2001). *Managing the side effects of chemotherapy and radiation therapy: A guide for patients and their families* (4th ed.). San Francisco: UCSF School of Nursing Press.

Fagerhaugh, S., Strauss, A., Suczek, B., & Wiener, C. (1987). *Hazards in hospital care: Ensuring patient safety.* San Francisco: Jossey-Bass.

Glaser, B. (1978). *Theoretical sensitivity.* Mill Valley, CA: Sociology Press.

Glaser, B., & Strauss, A. (1965). *Awareness of dying.* Chicago: Aldine.

Horner, S. D. (1997). Uncertainty in mothers' care for their ill children. *Journal of Advanced Nursing, 26,* 658-663.

Lazarus, R. S., & Folkman, S. (1984). *Stress, appraisal, and coping.* New York: Springer.

McCormick, K. M. (2002). A concept analysis of uncertainty in illness. *Journal of Nursing Scholarship, 34*(2), 127-131.

Miller, S. A., Dodd, M., Goodman, M. S., Pluth, N., & Ryan, L. (1984). *Cancer chemotherapy guidelines and recommendations for nursing education and practice.* Pittsburgh: Mead Johnson, Oncology Nursing Society.

Mishel, M. H. (1997). Uncertainty in acute illness. *Annual Review of Nursing Research, 15,* 57-80.

Nielsen, B., Dodd, M. J., Green, T., Johnson, J., Longman, A., Rickel, L., et al. (1984). *Outcome standards for public cancer education.* Pittsburgh: Oncology Nursing Society.

Oberst, M. T. (1993). Response to "Coping amid uncertainty: An illness trajectory perspective." *Scholarly Inquiry for Nursing Practice: An International Journal, 7*(1), 33-35.

Parry, C. (2003). Embracing uncertainty: An exploration of the experiences of childhood cancer survivors. *Qualitative Health Research, 13*(1), 227-246.

Strauss, A., Corbin, J., Fagerhaugh, S., Glaser, B., Maines, D., Suczek, B., et al. (1984). *Chronic illness and the quality of life.* St. Louis: Mosby.

Strauss, A., Fagerhaugh, S., Suczek, B., & Wiener, C. (1985). *Social organization of medical work.* Chicago: University of Chicago Press. (Republished 1997, New Brunswick, NJ: Transaction Books.)

West, C. M., Dodd, M. J., Paul, S. M., Schumacher, K., Tripathy, D., Koo, P., et al. (2003). The PRO-SELF: Pain control program—An effective approach for cancer pain management. *Oncology Nursing Forum, 30,* 65-73.

Wiener, C. (1981). *The politics of alcoholism: Building an arena around a social problem.* New Brunswick, NJ: Transaction Books.

Wiener, C. (2000). *The elusive quest: Accountability in hospitals.* New York: Aldine deGruyter.

Wiener, C. L., & Dodd, M. J. (1993). Coping amid uncertainty: An illness trajectory perspective. *Scholarly Inquiry for Nursing Practice: An International Journal, 7*(1), 17-31.

Wiener, C. L., & Dodd, M. J. (2000). Coping amid uncertainty: An illness trajectory perspective. In R. Hyman & J. Corbin (Eds.), *Chronic illness: Research and theory for nursing practice* (pp. 180-201). New York: Springer.

Wiener, C., & Strauss, A. (1997). *Where medicine fails* (5th ed.). New Brunswick, NJ: Transaction Books.

Wiener, C., & Wysmans, W. M. (1990). *Grounded theory in medical research: From theory to practice.* Amsterdam: Sivets and Zeitlinger.

BIBLIOGRAPHY
Primary Sources
Books

Brown, J., Dodd, M. J., Given, B., Grove, M., Hennessey, S., Hausdorff, J., et al. (1982). *Outcome standards for cancer patient education.* Pittsburgh: Oncology Nursing Society.

Cotanch, P., & Dodd, M. J. (1990). *Monograph of the advanced research sessions at the 14th Annual Oncology Nursing Society's Congress.* Pittsburgh: Oncology Nursing Society Press.

Dodd, M. J. (1978). *Oncology nursing case studies.* New York: Medical Publication Co.

Dodd, M. J. (1987). *Managing the side effects of chemotherapy and radiation therapy: A guide for patients and nurses.* Norwalk, CT: Appleton & Lange.

Dodd, M. J. (1988). *Monograph of the advanced research session at the 13th Annual Oncology Nursing Society's Congress.* Pittsburgh: Oncology Nursing Society Press.

Dodd, M. J. (1991). *Managing the side effects of chemotherapy and radiation: A guide for patients and their families* (2nd ed.). Englewood, NJ: Prentice-Hall.

Dodd, M. J. (1996). *Managing the side effects of chemotherapy and radiation therapy: A guide for patients and their families* (3rd ed.). San Francisco: UCSF School of Nursing Press.

Dodd, M. J. (2001). *Managing the side effects of chemotherapy and radiation therapy: A guide for patients and their families* (4th ed.). San Francisco: UCSF School of Nursing Press.

Fagerhaugh, S., Strauss, A., Suczek, B., & Wiener, C. (1987). *Hazards in hospital care: Ensuring patient safety.* San Francisco: Jossey-Bass.

Miller, S. A., Dodd, M., Goodman, M. S., Pluth, N., & Ryan, L. (1984). *Cancer chemotherapy guidelines and recommendations for nursing education and practice.* Pittsburgh: Mead Johnson, Oncology Nursing Society.

Nielsen, B., Dodd, M. J., Green, T., Johnson, J., Longman, A., Rickel, L., et al. (1984). *Outcome standards for public cancer education.* Pittsburgh: Oncology Nursing Society.

Strauss, A., Corbin, J., Fagerhaugh, S., Glaser, B., Maines, D., Suczek, B., et al. (1984). *Chronic illness and the quality of life.* St. Louis: Mosby.

Strauss, A., Fagerhaugh, S., Suczek, B., & Wiener, C. (1985). *Social organization of medical work.* Chicago: University of Chicago Press. (Republished 1997, New Brunswick, NJ: Transaction Books.)

Wiener, C. (1981). *The politics of alcoholism: Building an arena around a social problem.* New Brunswick, NJ: Transaction Books.

Wiener, C. (2000). *The elusive quest: Accountability in hospitals.* New York: Aldine deGruyter.

Wiener, C., & Strauss, A. (1997). *Where medicine fails* (5th ed.). New Brunswick, NJ: Transaction Books.

Wiener, C., & Wysmans, W. M. (1990). *Grounded theory in medical research: From theory to practice.* Amsterdam: Sivets and Zeitlinger.

Book Chapters

Dodd, M. J. (1997). Measuring self-care activities. In M. Frank-Stromborg & S. J. Olsen (Eds.), *Instruments for clinical health-care research* (pp. 378-385). Wilsonville, OR: Jones and Bartlett.

Dodd, M. J. (1999). Self-care and patient/family teaching. In S. L. Groenwald, M. H. Frogge, M. Goodman, & C. H. Yarbro (Eds.), *Cancer symptom management* (2nd ed., pp. 20-29). Wilsonville, OR: Jones and Bartlett.

Dodd, M. J., & Miaskowski, C. (2003). Symptom management, the PRO-SELF Program: A self-care intervention program. In B. Given, C. Given, & V. Champion (Eds.), *Evidence-based behavioral interventions for cancer patients: State of the knowledge across the cancer care trajectory* (pp. 218-241). New York: Springer.

Fagerhaugh, S., Strauss, A., Suczek, B., & Wiener, C. (1985). Safety work of patients in the technologized hospital. In K. King (Ed.), *Recent advances in nursing: Long-term care* (pp. 12-32). Edinburgh: Churchill Livingstone.

Fagerhaugh, S., Strauss, A., Suczek, B., & Wiener, C. (1986). Chronic illness, medical technology, and clinical safety in the hospital. In J. K. Roth (Ed.), *Research in the sociology of health care* (pp. 237-270). Greenwich, CT: JAI Press.

Larson, P., & Dodd, M. J. (1991). The cancer treatment experience: Family patterns of caring. In D. A. Gaut & M. M. Leininger (Eds.), *Caring: The compassionate healer* (pp. 61-78). National League of Nursing Publications.

Strauss, A., Fagerhaugh, S., Suczek, B., & Wiener, C. (1989). The hospital as multiple work sites. In P. Brown (Ed.), *Perspectives in medical sociology* (pp. 341-343). Belmont, CA: Wadsworth.

Journal Articles

Dodd, M. J., Dibble, S. L., & Thomas, M. L. (1992). Outpatient chemotherapy experience: Patients' and family members' concerns and coping strategies. *Journal of Public Health Nursing, 9*(1), 37-44.

Dodd, M. L., Dibble, S. L., Thomas, M. L. (1992). Self-care for patients experiencing cancer chemotherapy side effects: A concern for home care nurses. *Home Health-care Nurse, 9,* 21-26.

Dodd, M. J., Dibble, S. L., & Thomas, M. L. (1993). Predictors of concerns and coping strategies of cancer chemotherapy outpatients. *Journal of Applied Nursing Research, 6*(1), 2-7.

Dodd, M. J., Janson, S., Facione, N., Faucett, J., Froelicher, E. S., Humphreys, J., et al. (2001). Advancing the science of symptom management. *Journal of Advanced Nursing, 33*(5), 668-676.

Dodd, M. J., & Miaskowski, C. (2000). The PRO-SELF Program: A self-care intervention program for patients receiving cancer treatment. *Seminars in Oncology Nursing, 16*(4), 300-308.

Fagerhaugh, S., Strauss, A., Suczek, B., & Wiener, C. (1980). The impact of technology on patients, providers, and care patterns. *Nursing Outlook, 28,* 666-672.

Halliburton, P., Larson, P. J., Dibble, S. L., & Dodd, M. J. (1992). The recurrence experience: Family concerns during cancer chemotherapy. *Journal of Clinical Nursing, 1,* 275-281.

Jansen, C., Halliburton, P., Dibble, S., & Dodd, M. J. (1993). Family problems and challenges during cancer chemotherapy. *Oncology Nursing Forum, 20*(4), 689-696.

Larson, P., Dodd, M. J., & Aksamit, I. (1998). A symptom-management program for patients undergoing cancer treatment: The PRO-SELF Program. *Journal of Cancer Education, 13*(4), 248-252.

Mandrell, B. N., Ruccione, K., Dodd, M. J., Moore, J., Nelson, A. E., Pollock, B., et al. (2000). Consensus statements. Applying the concept of self-care to pediatric oncology patients. *Seminars in Oncology Nursing, 16*(4), 315-316.

Musci, E., & Dodd, M. J. (1990). Predicting self-care with patients and family members' affective states and family functioning. *Oncology Nursing Forum, 17*(3), 394-400.

Schumacher, K. L., Stewart, B., Archbold, P., Dodd, M., & Dibble, S. (2000). Family caregiving skill: Development of the concept. *Research in Nursing & Health, 23,* 191-203.

Strauss, A., Fagerhaugh, S., Suczek, B., & Wiener, C. (1981). Patients' work in the technologized hospital. *Nursing Outlook, 29,* 404-412.

Strauss, A., Fagerhaugh, S., Suczek, B., & Wiener, C. (1982). Sentimental work in the technologized hospital. *Sociology of Health and Illness, 4,* 254-278.

Strauss, A., Fagerhaugh, S., Suczek, B., & Wiener, C. (1982). The work of hospitalized patients. *Social Science and Medicine, 16,* 977-986.

Thomas, M. L., & Dodd, M. J. (1992). The development and testing of a nursing model of morbidity in cancer patients. *Oncology Nursing Forum, 19*(9), 1385-1396.

Wiener, C. (1975). The burden of rheumatoid arthritis: Tolerating the uncertainty. *Social Science and Medicine, 9,* 97-104.

Wiener, C., Fagerhaugh, S., Strauss, A., & Suczek, B. (1979). Trajectories, biographies and the evolving medical technology scene: Labor and delivery and the intensive care nursery. *Sociology of Health and Illness, 1,* 261-283. (Reprinted in A. Strauss & J. Corbin [Eds.]. [1997]. *Grounded theory in practice* [pp. 229-250]. Thousand Oaks, CA: Sage.)

Wiener, C., Fagerhaugh, S., Strauss, A., & Suczek, B. (1980). Patient power: Complex issues need complex answers. *Social Policy, 11,* 31-38.

Wiener, C., Fagerhaugh, S., Strauss, A., & Suczek, B. (1982). What price chronic illness? *Society, 19,* 22-30. (Reprinted in C. Wiener & A. Strauss [Eds.]. [1987]. *Where medicine fails* [5th ed., pp. 25-42]. New Brunswick, NJ: Transaction Books.)

Wiener, C., & Kayser-Jones, J. (1989). Defensive work in nursing homes: Accountability gone amok. *Social Science and Medicine, 28,* 37-44.

Secondary Sources

Horner, S. D. (1997). Uncertainty in mothers' care for their ill children. *Journal of Advanced Nursing, 26,* 658-663.

McCormick, K. M. (2002). A concept analysis of uncertainty in illness. *Journal of Nursing Scholarship, 34*(2), 127-131.

Mishel, M. H. (1997). Uncertainty in acute illness. *Annual Review of Nursing Research, 15,* 57-80.

Oberst, M. T. (1993). Response to "Coping amid uncertainty: An illness trajectory perspective." *Scholarly Inquiry for Nursing Practice: An International Journal, 7*(1), 33-35.

Parry, C. (2003). Embracing uncertainty: An exploration of the experiences of childhood cancer survivors. *Qualitative Health Research, 13*(1), 227-246.

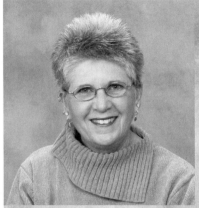

Photo credit: Center for Health Sciences Communication, Brody School of Medicine, East Carolina University, Greenville, NC.

Georgene Gaskill Eakes
1945-present

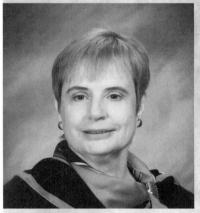

Photo credit: Olan Mills Portrait Studio, Centerdale, RI.

Mary Lermann Burke
1941-present

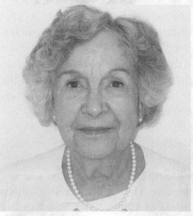

Photo credit: Shawn Hainsworth, New York.

Margaret A. Hainsworth
1931-present

Theory of Chronic Sorrow

Ann M. Schreier and Nellie S. Droes

CREDENTIALS OF THE THEORISTS
Georgene Gaskill Eakes

Georgene Gaskill Eakes was born in New Bern, North Carolina. She received a Diploma in Nursing from Watts Hospital School of Nursing in Durham, North Carolina, in 1966, and in 1977 she graduated Summa Cum Laude from North Carolina Agricultural and Technical State University with a baccalaureate in nursing. Eakes completed an M.S.N. at the University of North Carolina at Greensboro in 1980 and an Ed.D. from North Carolina State University in 1988. Eakes was awarded a federal traineeship for her graduate study at the master's level and a graduate fellowship from the North Carolina League for Nursing to support her doctoral studies. She was inducted into Sigma Theta Tau International Honor Society of Nurses in 1979 and Phi Kappa Phi Honor Society in 1988.

Early in her professional career, Eakes worked in both acute and community-based psychiatric and mental health settings. In 1980, she joined the faculty at East Carolina University School of Nursing, Greenville, North Carolina, and continues there today.

Eakes' interest in issues related to death, dying, grief, and loss dates to the 1970s when she sustained life-threatening injuries in an automobile crash. Her near-death experience heightened her awareness of how ill prepared health care professionals and lay people are to deal with individuals facing their mortality and the general lack of understanding of grief reactions experienced in response to loss situations. Motivated by this insight, she directed her early research efforts to the investigation of death anxiety among nursing personnel in long-term care settings and to the exploration of grief resolution among hospice nurses.

In 1983 Eakes established, as a community service, a twice-monthly support group for individuals diagnosed with cancer and their significant others, which she continues to co-facilitate. Her involvement with this group alerted her to the ongoing nature of grief reactions associated with diagnosis of potentially life-threatening, chronic illness. While presenting her dissertation research at a Sigma Theta Tau International research conference in Taipei, Taiwan, in 1989, she attended a presentation on chronic sorrow by Mary Lermann Burke and immediately made the connection between Burke's description of chronic sorrow in mothers of children with a myelomeningocele disability and her observations of grief reactions among the cancer support group members.

After the conference, Eakes contacted Burke to explore the possibility of collaborative research endeavors. Subsequent to their discussions, they scheduled a meeting that included Burke and her colleague, Margaret A. Hainsworth, and Carolyn Lindgren, a colleague of Hainsworth. The Nursing

Consortium for Research on Chronic Sorrow (NCRCS) was an outcome of this first meeting in the summer of 1989.

Subsequent to NCRCS's establishment, members conducted numerous collaborative qualitative research studies on populations of individuals affected with chronic or life-threatening conditions, on family caregivers, and on bereaved individuals. Eakes focused her individual studies on those diagnosed with cancer, family caregivers of adult mentally ill children, and individuals who have experienced the death of a significant other. From 1992 through 1997, Eakes received three research grant awards from East Carolina University School of Nursing and two research grants from Beta Nu Chapter of Sigma Theta Tau International to support her research endeavors.

In addition to her professional publications, Eakes has conducted numerous presentations on issues related to grief-loss and death and dying to professionals and lay groups at the local, state, national, and international levels. She has been heavily involved with the training of sudden infant death syndrome counselors for North Carolina and local and regional hospice volunteers. Eakes is also active in efforts to improve the quality of care at the end of life and, toward that end, serves as a member of the Board of Directors of the End of Life Care Coalition of Eastern North Carolina.

In 2002, Eakes received the East Carolina University Scholar Teacher Award in recognition of excellence in the integration of research into teaching practices. In 1999, Eakes received the Best of Image award for theory publication presented by Sigma Theta Tau International Honor Society of Nursing for the publication, "Middle-Range Theory of Chronic Sorrow." She was a finalist in the *Oncology Nursing Forum* Excellence in Writing award in 1994. Other honors and awards include selection as North Carolina Nurse Educator of the Year by the North Carolina Nurses Association in 1991 and as Outstanding Researcher by Beta Nu Chapter of Sigma Theta Tau International Honor Society for Nurses in 1994 and 1998. Eakes also serves as a reviewer for *Qualitative Health Research,* an international, interdisciplinary journal.

Eakes is a professor in the Department of Family and Community Nursing at East Carolina University School of Nursing, where she teaches undergraduate courses in psychiatric and mental health nursing and nursing research, a master's level course in nursing education, and an inter-disciplinary graduate course titled Perspectives on Death/Dying. Her current research efforts are directed toward further development of the Burke/Eakes Chronic Sorrow Assessment Tool, a quantitative instrument designed to assess for evidence of chronic sorrow and to identify effective coping mechanisms (G. Eakes, personal communication, 2005).

Mary Lermann Burke

Mary Lermann Burke was born in Sandusky, Ohio, where she received her elementary and secondary education. She was awarded her initial nursing diploma from Good Samaritan Hospital School of Nursing in Cincinnati in 1962, followed later that year by a post-graduate certification, from Children's Medical Center in District of Columbia. After several years of work experience in pediatric nursing, Burke graduated Summa Cum Laude from Rhode Island College, Providence, with a bachelor's degree in nursing. In 1982, she received her master's degree in parent-child nursing from Boston University. During this program, she was also awarded a Certificate in Parent-Child Nursing and Interdisciplinary Training in Developmental Disabilities from the Child Development Center of Rhode Island Hospital and the Section on Reproductive and Developmental Medicine, Brown University, in Providence. Her doctorate of nursing science in the Family Studies Cognate followed this in 1989 from Boston University.

Burke was inducted as a member of Theta Chapter, Sigma Theta Tau, during her master's program at Boston University in 1981 and as a charter member of Delta Upsilon Chapter-at-Large of Sigma Theta Tau at Rhode Island College in 1988. She received a Doctoral Student Scholarship Award from the Theta Chapter in 1988. She received the 1996 Delta Upsilon Chapter-at-Large Louisa A. White Award for Research Excellence.

During the period from 1991 through 1996, Burke received four Rhode Island College Faculty Research Grants for studies in the area of chronic sorrow. In 1998, she was awarded a grant from the Delta Upsilon Chapter-at-Large for initial quantitative instrument development for the study of chronic sorrow. Burke was principal investigator on the Transition to Adult Living Project, funded by a grant from the Department of Health and Human Services, Maternal and Child Health Bureau, Genetics Services Branch, from 1992 through 1995. A New England Regional Genetics Group Special Projects Grant, The Transition to Adult Living Project—System Dissemination of Information, supplemented this in 1995. Burke was co-principal investigator.

In her early career, Burke practiced in the pediatric nursing specialty in both acute and primary settings. She joined the faculty of Rhode Island College Department of Nursing as a clinical instructor in 1980 and became a full-time instructor in 1982, assistant professor in 1987, associate professor in 1991, and professor in 1996. During this period, she taught pediatric nursing in both theory and clinical courses. She also developed and taught a foundation nursing curriculum course encompassing nutrition, pharmacology, and pathophysiology. She retired from her Rhode Island College faculty position in December 2002.

Burke became interested in the concept of chronic sorrow during her master's degree program while engaged in a clinical practicum at the Child Development Center of Rhode Island Hospital. While working there with children with spina bifida and their parents, she developed the clinical hunch that the emotions displayed by the parents were consistent with chronic sorrow as first described by Olshansky (1962). Her master's thesis, *The Concerns of Mothers of Preschool Children with Myelomeningocele*, identified emotions similar to chronic sorrow. She then developed the Burke Chronic Sorrow Questionnaire for conducting her doctoral dissertation research, *Chronic Sorrow in Mothers of School-Age Children With Myelomeningocele*.

In June 1989, Burke presented her dissertation research at the Sigma Theta Tau International Research Congress in Taipei, Taiwan, where she interacted with Dr. Eakes of East Carolina University and Dr. Hainsworth of Rhode Island College. Subsequently, this group became the NCRCS, joined briefly by Dr. Carolyn Lindgren of Wayne State University. Together they developed a modified Burke/NCRCS Chronic Sorrow Questionnaire and conducted individually a series of studies that were analyzed collaboratively. Burke's individual studies in this series focused on chronic sorrow in infertile couples, adult children of parents with chronic conditions, and bereaved parents. The collaboratively analyzed studies resulted in the development of a middle range Theory of Chronic Sorrow, published in 1998. Members of the Consortium, both individually and collaboratively, presented numerous papers on chronic sorrow at local, state, national, and international conferences and wrote 10 articles published in refereed journals, receiving the Best of Image Award in the Theory Category from Sigma Theta Tau International for their article, "Middle-Range Theory of Chronic Sorrow." Most recently, Burke has collaborated with Dr. Eakes in the development of the Burke/Eakes Chronic Sorrow Assessment Tool.

Burke is active in numerous professional and community organizations. She is a member of the St. Joseph's Health Services of Rhode Island Board of Trustees. She has been awarded the Outstanding Alumna Award for Contributions in Nursing Education by Rhode Island College Department of Nursing and the Rhode Island College Alumni Honor Roll Award (L. Burke, personal communication, 2005).

Margaret A. Hainsworth

Margaret A. Hainsworth was born in Brockville, Ontario, Canada. She received her early elementary and secondary education in her hometown of Prescott, Ontario. Following high school graduation in 1949, she entered the diploma school of nursing at the Brockville General Hospital, Brockville, Ontario, graduating in 1953. In 1959, she immigrated to the United States to attend George Peabody College for Teachers in Nashville, Tennessee, receiving a diploma in public health nursing. In 1974 she continued her education at Salve Regina College, Newport, Rhode Island, and received a baccalaureate degree in nursing in 1973 and a master's degree in psychiatric and mental health nursing from Boston College in 1974. She received a doctoral degree in education administration from the University of Connecticut in 1986. In 1988, she was board certified as a clinical specialist in psychiatric and mental health nursing.

She was inducted into Sigma Theta Tau, Alpha Chi Chapter in 1978 and Delta Upsilon Chapter-at-Large in 1989. In 1976, she was awarded an outstanding faculty award at Rhode Island College. In 1992, she was selected to attend the Technical Assistance Workshop and Mentorship for Nurses in Implementation of the National Plan for Research in Child and Adolescent Mental Disorders that was sponsored by the National Institutes of Health. In 1991, she was selected to review manuscripts for the journal, *Qualitative Health Research, an Interdisciplinary Journal,* a Sage publication. In 1999, Hainsworth was accepted at the Royal Melbourne Institute of Technology in Melbourne, Australia, as a visiting fellow on a faculty exchange program.

Her practice in nursing was in the specialties of public health and psychiatric and mental health nursing. In 1974, she was accepted as a lecturer in the Department of Nursing at Rhode Island College and was promoted to full professor in 1992. Her major area of teaching was psychiatric care that consisted of both classroom lectures and clinical practice. She taught a course entitled *Death and Dying* that became an elective in the college's general studies program. Hainsworth always maintained her practice and was employed for 13 years as a consultant at Visiting Nursing Association. She entered into a private practice at Bay Counseling Association in 1993 and maintained this practice for 5 years.

Her interest in chronic illness and its relationship to sorrow began in her practice as a facilitator for a support group for women with multiple sclerosis. This practice led to her dissertation work, *An Ethnographic Study of Women With Multiple Sclerosis Using a Symbolic Interaction Approach.* This research was accepted for a presentation at the Sigma Theta Tau

Research Congress in Taipei, Taiwan, in 1989. At this conference she became familiar with the research on chronic sorrow after attending a presentation by Burke.

Building on Burke's work, the NCRCS was established in 1989 to expand the understanding of chronic sorrow. Hainsworth was one of the four co-founders and remained an active member until 1996. The research began with four studies that focused on chronic sorrow in individuals in chronic life situations, and the members of the consortium analyzed the data collaboratively. During the 7 years that she was a member, the consortium published 13 manuscripts and presented the findings from their studies at international, state, and regional conferences. In 1999, they were awarded the Best of Image Award in Theory from Sigma Theta Tau International (M. Hainsworth, personal communication, 2005).

THEORETICAL SOURCES

The NCRCS based the middle range Theory of Chronic Sorrow on two main sources. The work of Olshansky in 1962 was cited as the basis of the original concept of chronic sorrow (Eakes, Burke, & Hainsworth, 1998). Lazarus and Folkman's (1984) model of stress and adaptation formed the foundation for the conceptualization of how persons cope with chronic sorrow.

The concept of chronic sorrow originated with the work of Olshansky in 1962 (Lindgren, Burke, Hainsworth, & Eakes, 1992). The NCRCS theorists cite Olshansky's observations of parents with mentally retarded children that indicated these parents experienced recurrent sadness and his coining the term *chronic sorrow*. This original concept was described as "a broad, simple description of psychological reaction to a tragic situation" (Lindgren et al., 1992, p. 30).

During the 1980s other researchers began to examine the experience of parents of children who were either physically or mentally disabled. This work validated a recurrent sadness and a never-ending nature of grief experienced by these parents. Previous to this work, grief was conceptualized as a process that resolves over time and if unresolved, grief is abnormal according to Bowlby and Lindemann's work (Lindgren et al., 1992). In contrast to this time-bound conceptualization, inherent in the concept of chronic sorrow is that recurrent sadness is a normal experience, according to Wikler, Wasow, and Hatfield (Lindgren et al., 1992). Burke, in her study of children with spina bifida, defined chronic sorrow as "pervasive sadness that is permanent, periodic and progressive in nature" (Hainsworth, Eakes, & Burke, 1994, p. 59.)

The NCRCS did not confine their theory to the existence of chronic sorrow but sought to examine the response to the grief. They incorporated Lazarus and Folkman's 1984 work on stress and adaptation as the basis for effective management methods described in their model (Eakes et al., 1998). The disparity encountered and the response to re-grief stimulates individual coping mechanisms. There are categories of coping styles or management. Internal coping strategies include action-oriented, cognitive reappraisal, and interpersonal behaviors (Eakes et al., 1998). Thus, the middle range Theory of Chronic Sorrow extended the theoretical base of chronic sorrow to not only the experience of chronic sorrow in certain situations but also the coping responses to the phenomenon.

USE OF EMPIRICAL EVIDENCE
Chronic Sorrow

The empirical evidence supporting NCRCS's initial conceptual definition of chronic sorrow was derived from interviews with mothers of children with spinal bifida, which Burke conducted as part of her dissertation work. Through this research, Burke was able to define chronic sorrow as a pervasive sadness and found that the experience was permanent, periodic and potentially progressive (Eakes, Burke, Hainsworth, & Lindgren, 1993). Burke's initial work provided the foundation for subsequent series of studies, including the basis for interview guides used in these studies.

MAJOR CONCEPTS & DEFINITIONS

CHRONIC SORROW

Chronic sorrow is the ongoing disparity resulting from a loss characterized by pervasiveness and permanence. Symptoms of grief recur periodically and these symptoms are potentially progressive.

LOSS

Loss occurs as a result of disparity between the "ideal" and real situations or experiences. For example there is a "perfect child" and a child with a chronic condition who differs from that ideal.

TRIGGER EVENTS

Trigger events are situations, circumstances, and conditions that highlight the disparity or the recurrent loss and initiate or exacerbate feelings of grief.

MANAGEMENT METHODS

Management methods are means by which individuals deal with chronic sorrow. These may be internal (personal coping strategies) or external (health care practitioner or other persons' interventions).

Ineffective Management

Ineffective management results from strategies that increase the individual's discomfort or heighten the feelings of chronic sorrow.

Effective Management

Effective management results from strategies that lead to increased comfort of the affected individual.

These NCRCS studies involved the following:

- Individuals with cancer (Eakes, 1993), infertility (Eakes et al., 1998), multiple sclerosis (Hainsworth, Burke, Lindgren, & Eakes, 1993; Hainsworth, 1994), and Parkinson's disease (Lindgren, 1996)
- Spouse caregivers of persons with chronic mental illness (Hainsworth, Busch, Eakes, & Burke, 1995), multiple sclerosis (Hainsworth, 1995), and Parkinson's disease (Lindgren, 1996)
- Parent caregivers of adult children with chronic mental illness (Eakes, 1995)

Based on these studies, the theorists postulated that chronic sorrow occurs in any situation in which the loss is unresolved. These studies did not demonstrate consistently that the associated emotions worsened over time. However, the theorists concluded that the studies did support the "potential for progressivity and intensification of chronic sorrow over time" (Eakes et al., 1998, p. 180).

The NCRCS theorists extended their studies to individuals experiencing a single loss (bereaved). They found that this population experienced these same feelings of chronic sorrow (Eakes, Burke, & Hainsworth, 1999).

Based on this extensive empirical evidence, the NCRCS theorists refined the definition of chronic sorrow as the "periodic recurrence of permanent, pervasive sadness or other grief-related feelings associated with ongoing disparity resulting from a loss experience" (Eakes et al., 1998, p. 377).

Triggers

Using the empirical data from these series of studies, the NCRCS theorists identified primary events or situations that precipitated the reexperience of initial grief feelings. These events were labeled *chronic sorrow triggers* (Eakes et al., 1993). The NCRCS compared and contrasted the triggers of chronic sorrow in individuals with chronic conditions, family caregivers, and bereaved persons (Burke, Eakes, & Hainsworth, 1999). For all populations, comparisons with norms and anniversaries were found to trigger chronic sorrow. Both family caregivers and persons with chronic conditions

experienced triggering with management crises. One trigger unique for family caregivers was the requirement of unending caregiving. The bereaved population reported that memories and role change were unique triggers.

Management Strategies

The NCRCS posited that chronic sorrow is not debilitating when individuals effectively manage feelings. The management strategies were categorized as internal or external. Self-care management strategies were designated as internal coping strategies. The NCRCS further designated internal coping strategies as action, cognitive, interpersonal, and emotional.

Action coping mechanisms were used across all subjects-individuals with chronic conditions and their caregivers (Eakes, 1993, 1995; Eakes et al., 1993, 1999; Hainsworth, 1994, 1995; Hainsworth et al., 1995; Lindgren, 1996). The examples are like distraction methods commonly used to cope with pain. For instance, "keeping busy" and "doing something fun" are given as examples of action-oriented coping (Eakes, 1995; Lindgren et al., 1992). Cognitive coping was found to be used frequently and examples included "thinking positively," "making the most of it," and "not trying to fight it" (Eakes, 1995; Hainsworth, 1994; Lindgren, 1996). Interpersonal coping examples included "going to a psychiatrist," "joined a support group," and "talking to others" (Eakes, 1993; Hainsworth, 1994, 1995). Emotional strategy examples included "having a good cry" and expressing emotions (Eakes et al., 1998; Hainsworth, 1995). A management strategy was labeled effective when a subject described it as helpful in decreasing feelings of re-grief.

External management was described initially by Burke as interventions provided by health professionals (Eakes et al., 1998). Health care professionals assist affected populations to increase their comfort through roles of empathetic presence, teacher-expert, and caring and competent professional (Eakes, 1993, 1995; Eakes et al., 1993, 1999; Hainsworth, 1994, 1995; Hainsworth et al., 1995; Lindgren, 1996).

In summary, an impressive total of 196 interviews resulted in the middle range Theory of Chronic Sorrow. The theorists summarized a decade of research with individuals with chronic sorrow and found that this phenomenon frequently occurs in persons with chronic conditions, in family caregivers, and in bereaved persons (Burke et al., 1999; Eakes et al., 1998).

MAJOR ASSUMPTIONS
Nursing

Diagnosing chronic sorrow and providing inter-ventions are within the scope of nursing practice. Nurses can provide anticipatory guidance to individuals at risk. The primary roles of nurses include empathetic presence, teacher-expert, and caring and competent caregiver (Eakes, Burke, & Hainsworth, 1998).

Person

Humans have an idealized perception of life processes and health. People compare their experiences with both the ideal and with others around them. Although each person's experience with loss is unique, there are common and predictable features of the loss experience (Eakes, Burke, & Hainsworth, 1998).

Health

There is a normality of functioning. A person's health is dependent upon adaptation to disparities associated with loss. Effective coping results in a normal response to life losses (Eakes, Burke, & Hainsworth, 1998).

Environment

Interactions occur within a social context, which includes family, social, work, and health care environments. Individuals respond to their assessment of themselves in relation to social norms (Eakes, Burke, & Hainsworth, 1998).

THEORETICAL ASSERTIONS

1. Chronic sorrow is a normal human response related to ongoing disparity created by a loss situation.
2. Chronic sorrow is cyclical in nature.
3. Predictable internal and external triggers of heightened grief can be categorized and anticipated.
4. Humans have inherent and learned coping strategies that may or may not be effective in regaining normal equilibrium when experiencing chronic sorrow.
5. Health care professionals' interventions may or may not be effective in assisting the individual to regain normal equilibrium.
6. A human who experiences a single or an ongoing loss will perceive a disparity between the ideal and reality.
7. The disparity between the real and the ideal leads to feelings of pervasive sadness and grief (Eakes, Burke, & Hainsworth, 1998).

LOGICAL FORM

This theory is based on a series of qualitative studies. Through the analysis of 196 interviews, the middle range Theory of Chronic Sorrow evolved. With the empirical evidence, the NCRCS theorists described the phenomenon of chronic sorrow, identified common triggers of re-grief, and described internal coping mechanisms and the role of nurses in the external management of chronic sorrow. The theoretical assumptions are evidenced clearly in the empirical data.

ACCEPTANCE BY THE NURSING COMMUNITY
Practice

The series of studies by the NCRCS, which form the foundation of the middle range Theory of Chronic Sorrow (Eakes et al., 1998), are replete with implications for practice. Each article included a section that related the findings to clinical nursing practice (Burke et al., 1999; Eakes, 1993, 1995; Hainsworth, 1994, 1995; Hainsworth et al., 1993, 1994, 1995; Lindgren, 1996; Lindgren et al., 1992). In addition, the NCRCS work has provided other authors a basis for publications that are directed to a practice-focused audience.

NCRCS nursing practice implications. The major practice implications are suggestions for nurses in assisting individuals and family caregivers to effectively manage the milestones or triggering events. Roles outlined for nurses included: empathetic presence, teacher-expert, and caring and competent professional (Eakes, et al., 1993).

Other practice-focused literature. Several non-NCRCS nurse authors have written and published articles for nurses or physicians (Gedaly-Duff, Stoger, & Shelton, 2000; Krafft & Krafft, 1998; Scornaienchi, 2003). Other practice-focused literature, although not nurse authored, provided practice guidance that nurses would find useful (Doka, 2004; Miller, 1996).

Although the work listed here is described as relating to practice, it also can be considered educationally related. The next section presents additional evidence supporting NCRCS's work on chronic sorrow's relevance for the educational community.

EDUCATION

Two aspects of the use of the middle range Theory of Chronic Sorrow are outlined here. One is in use as a nursing diagnosis by the North American Nursing Diagnosis Association (NANDA) (NANDA International, 2003). The other is the use of the work of NCRCS in continuing education.

Chronic Sorrow: A Nursing Diagnosis

Review of the extant literature on chronic sorrow revealed that it was accepted as a nursing diagnosis by NANDA in 1998 (NANDA International, 2003). Comparison of the definitions used by NANDA and NCRCS (Eakes, et al., 1998) revealed essentially similar dimensions. Moreover, several widely used nursing diagnosis textbooks (Ackley & Ladwig, 2004; Carpenito, 2004) and undergraduate specialty textbooks cited the work of NCRCS (Lewis, Heitkemper, & Dirksen, 2004; Wong, Hockenberry-Eaton, Wilson, Winkelstein, & Schwartz, 2001).

Educational Implications

In addition to chronic sorrow's inclusion in the NANDA listing, more recent work by the research team at the University of Iowa in developing the Nursing Intervention Classification and the Nursing Outcome Classification included linkages among chronic sorrow and diagnostic category, interventions, and outcomes (Johnson, Bulechek, McCloskey Dochterman, Maas, & Moorhead, 2001). The linkages hold educational implications, because they provide guidance to nurse educators in teaching clinical decision making and designing curricula. Moreover, they refocus care planning to include attention to outcomes, an essential step in teaching evidence-based practice (Pesut & Herman, 1998).

Graduate research education. The work of NCRCS provided a theoretical basis for several master's theses and doctoral dissertations. The unpublished master's theses of Golden (1994) and Shumaker (1995) on chronic sorrow in mothers of chronically ill children and the doctoral dissertation–based articles of Hobdell (2004; Hobdell & Deatrick, 1996), Mallow (Mallow & Bechtel, 1999), and Northington (2000) attest to the use of the theoretical work of the NCRCS in graduate nursing education.

Continuing education. Three continuing education articles used the consortium's work on chronic sorrow. Meleski (2002) and Melnyk, Feinstein, Moldenhouer, and Small (2001) published continuing education courses designed for clinicians who work with families with chronically ill children. Drench's (2003) course for physical therapists and physical therapy assistants presented content on loss and grief that included NCRCS's work.

RESEARCH

A review of published research that has used NCRCS's work revealed that most articles were an extension of this work. They involved representatives of populations previously studied, as follows:

- Individuals with cancer (Eakes, 1993) multiple sclerosis (Hainsworth et al, 1993) infertility (Eakes, 1998) and Parkinson's disease (Lindgren, 1996)

- Caregivers of children with developmental delays (Burke, 1989) and adults with chronic mental illness (Eakes, 1995)
- Bereaved individuals (Eakes, Burke, & Hainsworth, 1999)

Several studies extended the work to new populations, individuals with human immunodeficiency virus (Lichtenstein, Laska, & Clair, 2002), mothers with human immunodeficiency virus (Ingram & Hutchinson. 1999), and caregivers of children with sickle cell disease (Northington, 2000), asthma (Matby, Kristjanson, & Coleman, 2003), and diabetes (Lowes & Lyne, 2000).

Although most of the authors were nurses from the United States, the literature indicated an international influence as reflected in publications by nurses from Australia (Matby et al., 2003), New Zealand (Carter, McKenna, MacLeod, & Green, 1998), Sweden (Pejlert, 2001), and the United Kingdom (Lowes & Lyne, 2000). Several studies were written by occupational therapists, and one was by sociologists, thereby providing support for the assertion that the NCRCS work has had an international and interdisciplinary influence on research.

FURTHER DEVELOPMENT

One area for further development is the variation in intensity of chronic sorrow. As suggested in a study of caregivers of adults with mental or chronic illness and children with chronic disabilities, role changes impact the intensity of chronic sorrow (Lee, Strauss, Wittman, Jackson, & Carstens, 2001). With a measurement of intensity, the middle range Theory of Chronic Sorrow would be useful as a framework for studies of the effectiveness of interventions. Some other possible nursing outcomes suggested by Ackley and Ladwig (2004) include acceptance, health status, and depression and mood equilibrium. Ackley and Ladwig suggested nursing interventions for clients with chronic sorrow. Through research, empirical support for these nursing interventions would add to evidence-based nursing practice.

Eakes and Burke (2002) are in the process of developing an assessment instrument for chronic sorrow and have reported preliminary data using the Burke/Eakes Chronic Sorrow Assessment Tool. The assessment tool and the theoretical model "will facilitate further expansion of research on chronic sorrow and provide opportunities to test the theory" (Eakes, 2004, p. 172).

CRITIQUE
Clarity

This theory clearly describes a phenomenon that is observed in the clinical area when loss occurs and it is clearly evident that it is accepted in nursing practice. As indicated previously, a nursing diagnosis of chronic sorrow appears in nursing textbooks and is defined as cyclical, recurrent, and potentially progressive and, as such, is consistent with the definition of these theorists. In each of the published works of these theorists, key concepts are defined, and this middle range theory describes the proposed relationship between these concepts. The relationship between concepts makes intuitive sense. For example, it is clear that effective management, whether internal or external, will lead to increased comfort and, conversely, ineffective management will lead to increased discomfort and intensity of chronic sorrow. As a middle range theory, the scope is limited to explanation of a single phenomenon, that of response to loss, and is congruent with clinical practice experience. As Eakes has stated, the beauty of this middle range theory is that it rings true with practitioners, students, and educators as is evident from the continued communication nationally and internationally (G. Eakes, personal communication, December 2004).

One unclear aspect of the theory is an explanation for why not all individuals with unresolved losses experience chronic sorrow. Some, albeit few, of the NCRCS's interviewees did not experience the symptoms labeled as chronic sorrow. No further data have been provided about these individuals. Do individuals who do not experience chronic sorrow have different personality characteristics, such as resiliency, or receive different health care interventions at the time of the loss? What would the data from these individuals suggest about coping with ongoing loss?

Another concept that needs clarification is the progression of chronic sorrow. Although chronic sorrow is described as potentially progressive, what is the progression and is this progression pathological in nature?

Clarification of the categories of internal management strategies is warranted. It is unclear to these reviewers how problem-oriented and cognitive strategies are different. Likewise, the emotive-cognitive, emotional, and interpersonal strategies are not clearly described. There is some obvious overlap between external versus internal management when the word *interpersonal* is used to describe seeking professional help.

Simplicity

The Theoretical Model of Chronic Sorrow (Figure 31-1) enhances the understanding of the relationship between the variables. With this model, it is clear that chronic sorrow is cyclical in nature, pervasive, and potentially progressive. Further, with the subconcepts of internal versus external management and ineffective versus effective management, it is clear what type of assessment and at what point appropriate intervention by nurses and other health care providers would be best to prevent chronic sorrow from becoming progressive. With a limited number of defined variables, the theory is succinct and readily understood. As a middle range theory, it is useful for research design and practice guidance.

Generality

The concept of chronic sorrow began with the study of parents of children with a physical or cognitive defect. Through the empirical evidence, the theory was expanded to include a variety of loss experiences. The theory clearly applies to a wide range of losses and is applicable to the affected individual as well as to the caregivers and the bereaved. In

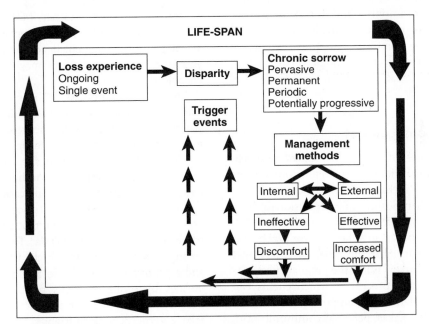

Figure **31-1 Theoretical Model of Chronic Sorrow.** (From Eakes, G. G. Burke, M. L., & Hainsworth, M. A. [1998]. Middle range theory of chronic sorrow. *Image: The Journal of Nursing Scholarship, 30*[2], 180.)

addition, the theory is useful to a variety of health care practitioners. With these concepts, the unique nature of the experience is captured with the broadness of the concepts such as triggers. The triggers and the management strategies are unique to the individual situation and thus allow the application to a wide variety of situations.

Empirical Precision

As is characteristic of middle range theory, the limited scope readily allows researchers to study the phenomenon. With a limited number of variables and defined relationships among the variables, researchers are able to generate hypotheses related to the study of nursing interventions that promote effective management strategies for chronic sorrow. These outcome studies provide and add to the foundation of evidence-based practice.

Because the theory was derived from empirical evidence, it has clear utility for further research. The clear definition of chronic sorrow allows the study of individuals with a variety of losses and those loss situations that commonly result in chronic sorrow. In their study of bereaved individuals, Eakes and colleagues (1999) identified symptoms of chronic sorrow in most subjects. Through further study, researchers can devise assessment tools for clinical practice.

Derivable Consequences

As a consequence of this rich body of research, chronic sorrow is a widely accepted phenomenon, as is evident by its inclusion in NANDA diagnoses. Nurses and other health care professionals have found validity for their experiences with loss in the clinical arena. Subsequently, health care practitioners are able to normalize the experience. As Eakes stated, "chronic sorrow is like the pregnancy experience, it is a normal process in which clients can benefit from guidance and support of health care professionals" (G. Eakes, personal communication, December 2004). Eakes further states that this experience is unique to each individual and to each situation.

SUMMARY

Loss is an experience common to all individuals. This middle range theory describes the phenomenon of chronic sorrow as a normal response to the ongoing disparity created by the loss. The major concepts are described and include disparity, triggers, and management strategies (internal and external). The theoretical sources and empirical evidence are described. The chapter presents evidence that the theory is accepted and used in practice, education, and research. It is referenced internationally by nurses and by providers in other disciplines. Suggestions for further development and research are presented. A thorough critique describes the clarity of concepts, and the simplicity and the usefulness of the theory for evidence-based research.

Case Study

Susan Jones is a 21-year-old woman who sustained a spinal cord injury at the age of 14 as a result of a diving accident. She is quadriplegic and attends a local college. Her mother, Mary Jones, is her primary caregiver. Mrs. Jones complains of difficulty sleeping and has frequent headaches. As the nurse, you suspect that Mrs. Jones may be experiencing chronic sorrow.

Using the Burke/NCRCS Chronic Sorrow Questionnaire (caregiver version) as an interview guide, you find evidence of chronic sorrow (Eakes, 1995). Mrs. Jones describes frequent feelings of being overwhelmed. She expresses that she feels both angry at times and heartbroken that her daughter will never have a normal life. She indicates that she has had these feelings off and on since her daughter's accident. Further, she tells you that she sees no end to her caregiving responsibilities. These feelings are strongest when her friend's children get married and get jobs away from home. She copes with these feelings by trying to focus on the positive (her daughter is alive and her sons are doing well) and talking with a few close friends.

You reassure Mrs. Jones that she is not alone in her situation and that it is normal to have these feelings. In the course of the interview, you find that

Mrs. Jones has not sought professional counseling help. Mrs. Jones tells you that she feels better, because this is the first time a health professional has asked her about her feelings. With Mrs. Jones you begin to strategize on finding respite care and a regular mental health counselor to assist her in coping with chronic sorrow.

CRITICAL THINKING *Activities*

1. Using the middle range Theory of Chronic Sorrow as a framework, devise one or more hypotheses about parents of children with diabetes who do or do not attend a support group.

2. Providing a support group is only one possible intervention strategy to assist individuals experiencing chronic sorrow. What outcome measures or objective evaluation would you use to validate the effectiveness of interventions?

3. Compare and contrast the middle range Theory of Chronic Sorrow to Kubler-Ross' stages of grief or to Bowlby's theory of loss.

4. Describe the experience of three individuals with a chronic condition such as multiple sclerosis. Do you think that the theoretical assertions of the middle range Theory of Chronic Sorrow apply in these situations? State your rationale.

REFERENCES

Ackley, B. J., & Ladwig, G. B. (2004). *Nursing diagnosis handbook: A guide to planning care* (6th ed.). St. Louis: Mosby.

Burke, M. L., Eakes, G. G., & Hainsworth, M. A. (1999). Milestones of chronic sorrow: Perspectives of chronically ill and bereaved persons and family caregivers. *Journal of Family Nursing, 5*(4), 374-387.

Carpenito, L. J. (2004). *Nursing diagnosis: Application to clinical practice.* Philadelphia: Lippincott Williams & Wilkins.

Carter, H., McKenna, C., MacLeod, R., & Green, R. (1998). Health professionals' responses to multiple sclerosis

and motor neuron disease. *Palliative Medicine, 12*(5), 383-394.

Doka, K. J. (2004). Grief and dementia. In K. J. Doka (Ed.), *Living with grief: Alzheimer's disease.* Washington DC: Hospice Foundation of America.

Drench, M. E. (2003). Loss, grief, and adjustment: A primer for physical therapy. Part I. *PT, 11*(6), 50-62.

Eakes, G. G. (1993). Chronic sorrow: A response to living with cancer. *Oncology Nursing Forum, 20*(9), 1327-1334.

Eakes, G. G. (1995). Chronic sorrow: The lived experience of parents of chronically mentally ill individuals. *Archives of Psychiatric Nursing, 9*(2), 77-84.

Eakes, G. G. (2004). Chronic sorrow. In S. J. Peterson & T. S. Bredow (Eds.), *Middle range theories: Application to nursing research* (pp. 165-175). Philadelphia: Lippincott Williams & Wilkins.

Eakes, G. G., & Burke, M. L. (2002). Development and validation of the Burke/Eakes chronic sorrow assessment tool. Unpublished raw data (eakesg@mail.ecu.edu).

Eakes, G. G., Burke, M. L., & Hainsworth, M. A. (1998). Middle-range theory of chronic sorrow. *Image: The Journal of Nursing Scholarship, 30*(2), 179-184.

Eakes, G. G., Burke, M. L., & Hainsworth, M. A. (1999). Chronic sorrow: The lived experience of bereaved individuals. *Illness, Crisis, and Loss, 7*(1), 172-182.

Eakes, G. G., Burke, M. L., Hainsworth, M. A., & Lindgren, C. (1993). Chronic sorrow: An examination of nursing roles. In S. G. Funk, E. Tornquist, & M. T. Champagne (Eds.), *Key aspects of caring for the chronically ill: Hospital and home* (pp. 231-236). New York: Springer.

Gedaly-Duff, V., Stoger, S., & Shelton, K. (2000). Working with families. In R. E. Nickel & L. W. Desch (Eds.), *The physicians' guide to caring for children with disabilities and chronic conditions* (pp. 31-75). Baltimore: Paul H. Brooks.

Golden, B. A. (1994). *The presence of chronic sorrow in mothers of children with cerebral palsy.* Unpublished master's thesis, University of Arizona, Tempe.

Hainsworth, M. A. (1994). Living with multiple sclerosis: The experience of chronic sorrow. *Journal of Neuroscience Nursing, 26*(4), 237-240.

Hainsworth, M. A. (1995). Helping spouses with chronic sorrow related to multiple sclerosis. *Journal of Gerontological Nursing, 21*(7), 29-33.

Hainsworth, M. A., Burke, M. L., Lindgren, C. L., & Eakes, G. G. (1993). Chronic sorrow in multiple sclerosis: A case study. *Home Healthcare Nurse, 11*(2), 9-13.

Hainsworth, M. A., Busch, P. V., Eakes, G. G., & Burke, M. L. (1995). Chronic sorrow in women with chronically mentally disabled husbands. *Journal of the American Psychiatric Nurses Association, 1*(4), 120-124.

Hainsworth, M. A., Eakes, G., & Burke, M. L. (1994). Coping with chronic sorrow. *Issues in Mental Health Nursing, 15*(1), 59-66.

Hobdell, E. (2004). Chronic sorrow and depression in parents of children with neural tube defects. *Journal of Neuroscience Nursing, 36*(2), 82-88.

Hobdell, E. F., & Deatrick, J. A. (1996). Chronic sorrow: A content analysis of parental differences. *Journal of Genetic Counseling, 5*(2), 57-68.

Ingram, D., & Hutchinson, S. A. (1999). Defensive mothering in HIV-positive mothers. *Qualitative Health Research, 9*(2), 243-258.

Johnson, M., Bulechek, G., McCloskey Dochterman, J., Maas, M., & Moorhead, S. E. (2001). *Nursing diagnoses, outcomes, and interventions: NANDA, NOC and NIC linkages.* St. Louis: Mosby.

Krafft, S. K., & Krafft, L. J. (1998). Chronic sorrow: Parents' lived experience. *Holistic Nursing Practice, 13*(1), 59-67.

Lazarus, R. S., & Folkman, S. (1984). *Stress, appraisal, and coping.* New York: Springer.

Lee, A. L., Strauss, L., Wittman, P., Jackson, B., & Carstens, A. (2001). The effects of chronic illness on roles and emotions of caregivers. *Occupational Therapy in Health Care, 14*(1), 47-60.

Lewis, S. M., Heitkemper, M. L., & Dirksen, S. R. (2004). *Medical surgical nursing: Assessment and management of clinical problems* (6th ed., Vol. 2). St. Louis: Mosby.

Lichtenstein, B., Laska, M. K., & Clair, J. M. (2002). Chronic sorrow in the HIV-positive patient: Issues of race, gender, and social support. *AIDS Patient Care and STDs, 16*(1), 27-38.

Lindgren, C. L. (1996). Chronic sorrow in persons with Parkinson's and their spouses. *Scholarly Inquiry for Nursing Practice, 10*(4), 351-370.

Lindgren, C. L., Burke, M. L., Hainsworth, M. A., & Eakes, G. G. (1992). Chronic sorrow: A lifespan concept. *Scholarly Inquiry for Nursing Practice, 6*(1), 27-42.

Lowes, L., & Lyne, P. (2000). Chronic sorrow in parents of children with newly diagnosed diabetes: A review of the literature and discussion of the implications for nursing practice. *Journal of Advanced Nursing, 32*(1), 41-48.

Mallow, G. E., & Bechtel, G. A. (1999). Chronic sorrow: The experience of parents with children who are developmentally disabled. *Journal of Psychosocial Nursing and Mental Health Services, 37*(7), 31-35.

Matby, H. J., Kristjanson, L., & Coleman, M. (2003). The parenting competency framework: Learning to be a parent of a child with asthma. *International Journal of Nursing Practice, 9*(6), 368-373.

Meleski, D. D. (2002). Families with chronically ill children. *American Journal of Nursing, 102*(5), 47-54.

Melnyk, B. M., Feinstein, N. F., Moldenhouer, Z., & Small, L. (2001). Coping in parents of children who are chronically ill: Strategies for assessment and intervention. *Pediatric Nursing, 27*(6), 548-558.

Miller, F. E. (1996). Grief therapy for relatives of persons with serious mental illness. *Psychiatric Services, 47*(6), 633-636.

NANDA International. (2003). *NANDA: Nursing diagnoses: Definitions & classification 2003-2004.* Philadelphia: NANDA International.

Northington, L. (2000). Chronic sorrow in caregivers of school age children with sickle cell disease: A grounded theory approach. *Issues in Comprehensive Pediatric Nursing, 23*(3), 141-154.

Olshanky, S. (1962). Chronic sorrow: A response to a mentally defective child. *Social casework, 43*, 191-193.

Pejlert, A. (2001). Being a parent of an adult son or daughter with severe mental illness receiving professional care: Parents' narratives. *Health and Social Care in the Community, 9*(4), 194-204.

Pesut, D., & Herman, J. (1998). OPT: Transformation of nursing process for contemporary practice. Outcome-Present State-Test. *Nursing Outlook, 46*(1), 29-36.

Scornaienchi, J. M. (2003). Chronic sorrow: One mother's experience with two children with lissencephaly. *Journal of Pediatric Health Care, 17*(6), 290-294.

Shumaker, D. (1995). *Chronic sorrow in mothers of children with cystic fibrosis.* Unpublished master's thesis, University of Tennessee, Memphis.

Wong, D. L., Hockenberry-Eaton, M., Wilson, D., Winkelstein, M. L., & Schwartz, P. (2001). *Wong's essentials of pediatric nursing* (6th ed.). St. Louis: Mosby.

BIBLIOGRAPHY
Primary Sources
Book Chapters

Eakes, G. G. (2004). Chronic sorrow. In S. J. Peterson & T. S. Bredow (Eds.), *Middle range theories: Application to nursing research* (pp. 165-175). Philadelphia: Lippincott Williams & Wilkins.

Eakes, G. G., Burke, M. L., Hainsworth, M. A., & Lindgren, C. (1993). Chronic sorrow: An examination of nursing roles. In S. G. Funk, E. Tornquist, & M. T. Champagne (Eds.), *Key aspects of caring for the chronically ill: Hospital and home* (pp. 231-236). New York: Springer.

Journal Articles

Burke, M. L., Eakes, G. G., & Hainsworth, M. A. (1999). Milestones of chronic sorrow: Perspectives of chronically ill and bereaved persons and family caregivers. *Journal of Family Nursing, 5*(4), 374-387.

Burke, M. L., Hainsworth, M. A., Eakes, G. G., & Lindgren, C. L. (1992). Current knowledge and research on chronic sorrow: A foundation for inquiry. *Death Studies, 16*(3), 231-245.

Eakes, G. G. (1993). Chronic sorrow: A response to living with cancer. *Oncology Nursing Forum, 20*(9), 1327-1334.

Eakes, G. G. (1995). Chronic sorrow: The lived experience of parents of chronically mentally ill individuals. *Archives of Psychiatric Nursing, 9*(2), 77-84.

Eakes, G. G., Burke, M. L., & Hainsworth, M. A. (1998). The middle-range theory of chronic sorrow. *Image: The Journal of Nursing Scholarship, 30*(2), 179-184.

Eakes, G. G., Burke, M. L., & Hainsworth, M. A. (1999). Chronic sorrow: The lived experience of bereaved individuals. *Illness, Crisis, and Loss, 7*(1), 172-182.

Eakes, G. G., Hainsworth, M. E., Lindgren, C. L., & Burke, M. L. (1991). Establishing a long-distance research consortium. *NursingConnections, 4*(1), 51-57.

Hainsworth, M. A. (1994). Living with multiple sclerosis: The experience of chronic sorrow. *Journal of Neuroscience Nursing, 26*(4), 237-240.

Hainsworth, M. A. (1995). Helping spouses with chronic sorrow related to multiple sclerosis. *Journal of Gerontological Nursing, 21*(7), 29-33.

Hainsworth, M. A., Burke, M. L., Lindgren, C. L., & Eakes, G. G. (1993). Chronic sorrow in multiple sclerosis: A case study. *Home Healthcare Nurse, 11*(2), 9-13.

Hainsworth, M. A., Busch, P. V., Eakes, G. G., & Burke, M. L. (1995). Chronic sorrow in women with chronically mentally disabled husbands. *Journal of the American Psychiatric Nurses Association, 1*(4), 120-124.

Hainsworth, M. A., Eakes, G., & Burke, M. L. (1994). Coping with chronic sorrow. *Issues in Mental Health Nursing, 15*(1), 59-66.

Lindgren, C. L. (1996). Chronic sorrow in persons with Parkinson's and their spouses. *Scholarly Inquiry for Nursing Practice, 10*(4), 351-370.

Lindgren, C. L., Burke, M. L., Hainsworth, M. A., & Eakes, G. G. (1992). Chronic sorrow: A lifespan concept. *Scholarly Inquiry for Nursing Practice, 6*(1), 27-42.

Dissertation

Burke, M. L. (1989). Chronic sorrow in mothers of school age children with a myelomeningocele disability (Doctoral dissertation, Boston University, 1989). *Dissertation Abstracts International, 50,* 233-234B.

Unpublished Data

Eakes, G. G., & Burke, M. L. (2002). Development and validation of the Burke/Eakes chronic sorrow assessment tool. Unpublished raw data (eakesg@mail.ecu.edu).

Secondary Sources
Books

Ackley, B. J., & Ladwig, G. B. (2004). *Nursing diagnosis handbook: A guide to planning care* (6th ed.). St. Louis: Mosby.

Carpenito, L. J. (2004). *Nursing diagnosis: Application to clinical practice.* Philadelphia: Lippincott Williams & Wilkins.

Johnson, M., Bulechek, G., McCloskey Dochterman, J., Maas, M., & Moorhead, S. E. (2001). *Nursing diagnoses, outcomes, and interventions: NANDA, NOC and NIC linkages.* St. Louis: Mosby.

Lazarus, R. S., & Folkman, S. (1984). *Stress, appraisal, and coping.* New York: Springer.

Lewis, S. M., Heitkemper, M. L., & Dirksen, S. R. (2004). *Medical surgical nursing: Assessment and management of clinical problems* (Vol. 2). St. Louis: Mosby.

NANDA International. (2003). *NANDA: Nursing diagnoses: Definitions & classification 2003-2004.* Philadelphia: NANDA International.

Walker, L. O., & Avant, K. C. (2005). *Strategies for theory construction in nursing.* Upper Saddle River, NJ: Pearson Prentice-Hall.

Wong, D. L., Hockenberry-Eaton, M., Wilson, D., Winkelstein, M. L., & Schwartz, P. (2001). *Wong's essentials of pediatric nursing.* St. Louis: Mosby.

Book Chapters

Doka, K. J. (2004). Grief and dementia. In K. J. Doka (Ed.), *Living with grief: Alzheimer's disease.* Washington DC: Hospice Foundation of America.

Gedaly-Duff, V., Stoger, S., & Shelton, K. (2000). Working with families. In R. E. Nickel & L. W. Desch (Eds.), *The physicians' guide to caring for children with disabilities and chronic conditions* (pp. 31-75). Baltimore: Paul H. Brooks.

Lindgren, C. L. (2000). Chronic sorrow in long-term illness across the life span. In J. M. Miller (Ed.), *Coping with chronic illness: Overcoming powerlessness* (3rd ed., pp. 125-143). Philadelphia: F. A. Davis.

Smith, M. J., & Liehr, P. (2003). Introduction: Middle range theory and the ladder of abstraction. In M. J. Smith & P. Liehr (Eds.), *Middle range theory for nursing* (pp. 1-23). New York: Springer.

Journal Articles

Carter, H., McKenna, C., MacLeod, R., & Green, R. (1998). Health professionals' responses to multiple sclerosis and motor neuron disease. *Palliative Medicine, 12*(5), 383-394.

Charles, K., Sellick, S. M., Montesanto, B., & Mohide, E. A. (1996). Priorities of cancer survivors regarding psychosocial needs. *Journal of Psychosocial Oncology, 14*(2), 57-72.

Dewar, A. L., & Lee, E. A. (2000). Bearing illness and injury. *Western Journal of Nursing Research, 22*(8), 912-926.

Doornbos, M. M. (1997). The problems and coping methods of caregivers of young adults with mental illness. *Journal of Psychosocial Nursing and Mental Health Services, 35*(9), 22-26.

Doornbos, M. M. (2000). King's systems framework and family health: The derivation and testing of a theory. *Journal of Theory Construction & Testing, 4*(1), 20-26.

Drench, M. E. (2003). Loss, grief, and adjustment: A primer for physical therapy. Part I. *PT, 11*(6), 50-62.

Gordon, M. (1998, September 30). Nursing nomenclature and classification system development. *Online Journal of Issues in Nursing.* Retrieved December 20, 2004, from *http://www.nursingworld.org/ojin/tpc7/tpc7_1.htm*

Hewson, D. (1997). Coping with loss of ability: "Good grief" or episodic stress responses. *Social Science & Medicine, 44*(8), 1129-1139.

Hobdell, E. (2004). Chronic sorrow and depression in parents of children with neural tube defects. *Journal of Neuroscience Nursing, 36*(2), 82-88.

Hobdell, E. F., & Deatrick, J. A. (1996). Chronic sorrow: A content analysis of parental differences. *Journal of Genetic Counseling, 5*(2), 57-68.

Howard, P. B. (1998). The experience of fathers of adult children with schizophrenia. *Issues in Mental Health Nursing, 19*(4), 399-413.

Ingram, D., & Hutchinson, S. A. (1999). Defensive mothering in HIV-positive mothers. *Qualitative Health Research, 9*(2), 243-258.

Johnsonius, J. R. (1996). Lived experiences that reflect embodied themes of chronic sorrow: A phenomenological pilot study. *Journal of Nursing Science, 1*(5/6), 165-173.

Kearney, P. M., & Griffin, T. (2001). Between joy and sorrow: Being a parent of a child with developmental disability. *Journal of Advanced Nursing, 34*(5), 582-592.

Krafft, S. K., & Krafft, L. J. (1998). Chronic sorrow: Parents' lived experience. *Holistic Nursing Practice, 13*(1), 59-67.

Langridge, P. (2002). Reduction of chronic sorrow: A health promotion role for children's community nurses. *Journal of Child Health Care, 6*(3), 157-170.

Lee, A. L., Strauss, L., Wittman, P., Jackson, B., & Carstens, A. (2001). The effects of chronic illness on roles and emotions of caregivers. *Occupational Therapy in Health Care, 14*(1), 47-60.

Lichtenstein, B., Laska, M. K., & Clair, J. M. (2002). Chronic sorrow in the HIV-positive patient: Issues of race, gender, and social support. *AIDS Patient Care and STDs, 16*(1), 27-38.

Liehr, P., & Smith, M. J. (1999). Middle range theory: Spinning research and practice to create knowledge for the new millennium. *ANS Advances in Nursing Science, 21*(4), 81-91.

Lindgren, C. L., Connelly, C. T., & Gaspar, H. L. (1999). Grief in spouse and children caregivers of dementia patients. *Western Journal of Nursing Research, 21*(4), 521-537.

Lowes, L., & Lyne, P. (2000). Chronic sorrow in parents of children with newly diagnosed diabetes: A review of the literature and discussion of the implications for nursing practice. *Journal of Advanced Nursing, 32*(1), 41-48.

Mallow, G. E., & Bechtel, G. A. (1999). Chronic sorrow: The experience of parents with children who are developmentally disabled. *Journal of Psychosocial Nursing and Mental Health Services, 37*(7), 31-35.

Matby, H. J., Kristjanson, L., & Coleman, M. (2003). The parenting competency framework: Learning to be a parent of a child with asthma. *International Journal of Nursing Practice, 9*(6), 368-373.

Meleski, D. D. (2002). Families with chronically ill children. *American Journal of Nursing, 102*(5), 47-54.

Melnyk, B. M., Feinstein, N. F., Moldenhouer, Z., & Small, L. (2001). Coping in parents of children who are chronically ill: Strategies for assessment and intervention. *Pediatric Nursing, 27*(6), 548-558.

Miller, F. E. (1996). Grief therapy for relatives of persons with serious mental illness. *Psychiatric Services, 47*(6), 633-636.

Northington, L. (2000). Chronic sorrow in caregivers of school age children with sickle cell disease: A grounded theory approach. *Issues in Comprehensive Pediatric Nursing, 23*(3), 141-154.

Parse, R. R. (1997). Joy-sorrow: A study using the Parse research method. *Nursing Science Quarterly, 10*(2), 80-87.

Pejlert, A. (2001). Being a parent of an adult son or daughter with severe mental illness receiving professional care: Parents' narratives. *Health and Social Care in the Community, 9*(4), 194-204.

Pesut, D. J., & Herman, J. (1998). OPT: Transformation of nursing process for contemporary practice. *Nursing Outlook, 46*(1), 29-36.

Phillips, M. (1991). Chronic sorrow in mothers of chronically ill and disabled children. *Issues in Comprehensive Pediatric Nursing, 14*(2), 111-120.

Scornaienchi, J. M. (2003). Chronic sorrow: One mother's experience with two children with lissencephaly. *Journal of Pediatric Health Care, 17*(6), 290-294.

Sumner, J. (2001). Caring in nursing: A different interpretation. *Journal of Advanced Nursing, 35*(6), 926-932.

Thorne, S., Paterson, B., Acorn, S., Canam, C., Joachim, G., & Jillings, C. (2002). Chronic illness experience: Insights from a metastudy. *Qualitative Health Research, 12*(4), 437-452.

Dissertations

Hobdell, E. F. (1993). The relationship between chronic sorrow and accuracy of perception of cognitive development in parents of children with neural tube defect (Doctoral dissertation, University of

Pennsylvania, 1993). *Dissertation Abstracts International, B 54/03,* 1333.

Northington, L. K. (1999). Chronic sorrow in caregivers of school age children with sickle cell disease: A grounded theory approach (Doctoral dissertation, Louisiana State University, Health Science Center, 1999). *Dissertation Abstracts International, B 59/10,* 5313.

Master's Theses

Golden, B. A. (1994). *The presence of chronic sorrow in mothers of children with cerebral palsy.* Unpublished master's thesis, University of Arizona, Tempe.

Shumaker, D. (1995). *Chronic sorrow in mothers of children with cystic fibrosis.* Unpublished master's thesis, University of Tennessee, Memphis.

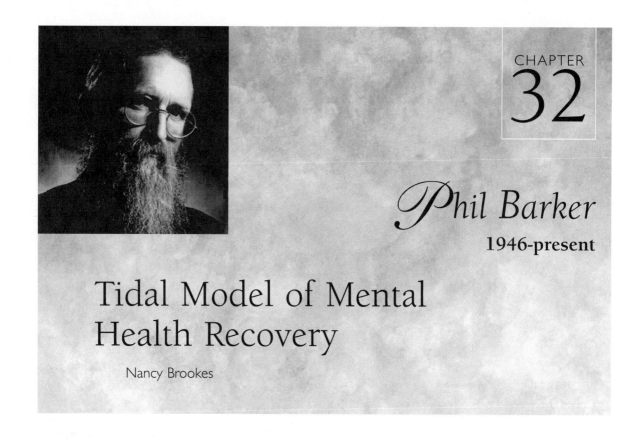

CHAPTER

32

Phil Barker

1946-present

Tidal Model of Mental Health Recovery

Nancy Brookes

CREDENTIALS OF THE THEORIST

Phil Barker was born in Scotland by the sea, and thus began the influence of and his interest in water, the ultimate metaphor of life (Barker, 1996a). He credits his father and grandfather with "the warmth of nurture and the discipline of boundaries," who helped him to appreciate that "life was an answer waiting for the right question." He, like them, became a philosopher (Barker, 1999b, p. xii). Life in this context also contributed to his enduring curiosity and the philosophy of the everyday, which resonate throughout the Tidal Model.

Barker trained as a painter and sculptor during the mid-1960s and won the prestigious Pernod Award for young painters in 1974, by which time he had already become a psychiatric nurse. He continues to paint word pictures in metaphor. Barker

credits art school with introducing him to "learning from reality," the reality of experience, which became the focus of his philosophical inquiries. His fascination with Eastern philosophies, which began at art school, flows through the Tidal Model with echoes of chaos, uncertainty, change, and the Chinese idea of crisis as opportunity. This early involvement in the arts also helps to explain Barker's view of nursing as "the craft of caring" (Barker, 2000c, 2000e; Barker & Whitehill, 1997).

After art school, Barker worked as a commercial artist and mural painter, supplementing his income with work as a laborer on the railroads and in factories. His "ocean of experience" surged in a new direction in 1970 when he took a position as an "attendant at the local asylum." His fascination with the human dimension, the lived experience, and the stories of people challenged by mental distress prompted him to transfer his interest in the arts and humanities to nursing.

Barker's early progress through nursing, although unusual, was typical of the times and context. Nursing, per se, was submerged temporarily when he began to study and practice various psychotherapies such as cognitive behavioral therapy and family and group therapy. Barker's doctoral research featured cognitive behavioral work with a group of women living with depression (Barker, 1987). However, around this time, Barker became uncomfortable with the application of therapies to people experiencing problems in living and the "uncertainty principle" reasserted itself. His curiosity about life and persons provoked questions about the people with whom he was working, their resilience, and their integrity. He was learning from them what it meant to experience distress, and he wondered what recovery meant to people? Questions also reemerged around what it is to be a person, what is the proper focus of nursing, and what are nurses needed for? During his tenure as Professor of Psychiatric Nursing Practice at the University of Newcastle, these questions framed his research agenda and culminated in the Tidal Model.

As the United Kingdom's first Professor of Psychiatric Nursing Practice, Barker continued to maintain a practice, and this was central to the development of the Tidal Model. Throughout his nursing career, Barker has wondered about the proper focus of psychiatric nursing and the role of care, compassion, understanding, and courage in helping people experiencing extreme distress, loss of self, or spiritual crises (Barker, 1999b). The Tidal Model developed within this context and history, and the story continues. The narrative knowledge base for the Tidal Model, although particular, is not exclusive and it leaves room both for development and for other viewpoints.

Barker has published in the area of psychiatric and mental health nursing since 1978. A prolific writer, he has written 14 books, more than 50 book chapters, and more than 150 academic papers. He has been assistant editor for the *Journal of Psychiatric and Mental Health Nursing* for the last 10 years. Barker was made a fellow of the Royal College of Nursing (United Kingdom) in 1995, only the fourth psychiatric nurse to be so honored. He received the Red Gate Award for Distinguished Professors at the University of Tokyo in 2000, and in 2001 he received an honorary doctorate from Oxford Brookes University in England and a room was named in his honor at the Health Care Studies Faculty at Homerton College, Cambridge. He has held visiting professorships at several international universities, including Australia (Sydney), Europe (Barcelona), and Japan (Tokyo).

Barker has traveled widely with his wife and professional partner, Poppy Buchanan-Barker, in response to interest in the recovery paradigm underlying the Tidal Model, conducting workshops and seminars in Australia, Canada, New Zealand, Japan, Finland, Ireland, and the United Kingdom. A popular commentator on the human condition, he brings to radio, television, and the popular press his passion for and curiosity about the recovery process and what it might mean to be a person.

Currently, Barker is a visiting professor in health science at Trinity College, Dublin, and an Honorary Professor at the University of Dundee, Scotland, where he maintains a private psychotherapy practice. With Poppy Buchanan-Barker he is developing a recovery paradigm at Clan Unity, their international mental health recovery and reclamation consultancy based in Scotland.

THEORETICAL SOURCES

The Tidal Model is a radical (focused upon nursing's fundamental care processes), catholic (universally applicable), and practical model to guide psychiatric and mental health nursing (Barker, 2001b). The theory is also radical in its reconceptualization of mental health problems and needs as unequivocally human, rather than psychological, social, or physical (Barker, 2002b). The Tidal Model "emphasizes the central importance of: developing understanding of the person's needs through collaborative working, developing a therapeutic relationship through discrete methods of active empowerment, establishing nursing as an educative element at the heart of interdisciplinary intervention" (Barker,

2000e, p. 4) and searching for solutions, resolving problems, and promoting mental health through narrative interventions (Stevenson, Barker, & Fletcher, 2002).

The Tidal Model is a philosophical approach to the recovery of mental health. It is not a model of care or treatment of mental illness, although people described as mentally ill do need and receive care. The Tidal Model represents a specific world view that helps the nurse begin to understand what mental health might mean for the particular person-in-care and how that person might be helped to map and begin the complex and demanding voyage of recovery.

The Tidal Model is not prescriptive, rather a set of principles—the 10 commitments—serve as the metaphorical compass for the practitioner. They guide the nurse in developing responses to meet the individual and contextually bound needs of the person who has become the patient. The experience of mental distress invariably is described in metaphorical terms. The Tidal Model employs the universal and culturally significant metaphors associated with the power of water and the sea, to represent the known aspects of human distress. Water is "the core metaphor for both the lived experience of the person . . . and the care system that attempts to mould itself around a person's need for nursing" (Barker, 2000e, p. 10).

Barker describes an "early interest in the human content of mental distress . . . and an interest in the human (phenomenological) experience of distress," which is viewed in contexts and wholes rather than isolated parts (Barker, 1999b, p. 13). The "whole" nature of being human is "re-presented on physical, emotional, intellectual, social and spiritual planes" (Barker, 2002b, p. 233). This phenomenological interest pervades the Tidal Model with an emphasis on the lived experience of persons, their stories (replete with metaphors), and narrative interventions. Nurses carefully and sensitively meet and interact with people in a "sacred space" (Barker, 2003a).

A key feature of Barker's nursing practice has been his exploration of the possibilities of genuine collaborative relationships with users of mental health services. In the 1980s he developed his interest in the concept of "caring with" people, learning that the professional-person relationship could be more mutual than the original nurse-patient relationship defined by Peplau (1952, 1997). Barker further developed this concept during the 1990s in a working relationship with Dr. Irene Whitehill and with other people who used mental health services (Barker & Whitehill, 1997). This work led to the "need for nursing" and "empowerment" studies, as well as a commitment to publish the stories of people's experience of madness and their voyage of recovery, complete with personal and spiritual meanings (Barker & Buchanan-Barker, 2004a, 2004b, 2004c; Barker, Jackson, & Stevenson, 1999a).

Barker's longstanding appreciation of Eastern philosophies pervades his work. The work of Shoma Morita is an example of how the philosophical assumptions of Zen Buddhism were integrated with psychotherapy (Morita, Kondo, Levine, & Morita, 1998). Morita's dictum to "do what needs to be done" resonates in many of the practical activities of the Tidal Model. People have the capacity to live and grow through distress, by doing what needs to be done. For people who are in acute distress, especially when they are at risk to self or others, it is vital that nurses try to relate directly to the person's ongoing experience. Originally Barker called this process *engagement,* but he has now redefined the specific interpersonal process as "bridging," emphasizing the need to build, creatively, a means of reaching the person, crossing the murky waters of mental distress in the process (Barker & Buchanan-Barker, 2004c).

The Tidal Model also can be viewed through the lens of social constructivism, recognizing that there are multiple ways of understanding the world. Meaning emerges through the complex webs of interaction, relationships, and social processes. Knowledge does not exist independently of the knower and all knowledge is situated (Stevenson, 1996). Change is the only constant, as meaning and social realities constantly are renegotiated or constructed through language and interaction. The potential of reauthoring, rewriting, or reconstructing the story with persons-in-care lies in dialogue.

In a critical sense, people make themselves up as they talk (Barker, 2003a).

Barker credits many thinkers with influencing his work, beginning with Annie Altschul and Thomas Szasz. His view of mental health problems as problems of living, as popularized by Szasz (1961, 2000) and later Podvoll (1990), is a perspective he prefers to diagnostic labeling and the biomedical construction of people and illness (Barker, 2001c). Travelbee's (1969) concept of the therapeutic use of self flows through the Tidal Model and provides an anchor for the "proper focus of nursing." Three main theoretical frameworks underpin the Tidal Model: Peplau's interpersonal relations theory, the theory of psychiatric and mental health nursing derived from the need for nursing studies, and empowerment within interpersonal relationships. The pragmatic emphasis on strength-based, solution-focused approaches acknowledges the important influence of Steve de Shazer (1994) and solution-focused therapy.

The Tidal Model draws its core philosophical metaphor from chaos theory, where the unpredictable, yet bounded, nature of human behavior and experience can be compared with the flow and power of water (Barker, 2000b). In constant flux, the tides ebb and flow; they exhibit nonrepeating patterns yet stay within bounded parameters (Vicenzi, 1994). Barker (2000b) acknowledges the "complexity [of] both the internal universe of human experience and the external universe, which is, paradoxically, within and beyond the individual, at one and the same time" (p. 52). Within this complex, nonlinear perspective, small changes can create unpredictable changes. This hopeful message directs nurses and persons to identify small changes and variations. Chaos theory suggests that there are limits to what we can know, and Barker invites nurses to cease the search for certainty, embracing instead the reality of uncertainty. Know that "change is constant;" one of the tidal commitments identifies and celebrates change in people, circumstances, relationships, and organizations (Barker, 2003b). This perspective also presents challenges in trying to understand people, relationships, and situations. It directs inquiry in qualitative, nonlinear ways, such

as action research, grounded theory, phenomenology, and critical theory (Barker, 1999a).

Annie Altschul, the grande dame of British psychiatric nursing (Barker, 2003a, p. 12), along with Hilda Peplau, was one of Barker's mentors. Altschul's influence, especially her early appreciation of systems theory, is evident in the Tidal Model, as is her interest in understanding rather than explaining mental distress and her belief that people need more straightforward help than many of the psychiatric theories suggest. The power of the nurse-person relationship and a therapeutic system where the whole life of the person is accommodated also flows through the theory (Barker, 1999b, 2003a). Altschul was the "voice of a generation concerned with helping people through 'ordinary' everyday interactions and found these ordinary interactions could be quite *extraordinary*" (Barker, 2002a, p. 127). Ordinary, everyday interactions or conversations are indeed the proper focus of nursing.

Barker credits Peplau, the mother of psychiatric nursing, with his becoming "an advocate for nursing as a therapeutic activity in its own right" (Barker, 2000a, p. 617). Peplau introduced her interpersonal paradigm for the study and practice of nursing during the early 1950s and defined nursing as "a significant, therapeutic, interpersonal process" (Peplau, 1952, p. 16). Both the nurse and the person participate in and contribute to the relationship, which itself can be therapeutic. Although persons and relationships are inherently complex, the nurse and the person "flow effortlessly, through each other's experience" and enjoy the infinite possibilities of interpersonal dialogue (Barker, 2000b, p. 53). A solution-orientation reframes nurse-person relationships. Although both participants in the relationship have expertise, persons are the experts in their own lives, with strengths and resources, which may need to be "uncovered" (Barker, 1998b; McAllister, 2003).

"Language influences thought; thought then influences action; thought and action together evoke feelings in relation to a situation or context" (Peplau, 1969, p. 267). Nurses work "in language," and this is a powerful medium (Barker, 1996b, p. 6). We engage in the collaborative exploration of the person's story and help create a coherent, respectful narrative in everyday language, the person's natural language. The stories include who this person is, what his or her experience has been, what the person needs in the form of nursing, and how to progress through his or her story or build a recovery story (Barker, Reynolds, & Ward, 1995). A defining characteristic of the Tidal Model is an emphasis on the narrative in the person's own voice.

The empirically derived empowering interactions framework suggests that improvement in the person's situation and lifestyle is possible, building on strengths is better than focusing on problems, collaboration is key, participation is the way, and self-determination is the ultimate goal (Barker & Buchanan-Barker, 2004a; Barker, Stevenson, & Leamy, 2000). Eight respectful, empowering interactions also bring generally invisible nursing interactions into the practice arena (Michael, 1994). de Shazer's (1994) influence is evident as he asserts that change and intervention "boils down to stories about the telling of stories, the shaping and reshaping of stories so that troubled people change their story" (p. xvii).

The strength base of the Tidal Model emphasizes searching for and revealing solutions and identifying resources. The theory integrates the need for nursing studies, collaboration, empowerment, interpersonal relationships, narrative, and systemic and solution-oriented approaches. The solution-focus, a model of questions, provides specific direction for nurses. In the holistic assessment, nurses explore the person's present problems or needs, the scale of these problems or needs, what is currently part of the person's life that might help to resolve problems or meet needs, and what needs to happen to bring about change (Barker, 2000e). Nurses help to identify and mobilize persons' strengths and resources, and the person's goals direct the work of the health care team (Barker, 2000e; Stevenson, Jackson, & Barker, 2003). The 10 commitments (Box 32-1) also support this perspective and direction. This is a significant reframing of the view of the person-in-care and the proper focus of nursing. It requires courage and creativity to "unlearn" our deficit models and the notion of the nurse as expert.

Box **32-1**

The Ten Commitments: Essential Values of the Tidal Model

The Tidal Model originally drew on our values about relating to people and trying to help them in their distress. The values embedded in the Tidal Model also reflect, not surprisingly, a philosophy of how we would wish or expect to be treated when we experience distress or difficulty in our lives.

As more and more people have become involved in exploring the potential of the Tidal Model for their work, in different settings, the need to reaffirm the core values of the Tidal Model have become more apparent. We have come to appreciate how both the helper (whether professional, friend or fellow traveler) and the person need to make a commitment to change. Rarely is this easy. However, this commitment is what binds them together.

Here we offer the following 10 commitments, which distill the essence of the practice of the Tidal Model. These commitments need to be firmly in place, in both the hearts and minds of the helping team if it wishes to say it is pursuing and developing the philosophy of the Tidal Model.

1. *Value the voice:* the person's story is the beginning and end point of the whole helping encounter. The person's story embraces not only the account of the person's distress, but also the hope for its resolution. This is the voice of experience. We need to guard it well, as the voice begins to help the person to make herself or himself anew. For this simple, yet powerful, reason we emphasize that the

Box 32-1

The Ten Commitments: Essential Values of the Tidal Model—cont'd

story of the recovery voyage—and all the care plans supporting it—should be written in the person's own voice.

2. *Respect the language:* the person has developed a unique way of expressing the life story, of representing to others that which the person alone can know. The language of the story, complete with its unusual grammar and personal metaphors, is the ideal medium for lighting the way. There is no need to colonize the person's story, substituting the often arcane, ugly, and awkward language of psychiatry, psychobabble, or the social sciences. People already own the most powerful language for describing, defining, and articulating their personal experience: their own language.

3. *Develop genuine curiosity:* the person is writing a life story but should not be confused with an "open book." Those who seek to be of assistance to the person need to develop ways of expressing genuine interest in the story, as written and as it continues to be written, so that they might better understand the storyteller and the human significance of the unfolding life story.

4. *Become the apprentice:* the person is the world expert on the life story. We can begin to learn something of the power of that story, but only if we apply ourselves diligently and respectfully to the task by becoming the apprentice.

5. *Reveal personal wisdom:* the person has developed a powerful storehouse of wisdom in the writing of the life story. One of the key tasks for the helper is to assist in revealing that wisdom, which will be used to

sustain the person and to guide the journey of reclamation and recovery.

6. *Be transparent:* both the person and the professional embody the opportunity to become a team. If this relationship is to prosper, both must be willing to let the other into confidence. The professional helper is in a privileged position and should model this confidence building by being transparent at all times, helping the person understand what is being done and why.

7. *Use the available toolkit:* the person's story contains numerous examples of what has worked or what might work for this person. These represent the main tools that need to be used to unlock or build the story of recovery.

8. *Craft the step beyond:* the helper and the person work together to construct an appreciation of what needs to be done "now." The first step is the crucial step, revealing the power of change and pointing toward the ultimate goal of recovery.

9. *Give the gift of time:* there is nothing more valuable than the time the helper and the person spend together. Time is the midwife of change. There is no value in asking "How much time do we have?" We have all the time there is. The question is, surely, how do we use this time?

10. *Know that change is constant:* the Tidal Model assumes that change is inevitable, for change is constant. This is the common story for all people. The task of the professional helper is to develop awareness of how that change is happening and how that knowledge might be used to steer the person out of danger and distress back onto the course of reclamation and recovery.

From Barker, P. J. (2003). *The 10 commitments: Essential values of the Tidal Model.* Newport on Tay, Scotland: Phil Barker. Retrieved April 18, 2004 from *http://www.tidal-model.co.uk/New%2010%20Commitments.htm*

MAJOR CONCEPTS *&* DEFINITIONS

THEORETICAL BASIS OF THE TIDAL MODEL

The Tidal Model begins from four simple, yet important, starting points:

1. *The primary therapeutic focus in mental health care lies in the community.* People live on an "ocean of experience" (their natural lives) and psychiatric crisis is only one thing, among many, that might threaten to "drown" them. Ultimately, the aim of mental health care is to return people to that "ocean of experience," so that they might continue with their life journeys.

2. *Change is a constant, ongoing, process.* Although people are constantly changing, this may be beyond their awareness. One of the main aims of the interventions used within the model is to help people develop their awareness of the small changes that, ultimately, will have a big effect on their lives.

3. *Empowerment lies at the heart of the caring process.* Nurses help people to identify how they might take greater charge of their lives, and all their related experiences.

4. *The nurse and the person are united (albeit temporarily) like dancers in a dance.* When effective nursing happens, as W.B. Yeats (1928) might have remarked, "How do we tell the dancer from the dance?" Nursing is something that involves caring with people, rather than for them or even just about them. This has implications not only for what goes on within the relationship, but also for the kind of support nurses might need from others to maintain the integrity of the caring process (Barker, n.d., *The Theoretical Basis of the Tidal Model*).

PERSONHOOD IN THREE DIMENSIONS

The person who lives within his or her world of experience is represented in three dimensions: world, self, and others. A series of solution-focused, strength-based assessments developed within these dimensions facilitate a narrative, person-centered approach.

The world dimension focuses upon persons' need to be understood and to have their perceptions validated. A holistic nursing assessment is documented in the person's own voice. This assessment focuses upon the person's world of experience and provides the opportunity to learn about the person's current problems or needs, the scale or an evaluation of these problems or needs, what resources in the person's life might help to resolve problems or meet the needs, and what needs to happen to bring about change (Barker, 2000e).

The self dimension emphasizes the person's need for both emotional and physical security. A collaborative security assessment addresses this need and results in a security plan, which identifies the support necessary to ensure personal security and decrease risk of harm to self or others (Barker, 2000e). The areas of suicide risk, violence, self-harm and self-neglect are targeted specifically, although the risk for suicide is the most robust.

The kind of support and services that the person might need to live an ordinary life is addressed in the others dimension. Interdisciplinary teamwork is highlighted in this dimension as specific medical, social, or psychological interventions are included, as are such things necessary for everyday living: finances, housing, and other determinants of health. Family, friends, and significant others also find a place in this dimension (Barker, 2000e).

WATER: A METAPHOR

The Tidal Model emphasizes the unpredictability of human experience through the core metaphor of water.

Life is a journey taken on an ocean of experience. All human development, including the experience of health and illness, involves discoveries made on that journey across the ocean of experience. At critical points in the journey people may experience storms or piracy. The ship may begin to take in water and the person may face the prospect of drowning or shipwreck. The person may need to be guided to a safe haven, to undertake repairs, or to recover from the trauma. Once the ship is made intact or the person has regained their sea legs, the journey may begin again, as the person sets again on course on the ocean of experience. This metaphor illustrates many of the elements of the psychiatric crisis and the necessary responses to this human predicament.

Storms at sea is a metaphor for problems of living; *piracy* evokes the experience of rape or the robbery of the self that severe distress can produce. Many users describe the overwhelming nature of the experience of distress as akin to drowning, and this often ends in a metaphorical shipwreck on the shores of the acute psychiatric unit. A proper "psychiatric rescue" should be akin to "lifesaving" and should lead the person to a genuine safe haven where the necessary human repair work can take place (Barker, 2000d).

GUIDING PRINCIPLES

- *Curiosity:* person is the world's leading authority on his or her life
- *Resourcefulness:* focus on and work with person's resourcefulness; individual resources, resources in interpersonal and social network
- *Respect for person's wishes:* wishes of person are human heart of caring process
- *Crisis as opportunity:* natural signal something needs to be done; opportunity for change, take new direction in life, review life
- *Think small:* initial goals are small and specific (versus the end point of care process)
- *Elegance:* simplest possible intervention for changes necessary to experience change (versus highly complex, multilevel interventions) (Barker, 2000e)

GETTING IN THE SWIM— ENGAGEMENT BELIEFS

When people are in serious distress they often feel as if they are drowning. In such circumstances, they need a "lifesaver." Of course, lifesavers need to engage with the person—they need to get close— to begin the rescue process. To get "in the swim" and to begin the engagement process, we need to believe that:

- Recovery is possible
- Change is inevitable; nothing lasts
- Ultimately, people know what is best for them
- Persons possess all the resources they need to begin the recovery journey
- The person is the teacher and we, the helpers, are the pupils
- We need to be creatively curious, to learn what needs to be done to help the person, now (Barker, n.d., *A Beginner's Guide to the Tidal Model*)

THERAPEUTIC PHILOSOPHY

This person-centered approach involves asking the following four questions:

1. *Why this? Why now?* Why is the person experiencing the particular difficulty, now, and what needs to be done now to address the problem?
2. *What works?* The Tidal Model aims to find out what has worked for the person in the past and what might work in the immediate future.
3. *What is the personal theory?* How does the person understand or explain his or her current problem?
4. *How to limit restrictions?* How little might the nurse do and how much might the person do to bring about therapeutic change, using the least restrictive interventions? (Barker, 2000e)

CONTINUUM OF CARE

As needs flow with the person across artificial boundaries, care is seamless, always with the

Continued

MAJOR CONCEPTS & DEFINITIONS—cont'd

intention of the person returning to his or her ocean of experience within his or her own community. Across the care continuum, people may need critical or immediate, transitional, or developmental care. Practical immediate care addresses searching for solutions to the person's problems, generally in the short term, and focuses upon what needs to be done, now. People enter the care continuum for immediate care when experiencing an initial mental health crisis, possibly entering the mental health system for the first time, or when a crisis occurs with people already familiar to the system. Transitional care addresses the smooth passage from one setting to another, when the person is moving from one form of care to another. Here, nursing responsibilities include liaising with colleagues and ensuring the person's participation in the transfer of care. The other end of the continuum is developmental care, where the focus is on more intensive and longer-term support or therapeutic intervention (Barker, 2000e).

USE OF EMPIRICAL EVIDENCE

Barker's longstanding curiosity about the nature and focus of psychiatric nursing and the stories of persons-in-care led to the development of a theoretical construction of psychiatric nursing, or a meta-theory, that could be further explored through empirical inquiry (Barker, Reynolds, & Stevenson, 1997). Over 5 years, from 1995, the Newcastle and North Tyneside research team developed an understanding of what people experiencing problems in living might need from nurses. They began to use their emergent findings in 1997 as the basis for the development of the Tidal Model.

Barker supports learning from, using, and integrating extant theory and research, as well as the experience of reality—"evidence from the most 'real' of real worlds" (Barker & Jackson, 1997). An example is the "need adapted" approach to caring with people with schizophrenia, developed from Alanen's (Alanen, Lehtinen, & Aaltonen, 1997) studies. One understanding that underpins Alanen's work and flows through the Tidal Model is that people and their families need to think of psychiatric situations, like admission to a psychiatric facility, as resulting from the problems of living they have encountered and not as a mysterious illness which is within the patient (Alanen et al., 1997).

The power of the nurse-patient relationship demonstrated through Altschul's pioneering research in the early 1960s and Peplau's paradigm of interpersonal relationships that derived in part from the study of human interactions contribute to the empirical base of the Tidal Model. Altschul's study of nurse-patient interactions in the 1960s provides empirical support for "the complex, yet paradoxically 'ordinary' nature of the relationship" (Barker, 2002a, p. 127). Altschul's study of community teams in the 1980s raised questions about the "proper focus of nursing" and the "need for nursing," and both Altschul and Peplau provided evidence related to interdisciplinary teamwork.

Two of Barker's theory-generating studies provide an empirical base for the Tidal Model. During the "need for nursing" studies (Barker et al., 1999a; Barker, Jackson, & Stevenson, 1999b), researchers examined the perceptions of service users, significant others, members of multidisciplinary teams, and nurses. They sought to clarify discrete roles and functions of nursing within a multidisciplinary care and treatment process and to learn what people value in nurses (Barker, 2001c). The studies demonstrated that both professionals and persons-in-care wanted nurses to relate to people in ordinary, everyday ways. There was universal acceptance of special interpersonal relationships between nurses and persons, echoing Peplau's (1952) work. "Knowing you, knowing me" emerged as the core concept in these studies. Three roles are identified as ordinary-me, pseudo-ordinary–

engineered-me, and professional-me. These relationships are fluid, requiring nurses to "toggle," or switch back and forth, between highly professional and distinctly ordinary presentations of self (Jackson & Stevenson, 1998, 2000). Sometimes people need someone to take care of them, other times someone to take care with them (Barker, et al., 1999a, 1999b). The studies also suggest that nurses need to respond sensitively to persons' and their families' often rapidly fluctuating human needs. They need to "tune in to what needs to be done now" to meet a person's needs (Barker, 2000e). Nurses are translators, for the person to the treatment team and others and the "glue" that holds the system together (Stevenson & Fletcher, 2002).

The second study focused on the nature of empowerment and how this is enacted in relationship between nurses and persons-in-care and resulted in the empowering interactions model (Barker, et al., 2000). This was developed through Flanagan's critical incident technique (Flanagan, 1954) within a cooperative inquiry method (Heron, 1996), using a modified grounded theory approach (Glaser & Strauss, 1967). It developed Peplau's assumptions about importance of specific interpersonal transactions, and it provides guidance and strategies for nurses within collaborative nurse-person relationships. Strategies include being respectful of people's knowledge and expertise about their own health and illness, putting the person in the driver's seat in relation to the interaction, seeking permission to explore the person's experience, valuing the person's contribution, being curious as a way of validating the person's experience, finding common language to describe the situation, taking stock and reviewing collaboratively, and inspiring hope through designing a realistic future.

MAJOR ASSUMPTIONS

Nurses are involved in the process of working with people, their environments, and their health status, as well as their need for nursing (Barker, 1996a). The Tidal Model rests on the assumptions that there are

such "things" as psychiatric needs and that nursing might in some way meet those needs (Barker & Whitehill, 1997). Persons and those around them already possess the solutions to their life problems; nursing is about drawing out these solutions (Barker, 1995).

Two basic assumptions underpin the Tidal Model. First, change is the only constant. Nothing lasts. All human experience involves flux and people are constantly changing. This suggests the value of helping people become more aware of how change is happening within and around them in the "now" (Barker & Buchanan-Barker, 2004a). Second, people are their stories. They are no more and no less than the complex story of their lived experience. The person's story always is framed in the first person, and the story of how this person came to be here experiencing this "problem of living" contains raw material for solutions. Ultimately, our problems belong to us and are unique. What we have to work with is the story, the most valuable form of evidence (Barker & Buchanan-Barker, 2004a).

The Tidal Model assumes that when people are caught in the psychic storm of "madness," it is "as if" they risk drowning in their distress or foundering on the rocks; it is "as if" they have been boarded by pirates and have been robbed of some of their human identity; it is "as if" they have been washed ashore on some remote beach, far from home and alienated from all that they know and understand. All persons in such circumstances need, first of all, a safe haven, to which they might retire to begin the necessary repair work on the ship of their lives. Having regained their sea legs and the confidence to set sail again on the ocean of their experience, persons need to begin the complex and challenging task of charting their recoveries.

Nursing

Nursing is changing continuously, internally and in relation to other professions, in response to changing needs and changing social structures. The nature of Barker's relationship with users of services confirms his appreciation of nursing as a social, rather than professional, construct. "If any one thing defines nursing, globally, it is the social construction of the nurse's role" (Barker, et al., 1995, p. 390). Nursing as nurturing, exists only when the conditions necessary for the promotion of growth or development are being put in place. Nursing is an enduring human interpersonal activity and involves a focus on the promotion of growth and development (Barker & Whitehill, 1997).

Nursing is a human service offered by one group of human beings to another. There is a power dynamic in the "craft of caring;" one person has a duty to care for another (Barker, 1996b). Nursing is a practical endeavor focused on identifying what people need now, collaboratively exploring ways of meeting those needs and developing appropriate systems of human care (Barker, 1995, 2003a). The proper focus of nursing is the need expressed by the person-in-care, which "can only be defined as a function of the relationship between a *person-with-a-need-for-nursing* and a *person-who-has-met-that-need*" (Barker, 1996a, p. 241; Barker et al., 1995, p. 389). These responses are the phenomenological focus of nursing (Barker, et al., 1995; Peplau, 1987). This focus is on human responses to actual or potential health problems (American Nurses Association, 1980) and may range across the person's relationship with the environment, behavior, emotions, beliefs, identity, capability, and spirituality (Barker, 1998a).

Nursing's exploration of the human context of being and caring suggests nursing as a form of human inquiry. Being with and caring with people is the process that underpins all psychiatric and mental health nursing, and this process distinguishes nurses from all other health and social care disciplines (Barker, 1997). Nursing complements other services and is congruent with the roles and functions of other disciplines in relation to the person's needs (Barker, 2001c).

Person

Within the Tidal Model, interest is directed toward the phenomenological view of the person's lived experience and his or her story or narrative. Persons are natural philosophers and meaning makers, devoting much of their lives to establishing the meaning and value of their experience and to constructing explanatory models of the world and their place in it (Barker, 1996b). Nurses are able to see and appreciate the world from the person's perspective and share this with the person. People are their stories. "The person's sense of self, and the world of experience—including the experience of others—is inextricably tied to their life stories and the various meanings they have generated" (Barker, 2001c, p. 219). People are in a constant state of flux, engaged in the process of becoming (Barker, 2000c). They live within their world of experience represented in three dimensions: world, self, and others. The Tidal Model "holds few assumptions about the proper course of a person's life" (Barker, 2001a, p. 235). Persons are defined in relation, as for example someone's mother, father, daughter, son, sister, brother, friend. They are also in relation with nurses.

Health

Barker provides the provocative definition of health put forth by Illich (1976) as follows:

> . . . the result of an autonomous yet culturally shaped reaction to socially created reality. It designates the ability to adapt to changing environments, to growing up . . . to healing when damaged, to suffering and to the peaceful expectation of death. Health embraces the future . . . includes the inner resources to live with it. (p. 273)

Health is a personal task for which success is "in large part the result of self-awareness, self-discipline, and inner resources by which each person regulates his/her own daily rhythms and actions, his/her diet, and his/her sexuality" (Illich, 1976, p. 274). Our personhood, connections, and fragility "make the experience of pain, of sickness, and of death an integral part of life" (Illich, 1976, p. 274). Illich's (1976) description illustrates both the chaotic and Zen sense of reality. "Health is not 'out-there,' it is not something to be pursued, gained or delivered (health-care). It is a part of the whole task of being and living" (Barker, 1999b, p. 240).

"Health means whole . . . and is likely linked to the way we live our lives, in the broadest sense. This 'living' includes the social, economic, cultural and spiritual context of our lives" (Barker, 1999b, p. 48). The experience of health and illness is fluid. Within a holistic view, people have their own individual meanings of health and illness that we value and accept. Nurses engage with people to learn their stories and their understanding of their current situations, including relationships with health and illness within their world views (Barker, 2001c). Appreciating the person's own meanings of health enables the nurse to stay focused on the person's definitions of desired outcome (Montgomery & Webster, 1993). This holistic, phenomenological, person-centered perspective leads to a wide range of possibilities.

Ill health or illness almost always involves a spiritual crisis or a loss of self (Barker, 1996a). A state of dis-ease is a human problem with social, psychological and medical relations—a whole life crisis. Nursing in the Tidal Model is pragmatic and focused upon persons' strengths, resources, and possibilities, maintaining a health orientation, a healthy theory.

Environment

The environment is largely social in nature, the context in which persons travel within their ocean of experience; nurses create "space" for growth and development. Therapeutic relationships are used in ways that enhance persons' relationships with their environments (Montgomery & Webster, 1993). Human problems may derive from complex person-environment interactions in the organized chaos of the everyday world (Barker, 1998b). "Persons live in a social and material world where their interaction with the environment includes other people, groups, and organizations" (Barker, 2003a, p. 67). Family, culture, and relationships are integral to this environment. Within the environment are vital areas of everyday living including housing, financing, occupation, leisure, a sense of place, and a sense of belonging (Barker, 2001c).

The artificial divide between community and institution is rejected as needs flow with the person across these boundaries. Much psychiatric nursing takes place in the most mundane of settings; from day rooms of hospital wards to the living room or kitchen of the person's own home (Barker, 1996b). With critical interventions, nurses need to make the person and the environment safe and secure. Engagement is critical and the social environment is critical for engagement. When people are deemed to be at risk, they may need to be detained in a safe and supportive environment, a safe harbor until they return to their ocean of experience in the community (Barker, 2003a). "Nurses organize the kind of conditions that help to alleviate distress and begin the longer term process of recuperation, resolution or learning. They help persons to feel the 'whole' of their experience . . . and engender the potential for healing" (Barker, 2003a, p. 9).

THEORETICAL ASSERTIONS

The Tidal Model is based upon four premises concerning practice, which were developed by Barker during the mid-1990s using an "expert nurse" focus group (Barker, 1997). These premises were validated by a group of former psychiatric patients, led by Barker's colleague of many years, the mental health service user and activist, Dr. Irene Whitehill.

Psychiatric nursing is an interactive, developmental human activity, more concerned with the future development of the person than the origins or cause of their present mental distress.

The experience of mental distress associated with psychiatric disorder is represented through public disturbance or reports of private events that are known only to the person concerned. Nurses help people access, review, and reauthor these experiences.

Nurses and the people-in-care are engaged in a relationship based upon mutual influence. Change is constant, and within relationships there are changes in the relationship and within the participants in the relationship.

The experience of mental illness is translated into a variety of disturbances of everyday living and human responses to problems in living (Barker & Whitehill, 1997).

These premises are framed within the wider philosophical and theoretical perspective, especially the phenomenological assertion that people own their experience, only the person can know his or her experience and what it means. Mental illness is a symbolic force, which is known only, in phenomenological terms, to the person involved. The lived experience is the medium through which we receive important messages about our life and its meaning (Barker, 2001c). Barker views mental distress as part of the whole that is the person, not something split off from the person's "normal" being.

In keeping with this phenomenological perspective, the Tidal Model assumes and asserts that people know what their needs are or can be helped to recognize or acknowledge them over time. From that minimally empowered position, people may be helped to meet these needs in the short term. Nurses and everyone else in the person's social world relate to the expressed behavior.

Barker's concept of "the need for nursing" flows with the person across artificial boundaries of dichotomies like community and hospital, acute and long-term care, and the various specialties, each of which risks reducing the person to a collection of disparate parts (Barker, 2001a).

Mental illness is disempowering and "people who experience any of the myriad threats to their personal or social identities, commonly called mental illness or mental health problems, experience a human threat that renders them vulnerable." However, "most people are sufficiently healthy to be able to act for themselves and to influence constructively the direction of their lives" (Barker, 2003a, pp. 6-7). Recovery is possible and people have the personal and interpersonal resources that enable this recovery process (Barker, 2001c).

LOGICAL FORM

The Tidal Model is presented in logical form. It is logically adequate, the structure of relationships is clear and concepts are precise, developed, and developing. It contains broad ideas, addresses many situations of persons with problems in living, follows the "logic of experience" (Barker, 1996b), and

develops "practice-based evidence" (P. Barker, personal communication, April 12, 2004).

Barker and his colleagues constructed a metatheory of psychiatric and mental health nursing. This developed from their collective education, experience, practice, and observations that formed generalizable wholes or principles. Questions about the nature of persons, problems in living, and nursing were followed by systematic inquiry. The theory both informs and is shaped by research. The Tidal Model flows from a particular philosophical perspective and world view, which provides the context for beliefs about persons and nursing. An integrative approach brought in other concepts and theories. Chaos theory, for example, helps one to understand and explain persons' lived experience. The solution orientation enriched the theoretical formulations. Within the framework the selected concepts—partnerships-collaboration, empowerment, narratives, and solutions—form logical and complete relationships.

The theory specifies nursing's focus of inquiry, identifies phenomena of particular interest to nursing, and provides a broad perspective for nursing research, practice, and education. Descriptions of nursing delineate it from medicine and other disciplines, specify the contribution of nursing to the health care team, and provide direction for interdisciplinary collaboration. The theory classifies a body of nursing knowledge which is largely narrative. The components are clearly presented and logically derived from clinical observation, theory, research, and philosophy.

The emergent evidence, from user evaluations in the United Kingdom, Ireland, Canada and New Zealand, confirm the importance of the simple affirmation of the personal narrative, with its emphasis on understanding what is happening for and to the person, and what this means for the person, in his or her own language. The story, written in the person's own voice, is not translated into professional jargon. The attempt to understand persons' constructions of their world is expressed through the holistic assessment, a product of several years of clinical development. This provides an elegant means of helping persons relate their story and of exploring what needs to be done now to address problems. Care planning is a collaborative exercise, with an emphasis on developing an awareness of change and revealing solutions rather than solving problems. The celebration of personhood and the holistic, narrative approach create a range of approaches toward working collaboratively with people. This emphasizes persons' inherent resources and acknowledges change as an enduring characteristic.

ACCEPTANCE BY THE NURSING COMMUNITY

The clear, conceptual base of the Tidal Model gives direction for nursing practice, education, and research. The Tidal Model has appeal for facilities committed to person-centered care and research-based practice. At the practice level it provides rationales for nursing actions. Those implementing the Tidal Model are encouraged to adapt the original philosophy and practice principles to their local circumstances. Acceptance of the theory is facilitated by the philosophical, theoretical, research, and practical base, along with clearly stated values and principles.

Practice

The Tidal Model was developed in practice between 1995 and 1997 and was introduced formally on two acute psychiatric wards in Newcastle, England, in 1998. It was adopted subsequently by the Mental Health Program and in 2000 rolled out across nine acute psychiatric wards, their associated community support teams, and one 24-hour facility in the community (Barker & Buchanan-Barker, 2004c). The Tidal Model is international in scope, because interest spread from the United Kingdom, to Ireland, then throughout the world.

Most of the Tidal Model developmental work is being undertaken in the United Kingdom, with projects ranging across hospital and community services, from acute, through rehabilitation, to specialist forensic services and community care.

These projects also range from metropolitan services in cities like central London and Birmingham, where the clinical populations are socially, culturally, and ethnically diverse, to Cornwall, Glamorgan, and Norfolk, where they serve people from more traditional English and Welsh towns and villages in the wide-ranging rural community. The biggest project to date is in Scotland, where the Glasgow mental health services operate a series of Tidal Model projects across the city, in the largest mental health trust in the United Kingdom.

The Republic of Ireland has more than 30 projects, most of these situated in County Cork, with other projects in County Mayo and Dublin, ranging across hospital and community settings. Cork City, Ireland, was the first to introduce and develop the Tidal Model within community mental health care at Tosnú (Gaelic for a *fresh start*) Holistic Centre, and now there are almost 20 projects bridging hospital and community services.

At the Royal Ottawa Hospital in Canada, three programs implemented the Tidal Model in September 2002. The Forensic and Mood programs include inpatient wards and outpatient components. The Substance Use and Concurrent Disorders Program includes an inpatient ward, outpatient nursing, day hospital, and a residential program in the community and is the first program of its kind to implement the Tidal Model. In February 2004, the Tidal Model was introduced to the remaining inpatient wards including geriatric, crisis and evaluation, general psychiatry in transition, psychosocial rehabilitation, schizophrenia, and youth.

In Australia, the model was first introduced in Sydney but now is the focus of a major development in Townsville, Queensland, where the lead nurse is attempting to build formal bridges between the professional and consumer perspectives on recovery. In New Zealand, nurses at the Rangipapa forensic service in Porirua have been developing their care around the Tidal Model for almost 3 years, and this was the first forensic service in the world to adopt the model. The Tidal Model's emphasis on narrative has proven particularly attractive to the indigenous Maori and Pacific Islands people, who greatly value the power of storytelling. This is reflected in a recent evaluation of the perceptions of Tidal Model care by some of the unit's residents.

In Japan, the model has been the focus of a major development program at the Kanto Medical Center, the largest private psychiatric facility in Tokyo, over the past 2 years. There, Dr. Tsuyoshi Akayama, the lead psychiatrist, translated all the Tidal Model training materials into Japanese and then taught his medical and nursing colleagues how to use it, following his short study tour in Newcastle with Barker. This was the first example of a formal collaboration between psychiatrists and nurses; in all of the earlier projects, nurses had led the implementation alone. The Japanese have set a trend for greater interdisciplinary collaboration, albeit with nursing taking the lead role.

Education

Barker provides a multimedia education package for those implementing the Tidal Model, and all sites use this program to prepare for implementation. This ensures a common perspective among and fidelity to the values, principles, and processes of the Tidal Model, yet it allows creative, locally relevant implementation. Nurses within the Tidal Model community have the opportunity to learn about the model before, during, and following its implementation. In the first wave at Newcastle upon Tyne, over 150 nurses participated in the formal training, and over the next 2 years almost 300 nurses participated in the multimedia education program.

The Tidal Model is integrated into the diploma, graduate, and postgraduate nursing programs at the University of York. Ian Beech, a mental health nurse and lecturer at the University of Glamorgan, developed the first educational program for practitioners in Wales. At University College Cork, the Tidal Model is linked between the university and various practice settings. At the University of Ottawa, Canada, the Tidal Model is included in the undergraduate theories and concepts course; it also frames the Community Mental Health Nursing course. The Tidal Model is included in the Mount Royal College community mental health course in Calgary, Canada. The holistic, strength-based, narrative Tidal

Model holds great promise for inclusion in educational programs concerned with research-based practice and person-centered care.

Research

The Tidal Model developed from a clinical research program. All international Tidal Model network members are encouraged to evaluate the model in practice. A research and development consultancy was established as a loose network for Tidal Model implementation and development projects. The consultancy provides a framework for evaluation of the Tidal Model in action from the perspective of organizational outcome, professional experience, and user-consumer experience (Barker & Buchanan-Barker, 2004c). The important task of evaluating the implementation, processes, and outcomes of the Tidal Model in practice is ongoing in Canada, Ireland, Japan, New Zealand, and across the United Kingdom.

Two evaluation studies (Fletcher & Stevenson, 2001; Stevenson & Fletcher, 2002) explored outcome measures that could be important in evaluating the Tidal Model and evaluated the impact of its assessment in practice (Stevenson & Fletcher, 2002). Results of both studies indicate an increase in the number of admissions and a decrease in the length of stays. There were decreases in the need for the highest level of observation, which correlated with the speed of assessment and decreased incidents of violence, self-harm, and use of restraints. Nurses, themselves, reported that the Tidal Model enhanced professional practice and encouraged fuller engagement with persons-in-care. It was useful in helping persons to fulfill care plans and enabled nurses to focus their interactions on persons' needs. Support workers were more able to help persons identify goals and targets for the day and carry them out; they described the Tidal Model as a way of raising their profiles and professional esteem (Stevenson & Fletcher, 2002). These studies provide support for the implementation of this person-centered theory in practice.

Barker and Walker (2000) studied senior nurses' views of multidisciplinary teamwork in 26 acute psychiatric admission units and the relationship to the care of persons and their families. Although nurses face challenges in implementing "working in partnership," the study provides some direction for further inquiry around the interdisciplinary nature of the theory.

The transition for nurses to a solution focus in interactions was the subject of study by the Newcastle team (Stevenson, et al., 2003). Nurses participated in a specially tailored solution education initiative, and the impact was assessed for both nurses and persons-in-care using multiple data sources. This study provides strong evidence of a significant improvement in nurses' solution-focused knowledge, performance, and use in practice. Persons-in-care also found the approach helpful.

The Royal Ottawa Hospital Tidal team replicated the Newcastle study in 2003, with similar results. The Tosnu team completed a user-focused evaluation of the Tidal Model implementation. In Birmingham, on the Tolkien ward, a 4-month evaluation has been completed. Evaluation work is ongoing at St. Tydfil Hospital in Wales. Irish nurses have been in the forefront on evaluation, presenting the first national conference on the Tidal Model in practice, in Dublin in 2003, where nurses from across the republic previewed the results of their evaluations of service change and consumer satisfaction (Barker, 2004).

In New Zealand a qualitative, hermeneutic phenomenological study followed the implementation of the Tidal Model in a secure treatment unit. The study explored the lived experience of four inpatients and four nurses. Five themes that reflected meanings attached to providing and receiving care emerged: relationships, hope, human face, leveling, and working together. This suggests positive experiences and outcomes with the implementation of the Tidal Model (Brian Phillips, personal communication, September 15, 2003).

The Tidal Model is set in a research base that provides the possibility of research utilization or the more contemporary knowledge transfer. Nurses practicing within the Tidal Model are actively using research in practice, as well as contributing to the development of nursing practice. The Tidal Model has potential for participatory action research, uncovering knowledge embedded in practice and developing new knowledge and understandings.

FURTHER DEVELOPMENT

The Tidal Model is clear; concepts are defined and relationships identified. This enables the identification of areas for further theory development. For example, Barker is reframing his original notion of the "logic of experience" as "practice-based evidence" (P. Barker, personal communication, April 12, 2004). "Practice-based evidence" represents the knowledge of what is possible in this particular situation and which might contribute further to our shared understanding of human helping.

Several other developments characterize the Tidal Model. It has evolved from the initial acute, inpatient use across the continuum of care, with critical, transitional, and developmental components. The theory has evolved to the Tidal Model of Mental Health Recovery and Reclamation, broadening both its scope and utility. Colleagues in other fields such as palliative care have expressed appreciation of the model and the desire to bring it into their practice settings. Other professions also support the values, philosophy, and utility of the Tidal Model. Mental health user-consumer-survivor communities around the world are involved in the continuing development of this mental health recovery theory (Barker & Buchanan-Barker, 2004c).

In the short time since its inception, the Tidal Model has gained national and international attention. It continues to be implemented, taught, and studied internationally, with new sites joining from around the world. In November 2003, the Tidal Model was launched in North America. As new sites implement and study the Tidal Model, the practical, theoretical, and research base will be enriched. Although psychiatric and mental health care is considered a specialty, it has almost limitless possibilities in geography, settings, and clinical populations.

In 2003, Barker reaffirmed the values underlying the Tidal Model in the 10 commitments (see Box 32-1). They provide the necessary guidance to pursue and develop the philosophy of the Tidal

Model. Although Barker expects fidelity to the principles and values of the Tidal Model (10 commitments) in its implementation, he cautions against slavish importation. Implementation needs to be tailored to fit the local context with the result that each implementation will be unique and will contribute to the theory's development. This reflects Barker's appreciation of the concept of "practice-based evidence," what he called the *art of the possible,* that is, developing philosophically and theoretically sound forms of practice, which are based on considerations of what is appropriate, meaningful, and potentially effective in any given practice context.

The Tidal Model is developing across cultures, with varied clinical populations, in a variety of settings. The body of knowledge framed within the Tidal Model continues to develop, acknowledging the wide range of complex factors, which define people and their human needs: personal history, personal preferences, values and beliefs, social status, cultural background, family affiliations, and community membership (Barker, 2003a).

CRITIQUE

The Tidal Model of Mental Health Recovery is directed toward understanding and explaining further the human condition. Central to this effort is helping people use their voices as the key instrument for charting their recovery from mental distress. The Tidal Model is a genuine person-centered model of mental health care delivery that also is respectful of culture and creed (Barker & Buchanan-Barker, 2004c). This practical theory identifies concepts necessary to understand the human needs of people with problems in living, and how and what nurses might do to address those needs. The theory systematically explains specific phenomena and suggests the nature of relationships within a particular world view. Barker, however, has asserted consistently that the theory is "no more than words on paper" (Barker, 2004). It is not a reified work or recipe for practice, but a practical and evolving guide for delivering collaborative, person-centered, strength-based, and empowering care through relationship.

Clarity

The concepts, subconcepts, and relationships are developed logically, are clear, and the assumptions are consistent with the theory's goals. Words have multiple meanings; however, these major concepts, subconcepts, and relationships are described carefully, specifically, and metaphorically if not necessarily concisely. The careful selection of the term *problems in living* or *mental distress* and the view of people experiencing these problems as persons directs nurses to their proper focus. The identification of human needs, rather than psychological, social, or physical needs, also provides clarity and focus. How nurses see persons and how persons want to be nursed are illustrated clearly through the core category of "knowing you, knowing me." Three subcategories, ordinary me, pseudo-ordinary or engineered me, and professional me, each have four dimensions, depth of knowing, power, time, and translation (Barker et al., 1999a).

In practice, using the person's own language, not translating into jargon or professional language, contributes to the theory's success. Major concepts, collaboration, empowerment, relationships and solution focus, empowering through relationships, narrative, and the use of problems in living, are sufficiently clear and open the theory for use in other areas of nursing and health care.

A number of concepts and relationships are presented elegantly and schematically within the Tidal Model. The person's unique lived experience is synergistic and reciprocal among the world, self, and others' domains. This is represented as a triangle (Figure 32-1). In the holistic assessment, the person's story is at the heart of care planning and is represented as a heart. The circle of security assessment and plan surrounds the heart, all of which is surrounded by the interdisciplinary team circle (Figure 32-2). Figure 32-3 demonstrates the intersection of the continuum of care (immediate, transitional, and developmental) and the focus of care (Barker, 2000e). This clear, easily understood theory is accessible both conceptually and linguistically through the use of everyday language.

Simplicity

The Tidal Model is based upon a few simple ideas about "being human" and "helping one another" (Barker, 2000e). It is comprehensive, elegant in its simplicity, and at a level of abstraction to guide practice, education, and research. However, the concepts are complex and the broad relationships among the concepts add to the complexity of the Tidal Model; people and relationships are complex.

Assumptions, concepts, and relationships are described in everyday language and illuminated through metaphor. For example, simply being respectful of persons' knowledge and expertise about their own health and illnesses and listening to persons' stories is empowering. Abstract and complex concepts or relationships, such as chaos

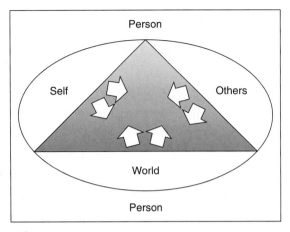

Figure **32-1 Three dimensions of personhood.** (From Barker, P. J. [2000]. *The Tidal Model theory and practice* [pp. 29-31]. Newcastle, UK: University of Newcastle. Copyright Phil Barker, 2000.)

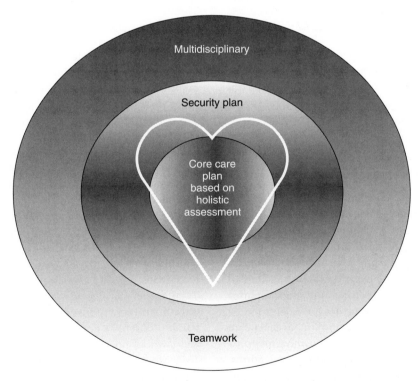

Figure **32-2 Structure of care.** (From Barker, P. J. [2000]. *The Tidal Model theory and practice* [p. 27]. Newcastle, UK: University of Newcastle. Copyright Phil Barker, 2000.)

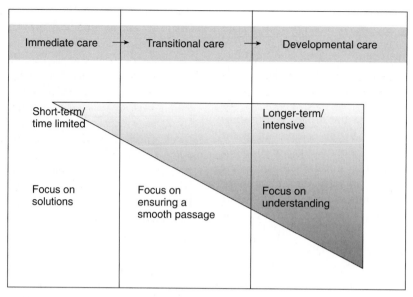

Figure **32-3 Tidal Model care continuum.** (From Barker, P. J. [2000]. *The Tidal Model theory and practice* [p. 22]. Newcastle, UK: University of Newcastle. Copyright Phil Barker, 2000.)

theory, are expressed metaphorically as in the ebb and flow of the tide. Practical and philosophical, the Tidal Model provides some direction in operationalizing or using some of the concepts, although not prescribing practice.

Generality

The Tidal Model is international in scope, suggesting its relevance cross-culturally and cross-nationally. By the beginning of 2004, there were almost 100 Tidal Model projects in progress in various clinical settings in countries around the world: Australia, Canada, England, Ireland, Japan, New Zealand, Scotland, and Wales (Barker & Buchanan-Barker, 2004c). A wide range of settings and clinical populations are represented in the Tidal Model projects: rural and urban, acute, crisis and longer-term care wards, private and public facilities, community programs, rehabilitation, forensic, youth, and adults. The Tidal Model has been successful across the continuum of psychiatric and mental health care and in a range of practice situations.

Universal characteristics of collaboration, empowerment, relationships, stories, and strengths appeal to nurses, service users, and colleagues in other disciplines and support general applicability. The Tidal Model is also consistent with the Ottawa Charter for Health Promotion description of the process of enabling people to increase control over and improve their health, in which the process of empowerment and participation is seen as fundamental to good health (World Health Organization, 1986). The 10 tidal commitments (Barker, 2003b) provide guidance and direction in using the theory.

Barker acknowledges that in order to practice within the Tidal Model we need to believe that recovery is possible and change is inevitable. "The Tidal Model *per se* does not work. The practitioner is the instrument or medium of change" (Buchanan-Barker, 2004, p. 1). Practitioners with different world views would not be comfortable with or accept the Tidal Model, and such diversity is respected. Because the Tidal Model was developed specifically for psychiatry and mental health care, the criterion of generality is met.

Empirical Precision

This substantive theory is grounded in the data that emerged inductively from the study of the need for nursing. Studies guided by the Tidal Model suggest its utility and precision and provide confidence that the theory is useful, practical, and accessible. Studies of the impact of the implementation of the theory in practice also support its utility and precision. The need for nursing, the proper focus of nursing, and the empowering interactions framework provide a strong empirical base for the Tidal Model.

Nurses working with diverse clinical populations and in a variety of settings are testing the Tidal Model in practice. The focus of inquiry is person-centered outcomes and the lived experience of persons collaborating in care. Studies addressing the solution orientation in empowering interactions contribute to the empirical adequacy of and confidence in this shared solution-focused perspective. Some theoretical underpinnings such as chaos theory are not amenable to study, although they contribute to the theoretical and conceptual basis of the model. The Tidal Model Web site at *http://www.tidal-model.co.uk* enables accessibility to and connection with the international Tidal Model community.

Derivable Consequences

The Tidal Model provides direction and focus for nursing. The theory is accessible conceptually and linguistically and lends itself to research. This research, relevant to nurses' work, contributes knowledge to guide and inform practice. Studies guided by the Tidal Model also explore its impact and a variety of outcomes. The narrative knowledge derived from the theory advances the practice of nursing, nursing education, nursing research, and policy. The Tidal Model is represented by a range of holistic (exploratory) and focused (risk) assessments, which generate person-centered interventions that emphasize the person's extant resources and capacity for solution finding (Barker, 2001b).

Working within the Tidal Model enables nurses to articulate their practice and for "invisible skills" to surface (Michael, 1994). For example, empowerment strategies such as respecting the person and inspiring hope give voice to nurses, themselves. Nurses gain confidence in working among interdisciplinary team members as their contribution and focus is more clearly articulated.

Challenges exist at a practical, personal, and system level with any change, and these are anticipated and addressed. However, the Tidal Model is an important and essential theory to develop and guide practice in psychiatry and mental health care. It is also an important theoretical context for facilities whose practitioners are committed to person-centered care and offers practical methods for its implementation.

SUMMARY

The Tidal Model developed from a discrete focus on psychiatric nursing in acute settings to a more flexible mental health recovery and reclamation model for any setting, relevant to any discipline. It emphasizes empowering forms of engagement, the importance of the lived experience, and an appreciation of the potential for healing that lies within the reauthoring of the narrative (Barker, 2004).

The Tidal Model provides an orientation to practice that is research based, holistic, and person centered. Keen describes a "deeply collaborative, person-centered, solution-focused, narrative-based, pragmatic and systemic theory" (Barker & Buchanan-Barker, 2004c, p. 391). The theory describes various assumptions about people, their inherent value, and the value of relating to people in particular ways. It describes how people might come to appreciate differently, perhaps better, their own value and the unique value of their experience. The Tidal Model opens possibilities of new ways of being in relation with people. Perhaps some of its appeal is that it harkens back to our roots and values that brought us to nursing in the first place. Although the theory provides direction for practice, education, and research, it is not easy. Nurses are aware of the challenge in making the shift to commit to change and to grow and develop in enacting the essence of the Tidal Model, the 10 tidal commitments.

Case Study

Scott was a young man described as having had a first episode of psychosis. He had beaten his father, who subsequently died. Scott was transferred to a secure unit, where his primary nurse began to explore his story with him through a holistic assessment, which represents Scott's world of experience, at this time.

How this began: "It all started when my father punched my mother again; he was totally drunk that night. It was so noisy in that room, the television, the banging, and those voices in my head. They kept yelling at me to do something fast to save my mother. I don't remember exactly what had happened after; I was so confused."

How this affected me: "I don't know. I was in jail for 4 months before coming here. They told me I killed my father. I don't remember much except that I kept hammering his head. I just remember I was standing in a pool of blood." "They told me my mother is still in the hospital. I haven't seen her since." "I'm scared. I can't sleep."

How I felt in the beginning: It "just devastated me, turned me upside down." "I felt awful even though I hated him so much, he never listened to me, no one ever listened to me or believes me." "I hate him because I watched him beating my mother all my life."

How things have changed over time: "It got worse when my stepbrother ran away. My father was a sinner, a drunk, wife beater, even conspired with the communists. I was not allowed to leave the house except school; my mother stayed in all day to do farm work; he was the only one that ran errands outside the house." "I've always been a bit scared and angry too."

The effect on my relationships: "I don't have any relationships with anyone; I don't like people because nobody likes me."

How I feel now: "Well, I feel nervous, very shaky and scared. I don't know what to expect; I don't know what is going to happen." "Confused, I guess, and I'm tired."

What I think this means: "I don't know, that was my question, maybe I will go back to jail, maybe it means I needed help." "It means I have a lot of challenges to meet."

What all this says about me as a person: "I just want to be a better person, I want to be well, and I want to take care of my mother."

What needs to happen now: "Well, I suppose I'm here for an assessment."

What I expect the nurse to do for me: "Continue to talk to me the way you are talking to me. No one ever talks to me like this. You are listening and it seems like you believe me. This is so different from jail and anywhere else."

The people who are important: "My mother is the only important person in this world. My stepbrother came back only for the money."

Things that are important: "Well, able to share with others." "My dog, Pepper, but he is at the humane society right now." "I have a really nice picture of me and my mom."

Ideas about life that are important: "To be able to fit in."

Evaluating the problems: "My main problems are loneliness and what's going to happen in my future. My whole life is complex!" "I would rate my loneliness as an 8 for distress, 8 for disturbance, and 2 for control. My future and what's going to happen would be a 10 for distress, 10 for disturbance, and I have no control, a zero."

How I'll know the problem has been solved: "I'll know the problem has been solved maybe when the voices stop talking to me, when I get out of jail and out of the hospital."

What needs to change for this to happen: "Maybe I need to take medication, maybe I just have to start talking to real people, not the voices."

The nurse recognized that Scott needed some help to feel more emotionally secure. She engaged him in a security assessment and they developed a security plan together.

Later in the week, the nurses noted that Scott was spending a lot of time in his room. Instead of encouraging Scott to participate in ward activities, his primary nurse shared her observation and asked Scott how it was helpful to him to spend so much time lying on his bed, alone in the room. Scott's reply was "the voices don't bother me so much."

This opened a conversation, helping the nurse begin to understand what this was like for Scott and what might be helpful for him.

In another conversation, the primary nurse asked "the miracle question." "Suppose that tonight, while you are asleep, the problem you have was miraculously solved. How would you know? What would be the first difference you noticed when you woke up?' Scott's unexpected reply was, "I'd have a friend." By exploring, rather than closing down, the narrative, the nurse began to involve Scott in "what needed to be done" to help him.

Questions that might be asked in a security assessment: The security plan has two questions: What can I do that will help me to deal with my present problems? And what help can others offer that I might find valuable? What might Scott's security plan look like?

CRITICAL THINKING *Activities*

1. There are 10 tidal commitments. Select three or four and consider how these might be realized in practice.

2. Where would you find support for each of the tidal commitments within your workplace?

REFERENCES

Alanen, Y., Lehtinen, K., & Aaltonen, J. (1997). Need-adapted treatment of new schizophrenic patients: Experience and results of the Turku project. *Acta Psychiatrica Scandanavica, 83,* 363-372.

American Nurses Association. (1980). *Nursing. A social policy statement.* Kansas City, MO: American Nurses Association.

Barker, P. J. (1987). *An evaluation of specific nursing interventions in the management of patients suffering from manic-depressive psychosis.* Unpublished doctoral thesis, Dundee Institute of Technology, University of Abertay, Scotland.

Barker, P. J. (1995). Promoting growth through community mental health nursing. *Mental Health Nursing, 15*(3), 12-15.

Barker, P. J. (1996a). Chaos and the way of Zen: Psychiatric nursing and the 'uncertainty principle.' *Journal of Psychiatric and Mental Health Nursing, 3,* 235-243.

Barker, P. J. (1996b). The logic of experience: Developing appropriate care through effective collaboration. *Australian and New Zealand Journal of Mental Health Nursing, 5,* 3-12.

Barker, P. J. (1997). Towards a meta-theory of psychiatric nursing. *Mental Health Practice, 1*(4), 18-21.

Barker, P. J. (1998a). It's time to turn the tide. *Nursing Times, 94*(46), 11-12.

Barker, P. J. (1998b). The future of the theory of interpersonal relations? A personal reflection on Peplau's legacy. *Journal of Psychiatric and Mental Health Nursing, 5,* 213-220.

Barker, P. J. (1999a). *Qualitative research in nursing and health care.* London: NT Books.

Barker, P. J. (1999b). *The philosophy and practice of psychiatric nursing.* Edinburgh: Churchill Livingstone.

Barker, P. J. (2000a). Commentaries and reflections on mental health nursing in the UK at the dawn of the new millennium: Commentary 1. *Journal of Mental Health, 9*(6), 617-619.

Barker, P. J. (2000b). From chaos to complex order: Personal values and resources in the process of psychotherapy. *Perspectives in Psychiatric Care, 36*(2), 51-57.

Barker, P. J. (2000c). Reflections on caring as a virtue ethic within an evidence-based culture. *International Journal of Nursing Studies, 37,* 329-336.

Barker, P. J. (2000d). *The Tidal Model—Humility in mental health care.* Newport on Tay, Scotland: Phil Barker. Retrieved April 15, 2005 from *http://www.clan-unity. co.uk/writing%206.htm*

Barker, P. J. (2000e). *The tidal model theory and practice.* Newcastle, UK: University of Newcastle.

Barker, P. J. (2001a). The tidal model: Developing an empowering, person-centred approach to recovery within psychiatric and mental health nursing. *Journal of Psychiatric and Mental Health Nursing, 8,* 233-240.

Barker, P. J. (2001b). The tidal model: Developing a person-centered approach to psychiatric and mental health nursing. *Perspectives in Psychiatric Care, 37*(3), 79-87.

Barker, P. J. (2001c). The tidal model: The lived experience in person-centred mental health nursing. *Nursing Philosophy, 2,* 213-223.

Barker, P. J. (2002a). Annie Altschul—An appreciation. *Journal of Psychiatric and Mental Health Nursing, 9,* 127-128.

Barker, P. J. (2002b). Doing what needs to be done: A respectful response to Burnard and Grant. *Journal of Psychiatric and Mental Health Nursing, 9,* 232-236.

Barker, P. J. (2003a). *Psychiatric and mental health nursing: The craft of caring.* London: Arnold.

Barker, P. J. (2003b). *The 10 commitments: Essential values of the tidal model.* Newport on Tay, Scotland: Phil Barker. Retrieved April 18, 2004 from *http://www.tidal-model.co.uk/New%2010%20Commitments.htm*

Barker, P. J. (2004, September/October). Uncommon sense—The tidal model of mental health recovery. *New Therapist, 33,* 14-19.

Barker, P. J. (n.d.). *A beginner's guide to the tidal model.* Newport on Tay, Scotland: Phil Barker. Retrieved April 18, 2004 from *http://www.tidal-model.co.uk/New%20beginner's%20Guide.htm*

Barker, P. J. (n.d.) *The theoretical basis of the tidal model.* Newport on Tay, Scotland: Phil Barker. Retrieved April 18, 2004 from *http://www.tidal-model.co.uk/New%20theory%203.htm*

Barker, P., Jackson, S., & Stevenson, C. (1999a). The need for psychiatric nursing: Toward a multidimensional theory of caring. *Nursing Inquiry, 6,* 103-111.

Barker, P. J. & Buchanan-Barker, P. (2004a). Beyond empowerment: Revering the story teller. *Mental Health Practice, 7*(5), 18-20.

Barker, P. J., & Buchanan-Barker, P. (2004b). *Spirituality and mental health: Breakthrough.* London: Whurr.

Barker, P. J., & Buchanan-Barker, P. (2004c). *The Tidal Model: A guide for mental health professionals.* London: Brunner-Routledge.

Barker, P. J., & Jackson, S. (1997). No apologies for "imperialist" view (Letter). *Nursing Standard, 11*(20), 10.

Barker, P. J., Jackson, S., & Stevenson, C. (1999b). What are psychiatric nurses needed for? Developing a theory of essential practice. *Journal of Psychiatric and Mental Health Nursing, 6,* 273-282.

Barker, P. J., Reynolds, W., & Stevenson, C. (1997). The human science basis of psychiatric nursing: Theory and practice. *Journal of Advanced Nursing, 25,* 660-667.

Barker, P. J., Reynolds, W., & Ward, T. (1995). The proper focus of nursing: A critique of the caring ideology. *International Journal of Nursing Studies, 32*(4), 386-397.

Barker, P. J., Stevenson, C., & Leamy, M. (2000). The philosophy of empowerment. *Mental Health Practice, 20*(9), 8-12.

Barker, P. J., & Walker, L. (2000). Nurses' perceptions of multidisciplinary teamwork in acute psychiatric settings. *Journal of Psychiatric and Mental health Nursing, 7,* 539-546.

Barker, P. J., & Whitehill, I. (1997). The craft of care: Towards collaborative caring in psychiatric nursing. In S. Tilley (Ed.), *The mental health nurse. Views of practice and education* (pp. 15-27). Oxford: Blackwell Science.

Buchanan-Barker, P. (2004). *Uncommon sense: The value base of the tidal model.* Newport on Tay, Scotland: Phil Barker. Retrieved April 18, 2004 from *http://www.tidal-model.co.uk/New%Uncommon%20sense.htm*

de Shazer, S. (1994). *Words were originally magic.* New York: Norton.

Flanagan, J. C. (1954). The critical incident technique. *Psychological Bulletin, 51,* 327-358.

Fletcher, E., & Stevenson, C. (2001). Launching the tidal model in an adult mental health programme. *Nursing Standard, 15*(49), 33-36.

Glaser, B. G., & Strauss, A. L. (1967). *The discovery of grounded theory: Strategies for qualitative research.* Chicago: Aldine-Atherton.

Heron, J. (1996). *Cooperative inquiry: Research into the human condition.* London: Sage.

Illich, I. (1976). *Limits to medicine: Medical nemesis—The expropriation of health.* London: Marion Boyars.

Jackson, S., & Stevenson, C. (1998). The gift of time from the friendly professional. *Nursing Standard, 12,* 31-33.

Jackson, S., & Stevenson, C. (2000). What do people need psychiatric and mental health nurses for? *Journal of Advanced Nursing, 31*(2), 378-388.

McAllister, M. (2003). Doing practice differently: Solution-focused nursing. *Journal of Advanced Nursing, 41*(6), 528-535.

Michael, S. P. (1994). Invisible skills: How recognition and value need to be given to the 'invisible skills' frequently used by mental health nurses, but often unrecognized by those unfamiliar with mental health nursing. *Journal of Psychiatric and Mental Health Nursing, 1,* 56-57.

Montgomery, C., & Webster, D. (1993). Caring and nursing's metaparadigm: Can they survive the era of managed care? *Perspectives in Psychiatric Care, 29*(4), 5-12.

Morita, M., Kondo, A., Levine, P., & Morita, S. (1998). *Morita therapy and the true nature of anxiety-based disorders (Shinkeishitsu).* Princeton, NJ: University of New York Press.

Peplau, H. (1987). Interpersonal constructs for nursing practice. *Nurse Education Today, 7,* 201-208.

Peplau, H. E. (1952). *Interpersonal relations in nursing.* New York: Putman. (Reissued 1988, London: Macmillan.)

Peplau, H. E. (1969). Professional closeness: As a special kind of involvement with a patient, client, or family groups. *Nursing Forum, 8,* 342-360.

Peplau, H. E. (1997). Peplau's theory of interpersonal relations. *Nursing Science Quarterly, 10*(4), 162-167.

Podvoll, E. M. (1990). *The seduction of madness: Revolutionary insights into the world of psychosis and a compassionate approach to recovery at home.* New York: Harper Collins.

Stevenson, C. (1996). The Tao, social constructivism and psychiatric nursing practice and research. *Journal of Psychiatric and Mental Health Nursing, 3,* 217-224.

Stevenson, C., Barker, P., & Fletcher, E. (2002). Judgment days: Developing an evaluation for an innovative nursing model. *Journal of Psychiatric and Mental Health Nursing, 9,* 271-276.

Stevenson, C., & Fletcher, E. (2002). The tidal model: The questions answered. *Mental Health Practice, 5*(8), 29-38.

Stevenson, C., Jackson, S., & Barker, P. (2003). Finding solutions through empowerment: A preliminary study of a solution-oriented approach to nursing in acute psychiatric settings. *Journal of Psychiatric and Mental Health Nursing, 10*, 688-696.

Szasz, T. S. (1961). *The myth of mental illness: Foundations of a theory of personal conduct.* New York: Hoeber-Harper.

Szasz, T. S. (2000). The case against psychiatric power. In P. J. Barker & C. Stevenson (Eds.), *The construction of power and authority in psychiatry.* Oxford: Butterworth Heinemann.

Travelbee, J. (1969). *Intervention in psychiatric nursing: Process in the one-to-one relationship.* Philadelphia: F. A. Davis.

Vicenzi, A. E. (1994). Chaos theory and some nursing considerations. *Nursing Science Quarterly, 7,* 36-42.

World Health Organization. (1986). *The Ottawa charter for health promotion.* Geneva: World Health Organization.

Yeats, W. B. (1928). *The tower.* New York: Macmillan.

BIBLIOGRAPHY
Primary Sources
Books

Barker, P. J. (1985). *Patient assessment in psychiatric nursing.* London: Croom Helm.

Barker, P. J. (1997). *Assessment in psychiatric and mental health nursing: In search of the whole person.* Cheltenham, UK: Stanley Thornes.

Barker, P. J. (1999). *The philosophy and practice of psychiatric and mental health nursing.* Edinburgh: Churchill Livingstone.

Barker, P. J. (1999). *The talking cures: A guide to the psychotherapies for health care professionals.* London: NT Books.

Barker, P. (2000). *Qualitative research in nursing and health care.* Nursing Times Clinical Monographs (No 13). London: NT Books.

Barker, P. J. (2000). *The tidal model theory and practice.* Newcastle, UK: University of Newcastle.

Barker, P. J. (2003). *Psychiatric and mental health nursing: The craft of caring.* London: Arnold.

Barker, P. J. (2004). *Assessment in psychiatric and mental health nursing: In search of the whole person* (2nd ed.). London: Nelson-Thornes.

Barker, P. J., & Baldwin, S. (1991). *Ethical issues in mental health.* London: Croom Helm.

Barker, P. J., & Buchanan-Barker, P. (2004). *Spirituality and mental health: Breakthrough.* London: Whurr.

Barker, P. J., & Buchanan-Barker, P. (2004). *The tidal model: A guide for mental health professionals.* London: Brunner-Routledge.

Barker, P. J., Campbell, P., & Davidson, B. (1999). *From the ashes of experience: The experience of recovery from psychosis.* London: Whurr.

Barker, P. J., & Davidson, B. (1998). *Psychiatric nursing: Ethical strife.* London: Edward Arnold.

Barker, P. J., & Kerr, B. (2001). *The process of psychotherapy.* Oxford: Butterworth Heinemann.

Barker, P. J., & Stevenson, C. (1999). *The construction of power and authority in psychiatry.* Oxford: Butterworth Heinemann.

Book Chapters

Barker, P. J. (1990). Cognitive therapy model: Principles and general applications. In W. Reynolds & D. F. S. Cormack (Eds.), *Psychiatric and mental health nursing: Theory and practice.* London: Chapman & Hall.

Barker, P. J. (1990). Professional stress. In D. F. S. Cormack (Ed.), *Developing your career in nursing.* London: Chapman & Hall.

Barker, P. J. (1991). The interview. In D. F. S. Cormack (Ed.), *The research process in nursing* (2nd ed.). Oxford: Blackwell Scientific.

Barker P. J. (1992). Professional and practice perspectives: Psychiatric nursing. In T. Butterworth & J. Faugier (Eds.), *Clinical supervision and mentorship in nursing.* London: Chapman & Hall.

Barker, P. J. (1992). Understanding people—Problems of development: Stress and distress. In H. Wright & M. Giddey (Eds.), *Mental health nursing: From first principles to professional practice* (pp. 103-115). London: Chapman & Hall.

Barker, P. J. (1993). Foreword. In D. Milne (Ed.), *Psychology and mental health nursing.* London: BPS Books.

Barker, P. J. (1996). The Interview. In D. F. S. Cormack (Ed.), *The research process in nursing* 3rd ed.). Oxford: Blackwell Scientific.

Barker, P. J. (1997). Counselling for behavioural change. In P. Burnard & I. Hulatt (Eds.), *Nurses counseling: The view from the practitioners.* Oxford: Butterworth Heinemann.

Barker, P. J. (1998). Advanced practice in mental health nursing: Developing the core. In G. Rolfe & P. Fulbrook (Eds.), *Advanced nursing practice.* Oxford: Butterworth Heinemann.

Barker, P. J. (1998). Depression. In M. Clinton & S. Nelson (Eds.), *Advanced practice in mental health nursing.* Oxford: Blackwell.

Barker, P. J. (1998). Psychiatric nursing. In A. C. Butterworth, J. Faugier, & P. Burnard (Eds.), *Clinical supervision and mentorship in nursing.* Cheltenham, UK: Stanley Thornes.

Barker, P. J. (1999). History, truth and the politics of madness. In P. J. Barker & C. Stevenson (Eds.), *The construction of power and authority in psychiatry.* Oxford: Butterworth Heinemann.

Barker, P. J. (1999). The construction of mind and madness: From Leonardo to the Hearing Voices Network. In P. J. Barker & C. Stevenson (Eds.), *The construction of power and authority in psychiatry.* Oxford: Butterworth Heinemann.

Barker, P. J. (2001). Working with the metaphor of life and death. In D. Kirklin & R. Richardson (Eds.). *Medical humanities: A practical introduction.* London: Royal College of Physicians.

Barker, P. J. (2002). Realising the promise of liaison mental health care. In S. Regel & D. Roberts (Eds.), *Mental health liaison: A handbook for nurses and health professionals.* London: Bailliere Tindall.

Barker, P. J. (2004). Who cares any more, anyway? In S. Wilshaw (Ed.), *Consultant nursing in mental health.* Sussex, UK: Kingsham Press.

Barker, P. J., & Baldwin, S. (1991). Change not adjustment: The ethics of psychotherapy. In P. J. Barker & S. Baldwin (Eds.), *Ethical issues in mental health.* London: Chapman & Hall.

Barker, P. J., & Buchanan-Barker, P. (2004). Spirituality and mental health: An integrated dimension. In S. Ramon & J. Williams (Eds.), *Mental health at the crossroads: The promise of the psychosocial approach.* Sussex, UK: Ashgate.

Barker, P. J., & Davidson, B. (1998). Epilogue: The heart of the ethical matter. In P. J. Barker & B. Davidson (Eds.), *Psychiatric nursing: Ethical strife.* London: Arnold.

Barker, P. J., Manos, E., Novak, V., & Reynolds, B. (1998). The wounded healer and the myth of mental well-being: Ethical issues concerning the mental health status of psychiatric nurses. In P. J. Barker & B. Davidson (Eds.), *Psychiatric nursing: Ethical strife.* London: Arnold.

Barker, P. J., & Whitehill, I. (1997). The craft of care: Towards collaborative caring in psychiatric nursing. In S. Tilley (Ed.), *The mental health nurse: Views of practice and education.* Oxford: Blackwell Science.

Stevenson, C., & Barker, P. J. (1996). Negotiating boundaries: Reconciling differences in mental health teamwork. In N. Cooper, C. Stevenson, & G. Hale (Eds.), *Integrating perspectives on health* (pp. 47-56). Buckingham, UK: Open University Press.

Journal Articles

Barker, P. J. (1988). Reasoning about madness: The long search for the vanishing horizon (Part 2). *Community Psychiatric Nursing Journal, 8*(5), 14-19.

Barker, P. J. (1989). Reflections on the philosophy of caring in mental health. *International Journal of Nursing Studies, 26*(2), 131-141.

Barker, P. J. (1990). Needs and wants and fairy-tale wishes: A Scottish impression of care in the community. *Architecture and Comportment: Architecture and Behaviour, 6*(3), 233-244.

Barker, P. J. (1990). The conceptual basis of mental health nursing. *Nurse Education Today, 10,* 339-348.

Barker, P. J. (1990). The philosophy of psychiatric nursing. *Nursing Standard 3*(12), 28-33.

Barker, P. J. (1990). Training to meet the new agenda. *Nursing Times, 86*(39), 71.

Barker, P. J. (1993). The Peplau legacy . . . Hildegard Peplau. *Nursing Times, 89*(11), 48-51.

Barker, P. J. (1995). Seriously misguided. *Nursing Times, 92*(34), 56-57.

Barker, P. J. (1996). Chaos and the way of Zen: Psychiatric nursing and the 'uncertainty principle.' *Journal of Psychiatric and Mental Health Nursing, 3,* 235-344.

Barker, P. J. (1996). The logic of experience: Developing appropriate care through effective collaboration. *Australian and New Zealand Journal of Mental Health Nursing, 5,* 3-12.

Barker, P. J. (1997). Towards a meta theory of psychiatric nursing. *Mental Health Practice, 1*(4), 18-21.

Barker, P. J. (1998). Creativity and psychic distress in writers, artists and scientists. *Journal of Psychiatric and Mental Health Nursing, 5*(2), 109-118.

Barker, P. J. (1998). Different approaches to family therapy. *Nursing Times, 94*(14), 60-62.

Barker, P. J. (1998). It's time to turn the tide. *Nursing Times, 18*(94), 70-72.

Barker, P. J. (1998). La Funcion Psicoterapeutica de la Enfermera en la Cuidado del Paciente Psicotico. *Avances en Salud Mental, 2,* 4-7.

Barker, P. J. (1998). Psychodynamic psychotherapy in nursing. *Nursing Times, 94*(2), 54-56.

Barker, P. J. (1998). Sharpening the focus of mental health nursing: Primary health care. *Mental Health Practice, 1*(7), 14-15.

Barker, P. J. (1998). Solution-focused therapies. *Nursing Times, 94*(19), 53-55.

Barker, P. J. (1998). The behavioural psychotherapies. *Nursing Times, 94*(10), 44-46.

Barker, P. J. (1998). The future of interpersonal relations theory: A personal reflection on Peplau's legacy. *Journal of Psychiatric and Mental Health Nursing, 5*(3), 213-220.

Barker, P. J. (1998). The humanistic therapies. *Nursing Times, 94*(6), 52-53.

Barker, P. J. (2000). Commentaries and reflections on mental health nursing in the UK at the dawn of the new millennium. *Journal of Mental Health, 9*(6), 617-619.

Barker, P. J. (2000). The tidal model of mental health care: Personal caring within the chaos paradigm. *Mental Health Care, 4*(2), 59-63.

Barker, P. J. (2000). The tidal model: The lived experience in person-centred mental health care. *Nursing Philosophy, 2*(3), 213-223.

Barker, P. J. (2000). The virtue of caring. *International Journal of Nursing Studies, 37,* 329-336.

Barker, P. J. (2000). Working with the metaphor of life and death. *Journal of Medical Ethics, 26,* 97-102.

Barker, P. J. (2000, November/December). Turning the tide. *OpenMind, 106,* 10-11.

Barker, P. J. (2001). Psychiatric caring. *Nursing Times, 97*(10), 38-39.

Barker, P. J. (2001). Response to Duncan-Grant. *Journal of Psychiatric and Mental Health Nursing, 8,* 180-183.

Barker, P. J. (2001). The ripples of knowledge and the boundaries of practice. *International Journal of Psychotherapy, 6*(1), 11-23.

Barker, P. J. (2001). The tidal model: Developing an empowering, person-centred approach to recovery within psychiatric and mental health nursing. *Journal of Psychiatric and Mental Health Nursing, 8*(3), 233-240.

Barker, P. J. (2001). The tidal model: Developing a person-centred approach to psychiatric and mental health nursing. *Perspectives in Psychiatric Care, 37*(3), 79-87.

Barker, P. J. (2002). Annie Altschul: An appreciation. *Journal of Psychiatric and Mental Health Nursing, 9*(2), 127-128.

Barker, P. J. (2002). Doing what needs to be done: A respectful response to Burnard and Grant. *Journal of Psychiatric and Mental Health Nursing, 9,* 232-236.

Barker, P. J. (2002). End of an era? *Mental Health Practice, 5*(5), 26-27.

Barker, P. J. (2002). Inspiration: My cousin Vinnie. *Pendulum: The Journal of the Manic Depression Fellowship, 18*(4), 11.

Barker, P. J. (2002, July/August). Update: Acute care guidelines. *OpenMind, 116,* 24.

Barker, P. J. (2002). The tidal model: The healing potential of metaphor within the patient's narrative. *Journal of Psychosocial Nursing and Mental Health Services, 40*(7), 42-50, 54-55.

Barker, P. J. (2003). Putting acute care in its place. *Mental Health Nursing, 23*(1), 12-15.

Barker, P. J. (2003). The tidal model: Psychiatric colonization, recovery and the paradigm shift in mental health care. *International Journal of Mental Health Nursing, 12*(2), 96-102.

Barker, P. J. (2004). Commentary: Mental health recovery and occupational therapy in Australia and New Zealand. *International Journal of Therapy and Rehabilitation, 11*(2), 70.

Barker, P. J. (2004, September/October). Uncommon sense—The tidal model of mental health recovery. *The New Therapist, 33,* 14-19.

Barker, P. J., & Baldwin, S. (1993, February 24). Speaking out. *Nursing Times, 89*(8), 62.

Barker, P. J., Baldwin, S., & Ulas, M. (1989) Medical expansionism: Some implications for psychiatric nursing practice. *Nurse Education Today, 9,* 192-202.

Barker, P. J., & Buchanan-Barker, P. (2001, November/December). Apologising for our colonial past. *OpenMind, 112,* 10.

Barker, P. J., & Buchanan-Barker, P. (2003, November/December). Banning 'bonkers.' *OpenMind, 124,* 26.

Barker, P. J., & Buchanan-Barker, P. (2003). Beyond empowerment: Revering the storyteller. *Mental Health Practice, 7*(5), 18-20.

Barker, P. J., & Buchanan-Barker, P. (2003). Death by assimilation. *Asylum, 13*(3), 10-13.

Barker, P. J., & Buchanan-Barker, P. (2003, May/June). Not so NICE guidelines. *OpenMind, 14*(*121*).

Barker, P. J., & Buchanan-Barker, P. (2003). Schizophrenia: The 'not-so-nice' guidelines (Commentary). *Journal of Psychiatric and Mental Health Nursing, 10,* 372-378.

Barker, P. J., & Cutcliffe, J. (1999). Clinical risk: A need for engagement not observation. *Mental Health Practice, 2*(8), 8-12.

Barker, P. J., Glenister, D., Jackson, S., Parkes, T., Parson, S., & Ryan, D. (1998). End of the old pier show? *Mental Health Practice, 1*(7), 22.

Barker, P. J., & Jackson, S. (1996). No apology for "imperialist" views. *Nursing Standard, 11*(20), 10.

Barker, P. J., & Jackson, S. (1997). Mental health nursing: Making it a primary concern. *Nursing Standard, 11*(17), 39-41.

Barker, P. J., Jackson, S., & Stevenson, C. (1999). The need for psychiatric nursing: Towards a multidimensional theory of caring. *Nursing Inquiry, 6,* 103-111.

Barker, P. J., Jackson, S., & Stevenson, C. (1999). What are psychiatric nurses needed for? Developing a theory of essential nursing practice. *Journal of Psychiatric and Mental Health Nursing, 6*(4), 273-282.

Barker, P. J., Keady, J., Croom, S., Stevenson, C., Adams, T., & Reynolds, B. (1998). The concept of serious mental illness: Modern myths and grim realities. *Journal of Psychiatric and Mental Health Nursing, 5*(4), 247-254.

Barker, P. J., Leamy, M., & Stevenson, C. (2000). The philosophy of empowerment. *Mental Health Nursing, 20*(9), 8-12.

Barker, P. J., & Reynolds, W. (1994). "A critique: Watson's caring ideology, the proper focus of psychiatric nursing." *Journal of Psychosocial Nursing and Mental Health Services, 32*(5), 17-22.

Barker, P. J., & Reynolds, B. (1996). Rediscovering the proper focus of nursing: A critique of Gournay's position on nursing theory and models. *Journal of Psychiatric and Mental Health Nursing, 3,* 75-80.

Barker, P. J., Reynolds, B., & Stevenson, C. (1998). The human science basis of psychiatric nursing: Theory and practice. *Perspectives in Psychiatric Care, 34,* 5-14.

Barker, P. J., Reynolds, B., Whitehill, I., Delaval, S., & Novak, V. (1996) Working with mental distress. *Nursing Times, 92*(2), 25-27.

Barker, P. J., & Stevenson, C. (2002). Reply to Gamble and Wellman. *Journal of Psychiatric and Mental Health Nursing, 9*(6), 743-745.

Barker, P. J., & Walker, L. (2000). Nurses' perceptions of multidisciplinary teamwork in acute psychiatric settings. *Journal of Psychiatric and Mental Health Nursing, 7*, 539-546.

Barker, P. J., Walker, L., & Pearson, P. (1998). Extending the role of the community mental health nurse. *British Journal of Community Nursing, 3*(10), 496-500.

Buchanan-Barker, P., & Barker, P. J. (2002). Lunatic language. *OpenMind, 115*, 23.

Buchanan-Barker, P., & Barker, P. J. (2003). NICE: Does the gold standard have feet of clay? *Mental Health Nursing, 23*, 9-11.

Cutcliffe, J., & Barker, P. J. (2002). Considering the care of the suicidal client and the case for "engagement and inspiring hope" or "observations." *Journal of Psychiatric and Mental Health Nursing, 9*(5), 611-621.

Parsons, S., & Barker, P. J. (2001). The Phil Hearne Course: An evaluation of a multidisciplinary mental health education programme. *Journal of Psychiatric and Mental Health Nursing, 7*(2), 101-108.

Stevenson, C., Barker, P. J., & Fletcher, E. (2002). Judgment days: Developing an evaluation for an innovative nursing model. *Journal of Psychiatric and Mental Health Nursing, 9*(3), 271-276.

Stevenson, C., Jackson, S., & Barker, P. (2003). Finding solutions through empowerment: A preliminary study of a solution-oriented approach to nursing in acute psychiatric settings. *Journal of Psychiatric and Mental Health Nursing, 10*(6), 688-696.

Walker, L., & Barker, P. J. (1998). The required role of the CPN: Uniformity or flexibility? *Clinical Effectiveness in Nursing, 2*, 21-29.

Wilkin, P., & Barker, P. (2002). A conversation with Phil Barker. Sacred space. *International Journal of Spirituality and Health, 3*(4), 15-23.

Dissertation

Barker, P. J. (1987). *An evaluation of specific nursing interventions in the management of patients suffering from manic depressive psychosis.* Unpublished doctoral thesis, Dundee Institute of Technology, University of Abertay, Scotland.

Papers Presented

Barker, P. J. (1999, Feb.). *Mental health solidarity.* Paper presented to the European Mental Health Nursing Conference, Jersey, UK.

Barker, P. J. (1999, April). *The Stanley Moore memorial lecture.* Paper presented to the CPNA Annual Conference, Edinburgh, Scotland.

Barker, P. J. (2000, May 5). *The interpersonal politics of engagement.* Paper presented in Cambridge, UK. Accessed January 7, 2005 at: *http://www.clan-unity. co.uk/writing%201.htm*

Barker, P. J. (2003, April). *The philosophical basis of effective care and treatment in psychiatry.* Paper presented to the conference, "Kvalitet, effekt og produktivitet—Hvordan kombinere?" Psykiatriens arlige lederkonferanse, Stavanger, Norway.

Ryan, T., & Barker, P. J. (2003, September). *Not rocket science: Tidal movement in the tropics.* Paper presented at the Australian and New Zealand Mental Health Nurses 29th International Conference, Rotorua, New Zealand.

Reports

Cutcliffe, J., Stevenson, C., Jackson, S., Barker, P. J., & Smith, P. (2003). *Meaningful, caring responses to suicidality.* Report for Trent NHS Executive, Sheffield, UK.

Stevenson, C., Jackson, S., & Barker, P. J. (2002). *Developing solution-oriented interventions within a nursing model in acute psychiatric settings in Newcastle, North Tyneside and Northumberland Mental Health NHS trust.* Report for the Foundation of Nursing Studies, London.

Videotapes

Glover, T. (Producer), & Barker, P. J. (Writer/Director). (2003). *The scary reality of madness* (Videotape). Newcastle, UK: Tony Glover Film and Video Limited. Available from tony@glover1057.fsnet.co.uk

Glover, T. (Producer), Whitehill, I., & Barker, P. J. (Writers). (2002). *Irene's story* (Videotape). Newcastle, UK: Tony Glover Film and Video Limited. Available from tony@glover1057.fsnet.co.uk

Secondary Sources
Books

Morita, M., Kondo, A., Levine, P., & Morita, S. (1998). *Morita therapy and the true nature of anxiety-based disorders (Shinkeishitsu).* Princeton, NJ: University of New York Press.

Newnes, C., Holmes, G., & Dunn, C. (2000). *This is madness. A critical look at psychiatry and the future of mental health services.* Ross-on-Wye, UK: PCCS Books.

Journal Articles

Adam, R., Tilley, S., & Pollock, L. (2003). Person first: What people with enduring mental disorders value about community psychiatric nurses and CPN services. *Journal of Psychiatric and Mental Health Nursing, 10*, 203-212.

Anthony, P., & Crawford, P. (2000). Service user involvement in care planning: The mental health nurse's perspective. *Journal of Psychiatric and Mental Health Nursing, 7,* 425-434.

Beech, P., & Norman, I. J. (1995). Patients' perceptions of the quality of psychiatric nursing care: Findings from a small study. *Journal of Clinical Nursing, 4,* 117-123.

Burnard, P. (2002). Not waving but drowning: A personal response to Barker and Grant. *Journal of Psychiatric and Mental Health Nursing, 9,* 221-232.

Bowles, A. (2000). Therapeutic nursing care in acute psychiatric wards: Engagement over control. *Journal of Psychiatric and Mental Health Nursing, 7,* 179-184.

Casey, B., & Long, A. (2003). Meanings of madness: A literature review. *Journal of Psychiatric and Mental Health Nursing, 10,* 89-99.

Cleary, M., Horsfall, J., & Hunt, G. (2003). Consumer feedback on nursing care and discharge planning. *Journal of Advanced Nursing, 42*(3), 269-277.

Collins, S., & Cutcliffe, J. (2003). Addressing hopelessness in people with suicidal ideation: Building upon the therapeutic relationship utilizing a cognitive behavioural approach. *Journal of Psychiatric and Mental Health Nursing, 10,* 175-185.

Cutcliffe, J. R., & Goward, P. (2000). Mental health nurses and qualitative research methods: A mutual attraction? *Journal of Advanced Nursing, 31*(3), 590-598.

Cutcliffe, J. R., & Grant, G. (2001). What are the principles and processes of inspiring hope in cognitively impaired older adults within a continuing care environment? *Journal of Psychiatric and Mental Health Nursing, 8,* 427-436.

Deacon, M. (2003). Caring for people in the 'virtual ward.' *Journal of Psychiatric and Mental Health Nursing, 10,* 465-471.

Dodds, P., & Bowles, N. (2001). Dismantling formal observation and refocusing nursing activity in acute inpatient psychiatry: A case study. *Journal of Psychiatric and Mental Health Nursing, 8,* 183-188.

Felton, A., & Stickley, T. (2004). Pedagogy, power and service user involvement. *Journal of Psychiatric and Mental Health Nursing, 11*(1), 89-98.

Forchuk, C., Jewell, J., Tweedell, D., & Steinnagel, L. (2003). Reconnecting: The client experience of recovery from psychosis. *Perspectives in Psychiatric Care, 39*(4), 141-150.

Gamble, C., & Wellman, N. (2002). Judgment impossible. *Journal of Psychiatric and Mental Health Nursing, 9,* 741-742.

Grant, A. (2001). Knowing me knowing you: Towards a new relational politics in 21st century mental health nursing (Commentary). *Journal of Psychiatric and Mental Health Nursing, 8,* 269-275.

Grant, A. (2001). Psychiatric nursing and organizational power: Rescuing the hidden dynamic (Commentary). *Journal of Psychiatric and Mental Health Nursing, 8,* 173-177.

Grant, A. (2001). Rejoinder to Barker and Clarke. *Journal of Psychiatric and Mental Health Nursing, 8,* 463-465.

Hall, J. E. (2004). Restriction and control: The perceptions of mental health nurses in a UK acute inpatient setting. *Issues in Mental Health Nursing, 25,* 539-552.

Hannigan, B., & Cutcliffe, J. (2002). Challenging contemporary mental health policy: Time to assuage the coercion? *Journal of Advanced Nursing, 37*(5), 477-484.

Hayne, Y. M. (2003). Experiencing psychiatric diagnosis: Client perspectives on being named mentally ill. *Journal of Psychiatric and Mental Health Nursing, 10,* 722-729.

Holst, H., & Severinsson, E. (2003). A study of collaboration inpatient treatment between the community psychiatric health services and a psychiatric hospital in Norway. *Journal of Psychiatric and Mental Health Nursing, 10,* 650-658.

Hopton, J. (1996). Reconceptualizing the theory-practice gap in mental health nursing. *Nurse Education Today, 16,* 227-232.

Hostick, T., & McClelland, F. (2002). 'Partnership': A co-operative inquiry between community mental health nurses and their clients. 2. The nurse-client relationship. *Journal of Psychiatric and Mental Health Nursing, 9,* 111-117.

Hummelvoll, J., & Severinsson, E. (2001). Coping with everyday reality: Mental health professionals' reflections on the care provided in an acute psychiatric ward. *Australian and New Zealand Journal of Mental Health Nursing, 10,* 156-166.

Jackson, S., & Stevenson, C. (1998). The gift of time from the friendly professional. *Nursing Standard, 12*(51), 31-33.

Jackson, S., & Stevenson, C. (2000). What do people need psychiatric and mental health nurses for? *Journal of Advanced Nursing, 31*(2), 378-388.

Jones, A. (1996). The value of Peplau's theory for mental health nursing. *British Journal of Nursing, 5*(14), 877-881.

Keen, T. M. (2003). Post-psychiatry: paradigm shift or wishful thinking? A speculative review of future possibles for psychiatry. *Journal of Psychiatric and Mental Health Nursing, 10,* 29-37.

Kettles, A. M., Moir, E., Woods, P., Porter, S., & Sutherland, E. (2004). Is there a relationship between risk assessment and observation? *Journal of Psychiatric and Mental Health Nursing, 11*(2), 156-164.

Kilkku, N., Munnukka, T., & Lehtinen, K. (2003). From information to knowledge: The meaning of information-giving to patients who had experienced first-episode psychosis. *Journal of Psychiatric and Mental Health Nursing, 10,* 57-64.

Kitson, A. (2004). The state of the art and science of evidence-based nursing in UK and Europe. *Worldviews on Evidence-Based Nursing, 1*(1), 6-8.

Koivisto, K., Janhonen, S., & Vaisanen, L. (2003). Patients' experiences of psychosis in an inpatient setting. *Journal of Psychiatric and Mental Health Nursing, 10,* 221-229.

Lacey, D. (1993). Discovering theory from psychiatric nursing practice. *British Journal of Nursing, 2*(15), 763-766.

Lakeman, R. (1998). Beyond glass houses in the desert: A case for a mental health 'care' system. *Journal of Psychiatric and Mental Health Nursing, 5,* 324-328.

McAllister, M., & Walsh, S. (2003). CARE: A framework for mental health practice. *Journal of Psychiatric and Mental Health Nursing, 10,* 39-48.

McCann, T., & Hemingway, S. (2003). Models of prescriptive authority for mental health nurse practitioners (Commentary). *Journal of Psychiatric and Mental Health Nursing, 10,* 743-749.

McCann, T. V., & Clark, E. (2004). Advancing self-determination with young adults who have schizophrenia. *Journal of Psychiatric and Mental Health Nursing, 11*(1), 12-20.

Musker, M. (1997). Applying empowerment in mental health practice. *Nursing Standard, 11*(31), 45-47.

Noak, J. (2001). Do we need another model for mental health care? *Nursing Standard, 16*(8), 33-35.

Patton, D. (2004). An analysis of Roy's adaptation model of nursing as used within acute psychiatric nursing. *Journal of Psychiatric and Mental Health Nursing, 11*(2), 221-228.

Repper, J. (2000). Adjusting the focus of mental health nursing: Incorporating service users' experiences of recovery. *Journal of Mental Health, 9*(6), 575-587.

Rolfe, G. (1999). What to do with psychiatric nursing (Commentary). *Journal of Psychiatric and Mental Health Nursing, 3,* 330-333.

Rycroft-Malone, J., Seers, K., Titchen, A., Harvey, G., Kitson, A., & McCormack, B. (2004). What counts as evidence in evidence-based practice? *Journal of Advanced Nursing, 47*(1), 81-90.

Saunders, J. (1997). Walking a mile in their shoes . . . Symbolic interactionism for families living with severe mental illness. *Journal of Psychosocial Nursing, 35*(6), 8-13.

Stevenson, C., & Fletcher, E. (2002). The tidal model: The questions answered. *Mental Health Practice, 5*(8), 29-38.

Stickley, T. (2002). Counseling and mental health nursing: A qualitative study. *Journal of Psychiatric and Mental Health Nursing, 9,* 301-308.

Tilley, S. (1995). Notes on narrative knowledge in psychiatric nursing. *Journal of Psychiatric and Mental Health Nursing, 2,* 217-226.

Tilley, S. (1999). Altschul's legacy in mediating British and American psychiatric nursing discourses: Common sense and the 'absence' of the accountable practitioner. *Journal of Psychiatric and Mental Health Nursing, 6,* 283-295.

Vuokila-Oikkonen, P., Janhonen, S., & Vaisanen, L. (2004). "Shared-rhythm cooperation" in cooperative team meetings in acute psychiatric inpatient care. *Journal of Psychiatric and Mental Health Nursing, 11*(2), 129-140.

Whittington, D., & McLaughlin, C. (2000). Finding time for patients: An exploration of nurses' time allocation in an acute psychiatric setting. *Journal of Psychiatric and Mental Health Nursing, 7,* 259-268.

Peer-Reviewed Presentations

Brookes, N., & Tansey, M. (2004, May). *The tidal model of mental health recovery: An evaluation.* Paper presented at the Second Annual Clinical Nursing Research Conference, University of Ottawa and Tau Gamma Chapter Sigma Theta Tau International, Ottawa, Canada.

Brookes, N., & Tansey, M. (2004, May). *The tidal model of mental health recovery: Research into practice.* Paper presented at the Second Annual Clinical Nursing Research Conference, University of Ottawa and Tau Gamma Chapter Sigma Theta Tau International, Ottawa, Canada.

Brookes, N., Tansey, M., & Murata, L. (2003, June). *Celebrating narrative knowledge: The tidal model of psychiatric & mental health nursing.* Paper presented at Championing Nursing Knowledge: Making a Difference in Patient Outcomes, 2nd Biennial International Conference on Nursing Best Practice Guidelines, Toronto-Markham, Canada.

Brookes, N., Tansey, M., & Murata, L. (2003, May). *The tidal model of psychiatric and mental health nursing practice: Research into practice, practice into research.* Poster presented at the First National Clinical Research Day, University of Ottawa, Ottawa, Canada.

Brookes, N., Tansey, M., & Murata, L. (2003, October). *Sharing stories of the tidal model of psychiatric and mental health nursing practice.* Paper presented at The Art, the Science, and the Ethics of Psychiatric and Mental Health Nursing, International Mental Health Nursing Conference, Toronto, Canada.

Cook, N., Sadler, D., & Phillips, B. (2003, September). *Practice innovation: The tidal model pilot in a regional forensic unit.* Paper presented at the Australian and New Zealand Mental Health Nurses 29th International Conference, Rotorua, New Zealand.

Davidson, L. (2002, April). *Recovery, the tidal model and person-centred mental health.* Commentary on the Tidal Model Conference, Exeter, UK.

Fowler, K. (2003, October 30). *Ready or not—Engagement, readiness development, choosing, achieving, provide alternative services.* Poster presentation at The Art, the Science, and the Ethics of Psychiatric and Mental Health Nursing, International Mental Health Nursing Conference, Toronto, Canada.

Stevenson, C. (2001, September). *Evaluating the tidal model.* Paper presented at the First Annual Tidal Model Conference, Newcastle upon Tyne, UK.

Stevenson, C., & Fletcher, E. (2002, May). *Delivering patient-centred care: A case study of the tidal model.* Paper presented at Mental Health 2002, London.

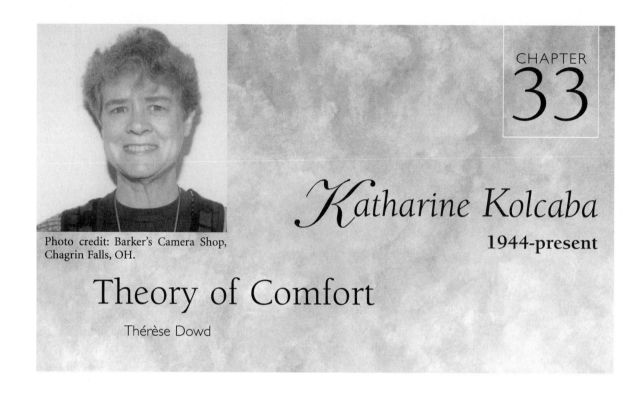

CHAPTER

33

Katharine Kolcaba
1944-present

Photo credit: Barker's Camera Shop, Chagrin Falls, OH.

Theory of Comfort

Thérèse Dowd

CREDENTIALS AND BACKGROUND OF THE THEORIST

Katharine Kolcaba was born in Cleveland, Ohio, where she spent most of her life. In 1965, she received a diploma in nursing from St. Luke's Hospital School of Nursing in Cleveland. She practiced part time for many years in medical-surgical nursing, long-term care, and home care before returning to school. In 1987, she graduated in the first R.N. to M.S.N. class at the Frances Payne Bolton School of Nursing, Case Western Reserve University (CWRU), with a specialty in gerontology. While going to school, Kolcaba job-shared a head nurse position on a dementia unit. In the context of that unit, she began theorizing about the outcome of comfort.

The author wishes to thank Katharine Kolcaba for her assistance.

After graduating with her master's degree in nursing, Kolcaba joined the faculty at The University of Akron College of Nursing. Since that time, she has maintained American Nurses Association (ANA) certification in gerontology. She returned to CWRU to pursue her doctorate in nursing on a part-time basis while continuing to teach full time. Over the next 10 years, she used course work from her doctoral program to develop and explicate her theory. During that time, Kolcaba published a concept analysis of comfort with her philosopher-husband (Kolcaba & Kolcaba, 1991), diagrammed the aspects of comfort (Kolcaba, 1991), operationalized comfort as an outcome of care (Kolcaba, 1992a), contextualized comfort in a middle range theory (Kolcaba, 1994), and tested the theory in an intervention study (Kolcaba & Fox, 1999).

Professors to whom Kolcaba is indebted include Beverly Roberts, May Wykle, Wilma Phipps, Mary Adams, Betty Adams, Rosemary Ellis, Joanne

Youngblut, Shirley Moore, and Jaclene Zauszniewski. She also wants to thank her students who gave her valuable feedback over the years as they applied the Theory of Comfort in their gerontological nursing courses and assisted her in refining the theory, making it user friendly (Kolcaba, 1995). Ongoing presentations about comfort at research societies helped to refine her theory further. Her theory continues to evolve through personal and Web site interactions with colleagues and students.

Kolcaba received a Predoctoral Fellowship for Interdisciplinary Health from CWRU and an ANA scholarship to complete her dissertation. In 1995, she received the Honor a Researcher Award from the Midwest Nursing Research Society and the Lillian De Young Research Award from The University of Akron College of Nursing for outstanding merit in research in development. Kolcaba graduated with her Ph.D. in nursing in 1997 and received her Certificate of Authority (clinical nurse specialist) at that time. She also received the Marie Haug Student Award for excellence in aging studies from CWRU, is a member of the ANA Society of Scholars, and is in *Who's Who in American Nursing* (1991) and *The Encyclopedia of Nursing Research* (Kolcaba, 1998).

Currently, Kolcaba is an associate professor of nursing at The University of Akron College of Nursing, where she teaches nursing theory and nursing research. Her areas of interest include interventions and measurements for urinary incontinence (UI), measurement of comfort at end of life, and outcomes research. She continues to reside in the Cleveland area with her husband, and she enjoys being near her grandchildren and her mother. She is founder and coordinator of her local parish nurse program and is a member of ANA, Sigma Theta Tau, Midwest Nursing Research Society, Health Ministries Association, and League of Women Voters.

THEORETICAL SOURCES

Kolcaba began her theoretical work when she diagrammed her nursing practice early in her doctoral work. This is described in detail later in this chapter. When Kolcaba presented her framework for demen-

tia care (Kolcaba, 1992a), an audience member asked, "Have you done a concept analysis of comfort?" Kolcaba's reply was, "No, but that is my next step" (K. Kolcaba, personal communications, 1995-2005). This began her long investigation into the concept of comfort.

The first step, the promised concept analysis, began with an extensive review of the literature about comfort from the disciplines of nursing, medicine, psychology, psychiatry, ergonomics, and English (specifically Shakespeare's use of comfort and the *Oxford English Dictionary*, which traces origins of words). In various articles, she gives a historical account of the use of comfort in nursing. For example, Nightingale (1859) exhorted, "It must never be lost sight of what observation is for. It is not for the sake of piling up miscellaneous information or curious facts, but for the sake of saving life and increasing health and comfort" (p. 70).

From 1900 to 1929, comfort was the central goal of nursing and medicine because, through comfort, recovery was achieved (McIlveen & Morse, 1995). The nurse was duty bound to attend to details influencing patient comfort. Aikens (1908) stated that there was nothing concerning the comfort of the patient that was small enough to ignore. Comfort of the patient was the nurse's first and last consideration. A good nurse made patients comfortable and the provision of comfort was a primary determining factor of a nurse's ability and character (Aikens, 1908).

Harmer (1926) stated that nursing care was concerned with providing a "general atmosphere of comfort" and that personal care of patients included attention to "happiness, comfort, and ease, physical and mental" in addition to "rest and sleep, nutrition, cleanliness, and elimination" (p. 26). Goodnow (1935) devoted a chapter in her book, *The Technique of Nursing*, to the patient's comfort. She wrote, "A nurse is judged always by her ability to make her patient comfortable. Comfort is both physical and mental, and a nurse's responsibility does not end with physical care" (p. 95). In textbooks dated 1904, 1914, and 1919, emotional comfort was called *mental comfort* and was achieved mostly by providing physical comfort and modifying the environment for patients (McIlveen & Morse, 1995).

In these examples, comfort is positive, it is achieved with the help of nurses and, in some cases, it indicates an improvement from a previous state or condition. Intuitively, comfort is associated with a nurturing activity. From its origins, Kolcaba explicated its strengthening features and, from ergonomics, comfort's direct link to job performance. However, often its meaning is implicit, hidden in context, and ambiguous. The concept varies semantically as a verb, noun, adjective, adverb, process, and outcome.

Three early nursing theorists' ideas were used to synthesize or derive the types of comfort in Kolcaba's concept analysis (Kolcaba & Kolcaba, 1991). Relief was synthesized from the work of Orlando (1961), who stated that nurses relieved the needs expressed by patients. Ease was synthesized from the work of Henderson (1966), who described 13 basic functions of human beings that had to be maintained in homeostasis. Transcendence was derived from Paterson and Zderad (1975), who believed that patients could rise above their difficulties with the help of nurses.

In her theory of caring, Watson (1979) claimed that the patient's environment was critical for mental and physical well-being. Therefore, when possible, nurses provided comfort through environmental interventions. Watson identified comfort measures that nurses used in that regard (*Who's Who in American Nursing*, 1991). She used the term *comfort measures* synonymously with *interventions*.

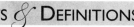

MAJOR CONCEPTS *&* DEFINITIONS

In Kolcaba's Theory of Comfort, recipients of comfort measures are known in a variety of ways such as patients, students, prisoners, workers, older adults, communities, and institutions.

HEALTH CARE NEEDS

Kolcaba defines health care needs as needs for comfort, arising from stressful health care situations, that cannot be met by recipients' traditional support systems. These needs include physical, psychospiritual, social, and environmental needs made apparent through monitoring and verbal or nonverbal reports, needs related to pathophysiological parameters, needs for education and support, and needs for financial counseling and intervention (Kolcaba, 1994).

COMFORT MEASURES

Comfort measures are defined as nursing interventions designed to address specific comfort needs of recipients, including physiological, social, financial, psychological, spiritual, environmental, and physical interventions (Kolcaba, 1994).

INTERVENING VARIABLES

Intervening variables are defined as interacting forces that influence recipients' perceptions of total comfort. These consist of variables such as past experiences, age, attitude, emotional state, support system, prognosis, finances, and the totality of elements in recipients' experience (Kolcaba, 1994).

COMFORT

Comfort is defined as the state that is experienced by recipients of comfort measures. It is the immediate and holistic experience of being strengthened through having the needs met for the three types of comfort (relief, ease, and transcendence) in four contexts of experience (physical, psychospiritual, social, and environmental) (Kolcaba, 1994; Kolcaba & Fox, 1999). Types of comfort are defined as follows (Kolcaba, 2001):

- *Relief:* the state of a recipient who has had a specific need met
- *Ease:* the state of calm or contentment
- *Transcendence:* the state in which an individual rises above his or her problems or pain

Kolcaba (2003) derived the contexts in which comfort is experienced from the literature on holism and she defined them as follows:

- *Physical:* pertaining to bodily sensations
- *Psychospiritual:* pertaining to internal awareness of self, including esteem, self-concept, sexuality,

MAJOR CONCEPTS & DEFINITIONS—cont'd

and meaning in life; relationship to a higher order or being

- *Environmental:* pertaining to external surroundings, conditions, and influences
- *Social:* pertaining to interpersonal, family, and societal relationships

HEALTH-SEEKING BEHAVIORS

The concept of HSBs was synthesized by Dr. Rozella Schlotfeldt (1975) and represents the broad category of subsequent outcomes related to the pursuit of health as defined by the recipient(s), in consultation with the nurse. Schlotfeldt stated that HSBs could be internal, external, or a peaceful death.

INSTITUTIONAL INTEGRITY

Kolcaba (2001) provides the following technical definition of institutional integrity: corporations, communities, schools, hospitals, churches, reformatories, and so on, that possess qualities or states of being complete, whole, sound, upright, appealing, honest, and sincere. This definition was derived from the literature on outcomes research and entails both normative and descriptive components. The institution can have, but does not need to have, walls. The relationship between comfort and institutional integrity is recursive.

USE OF EMPIRICAL EVIDENCE

The seeds of modern inquiry about comfort were sown in the 1980s, marking a period of collective, but separate, awareness about the concept of holistic comfort. Morse (1983) began observing the comforting actions of nurses and described comfort as "the most important nursing action in the provision of nursing care for the sick" (p. 6). Hamilton (1989) made a leap forward by exploring the meaning of comfort from the patient's perspective. She used interviews to ascertain how each patient in a long-term care facility defined comfort. The theme that emerged most frequently was relief from pain, but patients also identified good position in well-fitting furniture and a feeling of being independent, encouraged, worthwhile, and useful. At the end of the article, Hamilton (1989) stated, "The clear message is that comfort is multi-dimensional, meaning different things to different people" (p. 32).

Morse continued to focus on comforting as a nursing action and believed that this action was central to nursing and must be described. She used a qualitative, observational approach to study nurses

at work. The comforting actions that Morse (1983) described consisted of touching and talking and, to a lesser extent, listening. Although she did not specify semantic senses or definitions and often used the terms *comfort, comforting, comfortable,* and *comforted* interchangeably, she was describing the process of comfort by nurses. In and of itself, this process can be called a *comfort measure* if the outcome of that process is enhanced comfort compared with a baseline. After Kolcaba developed her theory, she tested it in an experimental design for her dissertation (Kolcaba & Fox, 1999). In this study, health care needs were those stressors (comfort needs) associated with a diagnosis of early breast cancer. The holistic intervention was guided imagery, designed specifically for this population to meet their comfort needs, and the desired outcome was comfort. The findings revealed a significant difference in comfort over time between women receiving guided imagery and the usual care group (Kolcaba & Fox, 1999). Other empirical tests of the first part of Comfort Theory have been conducted by Kolcaba and associates and are detailed in her book (Kolcaba, 2003, pp. 113-124) and cited on her award-winning Web site (Kolcaba, 1997). These comfort studies demonstrated significant differences between treatment and comparison groups on comfort over time. The following interventions were tested:

- Types of immobilization for persons after coronary angiography
- Cognitive strategies for persons with urinary frequency and incontinence
- Generalized comfort measures for women during first and second stages of labor

Kolcaba, Dowd, Steiner, and Mitzel (2004) tested the effects of hand massage for persons near the end of life. In each study, interventions were targeted to all attributes of comfort relevant to the research settings, comfort instruments were adapted from the General Comfort Questionnaire (Kolcaba, 1997, 2003) using the toxonomic structure (TS) of comfort as a guide, and there were at least two measurement points, usually three, to capture change in comfort over time.

Evidence in support of the Theory of Comfort was found in a theoretical study that looked at the following four major tenets about the nature of holistic comfort (Kolcaba & Steiner, 2000):

1. Comfort is generally state specific.
2. The outcome of comfort is sensitive to changes over time.
3. Any consistently applied holistic nursing intervention with an established history for effectiveness enhances comfort over time.
4. Total comfort is greater than the sum of its parts.

The results of tests for each tenet, using data from Kolcaba and Fox's (1999) study of women with breast cancer, supported each one. Other areas of study that have been discussed with Kolcaba via her Web site include burn units, nursing homes, home care, chronic pain, massage therapy, pediatrics, oncology, dental hygiene, transport nursing, prisons, and mental disabilities.

MAJOR ASSUMPTIONS

METAPARADIGM CONCEPTS

Kolcaba's (2001) definitions are detailed in the following sections.

Nursing

Nursing is the intentional assessment of comfort needs, design of comfort measures to address those needs, and reassessment of comfort levels after implementation compared with the baseline. Assessment and reassessment can be intuitive or subjective or both, such as when a nurse asks if the patient is comfortable, or objective, such as in observations of wound healing, changes in laboratory values, or changes in behavior. Assessment can be achieved through the administration of visual analog scales or traditional questionnaires, both of which Kolcaba (2001) has developed.

Patient

Recipients of care can be individuals, families, institutions, or communities in need of health care.

Environment

The environment is any aspect of patient, family, or institutional surroundings that can be manipulated by nurse(s) or loved one(s) to enhance comfort.

Health

Health is optimal functioning, as defined by the patient or group, of a patient, family, or community.

ASSUMPTIONS

1. Human beings have holistic responses to complex stimuli (Kolcaba, 1994).
2. Comfort is a desirable holistic outcome that is germane to the discipline of nursing (Kolcaba, 1994).
3. Human beings strive to meet their basic comfort needs or to have them met. It is an active endeavor (Kolcaba, 1994).
4. Enhanced comfort strengthens patients to engage in health-seeking behaviors (HSBs) of their choice (Kolcaba & Kolcaba, 1991).

5. Patients who are empowered to actively engage in HSBs are satisfied with their health care (Kolcaba, 1997, 2001).

6. Institutional integrity is based on a value system oriented to the recipients of care (Kolcaba, 1997, 2001).

THEORETICAL ASSERTIONS

1. Nurses identify unmet comfort needs of their patients, design comfort measures to address those needs, and seek to enhance their patients' comfort, which is the immediate desired outcome (Kolcaba, 1994).

2. Enhanced comfort is directly and positively related to engagement in HSBs, which is the subsequent desired outcome (Kolcaba, 1994).

3. When persons have the proper support to engage fully in HSBs, such as their rehabilitation or recovery program or regimen, institutional integrity is enhanced, as well (Kolcaba, 1997, 2001).

LOGICAL FORM

Kolcaba (2003) states that she developed the Theory of Comfort through the following three types of logical reasoning: (1) induction, (2) deduction, and (3) retroduction.

Induction

Induction occurs when generalizations are built from a number of specific observed instances (Bishop, 2002). When nurses are earnest about their practice and earnest about nursing as a discipline, they become familiar with implicit or explicit concepts, terms, propositions, and assumptions that underpin their practice. When nurses are in graduate school, they may be asked to diagram their practice (as Dr. Rosemary Ellis asked Kolcaba to do), which is a deceptively easy-sounding assignment.

Such was the scenario during the late 1980s. Kolcaba was head nurse on an Alzheimer's unit at the time and knew some of the terms then used to describe the practice of dementia care, such as *facilitative environment, excess disabilities,* and *optimum function.* When she drew relationships among them, she recognized that these three terms did not fully describe her practice. An important nursing piece was missing, and she pondered about what nurses were doing to prevent excess disabilities (later naming those actions *interventions*) and how to judge if the interventions were working. Optimum function had been conceptualized as the ability to engage in special activities on the unit, such as setting the table, preparing a salad, or going to a program and sitting through it. These activities made the residents feel good about themselves, as if it were the right activity at the right time. These activities did not happen more than twice a day, because the residents couldn't tolerate much more than that. What were they doing in the mean time? What behaviors did the staff hope they would exhibit that would indicate an absence of excess disabilities? Should the term *excess disabilities* be delineated further for clarity?

Partial solutions to these questions were to (1) divide excess disabilities into physical and mental, (2) introduce the concept of comfort to the original diagram, because this word seemed to convey the desired state for patients when they were not engaging in special activities, and (3) note the nonrecursive relationship between comfort and optimum functioning. These efforts marked the first steps toward a theory of comfort and thinking about the complexities of the concept (Kolcaba, 1992a).

Deduction

Deduction is a form of logical reasoning in which specific conclusions are inferred from more general premises or principles; it proceeds from the general to the specific (Bishop, 2002). The deductive stage of theory development resulted in comfort being related to other concepts to produce a theory. The work of three nursing theorists were entailed in the definition of comfort; therefore Kolcaba had to look elsewhere for the common ground that was needed to unify relief, ease, and transcendence. What was needed, she realized, was a more abstract and general conceptual framework that was congruent with comfort and contained a manageable number of highly abstract constructs.

The work of psychologist Henry Murray (1938) met these criteria for a framework upon which to hang Kolcaba's nursing concepts. His theory was about human needs; therefore, it was applicable to patients who experience multiple stimuli in stressful health care situations. This was the deductive stage of theory development, beginning with an abstract, general theoretical construction and substructing downward to more specific levels that included concepts for nursing practice.

Murray's intent was to synthesize a grand theory for psychology from existing, lesser psychological theories of his time. His concepts are found in *Lines 1, 2,* and *3* of Figure 33-1. Comfort was perceived by patients; therefore, it was logically substructed under Murray's concept of perception. Obstructing forces were substructed for nursing as health care needs, facilitating forces were comfort measures, and interacting forces were intervening variables.

The second and practical part of the theory addressed the question, "Why comfort?" For

nursing, unitary trend was substructed to health thema, which was further substructed to HSBs. Some examples of HSBs are decreased length of stay, improved functional status, better response (or effort) to therapy, faster healing, and increased patient satisfaction (Schlotfeldt, 1975).

Retroduction

Retroduction is a form of reasoning that originates ideas. It is useful for selecting phenomena that can be developed further and tested. This type of reasoning is applied in fields in which there are few available theories (Bishop, 2002). Such is the case with outcomes research which, to date, is centered on collecting large databases for measuring selected outcomes and relating those outcomes to types of nursing, medical, institutional, or community protocols. Adding a nursing theoretical framework to outcomes research would enhance this area of nursing investigation, because theory-based practice enables nurses to design interventions that are congruent with desired outcomes, increasing the

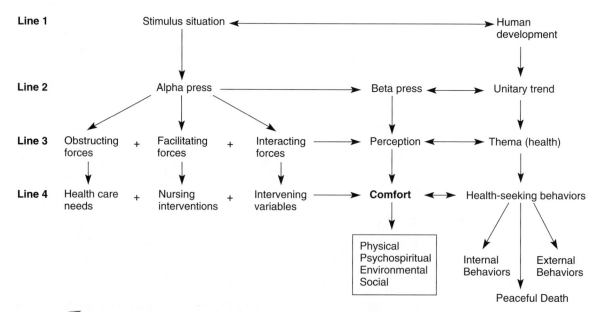

Figure **33-1** **(Middle Range) Theory of Comfort.** (From Kolcaba, K. Y. [1994]. A theory of holistic comfort for nursing. *Journal of Advanced Nursing, 19,* 1178-1184.)

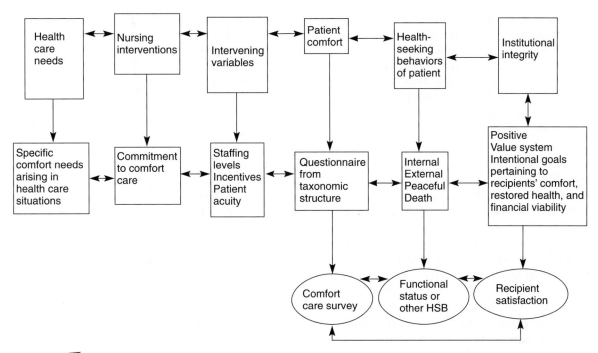

Figure **33-2 Comfort Theory adapted for outcomes research.** (From Kolcaba, K. [2001]. Evolution of the mid-range theory of comfort for outcomes research. *Nursing Outlook, 49*[2], 86-92.)

likelihood of finding significant results (Figure 33-2). Significant results for desired outcomes would provide data to respective institutions and policy makers about the importance of nursing in the present competitive market.

Murray's twentieth-century framework could not account for twenty-first–century emphasis on institutional and community outcomes. However, using retroduction, Kolcaba added the concept of institutional integrity to the middle range Theory of Comfort at the end of *Line 4* (see Figure 33-1). Adding the term to the Theory of Comfort extends the theory to considering relationships between HSBs and institutional integrity.

Line 4 (see Figure 33-1) of the diagram represents the middle range Theory of Comfort and can be applied further to any specific health care situation or research problem at the practice level. More narrow concepts congruent with a specific setting

can be derived from *Line 4* to form a new *Line 5* (microlevel or practice level theories). These microlevel comfort theories can serve as conceptual frameworks for practice, education, and research and would be publishable as such. The Theory of Comfort can be tested in parts or as a whole.

ACCEPTANCE BY THE NURSING COMMUNITY
Practice

This theory is still quite new. It is being recognized increasingly by students who are choosing it as a guiding frame for their studies, such as in nurse midwifery (Schuiling & Sampselle, 1999), labor and delivery (Koehn, 2000), cardiac catheterization (Hogan-Miller, Rustad, Sendelbach, & Goldenberg, 1995), critical care (Jenny & Logon, 1996; Kolcaba

& Fisher, 1996), hospice (Vendlinski & Kolcaba, 1997), infertility (Schoerner & Krysa, 1996), radiation therapy (Cox, 1998; Kolcaba & Fox, 1999), orthopedic nursing (Panno, Kolcaba, & Holder, 2000), perioperative nursing (Wilson & Kolcaba, 2004), hospitalized elderly (Robinson & Benton, 2002), and UI (Dowd, Kolcaba, & Steiner, 2000).

A qualitative approach has been used to describe comfort from a patient's perspective and as an outcome of holistic nursing strategies in the emergency room (Hawley, 2000), in orthopedics (Santy, 2001), in postsurgical areas (McCaffrey & Good, 2000), and in postpartum (Collins, McCoy, Sale, & Weber, 1994).

Kolcaba states that comfort care entails at least the following three types of comfort interventions:

1. Technical comfort measures are those interventions designed to maintain homeostasis and manage pain, such as the monitoring of vital signs and blood chemistry results. It also includes administration of pain medications. These comfort measures are designed to (1) help the patient maintain or regain physical function and comfort, and (2) prevent complications.

2. Coaching includes interventions designed to relieve anxiety, provide reassurance and information, instill hope, listen, and help plan realistically for recovery, integration, or death in a culturally sensitive way. For coaching to be effective, it must be timed well to capture a patient's readiness to accept new thoughts (Benner, 1984).

3. "Comfort food" for the soul includes interventions that are unexpected by today's patient but so very welcome, because they entail old-fashioned and basic nursing care. Like comfort food that you eat, these comfort interventions make patients feel strengthened in an intangible, personalized sort of way. Comfort food interventions target transcendence through presencing and memorable connections between nurse and recipient, who might be one patient, a patient and family, or a group. Suggestions for "comfort food" for patients include massage, environmental adaptations to enhance peace and tranquility, guided imagery, music therapy, reminiscence, and hand-holding. These interventions fortify patients for difficult tasks. Today's nurse often doesn't have time to provide "comfort food" for the soul, but these types of comfort interventions are facilitated by a commitment by the institution to comfort care (Kolcaba, 2003). Kolcaba believes this is how nurses really want to practice and, if given the opportunity to do so, promotes greater nurse creativity and satisfaction as well as high patient satisfaction.

In order to enhance comfort, the nurse must deliver the appropriate intervention in a caring manner. However, when the appropriate intervention is delivered in an intentional and comforting manner, comfort still may not be enhanced sufficiently. When this happens, the nurse looks at the intervening variables for reasons that comfort care is not working. Such variables as abusive homes, lack of financial resources, devastating diagnoses, or cognitive impairments may render ineffective the most appropriate interventions and comforting actions.

As stated previously, the construct of comfort care includes interventions, comforting actions, and the goal of enhanced comfort. It is intentional. This is much different than the usual connotation of comfort care as an advance directive, thought of as a last resort in many institutions. This comfort care is proactive, energized, intentional, and longed for by patients and families in all settings.

Education

Following the guidelines for teaching comfort in baccalaureate nursing programs, the Theory of Comfort was applied to the nursing care of patients receiving radiation therapy and reported by Cox (1998). The theory proved easy for student nurses to understand and apply and provided an effective method to assess and address holistic comfort needs in elders in an acute care setting. There is a subchapter about comfort theory in *Core Concepts in Advanced Nursing Practice* (Robinson & Kish, 2001). The theory is not limited to gerontological or advanced practice education. It would be difficult to bring to mind a nursing setting or practice in which comfort would not be appropriate.

Research

An entry in *The Encyclopedia of Nursing Research* speaks to the importance of measuring comfort as a nursing-sensitive outcome (Kolcaba, 1998). Nurses can provide evidence to influence decision making at institutional, community, and legislative levels only through comfort studies that demonstrate the effectiveness of holistic nursing care. The measurement of comfort in large hospital and home care data sets has been advocated to add to the literature on outcomes research (Kolcaba, 1997, 2001).

Using the taxonomic structure of comfort (Figure 33-3) as a guide, Kolcaba (1991, 1992a; Kolcaba & Fisher, 1996; Vendlinski & Kolcaba, 1997) developed the General Comfort Questionnaire to measure holistic comfort in a sample of hospital and community participants. To do this, positive and negative items were generated for each cell in the grid. Twenty-four positive items and twenty-four negative items were compiled with a Likert-type format ranging from strongly agree to strongly disagree. Higher scores indicated higher comfort. At the end of the instrumentation study with 206 one-time participants from all types of units in two hospitals and 50 people from the community, the General Comfort Questionnaire demonstrated a Cronbach alpha of 0.88 (Kolcaba, 1992b).

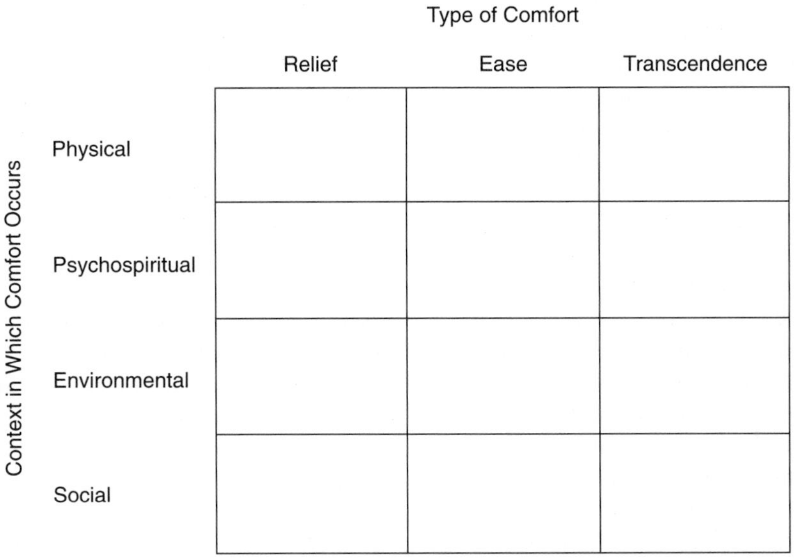

Type of Comfort:
Relief: The state of a patient who has had a specific need met
Ease: The state of calm or contentment
Transcendence: The state in which one rises above one's problems or pain

Context in Which Comfort Occurs:
Physical: Pertaining to bodily sensations
Psychospiritual: Pertaining to internal awareness of self, including esteem, concept, sexuality, and meaning in one's life; one's relationship to a higher order or being
Environmental: Pertaining to the external surroundings, conditions, and influences
Social: Pertaining to interpersonal, family, and societal relationships

Figure **33-3** **Taxonomic structure of comfort.** (From Kolcaba, K., & Fisher, E. [1996]. A holistic perspective on comfort care as an advance directive. *Critical Care Nursing Quarterly,* *18*[4], 66-76.)

The taxonomic structure of comfort provides a map of the content domain of comfort so that future researchers can use it to design their own comfort instruments. Testing of a questionnaire developed from the taxonomy is described for the end-of-life instrument (Novak, Kolcaba, Steiner, & Dowd, 2001). Kolcaba (online) has listed steps for adapting the General Comfort Questionnaire for new research problems on her Web pages. Therefore it is very easy for researchers to generate comfort questionnaires specific to their areas of research. Visual analog scales and other traditionally formatted questionnaires can be downloaded from Kolcaba's Web site. Kolcaba believes that her Internet presence and responsiveness to inquiries that arise from her Web pages has enhanced the popularity of her theory. In addition, it is very easy to acquire and use existing questionnaires, or develop new questionnaires if necessary, given the instructions on the Web site. The theory may also be popular because comfort seems to be a universally desirable outcome of nursing care, at least for patients.

FURTHER DEVELOPMENT

Kolcaba has persisted in the development of her theory from its conception as the root of her practice, to the concept analysis that provided taxonomic structure of comfort, to the development of ways to measure the concept, and currently in its use for practice, education, and research. She has used a full array of approaches to develop her concept. Through qualitative work, Kolcaba identified the concept's historical use in nursing and strongly supported her rationale for her claim to its centrality for nursing. The three types of comfort—relief, ease, and transcendence—that were synthesized from Orlando (1961), Henderson (1966), and Paterson and Zderad (1975), respectively, are integral to the theory and were validated through factor analysis of the instrument developed with the guidance of the taxonomic structure (Kolcaba, 1992a, 1994). These three types of comfort emerged in the literature review and were confirmed by factor analysis (Kolcaba, 1992a).

The methodical development of the concept resulted in a strong, clearly organized, and logical theory that is readily applied in many settings for education, practice, and research. Kolcaba has developed templates for instrument development so that individuals can measure the concept in new settings. Kolcaba has also provided comfort care templates for use in practice settings. Students have identified how useful the concept is in practice. Research outcomes have shown the appropriateness of this concept for measuring whole-person changes that have been difficult to glean from standard, narrow measures, such as those for UI.

So far, the first part of the Theory of Comfort has stood up to empirical testing. When a comfort measure (intervention) is targeted to meet the holistic comfort needs of patients in specific health care situations, patients' comfort can be enhanced over a baseline measurement (given a strong study design and carefully adapted comfort instruments). Also, enhanced comfort has been correlated with engagement in HSBs (Schlotfeldt, 1975). Testing which of the variables come first (comfort or HSBs) can be, but has not yet been, tested with path analysis.

To demonstrate that comfort is an important mission for nursing, tests of the second and third parts of Theory of Comfort should be conducted. Choices for desirable HSBs could include increased functional status, faster progress during rehabilitation, faster healing, or peaceful death when appropriate. Institutional outcomes could include decreased length of stay for hospitalized patients, smaller number of readmissions, and higher patient satisfaction.

It is postulated that an intentional emphasis on and support for comfort care by an institution or community will be rewarded by increased satisfaction, because persons are healed, strengthened, and motivated to be healthier. If this scenario stands up to testing, institutions and communities will have more evidence that comfort care matters, not only for recipients of care, but for the viability of those institutions.

Extending the Theory of Comfort to the community is of current interest. It is well known that some communities are more comfortable to live in, grow old in, and go to school in than are others. Can the comfort of a community be enhanced with nursing interventions? Can the comfort of a community be measured? These are questions that Kolcaba is mulling over; input on answers or insights regarding these questions is eagerly requested through her Web pages or personal contact.

Another area of interest for further development is the universal nature of comfort. Currently, the General Comfort Questionnaire has been translated into Taiwanese and Spanish. A pending study is a translation into Turkish. Kolcaba is very interested in measuring comfort in children and is negotiating with pediatric nurses and researchers to develop a comfort instrument for self-assessment by children. Trying to determine the age-appropriateness for understanding the complexities of comfort is a challenge to those in this line of research.

The Theory of Comfort has already made significant contributions to nursing and is poised for greatly expanded use in the discipline. Kolcaba's energy for disseminating her theory through presentations, publications, and Web sites is as great as her energy for developing and applying her theory. This committed theoretician is a model of excellence for the nursing community in her drive to further the discipline's domain of knowledge and to promote patient-focused care.

CRITIQUE
Clarity

Some of the early articles, such as the concept analysis piece, are difficult to read but are consistent in terms of definitions, derivations, assumptions, and propositions. The seminal article explicating the Theory of Comfort is easier to read and, in subsequent articles, Kolcaba applies the theory to specific practices using academic, but understandable, language. All research concepts are defined theoretically and operationally.

Simplicity

The Theory of Comfort is simple because it goes back to basic nursing care and the traditional mission of nursing. Its language and application are

of low technology, but this does not preclude its use in highly technological settings. There are few variables in the theory, and not all of the variables have to be used for any research or educational project. The main thrust of the theory is to return nursing to a practice focused on needs of patients, inside or outside institutional walls. Its simplicity allows students and practicing nurses to learn and practice the theory easily (Kolcaba, 1995; Panno et al., 2000).

Generality

Kolcaba's theory has been applied in numerous research settings, cultures, and age groups. The only limiting factor for its application is how much commitment nurses and administrators are willing to make in meeting the comfort needs of patients. If both the nurse and the institution or community are committed to this type of nursing care, the Theory of Comfort enables nurses to practice in efficient, individualized, holistic patterns. The taxonomic structure of comfort allows researchers to develop their own comfort instruments for new settings (Kolcaba, 1991).

Empirical Precision

The first part of the theory, predicting that effective nursing interventions offered over time will demonstrate enhanced comfort, has been tested and supported with women with breast cancer (Kolcaba & Fox, 1999) and persons with UI (Dowd et al., 2000). In the UI study, enhanced comfort was related to an increase in HSBs, supporting the second part of the comfort theory. The relationship between comfort and institutional integrity has yet to be tested.

For patients with breast cancer and UI and for those at end of life (Vendlinski & Kolcaba, 1997), the adapted comfort instruments have demonstrated strong psychometric properties, which means that those questionnaires are good measurements of comfort and can reveal changes in comfort over time. These findings support the theoretical foundation for the taxonomic structure of comfort.

Derivable Consequences

The Theory of Comfort can describe a patient-centered practice and explain how to determine if comfort measures matter to patients, their health, and the viability of institutions. The theory can predict the benefits of effective comfort measures (interventions) for enhancing comfort and engagement in HSBs. The Theory of Comfort is dedicated to strengthening nursing while bringing the discipline back in contact with its roots.

SUMMARY

From its inception, the Theory of Comfort has focused on what nursing does for the patient. As it has evolved over time, the definition was derived from a concept analysis, has expanded to include broader aspects of the patient such as cultural and spiritual, but the basic format of the 12 cells remains the same. The development of the General Comfort Questionnaire was seminal to validating that this concept can be measured and that it is an outcome unique and separate from other outcomes of nursing care.

The concept has relevancy for practice and easily guides nursing in its planning and design of nursing care in any setting. Its usefulness in education has been described as providing novices with a framework that enables them to organize their assessments and plans for care and yet to learn about the art of nursing as well as the science. It is also useful for expert nurses in their delivery of care and as they explain what they do beyond the technical aspects of nursing. In research the theory provides a way to validate that there has been improvement in patient comfort after comforting interventions. The concept of comfort accounts for that quality in which the patient describes "feeling better." Kolcaba has made consistent and persistent efforts to develop and expand the concept into all realms of nursing. Through her own thinking and in interaction with nurses and other person-oriented professionals, the concept has evolved continually, including into patient care products.

Through Kolcaba's prolific writing and active Internet activities, the Theory of Comfort is known worldwide.

Comfort is understood readily by persons from all walks of life and its complexity can account for the whole patient response. It is an elegant, flexible, and highly useful concept for nursing.

Case Study

A 32-year-old African-American mother of three toddlers who is 28 weeks pregnant is admitted to the high-risk pregnancy unit with regular contractions. She is concerned because plans for her family are not finalized. She has many comfort needs, which are diagramed in Table 33-1. When nurses assess for comfort needs in any of their patients, they can use the taxonomic structure, or comfort grid, to identify and organize all known needs. Using the comfort grid as a mental guide, nurses can design interrelated comforting interventions that can be implemented in one or two nurse-patient-family interactions. For this case study, suggestions for individualizing the three types of comfort interventions are listed in Table 33-2.

To determine through research if the comforting interventions listed in Table 33-2 achieved their goal of enhancing this patient's holistic comfort, a comfort questionnaire could be developed, by writing items for each cell in the comfort grid (see Table 33-1). Complete directions for doing so are in *Comfort Theory and Practice: A Vision for Holistic Health Care and Research* (Kolcaba, 2003). A Likert-type scale with responses ranging from 1 to 6 would facilitate a total comfort score. Such a questionnaire would be given to the patient before and after the interventions are implemented, and an increase in comfort would demonstrate enhanced comfort. For clinical use, the nurse could ask the patient to rate her comfort before and after receiving the interventions on a scale from 0 to 10, with 10 being highest level possible.

Table 33-1

Taxonomic Structure of Comfort Needs

CONTEXT OF COMFORT	RELIEF	EASE	TRANSCENDENCE
Physical	Aching back Early strong contractions	Restlessness and anxiety	Patient thinking, "What will happen to my family and to my babies?"
Psychospiritual	Anxiety and tension	Uncertainty about prognosis	Need for emotional and spiritual support
Environmental	Roommate is a primigravida Room small, clean, and pleasant	Lack of privacy Phone in room Feeling of confinement with bed rest	Need for calm, familiar environmental elements and accessibility of distraction
Sociocultural	Absence of family and culturally sensitive care	Family not present Language barriers	Need for support from family or significant other Need for information, consultation

Table 33-2

Comfort Care Actions and Interventions

TYPE OF COMFORT CARE ACTION OR INTERVENTION	EXAMPLE
Standard comfort interventions	Vital signs Laboratory test results Patient assessment Medications and treatments Social worker
Coaching	Emotional support Reassurance Education Listening Clergy
Comfort food for the soul	Energy therapy such as healing touch if it is culturally acceptable Music therapy or guided imagery (patient's choice of music) Spending time Personal connections Reduction of environmental stimuli

CRITICAL THINKING *Activities*

1. Does the Theory of Comfort offer a comprehensive framework for practice? Why or why not?

2. Do you believe that comfort is a universal need? How could you demonstrate that comfort theory is transcultural?

3. How would you apply comfort theory in the community? A country? What types of interventions could you design to enhance comfort in an aggregate group? How would you measure if your intervention was effective compared with a baseline?

4. How can comfort theory influence policy change?

5. If you were asked to diagram your practice, what concepts would you include as desirable outcomes? As intervening variables? As nursing interventions? What would your diagram look like, including directional arrows and positive or negative relationships? Are there any concepts needing further exploration (that do not have a nursing history)?

6. What should be added to Kolcaba's Web site? Is there anything you don't understand? Feel free to send your suggestions to her by e-mail.

REFERENCES

Aikens, C. (1908). Making the patient comfortable. *The Canadian Nurse, 4*(9), 422-424.

Benner, P. (1984). *From novice to expert.* Reading, MA: Addison-Wesley.

Bishop, S. (2002). Logical reasoning. In A. Marriner Tomey & M.A. Alligood (Eds.), *Nursing theorists and their work* (5th ed., pp. 22-41). St. Louis: Mosby.

Collins, B. A., McCoy, S. A., Sale, S., & Weber, S. E. (1994). Descriptions of comfort by substance-using and nonusing postpartum women. *Journal of Obstetric, Gynecologic, & Neonatal Nursing, 23*(4), 293-300.

Cox, J. (1998). Assessing patient comfort in radiation therapy. *Radiation Therapist, 5*(2), 119-125.

Dowd, T., Kolcaba, K., & Steiner, R. (2000). Using cognitive strategies to enhance bladder control and comfort. *Holistic Nursing Practice, 14*(2), 91-103.

Goodnow, M. (1935). *The technique of nursing* (p. 95). Philadelphia: W. B. Saunders.

Harmer, B. (1926). *Methods and principles of teaching the principles and practice of nursing.* New York: Macmillan.

Hamilton, J. (1989). Comfort and the hospitalized chronically ill. *Journal of Gerontological Nursing, 15*(4), 28-33.

Hawley, M. P. (2000). Nurse comforting strategies: Perceptions of emergency department patients. *Clinical Nursing Research, 9*(4), 441-459.

Henderson, V. (1966). *The nature of nursing.* New York: Macmillan.

Hogan-Miller, E., Rustad, D., Sendelbach, S., & Goldenberg, I. (1995). Effects of three methods of femoral site immobilization on bleeding and comfort after coronary angiogram. *American Journal of Critical Care, 4*(2), 143-148.

Jenny, J., & Logon, J. (1996). Caring and comfort metaphors used by patients in critical care. *Image: The Journal of Nursing Scholarship, 28*(4), 349-352.

Koehn, M. L. (2000). Alternative and complementary therapies for labor and birth: An application of Kolcaba's theory of holistic comfort. *Holistic Nursing Practice, 15*(1), 66-77.

Kolcaba, K. (1991). A taxonomic structure for the concept comfort. *Image: The Journal of Nursing Scholarship, 23*(4), 237-240.

Kolcaba, K. (1992a). Holistic comfort: Operationalizing the construct as a nurse-sensitive outcome. *ANS Advances in Nursing Science, 15*(1), 1-10.

Kolcaba, K. (1992b). The concept of comfort in an environmental framework. *Journal of Gerontological Nursing, 18*(6), 33-38.

Kolcaba, K. (1994). A theory of holistic comfort for nursing. *Journal of Advanced Nursing, 19,* 1178-1184.

Kolcaba, K. (1995). The art of comfort care. *Image: The Journal of Nursing Scholarship, 27*(4), 287-289.

Kolcaba, K. (1997). *TheComfortLine.com.* Akron, OH: The University of Akron College of Nursing.

Kolcaba, K. (1998). Comfort. In J. Fitzpatrick (Ed.), *The encyclopedia of nursing research* (pp. 102-104). New York: Springer.

Kolcaba, K. (2001). Evolution of the midrange theory of comfort for outcomes research. *Nursing Outlook, 49*(2), 86-92.

Kolcaba, K. (2003). *Comfort theory and practice: A vision for holistic health care and research* (pp. 113-124). New York: Springer.

Kolcaba, K., Dowd, T., Steiner, R., & Mitzel, A. (2004). Hand massage to enhance comfort for hospice patients. *Journal of Hospice and Palliative Care, 6*(2), 91-102.

Kolcaba, K., & Fisher, E. (1996). A holistic perspective on comfort care as an advance directive. *Critical Care Nursing Quarterly, 18*(4), 66-76.

Kolcaba, K., & Fox, C. (1999). The effects of guided imagery on comfort of women with early stage breast cancer undergoing radiation therapy. *Oncology Nursing Forum, 26*(1), 67-92.

Kolcaba, K., & Kolcaba, R. (1991). An analysis of the concept of comfort. *Journal of Advanced Nursing, 16,* 1301-1310.

Kolcaba, K., & Steiner, R. (2000). Empirical evidence for the nature of holistic comfort. *Journal of Holistic Nursing, 18*(1), 46-62.

McCaffrey, R. G., & Good, M. (2000). The lived experience of listening to music while recovering from surgery. *Journal of Holistic Nursing, 18*(4), 378-390.

McIlveen, K., & Morse, J. (1995). The role of comfort in nursing care: 1900-1980. *Clinical Nursing Research, 4*(2), 127-148.

Morse, J. (1983). An enthnocentric analysis of comfort: A preliminary investigation. *Nursing Papers, 15*(4), 6-19.

Murray, H. (1938). *Explorations in personality.* New York: Oxford Press.

Nightingale, F. (1859). *Notes on nursing* (p. 70). London: Harrison.

Novak, B., Kolcaba, K., Steiner, R., & Dowd, T. (2001). Instrumentation study for end-of-life comfort questionnaires. *American Journal of Palliative Care, 18*(3), 170-180.

Orlando, I. (1961). *The dynamic nurse-patient relation-ship: Function, process, and principles.* New York: Putnam.

Panno, J., Kolcaba, K., & Holder, C. (2000). Acute care for elders (ACE): A holistic model for geriatric orthopaedic nursing care. *Journal of Orthopaedic Nursing, 19*(6), 53-60.

Paterson, J., & Zderad, L. (1975). *Humanistic nursing* (2nd ed.). New York: National League for Nursing. [Reprinted in 1988.]

Robinson, S., & Benton, G. (2002) Warmed blankets: An intervention to promote comfort for elderly hospitalized patients. Geriatric Nursing, *23*(6), 320-323.

Robinson, D., & Kish, C. (2001). *Core concepts in advanced nursing practice.* St. Louis: Mosby.

Santy, J. (2001). An investigation of the reality of nursing work with orthopaedic patients. *Journal of Othopaedic Nursing, 5*(1), 22-29.

Schlotfeldt, R. (1975). The need for a conceptual framework. In P. Verhovic (Ed.), *Nursing research* (pp. 3-25). Boston: Little & Brown.

Schoerner, C., & Krysa, L. (1996). The comfort and discomfort of infertility. *Journal of Obstetrical, Gynecological, & Neonatal Nurses, 25*(2), 167-172.

Schuiling, K., & Sampselle, C. (1999). Comfort in labor and midwifery art. *Image: The Journal of Nursing Scholarship, 31*(1), 77-81.

Vendlinski, S., & Kolcaba, K. (1997). Comfort care: A framework for hospice nursing. *The American Journal of Hospice and Palliative Care, 14*(6), 271-276.

Watson, J. (1979). *Nursing: The philosophy and science of caring.* Boulder, CO: Associated University Press.

Who's Who in American Nursing. (1991). Washington, DC: The Society of Nursing Professionals.

Wilson, L., & Kolcaba, K. (in press). Practical application of comfort theory in the perianesthesia setting (Invited article). *Journal of PeriAnesthesia Nursing, 19*(3), 164-173.

BIBLIOGRAPHY
Primary Sources
Book

Kolcaba, K. (2003). *Comfort theory and practice.* New York: Springer.

Book Chapters

Kolcaba, K. (2001). Holistic care: Is it feasible in today's health care environment? In H. Feldman (Ed.), *Nursing leaders speak out* (pp. 49-54). New York: Springer.

Kolcaba, K. (2001). Kolcaba's theory of comfort. In D. Robinson & C. Kish (Eds.), *Core concepts for advanced nursing practice* (pp. 418-422). St. Louis: Mosby.

Kolcaba, K. (2003). The theory of comfort. In S. J. Peterson & T. S. Brednow (Eds.), *Middle range theories: Application to nursing research* (pp. 255-273). Philadelphia: Lippincott Williams & Wilkins.

Kolcaba, K. (2005). Comfort (including definition, theory of comfort, relevance to nursing, review of comfort studies, and future directions.) In J. Fitzpatrick (Ed.), *The encyclopedia of nursing research* (2nd ed.). New York: Springer.

Journal Articles

Dowd, T., Kolcaba, K., & Steiner, R. (2000). Cognitive strategies to enhance comfort and decrease episodes of urinary incontinence. *Holistic Nursing Practice, 14*(2), 91-102.

Fox, C., & Kolcaba, K. (1995). Unsafe practice: A lack of strategies for effective decision making. *Nurse Educator, 20*(5), 3-4.

Fox, C., & Kolcaba, K. (1996, Spring). Decision making in unsafe practice situations. *Revolution: The Journal of Nurse Empowerment, 6*(1/2), 68-69.

Kinion, E., & Kolcaba, K. (1992). Plato's model of the psyche. *Journal of Holistic Nursing, 10,* 218-230.

Kolcaba, K. (1987). Reaching optimum function is realistic goal for elderly (Letter to the editor). *Journal of Gerontological Nursing, 13*(12), 36.

Kolcaba, K. (1988). A framework for the nursing care of demented patients. *Mainlines, 9*(6), 12-13.

Kolcaba, K. (1991). A taxonomic structure for the concept comfort: Synthesis and application. *Image: The Journal of Nursing Scholarship, 23,* 237-240.

Kolcaba, K. (1992a). Holistic comfort: Operationalizing the construct as a nurse-sensitive outcome. *ANS Advances in Nursing Science, 15*(1), 1-10.

Kolcaba, K. (1992b). The concept of comfort in an environmental framework. *Journal of Gerontological Nursing, 18*(6), 33-38.

Kolcaba, K. (1995). Process and product of comfort care, merged in holistic nursing art. *Journal of Holistic Nursing, 13*(2), 117-131.

Kolcaba, K. (1995). The art of comfort care. *Image: The Journal of Nursing Scholarship, 27,* 293-295.

Kolcaba, K. (2001). Evolution of the mid range theory of comfort for outcomes research. *Nursing Outlook, 49*(2), 86-92.

Kolcaba, K., & Dowd, T. (2000). Kegel exercises: Strengthening the weak pelvic floor muscles that cause urinary incontinence. *American Journal of Nursing, 100*(11), 59.

Kolcaba, K., Dowd, T., Steiner, R., & Mitzel, A. (2004, April/June). Efficacy of hand massage for enhancing comfort of hospice patients. *Journal of Hospice and Palliative Care, 6*(2), 91-102.

Kolcaba, K., & Fisher, E. (1996). A holistic perspective on comfort care as an advance directive. *Critical Care Nursing Quarterly, 18*(4), 66-76.

Kolcaba, K., & Fox, C. (1999). The effects of guided imagery on comfort of women with early-stage breast cancer going through radiation therapy. *Oncology Nursing Forum, 26*(1), 67-71.

Kolcaba, K., & Kolcaba, R. (1991). An analysis of the concept comfort. *Journal of Advanced Nursing, 16,* 1301-1310.

Kolcaba, K., & Kolcaba, R. (2003). Fiduciary decision-making using comfort care. *Philosophy in the Contemporary World, 10*(1), 81-86.

Kolcaba, K., & Miller, C. (1989). Geropharmacology: A nursing intervention. *Journal of Gerontological Nursing, 15*(5), 29-35.

Kolcaba, K., Panno, J., & Holder, C. (2000) Acute care for elders (ACE): A holistic model for geriatric orthopaedic nursing care. *Journal of Orthopaedic Nursing, 19*(6), 53-60.

Kolcaba, K., & Steiner, R. (2000). Empirical evidence for the nature of holistic comfort. *Journal of Holistic Nursing, 18*(1), 46-62.

Kolcaba, K., & Wilson, L. (2002). The framework of comfort care for perianesthesia nursing (with post-test for 1.2 contact hours). *Journal of Perianesthesia Nursing, 17*(2), 102-114.

Kolcaba, K., & Wykle, M. (1996). Comfort research: Spreading comfort around the world. *Reflections: Sigma Theta Tau International, 23*(2), 12-13.

Novak, B., Kolcaba, K., Steiner, R., & Dowd, T. (2001). Measuring comfort in families and patients during end of life care. *American Journal of Hospice and Palliative Care, 13*(3), 170-180.

Vendlinski, S., & Kolcaba, K. (1997). Comfort care: A framework for hospice nursing. *The American Journal of Hospice and Palliative Care, 11,* 271-276.

Wilson, L., & Kolcaba, K. (2004). Practical application of comfort theory in the perianesthesia setting [Invited article]. *Journal of PeriAnesthesia Nursing, 19*(3), 164-173.

Secondary Source
Book Chapter

Sitzman, K., & Eichelberger, L. (2004). *Understanding the work of nurse theorists: A creative beginning* (pp. 117-122). Sudbury, MA: Jones and Bartlett.

Web Site

Kolcaba, K. (1997). *TheComfortLine.com.* Akron, OH: The University of Akron College of Nursing. Retrieved January 12, 2005, from: *http://www.thecomfortline.com*

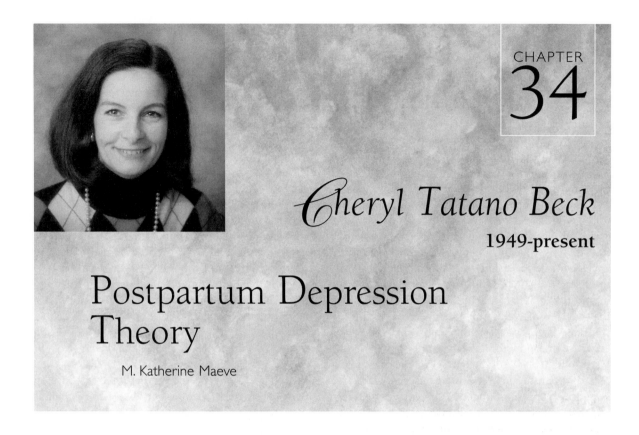

Cheryl Tatano Beck

1949-present

Postpartum Depression Theory

M. Katherine Maeve

CREDENTIALS AND BACKGROUND OF THE THEORIST

Cheryl Tatano Beck graduated from the Western Connecticut State University with a baccalaureate in nursing in 1970. She recognized during her first clinical rotation that obstetrical nursing was to be her lifelong specialty. After graduation, Beck worked as a registered nurse at the Yale New Haven Hospital on the postpartum and normal newborn nursery unit. By 1972, Beck had graduated from Yale University with a master's degree in maternal-newborn nursing and a certificate in nurse midwifery. In

The author wishes to thank Dr. Cheryl Tatano Beck for her generosity of spirit in allowing liberties with the interpretation of her life's work, and to follow some theoretical leaps and paths we had not thought of before. Thanks are also extended to Dr. Peggy L. Chinn, who happily has not retired as a mentor.

1982, she received a doctorate in nursing science from Boston University.

Beginning at the rank of instructor in 1973, Beck has held academic appointments with increasing rank at several major universities, including University of Maryland, University of Michigan, Florida Atlantic University, University of Rhode Island, Yale University, and as professor at the University of Connecticut where she holds a joint appointment in the School of Nursing and the School of Medicine. Beck has served as consultant on numerous research projects for universities and state agencies in the northeastern United States. During her career, Beck has been given more than 30 awards, including Distinguished Researcher of the Year by the Eastern Nursing Research Society in 1999. She was inducted as a fellow in the American Academy of Nursing in 1993.

A prolific author and disseminator of her research, Beck has authored more than 100 journal articles and given scores of research presentations locally, nationally, and internationally. She has served on the editorial boards of many nursing journals, including *Advances in Nursing Science, Nursing Research,* and the *Journal of Nursing Education.* Beck served on the executive board for the Marce Society, an international society for the understanding, prevention, and treatment of mental illness associated with childbirth and on the advisory committee of the Donaghue Medical Research Foundation in Connecticut.

Beck has written several articles regarding statistical analysis strategies and approaches to qualitative analysis strategies. Many in nursing will recognize the classic Polit and Hungler research text, a fixture in countless graduate nursing programs. Beck is now the coauthor of Polit's book for the seventh edition (Polit & Beck, 2003), indicating Beck's level of expertise in conducting research.

Although Beck conducted seven major studies regarding educational and caring issues with undergraduate nursing students, for over 3 decades she has retained her dedication to knowledge development in obstetrical nursing. Fittingly, she began her research career with women in labor, examining their cognitive and emotional responses to fetal monitoring (Beck, 1980). Beck's research wound its way through the labor and birth process and became firmly planted in the postpartum period, with a specific focus on postpartum mood disorders.

This body of work has resulted in a substantive theory of postpartum depression (Beck, 1993) and the development of the Postpartum Depression Screening Scale (PDSS) (Beck, 2002c; Beck & Gable, 2000) and the Postpartum Depression Predictors Inventory (PDPI) (Beck, 1998, 2001, 2002b). The sum of this work will be interpreted as a prescriptive situation-specific theory (Chinn & Kramer, 2004; Im & Meleis, 1999; Meleis, 1997). The time line of Beck's research is outlined in Table 34-1, demonstrating the logical progression of her work.

THEORETICAL AND PHILOSOPHICAL SOURCES

Although Beck does not address caring as a theoretical or philosophical construct specific to her research, she has conducted several studies that evidence her belief that "caring is the essence of nursing" (Beck, 1999, p. 629). Beck's use of the ideas of Jean Watson with regard to caring theory endorses caring as central to nursing, while acknowledging Watson's concern that quantitative methodologies may not be able to reflect adequately the ideal of transpersonal caring. However, Beck also acknowledges the imperative that nursing science has to demonstrate aspects of caring that withstand scientific scrutiny from various perspectives. It is obvious that throughout Beck's writings (including research reports using both quantitative and qualitative methods) that the notion of advancing nursing as a caring profession and living caring through our practice is desirable and achievable in practice, research, and education.

Because many of the studies used to develop Beck's Postpartum Depression Theory were qualitative in nature, various theoretical sources have been cited by Beck reflecting the philosophical and theoretical roots of those methodologies and how they were important for the kind of knowledge developed in each study. Phenomenology was used in the first major study of how women experienced postpartum depression, using Colaizzi's (1978) approach. In her next study, Beck used grounded theory as influenced by the theoretical and philosophical ideas of Glaser (1978), Glaser and Strauss (1967), and Hutchinson (1986). Grounded theory is based on symbolic interactionism, which focuses on human behaviors and interactions that explain the dynamic and complex nature of human problems and the processes involved as humans encounter and move through these problems.

Although Beck does not explicitly identify feminist theory as foundational to her work, she has identified it as an important theoretical perspective for understanding how postpartum depression approached from a medical or disease model can

Table 34-1

Time Line of Beck's Perinatal Research

YEAR	FOCUS OF RESEARCH
1972	Women's cognitive and emotional responses to fetal monitoring (master's thesis)
1977	Replication of master's thesis
1982	Parturients' temporal experiences during labor (doctoral dissertation)
1985	Mothers' temporal experiences in postpartum period after vaginal and caesarian deliveries
1988	Postpartum temporal experiences of primiparas
1989	Incidence of maternity blues in primiparas and length of hospital stay
1990	Teetering on the edge: a grounded theory study of PPD
1992	The lived experience of PPD
1994	Nurses' caring with postpartum depressed mothers
1995	Screening methods for PPD
1995	PPD and maternal-infant interaction
1995	Mothers with PPD perceptions of nurses' caring
1996	The relationship between PPD and infant temperament
1996	Predictors of PPD meta-analysis
1996	Mothers with PPD and their experiences interacting with children
1996	Concept analysis of panic
1997	Developing research programs using qualitative and quantitative approaches
1998	Effects of PPD on child development
1998	Checklist to identify women at risk for PPD
1999	Maternal depression and child behavioral problems
2000	PDSS: Development and psychometric testing
2001	Comparative analysis between PDSS and two other depression instruments
2001	Item response theory in affective instrument development
2001	Ensuring content validity
2002	PPD—metasynthesis
2002	Revision of PDPI
2002	Mothering multiples
2003	PPD in mothers of babies in NICU
2003	PDSS—Spanish version
2004	Birth trauma
2004	Posttraumatic stress disorder after childbirth
In progress	PDSS—telephone version
In progress	South African women's experiences of postnatal depression

NICU, Neonatal intensive care unit; *PDPI*, Postpartum Depression Predictors Inventory; *PDSS*, Postpartum Depression Screening Scale; *PPD*, postpartum depression.

effectively obscure the social nature of women's problems. Throughout all of Beck's work (and consistent with feminist theory), there is an explicit valuing of the importance of understanding pregnancy, birth, and motherhood through "the eyes of women" (Beck, 2002a). Furthermore, Beck acknowledges that childbirth occurs in many simultaneous contexts (medical, social, economic) and that mothers' reactions to childbirth and motherhood are shaped by their responses to these contexts.

A more unusual theoretical source of influence came from the work of Sichel and Driscoll (1999). These authors developed an earthquake model to conceptualize how interactions between biology and life result in what they term *biochemical loading*, wherein a woman's brain must repeatedly respond chemically to various stressors. Over time, with constant chemical challenges related to stresses, women's brains may develop a kind of "fault line" that perhaps is less likely to remain intact during critical moments in women's lives, such as the challenges women face around childbirth, resulting in a kind of "earthquake." Beck understood Sichel and Driscoll's model to "suggest that a woman's genetic makeup, hormonal and reproductive history, and life experiences all combine to predict her risk of 'an earthquake' which occurs when her brain cannot stabilize and mood problems erupt" (Beck, 2001, p. 276). It is easy to understand physiologically the

hormonal challenges of all pregnancies to all women. However, Sichel and Driscoll's earthquake model was important in helping Beck holistically conceptualize the length and breadth of phenomena that could affect the development of postpartum depression for individual women and groups of women within similar contexts. Although Beck states she never experienced postpartum depression after the births of her own children, anyone who has can relate to the metaphor of an earthquake, complete with its tremors and associated terrors, perhaps culminating in complete and devastating postpartum depression or, worse, postpartum psychosis.

Beck has identified Robert Gable as a particularly important source in her work. Now Professor Emeritus at the Neag School of Education, University of Connecticut, Gable coauthored an important text called *Instrument Development in the Affective Domain* (Gable & Wolf, 1993). After developing a wealth of knowledge about postpartum depression, the next logical steps for Beck became developing instruments that could predict and screen for postpartum depression. Gable assisted Beck with the theoretical and practical skills to operationalize her theory for practical use. Gable has remained directly involved through the step-by-step development of the PDSS, including the Spanish version (Beck & Gable, 2003).

Text continued on p. 750

MAJOR CONCEPTS & DEFINITIONS

Concepts should not be considered either permanent or static (Chinn & Kramer, 2004). Rather, they should be considered dynamic in that they are always open to new knowledge, experiences, perceptions, and data. From a human science orientation, it is important that participants involved in the development and use of the theory have the continuing ability to rearticulate understandings, label new concepts, and redefine existing concepts. This idea of constant reshaping is consistent with

the definition of theory used for this study, particularly with regard to the tentative nature of theory. Each of the major concepts noted in the following have undergone refinement and clarification since Beck's work began during the early 1990s.

CONCEPTS 1 AND 2

The first two concepts, postpartum mood disorders and loss of control, represent concepts that developed through Beck's earlier studies utilizing phenomenology and grounded theory methods.

1. Postpartum Mood Disorders

The definitions of postpartum depression and maternity blues were present in the beginning of Beck's work but have become better delineated over time, as has our general understanding of postpartum psychosis. Two other perinatal mood disorders, postpartum obsessive-compulsive disorder and postpartum-onset panic disorder, have been identified. Beck considers it important to understand more precisely each disorder, how they are different and how they are interrelated (Beck, 2002c).

Postpartum Depression. A nonpsychotic major depressive disorder with distinguishing diagnostic criteria, postpartum depression often begins as early as 4 weeks after birth. It may also occur anytime within the first year after childbirth. Postpartum depression is not self-limiting and is more difficult to treat than simple depression. Prevalence rates are 13% to 25%, with more women affected who are poor, live in the inner city, or are adolescents. Approximately 50% of all women suffering from postpartum depression have episodes lasting 6 months or longer.

Maternity Blues. Also known as *postpartum blues* and *baby blues,* maternity blues is a relatively transient and self-limited period of melancholy and mood swings during the early postpartum period. Maternity blues affects up to 75% of all women in all cultures.

Postpartum Psychosis. A psychotic disorder, postpartum psychosis is characterized by hallucinations, delusions, agitation, inability to sleep, along with bizarre and irrational behavior. Although postpartum psychosis is relatively rare (1 to 2 women per 1000 births), it represents a true psychiatric emergency, because both mother and baby (and perhaps other children) are in grave

danger of harm. Although postpartum psychosis often begins to appear during the first week postpartum, it frequently is not detected until serious harm has occurred.

Postpartum Obsessive-Compulsive Disorder. Only recently identified, the prevalence rates of postpartum obsessive-compulsive disorder have not been reported. Symptoms include repetitive, intrusive thoughts of harming the baby, a fear of being left alone with the infant, and hypervigilance in protecting the infant.

Postpartum-Onset Panic Disorder. This postpartum disorder has been identified only recently and is also without reported prevalence rates. It is characterized by acute onset of anxiety, fear, rapid breathing, heart palpitations, and a sense of impending doom.

2. Loss of Control

Loss of control was identified as the basic psychosocial problem in the 1993 substantive theory development phase of Beck's work. This descriptive theory captured the process women go through as they experience postpartum depression. Loss of control was an aspect women experienced in all areas of their lives. The particulars of the circumstances and life situations among the women who participated in this study may be different from those of other women. For instance, not all groups of women would have knowledge of, or access to, support groups. However, the concept of loss of control fits with extant literature and experience. The process of loss of control left women "teetering on the edge" and consisted of the following four stages:

1. *Encountering terror:* consisted of horrifying anxiety attacks, enveloping fogginess, and relentless obsessive thinking
2. *Dying of self:* consisted of alarming unrealness, contemplating and attempting self-destruction, isolating oneself

Continued

MAJOR CONCEPTS *&* DEFINITIONS—cont'd

3. *Struggling to survive:* consisted of battling the system, seeking solace at support groups, praying for relief
4. *Regaining control:* consisted of unpredictable transitioning, guarded recovery, mourning lost time

CONCEPTS 3 THROUGH 9

All of the conceptual ideas and definitions described above were used to develop specific foci for development and testing. Initially, Beck (1998) identified eight risk factors for postpartum depression. These were expanded upon in areas in which Beck heuristically determined that more conceptual clarity was needed. For instance, initially Beck subsumed infant temperament within the concept of child care stress. Therefore, Beck undertook a study to determine if there was a specific relationship between infant temperament and postpartum depression. Because of her own study and as part of the meta-analysis of other studies, infant temperament ultimately was identified as a separate risk factor and predictor for postpartum depression (Beck, 1996b).

Another important example of change is marriage. In Beck's original studies, women tended to be white, middle class, and married. In those first studies, marital satisfaction was noted to be the issue. Through subsequent research, it was noted that there were two marital factors of concern, marital status and the nature of the marital relationship satisfaction (Beck, 2002b). Two other risk factors were also identified through both quantitative and qualitative meta-analyses and metasyntheses of extant literature, socioeconomic status and issues of unplanned and unwanted pregnancies.

The Postpartum Depression Prediction Inventory (PDPI) has not yet reached the level of testing and statistical development that the PDSS has reached. However, PDPI has been found valid and reliable in recent studies (Beck, 2002b; Hanna, Jarman, Savage, & Layton, 2004).

CONCEPTS 3 THROUGH 15

These concepts represent the major concepts found to be significant predictors or risk factors for postpartum depression (Beck, 2002b). The most current interpretation of effect size was assigned after a meta-analysis of 138 extant studies and is reported at the end of each concept definition (Beck, 2002b).

3. Prenatal Depression

Depression during pregnancy was found to be the strongest predictor of postpartum depression. Prenatal depression occurs any or all of the trimesters of pregnancy.
   (Effect size = Medium)

4. Child Care Stress

Stressful events related to child care involve factors such as infant health problems and difficulty in infant care pertaining to feeding and sleeping.
   (Effect size = Medium)

5. Life Stress

Life stress is an index of stressful life events during the pregnancy and postpartum. The number of life experiences along with the amount of stress created by each of the life events are combined to determine the amount of life stress a woman is experiencing. Stressful life events can be either negative or positive and can include experiences such as the following:
- Marital changes (e.g., divorce, remarriage)
- Occupational changes (e.g., job change)
- Crises (e.g., accidents, burglaries, financial crises, and illness requiring hospitalization)
   (Effect size = Medium)

6. Social Support

Social support consists of receiving both in-strumental support (e.g., babysitting, help with

MAJOR CONCEPTS & DEFINITIONS—cont'd

household chores) and emotional support. Structural features of a woman's social network (husband or mate, family, and friends) include proximity of its members, frequency of contact, and number of confidants with whom the woman can share personal matters. Lack of social support occurs when a woman perceives she is not receiving the amount of instrumental or emotional support she expected.

(Effect size = Medium)

7. Prenatal Anxiety

Prenatal anxiety can occur during any trimester or throughout the pregnancy. Anxiety refers to feelings of uneasiness or apprehension concerning a vague, nonspecific threat.

(Effect size = Medium)

8. Marital Satisfaction

The degree of satisfaction with a marital relationship is assessed and includes how happy or satisfied the woman is with certain aspects of her marriage, such as communication, affection, similarity of values (e.g., finances, child care), mutual activity and decision making, and global well-being.

(Effect size = Medium)

9. History of Depression

Any report by a mother of having had a bout of depression before this pregnancy must be noted.

(Effect size = Medium)

10. Infant Temperament

Temperament refers to the infant's disposition and personality. Difficult temperament describes an infant who is irritable, fussy, unpredictable, and difficult to console.

(Effect size = Medium)

11. Maternity Blues

Maternity blues was defined previously as a non-pathological condition found in many women after birth. Prolonged episodes of maternity blues (lasting more than 10 days) can be predictive of postpartum depression.

(Effect size = Small to medium)

12. Self-Esteem

Self-esteem refers to a woman's global feelings of self-worth and self-acceptance. It is her confidence and satisfaction in herself. A low self-esteem reflects a negative self-evaluation and feelings about oneself or one's capabilities.

(Effect size = Medium)

13. Socioeconomic Status

Socioeconomic status is a person's rank or status in society, involving a combination of social and economic factors such as income, education, and occupation.

(Effect size = Small)

14. Marital Status

This demographic characteristic focuses on a woman's standing in regard to marriage. The ranking denotes whether a woman is single, married or cohabiting, divorced, widowed, separated, or partnered.

(Effect size = Small)

15. Unplanned or Unwanted Pregnancy

This refers to a pregnancy that was not planned or wanted by the woman. Many pregnancies in the United States are unplanned. Of particular note is the issue of pregnancies that remain unwanted after initial ambivalence.

(Effect size = Small)

CONCEPTS 16 THROUGH 22

These last concepts represent the distillation of all predictor and risk concepts that are used to screen women for postpartum depression symptomatology in the PDSS (Beck, 2002c).

Continued

MAJOR CONCEPTS & DEFINITIONS—cont'd

16. Sleeping and Eating Disturbances

These disturbances consist of an inability to sleep even when the baby is asleep, tossing and turning before actually falling asleep, waking up in the middle of the night with difficulty going back to sleep, loss of appetite, consciously being aware of the need to eat but still being unable to eat.

17. Anxiety and Insecurity

Anxiety and insecurity manifests in hyperattention to relatively minor issues, feeling as if one is jumping out of her skin and feeling the need to keep moving or pacing. In addition, there is an ever present feeling of insecurity and a sense of being overwhelmed in the new role of mother.

18. Emotional Lability

Emotional lability refers to a woman's sense that her emotions are unstable and out of her control, commonly characterized as crying for no particular reason, irritability, explosive anger, and fear that she may never be happy again.

19. Mental Confusion

Mental confusion is a marked inability to concentrate, focus upon a singular task, or make decisions. There is a general feeling of being unable to regulate one's own thought processes.

20. Loss of Self

Women sense that those aspects of self that reflected their personal identity have changed since the birth, so that women cannot identify who they really are and become fearful that they might never be able to become their real selves again.

21. Guilt and Shame

Feelings of guilt and shame are related to a woman's perception that she is performing poorly as a mother and has negative thoughts regarding her infant. This shame and guilt results in an inability to be open with others about how she feels and contributes to delay in diagnosis and intervention.

22. Suicidal Thoughts

Suicidal thoughts concern women's frequent thoughts of harming themselves or ending their own lives to escape the living nightmare of postpartum depression.

USE OF EMPIRICAL EVIDENCE

When Beck began to examine postpartum depression in 1993, she noted that only two qualitative studies contributed to the knowledge base of the disorder. Most studies were based upon knowledge developed in disciplines other than nursing. Beck's background as a nurse midwife undoubtedly gave her a view of women throughout the postpartum period not commonly available to those in other nursing disciplines involved with women during the perinatal period.

In 1993, after four major studies regarding women in the postpartum period (see Table 34-1),

Beck developed a substantive theory of postpartum depression using grounded theory methodology. The substantive theory developed was entitled "teetering on the edge," with the basic psychosocial problem identified as loss of control (Beck, 1993). The four-stage process of teetering on the edge was identified as follows:

1. Encountering terror
2. Dying self
3. Struggling to survive
4. Regaining control

Since development of the substantive theory, Beck has completed 14 other studies designed to refine the theory by examining the experiences of postpartum depression on mother-child inter-actions, postpartum panic, posttraumatic stress disorder (PTSD), and birth trauma to tease out differences among postpartum mood disorders (postpartum depression, maternity blues, postpartum psychosis, postpartum obsessive-compulsive disorder, postpartum-onset panic disorder). Also during this period, meta-analyses were conducted on predictors of postpartum depression, the relationship between postpartum depression and infant temperament, and the effects of postpartum depression on mother-infant interaction. In addition, two qualitative metasyntheses were conducted on postpartum depression and mothering multiples.

MAJOR ASSUMPTIONS
Nursing

Beck has consistently described nursing as a caring profession with caring obligations to persons we care for, students, and each other. In addition, interpersonal interactions between nurses and those for whom we care are the primary ways nursing accomplishes goals of health and wholeness.

Person

In Beck's writings, persons are described in terms of wholeness. Persons have biological, sociological, and psychological components. Further, there is a strong commitment to the idea that persons, or personhood, must be understood within the context of family and within the context of community.

Health

Beck does not offer an explicit definition of health. However, throughout her writings she considers traditional ideas of physical and mental health. Health is also the consequence of women's responses to the contexts of their lives and to the contexts of their environments. All contexts of health, then, are vital to understanding any singular issue of health.

Environment

Like many nursing scholars, Beck writes about the environment in broad terms that might include individual factors, but also includes the world outside of each person. The outside environment includes events, situations, culture, physicality, ecosystems, and sociopolitical systems. In addition, there is an acknowledgment that women in the childbearing period receive care within a health care environment structured in the medical model and permeated with patriarchal ideology.

THEORETICAL ASSERTIONS

The theoretical assertions within Beck's theory are well represented throughout her writings. She acknowledges the importance of Sichel and Driscoll's (1999) work related to the biological factors involved in postpartum depression in the following assertions:

- The brain can biochemically accommodate various stressors, whether related to internal biology or external events.
- Stressful events (internal or external), particularly over long periods, cause disruption of the biochemical regulation in the brain. The more insults to the brain, the more chronically disregulated the brain becomes. Because an already disregulated brain is again challenged with new stressors (internal or external), it is likely that serious mood and psychiatric disorders will result.
- Women's unique and normal brain and hormonal chemistry result in a vulnerability to mood disorders at critical times in their lives, including after giving birth.
- Postpartum depression is caused by a combination of biological (including genetic), psychological, social, relational, economic, and situational life stressors.
- Postpartum depression is not a homogenous disorder. Women may express postpartum depression with a single symptom but are more likely to have a constellation of varying symptoms. This is related to varying life histories of internal and external stressors.

- Culturally, women are expected to feel happy, look happy, act happy, understand how to be a mother naturally, and experience motherhood with a sense of fulfillment. These expectations make it difficult for women to express genuine feelings of distress.

- The stigma attached to mental illness increases dramatically when a mental illness is related to the birth of a child, leading women to suffer in silence.

- Within a levels of prevention framework, postpartum depression can be prevented through identification and mitigation of risk factors during the prepartum period. Postpartum depression, itself, can be identified early with careful screening and can be treated effectively. Prevention can alleviate months of suffering and decrease the harmful effects on women, their infants, and their families.

- A number of biological, sociological, and psychological issues and challenges are entirely normal in all pregnancies. These may include fatigue, sleep alterations, questioning one's abilities, and the like. Comprehensive prenatal and postnatal care can eliminate troublesome pathological symptoms and help women normalize expected symptoms, thus reducing the degree of stress they actually experience.

LOGICAL FORM

Chinn and Kramer (2004) identify inductive logic as foundational to qualitative methods, with reasoning from the particular to the general. In contrast, deductive reasoning moves from the general to the particular, drawing conclusions that represent the general. Beck's Postpartum Depression Theory, as described in previous sections of this chapter, identifies how both inductive and deductive logic significantly contributed to the development of the theory.

There are different ways to define and categorize theories. Because Beck's theory reflects a very complex and focused path in its evolution, it is helpful to be clear about what criteria were used to understand and present the theory. The definition of theory currently used is "a creative and rigorous structuring of ideas that projects a tentative, purposeful, and systematic view of phenomena" (Chinn & Kramer, 2004, p. 91). Im and Meleis (1999) describe three kinds of theories: grand theories, middle range theories, and situation-specific theories (SSTs). Literature often implies a hierarchal ranking of theories, perhaps endorsed by the notion that theories could be seen as higher versus lower, particularly with regard to levels of abstraction. However, in this discussion the three types of theories merely represent their respective uses and purposes, providing strengths and weaknesses within differing contexts.

Grand theories represent more global, abstract ideas about the nature, mission, and general goals of nursing, such as those of Peplau, Rogers, Henderson, and many others. Grand theories are also those that develop philosophies of nursing and that define nursing. For instance, Watson used theoretical reasoning derived from an explicit philosophical stance to ground the essence of nursing in caring. Using Watson's ideas about caring can be useful in all contexts of nursing. Her theory has less specificity, however, in a practice situation that may be grounded in caring, but it requires specific information by which to competently provide care. For instance, ideas about caring for women suffering from postpartum depression is an important foundational approach, one both explicitly and implicitly noted by Beck throughout her work.

Middle range theories are focused on concepts of interest that may be of importance in many contexts such as uncertainty, grief, or caregiving. These are concepts of interest for all age groups, genders, and social contexts and, therefore, may be generalizable across populations (Chinn & Kramer, 2004). Middle range theories often are derived using grounded theory methodologies, also termed *substantive theories*. Beck's substantive theory of postpartum depression found that loss of control was the basic psychosocial problem facing women. This problem could occur in many contexts other than the postpartum period.

The idea of SSTs was developed by Meleis (1997) and advanced by Im and Meleis (1999), who defined them as "theories that focus on specific nursing phenomena that reflect clinical practice and that are limited to specific populations or to particular fields of practice" (p. 13). SSTs are developed to provide a framework by which to approach particular problems, in particular contexts, with immediate clinical significance. In addition, because of their specificity, SSTs must consider "sociopolitical, cultural and/or historic contexts" (Im & Meleis, 1999, p. 13).

Beck never explicitly conceptualized her work in terms of being an SST. Through the heuristic processes involved in writing this chapter and the intention to use Beck's work as the theoretical framework for an upcoming study with incarcerated women, it became increasingly apparent that seen as a whole, her work fulfills criteria for an SST (Chinn & Kramer, 2004; Im & Meleis, 1999).

The evolution of Beck's theory is instructional for several reasons. First, the SST developed wholly because of Beck's unceasing, linear, and logical efforts to develop the theory for pragmatic practice concerns. Because her theory is relatively new, there are few contributors to the substance of the theory. Therefore, we have an opportunity to follow a very clear and focused process of theory development by a scholar who began the work as a young woman and who is still relatively young; there is much yet to come. Beck does not need to wait for others to test her theory, use it with various populations, test instruments, and the like. She has done and continues to expand and develop the theory through her own efforts.

Second, Beck's theory of postpartum depression is remarkable because it goes against the traditionally understood hierarchy of theories. Although Beck began her work with a global understanding of caring, her focused work on postpartum depression was advanced through the development of a substantive, middle range theory and has been advanced further into what is now understood in this discussion as an SST. It would be a mistake, however, to view this journey from the top (grand theory) down to an SST theory. Rather, Beck's was built from the ground up—where people really live and where nurses really practice.

Third, most theorists develop a grand theory, or a middle range theory, and continue their contributions to those theories, but usually within the same theory type. Beck's research, however, was always outcome oriented. From the beginning, Beck's goal has been to understand postpartum depression in a way that would allow professionals to develop adequate prevention strategies, develop screening programs for early intervention, and to develop adequate treatment strategies to prevent harm to women, their children, and their families. True to her research aims, what began as a descriptive substantive theory of postpartum depression has now evolved into a prescriptive SST. What follows is the story of this evolution of Beck's Postpartum Depression Theory, uniquely approached, and uniquely understood by me.

ACCEPTANCE BY THE NURSING COMMUNITY
Practice

As Beck's research findings have been disseminated more widely, the theory (and the instruments that reflect the theory) has been utilized increasingly throughout the United States. In addition, the PDSS is in use (and translated as appropriate) in Canada, Australia, New Zealand, Ireland, South Africa, Germany, Russia, Turkey, and Israel. Three practice sites that utilize Beck's theory and instruments in unique ways are discussed in the following. Importantly, these programs are directed by a nurse, a social worker, and a mother who lost her daughter to postpartum depression.

Nurse Angela Raney has indicated that the PDSS has become a standard of care for the women she works with in the high-risk obstetrical clinic of the Medical University of South Carolina Hospital for more than 2 years (A. Raney, personal communication, April 28, 2004). The clients in this clinic vary in age across the spectrum, come from various ethnic backgrounds, and have a wide range of medical risk factors. Raney reports a high correlation between high scores on the PDSS and women who are actually clinically depressed. In addition, she has noted that the tool itself has become a vehicle for opening discussions with women, discussions that had not occurred prior to implementation of the tool. Further, high scores on the PDSS have given physicians concrete information by which to understand how postpartum depression is expressed in their patients, increasing the physicians' own sensitivity and awareness. Very predictably, marshalling of community resources to meet the specific needs of individual clients has been a challenge. However, Raney is a determined young woman who has dramatically changed the landscape for the Charleston community in understanding and responding to the special needs of women during this time of vulnerability.

Public health initiatives that involve working with new mothers and babies are also utilizing Beck's theory of postpartum depression via the PDSS. For example, the Healthy Start CORPS: Inter-Conceptual Care Case Management Project in North Carolina begins to follow women when they are 6 weeks postpartum. All new clients, many of whom are Native American, are given the PDSS so that intervention and management strategies can be built into plans of care for individual women and their families (L. Baker, personal communication, April 29, 2004). The director of the program, Lisa Baker, emphasizes the ease with which women are able to discuss symptoms of postpartum depression after the tool has been administered.

Beck's work has also been instrumental in community intervention and education projects such as the Ruth Rhoden Craven Foundation for Postpartum Depression Awareness located in South Carolina. Helena Bradford founded this organization because of a tragic postpartum mood disorder within her own family. Ms. Bradford advocates for postpartum awareness within her community but focuses particularly on educating area physicians. Ms. Bradford conducts support groups whose members frequently bring serial results from their PDSSs to provide their own physicians with visible scientific evidence that their postpartum depression existed and has been improving (H. Bradford, personal communication, April 28, 2004).

Education

Beck is a frequently invited guest to professional educational conferences and workshops. Her work is cited frequently in nursing texts concerning maternal and newborn nursing, such as that of Ladewig, London, and Olds (2001). At both undergraduate and graduate levels, Beck's work sets the standard for knowledge and understanding about postpartum depression. In addition, Beck's work has been used to educate members of other disciplines, such as physicians, mental health workers, public health professionals, social workers, and those who work in social service agencies that provide protective care for women and children. Beck also brings her work to the general public and policy makers through active community involvement at the local, state, national, and international levels.

Research

The long research development of Beck's theory is evident in Table 34-1. As previously noted, she has received numerous awards recognizing the importance of her research. Although the bulk of research was conducted by Beck herself, nurses increasingly are using Beck's work for master's and doctoral level research. In addition, Beck facilitates practice implementation research for academic and nonacademic sites.

FURTHER DEVELOPMENT

Beck has identified what will likely become another major concept in her theory, as well as a restructuring of postpartum mood disorder definitions (Beck, 2004a, 2004b). Because of increasing reports of PTSD after childbirth, she examined women's experiences of traumatic births (Beck, 2004a). In this beginning work, birth trauma was defined as "an event occurring during the labor and delivery process that involves actual or threatened serious injury or death to the mother or her infant. The birthing woman experiences intense fear, helplessness, loss of control, and horror" (Beck, 2004a, p. 28).

Beck noted that women who actually had been suffering from PTSD were misdiagnosed as having postpartum depression and were treated incorrectly with antidepressant medications. She suggests that the first major concept reported in this chapter, postpartum mood disorders, should be changed to postpartum mood and anxiety disorders (Beck, 2004b). PTSD would then be differentiated as a distinct diagnosis with different treatment approaches. Birth trauma, as a concept, will be examined empirically and included in predictor and screening instruments as appropriate.

Currently, Beck is conducting a phenomenological study with very poor, indigent black women who live in Khayelitsha, South Africa. The purpose of this research is to develop a screening scale specific for this particular population. Importantly, Beck began her work with American women in the same manner. To date, she notes that the women in this study tend to describe their depression in somatic terms, like having a "heavy heart," focusing on the way it feels physically to suffer depression.

CRITIQUE
Clarity

Beck's theory evidences a large amount of semantic clarity as concepts are defined clearly and consistently. Within and between research reports, Beck uses terms, ideas, definitions, and concepts in a way that reflect growth, yet are easily understood. Although her research and writings use both inductive and deductive language, her verbiage is both economical and clear.

Simplicity

Because this is a prescriptive SST, it is necessarily complex. Nothing about postpartum depression is simple, experientially or theoretically. Yet, everything about Beck's theory of postpartum depression follows a simple and logical progression. It is accessible empirically, and it is accessible theoretically. In other words, it makes sense, simply. Importantly,

concepts and definitions used for predicting a woman's risk for postpartum depression and concepts and definitions used to screen women for postpartum depression symptomatology are directly meaningful for women, the lay public, and practitioners from many disciplines.

Generality

Chinn and Kramer (2004) note that generality refers to a theory's ability to remain conceptually simple, yet account for a broad range of empirical experiences. Postpartum depression is a relatively narrow experience; however, its causation is especially complex. Beck has accounted for the complexity of postpartum depression within the entirety of the theory. Generality issues of importance relate to how the theory is applicable in different cultural contexts. Although the theory originally was developed with primarily white middle class married women, the theory has been used successfully with Hispanic women and Native American women. However, it has yet to be widely examined for use with African-American women, chronically poor women, and women who live chronically chaotic lives, although an increasing number of nurse scholars are developing projects with women in these areas.

Empirical Precision

The PDSS has been subjected to rigorous statistical processes toward development and standardization. Beck and Gable (2000) examined psychometric properties of the scale with regard to reliability of the measure within developmental and diagnostic samples. Validity analyses were conducted with the two samples, as were procedures used to establish cutoff scores for clinical interpretations. These studies indicated that the PDSS is a reliable and valid screening instrument for detection of postpartum depression (Beck & Gable, 2000, 2001a, 2001b, 2001c, 2001d). As previously noted, the theory as well as the PDSS are relatively new and have therefore not been critiqued empirically by a wide variety of scholars.

Derivable Consequences

The value of Beck's work is of growing importance within nursing and within other disciplines. The sequence of events in the life of our fellow nurse, Andrea Yates (along with too many others) (Meier, 2002), points to the extraordinary need for a greater awareness and use of Beck's Postpartum Depression Theory for prevention, identification, early intervention, and treatment. Perinatal mood disorders are obviously more than transient inconveniences for women and their families.

There is a growing awareness that identification and early intervention of postpartum depression belongs to more than those who are primarily responsible for caring for women during pregnancy and immediately after birth (Beck, 2003; Kennedy, Beck, & Driscoll, 2002). Because of consistent interactions with mothers, pediatric and neonatal nurses can make valuable contributions to successful interventions with mothers suffering from postpartum depression. Psychiatric nurses might also be able to identify problems in women (or their children) that do not immediately indicate postpartum depression.

However, knowledge about postpartum depression is developing in a way that sheds light on less obvious consequences. Recently postpartum depression has been linked to adverse effects on children's cognitive and emotional development and behavior problems of older children in school (Beck, 1996a, 1999). Postpartum depression could have a negative effect upon situations such as substance use, traffic accidents, criminal behaviors, domestic violence, progress in school, employment and income, and many others. A growing awareness within nursing, other health care professionals, and the general public will allow greater identification of the influence of postpartum depression on the many contexts within which people live their lives.

SUMMARY

The development of Beck's Postpartum Depression Theory is the quintessential example of how nursing knowledge is developed from nursing problems, utilizing multiparadigmatic methods, with rigorous testing. The theory was influenced by diverse theoretical and philosophical stances, adding both breadth and texture. The most important features of Beck's theory are its immediate accessibility and its dynamic nature. Most nurses would be able to read the theory and understand how it might be applicable within their own practice settings. Beck and others continue to expand the theory by exploring its applicability to different populations and by exploring potential subjects and connections suggested by experience and research.

Increasingly, nurses and the wider society are recognizing that issues of postpartum depression have not been adequately understood or acknowledged. Like other health care professions, nursing did not anticipate Andrea Yates, a 36-year-old Texas mother with postpartum depression who methodically drowned all five of her children ages 6 months to 7 years, nor any of the other unfortunate women and families who have found their way onto the evening news. Dr. Cheryl Tatano Beck has changed that. Beck has demonstrated how all levels of prevention may be applied to the problems of postpartum depression. We have the knowledge and the instruments for understanding prevention, early intervention, and treatment of this disorder.

Case Study

At the tender age of 11, Kim was "sold" by her mother to three adult men for an evening of sex and drugs. Kim related that as her mother went out the door she advised her to "do what they tell you and I'll be back in the morning." Although Kim did well during the sporadic times she went to school, her life was a series of drug and sex binges. At 17, Kim was in jail and pregnant. Kim had been arrested several times and released, but the judge insisted that this time she stay incarcerated until after the baby was born to guarantee the baby would be crack-free at birth. Kim's prenatal records, however, did not indicate drug or alcohol use, and neither did her jail records. She adamantly insisted that she never used drugs or alcohol once she found out she was pregnant (late in the first trimester). Through a series of misunderstandings, she was released 2 weeks before the baby's birth. However, Kim did well, continued to stay drug-free, even refused medication during labor, and delivered a beautiful healthy baby—a baby whose blood test results were negative for drugs.

Kim recalls that she began motherhood believing this would be the event that would turn her own life around. It did for several weeks, but slowly Kim became involved in her old life. She received money to buy clothes and food for her baby. In spite of that help, however, Kim had no place to live and no money to support herself. She never had held a legal job. She qualified for postpartum medical care for 6 weeks, but after that she was on her own.

When the baby was 7 months old, a nurse received a call from Kim asking to help her give it up for adoption, because she believed she could no longer give her baby the life she knew it deserved. She was using drugs again, and the baby was being kept by whoever was in the mood to do so.

Kim chose a local Christian adoption agency. Staff there gave her the opportunity to choose the family she wanted to raise her baby. Eighteen months later, Kim gave birth to another baby. This time, she swore things would be different. When this new baby was also about 7 months old, Kim found herself deeply involved in crack use, with her baby being passed around from relative to relative and from friend to friend. Unfortunately, Kim was present during the commission of a violent crime with a tragic ending. Although Kim did not actually commit this crime, she was present and likely will be punished.

Kim once remarked that she loved being pregnant, loved giving birth, and loved the idea of being a mother. She said, "It would be great in the beginning, but after a couple of months I'd start feeling bad. It seems like with both my babies that around 6 or 7 months, I just couldn't handle anything."

Although Kim took the baby to a pediatrician for follow-up care, none of those care providers knew her or knew her history. Kim's affect is usually very upbeat; she smiles easily. It is not likely that anyone ever asked her any important questions about her life or her experience of being a mother. Kim was, for all intents and purposes, "lost to follow-up."

Kim's story illustrates the kinds of complexities that can make postpartum depression especially challenging for women who live amid drugs and chaos. In the midst of that, they still want to be mothers with the same hopes and same dreams we all have. Drugs, alcohol, crimes, and all the other ways Kim's life was chaotic were the only avenues by which she received services—after-the-fact services.

Interventions by others could have made a difference at many points in Kim's life. One of those points was during her prenatal period. She clearly evidenced most of the risk factors for postpartum depression, despite her cheerful attitude toward the pregnancy. If you had been one of Kim's nurses during her prenatal care and identified her to be at risk for postpartum depression, what kind of care plan would you have developed before or after her baby's birth?

CRITICAL THINKING *Activities*

1. Compare and contrast Beck's PDSS with other scales that screen for depression and postpartum depression. How are they different? Does Beck's instrument reflect nursing values and, if so, how?

2. Interview a friend or family member about her prenatal and postnatal experiences. What kinds of feelings did she have that you would have expected and what kinds of feelings did she have that surprised you? Might she have been at risk for postpartum depression?

REFERENCES

Beck, C. T. (1980). Patient acceptance of fetal monitoring as a helpful tool. *Journal of Obstetric, Gynecologic, & Neonatal Nursing, 9,* 350-353.

Beck, C. T. (1993). Teetering on the edge: A substantive theory of postpartum depression. *Nursing Research, 42,* 42-48.

Beck, C. T. (1996a). Postpartum depressed mothers' experiences interacting with their children. *Nursing Research, 45*(2), 98-104.

Beck, C. T. (1996b). The relationship between postpartum depression and infant temperament: A meta-analysis. *Nursing Research, 45*, 225-230.

Beck, C. T. (1998). A checklist to identify women at risk for developing postpartum depression. *Journal of Obstetric, Gynecologic, & Neonatal Nursing, 27*, 39-46.

Beck, C. T. (1999). Quantitative measurement of caring. *Journal of Advanced Nursing, 30*, 24-32.

Beck, C. T. (2001). Predictors of postpartum depression: An update. *Nursing Research, 50*(5), 275-285.

Beck, C. T. (2002a). A meta-synthesis of qualitative research. *MCN: The American Journal of Maternal Child Nursing, 27*(4), 214-221.

Beck, C. T. (2002b). Revision of the Postpartum Depression Predictors Inventory. *Journal of Obstetric, Gynecologic, & Neonatal Nursing, 31*(4), 394-402.

Beck, C. T. (2002c). *Postpartum depression screening scale (PDSS): Manual.* Los Angeles: Western Psychological Services.

Beck, C. T. (2003). Recognizing and screening for postpartum depression in mothers of NICU infants. *Advances in Neonatal Care, 3*, 37-46.

Beck, C. T. (2004a). Birth trauma: In the eye of the beholder. *Nursing Research, 53*, 28-35.

Beck, C. T. (2004b). Post traumatic stress disorder due to childbirth: The aftermath. *Nursing Research, 53*(4), 216-224.

Beck, C. T., & Gable, R. K. (2000). Postpartum depression screening scale: Development and psychometric testing. *Nursing Research, 49*(5), 272-282.

Beck, C. T., & Gable, R. K. (2001a). Item response theory in affective instrument development: An illustration. *Journal of Nursing Measurement, 9*, 5-22.

Beck, C. T., & Gable, R. K. (2001b). Comparative analysis of the performance of the Postpartum Depression Screening Scale with two other depression instruments. *Nursing Research, 50*, 242-250.

Beck, C. T., & Gable, R. K. (2001c). Further validation of the postpartum depression screening scale. *Nursing Research, 50*(3), 155-164.

Beck, C. T., & Gable, R. K. (2001d). Ensuring content validity: An illustration of the process. *Journal of Nursing Measurement, 9*(2), 201-215.

Beck, C. T., & Gable, R. K. (2003). Postpartum Depression Screening Scale—Spanish version. *Nursing Research, 52*, 296-306.

Chinn, P., & Kramer, M. (2004). *Integrated knowledge development in nursing* (6th ed.). St. Louis: Mosby.

Colaizzi, P. (1978). Psychological research as the phenomenologist views it. In R. Valle & M. King (Eds.), *Existential phenomenological alternative for psychology* (pp. 48-71). New York: Oxford University Press.

Gable, R., & Wolf, M. (1993). *Instrument development in the affective domain.* Boston: Kluwer Academic.

Glaser, B. (1978). *Theoretical sensitivity: Advances in the methodology of grounded theory.* Mill Valley, CA: Sociology Press.

Glaser, B., & Strauss, A. (1967). *The discovery of grounded theory.* Chicago: Aldine.

Hanna, B., Jarman, H., Savage, S., & Layton, K. (2004). The early detection of postpartum depression: Midwives and nurses trial a checklist. *Journal of Obstetric, Gynecologic, & Neonatal Nursing, 33*, 191-197.

Hutchinson, S. (1986). Grounded theory: The method. In P. Munhall & C. Oiler (Eds.), *Nursing research: A qualitative perspective* (pp. 111-130). Norwalk, CT: Appleton-Century-Crofts.

Im, E. O., & Meleis, A. (1999). Situation-specific theories: Philosophical roots, properties, and approach. *ANS Advances in Nursing Science, 22*(2), 11-14.

Kennedy, H., Beck, C., & Driscoll, J. (2002). A light in the fog: Caring for women with postpartum depression. *Journal of Midwifery & Women's Health, 47*(5), 318-330.

Ladewig, P., London, M., & Olds, S. (2001). *Contemporary maternal-newborn nursing care* (5th ed.). Philadelphia: Prentice Hall.

Meier, E. (2002). Pediatric ethics, issues & commentary. Andrea Yates: where did we go wrong? *Pediatric Nursing, 28*(3), 299.

Meleis, A. (1997). *Theoretical nursing: Development and progress* (3rd ed.). Philadelphia: Lippincott.

Polit, D., & Beck, C. T. (2003). *Nursing research: Principles and methods* (7th ed.). Philadelphia: Lippincott Williams & Wilkins.

Sichel, D., & Driscoll, J. (1999). *Women's moods.* New York: Harper Collins.

BIBLIOGRAPHY
Primary Sources
Books

Beck, C. T. (1999). *Postpartum depression: Case studies, research, and nursing care.* Washington, DC: Association of Women's Health, Obstetric and Neonatal Nurses.

Beck, C. T., & Gable, R. K. (2002). *Postpartum Depression Screening Scale manual.* Los Angeles: Western Psychological Services.

Polit, D., & Beck, C. T. (2003). *Nursing research: Principles and methods* (7th ed.). Philadelphia: Lippincott Williams & Wilkins.

Polit, D., & Beck, C. T. (2003) *Study guide to accompany nursing research: Principles and methods.* Philadelphia: Lippincott Williams & Wilkins.

Polit, D. F., Beck, C. T., & Hungler, B. P. (2001). *Essentials of nursing research: Methods, appraisal, and utilization.* Philadelphia: Lippincott.

Polit, D. F., Beck, C. T., & Hungler, B. P. (2001). *Study guide to accompany essentials of nursing research: Methods, appraisal, and utilization.* Philadelphia: Lippincott.

Polit, D. F., Beck, C. T., & Hungler, B. P. (2001). *Instructor's resource manual and textbook to accompany essentials of nursing research: Methods, appraisal, and utilization.* Philadelphia: Lippincott.

Book Chapters

Beck, C. T. (1994). Researching the lived experience of caring. In A. Boykin (Ed.), *Living a caring based program* (pp. 93-126). New York: National League for Nursing Publications.

Beck, C. T. (1998). Meta-analysis. In J. Fitzpatrick (Ed.), *Encyclopedia of nursing research* (pp. 308-310). New York: Springer.

Beck, C. T. (1998). Phenomenology. In J. Fitzpatrick (Ed.), *Encyclopedia of nursing research* (pp. 431-433). New York: Springer.

Beck, C. T. (1998). Replication research. In J. Fitzpatrick (Ed.), *Encyclopedia of nursing research* (pp. 485-486). New York: Springer.

Beck, C. T. (1999). Grounded theory research. In J. Fain (Ed.), *Reading, understanding, and applying nursing research* (pp. 205-225). Philadelphia: F. A. Davis.

Journal Articles

Beck, C. T. (1979). The occurrence of depression in women and the effect of the women's movement. *Journal of Psychiatric Nursing and Mental Health Services, 17,* 14-16.

Beck, C. T. (1980). Patient acceptance of fetal monitoring as a helpful tool. *Journal of Obstetric, Gynecologic, & Neonatal Nursing, 9,* 350-353.

Beck, C. T. (1982). The conceptualization of power. *ANS Advances in Nursing Science, 4,* 1-17.

Beck, C. T. (1983). Parturients' temporal experiences during the phases of labor. *Western Journal of Nursing Research, 5,* 283-295.

Beck, C. T. (1984). Subject mortality: It is inevitable? *Western Journal of Nursing Research, 6,* 331-339.

Beck, C. T. (1985). Teaching strategy for an undergraduate research course: Student exercises. *Nurse Educator, 10,* 6.

Beck, C. T. (1985). Theoretical frameworks cited in *Nursing Research* from 1974-1985. *Nurse Educator, 10,* 36-39.

Beck, C. T. (1986). Research attitudes in baccalaureate nursing students. *Nurse Educator, 11,* 6-7.

Beck, C. T. (1986). Strategies for teaching nursing research: Small group games. *Western Journal of Nursing Research, 8,* 233-238.

Beck, C. T. (1986). Teaching practicum with an educational nurse specialist. *Nurse Educator, 11,* 5.

Beck, C. T. (1986). Use of nonparametric statistics in graduate student research projects. *Journal of Nursing Education, 25,* 41-42.

Beck, C. T. (1987). Vaginal and cesarean birth mothers' temporal experiences during the postpartum period. *Journal of Obstetric, Gynecologic, & Neonatal Nursing, 16,* 366-367.

Beck, C. T. (1988). Creating a research atmosphere for the student body of a nursing department: The use of small group projects. *Nurse Educator, 13,* 5-6.

Beck, C. T. (1988). Norm setting for the verbal estimation of a 40-second interval by women of childbearing age. *Perceptual and Motor Skills, 67,* 557-578.

Beck, C. T. (1988). Pediatric nursing research published from 1977-1986. *Issues in Comprehensive Pediatric Nursing, 11,* 261-270.

Beck, C. T. (1988). Review of strategies for teaching nursing research 1979-1986. *Western Journal of Nursing Research, 10,* 222-225.

Beck, C. T. (1989). A teaching strategy: Mini publication workshop. *Nurse Educator, 14,* 28.

Beck, C. T. (1989). Fundamentals of obstetric, gynecologic, and neonatal nursing research. Part I. *Journal of Obstetric, Gynecologic, & Neonatal Nursing, 18,* 216-221.

Beck, C. T. (1989). Fundamentals of obstetric, gynecologic, and neonatal nursing research. Part II. *Journal of Obstetric, Gynecologic, & Neonatal Nursing, 18,* 288-294.

Beck, C. T. (1989). Fundamentals of obstetric, gynecologic, and neonatal nursing research. Part III. *Journal of Obstetric, Gynecologic, & Neonatal Nursing, 18,* 385-389.

Beck, C. T. (1989). Maternal newborn nursing research published from 1977-1986. *Western Journal of Nursing Research, 11,* 621-626.

Beck, C. T. (1990). The research critique: General criteria for evaluating a research project. *Journal of Obstetric, Gynecologic, & Neonatal Nursing, 19,* 18-22.

Beck, C. T. (1990). Qualitative research: Methodologies and use in pediatric nursing. *Issues in Comprehensive Pediatric Nursing, 13*(3), 193-201.

Beck, C. T. (1991). Early postpartum discharge: Literature review and critique. *Women and Health, 17,* 125-138.

Beck, C. T. (1991). How students perceive faculty caring: A phenomenological study. *Nurse Educator, 16*(5), 18-22.

Beck, C. T. (1991). Maternity blues research: A critical review. *Issues in Mental Health Nursing, 12,* 291-300.

Beck, C. T. (1991). Nursing students' lived experience of health: A phenomenological study. *Journal of Nursing Education, 30*(8), 371-374.

Beck, C. T. (1992). Caring between nursing students and physically/mentally handicapped children: A phenomenological study. *Journal of Nursing Education, 31,* 361-366.

Beck, C. T. (1992). The lived experience of postpartum depression: A phenomenological study. *Nursing Research, 41,* 166-170.

Beck, C. T. (1992). Caring among nursing students: A phenomenological study. *Nurse Educator, 17,* 22-27.

Beck, C. T. (1993). Caring relationships between nursing students and their patients. *Nurse Educator, 18,* 28-32.

Beck, C. T. (1993). Integrating research into an RN to BSN clinical course, a phenomenological method. *Western Journal of Nursing Research, 15,* 118-121.

Beck, C. T. (1993). Nursing students' initial clinical experience: A phenomenological study. *International Journal of Nursing Studies, 30,* 489-497.

Beck, C. T. (1993). Qualitative research: The evaluation of its credibility, fittingness and auditability. *Western Journal of Nursing Research, 15,* 263-266.

Beck, C. T. (1994). Achieving statistical power through design sensitivity. *Journal of Advanced Nursing, 20,* 912-916.

Beck, C. T. (1993). Teetering on the edge: A substantive theory of postpartum depression. *Nursing Research, 42,* 42-48.

Beck, C. T. (1994). Phenomenology: Its use in nursing research. *International Journal of Nursing Studies, 31,* 499-510.

Beck, C. T. (1994). Reliability and validity issues in phenomenological research. *Western Journal of Nursing Research, 16,* 254-267.

Beck, C. T. (1994). Replication strategies and their use in nursing research. *Image: The Journal of Nursing Scholarship, 26,* 191-194.

Beck, C. T. (1994). Statistical power analysis in pediatric nursing research. *Issues in Comprehensive Pediatric Nursing, 17,* 73-80.

Beck, C. T. (1994). Women's temporal experiences during the delivery process: A phenomenological study. *International Journal of Nursing Studies, 31,* 245-252.

Beck, C. T. (1995). Burnout in undergraduate nursing students. *Nurse Educator, 20,* 19-23.

Beck, C. T. (1995). Meta-analysis: Overview and application to clinical nursing research. *Journal of Obstetric, Gynecologic, & Neonatal Nursing, 27,* 39-46.

Beck, C. T. (1995). Perceptions of nurses' caring by mothers experiencing postpartum depression, *Journal of Obstetric, Gynecologic, & Neonatal Nursing, 24,* 819-825.

Beck, C. T. (1995). Screening methods for postpartum depression. *Journal of Obstetric, Gynecologic, & Neonatal Nursing, 24,* 308-312.

Beck, C. T. (1995). The effect of postpartum depression of maternal-infant interaction: A meta-analysis. *Nursing Research, 44,* 298-304.

Beck, C. T. (1996). A concept analysis of panic. *Archives of Psychiatric Nursing, 10,* 265-275.

Beck, C. T. (1996). Nursing students' experiences caring for cognitively impaired elders. *Journal of Advanced Nursing, 23,* 992-998.

Beck, C. T. (1996). Postpartum depressed mothers' experiences interacting with their children. *Nursing Research, 45,* 98-104.

Beck, C. T. (1996). Predictors of postpartum depression: A meta-analysis. *Nursing Research, 45,* 297-303.

Beck, C. T. (1996). The relationship between postpartum depression and infant temperament: A meta-analysis. *Nursing Research, 45,* 225-230.

Beck, C. T. (1996). Use of a meta-analytic database management system. *Nursing Research, 45,* 181-184.

Beck, C. T. (1997). Developing a research program using qualitative and quantitative approaches. *Nursing Outlook, 45,* 265-269.

Beck, C. T. (1997). Humor in nursing practice: A phenomenological study. *International Journal of Nursing Studies, 34,* 346-352.

Beck, C. T. (1997). Nursing students' experiences caring for dying patients. *Journal of Nursing Education, 36,* 408-415.

Beck, C. T. (1997). Use of meta-analysis as a teaching strategy in nursing research courses. *Journal of Nursing Education, 36,* 87-90.

Beck, C. T. (1998). A checklist to identify women at risk for developing postpartum depression. *Journal of Obstetric, Gynecologic, & Neonatal Nursing, 27,* 39-46.

Beck, C. T. (1998). A review of research instruments for use during the postpartum period. *MCN: The American Journal of Maternal Child Nursing, 23,* 254-261.

Beck, C. T. (1998). Effects of postpartum depression on child development: A meta-analysis. *Archives of Psychiatric Nursing, 12,* 12-20.

Beck, C. T. (1998). Intuition in nursing practice. Sharing graduate students' exemplars with undergraduate students. *Journal of Nursing Education, 37,* 169-172.

Beck, C. T. (1998). Postpartum onset of panic disorder. *Image: The Journal of Nursing Scholarship, 30,* 131-135.

Beck, C. T. (1998). Screening for postpartum depression. *OB/GYN Nursing Forum, 6,* 1-8.

Beck, C. T. (1999). Available instruments for research on prenatal attachment and adaptation to pregnancy. *MCN: The American Journal of Maternal Child Nursing, 24,* 25-32.

Beck, C. T. (1999). Content validity exercises for nursing students. *Journal of Nursing Education, 38,* 133-135.

Beck, C. T. (1999). Facilitating the work of a meta-analyst. *Research in Nursing and Health, 22,* 523-530.

Beck, C. T. (1999). Maternal depression and child behavioral problems: A meta-analysis. *Journal of Advanced Nursing, 29,* 623-629.

Beck, C. T. (1999). Opening students eyes: The process of selecting a research instrument. *Nurse Educator, 24,* 21-23.

Beck, C. T. (1999). Postpartum depression: Stopping the thief that steals motherhood. *AWHONN Lifelines, 3,* 41-44.

Beck, C. T. (1999). Quantitative measurement of caring. *Journal of Advanced Nursing, 30,* 24-32.

Beck, C. T. (2000). Choosing nursing as a career. *Journal of Nursing Education, 39,* 320-322.

Beck, C. T. (2000). Trends in nursing education since 1976. *MCN: The American Journal of Maternal Child Nursing, 25,* 290-295.

Beck, C. T. (2001). Caring within nursing education: A meta-synthesis. *Journal of Nursing Education, 40,* 101-109.

Beck, C. T. (2001). Comparative analysis of the performance of the Postpartum Depression Screening Scale with two other depression instruments. *Nursing Research, 50*(4), 242-250.

Beck, C. T. (2001). Maternal depression and problematic behavior in children. *Understanding Mental Health* (Online journal). Accessed January 12, 2004, at: *http://www.depression.org.uk*

Beck, C. T. (2001). Predictors of postpartum depression: An update. *Nursing Research, 50,* 275-285.

Beck, C. T. (2002). Mothering multiples: A meta-synthesis of the qualitative research. *MCN: The American Journal of Maternal Child Nursing, 27,* 214-221.

Beck, C. T. (2002). Postpartum depression: A meta-synthesis of qualitative research. *Qualitative Health Research, 12,* 453-472.

Beck, C. T. (2002). Releasing the pause button: Mothering twins during the first year of life. *Qualitative Health Research, 12,* 593-608.

Beck, C. T. (2002). Revision of the Postpartum Depression Predictors Inventory. *Journal of the Obstetric, Gynecologic, & Neonatal Nursing, 31,* 394-402.

Beck, C T. (2002). Theoretical perspectives of postpartum depression. *MCN: The American Journal of Maternal Child Nursing, 27,* 282-287.

Beck, C. T. (2003). Initiation into qualitative data analysis. *Journal of Nursing Education, 42,* 231-234.

Beck, C. T. (2003). Recognizing and screening for postpartum depression in mothers of NICU infants. *Advances in Neonatal Care, 3,* 37-46.

Beck, C. T. (2003). Seeing the forest for the trees: A qualitative synthesis exercise. *Journal of Nursing Education, 42,* 231-234.

Beck, C. T. (2004). Birth trauma: In the eye of the beholder. *Nursing Research, 53,* 28-35.

Beck, C. T. (2004). Post traumatic stress disorder due to childbirth: The aftermath. *Nursing Research, 53*(4), 216-224.

Beck, C. T., Bernal, H., & Froman, R. D. (2003). Methods to document the semantic equivalence of a translated scale. *Research in Nursing & Health, 26,* 64-73.

Beck, C. T., & Gable, R. K. (2000). Postpartum Depression Screening Scale: Development and psychometric testing. *Nursing Research, 49,* 272-282.

Beck, C. T., & Gable, R. K. (2001). Item response theory in affective instrument development: An illustration. *Journal of Nursing Measurement, 9,* 5-22.

Beck, C. T., & Gable, R. K. (2001). Comparative analysis of the performance of the Postpartum Depression Screening Scale with two other depression instruments. *Nursing Research, 50,* 242-250.

Beck, C. T., & Gable, R. K. (2001). Ensuring content validity: An illustration of the process. *Journal of Nursing Measurement, 9,* 201-215.

Beck, C. T., & Gable, R. K. (2001). Further validation of the Postpartum Depression Screening Scale. *Nursing Research, 50,* 155-164.

Beck, C. T., & Gable, R. K. (2003). Postpartum Depression Screening Scale—Spanish version, *Nursing Research, 52,* 296-306.

Beck, C. T., Reynolds, M., & Rutowski, P. (1992). Maternity blues and postpartum depression. *Journal of Obstetric, Gynecologic, & Neonatal Nursing, 21,* 287-293.

Beck, C. T., Reynolds, M., & Rutowski, P. (1992). Women's verbal estimation of a 40-second interval during the first week postpartum: A replication. *Perceptual and Motor Skills, 74,* 321-322.

Clemmens, D., Driscoll, J., & Beck, C. T. (2004). Postpartum depression as profiled through the Postpartum Depression Screening Scale. *MCN: The American Journal of Maternal Child Nursing, 29*(3), 180-185.

Kennedy, H., Beck, C. T., & Driscoll, J. (2002). A light in the fog: Caring for women with postpartum depression. *Journal of Midwifery & Women's Health, 47,* 318-330.

Beck Instruments

Beck, C. T. (1998). Postpartum Depression Predictors Inventory (PDPI). Available from *Journal of Obstetric, Gynecologic, & Neonatal Nursing,* published on behalf of the Association of Women's Health, Obstetrics and Neonatal Nurses, by Sage Science Press, an imprint of Sage Publications; Print ISSN: 0884-2175.

Beck, C. T., & Gable, R. K. (2002). *Postpartum Depression Screening Scale (PDSS).* Available through Western Psychological Services, 12031 Wilshire Blvd., Los Angeles, CA 90025-1251.

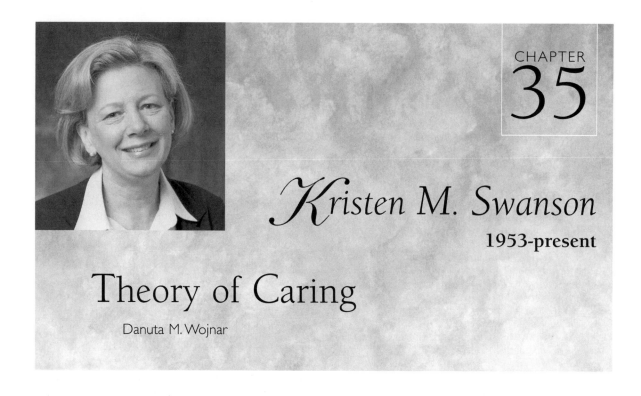

$\mathcal{K}$risten M. Swanson
1953-present

Theory of Caring

Danuta M. Wojnar

CREDENTIALS AND BACKGROUND OF THE THEORIST

Kristen M. Swanson, R.N., Ph.D., F.A.A.N., was born on January 13, 1953, in Providence, Rhode Island. She earned her baccalaureate degree (magna cum laude) from the University of Rhode Island College of Nursing in 1975. After graduation, Swanson began her career as a registered nurse at the University of Massachusetts Medical Center in Worcester. She later recalled that she was drawn to that institution because the founding nursing administration clearly articulated a vision for professional nursing practice and actively worked with nurses to apply these ideals while working with clients (Swanson, 2001).

As a novice nurse, more than anything Swanson wanted to become a knowledgeable and technically skillful practitioner with an ultimate goal of teaching these skills to others. Hence, she pursued graduate studies in Adult Health and Illness Nursing

Program at the University of Pennsylvania in Philadelphia. After receiving a master's degree in nursing (1978), Swanson worked for a year as a clinical instructor of medical-surgical nursing at the University of Pennsylvania School of Nursing and subsequently enrolled in the Ph.D. in nursing program at the University of Colorado in Denver. There she studied psychosocial nursing with an emphasis on exploring the concepts of loss, stress, coping, interpersonal relationships, person and personhood, environments, and caring.

While a doctoral student, as part of a hands-on experience with a self-selected health promotion activity, Swanson participated in a caesarian birth support group. At one of the meetings, which focused on miscarriage, she observed that although the guest speaker, a physician, focused on the incidence and health problems prevalent after miscarriage, women who attended the meeting were more interested in talking about their personal experiences with pregnancy loss. From that day on,

Swanson decided to learn more about the human experience and responses to miscarrying. Hence, caring and miscarriage became the focus of her doctoral dissertation and, subsequently, her program of research.

After earning her Ph.D. in nursing science, Swanson applied for and received an individually awarded National Research Service postdoctoral fellowship from the National Center for Nursing Research, which she completed under the direction of Dr. Kathryn E. Barnard at the University of Washington in Seattle. Afterward, she joined the faculty at the University of Washington School of Nursing, where she continues scholarly work to this day as a professor and chairperson of the Department of Family Child Nursing. In addition to teaching and administrative responsibilities, Swanson conducts research funded by the National Institutes of Health and National Institutes of Nursing Research, publishes, mentors master's and doctoral students, and serves as a consultant at national and international levels. In recognition of the many outstanding contributions to the development of nursing discipline, among other honors, Swanson was inducted as a fellow in the American Academy of Nursing (1991) as an assistant professor, and received a Distinguished Alumnus Award from the University of Rhode Island (2002).

THEORETICAL SOURCES

Swanson has drawn on various theoretical sources while developing her Theory of Caring. She recalls that from the beginning of her nursing career, knowledge obtained from book learning and clinical experience made her acutely aware of the profound difference caring made in the lives of people she served:

> Watching patients move into a space of total dependency and come out the other side restored was like witnessing a miracle unfold. Sitting with spouses in the waiting room while they entrusted the heart

(and lives) of their partner to the surgical team was awe inspiring. It was encouraging to observe the inner reserves family members could call upon in order to hand over that which they could not control. It warmed my heart to be so privileged as to be invited into the spaces that patients and families created in order to endure their transitions through illness, recovery, and, in some instances, death. (Swanson, 2001, p. 412)

In addition, Swanson credits several nursing scholars for the insights that shaped her beliefs about the nursing discipline and influenced her program of research. She acknowledges that taking Dr. Jacqueline Fawcett's course on the conceptual basis of nursing practice as a master's-prepared nurse not only made her better understand the differences between the goals of nursing and other health disciplines, but also made her realize that caring for others, as they go through life transitions of health, illness, healing, and dying, was congruent with her personal values (Swanson, 2001). Hence, Swanson chose Dr. Jean Watson as a mentor during her doctoral studies. She attributes the emphasis on exploring the concept of caring in her doctoral dissertation to Dr. Watson's influence. Despite the close working relationship and emphasis on caring in Swanson's dissertation work, neither Swanson nor Watson has ever seen Swanson's program of research as application of Watson's Theory of Human Caring (Watson, 1979, 1988, 1999). Instead, both Swanson and Watson assert that compatibility of findings on caring in their individual programs of research add credibility to their theoretical assertions (Swanson, 2001).

Swanson also acknowledges Dr. Kathryn E. Barnard for encouraging her to make the transition from the interpretive to contemporary empiricist paradigm, to transfer what she learned and postulated about caring through several phenomenological investigations to guide intervention research and, hopefully, clinical practice with women who have miscarried.

MAJOR CONCEPTS & DEFINITIONS

CARING

Caring is a nurturing way of relating to a valued other toward whom one feels a personal sense of commitment and responsibility (Swanson, 1991).

KNOWING

Knowing is striving to understand the meaning of an event in the life of the other, avoiding assumptions, focusing on the person cared for, seeking cues, assessing meticulously, and engaging both the one caring and the one cared for in the process of knowing (Swanson, 1991).

BEING WITH

Being with means being emotionally present to the other. It includes being there in person, conveying availability, and sharing feelings without burdening the one cared for (Swanson, 1991).

DOING FOR

Doing for means to do for others what one would do for self if at all possible, including anticipating needs, comforting, performing skillfully and competently, and protecting the one cared for while preserving his or her dignity (Swanson, 1991).

ENABLING

Enabling is facilitating the other's passage through life transitions and unfamiliar events by focusing on the event, informing, explaining, supporting, validating feelings, generating alternatives, thinking things through, and giving feedback (Swanson, 1991).

MAINTAINING BELIEF

Maintaining belief is sustaining faith in the other's capacity to get through an event or transition and face a future with meaning, believing in other's capacity and holding him or her in high esteem, maintaining a hope-filled attitude, offering realistic optimism, helping to find meaning, and standing by the one cared for no matter what the situation (Swanson, 1991).

USE OF EMPIRICAL EVIDENCE

Swanson formulated her Theory of Caring inductively as a result of several investigations. For her doctoral dissertation, using descriptive phenomenology, Swanson analyzed data obtained from in-depth interviews with 20 women who had recently miscarried. The following two models were proposed by Swanson as a result of this phenomenological investigation:

1. The Human Experience of Miscarriage Model
2. The Caring Model

The Caring Model, in which Swanson proposed that five basic processes (knowing, being with, doing for, enabling, and maintaining belief) give meaning to acts labeled as caring (Swanson-Kauffman, 1985, 1986, 1988a, 1988b), later became the foundation for Swanson's (1991) middle range Theory of Caring.

While a postdoctoral fellow, Swanson conducted another phenomenological study, which explored what it was like to be a provider of care to vulnerable infants in the neonatal intensive care unit (NICU). As a result of this investigation, Swanson (1990) discovered that the caring processes she identified with women who miscarried were also applicable to mothers, fathers, physicians, and nurses who were responsible for taking care of infants in the NICU. Hence, she retained the wording that described the acts of caring and proposed that all-inclusive care in a complex environment embraces balance of caring (for self and the one cared for), attaching (to others and roles), managing responsibilities (assigned by self, others, and society), and avoiding bad outcomes (Swanson, 1990).

In a subsequent phenomenological investigation conducted with socially at-risk mothers, Swanson

(1991) explored what it had been like for these mothers to receive an intense, long-term nursing intervention. Swanson recalls that as a result of this study she was finally able to define caring and further refine the understanding of caring processes. Collectively, phenomenological inquiries with women who miscarried, with caregivers in the NICU, and with socially at-risk mothers provided the basis for developing the Caring Model into the middle range Theory of Caring (Swanson, 1991, 1993).

Later, Swanson tested her Theory of Caring with women who miscarried in several investigations funded by the National Institutes of Health, National Institutes of Nursing Research, and other funding sources. Swanson's (1999a, 1999b) intervention research ($N = 242$) focused on examining the effects of caring-based counseling sessions on the women's coming to terms with loss and emotional well-being during the first year after miscarrying. Additional aims of the project were to examine the effects of the passage of time on healing during that first year and to develop strategies to monitor caring interventions. The main findings of this study showed that caring was effective in decreasing the participants' overall disturbed mood, depression, and anger. Furthermore, she found that with time all women, treated or not, assigned less personal significance to miscarrying, had higher levels of self-esteem, and had less anxiety, anger, and confusion.

To sum it up, the study demonstrated that although passing of time had positive effects on women's healing after miscarriage, caring interventions had a positive impact on decreasing the overall disturbed mood, anger, and level of depression.

The second aim of this investigation was to monitor the caring variable and identify whether caring was delivered as intended. Hence, caring was monitored in the following three ways:

1. Approximately 10% of counseling sessions were transcribed and data were analyzed using inductive and deductive content analysis.
2. Before each caring session, the counselor completed McNair, Lorr, and Droppleman's (1981) Profile of Mood States to monitor whether the counselor's mood was associated with women's ratings of caring after each session, using an investigator-developed Caring Professional Scale.
3. After each session, the counselor completed an investigator-developed Counselor Rating Scale and took narrative notes about her own counseling. The most noteworthy finding of monitoring caring was that, overall, the clients were highly satisfied with caring received during counseling sessions, suggesting that caring was delivered and received.

Swanson's (1999c) subsequent investigation was a literary meta-analysis on caring. An in-depth review of approximately 130 investigations on caring led Swanson to propose that knowledge about caring may be categorized into five hierarchical domains (levels) and that research conducted in any one domain assumes the presence of all previous domains (Swanson, 1999c). The first domain refers to the persons' capacities to deliver caring; the second domain refers to individuals' concerns and commitments that lead to caring actions; the third domain refers to the conditions (nurse, client, organizational) that enhance or diminish likelihood of delivering caring; the fourth domain refers to actions of caring; and the fifth domain refers to the consequences or the intentional and unintentional outcomes of caring for both the client and the provider (Swanson, 1999c). Conducting this literary meta-analysis clarified the meaning of the concept of caring as it is used in nursing discipline and validated transferability of Swanson's middle range Theory of Caring beyond perinatal context.

Currently, Swanson is conducting an intervention study funded by the National Institutes of Health called Couples Miscarriage Healing Project. The purpose of this investigation is to better understand the effects of miscarriage on men and women as individuals and as couples, to explore the effects of miscarriage on couple relationships, and to identify best ways of helping men and women heal as individuals and as couples after unexpected pregnancy loss. Hence, study participants (couples) are randomly assigned to one of the following three treatment groups: (1) nurse caring, three counseling sessions with a nurse, (2) self-caring, three videos and workbooks, or (3) combined caring, one nurse caring session and three videos and workbooks, to determine the most effective ways of supporting couples after miscarriage. All interventions are designed and delivered within Swanson's Theory of Caring framework.

MAJOR ASSUMPTIONS

In 1993, Swanson further developed her theory of informed caring by making explicit her major assumptions about the four main phenomena of concern to the nursing discipline: nursing, person-client, health, and environment.

Nursing

Swanson (1991, 1993) defines nursing as informed caring for the well-being of others. She asserts that the nursing discipline is informed by empirical knowledge from nursing and other related disciplines, as well as "ethical, personal and aesthetic knowledge derived from the humanities, clinical experience, and personal and societal values and expectations" (Swanson, 1993, p. 352).

Person

Swanson (1993) defines persons as "unique beings who are in the midst of becoming and whose wholeness is made manifest in thoughts, feelings, and behaviors" (p. 352). She posits that the life experiences of each individual are influenced by a complex interplay of "a genetic heritage, spiritual endowment and the capacity to exercise free will" (Swanson, 1993, p. 352). Hence, persons both shape and are shaped by the environment in which they live.

Swanson (1993) views persons as dynamic, growing, self-reflecting, yearning to be connected with others, and spiritual beings. She suggests the following:

... spiritual endowment connects each being to an eternal and universal source of goodness, mystery, life, creativity, and serenity. The spiritual endowment may be a soul, higher power/Holy Spirit, positive energy, or, simply grace. Free will equates with choice and the capacity to decide how to act when confronted with a range of possibilities. (p. 352)

Swanson (1993) noted, however, that limitations set by race, class, gender, or access to care might prevent individuals from exercising free will. Hence, acknowledging free will mandates nursing discipline to honor individuality and consider a whole range of possibilities that are acceptable or desirable to those whom the nurses attend.

Moreover, Swanson posits that the other, whose personhood nursing discipline serves, refers to families, groups, and societies. Thus, with this understanding of personhood, nurses are mandated to take on leadership roles in fighting for human rights, equal access to health care, and other humanitarian causes. Lastly, when nurses think about the other to whom they direct their caring, they also need to think of self and other nurses and their care as that cared-for other.

Health

According to Swanson (1993), to experience health and well-being is:

... to live the subjective, meaning-filled experience of wholeness. Wholeness involves a sense of integration and becoming wherein all facets of being are free to be expressed. The facets of being include the many selves that make us a human: our spirituality, thoughts, feelings, intelligence, creativity, relatedness, femininity, masculinity, and sexuality, to name just a few. (p. 353)

Hence, Swanson sees reestablishing well-being as a complex process of curing and healing that includes "releasing inner pain, establishing new meanings, restoring integration, and emerging into a sense of renewed wholeness" (Swanson, 1993, p. 353).

Environment

Swanson (1993) defines environment situationally. She maintains that for nursing it is "any context that influences or is influenced by the designated client" (p. 353). Swanson states that there are many kinds of influences on environment, such as the cultural, social, biophysical, political, and economic realms, to name only a few. According to Swanson (1993), the terms *environment* and *person-client* in nursing may be viewed interchangeably. For example, Swanson posits, "for heuristic purposes the lens on environment/designated client may be specified to the intra-individual level, wherein the 'client' may be at the cellular level and the environment may be the organs, tissues or body of which the cell is a component" (p. 353). Therefore, what is considered an environment in one situation may be considered client in another.

THEORETICAL ASSERTIONS

A fundamental and universal component of good nursing is caring for the client's biopsychosocial and spiritual well-being. Swanson's Theory of Caring (Swanson, 1991, 1993, 1999b) was empirically derived through phenomenological inquiry. It offers clear explanation of what it means for nurses to practice in a caring manner. It emphasizes that the goal of nursing is to promote well-being of others. Swanson (1991) defines caring as "a nurturing way of relating to a valued other toward whom one feels a personal sense of commitment and responsibility" (p. 162).

In summarizing the caring relationships between nurses and clients, Swanson (1993) noted that the repertoire of caring therapeutics of novice nurses might be somewhat limited and restricted by inexperience. Conversely, the techniques and knowledge imbedded in caring of experienced nurses are so

elaborate and subtle that caring might go unnoticed by an uninformed observer.

However, Swanson (1993) posits that, regardless of the years of nursing experience, caring is delivered as a set of sequential processes (subconcepts) that are created by the nurse's own philosophical attitude (maintaining belief), understanding (knowing), verbal and nonverbal messages conveyed to the client (being with), therapeutic actions (doing for and enabling), and the consequences of caring (intended client outcome). Swanson (1993) proposed that the caring processes are overlapping, may not exist in separation from each other, and that each of them is an integral component of the overarching structure of caring (Figure 35-1). Hence, according to Swanson, caring is grounded in maintenance of a basic belief in human beings, supported by knowing the client's reality, conveyed by being emotionally and physically present, and enacted by doing for and enabling the client.

LOGICAL FORM

Swanson's middle range Theory of Caring was developed empirically using inductive methodology. Chinn and Kramer (2004) assert that with inductive reasoning, hypotheses and relationships are induced by experiencing or observing phenomena and reaching conclusions. Swanson's theory was generated from phenomenological investigations with women who experienced unexpected pregnancy loss, caregivers to premature and ill babies in the NICU, and socially at-risk mothers who received long-term care from master's-prepared nurses. Swanson (1991) posits that caring, as a nurturing way of relating to another human being, is not the sole domain of perinatal nursing. In fact, she purports that knowing, being with, doing for, enabling, and maintaining belief are essential components of any nurse-client relationship. She claims that her in-depth meta-analysis of research on caring supports the generality of her theory beyond perinatal context (Swanson, 1999c).

The Structure of Caring

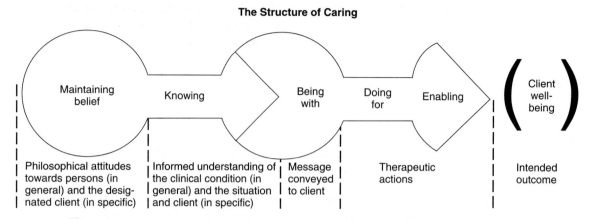

Figure 35-1 The structure of caring as linked to the nurse's philosophical attitude, informed understandings, message conveyed, therapeutic actions, and intended outcome. (From Swanson, K. M. [1993]. Nursing as informed caring for the well-being of others. *Image: The Journal of Nursing Scholarship, 25*[4], 352-357.)

ACCEPTANCE BY THE NURSING COMMUNITY

Practice

The usefulness of Swanson's Theory of Caring has been demonstrated in research, education, and clinical practice. The proposition that caring is central to nursing practice had its beginning in the theorist's own insights into the importance of caring in professional nursing practice and in the findings from Swanson's phenomenological investigations. Her subsequent investigations demonstrated applicability of the Theory of Caring in clinical nursing practice and research. Hence, Swanson's theory has been embraced as a framework for professional nursing practice by various organizations in the United States, Canada, and Sweden. An example is the Dalhousie University School of Nursing in Halifax, Nova Scotia, Canada, which selected Swanson's Theory of Caring to guide development of future generations of nurses as caring professionals. Likewise, nurses at IWK Health Centre, a tertiary care hospital for women, children, and families in Halifax, Nova Scotia, recognized that caring exemplifies the traditional legacy of nursing as a caring-healing discipline and that concepts presented in Swanson's theory are applicable in their clinical practice. Thus, in 1998, the Nursing Practice Council at IWK selected Swanson's Theory of Caring as a framework for professional nursing practice.

Reynolds (1971) suggests that a useful theory provides a sense of understanding and applicability in practice. Nurse caring may be manifested in a variety of ways and in many practice contexts. For example, in a postpartum context, demonstrating how to do a baby bath to new parents with competence and sensitivity incorporates all five caring processes. The act involves doing for (demonstrating bathing the newborn as parents would otherwise have done if they had the skill); the unrushed timing of the bath to make sure that infant is in an awake state and parents are present conveys willingness to be with; and the observing, querying, and involving parents in the task engages them in their own infant's care (enabling) while acknowledging that they are perfectly capable of caring for their new child and that their preferences matter (maintaining belief and knowing). In carrying out this seemingly simple act, the nurse can create an optimal environment for learning and enabling new parents to make decisions about infant care, while leveraging the task as an opportunity to engage in a meaningful social encounter and developing a trusting relationship.

Education

Caring is a concept difficult to embrace without understanding. Humane and altruistic caring that occurs when the theory is used in practice ranges from the simplicity of feeding or grooming an incapacitated elder, to the complexity of monitoring and managing the recovery of a patient who suffered a stroke, and to enhancing infant care skills of new parents. Nurse caring, as demonstrated by Swanson in research with women who miscarried, caregivers in the NICU, and socially at-risk mothers, recognizes the importance of attending to the wholeness of humans in their everyday lives. Thus Swanson's theory offers teachers of modern day nursing a simple way of initiating students into the profession by immersing them in the language of what it means to be caring and cared for to promote, restore, or maintain optimal wellness of individuals.

Research

Swanson has persisted in the development of her theory, from describing and defining the concept of caring and basic caring processes, to instrument development and testing in intervention research with women and men who experienced unexpected pregnancy loss. Recent review of computerized databases (MEDLINE, CINHAL, and Digital Dissertations) indicated that Swanson's work on caring and miscarriage has been cited or otherwise utilized in over 160 data-based publications.

FURTHER DEVELOPMENT

Swanson implies that she is more interested in testing and application of her theory in clinical practice than in its further development. Yet, there is much potential for further development and testing of Swanson's Theory of Caring in diverse contexts of health and illness. Conceivably, her claim about

what constitutes caring may be applicable in other helping disciplines such as teaching, social work, and medicine and in various life situations beyond nursing.

CRITIQUE
Clarity

Clarity refers to how well the theory can be understood and how clearly and consistently the concepts are presented and conceptualized (Walker & Avant, 1995). Meleis (1997) states that "precision of boundaries, a communication of a sense of orderliness, vividness, and consistency throughout the theory" (p. 262) are indicators of clarity. The concept of caring, central to the theory, and caring processes (knowing, being with, doing for, enabling, and maintaining belief) are clearly defined and arranged in a logical sequence that describes how caring is delivered. Moreover, Swanson's theory offers clear definitions of the main domains of nursing discipline (person, nurse, environment, and health) and describes them indirectly in various contexts in which the nurse-client interactions take place. By doing so, Swanson further explicates the definitions.

Simplicity

A simple theory has a minimal number of concepts. Complexity, on the other hand, refers to the explanations and relationships among variables (Chinn & Jacobs, 1987; Meleis, 1997). The appropriateness of the level of complexity within a theory depends on the nature of concepts and relationships they are set to explain or predict (Meleis, 1997). Swanson's Theory of Caring is simple yet elegant. It brings to the forefront the importance of caring, which exemplifies the discipline's traditional and modern values. Its main purpose is to help practitioners deliver nursing care that focuses on the needs of the individuals in a way that fosters their dignity, respect, and empowerment. Simplicity and consistency of language used to define the concepts allows students and nurses to understand and apply Swanson's theory in practice.

Generality

According to Chinn and Kramer (2004), the situations in which the theories may be applied should not be limited. Swanson's Theory of Caring may be applied in research and clinical work with diverse populations. The conditions essential for delivering caring that promotes individuals' wholeness across the life-span have been described clearly (Swanson, 1999c). Hence, the theory is generalizable to any nurse-client relationship and any clinical setting.

Empirical Precision

The assumptions of Swanson's Theory of Caring that applying caring processes in therapeutic communication with clients will enhance comfort and accelerate healing have been tested in clinical research. The concepts and assumptions are grounded in clinical nursing practice and research and are congruent. The completeness and simplicity of operational definitions strengthen empirical precision of this theory. Ellis (1968) proposed that theories are tentative and subject to change. Swanson (1999a, 1999b) has successfully applied and tested her Theory of Caring in a clinical trial with women and couples (ongoing). Furthermore, she has developed self-report measures to measure caring as delivered by health care professionals and by couples to each other. Both the template for delivering caring-based interventions and the development of research-based measures opens possibilities for use and further testing with other populations.

Derivable Consequences

Fawcett (1984) suggests that nursing theories should differentiate the focus of nursing from other helping disciplines. Swanson's theory of caring describes nurse-client relationships that promote wholeness and healing. Hence, the theory offers a framework for enhancing contemporary nursing practice while bringing the discipline to its traditional caring-healing roots. However, because Swanson, herself, purports that the Theory of Caring may be applied to caring relationships beyond the nurse-client encounters, it may not meet the criteria of differentiating caring as solely nursing's domain.

Case Study

The birth of a child is one of the most memorable experiences in a woman's life. You are a birth unit nurse, and at the change of a shift you are assigned to care for a teen mother who came to hospital alone and is now in active labor. When you arrive in her room, you notice that she is teary and appears frightened. Describe how you would apply Swanson's theory to connect emotionally and deliver caring in your work with this young mother.

CRITICAL THINKING *Activities*

1. Consider Swanson's caring theory as a framework for your own nursing practice. It what ways is it applicable?

2. Think about a time when you felt that someone cared about you deeply. What was it like for you to experience caring? What was most special in your interactions with that person?

3. Think about an interaction with a client-family in your clinical practice that you wish you could change or improve. Use the processes of the Theory of Caring to think critically about where you might have made more appropriate choices. If it were possible to improve this interaction, what would you change and why?

REFERENCES

Chinn, P. L., & Jacobs, M. K. (1987). *Theory and nursing: A systematic approach.* St. Louis: Mosby.

Chinn, P. L., & Kramer, M. (2004). *Integrated knowledge development in nursing* (6th ed.). St. Louis: Mosby.

Ellis, R. (1968). Characteristics of significant theories. *Nursing Research, 17*(5), 217-222.

Fawcett, J. (1984). The metaparadigm of nursing: Current status and future refinements. *Image: The Journal of Nursing Scholarship, 16,* 84-87.

McNair, D. M., Lorr, M., & Droppleman, L. F. (1981). *Profile of mood states: Manual.* San Diego: Educational and Industrial Testing Service.

Meleis, A. I. (1997). *Theoretical nursing: Development and progress.* Philadelphia: Lippincott-Raven.

Reynolds, P. D. (1971). *A primer of theory construction.* Indianapolis: Bobbs-Merrill.

Swanson, K. M. (1990). Providing care in the NICU: Sometimes an act of love. *ANS Advances in Nursing Science, 13*(1), 60-73.

Swanson, K. M. (1991). Empirical development of a middle range theory of caring. *Nursing Research, 40*(3), 161-166.

Swanson, K. M. (1993). Nursing as informed caring for the well-being of others. *Image: The Journal of Nursing Scholarship, 25*(4), 352-357.

Swanson, K. M. (1999a). Research-based practice with women who have had miscarriages. *Image: The Journal of Nursing Scholarship, 31*(4), 339-345.

Swanson, K. M. (1999b). The effects of caring, measurement, and time on miscarriage impact and women's well-being in the first year subsequent to loss. *Nursing Research, 48*(6), 288-298.

Swanson, K. M. (1999c). What's known about caring in nursing: A literary meta-analysis. In A. S. Hinshaw, J. Shaver, & S. Feetham (Eds.), *Handbook of clinical nursing research* (pp. 31-60). Thousand Oaks, CA: Sage.

Swanson, K. M. (2001). A program of research on caring. In M. E. Parker (Ed.), *Nursing theories and nursing practice* (pp. 411-420). Philadelphia: F. A. Davis.

Swanson-Kauffman, K. M. (1985). Miscarriage: A new understanding of the mother's experience. *Proceedings of the 50th Anniversary Celebration of the University of Pennsylvania School of Nursing,* 63-78.

Swanson-Kauffman, K. M. (1986). Caring in the instance of unexpected early pregnancy loss. *Topics in Clinical Nursing, 8*(2), 37-46.

Swanson-Kauffman, K. M. (1988a). The caring needs of women who miscarry. In M. M. Leininger (Ed.), *Care, discovery and uses in clinical and community nursing* (pp. 55-71). Detroit: Wayne State University Press.

Swanson-Kauffman, K. M. (1988b). There should have been two: Nursing care of parents experiencing the perinatal death of a twin. *Journal of Perinatal and Neonatal Nursing, 2*(2), 78-86.

Walker, L. O., & Avant, K. C. (1995). *Strategies for theory construction in nursing.* Norwalk, CT: Appleton & Lange.

Watson, J. (1979). *Nursing: The philosophy and science of caring.* Boston: Little & Brown.

Watson, J. (1988). New dimensions of human caring theory. *Nursing Science Quarterly, 1,* 175-181.

Watson, J. (1999). *Nursing: Human science and human care: A theory of nursing.* Sudbury, MA: Jones and Bartlett.

BIBLIOGRAPHY
Primary Sources
Book Chapters

Swanson-Kauffman, K. M. (1987). Overview of the balancing act: Having it all. In K. Swanson-Kauffman (Ed.), *Women's work, families and health.* New York: Hemisphere. (Reprint of Swanson-Kauffman, K. M. [1987]. Overview of the balancing act: Having it all. *Health Care of Women International, 8*[2-3], 101-108.)

Swanson-Kauffman, K. M. (1988). The caring needs of women who miscarry. In M. M. Leininger (Ed.), *Care, discovery and uses in clinical and community nursing* (pp. 55-71). Detroit: Wayne State University Press.

Swanson-Kauffman, K. M., & Roberts, J. (1990). Caring in parent and child nursing. In *Knowledge about care and caring: State of the art and future development.* Washington, DC: American Academy of Nursing.

Swanson-Kauffman, K. M., & Schonwald, E. (1988). Phenomenology. In B. Sarter (Ed.), *Paths to knowledge: Innovative research methods for nursing* (pp. 97-105). New York: National League for Nursing Publications.

Swanson, K. M. (1992). Foreword. In S. Wheeler & M. Pike (Eds.), *Grief ltd. manual.* Covington, IN: Grief Limited.

Swanson, K. M. (1999). What's known about caring in nursing: A literary meta-analysis. In A. S. Hinshaw, J. Shaver, & S. Feetham (Eds.), *Handbook of clinical nursing research* (pp. 31-60). Thousand Oaks, CA: Sage.

Swanson, K. M. (2001). A program of research on caring. In M. E. Parker (Ed.), *Nursing theories and nursing practice* (pp. 411-420). Philadelphia: Davis.

Swanson, K. M. (2002). Caring Professional Scale. In J. Watson (Ed.), *Assessing and measuring caring in nursing and health science* (pp. 203-206). New York: Springer.

Journal Articles

Quinn, J., Smith, M., Ritenbaugh, C., & Swanson, K. M. (2003). Research guidelines for assessing the impact of the healing relationship in clinical nursing. *Alternative Therapies, 9*(31), 69-79.

Swanson-Kauffman, K. M. (1981). Echocardiography: An access route to the heart. *Critical Care Nurse, 1*(6), 20-26.

Swanson-Kauffman, K. M. (1986). A combined qualitative methodology for nursing research. *ANS Advances in Nursing Science, 8*(3), 58-69.

Swanson-Kauffman, K. M. (1986). Caring in the instance of unexpected early pregnancy loss. *Topics in Clinical Nursing, 8*(2), 37-46.

Swanson-Kauffman, K. M. (1987). Overview of the balancing act: Having it all. *Health Care for Women International, 8*(2-3), 1-8.

Swanson-Kauffman, K. M. (1988). There should have been two: Nursing care of parents experiencing the perinatal death of a twin. *Journal of Perinatal and Neonatal Nursing, 2*(2), 78-86.

Swanson, K. M. (1990). Providing care in the NICU: Sometimes an act of love. *ANS Advances in Nursing Science, 13*(1), 60-73.

Swanson, K. M. (1991). Empirical development of a middle range theory of caring. *Nursing Research, 40*(3), 161-166.

Swanson, K. M. (1993). Commentary: The phenomena of doing well in people with AIDS. *Western Journal of Nursing Research, 15*(1), 56.

Swanson, K. M. (1993). Nursing as informed caring for the well-being of others. *Image: The Journal of Nursing Scholarship, 25*(4), 352-357.

Swanson, K. M. (1995). Commentary, the power of human caring: Early recognition of patient problems. *Scholarly Inquiry for Nursing Practice, 9*(4), 319-321.

Swanson, K. M. (1998). Caring made visible. *Creative Nursing Journal, 4*(4), 8-11, 16.

Swanson, K. M. (1999). Research-based practice with women who have had miscarriages. *Image: The Journal of Nursing Scholarship, 31*(4) 339-345.

Swanson, K. M. (1999). The effects of caring, measurement, and time on miscarriage impact and women's well-being in the first year subsequent to loss. *Nursing Research, 48*(6), 288-298.

Swanson, K. M. (2000). Predicting depressive symptoms after miscarriage: A path analysis based on Lazarus' paradigm. *Journal of Women's Health & Gender-Based Medicine, 9*(2), 191-206.

Swanson, K. M., Connor, S., Jolley, S., Pettinato, M., & Wang, T. (in revision). Multi-method exploration of women's responses to miscarriage during the first year after loss.

Swanson, K. M., Karmali, Z., Powell, S., & Pulvermakher, F. (2003). Miscarriage effects on couples' interpersonal and sexual relationships during the first year after loss: Women's perceptions. *Psychosomatic Medicine, 65*(5), 902-910.

Swanson, K. M., Shipman, J., Shipman, L., Spoor, L., Taylor, G, Zillyet, K. (in revision). Miscarriage and healing amongst the Shoalwaters tribe: A community-based participatory action research study.

Swanson, K. M., & Wojnar, D. (2004). Optimal healing environments in nursing. *Journal of Alternative and Complementary Medicine, 10*(1), 43-48.

Yorkston, K. M., Klasner, E. R., & Swanson, K. M. (2001). Communication in multiple sclerosis: Understanding the insider's perspective. *American Journal of Speech Language Pathology, 10*, 126-137.

Dissertation

Swanson-Kauffman, K. M. (1983). *The unborn one: A profile of the human experience of miscarriage.*

Unpublished doctoral dissertation, University of Colorado, Denver.

Newsletters and Reprints

Swanson-Kauffman, K. M. (1984, Spring). A methodology for the study of nursing as a human science. *Alpha Kappa Chapter at Large News,* 3.

Swanson-Kauffman, K. M. (1987). Caring in the instance of unexpected early pregnancy loss. *Counselor Connection, 3*(2), 2-5. (Reprint of Swanson-Kauffman, K. M. [1986]. Caring in the instance of unexpected early pregnancy loss. *Topics in Clinical Nursing, 8*[2], 37-46.)

Swanson-Kauffman, K. M. (1988). Miscarriage: An often-overlooked maternal loss. *Perinatal Newsletter, 2*(3), 1.

Published Abstracts

Swanson, K. M. (1993). Caring as intervention (Abstract). *Communicating Nursing Research, 26,* 299.

Swanson, K. M. (1993). Caring theory: Structure and assumptions (Abstract). *Communicating Nursing Research, 26,* 255.

Swanson, K. M. (1995). Effects of caring on healing post miscarriage (Abstract). *Communicating Nursing Research, 28,* 281.

Swanson, K. M., Kieckhefer, G., Henderson, D., Powers, P., Leppa, C. & Carr, K. (1991). Miscarriage: Patterns of meaning (Abstract). *Communicating Nursing Research, 24,* 110.

Swanson, K. M., Kieckhefer, G., Powers, P., & Carr, K. (1990). Meaning of miscarriage scale: Establishment of psychometric properties (Abstract). *Communicating Nursing Research, 23,* 89.

Swanson, K. M., Klaich, K., & Leppa, C. (1992). A caring intervention to promote well-being in women who miscarry (Abstract). *Communicating Nursing Research, 25,* 365.

Swanson, K. M., Pulvermakher, F., Karmali, Z., & Powell, S. (2001). Effects of miscarriage on couple relationships (Abstract). *Communicating Nursing Research, 34,* 339.

Swanson, K. M., Taylor, G., Shipman, L., Spoor K., & Zillyet, K. (2002). Miscarriage and healing amongst the Shoalwater (Abstract). *Communicating Nursing Research, 35,* 135.

Swanson-Kauffman, K. M. (1984). A profile of the human experience of miscarriage (Abstract). *Communicating Nursing Research, 6*(3), 46.

Swanson-Kauffman, K. M. (1985). A combined qualitative methodology for nursing research (Abstract). *Communicating Nursing Research, 18,* 57.

Swanson-Kauffman, K. M. (1985). Miscarriage: A new understanding of the mother's experience. *Proceedings of the 50th anniversary celebration of the University of Pennsylvania School of Nursing,* 63-78.

Swanson-Kauffman, K. M. (1986). Work and family: The delicate balance. Symposium (Abstract). *Communicating Nursing Research, 19,* 153-156.

Swanson-Kauffman, K. M. (1988). Empirical development and refinement of a model of caring (Abstract). *Communicating Nursing Research, 21,* 80.

Swanson-Kauffman, K. M. (1989). From phenomenological to experimental design: Qualitative inquiry as a framework for the intervention (Abstract). *Communicating Nursing Research, 22,* 147.

Swanson-Kauffman, K. M., Powers, P., Klaich, K., Lethbridge, D. & Jarrett, M. (1990). Success: As women view it (Abstract). *Communicating Nursing Research, 23,* 59.

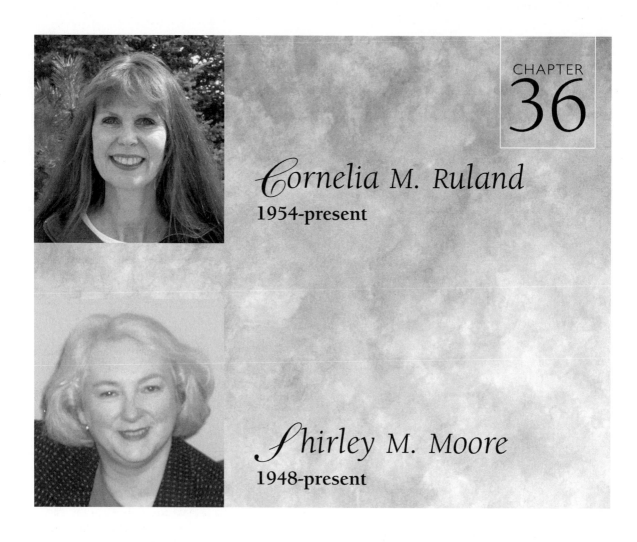

Cornelia M. Ruland

1954-present

Shirley M. Moore

1948-present

Peaceful End of Life Theory

Patricia A. Higgins

CREDENTIALS AND BACKGROUND OF THE THEORISTS

Cornelia M. Ruland

Cornelia M. Ruland received her Ph.D. in nursing from Case Western Reserve University, Cleveland, Ohio, in 1998. She is now the Director of the Center for Shared Decision Making and Nursing Research at Rikshospitalet University Hospital in Oslo, Norway. She also holds an appointment as adjunct faculty at the Department of Biomedical Informatics at Columbia University in New York. Ruland has established an extensive research program on improving shared decision making and patient-provider partnerships in health care, and the development, implementation, and evaluation of information systems to support it. Her focus is on aspects of and tools for shared decision making in clinically challenging situations: (1) when patients are confronted with difficult treatment or screening decisions for which they need help to understand the potential benefits and harms of alternative options and elicit their values and preferences and (2) preference-adjusted management of chronic or serious long-term illness over time. Ruland has been the primary investigator on a number of research projects and received several awards for her work.

The author wishes to express her appreciation to Cornelia Ruland and Shirley Moore for their contributions to the chapter.

Shirley M. Moore

Shirley M. Moore is Associate Dean for Research and Professor, School of Nursing, Case Western Reserve University. She received her diploma in nursing from the Youngstown Hospital Association School of Nursing (1969) and her bachelor's degree in nursing from Kent State University (1974). At Case Western Reserve University she earned a master's degree in psychiatric and mental health nursing (1990) as well as a Ph.D. in nursing science (1993). She has taught nursing theory and nursing science to all levels of nursing students and conducts a program of research and theory development that addresses recovery after cardiac events. Early in her own doctoral study, Moore was encouraged by nurse theorists Joyce J. Fitzpatrick, Jean Johnson, and Elizabeth Lenz not only to use theory but to develop theory as well. The Rosemary Ellis Theory Conference held annually for several years at Case Western Reserve University offered Moore another opportunity to explore theory as a practical tool for practitioners, researchers, and teachers. Influenced by these experiences, Moore has assisted in the development and publication of several theories (Good & Moore, 1996; Huth & Moore, 1998; Ruland & Moore, 1998) and has considered theory construction a skill essential to doctoral students.

THEORETICAL SOURCES

The Peaceful End of Life (EOL) Theory is informed by a number of theoretical frameworks. It is based primarily on Donabedian's classic model of structure, process, and outcomes (Ruland & Moore, 1998) which, in part, was developed from the grand theory of general systems. The influence of general systems theory is pervasive in all levels of nursing theory, from conceptual models to middle and microrange theories, an indicator of its usefulness in explaining the complexity of health care interactions and organizations. In the EOL theory, the structure-setting is the family system (terminally ill patient and all significant others) that is receiving care from professionals on an acute care hospital unit, and process is defined as those actions (nursing interventions) designed to promote the positive outcomes of the following: (1) being free from pain, (2) experiencing comfort, (3) experiencing dignity and respect, (4) being at peace, and (5) experiencing a closeness to significant others and those who care.

A second theoretical underpinning is that of preference theory (Brandt, 1979), used in part by philosophers to explain and define quality of life (Sandoe, 1999), a concept that is significant in EOL research and practice. In preference theory, the good life is defined as getting what one wants, an approach that seems particularly appropriate in EOL care. It can be applied to both sentient persons and to incapacitated persons who have previously provided documentation related to EOL decision making. Quality of life, therefore, can be evaluated as a manifestation of satisfaction through empirical assessment of such outcomes as symptom relief and satisfaction with interpersonal relationships. Incorporating patient preferences into health care decisions is considered both appropriate (Ruland & Bakken, 2001; Ruland, Kresevic, & Lorensen, 1997) and necessary for successful processes and outcomes (Ruland & Moore, 2001).

This theory was derived in a very pragmatic way. It happened in a doctoral theory course in which Ruland was a student and Moore was the faculty. Middle range theories were just emerging, and there were few good definitions or examples. The class was challenged to think about the future use and development of middle range theory for nursing science and practice. The students discussed knowledge sources from which they could derive middle range theory, such as empirical knowledge, clinical practice knowledge, and synthesized knowledge. Each student was asked to derive a middle range theory from a knowledge source of choice. Ruland had just completed a major project to develop a clinical practice standard for peaceful EOL with a group of cancer nurses in Norway. The standard was synthesized into the theory of peaceful EOL by Ruland and later refined with Moore's assistance. This theory became one of the earliest examples of use of a standard of practice as a source for middle range theory development.

MAJOR CONCEPTS *&* DEFINITIONS

NOT BEING IN PAIN

Being free of the suffering or symptom distress is the central part of many patients' EOL experience. Pain is considered an unpleasant sensory or emotional experience associated with actual or potential tissue damage (Lenz, Suppe, Gift, Pugh, & Milligan, 1995; Pain terms, 1979).

EXPERIENCE OF COMFORT

Comfort is defined inclusively, using Kolcaba and Kolcaba's (1991) work as "relief from discomfort, the state of ease and peaceful contentment, and whatever makes life easy or pleasurable" (Ruland & Moore, 1998, p. 172).

MAJOR CONCEPTS *&* DEFINITIONS—cont'd

EXPERIENCE OF DIGNITY AND RESPECT

Each terminally ill patient is "respected and valued as a human being" (Ruland & Moore, 1998, p. 172). This concept incorporates the idea of personal worth, as expressed by the ethical principle of autonomy or respect for persons, which states that individuals should be treated as autonomous agents, and persons with diminished autonomy are entitled to protection (United States, 1978).

BEING AT PEACE

Peace is a "feeling of calmness, harmony, and contentment, (free of) anxiety, restlessness, worries, and fear" (Ruland & Moore, 1998, p. 172). A peaceful state includes physical, psychological, and spiritual dimensions.

CLOSENESS TO SIGNIFICANT OTHERS

Closeness is "the feeling of connectedness to other human beings who care" (Ruland & Moore, 1998, p. 172). It involves a physical or emotional nearness that is expressed through warm, intimate relationships.

USE OF EMPIRICAL EVIDENCE

The theory of peaceful EOL is based on empirical evidence coming from both direct experience of expert nurses and a thorough review of the literature addressing several components of the theory. The group of expert practitioners who developed the standard of care for peaceful EOL had at least 5 years of clinical experience caring for terminally ill patients. The standard of care consisted of best practices based on research-derived evidence in the areas of pain management, comfort, nutrition, and relaxation. This prescriptive theory comprises several proposed relational statements for which more empirical evidence is needed, as well. Importantly, explicit hypotheses can be derived easily from these relational statements to be tested for their usefulness. It should be noted that the authors (both of the standard of care and the resulting theory) attempted to incorporate clearly described, observable concepts and relationships that express the notion of caring.

MAJOR ASSUMPTIONS
Nursing, Person, Environment, and Health

Because the theory of peaceful EOL was derived from standards of care written by a team of expert nurses who were addressing a practice problem, the metaparadigm concepts were inherent in the nursing phenomena addressed, the complex and holistic care required to support peaceful EOL.

The two identified assumptions of Ruland and Moore's (1998) theory are as follows:
1. The occurrences and feelings at the EOL experience are personal and individualized.
2. Nursing care is crucial for creating a peaceful EOL experience. Nurses assess and interpret cues that reflect the person's EOL experience and intervene appropriately to attain or maintain a peaceful experience, even when the dying person cannot communicate verbally.

Following are two additional, implicit assumptions:
1. Family, a term that includes all significant others, is an important part of EOL care.
2. The goal of EOL care is not to optimize care, in the sense that it must be the best, most technologically advanced treatment, a type of care that frequently results in overtreatment. Rather, the goal in EOL care is to maximize treatment; that is, best possible care will be provided through the judicious use of technology and comfort measures, in order to enhance quality of life and achieve a peaceful death.

THEORETICAL ASSERTIONS

Ruland and Moore (1998) identified six explicit relational statements (theoretical assertions) for their theory, as follows:

1. Monitoring and administering pain relief and applying pharmacologic and nonpharmacologic interventions contribute to the patient's experience of not being in pain.
2. Preventing, monitoring and relieving physical discomfort, facilitating rest, relaxation, and contentment, and preventing complications contribute to the patient's experience of comfort.
3. Including the patient and significant others in decision making regarding patient care, treating the patient with dignity, empathy and respect, and being attentive to the patient's expressed needs, wishes, and preferences contribute to the patient's experience of dignity and respect.
4. Providing emotional support, monitoring and meeting the patient's expressed needs for antianxiety medications, inspiring trust, providing the patient and significant others with guidance in practical issues, and providing physical presence of another caring person if desired contribute to the patient's experience of being at peace.
5. Facilitating participation of significant others in patient care, attending to significant other's grief, worries, and questions, and facilitating opportunities for family closeness contribute to the patient's experience of closeness to significant others or persons who care.
6. The patient's experiences of not being in pain, comfort, dignity, and respect, being at peace, closeness to significant others or persons who care contribute to the peaceful end of life. (p. 174)

LOGICAL FORM

The Peaceful EOL Theory was developed using both inductive and deductive methodology. A unique feature of the theory is its development from a standard of care. The peaceful EOL standard was created by expert nurses in response to a lack of direction for managing the complex care of terminally ill patients. The standard was developed for the surgical gastroenterological care unit in a university hospital in Norway. Thus, the standard served as a logical intermediary step between practice and theory. Standards of care are intended to serve as credible, authoritative statements that describe a practitioner's roles and responsibilities and an expected performance or level of nursing care by which the quality of practice can be evaluated (AACN, 1998). In this instance of knowledge development, the standard of care can be considered an interim step that effectively links clinical practice to theory.

For their theory, Ruland and Moore (2001) detailed the steps in the development of the standard for peaceful EOL, which included a review of the relevant literature and clarification of important concepts (deductive methodology) and the incorporation of clinical experience (inductive methodology). All of these steps are analogous to those used in theory development. The levels of the standard closely parallel the nursing process (assess, identify goals [outcomes], plan, implement, evaluate), which are analogous to the system functioning in Donabedian's structure-process-outcome theory. Thus, the logic of the development of this theory is straightforward and congruent.

ACCEPTANCE BY THE NURSING COMMUNITY
Practice

Two review articles cited the Peaceful EOL Theory. Liehr and Smith (1999) refer to the theory's development of a practice standard as a foundation for developing theory, and in the second article, Baggs and Schmitt (2000) discuss the potential usefulness of the theory as a means to improve EOL decision making for critically ill adults.

Education

No published reports were located describing use of this theory for education.

Research

No published reports were located describing use of this theory for research investigations. The theory's relatively recent publication may partially explain this gap in the literature. Additionally, neither author is currently using the theory as part of her research program, but both report that they routinely receive inquires about using the theory, particularly from graduate students.

FURTHER DEVELOPMENT

The Peaceful EOL Theory is a new theory that used an original source and, as such, Ruland and Moore acknowledge that it needs further refinement and development. A number of steps could be used to advance its development. One would be to test relationships among the five major concepts. To do this most economically, one could consider merging some of the process criteria from three of the concepts (pain, comfort, peace), creating a single concept related to physical-psychological symptom management. Concept analysis or mapping could be used to determine if some of the process criteria associated with the three concepts are sufficiently alike to allow merging. For instance, for the concept of pain, two process criteria (monitoring and administering pain relief and applying pharmacological and nonpharmacological interventions) are closely related to the comfort process criterion (preventing, monitoring, and relieving physical discomfort) and the peace process criterion (monitoring and meeting patient's needs for antianxiety medication). Nonpharmacological interventions (e.g., music, humor, or relaxation) that serve to distract a dying patient are useful for the relief of pain, anxiety, and general physical discomfort. This revision would also serve to link the Peaceful EOL Theory to the middle range theories of Good and Moore (1996), Good (1998), and Lenz and colleagues (Lenz, Pugh, Milligan, Gift, & Suppe, 1997; Lenz et al., 1995).

CRITIQUE
Clarity

All elements of the theory are stated clearly, including the setting, assumptions, and concepts and relational statements. These concepts vary considerably in their level of abstraction, from the more concrete (pain and comfort) to the more abstract (dignity).

Simplicity

Despite its uncomplicated terms and clear expression of ideas, the theory is one of the higher level middle range theories (Higgins & Moore, 2000), primarily because of the level of abstraction of the outcome criteria and the multidimensional complexity expressed in its relational statements.

Generality

The Peaceful EOL Theory has specific boundaries related to time, setting, and patient population. It was developed for use with terminally ill adults and their families who are receiving care in an acute care setting. The concept of peaceful EOL came from a Norwegian context and, thus, may not be appropriate for all cultures. Nevertheless, its concepts and relationships resonate with many nurses and it comprehensively addresses the multidimensional aspects of EOL care. For example, the outcome indicators associated with the five concepts address the technical aspect of care (providing both pharmacological and nonpharmacological interventions for the relief of symptoms), communication (decision making), the psychological aspect (emotional support), and dignity and respect (treating the patient with dignity, empathy, and respect) (Figure 36-1).

Empirical Precision

The deductive and inductive logic used to develop this theory provides a solid basis for developing testable hypotheses among the five concepts of the theory. Theoretical congruency is demonstrated through the outcome indicators, all of which are

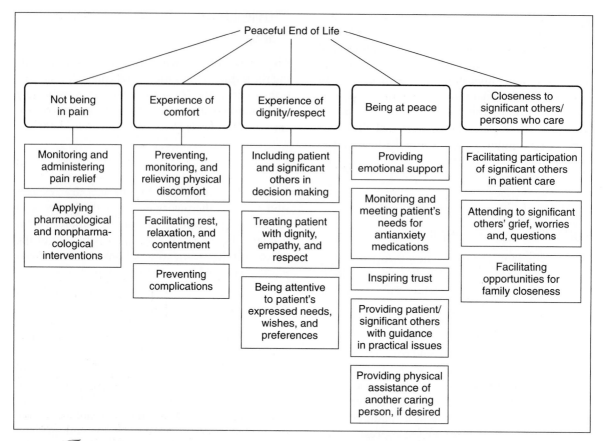

Figure **36-1** Relationships among the concepts of the Peaceful End of Life Theory.
(From Ruland, C. M., & Moore, S. M. (1998). Theory construction based on standards of care: A proposed theory of the peaceful end of life. *Nursing Outlook, 46*(4), 174.)

conceptualized from the perspective of the patients and their families.

Derivable Consequences

As a successful synthesis of clinical practice and scholarly theory development, the Peaceful EOL Theory is a framework, the development of which illustrates one way to bridge the theory-practice-research continuum. In addition to an identified need for a comprehensive middle range theory related to the EOL experience, Ruland and Moore (2001) developed it to illustrate the richness of practice as a source for the development of theory.

All of the outcome indicators are measurable, using qualitative or quantitative methodology or both (see Figure 36-1). Unlike some middle range theories, which have a specific instrument that measures a major concept, no particular instrument was developed, nor is required, for the Peaceful EOL Theory. Given the diversity and scope of the five concepts, multiple instruments would be needed to measure hypothesized relationships among the concepts. Mixed methods (Tashakkori & Teddlie, 2003) is a particularly appealing approach for measuring the concepts. For example, phenomenological methodology could be used to investigate patient and family perceptions of their opportunities for (and satisfaction with) family closeness or decision making or both. On the other hand, a number of existing instruments could be used to measure the outcome indicators associated with the five concepts (see Figure 36-1). For example, patient perception of symptoms could be measured by the Memorial Symptom Assessment Scale (Portenoy, Thaler, Kornblith, Lepore, Friedlander-Klar, et al., 1994) or the general comfort questionnaire developed by Kolcaba (2003).

Case Study

Mrs. Smith has been admitted to the oncology ward in the terminal stage of cancer. She is no longer conscious. She has indicated that she wants no heroic measures to save her life. There is discussion about starting intravenous fluids and tube feeding. There is a great deal of dissension among family members. Describe how the Peaceful EOL Theory will help you develop, implement, and evaluate appropriate nursing interventions.

CRITICAL THINKING *Activities*

1. Using professional practice standards from a national nursing organization, evaluate the correspondence of the concept "experience of dignity and respect" with the organization's standard(s) related to ethics. Discuss both similarities and differences related to relevance, significance, scope, usefulness, and adequacy.

2. Consider a clinical experience in which there is a great deal of dissension among family members of a terminally ill patient. Describe how the Peaceful EOL Theory will help you develop, implement, and evaluate appropriate nursing interventions. What are the theory's limitations?

3. Focusing on the concept "closeness to significant others," develop an evaluation

plan to assess the quality and effectiveness of care.

REFERENCES

American Association of Critical Care Nurses (AACN). (1998). *Standards for acute and critical care nursing practice.* Aliso Viejo, CA: AACN. Retrieved December 1, 2004, from *http://www.aacn.org/AACN/practice.nsf/ ad0ca3b3bdb4f33288256981006fa692/ 5e3c9805e57b3b0888256a6b00791f35*

Baggs, J. G., & Schmitt, M. H. (2000). End-of-life decisions in adult intensive care: Current research base 158 and directions for the future. *Nursing Outlook, 48*(4), 158-164.

Brandt, R. B. (1979). *A theory of the good and the right.* Oxford: Clarendon Press.

Good, M. (1998). A middle-range theory of acute pain management: Use in research. *Nursing Outlook, 46*(3), 120-124.

Good, M., & Moore, S. M. (1996). Clinical practice guidelines as a new source of middle-range theory: Focus on acute pain. *Nursing Outlook, 44*(2), 74-79.

Higgins, P. A., & Moore, S. M. (2000). Levels of theoretical thinking in nursing. *Nursing Outlook, 48*(4), 179-183.

Huth, M. M., & Moore, S. M. (1998). Prescriptive theory of acute pain management in infants and children. *Journal of the Society of Pediatric Nurses, 3*(1), 23-32.

Kolcaba, K. (2003). *Comfort theory and practice: A vision for holistic health care and research.* New York: Springer.

Kolcaba, K. Y., & Kolcaba, R. J. (1991). An analysis of the concept of comfort. *Journal of Advanced Nursing, 16*(11), 1301-1310.

Lenz, E. R., Pugh, L. C., Milligan, R. A., Gift, A., & Suppe, F. (1997). The middle-range theory of unpleasant symptoms: An update. *ANS Advances in Nursing Science, 19*(3), 14-27.

Lenz, E. R., Suppe, F., Gift, A. G., Pugh, L. C., & Milligan, R. A. (1995). Collaborative development of middle-range nursing theories: Toward a theory of unpleasant symptoms. *ANS Advances in Nursing Science, 17*(3), 1-13.

Liehr, P., & Smith, M. J. (1999). Middle range theory: Spinning research and practice to create knowledge for the new millennium. *ANS Advances in Nursing Science, 21*(4), 81-91.

Pain terms: A list with definitions and notes on usage. Recommended by the IASP Subcommittee on Taxonomy. (1979). *Pain, 6*(3), 249.

Portenoy, R. K., Thaler, H. T., Kornblith, A. B., Lepore, J. M., Friedlander-Klar, H., Coyle, N., et al. (1994). The Memorial Symptom Assessment Scale: An instrument for the evaluation of symptom prevalence, characteristics and distress. *European Journal of Cancer, 30A(9),* 1326-1336.

Ruland, C. M., & Bakken, S. (2001). Representing patient preference-related concepts for inclusion in electronic health records. *Journal of Biomedical Informatics, 34(6),* 415-422.

Ruland, C. M., Kresevic, D., & Lorensen, M. (1997). Including patient preferences in nurses' assessment of older patients. *Journal of Clinical Nursing, 6(6),* 495-504.

Ruland, C. M., & Moore, S. M. (1998). Theory construction based on standards of care: A proposed theory of the peaceful end of life. *Nursing Outlook, 46(4),* 169-175.

Ruland, C. M., & Moore, S. M. (2001). Eliciting exercise preferences in cardiac rehabilitation: Initial evaluation of a new strategy. *Patient Education and Counseling, 44(3),* 283-291.

Sandoe, P. (1999). Quality of life—Three competing views. *Ethical Theory and Moral Practice, 2(1),* 11-23.

Tashakkori, A., & Teddlie, C., (2003). *Handbook of mixed methods in social & behavioral research.* Thousand Oaks, CA: Sage.

United States, National Commission for the Protection of Human Subjects of Biomedical and Behavioral Research. (1978). *The Belmont report: Ethical principles and guidelines for the protection of human subjects of research* (Bethesda, MD). Washington, DC: The Commission. For sale by the Superintendent of Documents, U. S. Government Printing Office.

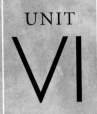

UNIT

VI

Future of Nursing Theory

- Theoretical systems are active and give direction to future research studies and administrative, educational, and practice applications.

- Theoretical works developed in a discipline affect the nature of the questions asked, the methods used to answer the questions, and the scope of knowledge addressed.

- Nursing models and theories exhibit characteristics of Kuhn's criteria for normal science; that is, a scientific community uses research based on scientific achievements as the foundation of practice.

- Expansion of philosophy of nursing science has increased the use of qualitative theory development in addition to quantitative methods and has greatly increased the development and use of middle range theories.

- Global communities of nurse scholars have emerged as a result of the expanded communication opportunities on the Internet.

State of the Art and Science of Nursing Theory

Martha Raile Alligood

From studying this text, it becomes obvious that the nursing theoretical works are active and growing as they point the way to future research studies and educational, administrative, and practice applications. Reviews of earlier editions of this text have been given careful consideration in the production of this sixth edition (Burns, 1999; Malinski, 1999; Reed, 1999). For example, inclusion of middle range theories continues to expand, with even more new middle range theories added to the theoretical works included. As Burns (1999) commented, "the more recent interest in middle range theories is seen as the result of an evolving understanding of theoretic thought and the growing recognition of the potential impact of theory on nursing practice" (p. 263). The authors responded to her suggestion that the middle range theory section be expanded and new chapters of that nature are included in this sixth edition. Furthermore, theory development and theory use is expanding at such a rapid rate that new nursing theoretical works have been added to every section of the text. Examples are

Martinsen's Philosophy of Caring in Chapter 10, Boykin and Schoenhofer's theory of Nursing Caring in Chapter 19, the Husteds' Symphonological Bioethical Theory in Chapter 26, and Reed's middle range Self-Transcendence Theory in Chapter 29.

The references of this text have been identified consistently as a major strength of the earlier editions. Malinski (1999) has said, "they provide a valuable resource for students" (p. 265). The references and the chapters are updated with each successive edition, reflecting the expansion of the literature as more and more nurses are coming to a working understanding of theory-based nursing for professional practice. Although theories are interesting to individuals as they learn the many unique ways that one can think about nursing, theories are more than just a unique creation to contemplate. Rather, they are vital for nurses to guide research, education, and administration and to know and apply in nursing practice (Alligood & Marriner Tomey, 1997, 2002, 2006). This becomes even more important as the number of nursing theoretical works increases. In this sixth edition, in order to deal with the growing body of nursing theoretical works and not wanting to eliminate significant theorists included in earlier editions, a new chapter has been created. Some of the early theorists have been grouped together noting their historical significance (see Chapter 5).

Reed (1999) was astute to observe that, "the book supports the momentum building within nursing to transcend the tired debate about the relevance of nursing models and apply this field of knowledge as a basis for understanding the substance and scholarship of nursing" (p. 268). In this sixth edition, our goal was to clarify the relevance of the nursing theoretical works, facilitate their recognition as systematic presentations of nursing substance, and stimulate their use as knowledge-building tools for future contributions to nursing scholarship and nursing science for practice, research, education, and administration. The theoretical works developed within a discipline determine the nature of the questions that are asked by the discipline, the methods of research used to answer the questions, and the scope of knowledge the questions address. How might nurses explore the state of the art and science of nursing theory? The answer to that question is found in the nursing literature from around the world that documents the use of nursing theoretical works.

This chapter addresses the continuing growth of nursing theory, followed by a discussion of the shift in the philosophy of nursing science and its impact resulting in theory development with both qualitative approaches and quantitative methods. Nursing theory is viewed in its new growth, as well as from a postmodern philosophical view that encourages reframing knowledge in a new light within an understanding of today (Morris, 2000). Morris (2000) suggests that the challenge implicit in this era, "is to understand our postmodern moment in ways that illuminate the current experience . . ." as "the postmodern era often co-opts or revises rather than reject outright the achievements of modernism . . ." (p. 8). Finally, the global nature of the appreciation of nursing theoretical works is presented by pointing to the growing bodies of communities of scholars, highlighting significant growth in selected organizations, and reminding the reader of the vital

nature of theory for the profession, discipline, and science.

NATURE OF NORMAL SCIENCE

Many of the nursing models and some theories included in this text have developed such that they exhibit characteristics of Kuhn's (1970) criteria for normal science (Wood & Alligood, 2002). Increasingly over the past 25 years, the conceptual models of nursing and nursing theories as presented by Fawcett (1984, 1989, 1993, 1995, 2000), Fitzpatrick and Whall (1984, 1989, 1996), George (1985, 1986, 1989, 1995, 2002), Meleis (1985, 1991, 1997, 2004), Marriner Tomey (1986, 1989, 1994) and, more recently, Alligood and Marriner Tomey (1997, 2002, 2006), McEwen and Wills (2002), Marriner Tomey and Alligood (1998, 2002, 2006), and Parker (2001) have led to paradigm-based education, administration, research, and practice. The communities of scholars continue to grow, becoming more formally organized as groups, addressing deeper questions, and sharing knowledge generated from their research and practice in newsletters and journals. Nursing models and theories provide nurses with perspectives of the central concepts of the discipline: person, environment, health, and nursing, known as the metaparadigm of nursing (Fawcett, 1984). Indeed, reference to these concepts as central to the discipline of nursing has such wide acceptance that they now commonly appear in print without a reference, evidence of consensus.

The theoretical works generate scholarship as frameworks for research projects and guides for decision making for theory-based nursing practice. Work within the communities of scholars that have formed around the models and theories has led to the development of many new research instruments unique to that perspective. Kuhn (1970) stated, "History suggests that the road to a firm research consensus is extraordinarily arduous" (p. 15). Conceptual models of nursing or "paradigms gain their status by being more successful than their competitors in solving a few problems that the group of practitioners have come to recognize as acute" (Kuhn, 1970, p. 23).

Kuhn (1970) defines normal science as "research firmly based upon one or more past scientific achievements, achievements that some particular scientific community acknowledges for a time as supplying the foundation for its further practice" (p. 10). Therefore, the characteristics of paradigms that give evidence of their nature and lead to normal science include a community of scholars who base their research and practice on the paradigm, the formation of specialized journals, the foundation of specialists' societies, and the claim for a special place in curricula (Kuhn, 1970). Each of the conceptual models of nursing included in this text have met these criteria. Each model is unique, so some have made more progress in certain of the criteria than others. For example, Rogers' Science of Unitary Human Beings (see Chapter 13) has generated numerous research studies, 13 research instruments, and 12 nursing process clinical tools for nursing practice (Fawcett, 2000; Fawcett & Alligood, 2001). In the mid-1980s, a community of scholars organized to form The Society of Rogerian Scholars. The organization supports a quarterly newsletter and a refereed journal, *Visions: The Journal of Rogerian Nursing Science,* to facilitate communication among the membership and foster the development of the science. There are many Rogerian texts, and Rogerian science has been used to structure curricula for undergraduate and graduate nursing programs. In 2002, the Society of Rogerian Scholars celebrated the accomplishments of the organization at their fall conference in Richmond: 20 years of Rogerian conferences, the 15-year anniversary for the society, and 10 years of publishing their journal.

Other conceptual models of nursing that have experienced similar growth are Orem's Self-Care Deficit Theory (see Chapter 14), the Neuman Systems Model (see Chapter 16), and Roy's Adaptation Model (see Chapter 17). Some nursing theories also exhibit characteristics of normal science, such as Erickson, Tomlin, and Swain's Theory of Modeling and Role-Modeling (see Chapter 25), Leininger's Theory of Culture Care (see Chapter 22), Parse's Theory of Human Becoming (see Chapter 24), and Margaret Newman's Theory of Health as Expanding Consciousness (see Chapter 23). Societies of nursing scholars keep increasing, and the volume of articles they publish from their research and practice is growing exponentially.

EXPANSION OF THEORY DEVELOPMENT

Johnson and Webber (2001) conclude their text on theory and reasoning in nursing with a chapter titled "The Impact of Theory on the Future of Nursing" (p. 215). In that chapter they ask the following three questions:

1. "Why is the development of theory important for the recognition of nursing as a profession?" (p. 220)
2. "Why is the development of theory important for the recognition of nursing as a discipline?" (p. 221)
3. "Why is the development of theory important for the recognition of nursing as a science?" (p. 227)

They identify the three significant areas affected by nursing knowledge and dependent on its continued development. Theory affects the recognition of nursing as a profession, a discipline, and a science. However, the future existence of nursing is dependent on the use of substantive nursing knowledge not just for recognition, but also to improve the quality of care to the patients whom we serve in the practice of nursing. Moving the practice of nursing to a professional delivery model requires movement beyond the vocational style that many nurses have been taught and to which they continue to cling. Nursing knowledge is the systematic presentation of nursing. That knowledge is what is transferred to those coming into the profession. Academe understands the importance of substance as a requirement in any field of learning. As more and more nurses work their way past "the tired debate about the relevance of nursing models and apply this field of knowledge as a basis for understanding the substance and scholarship of nursing" (p. 268), as Reed (1999) has suggested, nursing science will serve its purpose, improve the quality of care to those we serve and, yes, nursing will be recognized.

As a discipline, nursing has eagerly embraced qualitative research approaches to explore questions that quantitative research could not answer, and this expansion in philosophy of nursing science has resulted in qualitative theory development (Alligood, 2002; Alligood & May, 2000; Liehr & Smith, 1999; Smith & Liehr, 2003; Thorne, Kirkham, & MacDonald-Emes, 1997; Thorne, Kirkham, & O'Flynn-Magee, 2004). Concomitantly, the use of conceptual models of nursing and nursing theories has led to a greater understanding and expansion of the development of middle range or practice theory (Alligood, 2002b, 2002c). The open, freestyle thinking of contemporary postmodern philosophy has led to reconsideration of the wealth of knowledge in the early nursing theoretical writings (Alligood, 2002, 2004; Alligood & Fawcett, 1999; Alligood & May, 2000; Butcher, 1999). Early publications of the theorists are rich resources for interpreting new theory, such as the theory of nursing empathy discovered in King's Interacting Systems Framework (Alligood & May, 2000). Middle range theory has been defined as the "least abstract set of related concepts that propose a truth specific to the details of nursing practice" (Alligood & Marriner Tomey, 2002, p. 485). More recently, growth has occurred in development of nursing theories and middle range theories. This development is especially exciting because it clarifies the elusive practice theory that nurses have sought for so long (Alligood, 2002b). Liehr and Smith (1999) explored the nature of middle range theories in the nursing literature from 1988 to 1998 and identified 24 middle range theories. They noted that theory-generating approaches used to develop the 24 middle range theories were both quantitative and qualitative methods. Smith and Liehr (2003) have published their method of middle range theory development in a text. Although some have noted the shortfall of some middle range theories not being grounded or anchored in nursing science, their contributions outweigh this concern. The processes of science bring about necessary corrections over time as the whip lines in Chinn and Kramer's (2004) work has emphasized from the beginning.

Although the dialogue continues in the nursing literature about the myriad ways scholars classify the nursing theoretical works, it is important to remember that each work is unique and, therefore, any attempt to classify them uniformly is arbitrary at best and calls for judgment on the part of the person doing the classifying. Rather than focusing on classification of the works, a more useful emphasis would be on knowing the individual works, teaching them to students, and using them for the improvement of the professional practice of nursing.

Middle range theories and their use in nursing practice are encouraged for improving the quality of nursing practice whether developed quantitatively or qualitatively, because both are at the level of nursing practice. Rather than focus on the methodology, there is need to explore the relationship of the knowledge produced from both of these methods and approaches. Although they address different kinds of questions, all of the questions, whether studied with quantitative methods or qualitative approaches, are specific to nursing and generate nursing knowledge. Consideration of nursing theoretical works in relation to a generic structure of knowledge reveals that theory from the hypothetical-deductive method and theory from qualitative approaches eventually meet at a similar level of abstraction, that of middle range theory. However, they arrive there by different methods (Figure 37-1). Considering nursing knowledge in a generic structure moves discussions forward beyond the research method debates and theory classification disagreements to a focus on the knowledge or content of nursing science. It is helpful to understand that middle range theories are at various levels of abstraction within that category, just as all of the theoretical works in the other type classifications (philosophies, models, grand theories, and theories) have similarities and differences and vary in level of abstraction. Middle range theories are recognizable because they include the specifics of practice, such as the situation or health condition of the patient, patient population or age group, location of the patient or area of practice, and action of the nurse or intervention and the proposed outcome (Alligood, 2002a). Middle range theories are also developed by exploring and interpreting aspects of the lived experience of persons with a goal of

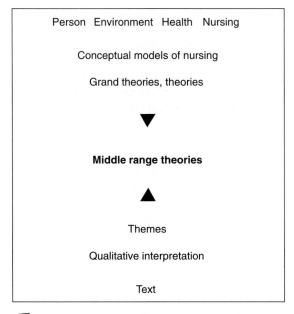

Person Environment Health Nursing

Conceptual models of nursing

Grand theories, theories

▼

Middle range theories

▲

Themes

Qualitative interpretation

Text

Figure **37-1** Middle range theory in a generic structure of nursing knowledge from quantitative research methods and qualitative research approaches. (Data from Fawcett, J. [2000]. *Contemporary nursing knowledge: Nursing models and theories.* Philadelphia: F. A. Davis.)

understanding the meaning of life events in relation to health and nursing.

GLOBAL COMMUNITIES OF NURSING SCHOLARS

In addition to the growth stimulated by a broader philosophy of nursing science, expansion of research methods and approaches, and the emergence of middle range theories, another major contribution to the state of the art and science of nursing theory is the global nature of communities of nurse scholars and their communication and information possibilities via the Internet. Most of the communities of scholars organized around the conceptual models of nursing have international memberships or organizations in their own countries. For example, the Orem organization is The International Orem

Society. It was founded in 1990 and sponsors biannual conferences in the United States and in other countries. The sixth conference was held in Bangkok, Thailand, in 2000. The 2002 conference was held in the United States in Atlanta, and the 8th Orem conference in 2004 was in Ulm, Germany. The International Orem Society has a semi-annual newsletter, maintains a Web site, and has recently launched a database, *Self-Care, Deficit Care, and Nursing.*

Similarly, the theme for the Eighth Biennial International Neuman Systems Model Symposium in 2001 was "Neuman Systems Model: Local to Global Connections." Among the attendees at the Ninth Biennial International Neuman Systems Model Symposium held in Philadelphia in 2003 were nine nurses from Holland, who explained that the Neuman model had been accepted as the framework for the delivery of nursing care in their country. This has come about largely through global communication with nurses on the Internet, increased possibilities for worldwide travel, and the publication of nursing theory textbooks in many languages. Nurses around the world are embracing nursing theory. For example, the second edition of *Nursing Theorists and Their Work* (Marriner Tomey, 1989) was translated into Italian, German, Finnish, and Japanese; the third edition (Marriner Tomey, 1994) was translated into Italian and Japanese; and the fifth edition (Marriner Tomey & Alligood, 2002) was translated and published in Spanish in 2003. This text is also distributed widely in English-speaking countries such as Canada, the United Kingdom, Australia, and New Zealand. The first edition of our other text, *Nursing Theory: Utilization and Application* (Alligood & Marriner Tomey, 1997), was translated and published in 2001 in classical Chinese, which is Taiwanese. Both texts have maintained consistent international circulations.

In consideration of this topic of global interest in conceptual models of nursing and nursing theory, reviewing the PubMed database for nursing theory articles in Spanish, French, and German verified the international use of nursing models and theories originating in the United States and identified theory development contributions from other countries using both quantitative and qualitative approaches.

The German publications numbered 164 and included articles based on work by Rogers, Orem, King, Leininger, and Erickson, Tomlin, and Swain, as well as qualitatively developed middle range theories. A nursing model, developed by Kappeli (1999) of the Department of Health of the State of Zurich in Switzerland, has been introduced in five Swiss hospitals (Anderregg-Tschudin, 1999). Kappeli (1999) presented at the symposium on nursing science at the University of Basel, examining the requirements for nursing science for the nursing service of a university hospital, and she concluded that nursing science is compatible with the ethos and goals of the nursing profession. The Spanish literature included 13 nursing theory articles referring to Orem, Peplau, and Henderson studies. The French literature included 94 nursing theory articles about the work of Orem, King, Rogers, Roy, Neuman, and Pender. These are only a few examples of the global use of nursing theory. We have included the theoretical work of Evelyn Adam, who is Canadian (see Chapter 5), since the first edition of this text and we added the work of Roper, Logan, and Tierney (see Chapter 5), who are nurse theorists from Scotland, with the nursing conceptual models in the fourth edition. Katie Eriksson is from Finland, and her work, philosophical theory on caring, is included in this sixth edition (see Chapter 11).

The development of global consciousness has arrived, as is evident because nursing articles from around the world are being shared in nursing journals in the United States and abroad. The development of Sigma Theta Tau International has been a part of this rapid expansion through their publications which embrace nursing worldwide. As the Internet facilitates communication among nurses around the world, more nurses are exposed to and share scientific knowledge at the professional level. For example, American nurses are publishing in a new peer-reviewed journal in Sweden, *Theoria: Journal of Nursing Theory*. It is published in English and is sponsored by the Swedish Society for Nursing Theories in Practice, Education, and Research.

Similarly, *Nursing Science Quarterly* has a regular global feature from countries such as Canada, Australia, New Zealand, England, Japan, Sweden, Korea, Germany, Turkey, and Taiwan.

Several general nursing theory Web sites have appeared, such as the Nursing Theory Page offered by Valdosta State University, College of Nursing; the Nursing Theory Link Page maintained by Clayton College and State University Department of Nursing; and the Nursing Theory Page that originally was designed and maintained by nursing faculty at University of Alberta in Edmonton, Canada. The latter is now maintained by the school of nursing at the University of San Diego in California. It is outstanding, because it links to home pages or Web sites for most theorists and their work. Another wonderfully informative site is the Australian nurses' site where nursing theory is number 1 in their list of top issues. Their site includes work from nursing theorists from around the world.

In conclusion, the state of the art and science of nursing theory is one of mushrooming growth. First, nursing theoretical works are used by communities of scholars who collaborate for the development of nursing science with a particular paradigm, and the nursing science that many are producing exhibits characteristics of normal science (Kuhn, 1970). Second, theory development is expanded with a broadened philosophy of nursing science and new research approaches that address unanswered nursing questions. The most exciting development in recent years is middle range theory and the understanding that it is the level of theory that guides nursing practice. Whether developed quantitatively or qualitatively, the level of abstraction facilitates understanding and application in practice as noted in Figure 37-1. Third, global communities of nursing scholars are forming around the world and sharing nursing theoretical works, which furthers development of nursing knowledge for global utility. Using the Internet, the nurses of the world are sharing ideas and knowledge, revisiting the earlier works of the nursing theorists, and generating new theories and new nursing knowledge. It is vital that nursing knowledge be learned, used, and applied in theory-based practice for the profession and the continued development of nursing as an academic discipline. It is true that "Theory without practice is empty and practice without theory is blind" (Cross, 1981).

REFERENCES

Alligood, M. R. (2002). A theory of the art of nursing discovered in Rogers' science of unitary human beings. *International Journal for Human Caring, 6*(2), 55-60.

Alligood, M. R. (2002a). Areas for further development of theory-based nursing practice. In M. Alligood & A. Marriner Tomey (Eds.), *Nursing theory: Utilization & application* (2nd ed., pp. 453-463). St. Louis: Mosby.

Alligood, M. R. (2002b). Philosophies, models, and theories: Critical thinking structures. In M. Alligood & A. Marriner Tomey (Eds.), *Nursing theory: Utilization & application* (2nd ed., pp. 41-61). St. Louis: Mosby.

Alligood, M. R. (2002c). The nature of knowledge needed for nursing practice. In M. Alligood & A. Marriner Tomey (Eds.), *Nursing theory: Utilization & application* (2nd ed., pp. 3-14). St. Louis: Mosby.

Alligood, M. R. (2004). The theoretical basis of professional nursing. In K. K. Chitty (Ed.), *Professional nursing* (3rd ed., pp. 271-298). Philadelphia: W. B. Saunders.

Alligood, M. R., & Fawcett, J. (1999). Acceptance of the invitation to dialogue: Examination of an interpretive approach for the science of unitary human beings. *Visions: The Journal of Rogerian Nursing Science, 7*(1), 5-13.

Alligood, M. R., & Marriner Tomey, A. (1997). *Nursing theory: Utilization & application.* St. Louis: Mosby.

Alligood, M. R., & Marriner Tomey, A. (2002). *Nursing theory: Utilization & application* (2nd ed.). St. Louis: Mosby.

Alligood, M. R., & Marriner Tomey, A. (2006). *Nursing theory: Utilization & application* (3rd ed.). St. Louis: Mosby.

Alligood, M. R., & May, B. A. (2000). A nursing theory of personal system empathy: Interpreting a conceptualization of empathy in King's interacting systems. *Nursing Science Quarterly, 13*(3), 243-247.

Anderregg-Tschudin, H. (1999). The complex interrelations between nursing diagnostic and nursing management [German]. *Pflege, 12*(4), 216-222.

Burns, N. (1999). [Review of the book *Nursing theorists and their work* (4th ed.)]. *Nursing Science Quarterly, 12*(3), 263-264.

Butcher, H. K. (1999). Rogerian ethics: An ethical inquiry into Rogers' life and science. *Nursing Science Quarterly, 12*(2), 111-118.

Chinn, P., & Kramer, M. (2004). *Integrated knowledge development in nursing* (6th ed.). St. Louis: Mosby.

Cross, P. (1981). *Adults as learners.* Washington, DC: Jossey-Bass.

Fawcett, J. (1984). *Analysis and evaluation of conceptual models of nursing.* Philadelphia: F. A. Davis.

Fawcett, J. (1989). *Analysis and evaluation of conceptual models of nursing* (2nd ed.). Philadelphia: F. A. Davis.

Fawcett, J. (1993). *Analysis and evaluation of nursing theories.* Philadelphia: F. A. Davis.

Fawcett, J. (1995). *Analysis and evaluation of conceptual models of nursing* (3rd ed.). Philadelphia: F. A. Davis.

Fawcett, J. (2000). *Analysis and evaluation of contemporary nursing knowledge: Nursing models and theories.* Philadelphia: F. A. Davis.

Fawcett, J., & Alligood, M. (2001). SUHB INSTRUMENTS: An overview of research instruments and clinical tools derived from the science of unitary human beings. *Theoria: Journal of Nursing Theory, 10*(3), 5-12.

Fitzpatrick, J. J., & Whall, A. L. (1984). *Conceptual models of nursing: Analysis and application.* Norwalk, CT: Appleton & Lange.

Fitzpatrick, J. J., & Whall, A. L. (1989). *Conceptual models of nursing: Analysis and application* (2nd ed.). Norwalk, CT: Appleton & Lange.

Fitzpatrick, J. J., & Whall, A. L. (1996). *Conceptual models of nursing: Analysis and application* (3rd ed.). Stamford, CT: Appleton & Lange.

George, J. B. (1985). *Nursing theories.* Norwalk, CT: Appleton & Lange.

George, J. B. (1986). *Nursing theories* (2nd ed.). Norwalk, CT: Appleton & Lange.

George, J. B. (1989). *Nursing theories* (3rd ed.). Norwalk, CT: Appleton & Lange.

George, J. B. (1995). *Nursing theories* (4th ed.). Upper Saddle River, NJ: Prentice Hall.

George, J. B. (2002). *Nursing theories* (5th ed.). Upper Saddle River, NJ: Prentice Hall.

Johnson, B., & Webber, P. (2001). *An introduction to theory and reasoning in nursing.* Philadelphia: Lippincott.

Kappeli, S. (1999). What sort of science does nursing require? [German]. *Pflege, 12*(3), 153-157.

Kuhn, T. S. (1970). *The structure of scientific revolutions* (2nd ed.). Chicago: University of Chicago Press.

Liehr, P., & Smith, M. J. (1999). Middle range theory: Spinning research and practice to create knowledge for the new millennium. *ANS Advances in Nursing Science, 21*(4), 81-91.

Malinski, V. (1999). [Review of the book *Nursing theorists and their work* (4th ed.)]. *Nursing Science Quarterly, 12*(3), 264-266.

Marriner Tomey, A. (1986). *Nursing theorists and their work.* St. Louis: Mosby.

Marriner Tomey, A. (1989). *Nursing theorists and their work* (2nd ed.). St. Louis: Mosby.

Marriner Tomey, A. (1994). *Nursing theorists and their work* (3rd ed.). St. Louis: Mosby.

Marriner Tomey, A., & Alligood, M. (1998). *Nursing theorists and their work* (4th ed.). St. Louis: Mosby.

Marriner Tomey, A., & Alligood, M. R. (2002). *Nursing theorists and their work* (5th ed.). St. Louis: Mosby.

McEwen, M., & Wills, E. (2002). *Theoretical basis for nursing.* Philadelphia: Lippincott Williams & Wilkins.

Meleis, A. I. (1985). *Theoretical nursing: Development and progress.* Philadelphia: Lippincott.

Meleis, A. I. (1991). *Theoretical nursing: Development and progress* (2nd ed.). Philadelphia: Lippincott.

Meleis, A. I. (1997). *Theoretical nursing: Development and progress* (3rd ed.). Philadelphia: Lippincott.

Meleis, A. I. (2004). *Theoretical nursing: Development and progress* (4th ed.). Philadelphia: Lippincott.

Morris, D. B. (2000). How to speak postmodern: Medicine, illness, and cultural change. *Hastings Center Report, 30*(6), 7-16.

Parker, M. (2001). *Nursing theories and nursing practice.* Philadelphia: F. A. Davis.

Reed, P. G. (1999). [Review of the book *Nursing theorists and their work* (4th ed.)]. *Nursing Science Quarterly, 12*(3), 266-268.

Smith, M. J., & Liehr, P. (2003). *Middle range theory for nursing.* New York: Springer.

Thorne, S., Kirkham, S. R., & MacDonald-Emes, J. (1997). Interpretive description: A noncategorical qualitative alternative for developing nursing knowledge. *Research in Nursing and Health, 20,* 169-177.

Thorne, S., Kirkham, S. R., & O'Flynn-Magee, K. (2004). The analytic challenge in interpretive description. *International Journal of Qualitative Methods, 3*(1), article 1. Retrieved May 21, 2004, from *http://www.ualberta.ca/aiiqm/backissues/3_1/pdf/thorneetal.pdf*

Wood, A., & Alligood, M. (2002). Nursing models: Normal science for nursing practice. In M. R. Alligood & A. M. Tomey (Eds.), *Nursing theory: Utilization & application* (2nd ed., pp. 15-39). St. Louis: Mosby.

Index

A

Abdellah, Faye Glenn, 50, 268
  background of, 56
  typology of nursing problems of, 58b
Acceptance, in Modeling and Role-Modeling Theory, 566
Acculturation health assessment enabler, in Culture Care Theory, 485
Achievement subsystem, in Johnson Behavioral System Model, 389
Achieving Methods of Intraprofessional Consensus, Assessment and Evaluation (AMICAE) Project, 148, 153
Ackley, B. J., 688
Acquired immunodeficiency syndrome
  and Self-Transcendence Theory, 651
Acquired immunodeficiency syndrome (AIDS), research in, 510
Action, in Health Promotion Model, 456
Activities of living (ALs), in Model for Learning, 64-65, 65f, 66f
Acton, G., 650, 651
Adam, Evelyn, 52, 63
Adams, Betty, 726
Adams, Mary, 726
Adaptation
  in Conservation Model, 229
  middle range theories of, 371-372
  in Modeling and Role-Modeling Theory, 567
  in Roy Adaptation Model, 357, 361
  in Uncertainty in Illness Theory, 625
Adaptation Model, Roy, 7, 31, 46, 787
  acceptance of, 365-372
  application of, 367
  case study in, 377
  concept and definitions of, 357-360
  critical thinking in, 377
  critique of, 373-374
  development of, 372-373
  empirical evidence for, 360
  logical form in, 364-365
  major assumptions in, 360-363
  scientific assumptions in, 361b
  summary of, 374-375, 375t-376t, 377
  theoretical assertions in, 363-364
  theoretical sources for, 356-357
Adaptation research instruments, 371
Adaptive modes, in Roy Adaptation Model, 375t-376t

Adaptive Potential Assessment Model (APAM), 565, 567, 568f, 570
Adaptive systems, human, 364, 364f
Adjustment, in Neuman Systems Model, 319
Administration, nursing
  in Nursing Process theory, 438-440
  relationship of caring to, 101
  in Symphonological Bioethical Theory, 595
Administrator, in Nursing as Caring theory, 415-416
Adolescents
  research on, 369-30, 569
  and Self-Care Deficit Theory, 276t
Advanced practice nursing, 54, 280, 330
Affiliated-individuation. in Modeling and Role-Modeling Theory, 564, 566
African-Americans
  and Culture Care Theory of Diversity and Universality, 487
  research in, 510
Agency
  definition of, 589
  nursing, 271
  in Symphonological Bioethical Theory, 587
Agent, in Self-Care Deficit Theory, 271
Aggressive-protective subsystem, in Johnson Behavioral System Model, 389
Aikens, C., 727
Alanen, Y., 704
Alanine aminotranferase (ALT), research in, 396
Alcoholism
  research in, 650
Alexander, J. W., 395
Algovia, Maite, 442
Alligood, 786
Alligood, M. R., 6, 132, 251, 306, 307, 325, 439, 615
Allison, S. E., 280, 283
Allport, C., 572
Allport, F. H., 300
Allport, Gordon, 268
Altschul, Annie, 699, 704
Alzheimer's disease, research in, 543, 568
Alzheimer's patients, research in, 573
AMICAE (Achieving Methods of Intraprofessional Consensus, Assessment and Evaluation) Project, 148, 153
Analysis
  defined, 1
  of theory, 1, 12-13

Anderson, B., 442
Anderson, E., 330
Anderson, K. G., 307
Anteparum stress, 611
Anthropology, 474
Anxiety, in Maternal Role Attainment Theory, 608
APAM (Adaptive Potential Assessment Model), in Modeling and Role-Modeling Theory, 565, 567, 568f, 570
"Applying the Art and Science of Human Caring" (video), 93
Appraisal of Self-Care Agency (ASA) scale, 281, 282
Apprentice, in Tidal Model of Mental Health Recovery, 701b
Araich, M., 367
Ardrey, R., 300
Arendt, Hannah, 170
Arnold, Magda, 268
Articulation research, 142, 150
Ashjian, Ann, 407
Assessment, in Neuman Systems Model, 323
Asthma, and Self-Care Deficit Theory, 279t
Atkinson, 390
Attachment, in Maternal Role Attainment Theory, 609
Attachment-affiliative subsystem, in Johnson Behavioral System Model, 388-389
Attention deficit-hyperactivity disorder (ADHD), research in, 371
Automatic nursing action, in Nursing Process Theory, 434, 437
Autonomy, as bioethical standard, 591b, 593f, 597
Avant, K. C., 12, 13, 31, 433, 437, 444
Axiomatic form, of theory organization, 41, 43-44, 43f
Axioms, in Caritative Caring Theory, 198

B
Baas, L. S., 573
Baccalaureate programs, 4, 8-9, 331
Bacon, A. C., 616
Baiardi, J., 371
Bailey, D. E., 631
Balance, in Neuman Systems Model, 319
Balasco, E. M., 152
Bandura, Albert, 454
Banfield, B. E., 281
Barker, E., 330
Barker, Phil
background of, 696
Tidal Model of Mental Health Recovery of
acceptance of, 709-711
case study for, 716-717
concepts and definitions in, 702-704
critical thinking in, 717
critique of, 712-715
development of, 711-712

Barker, Phil—cont'd
background of—cont'd
empirical evidence for, 704-705
major assumptions of, 705-707
summary of, 715
theoretical assertions of, 707-708
theoretical sources for, 697-700
Barnard, Chester, 268
Barnard, Kathryn E., 52, 763
background of, 62
Child Health Assessment Interaction Model of, 62-63, 64f
Barnum, B. J., 153
Barrett, E. A. M., 251, 252
Basic Needs Satisfaction Inventory, 570
Basic Psychiatric Concepts in Nursing (Leininger and Hofling), 473
Bates, M., 229
Batey, M. V., 9
Bauer, M., 443
Bauer, S., 443, 444
Bayley, E., 371
Beavin, J. W., 300
Beck, C., 650
Beck, Cheryl Tatano
background of, 743-744
perinatal research of, 745t
Postpartum Depression Theory of
acceptance of, 753-754
case study for, 756-757
concepts and definitions in, 746-750
critical thinking in, 757
critique of, 755-756
development of, 754-755
empirical evidence for, 750-751
major assumptions of, 751
summary of, 756
theoretical assertions of, 351-352
theoretical sources for, 744, 745t, 746
Becoming a mother
in Maternal Role Attainment Theory, 613
process of, 617
revised model for, 615f
Becoming a Mother: Research on Maternal Identity from Rubin to the Present (Mercer), 606, 611, 612, 616
Beginner, classification as advanced, 145
Behavior
and concept of caring, 97
in Health Promotion Model, 456, 457
in Johnson Behavioral System Model, 387
Behavioral assessment, in Johnson Behavioral System Model, 399
Behavioral System Model, Johnson
acceptance of, 393-395
concepts and definitions in, 387-389

Behavioral System Model, Johnson—cont'd
  critical thinking in, 400-401
  critique of, 397-398
  development of, 396-397
  empirical evidence for, 390
  logical form for, 393
  major assumptions in, 390-391
  subsystems in, 388-389
  summary of, 398
  theoretical assertions in, 391, 392f, 393
  theoretical sources for, 387
Behaviorism, 17
Being with, in Theory of Caring, 764
Beland, I., 227
Beliefs, cultural, 491. *See also* Culture
Bello, I. T. R., 306
Beneficence, as bioethical standard, 591b, 593f, 597
Benner, Patricia, 170
  background of, 140-143
  on clinical nursing practice
    concepts and definitions used by, 145-147
    critique of work of, 154-156
    and empirical evidence, 147-150
    and logical form, 152
    major assumptions in, 150-151
    summary of, 156-157
    theoretical assertions for, 151-152
    theoretical sources fir, 142-145
Benner, R. V., 145, 147, 148
Benson, D., 568
Benson, S., 394
Bentley, A., 300
Bentov, I., 500, 503, 505
Berdâev, Nikolaj, 194
Bereaved individuals, research on, 688
Berraco, Rocio, 442
Berry, T., 361
Bingham, V., 418
Biochemical loading, 746
Bioethical Decision Making Preference Scale for Patients, 596
Bioethical standards, 591b
Bioethics, defined, 586
Biography, in Illness Trajectory Theory, 667
Biology, in Bureaucratic Caring Theory, 121
Birth experience, perception of, 608
Bishop, S. M., 18
Bixenstine, E., 17
Bixler, G. K., 10
Bixler, R. W., 10
Black, A. S., 152
Black, P., 330
Blegen, M., 37
Bloch, C., 332
Blom, Ida, 169

Bochnak, M., 445
Bockenhauer, Barbara, 438, 443
Body, as natural attitude, 172
Body activities, in Illness Trajectory Theory, 667
Bohm, D., 120, 500
Bondy, 331
Boore, J. R., 420
Bosque, E. M., 31
Bournaki, M. C., 370
Bowlby, J., 564
Boykin, Anne, 118
  background of, 406
  and Nursing as Caring theory, 785
    acceptance of, 415-420
    case study in, 422-423
    concepts and definitions in, 408-412
    critical thinking in, 423
    critique of, 421
    development of, 420
    empirical evidence for, 412
    logical form for, 415
    major assumptions of, 412-413
    summary of, 422
    theoretical assertions in, 414-416
    theoretical sources for, 407-408
Boyle, Joyceen, 118
Braden, C. J., 626
Bradford, Helena, 754
Bramadat, I. J., 152
Brautigan, R., 330
Breast cancer
  and Self-Transcendence Theory, 651
  surviving, 631
Breast cancer patients
  research on, 730, 737
  resource kit for, 366-367
Breast cancer support groups, research on, 650
Breast-feeding mothers, research on, 442
Brecht, M., 395
Breckenridge, D. M., 334
Brester, M. H., 396
Breu, C., 442
Bridges. Introduction to the Methods of Caring Science (Eriksson), 204
Briggs, J., 119, 120
Brittin, M., 233
Bronfenbrenner, U., 607, 612, 614
Bronowski, J., 47
Brown, B., 594
Brown, H., 18, 19, 20, 21
Brown, Martha, 439
Brown, S. T., 306
Brownell, J., 408
Buchanan, D., 650
Buckley, 387

Bunn, H., 331
Bureaucratic Caring Theory, 118
    acceptance of, 126-129
    case study for, 134
    concepts and definitions in, 121
    critical thinking in, 134
    critique of, 129, 132-133
    development of, 129
    empirical evidence for, 122-124
    grounded theory in, 123, 123f
    as holographic theory, 124
    logical form for, 126
    major assumptions of, 124-125
    research publications related to, 130t-132t
    summarized, 133
    theoretical assertions of, 125-127
    theoretical sources for, 119
Burke, Mary Lermann, 679, 680
    background of, 681-382
    Chronic Sorrow Theory of, 682
        acceptance of, 686-687
        case study for, 690-691
        concepts and definitions in, 684
        critical thinking in, 691
        critique of, 688-690
        development of, 688
        empirical evidence in, 684-686
        major assumptions of, 686
        summary of, 690
        theoretical assertions for, 686
        theoretical sources for, 683-384
Burke, P. J., 613
Burke/Eakes Chronic Sorrow Assessment Tool, 681
Burns, C. M., 332
Burns, N., 785
Burr, H. S., 247
Burr, W. R., 607
Busen, N. H., 615

C
Call for nursing, in Nursing as Caring theory, 411
Calmness, in Peaceful End of Life Theory, 777
Cameron, J., 445
Campbell, J., 572
Cancer
    research in, 510
    and Self-Care Deficit Theory, 277t
Cancer care, research in, 672
Cancer pain, research in, 396
Cancer patients, research on, 443. *See also* Breast cancer
    patients
Cantril, H., 300
Capers, C. F., 332
Capitalism, 174

Caplan, G., 336
Caplan's conceptual model, 319
CAPSTI (Caring Attributes Professional Self-Concept-
    Technological Influence), 120b
Cardiac patients
    planning for, 569
    and Self-Care Deficit Theory, 278t
Care
    emic, 482
    etic, 482
    K. Martinsen's concept of, 175
    moral practice founded on, 176
    in Tidal Model of Mental Health Recovery, 713f
    in transcultural nursing, 476
    universality of, 481
Care: The Essence of Nursing and Health (Leininger),
    475
Caregivers
    of children with developmental delays, 688
    research on, 510, 569
    self-transcendence in, 651
    in Uncertainty in Illness Theory, 633
Caregiving, adaptation to, 372
Care management role, 280
Care providers, legitimate functional unity of, 285
Care-Q (Caring Assessment Instrument), 102b
Care system, components of, 285
Caring. *See also* Caring, Theory of; Nursing as Caring
    theory
    act of, 195
    artistic aspects of, 99
    as caritas, 199-200
    compared with curing, 99, 100
    conditions necessary for, 97-98
    defined, 99, 121, 764
    devaluation of, 182
    differential, 122-123, 123f, 125, 130t
    existential being, 172-173
    holographic theory of, 127
    interpretive analysis of, 180
    language of, 407-408
    K. Martinsen on, 178
    meaning of, 125-126, 131t
    motive for, 199
    for other, 175
    in Postpartum Depression Theory, 744
    relational, 131t
    spiritual-ethical, 124, 124f, 126
    structure of, 768
    transcultural, 124-125
    transpersonal, 99, 100
Caring: An Essential Human Need (Leininger), 475
*Caring, Nursing and Medicine, Historical Philosophical
    Essays* (Martinsen), 169, 170

Caring, philosophy of, 785
  acceptance of, 180-181
  case study for, 183
  concepts and definitions in, 176-177
  critical thinking in, 183
  critique of, 181-182
  development of, 181
  empirical evidence for, 177-178
  logical form in, 179-180
  major assumptions in, 178-179
  summary of, 182-183
  theoretical assertions in, 179
  theoretical sources for, 171-175
A Caring Approach in Nursing Administration (Nyberg),
    127
Caring Assessment Instrument (Care-Q), 102b
Caring Attributes Professional Self-Concept-
    Technological Influence (CAPSTI), 102b
Caring Behavior Inventory (CBI), 102b
Caring Behaviors Assessment (CBA), 102b
Caring communion, 195, 202
Caring culture, 197
Caring Dimensions Inventory (CDI), 102b
Caring-healing paradigm, cosmology of, 100
The Caring Imperative in Education (Leininger and
    Watson), 475
Caring inquiry, 129
Caring instruments, survey of use of, 102b
Caring Professional Scale (CPS), 102b
Caring science, 193
  as academic discipline, 194
  acceptance of, 100-102
  basic assumptions of, 195
  basic motive in, 194
  basic research in, 206
  case study for, 105
  critique of, 103-105
  in curriculum, 204
  development of, 102-103
  evidence for, 197
  logical form for, 100
  major assumptions in, 97
  in Nordic countries, 191, 192
  theoretical assertions in, 99-100
  values and, 98
Caring Theory. *See also* Bureaucratic Caring Theory
  acceptance of, 768-769
  case study for, 770
  concepts and definitions in, 764
  critical thinking in, 770
  critique of, 769
  development of, 769
  empirical evidence for, 764-766
  logical form for, 767

Caring Theory—cont'd
  major assumptions of, 766-767
  theoretical assertions for, 767
  theoretical sources for, 763
Caring Without Care? (Martinsen and Wærness), 169
Caritas, 195, 199
Caritas process, 103-104t, 105-106
Caritative Caring Theory, 192, 193
  acceptance of, 203-205
  case study, 207-208
  concepts and definitions in, 195-197
  critical thinking in, 208
  critique of, 206-207
  development of, 205-206
  empirical evidence in, 197-198
  ethics in, 195-196
  logical form for, 202-203
  major assumptions of, 198-201
  summary of, 207
  theoretical assertions in, 201-202
  theoretical sources for, 194-195
Caritative outlook, 199
Carper, B. A., 422
Case manager, 507
Case studies
  for Bureaucratic Caring Theory, 134
  in Caring Theory, 105, 770
  for Caritative Caring Theory, 207-208
  for Conservation Model, 235-237
  in Culture Care Theory, 490
  in Goal Attainment Theory, 309
  for Health as Expanded Consciousness Theory,
      512-513
  in Health Promotion Model, 462-463
  in Human Becoming Theory, 544
  in Illness Trajectory Theory, 674-675
  for Interacting Systems Framework, 309
  in Johnson Behavioral System Model, 398-400
  for Maternal Role Attainment Theory, 619
  for Neuman Systems Model, 336
  for novice to expert model, 157-159
  in Nursing as Caring theory, 422
  in Nursing Process theory, 438, 447
  for Peaceful End of Life Theory, 781
  in philosophy of nursing, 183
  for Postpartum Depression Theory, 756-757
  in Rogerian model, 256
  for Roy Adaptation Model, 377
  in Science of Unitary Human Beings, 256
  for Self-Care Deficit Nursing Theory, 285
  for Self-Transcendence Theory, 654
  for Uncertainty in Illness Theory, 634
  using F. Nightingale's theory, 84
Caspari, S., 205

Casual process theories, 42
  example of, 44, 45t
  features of, 44
Caudill, 390
Center for Epidemiological Studies Depression (CES-D)
    scale, 646
Center for Human Caring, at Univ. of Colorado, 92, 105
Certainty, in Symphonological Bioethical Theory, 592.
    See also Uncertainty in Illness Theory
Change, in Tidal Model of Mental Health Recovery, 698,
    699, 701b, 702
Chaos theory, 119, 124, 133, 247, 625
  and prolonged uncertainty, 628
  and Tidal Model of Mental Health Recovery, 698
Charity, idea of, 200
Chen, L., 330
Chesla, C. A., 141, 158
Childbirth, 746. *See also* Postpartum Depression Theory
Child Health Assessment Interaction Theory, K.E.
    Barnard's, 62-63, 64f
Childhood cancer, survivors of, 672
Childrearing attitudes, in Maternal Role Attainment
    Theory, 608
Children, and Self-Care Deficit Theory, 276t
Chinn, P. L., 12, 13, 74, 373, 387, 574, 752, 755, 767, 770,
    788
Chiou, C. P., 369
Chronic illness
  research in, 396
  and uncertainty, 627, 629
Chronic sorrow, theoretical model of, 698t
Chronic Sorrow Theory
  acceptance of, 686-688
  case study for, 690
  concepts and definitions in, 684
  critical thinking in, 691
  critique of, 688-690
  development of, 688
  empirical evidence for, 684-686
  logical form for, 686
  major assumptions of, 686
  summary of, 690
  theoretical assertions for, 686
  theoretical sources for, 683-384
"Circles of Knowledge," 93
Clarity
  in Bureaucratic Caring Theory, 129
  in Caring Theory, 103
  in Caritative Caring Theory, 206
  in Chronic Sorrow Theory, 688-689
  in Comfort Theory, 737
  of Conservation Model, 235
  in Illness Trajectory Theory, 673
  in Maternal Role Attainment Theory, 617-618
  in Modeling and Role-Modeling Theory, 573-574

Clarity—cont'd
  in Neuman Systems Model, 335
  in Nursing as Caring theory, 421
  in Nursing Process theory, 444
  in nursing theory, 12
  in Peaceful End of Life Theory, 779
  in Postpartum Depression Theory, 755
  in Roy Adaptation Model, 373
  in Self-Care Deficit Nursing Theory, 283
  in Self-Transcendence Theory, 652
  in Symphonological Bioethical Theory, 596
  in Theory of Caring, 769
  in Tidal Model of Mental Health Recovery, 712
Clark, B. S., 615
Clark, D., 650
Client system, in Neuman Systems Model, 321-322, 323,
    326b
Clifford, Joyce, 141
Clinical Experience in Nurse Education (Roper), 64
Clinical forethought, 150
Clinical nurse specialist role, 280
Clinical Nursing: A Helping Art (Wiedenbach), 57
Clinical practice development models (CPDMs), 142
*Clinical Wisdom and Interventions in Critical Care:
    A Thinking-in-Action Approach* (Benner,
    Hooper-Kyriakidis, and Stannard), 142
*Clinical Wisdom in Critical care: A Thinking-in-Action
    Approach* (Benner, Hooper-Kyriakidis, and
    Stannard), 141, 149, 153
Closeness to significant others, in Peaceful End of Life
    Theory, 777
Coaching, in Comfort Theory, 734
Coconstitution, defined, 524
Cocreating, in Human Becoming Theory, 526-527,
    532f
Cody, W. K., 47, 444
Coexistence, in Human Becoming Theory, 524
Coffman, Sherrilyn, 118
Coggiola, P., 330
Cognator, in Roy Adaptation Model, 358, 363-364, 363f,
    376t
Cognitive capacities, in Uncertainty in Illness Theory,
    625
Cognitive development, Piaget's theory of, 564
Cognitive functioning, Piaget's theory of, 19
Cognitive schema, in Uncertainty in Illness Theory,
    625
Cohen, I. B., 76
Cohen, S. M., 280
Coker, E., 306
Colaizzi, P., 744
Collaboration, in Tidal Model of Mental Health
    Recovery, 714
Colleges, nursing education in, 4. *See also* Baccalaureate
    programs; Master's programs

Comfort
  concept analysis of, 727
  defined, 728
  F. Nightingale on, 727
  taxonomic structure of, 735, 735f, 736
  universal nature of, 737
Comfort care, support for, 736
Comfort food, 734
Comfort measures, 728, 729
Comfort needs, taxonomic structure of, 739t
Comfort Theory
  acceptance of, 733-736
  case study for, 738
  concepts and definitions in, 728-729
  critical thinking in, 740
  critique of, 737-738
  development of, 736-737
  empirical evidence for, 729-730
  logical form for, 731-733
  major assumptions of, 730-731
  model of, 732f
  for outcomes research, 733f
  summary of, 738
  theoretical assertions in, 731
  theoretical sources for, 727-728
Commission on Accreditation in Physical Therapy
      Education (CAPTE), 332
Community
  in Theory of Comfort, 736-737
  in Tidal Model of Mental Health Recovery, 702
Community: A Human Becoming Perspective (Parse), 522
Community crisis centers, nurse counselor role in, 318
Community health, behavioral system framework for,
      397
Competencies
  in AMICAE Project, 148
  in P. Benner's philosophy of nursing, 154
  defined, 147
Competency-based testing, 153
Competent, classification as, 145-146
Complex caring dynamics, 129
Complexity, 119
  of P. Benner's theory of nursing practice, 154-155
  science, 132, 133
  theory, 124
Complex organizations, nursing in, 129
Comportment, defined, 147
Concepts
  abstract, 37
  analysis of, 38-39
  concrete, 37
  continuous, 37, 38
  discrete, 37
  nonvariable, 37
  in nursing theory, 36-39

Concepts development, Eriksson's model of, 197
Conceptual framework, Neuman Systems Model as, 333
Conceptual models, 225
  defined, 7
  grand theories of, 7
Conceptual Models for Nursing Practice (Johnson), 390
Connectedness, in Peaceful End of Life Theory, 777
Connecting-separating, in Human Becoming Theory,
      526-527, 532f
Consciousness
  absolute, 503, 505
  M. Newman's definition of, 502-503
  time as measure of, 505
Consensus, scientific, 21
Consequences, derivable
  in Bureaucratic Caring Theory, 133
  in Caring Theory, 105
  in Caritative Caring Theory, 207
  in Chronic Sorrow Theory, 690
  of Conservation Model, 235
  in Culture Care Theory, 489
  in Goal Attainment Theory, 309
  in Health as Expanded Consciousness Theory, 511
  in Health Promotion Model, 461-462
  in Human Becoming Theory, 543-544
  in Illness Trajectory Theory, 674
  in Johnson Behavioral System Model, 398
  in K. Martinsen's philosophy of caring, 182
  in Maternal Role Attainment Theory, 618
  in Modeling and Role-Modeling Theory, 574
  in Neuman Systems Model, 335-336
  of novice to expert model, 155-156
  in Nursing as Caring theory, 421
  in Nursing Process Theory, 446
  of nursing theory, 13
  in Peaceful End of Life Theory, 780
  in Postpartum Depression Theory, 756
  in Rogers' model, 255
  in Roy Adaptation Model, 374
  of Self-Care Deficit Nursing Theory, 284
  in Self-Transcendence Theory, 653
  in Symphonological Bioethical Theory, 597
  in Theory of Caring, 770
  in Theory of Comfort, 738
  in Tidal Model of Mental Health Recovery, 715
  in Uncertainty in Illness Theory, 633
Conservation
  defined, 230-231
  principles of, 231
Conservation Model, 227
  acceptance of, 233-235
  case study for, 235-237
  concepts and definitions in, 229-231
  critical thinking in, 237-238
  critique of, 235

Conservation Model—cont'd
  development of, 234-235
  empirical evidence for, 231
  logical form in, 233
  major assumptions of, 231-233
  summary of, 235
  theoretical assertions in, 233
  theoretical sources for, 229
Consistency, in Self-Transcendence Theory, 652
Constantine, J., 607
*Consultation and Community Organization in
    Community Mental Health Nursing* (Neuman),
    318
Consumer movement, 543
Contentment, in Peaceful End of Life Theory, 777
Context, in Symphonological Bioethical Theory, 587
Continuum of care, in Tidal Model of Mental Health
    Recovery, 703-704
Contract for nursing, in Self-Care Deficit Theory,
    285
Cook, E. T., 73
Cook, M., 233
Cook, N. F., 367
Cooley, C. H., 357
Cooley, M. E., 369
Cooper, D. H., 233
Cooperative inquiry, 510
Coping
  action-oriented, 685
  P. Benner's study of, 144
  in Chronic Sorrow Theory, 685
  defined, 144
  in Illness Trajectory Theory, 666
  in Roy Adaptation Model, 358
  in Uncertainty in Illness Theory, 632
Coping needs, in Roy Adaptation Model, 375t-376t
Corbin, J., 671
Corcoran-Perry, 420
Core, Care, and Cure Model, of L. Hall, 59, 62f
Cotranscendence, in Human Becoming Theory, 527,
    530, 532f
Counselor, nurse, 318
Couples Miscarriage Healing Project, 765
Coward, D. D., 650
Cowling, W. R., 251
Crandell, 390
Creation
  and sovereign life utterances, 176-177
  and vocation, 174
Creation theology, 173
Crisis. in Tidal Model of Mental Health Recovery,
    703
*The Crisis of Care: Affirming and Restoring Caring
    Practices in the Helping Professions,* (Phillips and
    Benner), 141-142

Crissman, S., 152
Critical analysis, in nursing theory, 35
Critical care nursing, domains of, 149
Critical care unit, meaning of caring in, 130t
Critical social theory, 625
Critical theory, 23
Critical thinking, 6, 11, 13
  in Bureaucratic Caring Theory, 134
  in Caring Theory, 105-106
  in Caritative Caring Theory, 208
  in Chronic Sorrow Theory, 691
  for Conservation Model, 237-238
  for Goal Attainment Theory, 310
  in Health as Expanded Consciousness Theory, 513
  in Health Promotion Model, 463
  in Human Becoming Theory, 544-546
  in Illness Trajectory Theory, 675
  for Interacting Systems Framework, 310
  in Johnson Behavioral System Model, 400-401
  in Maternal Role Attainment Theory, 619
  with Neuman Systems Model, 337
  and F. Nightingale's theory, 84
  and novice to expert model, 159
  in Nursing as Caring Theory, 423
  in Nursing Process Theory, 447
  in Peaceful End of Life Theory, 781
  in philosophy of nursing, 183
  in Postpartum Depression Theory, 757
  in Rogers' model, 251
  in Roy Adaptation Model, 377
  in Science of Unitary Human Beings, 256
  in Self-Care Deficit Nursing Theory, 287
  in Self-Transcendence Theory, 655
  in Theory of Caring, 770
  Theory of Comfort, 740
  in Uncertainty in Illness Theory, 634
Cross-cultural nursing, 476
Crowley, D. M., 9
Culbert, C., 233
Culture
  in Bureaucratic Caring Theory, 121
  caring, 197
  defined, 477, 478
  goal of, 480-481
  hospital, 130t
  and Nursing as Caring Theory, 418
  organizational, 119, 130t
  and science, 18
  in transcultural nursing, 476
Culture care
  accommodation in, 479, 487
  definition for, 478
  maintenance of, 479, 487
  negotiation in, 479, 487
  preservation of, 479, 487

Culture Care Diversity and Universality: A Theory of Nursing (Leininger and McFarland), 475
Culture Care Theory of Diversity and Universality, 473-475, 787
  acceptance of, 485-487
  case study in, 490
  clinical application of, 487
  concepts and definitions in, 478-479
  critical thinking in, 490-491
  critique of, 488-489
  development of, 488
  distinct features of, 477
  empirical evidence for, 479-481
  logical form in, 482-485, 484f
  major assumptions of, 481
  summary of, 489-490
  Sunrise Enabler in, 483, 484f
  theoretical assertions of, 481-482
  theoretical sources for, 475-477
Culture shock, 486
Curing, compared with caring, 99, 100
Curiosity, in Tidal Model of Mental Health Recovery, 701b, 703
Curl, E., 573
Curricula
  development of, 4
  in Human Becoming Theory, 540
  standardization of, 5, 9

D
Dalton, J. M., 31
Damus, K., 396
Dance of caring persons, 414, 414f, 416-417
Daniel, J. M., 306
Davidson, Alice, 118
Dawson, A., 443
Day, R. D., 607
Deaconesses, in Norway, 169
Dean, P. R., 307
De Chardin, Pierre Teilhard, 94, 319, 357
Decision making
  problem solving in, 96
  research in, 396
  in Symphonological Bioethical Theory, 592, 593f
DeClifford, J., 233
Deduction
  basic characteristics of, 32t-33t
  defined, 25
  examples, 26-27, 278
  in Theory of Comfort, 731-732
Dee, V., 395
Deeny, P., 330
Definitions
  operational, 39t
  theoretical, 39t

DeJoseph, J., 608, 610, 611
Deliberative nursing action, in Nursing Process Theory, 434, 437
Deliberative nursing process, 434
Demonstration of Caring-Based Model for Health Care Delivery, 417-418
Dennis, C. M., 284
Denver Nursing Project in Human Caring, 93
Denyes, M. J., 275, 280
Denyes Self-Care Agency Instrument (DSCAI), 280, 281, 282
Denyes Self-Care Practice Instrument (DSCPI), 280
Deontology, 586
Dependency subsystem, in Johnson Behavioral System Model, 388-389
Depression. *See also* Postpartum Depression Theory
  in Maternal Role Attainment Theory, 608
  postpartum, 747
Derdiarian, A. K., 394, 396
Derdiarian Behavioral System Model instrument, 394
Descartes, R., 172
De Shazer, S., 700
De Souza Toniolli, Ana Claudia CHECK, 442
A Developing Discipline: Selected Works of Margaret Newman (Newman), 498
Developmental Resources of Later Adulthood (DRLA) scale, 646
Developmental self-care requisites (DSCR), 270
Dever, M., 233
DeVillers, M. J., 366
Dewey, J., 300
Diabetes
  research in, 543
  and Self-Care Deficit Theory, 278t
Diagnoses, nursing
  chronic sorrow, 687
  in Johnson Behavioral System Model, 395
  in Neuman Systems Model, 328b-329b
  typology of, 368
Dickoff, J., 438
Diers, D., 300
Dignity
  in Caritative Caring Theory, 196
  in Peaceful End of Life Theory, 777
Dilthey, W., 150
DiMattio, M. J., 368
Direct invitation, in Nursing as Caring theory, 410-411
Discernment, professional, 176
Discipline
  defined, 8
  nursing as, 1, 8-10
  in Nursing as Caring theory, 413-414
The Discipline and Teaching of Nursing Process: An Evaluative Study (Orlando), 432, 437, 441, 444, 445

Disease, P. Benner on, 151
Disorders, in Johnson Behavioral System Model, 393-395
Distress, patient, in Nursing Process Theory, 445-446
Diversity, culture care, 478. *See also* Culture Care Theory of Diversity and Universality
Diversity of human field pattern scale (DHFPS), 255t
Dixon, E. L., 367
Doberneck, Barbara, 507
Dobratz, M. C., 367
Doctoral programs, nursing, 92
    development of, 5
    role of students in, 10
    transcultural nursing courses in, 486
Dodd, Marylin J., 396, 663
    background of, 664-666
    and Illness Trajectory Theory
        acceptance of, 671-672
        case study for, 674
        concepts and definitions in, 667-668
        critical thinking in, 675
        critique of, 673-674
        development of, 672-673
        empirical evidence for, 669
        major assumptions of, 670-671
        summary of, 674
        theoretical assertions of, 671
        theoretical sources for, 666
    oncology nursing focus of, 665
Dohrenwend, B. P., 356
Doing for, in Theory of Caring, 764
Domain
    in AMICAE project, 148
    in P. Benner's philosophy of nursing, 154
    of critical care nursing, 149
    defined, 147
Domain of inquiry enabler, in Culture Care Theory, 485
Donaldson, S. K., 9
Doornbos, M. M., 307
Dossey, B. M., 73
Dowd, T., 730
Dracup, 442
Dream experience, assessment of, 255t
Drench, M. E., 687
Dreyfus, Hubert, 143, 145
Dreyfus, Stuart, 143, 145
Dreyfus Model of Skill Acquisition, 143, 145, 146, 148, 152, 153, 154
Driever, M. J., 356
Driscoll, 746, 751
Driscoll, J., 756
Dubos, René, 229, 268
Duldt, B., 373
Dumas, R., 442
Dunlop, M. J., 154

Dunn, Halpert, 453
Dunn, K. S., 371
Dunphy, L. H., 420, 421
Dwyer, C. M., 330
Dye, Mimi, 438, 440, 445
Dying, culturally congruent care for, 483, 484f. *See also* Peaceful End of Life Theory
The Dynamic Nurse-Patient Relationship: Function Process and Principles of Professional Nursing (Orlando), 432, 434, 446

E
Eakes, Georgene Gaskill, 679
    background of, 680-681
    and Chronic Sorrow Theory, 680
        acceptance of, 686-687
        case study for, 690-691
        concepts and definitions in, 684
        critical thinking in, 691
        critique of, 688-690
        development of, 688
        empirical evidence for, 684-686
        major assumptions of, 686
        summary of, 690
        theoretical assertions for, 686
        theoretical sources for, 683-384
Earthquake model, 746
Ease, in Theory of Comfort, 728
Eckle, N. J., 158
Economics, in bureaucratic caring theory, 122
Edgil, A. E., 282, 334
Education. *See also* Colleges; Learning
    analysis in, 1
    P. Benner on, 153
    in bureaucratic caring theory, 121
    caring theory in, 101
    holistic, 100
    liberal, 100
    F. Nightingale on, 78, 80
    stage-based, 168, 169
Education, nursing
    Bureaucratic Caring Theory in, 127-128
    Caritative Caring Theory in, 203-204
    Chronic Sorrow Theory in, 687
    Comfort Theory in, 734
    Conservation Model in, 234
    Culture Care theory in, 486-487
    Goal Attainment Theory in, 306
    Health as Expanding Consciousness Theory, 508-509
    Health Promotion Model in, 460
    Human Becoming Theory in, 533-540
    Illness Trajectory Theory in, 672
    Interaction Systems Framework in, 306
    Johnson Behavioral System Model in, 395
    Maternal Role Attainment Theory in, 615-616

Education, nursing—cont'd
    Modeling and Role-Modeling Theory in, 572
    Neuman Systems Model in, 330-332
    Nursing as Caring Theory in, 416-417
    Nursing Process Theory in, 440
    philosophy of caring in, 180-181
    Postpartum Depression Theory in, 754
    and Rogers' model, 252
    Roy Adaptation Model in, 367
    Self-care Deficit Theory in, 280-281
    Self-Transcendence Theory in, 650
    Symphonological Bioethical Theory in, 594-595
    Theory of Caring in, 769
    Tidal Model of Mental Health Recovery in, 710
    Uncertainty in Illness Theory in, 630
Einstein, A., 247
Eisenberg, L., 151
Elder, R., 446
Elderly
    in Culture Care Theory, 487
    loneliness in, 650
    and mental health, 646-647
    research on, 509
    and Self-Care Deficit Theory, 276t
    in Self-Transcendence Theory, 645
Elegance, in Tidal Model of Mental Health Recovery, 703
The Elements of Nursing: A Model for Nursing Based on a Model of Living (Roper et al.), 64
Elements of Nursing (Roper), 64
Elias, Jose, 442
Eliminative subsystem, in Johnson Behavioral System Model, 388-389, 399
Ellis, Rosemary, 12, 13, 726
Emergency department, Nursing as Caring theory in, 418
Emergis (mental health program), 330
Empirical precision
    in Bureaucratic Caring Theory, 133
    in Caritative Caring Theory, 207
    in Chronic Sorrow Theory, 690
    in Comfort Theory, 737
    of Conservation Model, 235
    in Culture Care Theory, 489
    in Goal Attainment Theory, 308-309
    in Health as Expanded Consciousness Theory, 511
    in Health Promotion Model, 461
    in Human Becoming Theory, 542-543
    in Illness Trajectory Theory, 673
    in Johnson Behavioral System Model, 398
    in K. Martinsen's philosophy of caring, 182
    in Maternal Role Attainment Theory, 618
    in Modeling and Role-Modeling Theory, 574
    in Neuman Systems Model, 335
    of F. Nightingale's theory, 82
    in novice to expert model, 155

Empirical precision—cont'd
    in Nursing as Caring Theory, 421
    in Nursing Process Theory, 445-446
    in nursing theory, 13
    in Peaceful End of Life Theory, 779
    in Postpartum Depression Theory, 755
    in Roger's model, 254-255
    in Roy Adaptation Model, 373-374
    in science of caring, 103
    of Self-Care Deficit Nursing Theory, 284
    in Self-Transcendence Theory, 653
    in Symphonological Bioethical Theory, 597
    in Theory of Caring, 770
    in Tidal Model of Mental Health Recovery, 715
    in Uncertainty in Illness Theory, 633
Empiricism, 16, 17
Empiricists, of 20th-century, 18
Empowerment, in Tidal Model of Mental Health Recovery, 702, 714
Enabling, in Theory of Caring, 764
Enabling-limiting, in Human Becoming Theory, 526, 532f
Endo, E., 506, 508
End of life. *See also* Peaceful End of Life Theory
    and Comfort Theory, 737
    research on decisions of, 651
Endowment, in Modeling and Role-Modeling Theory, 567
Energy
    in conservation model, 231
    in Unitary Human Beings Theory, 246
Engagement beliefs, in Tidal Model of Mental Health Recovery, 703
Engel, G. S., 564, 565
Engle, V., 509
Enterostomal therapy (ET) nursing, 630
Entropy, in Neuman Systems Model, 321
Environment
    in Bureaucratic Caring Theory, 125
    and caring, 96
    in Chronic Sorrow Theory, 686
    in Conservation Model, 229-230, 232-233
    in Culture Care Theory, 477, 478
    in Goal Attainment Theory, 303
    in Health as Expanding Consciousness Theory, 500, 501f
    in Johnson Behavioral System Model, 391, 399-400
    in Maternal Role Attainment Theory, 611
    in Modeling and Role-Modeling Theory, 570
    in Neuman Systems Model, 321, 325
    F. Nightingale's theory of, 75-76
    in Nursing Process theory, 436
    in Peaceful End of Life Theory, 777
    in philosophy of caring, 179
    in Postpartum Depression Theory, 751

Environment—cont'd
  in Roy Adaptation Model, 356, 362-363
  in science of unitary human beings, 248
  in Self-Transcendence Theory, 647-648
  in Theory of Caring, 767
  in Theory of Comfort, 730
  in Tidal Model of Mental Health Recovery, 707
Environment-agreement, in Symphonological Bioethical
    Theory, 587-590
Environmental stimuli, adaptation to, 370
Epistemology, 16
  process in, 18
  rationalist, 17
Epstein, S., 357
Equilibrium, in Johnson Behavioral System Model, 389
Ergonomics, 728
Erickson, Helen C., 564, 565
  background of, 561-562
  and Modeling and Role-Modeling Theory, 562, 787
    acceptance of, 571-573
    case study for, 574-575
    concepts and definitions in, 565-567
    critical thinking in, 575
    critique of, 573-574
    development of, 573
    empirical evidence for, 567-570
    logical form for, 571
    major assumptions of, 570
    summary of, 574
    theoretical assertions of, 570-571
    theoretical sources for, 564-565
Erickson, Milton H., 564, 565
Erickson Maternal Bonding-Attachment Tool, 570
Erikson, E. H., 94, 100, 229, 357, 564
Erikson Psychosocial Stage Inventory, 570
Eriksson, Katie, 170, 181, 790
  background of, 191-194
  Caritative Caring Theory of
    acceptance of, 203-205
    case study for, 207-208
    concepts and definitions in, 195-197
    critical thinking in, 208
    critique of, 206-207
    empirical evidence for, 197-198
    ethics in, 195-196
    major assumptions of, 198-201
    major concepts and definitions for, 195-197
    summary of, 207
    theoretical sources for, 194-195
Ervin, S. M., 510
Escolona, 390
Ethical and Moral Dimensions of Care (Leininger), 475
*Ethical Decision Making in Nursing and Healthcare: The
    Symphonological Approach* (Husted and Husted),
    588, 596

Ethical Decision Making in Nursing (Husted), 588
Ethical Decision Making in Nursing (Husted and
    Husted), 596
Ethics
  in Bureaucratic Caring Theory, 121
  caring *vs.* nursing, 195-196
  in caritative caring, 194, 195-196, 206
  defined, 586
  ethos and, 200
  as primary, 173-174
  in Symphonological Bioethical Theory, 590-591
*Ethics, Discipline, and Refinement: Elizabeth Hagemann's
    Ethics Book—New Readings* (Martinsen and
    Wyller), 171
Ethnic, relational, 145
Ethnographic-ethnonursing, 119. *See also* Cross-cultural
    nursing
Ethnography, 122, 123, 126, 482
Ethnohistory, 477, 478
Ethnonursing method, 479, 480, 482
Ethos, in Caritative Caring Theory, 200
Evans, G. W., 307
Evers, G. C. M., 280
Evidence, empirical
  in P. Benner's work, 147-150
  in Bureaucratic Caring Theory, 122
  in Chronic Sorrow Theory, 684-686
  and concept of caring, 97
  in Conservation Model, 231
  in Health as Expanding Consciousness Theory,
    503-504
  in Health Promotion Model, 457-459
  in Human Becoming Theory, 528-529
  in Illness Trajectory Theory, 669-670
  in Johnson Behavioral System Model, 390
  in K. Martinsen's philosophy, 177-178
  in Maternal Role Attainment Theory, 610
  in Modeling and Role-Modeling Theory, 567-570
  in Nursing as Caring theory, 412
  in Nursing Process theory, 434
  in Postpartum Depression Theory, 750-751
  in Science of Unitary Human Beings, 247
  in Self-care Deficit Theory, 272
  in Self-Transcendence Theory, 646-647
  in Symphonological Bioethical Theory, 588-589
  in Theory of Caring, 764-766
  in Theory of Comfort, 729
  in Tidal Model of Mental Health Recovery, 704-705
  in Uncertainty in Illness Theory, 626-627
Excellence, notion of, 143
Exemplar, definition for, 147
Exercise Benefits-Barriers Scale (EBBS), 459
Exercise of Self-Care Agency (ESCA), 281, 282
Existential authenticity, 133
Existential being, as caring, 172

Existential-phenomenological forces, 96-97
Exosystem, in Maternal Role Attainment Theory, 612
Experience, defined, 144, 147
Expert, classification as, 146
Expertise
    development of, 144
    gaining, 149
Expertise in Nursing Practice: Caring, Clinical Judgment, and Ethics (Benner, Tanner, and Chesla), 141, 149, 153
The Eye and the Call, (Martinsen), 171
Eye of the heart, in philosophy of caring, 177

F
Faith-hope, in holistic nursing, 95
Family
    in Maternal Role Attainment Theory, 609
    in Peaceful End of Life Theory, 777
    research on, 367
    in Uncertainty in Illness Theory, 626-627
Family therapy, 19
Farley, Joanne, 80
Farnham, R. C., 510
Farrell, P., 152
Father, in Maternal Role Attainment Theory, 609
Faust, C., 439
Fawcett, Jacqueline, 6, 9, 45, 235, 254, 306, 307, 327, 332, 334, 336, 366, 369, 419, 433, 444, 763, 786
Feather, N. T., 390
Federowicz, M. L., 307
Feedback, in Neuman Systems Model, 320
Feelings
    of helplessness, 436
    sharing of, 96
Feinstein, N. F., 687
Feminism, 23
    history of, 169
    F. Nightingale on, 80
    and Postpartum Depression Theory, 744, 746
    theory, 94
Fenton, M. V., 152, 153
Ferketich, S., 608, 610, 611, 617
Ferran, C., 650
Feshbach, S., 389, 390
Fidelity, as bioethical standard, 591b, 593f, 597
Fight or flight syndrome, 230
Finch, D., 572
Finch, L. P., 419
First Time Motherhood: Experience from Teens to Forties (Mercer), 606, 616
Fitzpatrick, Joyce J., 77, 81, 234, 235, 433, 643, 644, 775, 786
Fitzpatrick, M. L., 11
Flannagan, J. M., 508
Fleischer, B. J., 281

Fleming, N., 233
Fleury, J., 631
Flexibility, in Maternal Role Attainment Theory, 608
Flexner, A., 408
Florida Atlantic Univ., 128
Focus of nursing, in Nursing as Caring Theory, 408
Folkman, S., 624, 672, 683
Foucault, Michel, 18, 174-175
Fox, C., 728, 730
Frame, K., 371
Frankl, V., 648
Frederickson, K., 372
Fredriksson, L., 205
Freedom
    as bioethical standard, 591b, 593f, 597
    in Human Becoming Theory, 524
Freud, Sigmund, 30
Frey, M. A., 281, 307
Froman, D., 307, 308
Fromm, Erich, 268
From Marx to Løgstrup: On Morality, Social Criticism and Sensuousness in Nursing (Martinsen), 170
From Novice to Expert: Excellence and Power in Clinical Nursing Practice (Benner), 141, 144, 145-147, 148, 149, 152, 156
Fruehwirth, S. E. S., 394
Fry, S., 23
Fryback, P. B., 510
Function, in Neuman Systems Model, 320
Functional requirements, in Johnson Behavioral System Model, 400

G
Gable, Robert K., 746, 755
Gadamer, H-G., 144, 197, 206
Gaffney. K. F., 280
Gale, G., 16, 19, 21
Gallagher, M. S., 370
Ganan, Rocio, 442
Gardner, B. D., 357
Gaut, D. A., 97, 408
Gavin, C., 443
Geden, E., 268, 281
Gender
    and Self-care Deficit Theory, 277t
    typology of, 38t
Generality, 12-13
    in Bureaucratic Care Theory, 132-133
    in Caritative Caring Theory, 206-207
    in Chronic Sorrow Theory, 689-690
    in Comfort Theory, 737
    in conservation model, 235
    in Culture Care Theory of Diversity and Universality, 488-489
    in Goal Attainment Theory, 308

Generality—cont'd
   in Health as Expanded Consciousness Theory,
      511
   in Health Promotion Model, 461
   in Human Becoming Theory, 542
   in Illness Trajectory Theory, 673
   in Johnson Behavioral System Model, 397-398
   in K. Martinsen's philosophy of caring, 182
   in Maternal Role Attainment Theory, 618
   in Modeling and Role-Modeling Theory, 574
   in Neuman Systems Model, 335
   of novice to expert skill acquisition model, 155
   in Nursing as Caring Theory, 421
   in Nursing Process Theory, 444-445
   in Peaceful End of Life Theory, 779
   in Postpartum Depression Theory, 755
   in M. Roger's model, 254
   in Roy Adaptation Model, 373
   in science of caring, 103
   in Self-Care Deficit Nursing Theory, 283
   in Self-Transcendence Theory, 652-653
   in Symphonological Bioethical Theory, 596
   in Theory of Caring, 770
   in Tidal Model of Mental Health Recovery, 714
   in Uncertainty in Illness Theory, 633
Generalizations, scientific, 29
General system theory, 319
George, J. B., 419, 433, 786
Gerstle, D. S., 307
Gestalt theory, in Neuman Systems Model, 319
Giangrande, S., 332
Gibbon, E. J., 508
Gibson, J. E., 229
Giere, R. N., 41
Giffin, K., 373
Gigliotti, E., 334
Giorgi, 523
Gjengdal, E., 182
Glaser, B., 117, 744
Global communities, of nursing scholars, 789-791
Global society, 587
Goal Attainment Theory, 297
   acceptance of, 305
   case study for, 309
   critical thinking in, 310
   critique of, 308-309
   development of, 302, 307-308
   empirical evidence for, 299, 300-302
   in interacting systems framework, 299, 301*f*
   logical form in, 303, 305
   propositions within, 304*b*
   relationship table for, 304*b*
   summary of, 309
   theoretical assertions of, 303, 304*b*, 304*f*
Goal Oriented Nursing Record (GONR), 306

Goals
   in Neuman Systems Model, 329b
   in Tidal Model of Mental Health Recovery, 703
Golden, B. A., 687
Goldstein, K., 229
Good, B., 151
Goodnow, M., 727
Goodwin, E. M., 307
Gordon, D. R., 153
Goto, H., 441
Gowan, N., 446
Graff, B. M., 280
Grafton, M. D., 331
Gramling, L. F., 31
Grand theories, 752
Gratification, in Maternal Role Attainment Theory, 608
Green, A., 419
Greene, Pamela, 440
Grey, M., 38
Grice, S. L., 394
Grieving and loss studies, in Human Becoming Theory,
   541. *See also* Middle range theories
Grinker, 390
Groer, M. W., 370
Grounded theory, 117, 122, 123, 126, 132, 133, 670
   inductive reasoning, 673
   methodologies, 752
   symbolic interactionism in, 744
Group psychotherapy, research on, 650, 651
Growth Through Uncertainty Scale (GTUS), 631
Grundtvig, Nikolaj Frederik Severin, 173
Guadiano, J. K., 509
Guided imagery, 729
*Guides for Developing Curriculum for the Education of
   Practical Nurses* (Orem), 268, 280-281
Gullifer, J., 269
Gunther, M. E., 307
Gustafson, W., 508

H
Haas, B. K., 39
Hage, J., 38, 41
Haggerty, L. A., 440, 442
Hainsworth, Margaret A., 679
   background of, 682-683
   and Chronic Sorrow Theory, 683
      acceptance of, 686-687
      case study for, 690-691
      concepts and definitions in, 684
      critical thinking in, 691
      critique of, 688-690
      development of, 688
      empirical evidence in, 684-686
      major assumptions of, 686
      summary of, 690

Hainsworth, Margaret A—cont'd
  theoretical assertions for, 686
  theoretical sources for, 683-384
Hall, E. T., 229
Hall, K. V., 234
Hall, Lydia, 51
  background of, 59
  Core, Care, and Cure model of, 59, 62f
Hamilton, J., 729
Hammond, H., 373
Hammond, K. R., 300
Hampe, S., 442
Hanchett, E., 442
Hand washing, F. Nightingale on, 76
Hanna, K. M., 307, 308
Hanson and Bickel's Perception of Self-Care Agency, 281
Hardt, M. E., 595
Hardy, M. E., 12, 81
Harmer, B., 727
Harmony, in Peaceful End of Life Theory, 777
Harms, M., 365
Harris, M. A., 281
Harrison, L. L., 370
Harter, 371
Hartman, R., 594
Hartrick, G. A., 613
Hassell, J. S., 330
Healing, transpersonal aspects of, 99
Healing web model, 509
Health
  in Acience of Unitary Human Beings, 248
  P. Benner on, 151
  in Bureaucratic Caring Theory, 125
  in Caritas Caring Theory, 201
  in Chronic Sorrow Theory, 686
  in Conservation Model, 232
  culturally congruent care for, 483, 484f
  in Culture Care Theory, 479
  as expanding consciousness, 502
  in Goal Attainment Theory, 303
  historical ideals of, 178-179
  in Interacting Systems Framework, 299
  in Johnson Behavioral System Model, 391, 392f
  in K. Martinsen's philosophy of caring, 178-179
  in Maternal Role Attainment Theory, 611
  in Modeling and Role-Modeling Theory, 570
  in Neuman Systems Model, 325, 334
  in Newman's theory of expanding consciousness, 500
  in Nursing Process Theory, 435-436
  in Peaceful End of Life Theory, 777
  in Postpartum Depression Theory, 751
  in Roy Adaptation Model, 362
  in Self-Transcendence Theory, 647
  social organization of, 125
  subjective nature of, 99

Health—cont'd
  in Symphonological Bioethical Theory, 588, 589
  in Theory of Caring, 766
  in Theory of Comfort, 730
  in Tidal Model of Mental Health Recovery, 706-707
Health as Expanding Consciousness (Newman), 498, 502, 505, 511
Health as Expanding Consciousness Theory, 252-253, 498, 787
  acceptance of, 507
  case study for, 512-513
  concepts and definitions in, 502-503
  critical thinking in, 513
  critique of, 511
  development of, 504-506, 511
  empirical evidence for, 503
  logical form for, 506-507
  major assumptions of, 503-504
  metaparadigm for, 499-500
  summary of, 511-512
  theoretical assertions in, 504-506
  theoretical sources for, 500-501
  and Young's stages of human evolution, 505, 506f
Health care, and bureaucratic caring, 120
Health care needs, in Theory of Comfort 728
Health care system, bioethical dilemmas in, 586
Health care teams, and Symphonological Theory, 594
Health-illness continuum, 367
Health practices, cultural, 491
Health Promoting Lifestyle Profile, 459
Health promotion, and Self-care Deficit Theory, 279t, 282
Health Promotion in Nursing Practice (Pender), 453, 457, 459
Health Promotion Model (HPM), 453, 455f
  acceptance of, 460-461
  case study for, 462-463
  critical thinking in, 463
  critique of, 461-462
  development of, 461
  empirical evidence in, 457-459
  logical form for, 460
  major assumptions of, 459
  major concepts and definitions of, 456-457
  revised, 457, 458-459, 458f
  summary of, 462
  theoretical assertions in, 459-460
  theoretical sources for, 454-455
Health-related quality of life (HRQOL), 368-369
Health-seeking behaviors, in Theory of Comfort, 729
Health status
  infant, 609
  in Maternal Role Attainment Theory, 608
Hegel, G. W. F., 119, 124, 126, 133, 500, 502

Heidegger, Martin, 94, 143, 144, 150, 151, 170, 172-173, 523, 529
Helicy, in homeodynamics, 249t
Helicy principle, Rogers', 644
Helping role, of nurse, 158
Helping-trust relationship, development of, 95-96
Helson, Harry, 356, 364
Helton, A., 330
Henderson, Virginia, 50, 54, 63, 141, 268, 441, 728, 752
    basic needs identified by, 56, 57b
    definition of nursing of, 55
    recognition of, 9
Herbert, J., 394
Hermeneutic dialectic, 511, 512
Hermeneutics, 23, 150
    critical, 175
    defined, 147
    in human becoming school of thought, 541
    and Nursing as Caring theory, 419
    in Tidal Model of Mental Health Recovery, 711
Hertz, J. E. G., 573
Hill, B. J., 368
Hilton, B. A., 630
Hilton, S. A., 331
Hirschfeld, M. J., 233
History
    and logical form, 179-180
    meaning of, 174-175
History, nursing
    curriculum era in, 4
    nursing knowledge in, 3
    nursing theory era in, 6
    research era in, 4
    and theory, 1, 4
    theory era in, 4-5
Hobdell, E., 687
Holaday, B., 394, 396
Holism, in Modeling and Role-Modeling Theory, 566
Holistic care, 95
Holland, K., 64
Hollingsworth, A. O., 280
Hologram, Theory of Bureaucratic Caring as, 120
Holographic theory, 121
Holography, 120
Home health nursing, and Nursing as Caring theory, 419
Homeodynamics, principles of, 248, 249t-250t, 253f
Hope: An International Human Becoming Perspective (Parse), 522
Hopey, K., 595
Hopkins Clinical Assessment of APAM, 570
Horn, B. J., 280
Horner, S. D., 672
Hospitals, magnet, 100-101
Houle, P., 438

The Human Becoming School of Thought: A Perspective for Nurses and Other Health Professionals (Parse), 522, 529, 531, 533
Human Becoming Theory
    acceptance of, 533-544, 534b-540b
    case study for, 544
    concepts and definitions in, 525-527
    critical thinking in, 544-546
    critique of, 541-544
    empirical evidence in, 528-529
    logical form for, 532-533
    major assumptions of, 529-532
    publications about, 534b-540b
    relationships in, 532f
    summary of, 544
    theoretical assertions in, 532
    theoretical sources for, 523-524
Human being. *See also* Person
    in Caritative Caring Theory, 194, 196, 198-199
    in conservation model, 232
    in Human Becoming Theory, 524
Human field image metaphor scale, 255t
Human field motion test (HFMT), 255 table
Human immunodeficiency virus (HIV)
    research on, 510, 688
    and Self-care Deficit Theory, 279t
    and Self-Transcendence Theory, 651
Humanism, 361
Humanities, 95
Humanness, in Nursing as Caring theory, 412-413
Human science theory, caring in, 99
Human-to-human relationship model, J. Travelbee's, 59, 62, 63f
Human-universe-health process, in Human Becoming Theory, 531-532
Husserl, Edmund, 170, 171, 172, 177
Husted, Gladys L.
    background of, 585
    Symphonological Bioethical Theory of, 785
        acceptance of, 594-595
        case study for, 597-598
        concepts and definitions in, 587-588
        critical thinking in, 598
        critique of, 596-597
        empirical evidence for, 588-589
        logical form for, 592-593
        major assumptions of, 589-590
        summary of, 597
        theoretical assertions of, 590-592
        theoretical sources for, 586-587
Husted, James
    background of, 585-586
    and Symphonlogical Bioethical Theory, 785
Hutchins, G., 418
Hutchinson, S., 744

I

The Idea of Caring (Eriksson), 193
Identity
    in Illness Trajectory Theory, 667
    maternal, 608
IFE (Index of field energy), 255t
Illich, I., 362, 706
Illness
    P. Benner on, 151
    in Johnson Behavioral System Model, 392f
    in Neuman Systems Model, 322
    social organization of, 125
Illness Trajectory Theory
    acceptance of, 671-672
    case study for, 674-675
    concepts and definitions in, 667-668
    critical thinking in, 675
    critique of, 673-674
    development of, 672-673
    empirical evidence for, 669-670
    logical form for, 671
    major assumptions of, 670-671
    summary of, 674
    theoretical assertions of, 671
    theoretical sources for, 666
    uncertainty in, 667, 668t
Illuminations: The Human Becoming Theory in Practice and Research (Parse), 522
Illusion, in Uncertainty in Illness Theory, 625
Im, E. O., 752
Imaging, in Human Becoming Theory, 525, 532f
Imbalance, in Neuman Systems Model, 319
Immobilization, research on, 730
Improvement, in Nursing Process Theory, 434
Induction
    basic characteristics of, 32t-33t
    defined, 27-29
    examples, 27-29
    in history of science, 17
    in Symphonological Bioethical Theory, 593
    in Theory of Comfort, 731
Industrialization, 174
Infant
    in Maternal Role Attainment Theory, 613
    and Self-care Deficit Theory, 276t
Infant temperament, in Maternal Role Attainment Theory, 609
Inference, in Uncertainty in Illness Theory, 625
Inflammatory response, defined, 230
Information-processing models, 624
Ingestive subsystem, in Johnson Behavioral System Model, 388-389
Inherent endowment, in Modeling and Role-Modeling Theory, 567
Input, in Neuman Systems Model, 320

Institutional integrity, in Theory of Comfort, 729
Instruments for Assessing and Measuring Caring in Nursing and Health Sciences (Watson), 97, 101, 106
Intent of nursing, in Nursing as Caring theory, 408
Interacting Systems Framework, 297, 788
    acceptance of, 306
    case study, 309
    concepts and definitions in, 299, 301f
    critical thinking in, 310
    development of, 300-302
    dynamic interacting systems in, 300f
    empirical evidence for, 299, 300-302
    Goal Attainment Theory developed from, 302
    major assumptions of, 302-303
    summarized, 309
    theoretical sources for, 298
Interactive, integrative participation, 510
Interdependence mode, in Roy Adaptation Model, 360, 364, 376t
International Association for Human Caring, 118, 406
International Neuman Systems Model Symposium, 789
International nursing, 441-442, 476
International Orem Society (IOS) for Nursing Science and Nursing Scholarship, 283, 789
Internet, 543
Interpersonal relations
    in Health Promotion Model, 456
    in Interacting Systems Framework, 301
    Peplau theory of, 54
Interventions, nursing
    comfort care actions and, 739t
    as comfort measures, 728
    holographic model of, 508, 509f
    in Johnson Behavioral System Model, 394
    in Neuman Systems Model, 322, 324f
    in Peaceful End of Life Theory, 779
    and role-modeling, 569
    in Roy Adaptation Model, 365
    self-care, 665
    in Self-Transcendence Theory, 646
    types of comfort and, 734
Introduction to Clinical Nursing (Levine), 228, 231-233, 234
Introduction to Nursing: An Adaptation Model (Roy), 356-357
An Introduction to the Theoretical Basis of Nursing (Rogers), 245
Inventory of Functional Status in the Elderly, 368
Invitation, in Caritative Caring Theory, 196
Irwin, M., 596
Isaramalai, S., 268
Isenberg, M. A., 369, 371
Issel, L. M., 330
Ittleson. W., 300

J

Jackson, D. D., 300
Jaco, Gartly, 268
Jacob, M., 74
Jacobs, M. K., 373, 574
Jacobson. H., 332
Jacono, B. J., 509
Jacono, J. J., 509
James, Jenny, 572
James, P., 438
Jelsma, N., 152
Jenkins, J., 64, 371
Jesek-Hale, S., 284
Jirovec, M. M., 371
Johns, C., 127
Johnson, B., 442
Johnson, Dorothy E., 63, 268, 355
  background of, 386-387
  Behavioral System Model of
    acceptance of, 393-395
    case study for, 398-400
    concepts and definitions in, 387-389
    critical thinking in, 400-401
    critique of, 397-398
    empirical evidence in, 390
    further development for, 396-397
    logical form for, 393
    major assumptions of, 390-391
    major concepts and definitions of, 387-389
    summary of, 398
    theoretical assertions in, 391, 392f, 393
    theoretical sources for, 387
Johnson, Jean, 775
Judgment
  clinical, 149
  professional, 176

K

Kagan, 390
Kaila, Eino, 194
Kalb, K. A., 508
Kalisch, B. J., 73
Kalisch, P. A., 73
Kameoka, T., 307, 308-309
Katz, Robert, 268
Kawamura, S., 441
Kearney, B., 281
Kearney, C., 420
Keenan, J., 38
Kelley, K. J., 300
Kelly, L., 371
Kemppainen, J. K., 306
Kennedy, H., 756
Kiehl, E. M., 307
Kierkegaard, Søren, 143, 173, 194, 198

Killeen, M. B., 307
Kim, H. S., 31
King, A., 408
King, Imogene, 268, 297 *See also* Interacting Systems
    Framework
  background of, 297-298
  and Goal Attainment Theory, 297
    case study for, 309
    critical thinking in, 310
    critique of, 308-309
    development of, 302
    and empirical evidence, 299, 300-302
    in interacting systems framework, 299, 301f
    logical form in, 303, 305
    propositions within, 304b
    relationship table for, 304b
    summary of, 309
    theoretical assertions of, 303, 304b, 304f
King International Nursing Group (KING), 298
Kirkevold, M., 180
Kiser-Larson, N., 420
Klein, M., 564
Kleinman, A., 151
Knafl, K. A., 38
Knowing, in Theory of Caring, 764
Knowledge
  embodied, 144
  emic, 477, 478
  etic, 477, 478
  practical, 144
  scientific, 22
  self-care, 567, 568, 569
  tacit, 587
Knowledge, nursing, 480
  as basis for nursing discipline, 10
  in clinical practice, 47
  compared with medical knowledge, 5
  development of, 3-4
  nature of, 9
  new paradigms in, 22
  synthesizing, 46
  systematic structure of, 6
Kobayshi, M., 441
Koertvelyessy, 334
Kokuyama, T., 441
Kolcaba, Katharine
  background of, 726-727
  Theory of Comfort of
    acceptance of, 733-736
    case study, 738
    concepts and definitions in, 728
    critical thinking in, 740
    critique of, 737-738
    development of, 736-737
    empirical evidence in, 729-730

Kolcaba, Katharine—cont'd
   Theory of Comfort of—cont'd
      major assumptions of, 730-731
      summary of, 738
      theoretical sources for, 727-728
Kolcaba, R., 730
Koniak-Griffin, D., 613
Koort, Peep, 194
Kramer, M., 12, 13, 147, 752, 755, 770, 788
Krieger, D., 300
Ku, N., 330
Kuhn, A., 300
Kuhn, Thomas S., 6, 10, 21, 22, 142, 194, 786-787
Kumata, M., 441

L
Laben, J. K., 306
Labor, research on, 730. *See also* Postpartum Depression
   Theory
Lachicotte, J. L., 395
Ladewig, P., 754
Ladwig, G. B., 688
Lamb, G. S., 508
Langer, Susan, 194
Language, 477
   and meaning, 175
   nurses' work in, 699-700
   poetic, 182
   in Tidal Model of Mental Health Recovery, 701b, 712
Languaging, in Human Becoming Theory, 525-526,
   532f
Lanouette, M., 394
Larson, P., 440
Lauder, W., 282
Law, in Bureaucratic Caring Theory, 121
Lazarus, Richard S., 94, 143, 144, 356, 624, 672, 683
Leadership, in Nursing Process theory, 438-440
Learning. *See also* Education
   interpersonal, 96
   of nursing skills, 149
Learning, clinical
   advanced beginner in, 145
   competent stage in, 146
   proficiency in, 146
   situation in, 146, 147
   stages of, 153
Learning outcomes, and Adaptation Model, 367
Leddy healthiness scale, 255t
Lee, B. T., 306
Lee, R. E., 542
Leigh, G. K., 607
Leininger, Madeleine M., 116, 117, 119
   background of, 472-475
   Culture Care Theory of Diversity and Universality of,
      473-475, 787

Leininger, Madeleine M—cont'd
   Culture Care Theory of Diversity and Universality
      of—cont'd
      acceptance of, 485-487
      case study in, 490
      clinical application of, 487
      concepts and definitions in, 478-479
      critical thinking in, 490-491
      critique of, 488-489
      development of, 488
      empirical evidence in, 479-481
      logical form in, 482-485, 484f
      major assumptions of, 481
      summary of, 489-490
      theoretical assertions of, 481-482
      theoretical sources for, 475-477
   definition of theory of, 477
Leitch, M., 390
Length of hospital stay, research on, 568, 569
Lenz, Elizabeth, 46, 775
Leonard, H., 442
Leonard, R., 442
Leu, J., 330
Lévinas, Emmanuel, 194, 195, 201
Levine, Myra Estrin, 268
   background of, 227-228
   Conservation Model of, *228*
      acceptance of, 233-235
      case study for, 235-237
      concepts and definitions of, 229-231
      critical thinking in, 237-238
      critique of, 235
      development of, 234-235
      empirical evidence for, 231
      logical form in, 233
      major assumptions of, 231-233
      summary of, 235
      theoretical assertions in, 233
      theoretical sources for, 229
Levy, K., 159
Lewin, Kurt, 268
Liehr, P., 46, 788
Life crisis, in Tidal Model of Mental Health Recovery,
   707
Life histories, 482
Life process, in Roy Adaptation Model, 358
Life satisfaction
   in elderly, 569
   and self-care resources, 568
Life stories, 482
Lifetime development, in Modeling and Role-Modeling
   Theory, 566
Lin, L., 330
Lin, M., 330
Linden, D., 420

Lindholm, L., 205
Linkages, in nursing theory, 41-44
Litchfield, M. C., 506
Living, model of, 64, 64t, 65f
Lock, S., 572
Locsin, R. C., 420, 421
Logan, 790
Logan, Janice, 440
Logan, Winifred W., 53, 64-65, 64t, 65f, 66f
Logic, 25
Logical empiricists, 18
London, M., 754
Lonergan, Bernard, 268
Lorenz, K., 389, 390
Loss, in Chronic Sorrow Theory, 684
Loss of control, in Postpartum Depression Theory, 747-748
Louis, M., 332
Lovejoy, N., 396
Lowry, L. W., 332
Lozano, Maria, 442
Luther, Martin, 174
Lynaugh, Joan, 141
Lynn, Christine E., 118
Løgstrup, Knud Eiler, 170, 173, 175, 180
Løgstrup, Rosemarie, 170

M

MacIntyre, Alasdair, 145
Macrae, J. A., 73
Magan, S. J., 508
Mahler, M. S., 564
Mahon, P. Y., 307
Maintaining belief, in Theory of Caring, 764
Majesky, S. J., 396
Malinski, V.
Mallow, G. E., 687
Malveiro, Paula, 442
Managed care
    in Johnson Behavioral System Model, 395
    USAF personnel and, 132t
Management, in Chronic Sorrow Theory, 684, 685-686
Man-Living-Health: A Theory of Nursing (Parse), 522, 533
Marchione, Joanne, 507
Mariolis, T., 509
Marital status, typology of, 38t
Marriner Tomey, A., 439, 542, 615, 786
Martin, S. A., 330, 331
Martinez, 356
Martinsen, Kari Marie
    background of, 167-171
    philosophy of caring of, 785
        acceptance of, 180-181
        case study for, 183

Martinsen, Kari Marie—cont'd
    philosophy of caring of—cont'd
        concepts and definitions in, 175-177
        critical thinking in, 181-182
        critique of, 181-182
        development of, 181
        empirical evidence for, 177-178
        logical form for, 179-180
        major assumptions of, 178-179
        summary of, 182-183
        theoretical assertions of, 179
        theoretical sources for, 171-175
Marx, Karl, 171-172, 319
Maslow, A., 94, 100, 564, 648
Mastal, M. F., 373
Master's programs, 9
    development of, 5
    in Human Becoming Theory, 540
    role of students in, 10
Mastsuo, M., 441
Maternal identity, in Maternal Role Attainment Theory, 608
Maternal Role Attainment Theory
    acceptance of, 614-616
    case study for, 619
    concepts and definitions in, 608-609
    critical thinking in, 619
    critique of, 617-618
    development of, 616-617
    empirical evidence for, 610
    logical form for, 614
    major assumptions of, 610-611
    model for, 607f
    original model for, 612-613
    process of, 616-617
    revised model for, 613-614, 615f
    stages of, 612-613
    summary of, 619
    theoretical assertions of, 611-614
    theoretical sources for, 606-607
Maternity, and Self-Care Deficit Theory, 278t
Maternity blues, 747, 749
Maxim, defined, 147
May, K. A., 608, 611, 615
Mayeroff, M., 407, 415
McBride, A. B., 613, 616, 618
McBride, L., 443, 444
McBride, S., 281
McCaleb, A. M., 282
McCance, Kathryn, 118
McCance, T. V., 420
McCorkle, R., 369
McCormick, K. M., 672
McCue, S., 371
McDonald, F. J., 365

McDonald, Lynn, 73
McElmurry, Beverly, 453
McEwen, M., 786
McFarland, J., 330
McFarland, M. R., 487
McGee, E., 650
McKenna, H. P., 330, 420
McKinney, N. L., 307
Mead, G. H., 357, 390, 607
Mead, Margaret, 473
Meaning
    embedded, 119, 148, 150
    embodied, 144
    in Health as Expanding Consciousness Theory,
        502
    of history, 174-175
    in Human Becoming Theory, 530
    in Tidal Model of Mental Health Recovery, 698
Mechanic, 356
Medical anthropology, 476
Medicine
    culture of, 175
    social history of, 169
Mefford, L. C., 233
Meighan, M., 615
Meleis, A., 5, 377, 752, 786
Meleski, D. D., 687
Melnyk, B. M., 687
Mendes, Ana, 442
Mental comfort, 727
Mental health. *See also* Tidal Model of Mental Health
        Recovery
    in elderly, 646-647
    recovery of, 698
    and Self-care Deficit Theory, 277t-278t
    and self-transcendence, 653
Mental Health Symptomatology (MHS) scores, 647
Mental illness, in Tidal Model of Mental Health
        Recovery, 708
Mental patterns, in Bureaucratic Caring Theory, 121
Mentzer, C., 509
Mercer, Ramona T., 608
    background of, 605-606
    and Maternal Role Attainment Theory
        acceptance of, 614-616
        case study for, 619
        concepts and definitions in, 608-609
        critical thinking in, 619
        critique of, 617-618
        development of, 616-617
        empirical evidence for, 610
        major assumptions of, 610-611
        summary of, 619
        theoretical assertions of, 611-614
        theoretical sources for, 606-607

Merleau-Ponty, M., 151, 171, 172, 173, 523, 529
Merton, R. K., 46, 571
Mertz, R., 442
Mesosystem, in Maternal Role Attainment Theory, 612
Meta-analysis, 369
Metaparadigm, 45
Metaphysics, 179, 180
Michaels, C., 508
Microsystem, in Maternal Role Attainment Theory,
        612
Middle range theories, 369, 633-634, 752, 785, 788
    of adaptation, 371-372
    of adaptation to caregiving, 372
    characteristics of, 690
    Chronic Sorrow Theory, 680-691
    globalization of, 789-790
    of goal attainment, 297, 298
    Maternal Role Attainment Theory, 605-619
    in nursing knowledge, 789f
    in nursing practice, 788-789, 790-791
    Peaceful End of Life Theory, 775-781
    Postpartum Depression Theory, 743-757
    SCDNT as, 282
    Self-Transcendence Theory, 643-655
    Theory of Caring, 762-770
    Theory of Comfort, 726-740
    Tidal Model of Mental Health Recovery, 696-717
Miller, K., 127
Mills, C. W., 47
Minckley, B. B., 300
Mind-body relationships, in Modeling and Role-
        Modeling Theory, 567
Ministration of help model, 61f
Miscarriage, research on, 541, 765
Mischo-Kelling, M., 442
Mishel, Merle H.
    background of, 626-624
    and Uncertainty in Illness Theory
        acceptance of, 630-631
        case study for, 634
        critical thinking in, 634
        critique of, 631-633
        development of, 631
        empirical evidence for, 626-627
        major assumptions of, 627-629, 628f
        summary of, 633-634
        theoretical assertions in, 629
        theoretical sources for, 624-625
Mishel Uncertainty in Illness Scale (MUIS-A), 623,
        626
Mishler, E. G., 22
Mitzel, A., 730
Modeling, act of, 565
*Modeling and Role-Modeling: A Theory and Paradigm for
    Nursing* (Erickson et al.), 571

Model of living, model of nursing based on, 64, 64t, 65f
Modeling and Role-Modeling Theory, 787
   acceptance by, 571-573
   case study for, 574-575
   concepts and definitions of, 565-567
   critical thinking in, 575
   critique of, 573-574
   development of, 573
   empirical evidence in, 567-570
   logical form for, 571
   major assumptions of, 570
   summary of, 574
   theoretical assertions of, 570-571
   theoretical sources for, 564-565
Modrcin-McCarthy, M. A., 371
Modrcin-Talbott, M. A., 369, 370
Moldenhouer, Z., 687
Monteiro, L. A., 80
Mood disorders, postpartum, 746-747. *See also*
   Postpartum Depression Theory
Moore, C., 372
Moore, J. B., 280, 282, 284
Moore, Shirley M., 727, 774
   background of, 775
   and Peaceful End of Life (EOL) Theory
      acceptance of, 778
      case study for, 781
      concepts and definitions in, 776-777
      critical thinking in, 781
      critique of, 779-780
      development of, 779
      empirical evidence for, 777
      major assumptions of, 777
      theoretical assertions of, 778
      theoretical sources for, 776
Moral practice, 176
Morita, Shoma, 698
Morris, M., 446
Morse, Janice, 102, 118, 729
Moss, R., 501
Mother-father relationship, in Maternal Role Attainment
   Theory, 609
Motherhood, research on, 746
Motive research, 194
Movement, in health as expanding consciousness theory,
   504, 505, 506f
Movement-space-time, in Health as Expanding
   Consciousness Theory, 503-504
Mrozek, R., 508
Murray, Henry, 732, 733
Murray, R., 75
Murrell-Amstrong, 371

N
Nåden, D., 204
Nagel, Ernest, 268

NANDA (North American Nursing Diagnosis
   Association), 498, 499, 687, 690
Nardi, P. M., 607
Narrative accounts, 155
National Institutes of Health, National Center for
   Nursing Research in, 453
National League for Nursing (NLN), accreditation
   criteria of, 5
Native American healers, 491
Natural Transcultural Nursing Society, 474
The Nature of Nursing: A Definition and Its Implications
   for Practice, Research, and Education
   (Henderson), 56
The Nature of Nursing: Reflections After 25 Years
   (Henderson), 56
Need-for-help
   identification of, 60f
   validation of, 62f
Need satisfaction, and affiliated-individuation, 564
Needs
   assistance with gratification of, 96
   Maslow 's theory of human, 564
   in Modeling and Role-Modeling Theory, 566
   in Nursing Process theory, 433
Neeson, J. D., 615
Negentropy
   in Neuman Systems Model, 321
   in system theory, 247
Nelson, A. M., 613
Nelson, S., 75
Neonatal intensive care unit (NICU), research on, 764
Neuman, Betty, 332, 334
   background of, 318-319
   Systems Model of, 324f, 787
      acceptance of, 325, 327, 332-333
      biennial symposia on, 327, 333
      case study for, 336
      concepts and definitions in, 320-323
      critical thinking in, 337
      critique of, 334-336
      development of, 333-334
      empirical evidence for, 323
      further development of, 333-334
      logical form of, 325
      major assumptions of, 323-325, 326b
      summary of, 336
      theoretical assertions of, 325, 326b
      theoretical sources for, 319-320
      web site, 332
Neuman Nursing Process Format, 327
The Neuman Systems Model: Application to Nursing
   Education and Practice (Neuman), 319, 332, 334
Neuman Systems Model Trustees Group, 334, 336
Nevada State College, nursing program in, 127, 128f
Neverveld, M. E., 152
Newman, D. M., 367

Newman, Margaret A., 252-253, 420
  background of, 497-498
  Health as Expanding Consciousness Theory of, 498, 787
    acceptance of, 507-511
    case study for, 511-512
    concepts and definitions in, 502-503
    critical thinking in, 513
    critique of, 511
    development of, 504-506, 511
    empirical evidence in, 503
    major assumptions of, 503-504
    metaparadigm for, 499-500
    summary of, 511-512
    theoretical assertions in, 504-506
    theoretical sources for, 500-501
Nightingale, Florence, 4, 5, 229, 268, 387
  acceptance by nursing community of, 79-81
  credentials and background of, 71-73
  critique of theory, 81-83
  empirical evidence used by, 76-77
  environmental focus of, 75-76
  environment defined by, 77-78
  and feminist theory, 80
  health defined by, 77
  logical form used by, 79
  major assumptions of, 77
  management style of, 80
  on nursing knowledge, 5
  philosophy of nursing of, 73-75
  recognition of, 9
  societal changes recognized by, 74
  as statistician, 76-77, 83
  theoretical assertions of, 78-79
  uniqueness of, 83
Nightingale Songs, 407
Nishio, K. T., 396
North American Nursing Diagnosis Association
    (NANDA), 498, 499
Northington, L., 687
Northrop, F.S.C., 247
Notes on Hospitals (Nightingale), 72
*Notes on Matters Affecting the Health, Efficiency, and
    Hospital Administration of the British Army
    Founded Chiefly on the Experience of the Late War*
    (Nightingale), 72, 76
Notes on Nursing (Nightingale), 75, 77, 78, 81, 83
Novice, classification as, 145
Novice to Expert Skill Acquisition Model
  acceptance of, 152-154
  case study for, 157-159
  concepts and definitions in, 145-147
  and critical thinking, 159
  critique of, 154-156
  development of, 154
  empirical evidence for, 147
  theoretical assertions for, 151-152

Nuamah, I. F., 369
Nuccio, S.A., 159
Nurse anthropologist, 116
Nurse-client relationship, 508
  in Culture Care Theory, 482
  experimental process of, 506
Nurse Educator Nursing Theory Conference (1978),
    9
Nurse-patient relationship, 698
  changing aspects of, 54, 55f
  as economic resource, 133
  in F. Nightingale's writings, 82
  phases and changing roles in, 56f
  phases of, 54, 55f
Nurse-Patient Relationship Resource Analysis, 129
Nurse-person relationship, in Tidal Model of Mental
    Health Recovery, 698, 702
Nurse researcher, 483
Nurse scientist program, 473
Nursing
  P. Benner on, 150
  Bureaucratic Caring Theory in, 124-125
  Chronic Sorrow Theory in, 686
  conceptual framework for, 274f
  defined, 652, 766
  in Goal Attainment Theory, 303
  Health as Expanding Consciousness Theory,
      499-500
  Human Becoming Theory in, 530-531
  Interacting Systems Framework, 299
  Johnson Behavioral System Model in, 390-391, 400
  K. Martinsen's philosophy of caring in, 178-179
  Maternal Role Attainment Theory in, 610-611
  Modeling and Role-Modeling Theory in, 565, 570
  Nursing Process Theory in, 435
  Peaceful End of Life Theory in, 777
  Postpartum Depression Theory in, 751
  Roy Adaptation Model in, 361-362
  Science of Unitary Human Beings in, 247
  Self-Transcendence Theory in, 647
  situation-dependent, 182
  in Symphonological Bioethical Theory, 588, 589
  theory-based, 785
  Theory of Caring in, 766
  Theory of Comfort in, 730
  as therapeutic activity in, 699
  Tidal Model of Mental Health Recovery in, 705-706
  transcultural, 485
*Nursing: Human Science and Human Care—A Theory of
    Nursing* (Watson), 93, 94, 98, 99, 101, 103
Nursing: The Philosophy and Science of Caring (1979)
    (Watson), 93, 97, 99, 101
Nursing and Anthropology: Two Worlds to Blend
    (Leininger), 473, 475
Nursing as Caring: A Model for Transforming Practice
    (Boykin and Schoenhofer), 406, 407, 408, 415

Nursing as Caring Theory, 785
  acceptance of, 415-420
  case study for, 422-423
  concepts and definitions in, 408-412
  critical thinking in, 423
  critique of, 421-422
  development of, 420
  empirical evidence for, 412
  logical form for, 415
  major assumptions of, 412-413
  summary of, 422
  theoretical assertions in, 414-416
  theoretical sources for, 407
Nursing care, culturally competent, 479
Nursing Care for Parents at Risk (Mercer), 606
Nursing Child Assessment Satellite Training Project, 62
Nursing clinician-case manager, 507
Nursing Concepts of Practice (Orem), 268, 269, 270, 275, 282
Nursing Consortium for Research on Chronic Sorrow (NCRCS), 680-681, 683, 684, 685, 687, 688
Nursing design, 271
Nursing Fundamentals (Parse), 522
Nursing History: Frank and Engaged Deaconesses: A Caring Profession Emerges 1860-1905 (Martinsen), 169
Nursing process
  defined, 436
  discipline, 434
  Roy's six-step, 365
Nursing Process Theory
  acceptance of, 437-443
  case study for, 438, 447
  concepts and definitions in, 433-434
  critical thinking in, 447
  critique of, 444-446
  development of, 443-444
  empirical evidence for, 434
  environment in, 436
  logical form in, 437
  major assumptions of, 434-436
  summary of, 446-447
  theoretical assertion of, 436-437
  theoretical sources for, 433
Nursing response, in Nursing as Caring theory, 411-412
Nursing Science: Major Paradigms, Theories, and Critiques (Parse), 522
Nursing science, *vs.* medical science, 367
Nursing shortage, 100
Nursing situation, in Nursing as Caring theory, 408-409, 409, 411, 422, 423
Nursing systems, 271
  basic, 273 f
  in Self-care Deficit Nursing Theory, 286-287
  theory of, 273

Nursing theorists, types of, 377
Nursing Theorists and Their Work (Marriner Tomey), 789
Nurturance, in Modeling and Role-Modeling Theory, 566
Nurturing relationships, in Nursing as Caring theory, 413
Nyberg, J. J., 127
Nygren, A., 194, 199, 201

O

Oberst, M. T., 670
Object attachment, and affiliated-individuation, 564
Objectivity, as bioethical standard, 591b, 593f, 597
Observation
  F. Nightingale on, 82
  theories and, 19-20
Observation participation reflection enabler, in Culture Care Theory, 485
Obsessive-compulsive disorder, postpartum, 747. *See also* Postpartum Depression Theory
Obstetrical nursing, 744
Occupational health nursing, 275
Olds, S., 754
Olsen, Ruth, 181
Olshansky, S., 683
Olson, J., 442
O'Malley, I. B., 73
Oncology nursing, 665, 670
Ontology, of nursing, 417
Open systems
  in Neuman Systems Model, 320-321
  universe of, 246
Ordering, in nursing theory, 41-44
Orem, Dorothea E., 789
  background of, 267-268
  Self-Care Deficit Nursing Theory of, 267, 787
    acceptance of, 275-283
    case study for, 285-287
    concepts and definitions in, 269-272
    critical thinking in, 287
    critique of, 283-284
    empirical evidence for, 272
    logical form for, 274
    major assumptions of, 272
    summary of, 284
    theoretical assertions of, 272-274
    theoretical sources for, 268-269
Orem Study Group, 282
Organismic response, defined, 230
Organizational caring tool, 129
Organizational culture, and Human Becoming Theory, 542
Originating, in Human Becoming Theory, 527, 532f

Orlando, Ida Jean, 7, 57, 59, 268, 728
  background of, 431-433
  Nursing Process Theory of, 432, 433
    acceptance of, 437-443
    case study for, 447
    critical thinking in, 447
    critique of, 444-446
    development of, 443-444
    empirical evidence in, 434
    logical form for, 437
    major assumptions of, 434-436
    major concepts and definitions of, 433-434
    summary of, 446
    theoretical assertions of, 436-437
    theoretical sources for, 433
  recognition of, 9
Orlando, J., 300
Orme, J. E., 300
Outcomes
  in Neuman Systems Model, 329b
  and role-modeling, 569
Outcomes, patient
  in Johnson Behavioral System Model, 395
  in Nursing as Caring theory, 414
Output, in Neuman Systems Model, 320
Ovarian cancer, research on, 282

P
Pagli, Lorita Marlena Freitag, 442
Pain, middle range theory of, 372
Pain control, research in, 396
Palencia, I., 372
Palmer, I.S., 77
Pandimensionality, in Science of Unitary Human Beings, 246
Panic disorder, postpartum-onset, 747. *See also* Postpartum Depression Theory
Paradigm case, defined, 147
Paradigms, 786
  in Modeling and Role-Modeling Theory, 571
  in nursing theory, 6
Parents at Risk (Mercer), 606
Parish nursing, 75, 508
Parker, Marilyn E., 407, 419, 786
Parry, C., 672
Parse, Rosemarie Rizzo, 253
  background of, 522-524
  Human Becoming Theory of, 787
    acceptance of, 533-544, 534b-540b
    case study for, 544
    concepts and definitions in, 525-527
    critical thinking in, 544-546
    critique of, 541-544
    empirical evidence for, 528-529
    logical form for, 532-533

Parse, Rosemarie Rizzo—cont'd
  Human Becoming Theory of—cont'd
    major assumptions of, 529-532
    summary of, 544
    theoretical assertions in, 532
    theoretical sources for, 523-524
Parsons, Talcott, 268, 387
Participant-observer, 509
Partner, in Maternal Role Attainment Theory, 609
Pateiro, Virginio, 442
Paterson, J. G., 300, 407, 728
Patient
  in Caritative Caring Theory, 196
  objectification of, 168
  in Symphonological Bioethical Theory, 589
  in Theory of Comfort, 730
Patient-Centered Approaches to Nursing (Abdellah et al.), 57
Patient education, and self-care deficit theory, 279t
Pattern recognition
  in Health as Expanding Consciousness Theory, 499-500, 501f
  human, 19
  Newman's theory of, 508
  research in, 510
Patterns
  and family interactions, 507
  in Health as Expanding Consciousness Theory, 503
  in Science of Unitary Human Beings, 246
Patterson, K. A., 615
The Pause: A Description of the Knowledge Object of Caring Science (Eriksson), 204
PDSS, 746, 753-754
Peaceful End of Life (EOL) Theory
  acceptance of, 778
  case study for, 781
  concepts and definitions in, 776-777
  critical thinking in, 781
  critique of, 779-780
  development of, 779
  empirical evidence for, 777
  logical form for, 778
  major assumptions of, 777
  relationships among concepts of, 780f
  theoretical assertions of, 778
  theoretical sources for, 776
Peat, F.D., 119, 120
Peitchinis, L., 438
Pelletier. *See* Orlando, Ida Jean
Pender, Nola J.
  background of, 452-454
  Health Promotion Model of, 453
    acceptance of, 460-461
    case study for, 462-463
    concepts and definitions in, 456-457

Pender, Nola J.—cont'd
  Health Promotion Model of—cont'd
    critical thinking in, 463
    critique of, 461-462
    development of, 461
    empirical evidence for, 457-459
    major assumptions of, 459
    summary of, 462
    theoretical assertions in, 459-460
    theoretical sources for, 454-455
Penhale, Helen, 452
People-truths, 479
Peplau, Hildegard E., 50, 59, 268, 300, 698, 704, 752
  Interpersonal Relations Theory of, 54
  recognition of, 9
Perceived Enactment of Autonomy Tool, 570
Perceived field motion (PFM) scale, 255 table
Perception, in Roy Adaptation Model, 360, 363-364
Perceptual awareness, 230
Perrin, C., 441
Person. *See also* Human being
  in Bureaucratic Caring Theory, 125
  in Chronic Sorrow Theory, 686
  in Conservation Model, 232
  defined, 766
  in Goal Attainment Theory, 303
  in Health as Expanding Consciousness Theory, 499,
    500, 501f
  in Human Becoming Theory, 523, 524
  in K. Martinsen's philosophy of caring, 178-179
  in Johnson Behavioral System Model, 390-391
  in Maternal Role Attainment Theory, 611
  in Modeling and Role-Modeling Theory, 566, 570
  in Nursing as Caring theory, 408, 413
  in Nursing Process theory, 435
  in Peaceful End of Life Theory, 777
  in Postpartum Depression Theory, 751
  in Roy Adaptation Model, 362, 363f
  in Science of Unitary Human Beings, 247
  self-interpreting being, 144
  as self-interpreting being, 150-151
  in Self-Transcendence Theory, 647
  in Symphonological Bioethical Theory, 589
  in Theory of Caring, 766
  in Tidal Model of Mental Health Recovery, 705
Personal factors, in Health Promotion Model, 456
Personal narrative, in Tidal Model of Mental Health
    Recovery, 708-709
Person-environment participation scale (PEPS), 255t
Person-environment relations, sequential patterns of, 501f
Personhood
  characteristics of, 412
  definition of, 410
  in Nursing as Caring Theory, 407, 410, 413
  in Tidal Model of Mental Health Recovery, 702, 713f

Person-patient, in Symphonological Bioethical Theory,
    588
Perspectives on Adolescent Health Care (Mercer), 606
Peterson, J. Z., 307
Phenix, P., 408
Phenomenological-hermeneutical process, in Nursing as
    Caring theory, 417. *See also* Hermeneutics
Phenomenology, 23, 122, 123, 143, 168, 173
  and Bureaucratic Caring Theory, 126
  and concept of caring, 97
  hermeneutic, 175
  methods, 482
  as natural attitude, 172
Phenomenology and Caring: Three Dialogues
    (Martinsen), 170
Phenomenology of the Social World (Schutz), 18
Phillips, J. R., 543
Philosophical assumptions, in Roy Adaptation Model,
    361b
Philosophies of nursing, 23
  of F.G. Abdellah, 57
  characteristics of, 69
  defined, 69
  L. Hall's, 59
  V. Henderson's, 56
  F. Nightingale's, 73-75, 83
  E. Wiedenbach's, 59
Philosophy, 16
  logic, 25
  and logical form, 179-180
  in nursing education, 168
*Philosophy and Nursing: A Marxist and Phenomenological
    Contribution* (Martinsen), 168
*The Philosophy of Caring in Practice: Thinking with Kari
    Martinsen in Nursing* (Austgard), 180-181
The Philosophy of Nursing (journal), 23
Phipps, Wilma, 726
Photography, 482
Physiological adaptive mode, in Roy Adaptation Model,
    375t-376t
Physiological-physical mode, in Roy Adaptation Model,
    358-359, 364
Piaget, J., 19, 564
Picard, C. A., 509
Pichler, V. H., 284
Pickrell, K. D., 542
Picton, C. E., 330
Pienschke, D., 442, 445
Pierce, 29
Pinheiro, Ana, 442
Podvoll, E. M., 699
Polanyi, Michael, 142, 587
Politics, in Bureaucratic Caring Theory, 122
Pollock, S. E., 372
Ponte-Reid, P. A., 443

Popper, Karl, 17, 22, 194
Positivism, 18, 20, 172
Poster, E. C., 395
Postmodern approach, to Theory of Caring, 100
Postmodernism, 22-23
Postmodern Nursing and Beyond (Watson), 93-94, 98,
    106
Postpartum depression
    defined, 747
    risk factors for, 748-749
Postpartum Depression Prediction Inventory (PDPI),
    748
Postpartum Depression Theory
    acceptance of, 753-754
    case study for, 756-757
    concepts and definitions in, 746-750
    critical thinking in, 757
    critique of, 755-756
    development of, 754-755
    empirical evidence for, 750-751
    logical form for, 752-753
    major assumptions of, 751
    summary of, 756
    theoretical assertions of, 351-352
    theoretical sources for, 744, 745t, 746
Postpositivism, 22
Poststructuralism, 23
Potter, M. L., 443, 446
Poush-Tedrow, CHECK, 356
Power-as-knowing participation-in-charge theory
    (PKPCT), 255t
Powering, in Human Becoming Theory, 527, 532f
Practical knowledge, defined, 144
Practice, nursing
    basis for, 5
    P. Benner on, 144-145, 150, 152-153, 156
    Bureaucratic Caring Theory in, 126-127
    and Caring Theory, 100-101, 768-769
    Caritas Caring Theory in, 203
    Chronic Sorrow Theory in, 686-687
    Comfort Theory in, 733-734
    Conservation Model in, 232, 233-234
    critical, 172
    Culture Care Theory in, 485-486
    Goal Attainment Theory in, 305
    Health as Expanding Consciousness Theory in, 507-
        508, 509f
    in Illness Trajectory Theory, 671-672
    impact of theory on, 785
    interaction with research and theory of, 46-47
    Johnson Behavioral System Model in, 393-395
    know-how of, 142-143
    knowledge embedded in, 148
    K. Martinsen on, 180
    Maternal Role Attainment Theory in, 614-615

Practice, nursing—cont'd
    middle range theories in, 788-789, 790-791
    Neuman Systems Model in, 327, 328b-329b, 330
    Nursing as Caring Theory in, 415-416
    nursing knowledge in, 11
    in Nursing Process Theory, 438-440, 439
    Peaceful End of Life Theory in, 778
    Postpartum Depression Theory in, 753-754
    and Rogerian model, 251-252
    in Roy Adaptation Model, 365-367
    Self-Care Deficit Theory in, 275, 280
    in Self-Transcendence Theory, 649-650
    skilled, 143-144
    spatial arrangements for, 175
    in Symphonological Bioethical Theory, 594
    systemic approach to, 11
    theory-based, 11
    theory in, 5
    in Tidal Model of Mental Health Recovery, 709-710
    Uncertainty in Illness Theory in, 630
Practice theory, 788. *See also* Middle range theories
Practice wisdom, 506
Praxis
    M. A. Newman's research as, 510
    and Nursing as Caring theory, 419
Preference theory, 776
Pregnancy, unplanned or unwanted, 749
Premature infants, research on, 370
Preparing for Nursing Research in the 21st Century;
    Evolution, Methodologies, and Challenges
    (Abdellah & Levine), 57
Prevention, in Neuman Systems Model, 319, 322-323,
    324f, 326b
Preventive nursing, 397
Price, B., 441
Prigogine, I., 501
The Primacy of Caring: Stress and Coping in Health and
    Illness (Benner and Wrubel), 141, 148
Primary care, 279t, 280
Probabilistic thinking, in Uncertainty in Illness Theory,
    626
Problem identification, in Neuman systems model, 319
Problem solving
    process, 443
    use of, 96
Process, in Neuman Systems Model, 320
Profession
    characteristics of, 10-11
    defined, 8
    nursing as, 8, 10
    in Nursing as Caring theory, 413-414
    theory in, 1
Profession, nursing, 35
    and nursing knowledge, 4
    and nursing practice, 5

Profession, nursing—cont'd
  paradigm shift in, 10
  role of theory in, 10
  transition from vocation to, 5
Professionalism, person-oriented, 176, 181
Professional-person relationship, 698
Proficiency, in clinical learning, 146
PRO-SELF Program, 665
Psychiatric nursing, 54, 697
  in Health as Expanding Consciousness Theory, 509
  in Tidal Model of Mental Health Recovery, 707
Psychology
  transpersonal, 94
  and uncertainty, 627
Psychosis, postpartum, 747. *See also* Postpartum
      Depression Theory
Psychotherapy, 698
Public health, Postpartum Depression Theory in, 754
Purpose of nursing, in Nursing Process Theory, 434

Q

Qualitative Inquiry: The Path of Sciencing (Parse), 522,
      529, 541
Qualitative Research Methods in Nursing (Leininger),
      475, 482
Qualitative theory development, 788
Quality of life, and uncertainty, 627
Quantitative content analysis, 369
Questionnaires
  Burke/NCRCS Chronic Sorrow, 690
  Child and Adolescent Self-Care Practice, 282
  General Comfort, 730, 735, 737
Quinn, J. F., 508

R

Randell, B., 356
Raney, Angela, 753-754
Rapkin, D., 615
Rapoport, 356, 387
Rationalism, 16, 17
Rawls, A., 394, 396
Ray, Marilyn Anne
  background of, 116-119
  Bureaucratic Caring Theory of, 118, 119
    acceptance of, 126-129
    case study for, 134
    concepts and definitions in, 121
    critical thinking in, 134
    critique of, 129, 132-133
    development of, 129
    empirical evidence for, 121-124
    grounded theory in, 123, 123f
    as holographic theory, 124
    logical form for, 126
    major assumptions of, 124-125

Ray, Marilyn Anne—cont'd
  Bureaucratic Caring Theory of—cont'd
    research publications related to, 130t-132t
    summarized, 133
    theoretical assertions of, 125-127
    theoretical sources for, 119
Reaction
  in Neuman Systems Model, 322, 324f
  in Nursing Process theory, 433, 437
Reasoning, logical
  deduction, 25-27, 32t-33t
  induction, 27-29, 32t-33t
  retroduction, 29-31, 32t-33t
Reciprocity
  in homeodynamics, 248, 249t
  in Nursing as Caring theory, 422
Reconciliation, in Caritative Caring Theory, 196-197
Reconstitution, in Neuman Systems Model, 323,
      324f
Redondo, Isabel, 442
Reed, P. G., 503, 786, 787
Reed, Pamela G., 785
  background of, 643
  Self-Transcendence Theory of
    acceptance of, 649-651
    case study for, 654
    concepts and definitions in, 645-646
    critical thinking in, 655
    critique of, 652-653
    development of, 651-652
    empirical evidence for, 646-647
    major assumptions of, 647-648
    summary of, 649, 653-654
    theoretical assertions in, 648-649
    theoretical sources of, 644-645
Reeder, Francelyn, 118
Reflexive principle, in Nursing Process theory, 439
Reform, health care, 101
Registering eye, in philosophy of caring, 177
Regulator, in Roy Adaptation Model, 358, 363-364, 363f,
      375t-376t
Rehabilitation nurse, and SCDNT, 282
Reidy, M., 442
Reilly, R., 441
Relational complexity, 133
Relational Complexity Theory, 131t
Relational statements
  axioms and propositions in, 43
  in nursing theory, 39-41
Relationships, in Tidal Model of Mental Health
      Recovery, 714
Relief, in Theory of Comfort, 728
Renal disease, and Self-care Deficit Theory, 279t
Renewal for Nursing (Levine), 228
Renpenning, K., 268, 280

Report on Measures Adopted for Sanitary Improvements in India from June 1869 to June 1870 (Nightingale), 72
Research
  P. Benner on, 153-154, 156
  on caring framework, 101-102, 102b
  early nursing, 102
  in educational programs, 9
  interdependence of theory and, 20
  K. Martinsen on, 181
  F. Nightingale on, 81
  in normal science, 787
  in nursing history, 4
  practice-based, 368-371
  qualitative, 787-788
  theory-based, 10
  theory-testing, 46
Research, nursing
  Bureaucratic Care Theory in, 128
  Caritas Caring Theory in, 204-205
  Chronic Sorrow Theory in, 687-688
  Comfort Theory in, 735-736
  Conservation Model in, 234
  Culture Care Theory in, 487
  Goal Attainment Theory in, 307
  Health as Expanding Consciousness Theory in, 509-511
  Health Promotion Model in, 461
  Human Becoming Theory in, 528, 541
  Illness Trajectory Theory in, 672
  Interaction Systems Framework in, 306-307
  interaction with practice and theory of, 46-47
  Johnson Behavioral System Model in, 395-396
  Maternal Role Attainment Theory in, 616
  by mid-1970s, 5
  Modeling and Role-Modeling Theory in, 572-573
  Nursing as Caring theory in, 417
  Nursing Process Theory in, 442-444
  Nursing Systems Model in, 332-333
  Peaceful End of Life Theory in, 779
  Postpartum Depression Theory in, 754
  Roy Adaptation Model in, 368-372
  Science of Human Beings in, 252-254
  Self-care Deficit Theory in, 281-282
  Self-Transcendence Theory in, 650-651
  Symphonological Bioethical Theory in, 595
  Theory of Caring, 769
  Tidal Model of Mental Health Recovery in, 710-711
  Uncertainty in Illness Theory in, 630-631
Resnik, 390
Resonancy, in homeodynamics, 248, 249t
Resourcefulness, in Tidal Model of Mental Health Recovery, 703
Respect
  in Peaceful End of Life Theory, 777
  in Tidal Model of Mental Health Recovery, 703

Response, in Roy Adaptation Model, 358
Responsibility, in Nursing Process theory, 433
Retroduction
  analysis of, 29-30
  basic characteristics of, 32t-33t
  defined, 29
  inference in, 30-31
  in Theory of Comfort, 732-733
Revealing-concealing, in Human Becoming Theory, 526, 532f
"Reversed care-law," 172
Reynolds, P. D., 12, 17, 42, 768
Rhythmicity, in Human Becoming Theory, 530
Ricoeur, Paul, 175
Riegel, B., 397
Riehl, 268
Righter, B. M., 630
Rights, in Symphonological Bioethical Theory, 588, 590
Riley, P., 280
Roach, M. S., 407, 415
Roberts, Beverly, 726
Roberts, C. S., 368
Roberts, K. L., 233
Robinson, D., 330, 573
Robinson Self-Appraisal Inventory, 570
Rogerian model
  case study, 256
  development of, 254
  in nursing practice, 251
  in nursing research, 252-254
  summary of, 256
Rogerian Nursing Science News, 245
Rogers, Carl, 100
Rogers, Martha E., 94, 229, 268, 500, 508, 523, 529, 644, 648, 652, 653, 752, 787. *See also* Unitary Human Beings Science
  background of, 244-245
  Science of Unitary Human Beings of
    acceptance of, 251
    case study for, 256
    concepts and definitions in, 246
    critical thinking in, 256
    critique of, 254-255
    development of, 254
    empirical evidence for, 247
    major assumptions of, 247-248, 250
    summary of, 256
    theoretical assertions in, 248, 250
    theoretical sources for, 245
Role function mode, in Roy Adaptation Model, 359-360, 364, 376t
Role-Modeling, art of, 565
Role strain-role conflict, in Maternal Role Attainment Theory, 608
Role theory, interactionist approach to, 607

Rooke, L., 306, 307
Roper, 790
Roper, Nancy, 52
    background of, 64
    model for nursing of, 64-65, 64t, 65f, 66f
*The Roper-Logan-Tierney Model of Nursing: Based on
    Activities of Living* (Roper et al.), 64
Rosenberg, J., 47
Rossi, L., 306
Roy, Sister Callista, 268, 369, 374
    Adaptation Model of, 787
        acceptance of, 365-372
        concepts and definitions in, 357-360
        critique of, 373-374
        development of, 372-373
        empirical evidence for, 360
        logical form in, 364-365
        major assumptions in, 360-363
        summary of, 374-375, 375t-376t, 377
        theoretical assertions in, 363-364
        theoretical sources for, 356-357*
    background of, 355-356
    six-step nursing process of, 365
The Roy Adaptation Model (Roy and Andrews), 356
Rubin, Jane, 143
Rubin, M. M., 280
Rubin, Reva, 606-607, 610
Ruland, Cornelia M., 774
    background of, 775
    and Peaceful End of Life (EOL) Theory
        acceptance of, 778
        case study for, 781
        concepts and definitions in, 776-777
        critical thinking in, 781
        critique of, 779-780
        development of, 779
        empirical evidence for, 777
        major assumptions of, 777
        theoretical assertions of, 778
        theoretical sources for, 776
Ruth Rhoden Craven Foundation for Postpartum
    Depression Awareness, 754

S
St. Augustine, 194
St. Thomas Hospital in London, school of nursing at, 4
Salience, defined, 147
Samarel, N., 366, 369
Sank, J. C., 616
Sartre, Jean-Paul, 94, 523, 529
Satisfaction, in Maternal Role Attainment Theory, 608
Sato, 356
Schaefer, K. M., 232
Schilling, L. S., 38
Schlotfeldt, Rozella, 729

Schmidt, R., 300
Schmieding, N. J., 439, 440, 441, 442, 443, 444, 445, 446
Schoenhofer, Savina O., 418
    background of, 406-407
    and Nursing as Caring theory, 785
        acceptance of, 415-420
        case study in, 422-423
        concepts and definitions in, 408-412
        critical thinking in, 423
        critique of, 421
        development of, 420
        empirical evidence for, 412
        logical form for, 415
        major assumptions of, 412-413
        major concepts and definitions of, 408-412
        summary of, 422-423
        theoretical assertions in, 414-416
        theoretical sources for, 407-408
Scholarship, nursing, 6
School-age children, pain-related responses in, 370
Schools, nursing, 4
Schorr, J. A., 509, 510
Schroeder, C. A., 509
Schubert, P. E., 508
Schumacher, L. P., 542
Schutz, A., 18
Science, 174. *See also* Caring science; Unitary Human
    Beings Science
    advancement of, 21
    and Conservation Model, 234
    development of, 16
    early 20th-century views of, 18
    history of, 16
    as interactive process, 20
    late 20th-century views of, 18-20
    normal, 21-22, 786-787
    of nursing theory, 786
    positivism, 172
    revolutionary, 22
    Rogerian, 245
    of self care, 282
    as social enterprise, 23
Science, nursing
    development of, 23
    nursing practice based on, 5
Scientific method, 22
Scientific process, 20
Sears, 390
Seidel, S. L., 306
Seip, Anne Lise, 169
Self
    in interacting systems framework, 299
    therapeutic use of, 698
Self-as-Carer Inventory (SCI), 281
Self-assertion, as bioethical standard, 591b, 593f, 597

Self-care
  assuming, 674
  defined, 269
  and dependent-care capabilities, 286
  developmental requisites for, 270
  exercise as, 282
  health deviation requisites, 270
  in Modeling and Role-Modeling Theory, 567
  F. Nightingale on, 77
  requisites for, 269-270
  research in, 543
  theory of, 273-274
  and therapeutic demand, 270-271
  universal requisites for, 270
Self Care, Dependent Care and Nursing (journal), 283
Self-care agency, 271
Self-care deficit, defined, 271
Self-Care Deficit Nursing Theory (SCDNT), 267, 268,
    787
  acceptance of, 275-283
  case study for, 285-287
  concepts and definitions in, 269-272
  critical thinking in, 287
  critique of, 283-284
  developmental requisites in, 286
  development of, 282-283
  documentation system, 275
  empirical evidence for, 272
  explained, 273
  health deviation requisites in, 286
  logical form for, 274
  major assumptions of, 272
  in nursing practice, 275
  summary of, 284
  theoretical assertions of, 272-274
  theoretical sources for, 268-269
  therapeutic demand in, 285-286
Self-care interventions, 665
Self-Care Inventory (SCI), 282
Self-Care Resource Inventory, 570
Self-concept, in Maternal Role Attainment Theory, 608
Self-concept-group identity mode, in Roy Adaptation
    Model, 359, 364
Self-concept mode, in Roy Adaptation Model, 376t
Self-confidence, in Maternal Role Attainment Theory,
    611
Self-discovery, 416
Self-efficacy
  in Health Promotion Model, 456
  in HPM, 454
Self-esteem
  in Maternal Role Attainment Theory, 608, 611
  and postpartum depression, 749
Self-help concepts, V. Henderson's, 55
Self-organization, relational, 132t, 133

Self-transcendence
  defined, 645, 648
  and mental health, 653
  themes of, 650
  and well-being, 650
Self-Transcendence Theory, 785
  acceptance of, 649-651
  case study for, 654
  concepts and definitions in, 645-646
  critical thinking in, 655
  critique of, 652-653
  development of, 651-652
  empirical evidence for, 646-647
  logical form in, 649
  major assumptions of, 647-648
  model of, 649f
  summary of, 649, 653-654
  theoretical assertions in, 648-649
  theoretical sources for, 644-645
Self-worth, in Conservation Model, 231
Selye, Hans, 94, 229, 230, 268, 319, 356, 390, 564, 565
Senesac, P., 365
Sensing, in philosophy of caring, 179
Sensitivity, cultivation of, 95
Set-of-laws approach, to theory building, 41-43
Sexual subsystem, in Johnson Behavioral System Model,
    389, 399
Sharts-Hopko, N. C., 307
Shea, N. M., 443
Sheafor, M., 443
Sherrington, A., 229
Shijiki, Y., 441
Shore, C. P., 613
Shultz, C., 650
Shumaker, D., 687
Sichel, D., 746, 751
Sickness Impact Profile, 368
Sieloff, C. L., 306, 307
Silver, M., 152
Sime, 420
Simmons, Leo W., 390
Simplicity
  of P. Benner's theory of nursing practice, 154-155
  in Bureaucratic Care Theory, 132
  in Caring Theory, 769
  in Caritative Caring Theory, 206
  in Chronic Sorrow Theory, 689
  in Comfort Theory, 737
  in Conservation Model, 235
  in Culture Care Theory, 488
  in Health as expanding Consciousness Theory, 511
  in Health Promotion Model, 461
  in Human Becoming Theory, 541-542
  in Illness Trajectory Theory, 673
  in Johnson Behavioral System Model, 397-398

Simplicity—cont'd
in K. Martinsen's philosophy of caring, 181-182
in Maternal Role Attainment Theory, 618
in Modeling and Role-Modeling Theory, 573-574
in Neuman Systems Model, 335
in Nursing as Caring theory, 421
in Nursing Process Theory, 444
in nursing theory, 12
in Peaceful End of Life Theory, 779
in Postpartum Depression Theory, 755
in Rogers' model, 254
in Roy Adaptation Model, 373
in science of caring, 103
in Self-care Deficit Nursing Theory, 283
in Self-Transcendence Theory, 652
in Symphonological Bioethical Theory, 596
in Tidal Model of Mental Health Recovery, 713-714
in Uncertainty in Illness Theory, 632-633
Sitma Theta Tau International, 790
Situated freedom, in Human Becoming Theory, 524
Situation
aspects of, 146
attributes of, 147
compared with environment, 151
in Health Promotion Model, 457
Situation-specific theories (SSTs), 752
Sivonen, K., 204
Skill acquisition, levels of, 143
Skinner, B. F., 17
Small, B., 396
Small, H., 73, 78
Small, L., 687
Smith, A. A., 332
Smith, C. A., 510
Smith, F. B., 73
Smith, M. C., 334, 420
Smith, M. J., 46, 788
Smoking cessation, research on, 366
Sneed, L. D., 306
Social cognitive theory, 454
Social crisis, for nursing, 172
Social integrity, conservation of, 231
Social relativism, 587
Social structure, in Theory of Culture Care Diversity
and Universality, 477, 478
Social support
in Maternal Role Attainment Theory, 609
uncertainty and, 626
Social system, 301
Society, in Bureaucratic Caring Theory, 121
Society for Advancement of Modeling and Role-
Modeling, 573
Socioeconomic status, and postpartum depression, 749
Sociology, in nursing education, 168
Sollid, D., 611

Solomon, J., 64
Sommer, R., 300
Sovereign life utterances, in philosophy of caring,
176-177
Space, in philosophy of caring, 179
Space nursing, 117
Space-time
in health as expanding consciousness theory, 505, 506f
Spinoza, Benedict, 585, 587
Spirituality, in Bureaucratic Caring Theory, 121
Stability, in Neuman Systems Model, 321
Stamler, C., 396
Steckler, J., 595
Stein, E., 29
Steiner, R., 730
Stempel, J. E., 508
Stevens, B., 30
Stimuli frame, in Uncertainty in Illness Theory, 625
Stimulus, in Roy Adaptation Model, 358
St-Jacques, A., 394
Stories
as method for knowing nursing, 409-410
in Tidal Model of Mental Health Recovery, 714
Storytelling, 156
Strachey, L., 73
Stranger to trusted friend enabler, in Culture Care
Theory, 485
Strauss, Anselm, 117, 670, 671, 744
Stress
P. Benner's study of, 144
defined, 144, 319
R. Lazarus' theory of, 144
in Maternal Role Attainment Theory, 609
and postpartum depression, 748
response to, 230
*Stress and Satisfaction on the Job: Work Meanings and
Coping of Mid-Career Men* (Lazarus), 144
Stressors
in Johnson Behavioral System Model, 389, 392f
in Neuman Systems Model, 322, 324f, 326b
uncertainty, 624
Structural components, in Johnson Behavioral System
Model, 400
Structure providers, in Uncertainty in Illness Theory,
625
Structuring, in Human Becoming Theory, 525-526, 532f
Styles, M. M., 11
Subjectivity, in Nursing as Caring theory, 422
Subsystems, in Johnson Behavioral System Model, 392f
Suchman, A., 330
Suffering
in Caritative Caring Theory, 196, 200-201
research related to, 205
Sullivan, H. S., 357
Sunrise Enabler, in Culture Care Theory, 483, 484f

Swain, Mary Ann P., 280, 564, 565
  background of, 563-564
  Modeling and Role-Modeling Theory of, 563, 787
    acceptance of, 571-573
    case study for, 574-574
    concepts and definitions in, 565-567
    critical thinking in, 575
    critique of, 573-574
    development of, 573
    empirical evidence for, 567-570
    logical form for, 571
    major assumptions of, 570
    summary of, 574
    theoretical assertions of, 570-571
    theoretical sources for, 564-565
Swanson, Kristen M.
  background of, 762-763
  Theory of Caring of, 767
    acceptance of, 768-769
    case study for, 770
    concepts and definitions in, 764
    critical thinking in, 770
    critique of, 769
    development of, 769
    empirical evidence for, 764-766
    major assumptions of, 766-767
    theoretical assertions for, 767
    theoretical sources for, 763
Swimme, B., 361
Symphonological Bioethical Theory
  acceptance of, 594-595
  case study for, 597-598
  concepts and definitions in, 587-588
  critical thinking in, 598
  critique of, 596-597
  development of, 595-596
  empirical evidence in, 588-589
  logical form for, 592-593
  major assumptions of, 589-590
  summary of, 597
  theoretical assertions of, 590-592
  theoretical sources for, 586-587
Symphonology, defined, 586
Synchrony, in homeodynamics, 250 table
Systems
  in Bureaucratic Caring Theory, 119
  in Johnson Behavioral System Model, 387-388
  in Roy Adaptation Model, 357
Systems Model, Neuman. *See* Neuman, Betty
Systems theory, 698
Szasz, Thomas, 699

T
Tak, S., 372
Tanner, C., 141

Taxonomy of Error, Root Cause and Practice (TERCAP)
    analysis audit tool, 142
Taylor, J. W., 233
Taylor, S. G., 268, 281, 282
Teaching, interpersonal, 96
Teamwork, in Tidal Model of Mental Health Recovery,
    710-711
Technology, in Bureaucratic Caring Theory, 122
Teleapprenticeship, 533
Temporal experience scale (TES), 255t
Temporality, in Illness Trajectory Theory, 667
Tension, in Johnson Behavioral System Model, 389, 392f
Tesler, M., 396
Textbook of the Principles and Practice of Nursing
    (Henderson), 55
Theoretical development, in F. Nightingale's work, 81
Theoretical works
  analysis of, 1
  conceptual frameworks for, 9
  middle range theory, 7 (*see also* Middle range
    theories)
  nursing conceptual models, 7
  and nursing knowledge, 8
  nursing philosophy, 6-7
  nursing theory, 7
  publishing, 9
  types of, 6-8, 7b
Theory
  construction of nursing, 16
  defined, 299, 476-477
  formal, 41-42
  interdependence of research and, 20-23
  and observation, 19-20
Theory, nursing. *See also specific theories*
  E. Adam's, 63
  analysis of, 12-13
  K. E. Barnard's, 63
  components of, 36t
    concepts and definitions, 36
    linkages and ordering, 41-44
    relational statements, 39-41
  history of, 4-8
  interaction with practice and research of, 46-47
  need for new, 181
  retroductive inference in, 31
  significance of, 8-12
  systematic view in, 6
  J. Travelbee's work on, 62
Theory development
  analogy in, 30
  contemporary issues in, 45-47
  creativity in, 47-48
  expansion of, 787-789
  middle range theories, 45, 46 (*see also* Middle range
    theories)

Theory development—cont'd
in nursing, 35
and nursing scholarship, 6
qualitative theory, 788
situation-specific theories, 45, 46
systematic, 35
Theory Development in Nursing (Newman), 498, 504
Theory for Nursing: Systems, Concepts, Process (King), 298, 303
Theory synthesis, 369
Theory-then-research strategy, for theory construction, 17
Therapeutic philosophy, in Tidal Model of Mental Health Recovery, 703
Therapeutic relationship, 438
Therapeutic touch, 508
Theses, in Caritative Caring Theory, 198
Thibaudeau, M., 442
Thomas, J. S., 280, 419
Thorne, S., 45
Thornton, R., 607
The Thoughtful Nurse (Martinsen), 171
Tidal Model of Mental Health Recovery
acceptance of, 709-711
care continuum in, 714f
case study for, 716-717
concepts and definitions in, 702-704
critical thinking in, 717
critique of, 712-715
development of, 711-712
empirical evidence for, 704-705
essential values of, 700b-701b, 711-712
logical form for, 708
major assumptions of, 705-707
summary of, 715
theoretical assertions of, 707-708
theoretical basis of, 702
theoretical sources for, 697-700
web site for, 715
Tierney, Alison J., 53, 64, 790
Time
in Health as Expanding Consciousness Theory, 504-505
in Tidal Model of Mental Health Recovery, 701b
Timelessness, in Health as Expanding Consciousness Theory, 505, 506f
To Be a Nurse (Adam), 63
Tomey, A. M., 6, 132, 325
Tomlin, Evelyn M., 564, 565
background of, 562-563
Modeling and Role-Modeling Theory of, 563, 787
acceptance of, 571-573
case study for, 574-575
concepts and definitions in, 565-567
critical thinking in, 575

Tomlin, Evelyn M.—cont'd
Modeling and Role-Modeling Theory of—cont'd
critique of, 573-574
development of, 573
empirical evidence for, 567-570
logical form for, 571
major assumptions of, 570
summary of, 574
theoretical assertions of, 570-571
theoretical sources for, 564-565
Toolkit, in Tidal Model of Mental Health Recovery, 701b
Total quality management framework, 130t
Toward a Theory for Nursing: General Concept of Human Behavior (King), 298
Transaction, model of, 302f
Transcendence
in Health as Expanding Consciousness Theory, 503
in Theory of Comfort, 728
Transcultural care
methodology in, 483
theory, 480
Transcultural Communicative Caring Tool, 127
Transcultural nurse generalist, 476
Transcultural nursing, 118, 472, 485-486, 491
compared with cross-cultural nursing, 476
defined, 476, 479
Transcultural Nursing: Concepts, Theories, and Practice (Leininger and McFarland), 473, 475
Transforming, in Human Becoming Theory, 527, 532f
Transparency, in Tidal Model of Mental Health Recovery, 701b
Travelbee, Joyce, 51, 181, 268
background of, 59, 62
human-to-human relationship model of, 59, 62, 63f
Trigger events, in Chronic Sorrow Theory, 684, 685
Tripp-Reimer, T., 37
TriService Nursing Research Program, 129
Trophicognosis, 230
Tsai, P. F., 31, 372
Tully, J. C., 613
Tulman, L., 366, 368
Turkel, Marian, 119, 127, 129, 130t, 133
Turner, J. H., 44, 607
Twigg, P., 542
Törnebohm, Håkan, 194

U
Uhl-Pierce, Joan, 118
Ulbrich, S. L., 282
Uncertainty
in chronic illness, 629
illness trajectory and, 666
in Illness Trajectory Theory, 667, 668t
as opportunity, 632
reality of, 698
in Uncertainty in Illness Theory, 625

Uncertainty Abatement Work, 664, 669t
Uncertainty in illness, perceived, 628f
Uncertainty in Illness Theory
    acceptance of, 630-631
    case study for, 634
    critical thinking in, 634
    critique of, 631-633
    development of, 631
    empirical evidence for, 626-627
    logical form in, 629-630
    major assumptions of, 627-629, 628f
    summary of, 633-634
    theoretical assertions in, 629
    theoretical sources for, 624-625
Unconditional acceptance, in Modeling and Role-
        Modeling Theory, 566
Unitary human being, defined, 247
Unitary Human Beings Science, 420, 523, 787
    acceptance of, 251
    case study for, 256
    concepts and definitions in, 246
    critical thinking in, 256
    critique of, 254-255
    development of, 254
    empirical evidence for, 247
    instruments developed for, 255 table
    logical form for, 250-251
    major assumptions of, 247-248, 250
    summary of, 256
    theoretical assertions in, 248, 250
    theoretical sources for, 245
    theory development within, 253f
Unitary-transformative paradigm, in Bureaucratic
        Caring Theory, 120
Universality. *See also* Culture Care Theory of Diversity
        and Universality
    of care, 481
    culture care, 478
Universities, nursing education in, 4
Untouchable zone, 177
Upchurch, S. L., 650
Urinary frequency, research on, 730
Urinary incontinence, research in, 737
Urine control, research in, 371
Urology, and Self-care Deficit Theory, 279t
Utilization, in nursing theory, 6

V
Vage, T. A., 233
Vaillancourt, V.M., 306
Valentine, S. O., 439
Values
    and concept of caring, 97
    cultural, 491
    humanistic altruistic system of, 95
    and science of caring, 98

Valuing, in Human Becoming Theory, 525, 532f
Van Kaam, 523
Van Landingham, 356
Van Manen, Max, 118
Van Servellen, G., 395
Vardiman, E. M., 282
Vasques, E., 615
Viera, C.S., 306
View of life, in Uncertainty in Illness Theory, 626,
        627
Villareal, E., 366
Villarruel, A. M., 275
Viola, Isabel, 442
Visintainer, M., 442
Visions: The Journal of Rogerian Nursing Science
        (Malinski and Barrett), 245
Visually impaired children, research on, 396
Vocation
    duty of, 174
    explication of, 174
    nature of, 177
    nursing practice as, 5
Voice, in Tidal Model of Mental Health Recovery, 700b-
        701b
Vojir, Carol, 118
Von Bertalanffy, Ludwig, 247, 268, 607
Von Post, I., 204
Von Wright, Georg, 194
Vulnerability, defined, 645, 648

W
Walike, B., 390
Walker, J., 371, 433
Walker, L. O., 12, 13, 31, 437, 444, 616, 710
Walker, P.H., 330
Wallace, William, 268
Walls, R., 650
Walton, C., 650
Wang, C., 275
Washington, L. J., 616
Water, metaphor of, 702-703
Watson, C.A., 306
Watson, Jean, 118, 127, 728, 744, 752, 763. *See also*
        Caring science; Caring Theory
    background of, 105
    caritative factors described by, 103, 104t, 105-106
    on nursing education, 101
    ontological shift of, 98
    postmodern approach of, 100
    publications of, 93
    on research, 101-102
    theoretical sources of, 93-95
Watson, Margaret Jean Harman. *See* Watson, Jean
Watzlawick, P., 300
Web sites, general nursing theory, 790
Webb, H., 233

Webber, Max, 174
Weber, N. A., 282
Weingourt, R., 508
Well-being
    culturally congruent care for, 483, 484f
    and self-transcendence, 650
    in Self-Transcendence Theory, 645, 648
Wellness
    in Neuman Systems Model, 322
    as nursing specialty, 460
Werner, H., 607
Western Commission of Higher Education in Nursing
    Conference (1977), 9
Whall, A. L., 77, 81, 235, 254, 307, 433, 786
Whall, Ann, 644
Whall, J. A., 234
Whitehead, A. N., 94
Whiting, J. F., 300
Whittemore, R., 372
Wholeness
    in Conservation Model, 229
    in Health as Expanding Consciousness Theory, 500
    in Nursing as Caring theory, 413
Wholistic approach, in Neuman Systems Model, 320,
    330-331, 335
Wicks, M. N., 307
Wiedenbach, Ernestine, 51, 268
    on clinical nursing, 57-58, 59f
    on ministration of help, 59, 61f
    patients' need-for-help identified by, 58-59, 60f
    recognition of, 9
    on validation of need-for-help being met, 59
    vision of nursing of, 57
Wiener, Carolyn L., 663
    background of, 664
    illness trajectory focus of, 664
    and Illness Trajectory Theory
        acceptance of, 671-672
        case study for, 674
        concepts and definitions in, 667-668
        critical thinking in, 675
        critique of, 673-674
        development of, 672-673
        empirical evidence in, 669
        major assumptions of, 670-671
        summary of, 674
        theoretical assertions of, 671
        theoretical sources for, 666
Wiklund, L., 205
Wilkie, D. J., 396
Williams, L. A., 306
Wills, E., 786
Wilt, D. L., 307

Winder, A., 441
Wingren, Gustaf, 195
Winker, C. K., 306
Winnicott, D. W., 564
Wisdom, in Tidal Model of Mental Health Recovery,
    701b
Wisdom and Skill (Kirkevold, Nortvedt, and Alvsvåg),
    181
Wisdom traditions, 94
Wise with Experience? On Sensation and Attention,
    Knowledge and Reflection in Practical Nursing
    (Olsen), 181
Wittneben, K., 442
Wolfer, J., 442
Wolff, 390
Women, and self-care deficit theory, 277t
Wongvatunyu, S., 268
Woodham-Smith, C. B., 73
Woods, S. J., 369
World view
    in Culture Care Theory, 477, 478
    holographic, 133
Wright, K., 650, 651
Wrubel, Judith, 143, 144, 148, 150, 151
Wurzbach, M. E., 630
Wykle, May, 726
Wärnå, C., 205
Wærness, Kari, 169

Y
Yale-sponsored Nursing Studies Index Project, 55
Yalom, 11 curative factors of, 95
Yeager, V., 420
Yeates-Giese, D., 233
Yeats, W. B., 702
Yeh, C. H., 368
Young, A. M., 500, 505, 506
Young, C. A., 651
Youngblut, Joanne, 727
Younger, M. S., 370
Young-McCaughan, S., 368

Z
Zauszniewski, Jaclene, 727
Zderad, L. T., 407, 728
Zeigler, S. M., 330
Zen Buddhism, 698
Zentner, J., 75
Zetterberg, H. L., 40
Zhan, L., 369
Zurakowski, T. L., 307